Hemodynamic Monitoring

INVASIVE AND NONINVASIVE CLINICAL APPLICATION

THIRD EDITION

GLORIA OBLOUK DAROVIC, RN, CCRN

Lecturer/Consultant, American Medical Education, Inc.
San Diego, California

SAUNDERS
An Imprint of Elsevier

SAUNDERS
An Imprint of Elsevier

The Curtis Center
Independence Square West
Philadelphia, Pennsylvania 19106-3399

NOTICE

Critical care is an ever-changing field. Standard safety precautions must be followed, but as new research and clinical experience broaden our knowledge, changes in treatment and drug therapy may become necessary or appropriate. Readers are advised to check the most current product information provided by the manufacturer of each drug to be administered to verify the recommended dose, the method and duration of administration, and contraindications. It is also advised that practitioners check with manufacturers of medical devices for the most current information regarding indications and guidelines, use, and warnings. It is the responsibility of the licensed prescriber, relying on experience and knowledge of the patient, to determine dosages and the best treatment for each individual patient. Neither the Publisher nor the editor assume any liability for any injury and/or damage to persons or property arising from this publication.

Library of Congress Cataloging-in-Publication Data

Darovic, Gloria Oblouk.
   Hemodynamic monitoring : invasive and noninvasive clinical application / Gloria Oblouk Darovic.-- 3rd ed.
      p. ; cm.
   Includes bibliographical references and index.
   ISBN 0-7216-9293-1 (softcover)
   1. Hemodynamic monitoring. 2. Cardiovascular system--Diseases--Diagnosis. I. Title.
   [DNLM: 1. Hemodynamics. 2. Cardiovascular Diseases--physiopathology. 3. Monitoring, Physiologic--methods. WG 106 D224h 2002]
   RC670.5.H45 D37 2002
   616.1'0754--dc21
                                                                                     2001057649

Vice President and Publishing Director, Nursing: Sally Schrefer

Executive Editor: Barbara Nelson Cullen

Associate Developmental Editor: Stacy Welsh

Publishing Services Manager: Catherine Jackson

Project Manager: Jeff Patterson

Designer: Amy Buxton

HEMODYNAMIC MONITORING: INVASIVE AND NONINVASIVE CLINICAL APPLICATIONS   ISBN 0-7216-9293-1

Printed in the United States of America

Last digit is the print number: 04 05 06 PIT/RDW 9 8 7 6 5 4 3

Contributors

Shaul Atar, MD
Director, Intensive Cardiac Care Unit
Ha'Emek Medical Center
Afula, Israel

Cory Franklin, MD
Director
Division of Medical Critical Care
Cook County Hospital
Chicago, Illinois

Gregory L. Freeman, MD
Professor of Medicine and Physiology
Chief of Cardiology
University of Texas Health Science Center
San Antonio, Texas

Patricia Graham, MS, RN, CCRN, CS
Critical Care Clinical Nurse Specialist
University of California at San Diego Medical Center
San Diego, California

Mary Fran Hazinski, RN, MSN, FAAN
Clinical Specialist, Division of Trauma
Departments of Surgery and Pediatrics
Vanderbilt University Medical Center
Consultant, Pediatric Critical Care
Vanderbilt Children's Hospital
Nashville, Tennessee

Robert J. Henning, MD, FACP, FACC, FCCP
Professor of Medicine
Director, Center for Cardiovascular Research
University of South Florida College of Medicine;
Director, Clinical Cardiology Services
James A. Haley Veterans Administration Hospital
Tampa, Florida

Lloyd W. Klein, MD
Professor of Medicine
Section of Cardiology
Rush Medical College of Rush University;
Co-Director, Cardiac Catheterization Laboratories;
Director, Interventional Cardiology
Rush Heart Institute
Rush Presbyterian—St. Luke's Medical Center
Chicago, Illinois

Elizabeth Krzywda, MSN, ANP
Adult Nurse Practitioner
Medical College of Wisconsin
Milwaukee, Wisconsin

Anand Kumar, MD
Assistant Professor of Medicine
Section of Critical Care Medicine
Section of Infectious Diseases
Rush University
Chicago, Illinois

Robert J. March, MD
Cardiovascular Surgeon
Rush Presbyterian—St. Luke's Medical Center
Chicago, Illinois

Henry J.L. Marriott, MD
Clinical Professor of Medicine (Cardiology)
Emory University School of Medicine
Atlanta, Georgia;
University of South Florida College of Medicine
Tampa, Florida

Barry Mizock, MD

Associate Director
Medical ICU
Cook County Hospital
Chicago, Illinois

Maryann F. Pranulis, RN, DNSc

Principal Consultant
M. F. Pranulis & Associates
Frederick, Maryland (formerly located in San Diego,
  California)

Robert J. Siegel, MD

Director, Cardiac Noninvasive Laboratory
Cedars-Sinai Medical Center
Los Angeles, California

Robert Simonelli, PharmD

Adjunct Professor
Duquesne University
Clinical Pharmacy Specialist
Mercy Hospital of Pittsburgh
Pittsburgh, Pennsylvania

Donna Stel, BSN, CCRN

SICU Staff Nurse
Rush Presbyterian—St. Luke's Medical Center
Chicago, Illinois

Karen L. Stratton, RN, C MSN

Medical Psychiatric Consultation Liaison Nurse
Rush Presbyterian—St. Luke's Medical Center
Chicago, Illinois

Joseph P. Zbilut, PhD, DNSc, APN/ANP

Professor, Adult Health Nursing
Professor, Molecular Biophysics and Physiology
Rush Presbyterian—St. Luke's Medical Center
Chicago, Illinois

Reviewers

Linda S. Baas, RN, PhD, ACNP, CCNS
Director, Acute Care Nurse Practitioner Program
Associate Professor
University of Cincinnati College of Nursing
Cincinnati, Ohio

Marianne Saunorus Baird, RN, MN
Saint Joseph's Hospital of Atlanta
Atlanta, Georgia

Paula M. Baker, RN, MSN
St. Vincent Hospital and Health Services
Indianapolis, Indiana

Cheryl L. Bittel, MSN, RN, CCRN
Saint Joseph's Hospital of Atlanta
Atlanta, Georgia

Elisabeth Glackin Bradley, MS, RN, APN, CCRN
Christiana Care Health System
Newark, Delaware

Nancy A. Davis, RN, BSN
North Ridge Medical Center
Fort Lauderdale, Florida

Gina Duncan, CCRN, RN, ACNP
University of Texas at Arlington
School of Nursing
Arlington, Texas

Paulette Morelli, RN, MSN, CNS, NP-C, CCRN
Christiana Care Health System
Newark, Delaware

Terry Savan, RN, BSN, MA, FNP-C, PA-C
Assistant Professor
Allenton College (De Sales University)
Center Valley, Pennsylvania

Laura D. Williams, RN, BSN, CCRN
Saint Joseph's Hospital of Atlanta
Atlanta, Georgia

The vision of this book inspired me.
The loving support of my family,
friends, and colleagues provided the sustenance required
to bring the vision to reality.

Preface

The third edition of this interdisciplinary text was written in response to the popularity of the first two editions, continued growth in the types and versatility of monitoring techniques, and greater insights into the strengths and shortcomings of specific monitoring technologies over the past several decades. Likewise, considerable expansion and change have occurred in the understanding of pathophysiology, assessment techniques, and related changes in the management of critically ill and injured patients. Because the fields of monitoring technologies and art and science of management of ICU patients are continually changing and evolving, the contributors and the author have made an effort to include the newest as well as some older techniques and equipment. This was done because of the considerable variability in the monitoring equipment available in different institutions and ICUs.

However, the focus of this text has not changed from that of the first two editions. The core of the text continues to concentrate on the educational needs of the clinician and care of the patient. To achieve this end, most contributors selected are actively involved in patient care. Consequently, they understand the needs of bedside practitioners. In each chapter, the contributors and the author have attempted to anticipate clinically relevant questions and present clear, practical answers whenever possible. Similarly, the descriptions of some techniques for monitoring-system setup and fidelity testing have been simplified for application to the clinical setting. The contributors and the author feel that the more complex, detailed, and time-consuming techniques for dynamic response testing of monitoring systems described in some critical care literature are suitable for the research setting but are not required for bedside care. In research laboratories, absolute consistency is required from test sample to test sample to eliminate as many variables in research-related outcomes as possible. In addition, the pressure stimuli applied to the research monitoring systems are typically controlled. At the bedside, the patient-related frequency response of pulsatile signals may change within seconds and cannot be controlled. Clinically, minor variations in frequency response and damping characteristics have minimal significance.

Some of the monitoring terms and abbreviations used, such as *pulmonary capillary wedge pressure* (PWP), are those chosen by the pioneers who developed the specific type of monitoring technique. Although several new terms have been suggested, such as *pulmonary artery wedge pressure* (PAWP) and *pulmonary artery occluded pressure* (PAOP), the differences in names are purely academic and do not change the principle and application of the technique. The abundance of medical names has the potential to confuse practitioners. Since PWP and other abbreviations are the most familiar and easy to say and write, they are used throughout this text.

The purpose of this text is to do the following:

1. Simply and comprehensively emphasize the most relevant technical points and appropriate clinical applications of monitoring techniques
2. Give the reader a sound, fundamental understanding of the anatomy and physiology of the cardiovascular and pulmonary systems
3. Provide the reader with important pathophysiologic, diagnostic, and management principles for common cardiopulmonary diseases, emphasizing the individuality of patient responses
4. Provide adequate illustrations to aid in conceptualization of the principles described in the text.

With the information provided, the clinician will be able to efficiently integrate all pathophysiologic, monitoring, assessment, and laboratory information into an effective, individualized patient management plan, thus avoiding a rote, recipe-book approach to patient care.

ACKNOWLEDGMENTS

A comprehensive, detailed textbook represents the cooperative effort of many people. These include the knowledgeable and experienced contributors who gave of their time and creative talents to create the matrix of the text.

Important also are the many physician and nurse colleagues who reviewed the original drafts and artwork and helped refine them with their suggestions and criticisms. Added to these are the various professionals at Mosby/ W.B. Saunders whose cooperative efforts transformed the piles of chapter drafts and crude author-drawn art into the attractive, finished product you hold in your hands. It is therefore with pleasure that I express gratitude to the many people who directly or indirectly contributed to the production of this text:

- To the contributors, for their talents, effort, and cooperation in the development of the chapters.
- To Dr. R. Phillip Dellinger, MD, FCCP; Dr. Charles E. Edmiston, PhD, CIC; Kim Garrett, MS, RN; and Erika Schwelnus, MSN, RN, for their time and generosity in reviewing specific chapters.
- To the artists and illustrators, Publishing Services Manager Catherine Jackson, and Project Manager Jeff Patterson.
- A very special thanks to Stacy Welsh and Barbara Nelson Cullen for their encouragement and support throughout the laborious writing of this text.
- A special acknowledgment to the late Barbara J. Agnew, RN, respected counselor, mentor, friend, and generous contributor of hemodynamic pressure tracings.

Gloria Oblouk Darovic

Contents

Hemodynamic Monitoring

INVASIVE AND NONINVASIVE CLINICAL APPLICATION

ANATOMY, PHYSIOLOGY, AND ASSESSMENT TECHNIQUES

1

GLORIA OBLOUK DAROVIC and KAREN L. STRATTON

Introduction to the Care of Critically Ill and Injured Patients

As recently as 100 years ago, only temperature, pulse, and respiration were monitored and recorded as part of patient evaluation regardless of the severity of the illness. Although the technology for auscultatory blood pressure measurement was available, routine measurement did not become a standard for circulatory assessment until the late 1920s. Before and including this time, patients with severe illness or injury typically died within hours or days of onset because assessment techniques were limited and effective therapies were nonexistent.

The introduction of antibiotics into clinical therapeutics during the 1940s had enormous impact on the outcome of infectious diseases (such as pneumonia, tuberculosis, bacterial endocarditis) that generally had fatal outcomes. Other new and refined medical and surgical therapies also held promise for improvement in the quality of life and prolongation of life in patients with chronic and acute illnesses.

Intensive therapy as a medical/nursing specialty evolved in tandem with the electronic revolution of the 1960s. Sophisticated hemodynamic and laboratory techniques vastly improved diagnosis, as well as evaluation of therapies specific to critically ill or injured patients. Devices now are commonly used to provide immediately available and continuous pressure measurements within the systemic and pulmonary circulations, central veins, pulmonary capillary bed, and right and left atria (which normally reflects the end-diastolic pressure of the respective ventricle), as well as flow measurements such as cardiac output.

The information obtained also can be used to calculate systemic and pulmonary vascular resistances and oxygen transport, as well as oxygen consumption. Nevertheless, directly obtained or calculated hemodynamic measurements have several clinical limitations. Some of these limitations are described in this chapter. The importance of recognition of the patient, the patient's family members, and the caregivers as vulnerable human beings is also presented, along with some stress prevention and stress reduction strategies.

CLINICAL LIMITATIONS OF HEMODYNAMIC MEASUREMENTS

Many factors may confound the accurate interpretation of hemodynamic and laboratory measurements and may also result in monitor display of inaccurate or misleading pressure measurements. These factors include patient-related variables; failure of monitor systems to indicate *adequacy* of regional blood flow and oxidative metabolism; appropriateness or inappropriateness of hemodynamic measurements to the patient's specific physiologic needs; and technical (monitoring system) variables that may result in the display of inaccurate pressure measurements and distorted waveforms.

Patient-Related Variables

A state of health is maintained by a complex, synchronous, and intricate balance of multiple systems' function. Disease or injury complicates physiology by two mechanisms. The first is the primary traumatic or pathologic insult to anatomic or physiologic integrity. The second develops as the organism attempts to maintain homeostasis and begin healing by initiating multiple, complex compensatory metabolic and hemodynamic mechanisms. However, the highly intricate machinery of the human body cannot be counted on to respond uniformly to a specific disease or injury in all people. The unpredictability of responses is complicated by the presence of coexisting disease, injury, and drug therapies that may either blunt or exaggerate the responses to the underlying problem(s) or may actually cause hemodynamic and laboratory measurements to shift opposite to the anticipated direction of change. Consequently, an isolated monitoring or laboratory measurement can be misleading and must be evaluated with consideration of (1) the patient's preexisting state of health; (2) the patient's age; (3) the rapidity of onset, stage, and severity of the underlying problem; and (4) the presence or absence of coexisting complications or drug therapies.

The "probable cause" for any unusual physical assessment, monitoring, or laboratory finding, based on each patient's history, must be sought when making diagnostic and therapeutic decisions. Each evaluation tool supplements and enlarges on the other. For example, during a severe asthmatic attack, an isolated blood gas analysis report may indicate an arterial pH and $PaCO_2$ within the "normal range" and may lull the unwary clinician into an unrealistic sense of security. However, the presence of severe dyspnea, use of all accessory muscles of ventilation, continued wheezing over both lung fields, and diminishing breath sounds should alert the clinician to the existence of a critical situation. In this case, the blood gas measurements represent the crossover point when severe airflow limitation or respiratory muscle fatigue overtakes the patient and the previous hyperventilation-induced respiratory alkalosis (decreased $PaCO_2$ and increased pH) is shifting through the normal range to respiratory acidosis (increased $PaCO_2$ and decreased pH).

The development of respiratory acidosis in patients with status asthmaticus is a harbinger of ventilatory collapse. Overall, if the patient is dyspneic and tachypneic and chest auscultatory findings are abnormal, "normal" pH and $PaCO_2$ measurements are not representative of an acceptable physiology and must be considered as an "abnormally normal measurement."

Failure of Hemodynamic Measurements to Indicate the Adequacy of Regional Blood Flow and Tissue Oxygenation

Currently, no computer or monitoring device can tell how cardiac output, whether high or low, is distributed or if specific organ system oxygen needs are being met. Normally, the distribution of cardiac output and regional blood flow is regulated by changes in the diameter of regional arterioles. Vascular tone, in turn, is determined by localized tissue oxygen needs (termed *autoregulation*).

Many conditions, such as sepsis and systemic inflammatory response syndrome, are associated with inappropriate systemic vasodilation. In affected patients, some tissue beds may receive blood flow in excess of metabolic demand and become hyperemic, whereas other tissue beds become underperfused and ischemic. Abnormalities in cellular oxygen uptake and utilization compound cellular dysfunction. For these two reasons, cellular hypoxia may exist despite normal blood oxygen content and cardiac output. The increased mixed venous oxygen saturation (greater than 75%) and narrow arteriovenous oxygen content difference (less than 30 to 50 ml/L) reveal that oxygen is not being metabolized normally by the body tissue. However, these measurements do not indicate which organ systems are most or least oxygen deprived. Overall, the maintenance of normal organ function depends on adequate local blood flow and oxidative metabolism. These can be evaluated only by bedside clinical and laboratory evaluation of major organ function.

Appropriateness of Hemodynamic Measurements to Patients' Physiologic Needs

Another important consideration is the *appropriateness* of the hemodynamic and laboratory measurements to the patient's underlying problem and the *effect* on the patient at that point in time. The standard values against which patients are evaluated were obtained from a sampling of "normal," healthy people at rest. However, critically ill and injured patients are rendered "abnormal" by their underlying condition. This means that the standard values may be physiologically and hemodynamically *unacceptable* in many intensive care unit (ICU) patients. For example, critically ill or injured patients generally require a compensatory increase in cardiac index about 50% greater than normal because of increased metabolic needs. A "normal" cardiac output would then result in significant systemic hypoperfusion. Likewise, a "normal" rate and depth of breathing observed in a "shocky" patient is not normal or acceptable. It would be associated with uncompensated metabolic acidosis and also warns of an impending "worst-case scenario"—combined circulatory failure and respiratory collapse.

Overall, hemodynamic or metabolic stability is not guaranteed because the patient's "numbers" are "good," regardless of how "good" is defined. If the patient looks clinically "bad" despite "good" numbers, the patient's physiologic status is probably bad.

Technical Shortcomings That May Produce Inaccurate Hemodynamic Measurements

Noninvasively obtained blood pressure measurements (auscultation, palpation) correlate poorly with intraarterial pressure in hypotensive and hypertensive patients. Invasive monitoring systems provide continuous pressure measurements and waveform displays. Accuracy remains constant over a wide range of pressures (if system setup and dynamic response characteristics are good). Invasive monitoring is therefore more advantageous and is considered the gold standard against which other pressure and flow monitoring systems are judged.

The term *direct pressure monitoring* is commonly applied to invasive systems because the in situ catheter is in "direct contact" with fluid within an anatomic structure such as the pulmonary artery. In situ pressure measurement, together with the technically sophisticated nature of monitoring systems, tends to inspire a "blind faith" in digital numeric and waveform displays or computer printouts. However, pressure and flow measurements are actually obtained *indirectly* through fluid-filled tubing, pressure transducers, filters, amplifiers, and monitoring consoles. Consequently, a number of factors can result in the display of data that bears little relationship to the patient's hemodynamic status. Such factors include the physical characteristics of fluid-filled monitoring systems; improper zeroing, leveling, or calibration of monitoring units; mechanical defects within the monitoring console and cables; malposition or occlusion of the sampling catheter tip; and patient-related factors, such as cardiac dysfunction and cyclic pressure effects of spontaneous or mechanical ventilation. These factors are discussed at length in Chapters 6, 7, and 10.

Reliability of Monitor Alarm Systems

All electronic monitoring systems have built-in automatic alarm systems. However, the reliability and sensitivity of alarms depend on the integrity of alarm system components, on the limit ranges set by caregivers, and on whether the alarm system is activated and functioning properly. Paralyzed or ventilator-dependent patients are *absolutely* dependent on functional, sensitive alarm systems because they are vulnerable to accidental "disconnect deaths." Because *absolute* reliability of electronic systems cannot be guaranteed, and the consequences of failure may be loss of life, *the most effective alarm system for any critically ill or injured patient is a vigilant clinician.*

All patient assessment techniques (laboratory, monitoring data, physical examination) are interdependent in effective patient evaluation. Accurate diagnosis and effective therapy depend on careful consideration and integration of all assessment techniques and interpretation of measurements by caregivers who are academically and clinically prepared for care of severely ill or injured patients.

OTHER IMPORTANT CONSIDERATIONS
The Patient as a Vulnerable Human Being

Most patients who are candidates for invasive hemodynamic monitoring have known or suspected cardiovascular disease or another major system disease or injury. As a result, attention is commonly focused on the underlying problem, cardiopulmonary function, and prevention and treatment of potential or actual complications, as well as the maintenance of the complex technology of critical care support and monitoring devices. The emotional and spiritual human being attached to the equipment may be easily overlooked.

Patients facing acute life-threatening illness, major surgery, or trauma are typically overwhelmed with fear, sense of entrapment, and depersonalization, as well as loss of autonomy. The very nature of the ICU environment with its peculiar-looking equipment, animated oscilloscope lights, hissing ventilators, and many alarms reflects the patient's underlying fear: "I really must be sick. Otherwise, I wouldn't be in a place like this." The feelings associated with entrapment in a life-threatening situation over which there is no control may produce or exacerbate complications such as cardiac arrhythmias, myocardial ischemic attacks, hypertension, stress ulceration, and so on (Figure 1-1).[1] It is therefore essential to care for the patient's emotional and spiritual heart as well as the physical heart in order to enhance healing and recovery. There is no rote formula. Rather, the clinician must exercise deliberate attention to patients' emotional needs. This requires sensitivity and intuition because patient situations and responses are not alike. Awareness and consideration of the patient's cultural background; listening attentively to what the patient says; and helping with the expression of fears, hopes, anxieties, or anger may facilitate an outpouring of pent-up emotions. Holding a patient's hand during uncomfortable or prolonged procedures (when possible) and including patients in bedside dialogue also may significantly contribute to a sense of inclusion and well-being.

Sometimes critically ill or injured patients are rendered mute by the nature of the disease or, more commonly, by the insertion of an artificial airway. This imposes another significant stress because the patient is unable to give voice to feelings and needs. Movements that may be interpreted by hospital personnel as restlessness or random, purposeless,

NO MEDICATION

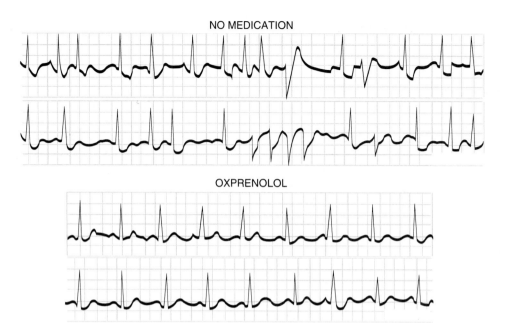

OXPRENOLOL

FIGURE 1-1 Public speaking normally evokes a potent stress response. ST segment depression and ectopic activity in a person with coronary artery disease are monitored while speaking before an audience *(top)*. The bottom electrocardiograph (ECG) tracing shows normal sinus rhythm, no ST-T wave changes, and no ectopic activity. This ECG was recorded from the same person on a separate but similar occasion before which he had taken an oral dose of 40 mg of oxprenolol. The drug blocked the effects of the stress response on the cardiovascular system. (From Taggert P, Carruthers M: Behavior pattern and emotional stress in the etiology of coronary heart disease: cardiological and biochemical correlates. In Wheatly D, editor: *Stress and the heart: interactions of the cardiovascular system, behavioral state, and psychotropic drugs,* New York, Raven Press, 1977.)

or confused behavior may be an attempt to communicate a basic need. The following excerpt from a letter written by the sister of a young, septicemic man who was dependent on many critical care support and monitoring devices exemplifies this problem:

> I wish he could tell me how he feels. The other day, he was trying very hard to get his hand free to do something. Everyone thought he was trying to pull something out. A nurse got brave and freed the restraint and all he'd wanted was to get his hair, now far too long, out of his eye.[2]

Other Psychosocial Support Measures for Patients and Family

Connected to the tubes and machines is the essence of our concern: the patient, the person. Also connected to this person are family and friends. It is these important aspects of care, the person and his or her family and friends, that are sometimes more difficult to diagnose and treat.

All patients, family members, and friends are stressed to some extent when a person is admitted to a critical care unit. The following are a few simple behavioral characteristics that can be identified in persons under elevated stress levels. Such persons *tend* to have the following characteristics:

1. They tend to be *self*-centered—not selfish. Need gratification is immediate and sometimes out of proportion to situation. They are "now" oriented.
2. They tend to see things as black and white. They see "you" in one of two ways: "You like me" or "You don't like me."
3. They tend to be more sensitive to *what* and *how* things are said to them.
4. They tend to have decreased attention span and decision-making abilities. They feel powerless, with a lost sense of security. Their focus may narrow to what they can accept, control, or understand. They may feel anxious, depressed, or apathetic.
5. They tend to have decreased concern about events outside of health issues and the health care environment. They are unconcerned about your problems and may see your giving reasons for why something was not done or done late as making "excuses."
6. They tend to want a forecast of their future health status. They "fill in the blanks" if not told, usually with more negative thoughts.
7. They tend to be more sensitive to pain (physical and emotional), especially at night, when things are quieter and they are alone with their thoughts.

Recognizing these behaviors can help the nurse understand the patient and family. The following strategies to reduce or prevent stress may then be introduced.

Anticipatory Teaching

The first and most important strategy is anticipatory teaching. Introduce yourself and give a brief update, every day and every shift, on what is going on now. Do not wait to be asked; it takes less time to teach now than to placate an angry or confused patient or family member later. For example, "All the tubes we talked about yesterday are draining fine, but this one has a little more blood today. That's why we are going to watch it closely and do a blood test to see if the counts are still the same." Note that a reference was made to one medical device (tubes) and one issue (more bloody drainage), but it was also mentioned what would be done about this issue (watch it and do blood test). Even things that are looking worse can and should be addressed, but it is necessary to provide a sense of being in charge of the event. For example, "Your dad's cardiac status is a little worse today. We have placed him on a new monitoring device and started him on a medication to make his heartbeat stronger." Do *not* teach to the point where the patient or family members begin to feel that the machine or the laboratory value is more important than anything else. When these areas are emphasized to patients and family members, they tend to focus *only* on these areas and want you to do so also. They have a hard time distinguishing the test or value from a life-threatening situation. It is hard for patients and family members to understand that our concern about the patient's leg edema yesterday is less important than his changing heart rhythm today.

Humor

The second strategy is humor. One opportunity to use humor is in teaching about the patient's daily schedules, which are often very nebulous or changeable. Understandably, patients and family members want to know what is going to happen next, and it is necessary to give them a sense of the hospital time schedules. For example, "The doctors have talked of sending you for a chest x-ray today or tomorrow, but they are not sure when. I will let you know as soon as a decision has been made." "You are scheduled for an angiogram at 8 AM tomorrow. It is not unusual for patients to be moved to a later time when an emergency comes in; we will certainly let you know if this should be necessary." "Dr. Jones is expected to see you at 2 PM, but that means he may get here between 1:30 PM and 5 PM."

These are good times to use humor. Share in a light way what tests will be done, but that delays or changes may occur. It is okay to make the hospital or yourself the "bad guy"; in this way difficult or unpleasant things can be made more bearable. For example, "You know us, one of our favorite things is to take blood or keep you waiting" (humor). "You have been very patient through all of this. Thank you for doing such a good job with all the tests, they can be very tiring" (supportive statement).

Listening and Reflective Empathy

The third strategy is in the use of listening to what the patient is saying and using reflective empathy. Listen to the tone of the voice and reflect back what you *think* you hear. Sometimes it is not *what* someone says, but *how* he or she says it. Ask the patient, "It sounds like all these tests, tubes, and numbers have got you scared, upset, or depressed. They certainly can be overwhelming at times. How have all these things been affecting you?" Even if your guess was wrong, the patient or family members will usually correct you and then tell you about their concern. They may not want to talk about the tubes, tests, or numbers. Do not attempt to take away the fears, worries, and concerns, which often are justified; reassure them that the staff is there to provide information and support them through this period.

Establishing Direct Eye Contact

The fourth strategy is the use of direct eye contact. First connect with people, then with objects. Hospital staff frequently enter a patient's room to do something to an intravenous line (IV), monitor, and so on. Pay attention to the person. First give direct eye contact to the person, then the IV. Eye contact is one reflection of attitude. When we are too busy to give eye contact, we appear disinterested to others, even if it is not true. They also may think we are not "good practitioners." They may respond to the practitioner with an "attitude," and the practitioner picks up the "attitude" and responds in the same manner. This vicious cycle is easy to get started. Attitudes, like measles and anxiety, are highly contagious.

Encouraging Self-Care

Families push their own personal endurance to the limit during the patient's critical state and commonly even during the patient's less critical state. They do not allow themselves to sleep, or cannot sleep; they eat poorly or not at all; they do not go home, or they spend long hours at the hospital just waiting or watching the monitors. It is those people who have overextended themselves, *but do not know it,* who often become overly involved in the medical management of the patient's care. They attempt to gain a sense of control over their feelings of powerlessness by overinvolvement in the patient's treatment. Thus they often use the things that we have taught them incorrectly or out of context in relation to the present set of priorities.

It is essential to encourage the patient's family members to care for themselves (the fifth strategy) with proper rest and nutrition. Encourage time away from the hospital to sleep, wash clothes, or have lunch with a friend. It may be necessary for some families with high levels of duty or guilt to institute special rest periods *for the patient* without visitors. Visiting is usually at the discretion of the clinician.

In summary, an old cliche says it best. Put yourself in the shoes of the patient or family members and treat them as you would want to be treated. Our work setting is commonplace to us; we see it every day. Patients and visitors do not see it daily, and it is usually frightening and filled with the prospect of pain and death. Meet them where they are, not where we think they should be.

The Caregiver as a Vulnerable Human Being

At the pressure input end of the monitoring system is a physiologically and emotionally vulnerable human being. It remains the responsibility of the clinicians (at the receiving end of monitoring devices) to look after the compelling, and sometimes overwhelming, physiologic and psychologic needs of patients. This is an awesome responsibility. Added to this is the responsibility of dealing with the emotional needs of family members who have varying degrees of denial, guilt, or unrealistic expectations.

People working with critically ill and injured patients are also vulnerable human beings with their own emotional and spiritual needs for validation and support. The physically, emotionally, and intellectually demanding nature of the work amplifies the need for acknowledgment. Unfortunately, this cannot come from patients who, upon recovery, rarely even have memory of the critical phase of their illness or injury. Whereas family and friends of clinicians may help meet the emotional needs of practitioners outside of the work area, the health care team also needs to work together to establish a symbiotic support system. Peer recognition and affirmation for "a job well done" nourish and inspire enthusiasm for future patient care challenges.

Suggestions for improvement are most effective when directly presented to the person in an objective, noncritical manner. A work environment in which each participant is acknowledged for contributing unique talents and in which suggestions for improvement are presented in a nonshaming manner helps create a professional experience that is nurturing and fulfilling and that facilitates personal and professional growth.

Preparation for Practice in Critical Care Units

Preparation for the responsibility of managing critically ill and injured patients mandates that clinicians receive specialized training in the art and science of critical care medicine or nursing. The basic didactic requirements of this specialty are as unique and complex as the physical equipment required for patient care. A caregiver who does not possess adequate technical skills and levels of understanding of physiology, pathophysiology, and principles of therapies negates the purpose of critical care units—to obtain the best possible outcome for patients who have major acute illness or injury.

Preparation for patient care continues beyond successful completion of a critical care course for two reasons:

1. The established body of knowledge related to critical care medicine and nursing is immense. Critical care courses generally prepare novices with only fundamental principles. There remains a vast area of information to learn to strengthen established skills or provide additional insights into currently understood principles.
2. It is the continuing responsibility of the professional critical care practitioner to keep current as new concepts in disease prevention, pathogenesis, and management continually unfold.

As practitioners of the art and science of healing, we frequently witness the entrance and exit of life, as well as some of its most poignant, intimate, and critical moments. It is befitting that we do so with great sensitivity and with great skill.

REFERENCES

1. Taggert P, Carruthers M: Behavior pattern and emotional stress in the etiology of coronary heart disease: cardiological and biochemical correlates. In Wheatly D, editor: *Stress and the heart: interactions of the cardiovascular system, behavioral state, and psychotropic drugs,* New York, Raven Press, 1977.
2. Richardson M: To Paul, wherever you may be. Unpublished manuscript.

2

GLORIA OBLOUK DAROVIC and JOSEPH P. ZBILUT

Pulmonary Anatomy and Physiology

Earliest medical records, as well as philosophic and theologic writings, indicated that humans recognized that breathing was synonymous with life: "And the Lord God formed man of the dust of the ground, and breathed into his nostrils the breath of life; and man became a living soul."[1] In the fifth century before the Christian era, Hippocrates stated that the heart "supplied the human body with life." The notion that *pneuma* (a spirit taken in with each breath) and blood meet in the heart for delivery to all parts of the body dates back to the ancient Greeks and Romans. Armed with this level of physiologic understanding, it would seem that insights into the vital interdependence between the heart and lungs would have been recognized at that time. But the following centuries were filled with academic swings moving closer to, and then further away from, present-day physiologic understanding.

The brilliant work of William Harvey, published in 1628,[2] postulated a continuous flow of blood within the closed circuit of the cardiovascular system. This work was a monumental contribution to physiology and medicine. Harvey was aware that the right heart pumped venous blood into the lungs from where it flowed to the left heart for delivery to the body. He mistakenly believed, however, that the heart manufactured "vital spirit," which, borne by blood, was equivalent to the soul and flowed into the body. At that time, the vital heart-lung connection was not yet appreciated.

Carbon dioxide was discovered in 1757, but its significance as a respiratory gas was not recognized. Approximately two decades later, Joseph Priestley isolated and described a gas that he named "dephlogisticated air."

He noted that a candle enclosed in a glass jar burned more intensely in a dephlogisticated air–enriched environment, then flickered and died when the gas was used up. In 1774, Antoine Lavoisier studied and gave the name "oxygen" to this newly discovered gas. Lavoisier also provided the first accurate description of respiratory dynamics: air is inhaled into the lungs, where oxygen is exchanged for the metabolic waste product, carbon dioxide. Lavoisier also stated that apart from causing burgundy venous blood to turn bright red, oxygen is necessary to normal organ function and the sustenance of life. Unfortunately, this revelation had no impact on clinical medicine, and the interdependence between lungs (oxygenation of blood) and the heart (pulse generator to drive oxygenated blood to body tissue) waited to be defined.

Despite the tremendous advances in the science and art of medicine in the twentieth century, the academic pendulum continued to swing rather than to move directly toward the concept that blood flow, blood oxygen content, and oxygen consumption are fundamental to life and are critical parameters in the evaluation and management of critically ill and injured patients. In the 1920s, a surgeon in Chicago began to measure arterial blood gases while the remainder of the world's medical community questioned their clinical value. Twenty years later, Cournand and co-workers[3] linked the heart and lungs as a single physiologic unit. The *cardiopulmonary unit* provides vital oxygen in adequate amounts over a varying spectrum of metabolic needs to maintain oxidative metabolism in order that the organism may function and survive.

Academic and clinical fracture of the cardiopulmonary link continued during the 35 years following the publication of Cournand's work. Cardiovascular specialists focused on continuous electrocardiogram (ECG) monitoring, arrhythmia management, and the "evolving myocardial infarction," while those physicians and nurses specializing in pulmonology centered attention on blood gases analysis, as well as new ventilator modes and adjustments of ventilator settings. Finally, awareness of the importance of oxygen delivery in critically ill and injured patients was ushered in by the landmark studies of Shoemaker and co-workers[4,5] and Finch and Lenfant,[6] which began early in the 1970s. They demonstrated that organ function and patient outcome relate to oxygen delivery as influenced by an interplay of the following factors: pulmonary gas exchange, blood flow as inferred by cardiac output measurements, hemoglobin's affinity for oxygen, and the hemoglobin level. Thus only recently has the delicate interdependence of the heart and lungs been fully recognized and its importance applied to patient management.

This chapter and Chapter 4 discuss the two systems separately for purely organizational purposes, although they function in unity for a single end-point essential to life—delivery of vital oxygen and removal of metabolic waste, such as carbon dioxide, from all body cells.

PULMONARY ANATOMY AND PHYSIOLOGY

The function of the pulmonary system is the exchange of oxygen and carbon dioxide between the atmosphere and the cells of the body. The term *respiration* refers to the movement of respiratory gas molecules across cell membranes, whereas the term *ventilation* refers to the exchange of air between the lungs and atmosphere. In other words, we breathe to ventilate and ventilate to ultimately respire at the cellular level. In clinical practice, the word "respiration" is sometimes used to describe the act of breathing, such as in counting "the respiratory rate," which may be variable and absent in breath holding. However, in physiologic fact, we continuously respire at the tissue level.

The four functional events leading to cellular respiration are

1. *Ventilation,* the bulk movement of gas in and out of the lungs
2. *Distribution* of these gases from the upper airways and tracheobronchial tree to the alveoli
3. *Diffusion,* the passive two-way transfer of respiratory gases from the alveoli, plasma, red blood cells, and body cells

4. *Perfusion/transport,* the movement of oxygenated blood through the pulmonary capillaries and veins and ultimate delivery to body cells

This chapter discusses these four processes respectively and separately, although physiologically they occur simultaneously. Anatomy and physiology are presented as an overview, and special ventilatory and respiratory considerations relating to acute or critical illness also are discussed.

VENTILATION
Breathing

Ventilation is the cyclic, rhythmic movement of the diaphragm and structures of the chest wall, which results in the bulk movement of gases in and out of the lungs.

The structures involved in ventilation include 12 ribs, the sternum, and the thoracic vertebrae, which form the bony cage of the thorax, as well as the ventilatory muscles, which act to expand or contract the volume of the chest cavity. The muscles of normal, quiet breathing include the diaphragm, which is the primary and strongest muscle of ventilation, and the external intercostal muscles. The accessory muscles are used when adequate ventilation cannot be achieved with normal breathing, such as during exercise or in patients with lung parenchymal disease or upper or lower airway obstruction.

The major accessory muscles of inspiration, such as the scalene, sternocleidomastoids, trapezius, and pectoralis muscles, elevate and raise the thorax. The minor inspiratory muscles include the alae nasi, which cause nasal flaring, and some small muscles of the head and neck.

Major accessory muscles of expiration are the internal intercostal muscles, which pull the ribs downward and inward, and the muscles of the abdominal wall. Upon contraction, the abdominal muscles force the diaphragm upward by raising intraabdominal pressure. The abdominal muscles also are necessary for coughing, defecation, sneezing, and the maintenance of good posture.

Overall, the structures of the chest wall have a tendency toward outward expansion. This can be noted in the operating room when, following creation of a midline sternotomy, the borders of the incised tissue spontaneously spring apart.

The two lungs fill a large part of the thoracic cavity; their prime function is gas exchange. The right lung has three lobes: upper, middle, and lower. The left lung has two lobes: upper and lower. The primary bronchi and pulmonary vessels enter each lung at its mediastinal surface, known as the hilum. Otherwise, the lungs lie free in their pleural cavities.

The pleural space is a potential space created by a visceral pleura attached to the lung and a parietal pleura attached to the chest wall. A film of fluid in the pleural space facilitates friction-free movement of the lungs during ventilation. The pressure within the intrapleural space remains subatmospheric and averages minus 4 to minus 8 mm Hg. This negative pressure acts as suction holding the elastic lungs, which have a tendency toward inward recoil, to the chest wall.

Mechanics of Ventilation

Between breaths, the recoil properties of the lung and chest wall are equal but oppositely directed. Pressures at the nostrils and mouth, tracheobronchial tree, and alveoli are atmospheric—760 mm Hg. Lung volume is static, and there is no airflow (Figure 2-1).

During *inspiration,* which is the active phase of breathing, the external intercostal muscles contract and pull the ribs upward and forward, and the dome-shaped diaphragm contracts to descend and flatten. The lungs, which are ad-

herent to the inside of the chest wall by the pleural seal, follow the outward movement of the chest and expand. The lower lung surfaces are pulled downward by the contracting diaphragm. As a consequence of the increased lateral, anteroposterior, and vertical dimensions of the chest cavity, pressures within the tracheobronchial tree and alveoli become subatmospheric—755 to 757 mm Hg—and air is drawn into the lungs (Figure 2-2). The negative intrathoracic pressure also creates a vacuum for venous blood, which facilitates and increases venous return to the heart.

During *expiration,* which is passive during quiet breathing, the external intercostal muscles relax and the elastic recoil properties of the lungs pull the chest wall to a contracted position. At the same time, the diaphragm relaxes and ascends to its resting dome shape. The dimensions and volume of the chest cavity are reduced, and as a result the pressures within the tracheobronchial tree and alveoli exceed atmospheric pressure—763 to 765 mm Hg. Air then flows out of the lungs because of the pressure gradient (Figure 2-3).

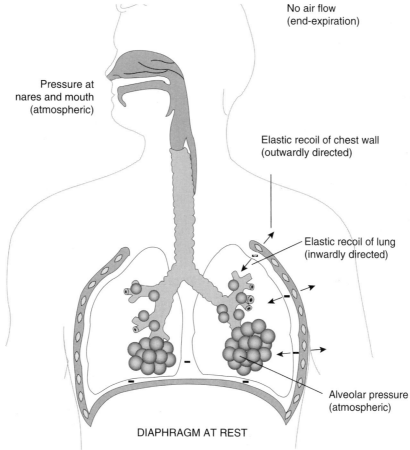

No air flow
(end-expiration)

Pressure at
nares and mouth
(atmospheric)

Elastic recoil of chest wall
(outwardly directed)

Elastic recoil of lung
(inwardly directed)

Alveolar pressure
(atmospheric)

DIAPHRAGM AT REST

FIGURE 2-1 Ventilatory mechanics at rest.

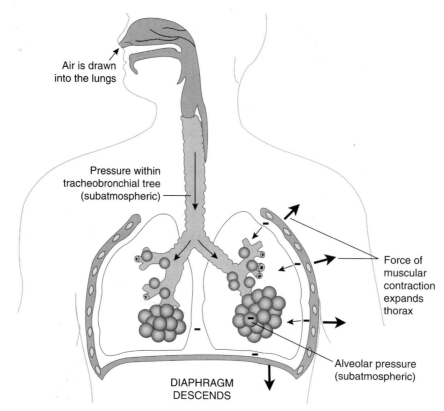

Air is drawn
into the lungs

Pressure within
tracheobronchial tree
(subatmospheric)

Force of
muscular
contraction
expands
thorax

Alveolar pressure
(subatmospheric)

DIAPHRAGM
DESCENDS

FIGURE 2-2 Ventilatory mechanics during inspiration. Size of arrows correlates with magnitude of expanding or contracting force.

In summary, normal, spontaneous breathing is negative pressure breathing. The thorax acts as a simple bellows pump, similar to an accordion. Expanding the size and volume of the thorax (inspiration) creates a negative intrathoracic pressure and draws air in. Contraction of thoracic size and volume (expiration) forces air out.

Breathing Supported by Mechanical Ventilators

Mechanical ventilation is used to support breathing in patients with apnea, ventilatory failure (inability to eliminate carbon dioxide), or oxygenation deficits. The types of mechanical ventilators most commonly used in clinical practice facilitate alveolar ventilation by applying a positive pressure to the patient's airway, typically via an artificial airway such as an endotracheal or a tracheostomy tube. During the inspiratory phase of the ventilatory cycle, the prescribed gas mixture flows into the patient's lungs because the terminal airways and alveoli are at lower pressure than the upper artificial airway. When the positive upper airway pressure is released, expiration occurs passively. Therefore mechanical ventilation is positive pressure breathing; the inspiratory force is a mechanically generated positive pressure

breath that pushes the prescribed gas mixture into the patient's lungs.

As mentioned previously, natural, spontaneous breathing is negative pressure breathing; the expanded thorax generates a negative intrathoracic pressure, which draws air into the lungs. (See Chapter 10, Figures 10-15, 10-24, and 10-25, for typical airway pressure curves associated with modes of ventilatory support compared with those of spontaneous breathing).

Control of Normal Ventilation

Total body tissue oxygen consumption and carbon dioxide production (respiration) are matched by immediate adjustments in the rate and depth of breathing (ventilation) to maintain arterial blood gases and pH at stable, physiologically acceptable levels. This ventilatory response is entirely dependent on nervous system control. Specialized neurons in the upper and lower pons and medulla (the respiratory center) alternately discharge inspiratory and expiratory signals to the muscles of ventilation. The neurons of the respiratory center, in turn, are excited or inhibited by islets of nervous tissue, termed *chemoreceptors,* that are located within the central and peripheral nervous systems. These chemosensitive

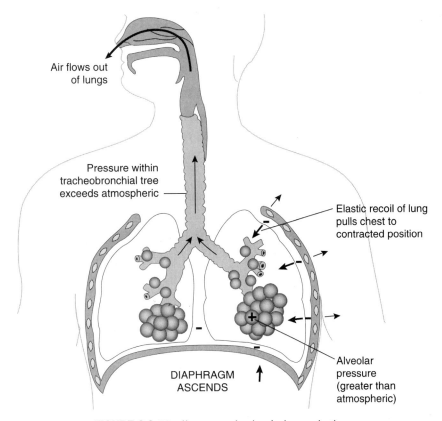

FIGURE 2-3 Ventilatory mechanics during expiration.

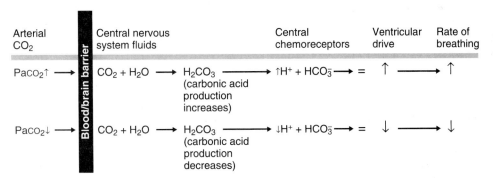

FIGURE 2-4 Within the central nervous system, carbon dioxide combines with water to form carbonic acid, which, in turn, dissociates into hydrogen and bicarbonate ions. The resulting pH shift directly affects the ventilatory drive and rate of breathing.

receptors immediately respond to changes in the chemistry of surrounding blood or fluid.

Central Nervous System Chemoreceptors. Hydrogen ions have a direct, potent stimulating effect on the central chemoreceptors, but the blood-brain barrier and blood–cerebrospinal fluid barrier are almost completely impermeable to hydrogen ions. However, carbon dioxide diffuses freely between the blood and cerebrospinal fluid (which is poorly buffered), and an increase or decrease in Pa_{CO_2} will result in a corresponding hydrogen ion change (pH) in both the interstitial fluid of the medulla and cerebrospinal fluid. In both of these fluids, the carbon dioxide immediately reacts with water to form carbonic acid and then free hydrogen ions (Figure 2-4). In other words, the arterial CO_2 potently influences the hydrogen ion concentration of central nervous system fluids. However, it is the hydrogen ion concentration in the cerebrospinal fluid (CSF) that primarily influences the brainstem chemoreceptors and controls breathing.

Elevations in $PaCO_2$ with a resulting CSF pH shift toward acidity (increased hydrogen ion concentration) excites the chemoreceptors, which in turn stimulate the respiratory center and ventilatory drive within seconds to minutes. Conversely, decreases in $PaCO_2$ with a resulting CSF pH shift toward alkalinity (decreased hydrogen ion concentration) in the brain and its fluids reduce chemoreceptor excitability and depress the respiratory center and rate and depth of breathing. For example, if a person hypoventilates and the $PaCO_2$ rises above 40 mm Hg, the resulting increase in CSF hydrogen ion concentration causes the central respiratory control mechanism to fire signals to respiratory muscles at an increased frequency. The resulting hyperventilation, in turn, immediately reduces the $PaCO_2$ in the arterial blood and CSF. The associated decrease in central nervous system hydrogen ions then blunts the ventilatory drive.

This rapid-acting feedback mechanism maintains arterial carbon dioxide levels and pH within the physiologically acceptable range (35 to 45 mm Hg and 7.35 to 7.45, respectively) over wide ranges of physical activity or metabolically altered states such as fever.

Peripheral Nervous System Chemoreceptors. The peripheral chemoreceptors located at the bifurcation of the carotid artery (carotid bodies) and aortic arch (aortic bodies) transmit excitatory signals to the central respiratory center in the brainstem in response to decreases in arterial oxygenation; this response is most potent in a PaO_2 range of 60 to 30 mm Hg. The peripheral chemoreceptors also respond weakly to increased $PaCO_2$, low perfusion states, metabolic or respiratory acidosis, anemia, or decreased hemoglobin concentration or saturation.

Overall, the central chemoreceptors are most influenced by and primarily regulate arterial $PaCO_2$. The peripheral chemoreceptors are primarily affected by blood O_2 content and thereby maintain ventilatory effects on blood oxygenation.

Other Ventilatory Responses

A number of other factors affect the rate and depth of breathing.

Stretch Receptors

The lung contains receptors that are sensitive to stretch. Stimulation of the receptors of the *Hering-Breuer reflex* results in inhibition of inspiration with lung infla-

tion beyond 800 to 1000 ml. This protects the lung from excessive inflation, particularly during exercise.

Pulmonary stretch receptors also are stimulated by decreased lung compliance (increased lung stiffness) and cause an increase in respiratory rate. This is seen in patients with chronic lung diseases such as pulmonary fibrosis, as well as acute conditions such as pulmonary embolism and edema. Sensory nerves termed *J receptors,* located in alveolar walls adjacent to capillaries, become stimulated when pulmonary capillaries become congested with blood or lung tissue becomes edematous. Excitation of the J receptors increases the rate of breathing. For example, tachypnea as a result of J receptor excitation heralds the onset of pulmonary edema before any other clinical signs of pulmonary edema become apparent. J receptor stimulation also contributes to the sensation of dyspnea.

Receptors from the Body

Stimulation of proprioceptors located in skeletal muscle, tendons, and joints, as well as pain receptors in muscle and skin, results in increases in both the rate and depth of breathing (hyperpnea). This is why moving of patients or painful stimuli such as pinching or slapping can stimulate breathing in patients with respiratory depression or apnea.

Voluntary (Cortical) Control of Breathing

Conscious control of breathing is essential for speech and breath control during activities such as swimming. A person can voluntarily hyperventilate or hypoventilate to levels that may produce serious blood gas and pH derangements. This effect is limited because when consciousness is lost from the effects of brain hypoxia (breath holding) or extreme respiratory alkalosis (forced hyperventilation), the autonomic centers again regain control. Intense emotions, especially rage and fear, also are potent ventilatory stimulants.

Alterations in Body Temperature

The rate of breathing increases proportionately with increases in body temperature and decreases with hypothermia below 94° F. This is due to the direct temperature effect on respiratory center activity, as well as the indirect effect of increasing or decreasing metabolism and oxygen demand throughout the body.

Sepsis

The endotoxins of gram-negative bacteria are potent stimuli to breathing. The resulting increase in minute volume (the total air volume inhaled or exhaled each minute) that is inappropriate to metabolic need usually produces a respiratory alkalosis.

In reviewing the list of factors that affect ventilatory responses, we can appreciate that patients at rest who begin to hyperventilate should be suspected of having acute pulmonary embolism, sepsis, circulatory failure, early pulmonary edema, or pain, and their condition should be immediately and carefully investigated.

Abnormalities of Ventilatory Control

A number of diseases and conditions are accompanied by abnormalities in ventilatory control. In some cases the abnormality in ventilatory control is an adaptive mechanism to the particular disease; in other cases the abnormality is a direct consequence of the underlying condition.

Chronic Obstructive Pulmonary Disease

Normally, excitation of the central chemoreceptors by hypercarbia is very strong within the first few hours of acute hypercarbia. However, if hypercarbia is sustained, the sensitivity decreases within 1 to 2 days. Gradual and progressive ventilatory insensitivity to carbon dioxide occurs in tandem with the gradual and progressive carbon dioxide retention characteristic of chronic obstructive pulmonary disease (COPD). One possible explanation of the decreased sensitivity to hypercarbia is that, over time, bicarbonate ions enter the CSF to buffer and normalize the pH in the medullary area, and this reduces the hypercarbic-related ventilatory drive.

The level of arterial oxygenation also tends to fall with the progression of COPD. However, peripheral chemoreceptor sensitivity to hypoxemia and the resulting hypoxic ventilatory stimulatory response remain intact for life. This is clinically significant because persons with chronic severe hypercarbia rely on the hypoxic drive for sufficient ventilation. Administration of oxygen in an amount that eliminates the hypoxic drive (a PaO_2 greater than 55 to 60 mm Hg) may result in sudden, severe respiratory depression in some spontaneously breathing COPD patients. Other ideas have been proposed for respiratory depression secondary to oxygen administration, but there are currently no fully accepted alternative ideas for the mechanism.

Other conditions known to be associated with ventilatory insensitivity to carbon dioxide include increased age, use of drugs that depress the central nervous system, and conditions associated with increased work of breathing. Advanced age and chronically increased work of breathing may be additive factors to the carbon dioxide insensitivity in patients with severe COPD.

Cerebrovascular Disease and Increases in Intracranial Pressure

Damage to the respiratory center following stroke is a common cause of long-term respiratory depression in older people. Acute increases in intracranial pressure may be associated with marked alterations of the breathing pattern and rate that profoundly influence arterial blood gases and pH.

DISTRIBUTION

Distribution is the delivery of fresh air to the gas-exchanging units (alveoli), via the upper and lower airways, made possible by ventilatory movements. Adequate distribution of inspired air ensures maximal gas partial pressure levels at the alveolus for efficient diffusion across the alveolar-capillary membrane.

Structure and Characteristics of the Airways

Structures of the *upper airway* include the nose, pharynx, and larynx wherein lie the vocal cords. The opening between the vocal cords is the narrowest portion of the upper airway and the most common site of upper airway obstruction. The *lower airway* consists of tubes that progressively divide by two, becoming narrower, shorter, and more numerous as they extend to the periphery of the lung. These structures, termed *conducting airways,* include the trachea, bronchi, bronchioles, and terminal bronchioles. Starting at the trachea, the progressively dividing airways resemble an inverted tree, hence the term *tracheobronchial tree* (Figure 2-5).

Cartilaginous plates are incorporated into the structure of the trachea and bronchi to prevent airway collapse. Approximately 20 C-shaped plates of cartilage support the anterior and lateral wall of the trachea; the posterior wall is made of smooth muscle and fibrous and elastic tissue. Hyperinflation of an endotracheal or a tracheostomy tube cuff or malposition of an artificial airway may result in compression of the vascular tissue underlying the relatively rigid cartilage plates and may result in ischemic necrosis of the tracheal wall. The scar tissue that replaces the damaged tracheal tissue may retract over time (months to years) and eventually may result in symptomatic tracheal stenosis. Allowing for a small cuff air leak and evaluation for proper tube position help prevent tracheal pressure necrosis.

The walls of the bronchi have less extensive cartilage so that these airways maintain an adequate amount of rigidity but are sufficiently mobile for lung expansion and deflation; bronchioles less than 1 to 1.5 mm in diameter do not have cartilaginous plates and therefore readily collapse during exhalation. Smooth muscle encircles the entire wall of bronchi within the lung; therefore bronchial

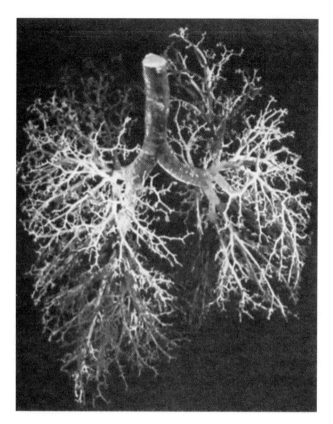

FIGURE 2-5 Tracheobronchial tree. Cast of the airways of a human lung; the alveoli are pruned away. In situ, the right main bronchus is more vertically positioned and larger in diameter than the left main bronchus. For this reason, aspirated material typically enters the right lung, and advancement of an endotracheal tube may result in right main bronchus intubation. (From West JB: *Respiratory physiology—the essentials,* ed 4, Baltimore, 1990, Williams & Wilkins.)

constriction may result in complete obliteration of the noncartilaginous terminal airway lumen.

Immediately distal to the terminal bronchioles are the respiratory bronchioles that have alveoli budding from their walls. Distal to these are the alveolar ducts and sacs, which are completely lined with alveoli. The composite of these structures is termed the *acinus* and is considered to be the basic pulmonary unit (Figure 2-6). The alveolated area is where gas exchange between inhaled air and pulmonary capillary blood occurs (pulmonary respiration) and is appropriately termed the *respiratory zone.* This area makes up most of the lung.

Mucociliary Clearance of Inhaled Debris

A moist mucous blanket lines the passages of the upper airways, as well as the tracheobronchial tree, providing an important cleansing and defense mechanism for the upper and lower airways. The mucus is secreted by goblet cells located in the lining of the air passages and by small submucosal glands.

The entire surface of the airways, as far down as the terminal bronchioles, is lined with ciliated epithelium; approximately 200 cilia are on each epithelial cell. The cilia beat in synchrony to move the mucoid secretions at a velocity of about 1 cm per minute. In the upper airways, mucus moves downward from the nose and sinuses to the pharynx, where it is swallowed. Through upward movement of the mucous blanket toward the pharynx, captured debris and particulate matter are cleared from the lower airways and lungs. Factors such as dehydration, cigarette smoking, alcohol ingestion, or a high inspired oxygen fraction (FiO_2) may impair mucociliary clearance and thus render the lungs more susceptible to infection.

Dead Space Volume

A significant portion of inhaled air normally never reaches the gas-exchanging areas and merely fills portions of the pulmonary system where gas exchange does not occur. This portion of inhaled air is termed *dead space air.* Dead space air is in the airways and may also be in the alveoli.

Dead Space Air in the Airways (Anatomic Dead Space)

The *anatomic dead space* is that portion of inhaled gases that fills the conducting airways and never reaches the alveolar membrane to participate in gas exchange. This fraction of "wasted ventilation" is equal to approximately 1 ml per 1 lb of ideal body weight. Anatomic dead space volume is fixed because the tracheobronchial tree does not change in size once full growth is attained. Thus a person whose ideal weight should be 150 lb (regardless of what it actually is) has a fixed anatomic dead space of 150 ml. Tidal volume is the amount of air inhaled or exhaled with each breath and is approximately 450 to 800 ml in a normal adult. Therefore:

    500 ml tidal volume
  − 150 ml anatomic dead space (wasted) ventilation
    350 ml alveolar ventilation (fresh inhaled air available for
         gas exchange)

In healthy persons, the dead space to tidal volume ratio is approximately 0.3. That is, approximately one third of the inhaled air normally does not participate in gas exchange and is wasted.

The rapid ventilatory rate or shallow breathing observed in some patients, particularly those critically ill or injured, may unfavorably alter the dead space to tidal vol-

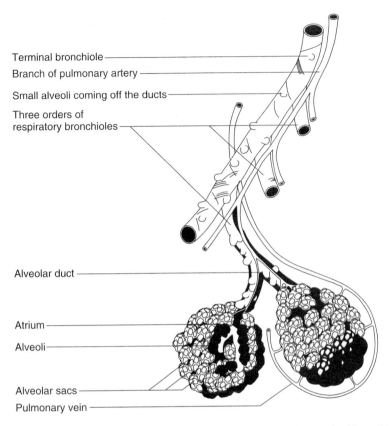

Terminal bronchiole

Branch of pulmonary artery

Small alveoli coming off the ducts

Three orders of
respiratory bronchioles

Alveolar duct

Atrium

Alveoli

Alveolar sacs

Pulmonary vein

FIGURE 2-6 The acinus, the basic pulmonary unit, begins just distal to the terminal bronchioles. (Redrawn from Wilson RF: *Critical care manual: applied physiology and principles of therapy,* ed 2, Philadelphia, 1992, Davis.)

ume ratio. Generally, as the rate of breathing increases (heart failure, fever), tidal volume tends to decrease; or as tidal volume falls (COPD, trauma, or surgery to the thorax or upper abdomen), there is a compensatory increase in the rate of breathing. Because anatomic dead space volume is constant, any decrease in tidal volume may potentially decrease alveolar ventilation even though minute volume (the total amount of air inhaled or exhaled in 1 minute) does not change. For example, a healthy adult may have a minute volume of 6 L according to the following measurements:

Tidal volume
    600 ml × respiratory rate 10 breaths/min = minute
            volume 6 L
−150 ml anatomic dead space (wasted) ventilation
    450 ml alveolar ventilation that exchanges with blood ×
        10 breaths/min = 4500 ml/min alveolar ventilation

If, for example, this person suffers thoracic trauma with rib fracture, the pain incurred with breathing will limit chest expansion and tidal volume. Thus:

Tidal volume 200 ml × respiratory rate 30 breaths/min
                    = minute volume 6 L
    −150   anatomic dead space
    50 ml   alveolar ventilation × 30 breaths/min
                = 1500 ml/min alveolar ventilation

This fact has important clinical significance because tachypneic patients have increased metabolic oxygen requirements (due to the increased work of breathing) but may not be oxygenating blood well. Overall, slow, deep breathing is more energy efficient and effective than rapid, shallow breathing.

Dead Space in the Alveoli (Alveolar Dead Space)

The *alveolar dead space* is that portion of inhaled gas delivered to alveolar units that are not functional because of an absence of blood flow to the adjacent capillaries. Although insignificant in health, alveolar dead space volume may increase with embolic occlusion of the pulmonary arterial vessels or with hyperinflation of alveoli because of the addition of positive end-expiratory pressure (PEEP) with mechanical ventilation or in a disease such as COPD (termed *intrinsic PEEP*) associated with intraalveolar air trapping. However, the most common cause of alveolar dead space is decreased cardiac output. In all of these clinical situations, regional or global pulmonary blood flow may be significantly reduced. In such patients, the increased alveolar dead space may result in hypoxia or an elevation in arterial carbon dioxide as a consequence of ventilation/perfusion imbalances. (Ventilation/perfusion imbalances are discussed later in this chapter.)

Anatomic and alveolar dead spaces are collectively termed *physiologic dead space*. In persons with healthy lungs, physiologic dead space volume is nearly equal to anatomic dead space volume. This is because nearly all alveoli are functional and minimally contribute to total dead space volume.

The dead space volume may be determined in the pulmonary function laboratory by measuring the partial pressure of CO_2 in arterial blood ($Paco_2$) and the average expired gas CO_2 ($Peco_2$) and applying those values to the following formula:

Dead space volume $= (Paco_2 - Peco_2) \div Paco_2$

For example, for a normal person with a $Peco_2$ of 28 mm Hg and a $Paco_2$ of 40 mm Hg:

$40 - 28 = 12$, and $12 \div 40 =$ Dead space volume of 0.3 L

If alveolar dead space increases, the arterial CO_2 will be higher than the end-tidal alveolar Pco_2. Following determination of tidal volume, the volume of alveolar dead space may then be calculated by subtracting the percent of anatomic dead space volume from the percent of total dead space volume.

Factors That Affect Efficiency of Ventilation, Distribution of Gas, and Work of Breathing

To make air flow from the nares to the gas-exchanging alveolar-capillary units, the inspiratory muscles must generate sufficient force to overcome the resistant elastic tissues of the lung and chest wall, as well as the frictional resistance to air flowing through the tracheobronchial tree. Expiration is normally passive. Changes in the following factors caused by disease increase inspiratory work and may significantly adversely influence distribution of gases and increase the work of breathing.

Compliance

The term *compliance* refers to the distensibility (stretchability) of the lung and surrounding chest wall.

Compliance is measured in terms of the volume of gas in milliliters, from end-expiration to end-inspiration, that can move into the lung for each unit of pressure increase measured in cm H_2O.

The normal lung expands approximately 200 ml for each cm H_2O pressure increase. Therefore, to inhale a normal resting tidal volume of 450 to 800 ml, a healthy person generates an expanding (intrathoracic) pressure of minus 2 to minus 10 cm H_2O. Approximately 70% of the work of breathing is consumed in overcoming the resistance to stretch of the elastic tissues of the lungs and chest wall.

Reduced Pulmonary Compliance (Stiff Lungs). This condition may be due to cardiogenic pulmonary edema because the pulmonary capillaries become engorged with blood and alveolar edema inhibits inflation of the involved alveoli. Similarly, pneumonia reduces lung compliance because the exudate-filled alveoli resist expansion. Disease associated with pulmonary fibrosis also decreases lung compliance, as does atelectasis. Noncompliant lungs increase the work of breathing because a negative inspiratory force greater than minus 10 cm H_2O is required to draw in a normal tidal volume. If the patient is being mechanically ventilated, a peak inspiratory pressure greater than 25 to 30 cm H_2O is required to push the prescribed tidal volume into nonyielding lungs. In severe disease such as adult respiratory distress syndrome (ARDS), peak inspiratory pressures may reach levels as high as 100 cm H_2O.

Increased Pulmonary Compliance (Flabby Lungs). This condition may be due to advanced age or emphysema because both conditions are associated with a progressive loss of the elastic recoil property of the lung tissue. Patients with pulmonary emphysema typically have a barrel-shaped thorax because the tendency toward outward expansion of the chest wall is unopposed by the flabby lungs. The work of breathing, however, is increased in these patients because muscular effort is required for expiration (active expiration). The hyperinflated, emphysematous lungs place the stretched inspiratory muscles at a mechanical disadvantage for efficient contraction; therefore inspiratory work is also increased.

Surface Tension, Lung Compliance, and Function. When water forms a surface with air, the molecules of water at the surface form a strong attraction to each other. This principle applies to any fluid-air surface. *Surface tension* is defined as the contracting force acting across the surface of a liquid. The effect of surface tension explains how a spider can walk over water and why falling raindrops do not split and disperse.

The surface tension of the liquid film lining the alveoli is another important factor contributing to the recoil properties of the lung. The attractional forces between the adjacent water molecules of the fluid lining of the alveolar walls are stronger than those between the molecules of alveolar air. Consequently, the fluid film becomes as small and tight as possible and the alveolar surface tension forces tend to resist expansion of the lungs. In other words, alveoli may be considered as a vast number of interconnected bubbles that tend to minimize the surface area and collapse.

Pulmonary surfactant is a surface tension–reducing agent composed of a complex mixture of proteins, ions, and several phospholipids. Secreted directly into the alveolus by type II pneumocytes, which partially line the alveolar wall, surfactant is physiologically advantageous for several reasons:

1. Lowering of alveolar surface tension, which then allows the lung to inflate more easily (decreases compliance)
2. Helping prevent the entry of lung water into the alveoli
3. Stabilizing alveoli, which are intrinsically unstable and tend to collapse or overinflate

In the absence of surfactant, small alveoli (with a high surface tension) would shrink or collapse while blowing up larger alveoli (which have a lower surface tension).[7] If this were to occur, no effective distribution of gases would take place and maldistribution of inhaled gases would, in turn, result in severe blood gas abnormalities.

Decreased surfactant production is associated with a variety of conditions, including cardiopulmonary bypass, prolonged high concentrations of inhaled oxygen (Fio_2), prolonged ventilatory assistance, ARDS, and neonatal hyaline membrane disease. Below-normal amounts of surfactant manifest pathophysiologically as stiff lungs, diffuse microatelectasis, and fluid-filled alveoli.

Chest Wall Compliance. The compliance of the tissue of the thorax also has an impact on the efficiency of ventilation and the work of breathing. Therefore spasm or swelling of the muscles of the thorax due to trauma (especially in muscular persons); circumferential deep-, partial-, or full-thickness burns; extreme obesity; or external binders may significantly decrease chest wall compliance and distribution of gas, as well as increase the work of breathing.

Airflow Resistance

We have seen that one significant portion of the work of breathing is to overcome the recoil properties of the lungs and chest wall. Another important portion of inspiratory work is to overcome resistance to airflow from the nostrils or mouth to the alveoli. Laminar (streamlined) flow occurs in the very small bronchi, which, by their vast number, provide the greatest surface area for gas flow. The pressure-flow characteristics of laminar flow are such that the rate of flow depends on the tube length and the cross-sectional tube diameter. The longer the tube or the smaller the tube diameter, the greater the resistance to flow. Bronchial length is not affected by any factor other than breathing. However, if the diameter of the airway is halved by bronchoconstriction, bronchial mucosal swelling, mucous plug, or tumor, the resistance to airflow in the involved area increases 16 times. Consequently, airway narrowing may profoundly impair distribution of inhaled gases and increase the work of breathing.

Expiration is normally passive (similar to a balloon deflating), because of the elastic energy stored in the chest during inspiration. When resistance to expiratory airflow is greater than stored elastic energy, the expiratory muscles are enlisted and the person's work of breathing increases. Clinically, this is encountered in patients with chronic airway disease or status asthmaticus (increased resistance to airflow) or pulmonary emphysema (decrease in stored elastic energy).

Overall, chest wall abnormalities and airway or pulmonary diseases may markedly alter the distribution of gases and increase the work of breathing. The excessive workload may ultimately lead to ventilatory muscle failure and death (see Chapter 18).

Effect of Artificial Airways

The addition of an endotracheal tube to the patient's airway imposes additional airflow resistance that increases as the cross-sectional diameter of the tube decreases. Stated another way, the smaller the internal diameter of the artificial airway, the greater the resistance to airflow. This may significantly add to the work of breathing if a patient is breathing unassisted through a T tube or is receiving ventilatory support utilizing spontaneous breathing systems such as intermittent mandatory ventilation. One study examined flow resistance in endotracheal tubes ranging from 5 to 10 mm at varying ventilatory rates and tidal volumes. This research demonstrated that "every millimeter decrease in tube size is accompanied by a large increase in resistance, in the range of 25–100%" and "a 1 mm decrease in tube size increases work by 34–154% depending upon the ventilatory rate and tidal volume."[8]

DIFFUSION

Two-way Transfer of Respiratory Gases

The preceding two sections have described the processes by which fresh air is brought to the alveolated area, which is the physiologic "site of action" in the lungs. Discussion now focuses on the factors that facilitate the two-way transfer of respiratory gases at the alveolar-capillary (respiratory) membrane and at the tissue level, as well as conditions that may impair diffusion.

Diffusion is defined as the passive movement of molecules (which are continually undergoing independent random motion) from an area of high to low concentration. Applied to pulmonary physiology, diffusion is the movement of respiratory gases from an area of high to low partial pressures. The primary gases involved are oxygen and carbon dioxide; each gas always moves in an opposite direction to the other. This gaseous movement occurs at the alveolar-capillary membrane (air-blood interface) and at the tissue level (blood-cell interface).

Diffusion at the Alveolar-Capillary Membrane (Air-Blood Interface)

The alveolus is the primary structure of gas exchange. The lungs contain between 200 and 600 million alveoli. The alveolar walls are composed of two types of cells attached to a basement membrane. Type I cells line most of the alveolar wall. The other alveolar cells are the type II cells, which produce surfactant, the surface tension–reducing agent described previously. Surfactant plays a major role in preventing alveolar collapse. Each alveolus is embraced by and wedded to an almost solid network of delicate pulmonary capillaries. The alveolar-capillary interface (respiratory membrane) consists of the alveolar cell membrane, basement membrane, interstitial space, capillary basement membrane, and capillary endothelial cell membrane (Figure 2-7).

The distance between air in the alveoli and blood in the pulmonary capillary is minimal—1/500 mm. Throughout the remainder of this chapter the terms *alveolar-capillary membrane* and *respiratory membrane* are used interchangeably.

Factors that govern the rate of gaseous diffusion across the respiratory membrane include the following:
* *The diffusion coefficient for the movement of each gas across the membrane.* This depends on the individual gas's solubility in the membrane; it is also inversely proportional to the square root of the gas's molecular weight. Applied to lung physiology, this means that carbon dioxide diffuses through the respiratory membrane about 20 times more rapidly than oxygen. For this reason, hypercarbia due purely to diffusion abnormalities does not occur, but mild arterial oxygen deficits due to "diffusion block" do occur. Although significant hypoxemia due to pure diffusion block is rarely present when the affected person is at rest, the PaO_2 may decrease significantly if cardiac output in-

creases (exercise, shivering, seizure activity, sepsis). The decrease in PaO_2 occurs because, as cardiac output increases, red blood cell rate of passage through the pulmonary capillaries is accelerated and this reduces the contact time with alveolar air.
* *The surface area of the respiratory membrane.* The alveolar surface area is approximately 70 square meters (the size of a tennis court) in the average healthy adult. The very large surface area for gas exchange, the small diameter of the pulmonary capillary (just large enough for red blood cells to pass single file), and the small blood volume in the pulmonary capillary bed at any time (70 ml) allow a continuously moving thin sheet of blood to interface with inhaled air. Even slight decreases in surface area can seriously affect gas exchange during stress induced by disease or exercise. If this surface area is reduced to one fourth to one third of its normal size (massive atelec-

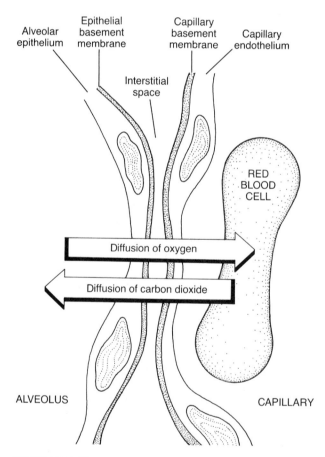

FIGURE 2-7 The structures of the alveolar-capillary membrane over which reciprocal diffusion of oxygen and carbon dioxide occurs.

tasis, surgical resection of part or all of the lung, or emphysema), diffusive gas exchange becomes significantly affected, even at rest.

- *The thickness of the respiratory membrane.* The rate of gaseous diffusion falls proportionate to increases in thickness of the respiratory membrane. Therefore increased membrane thickness (cardiogenic pulmonary edema, ARDS, pulmonary fibrosis) has the potential to interfere with diffusion of gases (diffusion block), but significant hypoxemia rarely is due to isolated diffusion block. In most lung diseases, coexisting ventilation/perfusion (V/Q) mismatches play a greater role in oxygenation deficits. (V/Q mismatches are discussed later in this chapter.)

- *The pressure gradient between the partial pressure of gases in the alveoli, plasma, and cells.* The weight of the layer of gases that surrounds our planet exerts an average force on the surface of the earth of 760 mm Hg at sea level. This is termed *atmospheric pressure* and is the sum of all the various pressures of gases that make up the atmosphere. The pressure exerted by one gas alone is termed the *partial pressure* because it accounts for only part of the total atmospheric pressure. For example, the atmosphere contains 21% oxygen; therefore the partial pressure of oxygen in the ambient air is 159 mm Hg (21% of 760 mm Hg = 159 mm Hg).

Alveolar air gas concentration is considerably different from that of the environment (Table 2-1). The reasons for the differences in alveolar and environmental gas concentrations are as follows:

1. Water vapor dilutes all other inspired gases. As air flows through the respiratory tract, it is exposed to the moist airway mucosa and becomes fully saturated with water before entering the alveoli.
2. Inhaled air mixes with the carbon dioxide that is exiting the alveoli.
3. Inspired oxygen is constantly being absorbed into pulmonary capillary blood.

4. Only approximately 350 ml of fresh inspired air reaches the alveoli with each breath; thus stale alveolar air is only partially replaced. The total volume of air in the lung available for gas exchange is about 3000 ml.

Diffusion at the Respiratory Membrane (Alveolar-Blood Interface)

Diffusion of Oxygen

A large oxygen pressure gradient exists across the alveolar-capillary membrane; the partial pressure of oxygen in venous blood is 40 mm Hg, whereas alveolar oxygen partial pressure is 104 mm Hg. Oxygen molecules rush down the large pressure gradient of 60 mm Hg and almost fully saturate the hemoglobin when the red blood cell is only one third past the respiratory membrane (Figure 2-8).

Evaluation of a patient's arterial P_{O_2} relative to that which would be expected for the percent of therapeutically oxygen-enriched gas mixture inhaled (F_{IO_2}) is helpful in evaluating deficits in arterial oxygenation as a result of pulmonary dysfunction (Table 2-2). For example, a Pa_{O_2} of 98 mm Hg is considered to be in the normal range if the person is breathing room air. If, however, the patient is inhaling a fraction of inspired oxygen (F_{IO_2}) of 60% and the Pa_{O_2} is 98 mm Hg, there must be some cause for pulmonary dysfunction, because the anticipated Pa_{O_2} should be 350 to 378 mm Hg. The disparity between the obtained and anticipated Pa_{O_2} measurements should be promptly investigated.

Diffusion of Carbon Dioxide

The partial pressure of carbon dioxide in mixed venous blood (Pv_{CO_2}) is about 47 mm Hg, whereas alveolar CO_2 is 40 mm Hg. Driven by the pressure gradient, some carbon dioxide molecules are yielded up to the alveolus, where they ultimately will be exhaled into the air (see Figure 2-8).

Diffusion at the Tissue Level (Blood-Cell Interface)

The laws of diffusion also apply at the blood-cell interface. Factors that tend to slow the rate of diffusion and impair oxygen delivery to and carbon dioxide removal from cells include (1) tissue edema because the respiratory gases have a greater distance to travel to and from cells and (2) a decreased arterial oxygen partial pressure or increased arterial carbon dioxide partial pressure because these narrow the pressure gradient for diffusion of these gases at the blood-cell interface.

When oxygenated blood reaches the capillary bed, the P_{O_2} is about 90 to 100 mm Hg, whereas the P_{O_2} in the interstitial space is about 40 mm Hg. This large pressure

TABLE 2-1
Partial Pressures of Environmental, Alveolar, and Arterial Gases

Gas	Air	Alveolus	Arterial Blood
Nitrogen	601 mm Hg	572 mm Hg	—
Oxygen	159 mm Hg	104 mm Hg	90–100 mm Hg
Carbon dioxide	0.3 mm Hg	40 mm Hg	40 mm Hg
Water as vapor	Variable	44 mm Hg	—

TABLE 2-2

Anticipated Pao$_2$ in Healthy Persons*

Fraction of Inspired Oxygen (%Fio$_2$)	Expected Pao$_2$ (mm Hg)
21	90–100
40	200–235
60	350–378
80	500–520
100	560–650

*Approximation of the anticipated Pao$_2$ in healthy persons while breathing oxygen-enriched gas mixture. Values below these listed suggest a disturbance in ventilation or perfusion (or both) and should be investigated.

gradient causes oxygen to rapidly diffuse from the blood into the interstitial space. The intracellular Po$_2$ is less than that of the surrounding interstitial space because the cells are constantly metabolizing oxygen. Because cells metabolize at different rates, the intracellular Po$_2$ averages about 23 mm Hg but may be as low as 1 mm Hg in tissues with high metabolic activity. The pressure gradient of approximately 17 mm Hg (40 mm Hg interstitial Po$_2$ minus 23 mm Hg intracellular Po$_2$ equals a Po$_2$ diffusion gradient of 17 mm Hg) causes oxygen to diffuse into the cells (Figure 2-9). Intracellular CO$_2$ levels also vary according to local metabolic activity but are always higher than those of the interstitial space and blood. Therefore carbon dioxide diffuses down the gradient from cell to interstitium to systemic capillary blood (see Figure 2-9).

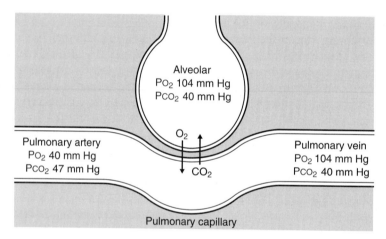

FIGURE 2-8 Diffusion and equilibration of oxygen and carbon dioxide across the respiratory membrane. The Po$_2$ of plasma in the pulmonary capillary normally equilibrates with the alveolar Po$_2$ within one third of the pulmonary capillary transit time when the person is at rest.

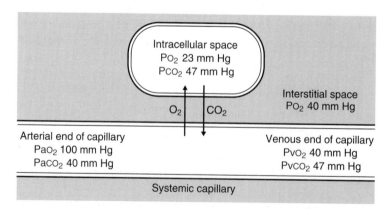

FIGURE 2-9 Diffusion and equilibration of oxygen and carbon dioxide at the tissue level. Increasing the respiratory gas gradient from the systemic capillary to the cells increases the rate of diffusion of respiratory gases from plasma to cells.

Overall, when blood reaches the pulmonary venous end of the capillary bed, the P_{O_2} is about 104 mm Hg because oxygen undergoes complete equilibration across the respiratory membrane. However, the P_{O_2} obtained from the systemic arteries is slightly less (normally no less than 6 mm Hg) because of the mixture of venous blood, termed *venous admixture*, to arterial blood via anatomic shunts.

Anatomic Shunt

The otherwise purely oxygenated blood coming from the lungs is mixed by deoxygenated blood before entering the aorta because the bronchial veins drain into the pulmonary veins and the thebesian veins (which drain the myocardium) ultimately channel into the left side of the heart. The term *venous admixture* designates that portion of cardiac output that has gone from the right to the left side of the heart without having been oxygenated. This deoxygenated blood, which is only 1% to 2% of total cardiac output, is a normal physiologic phenomenon and has minimal effect on lowering the arterial Pa_{O_2} (Figure 2-10).

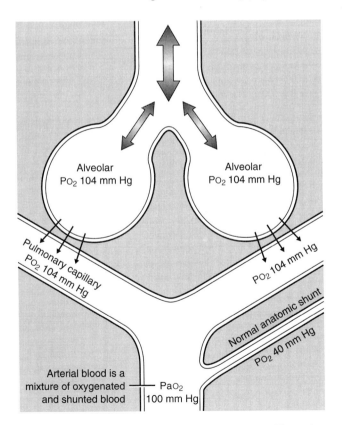

Alveolar
P_{O_2} 104 mm Hg

Alveolar
P_{O_2} 104 mm Hg

Pulmonary capillary
P_{O_2} 104 mm Hg

P_{O_2} 104 mm Hg

Normal anatomic shunt
P_{O_2} 40 mm Hg

Arterial blood is a mixture of oxygenated and shunted blood

Pa_{O_2}
100 mm Hg

FIGURE 2-10 Anatomic shunt. Schematic diagram illustrating the postpulmonary location of the right-to-left anatomic shunt in normal persons. Deoxygenated blood mixes with oxygenated blood in the pulmonary veins and left ventricular cavity. *Arrows* illustrate the direction and magnitude (size of arrows) of gas flow.

Anatomic shunting is increased in patients with structural abnormalities such as atrial or ventricular septal defects associated with right-to-left flow, arteriovenous malformations, and fistulas. As a consequence of the abnormal increase in anatomic shunting, the arterial P_{O_2} falls relative to the size of the defect and therefore the volume of blood flow through the defect.

PERFUSION/TRANSPORT

Perfusion/transport is the movement of oxygenated blood through the pulmonary capillaries and veins with ultimate delivery to body cells. These individual components of cardiopulmonary function (perfusion and transport) are extensive and complex and are therefore discussed separately.

Perfusion

Perfusion is the means by which mixed venous blood is brought to the alveolar-capillary membrane for oxygenation, carbon dioxide removal, sustenance of lung tissue, and ultimate delivery to the left side of the heart for transport to body cells. The anatomy and characteristics of the pulmonary circulation are presented first, followed by a discussion of the relationship of ventilation to perfusion in normal and diseased lungs.

Blood Supply to the Lungs

The lungs receive a double blood supply—the bronchial and pulmonary circulations.

Bronchial Circulation. The bronchial arteries come directly from the aorta and provide an oxygenated blood supply (approximately 1% to 2% of cardiac output) to the supporting tissues of the lung but have no role in oxygenating blood. If a pulmonary artery branch becomes obstructed by an embolism, the bronchial arterial circulation can sustain regional viability of lung tissue. If, however, the patient has significant heart failure or pulmonary fibrosis (which may compromise the adequacy of both the bronchial and pulmonary circulations), a pulmonary embolism is likely to be associated with necrosis of the involved lung tissue. The bronchial veins drain blood into the pulmonary veins.

Pulmonary Circulation. This is the circulation through which respiratory gas exchange occurs, and the circulation that receives the vastly greater portion of blood flow through the lungs. Pulmonary blood flow is powered by the relatively thin-walled right ventricle and, at any one time, is equal to left ventricular output or systemic blood flow.

Anatomy of the Pulmonary Circulation. From the right ventricle, mixed venous blood flows into the main pulmonary trunk, which then divides into the right and left main pulmonary artery branches. These arteries deliver blood to the two respective lungs and continue to divide for approximately 24 successive generations, becoming progressively narrower and shorter. Ultimately, the pulmonary arterioles join the pulmonary capillary network that surrounds, and is wedded to, the alveolar membranes. The capillary network is so dense that it can be conceptualized as an exceedingly thin, flowing sheet of blood interrupted by bands of connective tissue. At rest, blood transit time across this vital network is approximately three fourths of a second, during which time each red blood cell traverses two to three alveoli. Red blood cell transit time decreases as cardiac output increases, and thus, in high cardiac output states, the red blood cell may stay in the capillary only one third of a second.

Oxygenated pulmonary capillary blood is then collected by the small pulmonary veins, which progressively unite to form the four large pulmonary veins that, in turn, drain into the left atrium (Figure 2-11).

From the preceding anatomic description, the pulmonary circulation might seem to be a scaled-down version of the systemic circulation. However, several important differences are described in the following section.

Pulmonary Vascular Characteristics and Pressures (see also Chapter 4). The pulmonary artery branches are short and thin walled, with very little smooth muscle; are highly distensible; and have relatively large diameters. These physical characteristics are quite different from those of the systemic arteries, which are thick walled, are abundantly muscled, are less distensible, and have narrower lumens.

The reasons for these differences are that the systemic arteries regulate regional blood supply to body tissue (by constricting or dilating) according to changing local metabolic need and adjust vascular tone appropriate to postural changes, such as that from a supine to an upright position.

The pulmonary circulation accepts the same quantity of blood as does the systemic circulation, but its job is to continuously distribute cardiac output as evenly and efficiently as possible over the large alveolar-capillary membrane surface for exchange of respiratory gases. Heavily muscled, stiff pulmonary arterial walls would be counterproductive to this purpose (because these characteristics would increase resistance to blood flow) and are not necessary because the pulmonary arteries do not normally function to direct pulmonary blood from one lung area to another. The high distensibility characteristics of the pulmonary arteries

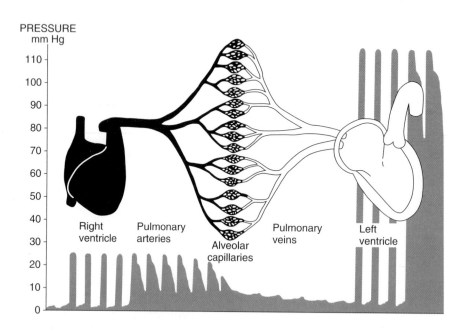

FIGURE 2-11 Pulmonary circulation. Because the pulmonary arterial system offers slight resistance to blood flow, the mean pressure difference between pulmonary artery and left atrium amounts to only 4 to 6 mm Hg. This low-pressure head drives the same volume of blood through the pulmonary circuit as flows through the systemic circulation with a pressure gradient of about 90 mm Hg. (From Rushmer RF: *Organ physiology: structure and function of the cardiovascular system,* ed 2, Philadelphia, 1976, W.B. Saunders.)

allow them to receive the pulsatile right ventricular output under remarkably low systolic and diastolic pressures. Pulmonary arterial pressures are only as high as those required to raise blood to the top of the lung. Therefore mean pulmonary artery pressure (15 mm Hg) is about one sixth of the mean aortic pressure (90 mm Hg) that is needed to drive the same amount of blood through the high-resistance systemic circulation. The driving pressure across the pulmonary circulation (pressure gradient) is one tenth that of the systemic circulation—approximately 9 mm Hg and 90 mm Hg, respectively. The relatively low mean pulmonary artery pressures keep right ventricular work and oxygen consumption at low levels as compared with those of the left ventricle. (See Table 2-3 for comparison of the pulmonary and systemic circulations.)

The pulmonary veins are also short, but their wall thickness and distensibility are similar to those of the systemic veins.

Pulmonary Vascular Resistance (see also Chapter 10). Resistance to blood flow through the pulmonary circulation is largely influenced by the degree of tone or caliber of the pulmonary arteries, capillaries, and veins. Pulmonary vascular resistance is normally very low due to the high distensibility of these blood vessels. As mentioned, the highly compliant pulmonary arteries facilitate the distribution of right ventricular output over the vast surface of the alveolar walls with minimal work for the right ventricle.

The distribution of blood flow through the lungs is determined largely by gravitational forces, whereas rate and volume of blood flow through the lungs are determined largely by the inflow (mean pulmonary artery pressure) minus outflow (left atrial pressure) difference. If the pressure gradient across the circulation decreases (the inflow pressure decreases [pulmonary hypotension] or if the outflow pressure increases [elevated left atrial pressure]), blood flow through the circulation decreases.

However, by altering the caliber of the pulmonary arterioles (dilation versus constriction), vasoactive stimuli acting on the arterioles may profoundly affect pulmonary vascular resistance and the distribution or rate of pulmonary blood flow. Likewise, vasoactive stimuli affect pulmonary venous tone, which increases pulmonary capillary pressure. The smooth muscle in pulmonary arterioles and veins responds to a number of vasoactive stimuli.

Factors That Affect Pulmonary Vascular Resistance. Increases or decreases in pulmonary vascular resistance may occur as a normal variant to the stresses and activities of life or may be related to systemic or pulmonary disease or administration of vasoactive agents.

Autonomic Nervous System. Autonomic nervous system activity has minimal effect on the pulmonary vasculature. Parasympathetic stimulation results in a minimal decrease in pulmonary vascular tone and resistance; sympathetic stimulation results in only a slight increase in pulmonary vascular tone and resistance.

Vasoactive Agents. Numerous humoral and pharmacologic agents affect pulmonary vascular resistance. Generally, the vascular effect (vasoconstriction or vasodilation) on the pulmonary circulation is similar to the effect on the systemic circulation, although generally less potent (Table 2-4). Overall, vasoconstrictor drugs increase pulmonary vascular resistance and are associated with elevations in pulmonary artery systolic and diastolic pressures with proportionate widening of the pulmonary artery diastolic to wedge pressure gradient. Vasodilator drugs decrease pulmonary vascular resistance and lower pulmonary artery systolic and diastolic pressures and are associated with approximation of pulmonary artery diastolic and wedge pressures. Humoral agents such as angiotensin II, brady-

TABLE 2-3
Comparison of Pulmonary and Systemic Circulations

	Systemic	Pulmonary
Vascular/Physical Characteristics	Thick walled	Thin walled
	Heavily muscled	Scant smooth muscle
	Relatively stiff	Distensible
	Narrow lumina	Wide lumina
Physiologic Characteristics	Dilate in response to acidemia and hypoxemia	Constrict in response to acidemia and hypoxemia
Pressures and Blood Flow		
Arterial mean (mm Hg)	120/80 90	25/8 15
Pressure gradient driving flow (mm Hg)	90	9
Mean capillary (mm Hg)	18	8
Mean venous (mm Hg)	0–8	4–12
Blood flow (L/min)	5	5
Vascular resistance	High	Low

TABLE 2-4
Pulmonary Vasoactive Drugs

Drug	Hemodynamic Effect
Vasoconstrictor	
Epinephrine (Adrenalin)	Increase pulmonary vascular resistance
Norepinephrine (Levophed)	Elevate pulmonary artery systolic and diastolic pressure
Metaraminol (Aramine)	
Vasodilator	
Isoproterenol (Isuprel)	Decrease pulmonary vascular resistance
Phentolamine (Regitine)	Decrease pulmonary artery systolic and diastolic pressure
Nifedipine (Procardia)	
Diltiazem (Cardizem)	
Hydralazine (Apresoline)	
Sodium nitroprusside (Nipride)	
Intravenous adenosine	
Inhaled nitric oxide	
Intravenous prostacylin (epoprostenol [Flolan])	

TABLE 2-5
Estimated Relationship of Mean Pulmonary Artery Pressure to Arterial Blood Oxygen Saturation and pH

	Arterial Oxygen Saturation (%)	pH	Estimated Mean Pulmonary Artery Pressure (mm Hg)
Normal	97–99	7.35–7.45	15
	93	7.53–7.22	20
	90	7.40	24
	85	7.40	28
	85	7.22	50
	80	7.40	34
	80	7.22	64
	70	7.40	47
	70	7.30	70
	60	7.40	55

Data from Ferrer MI: Management of patients with cor pulmonale, *Med Clin North Am* 63:255, 1979.

kinin, histamine, thromboxane, vasopressin, endothelin, and adenosine have variable effects on vascular tone relative to their action on specific receptor subtypes in the smooth muscle in pulmonary arteries and veins.

Hypoxemia. The potent pulmonary vasoconstrictive reaction in response to hypoxemia is in direct contrast to the hypoxemia-induced vasodilation that occurs in the systemic vascular beds. The contraction of smooth muscle in the pulmonary arteriolar walls in hypoxic regions of lung occurs in response to a decreased Po_2 of alveolar gas, not to the Po_2 of blood perfusing the vessels. Hypoxemia-induced pulmonary vasoconstriction is fundamentally a protective mechanism. In the presence of low alveolar oxygen concentrations (atelectasis, bronchitis, pneumonia), the adjacent blood vessels constrict and shunt blood away from the poorly ventilated alveoli to areas of lung that are better oxygenated. Unfortunately, with generalized low alveolar oxygen concentrations (high altitude, diffuse airway disease, diffuse microatelectasis), generalized pulmonary vasoconstriction occurs. The associated increase in pulmonary vascular resistance is reflected in elevated pulmonary artery systolic and diastolic pressures. Pulmonary hypertension may substantially increase the work of the right ventricle and ultimately cause it to fail.

Hydrogen Ion Concentration. An increased hydrogen ion concentration of blood perfusing the pulmonary arteries has a vasoconstrictor effect—pulmonary vascular resistance increases approximately 50% for each 0.1 unit pH drop. For example, if the pH drops from 7.40 to 7.30, a 50% increase in pulmonary vascular resistance can be anticipated. There is also a multiplier effect of acidemia on the hypoxic pulmonary vasoconstrictor response. This means that hypoxic pulmonary vasoconstriction becomes three times more potent when there is a simultaneous decrease in pH of approximately 0.1 unit (Table 2-5). High $Paco_2$ levels also enhance the hypoxic vasoconstrictor response, whereas low $Paco_2$ levels and alkalemia generally oppose the response. This has significant clinical relevance because these three conditions (hypoxemia, acidemia, hypercapnea) commonly coexist in poorly ventilated lungs, and the amplified vasoconstrictor response may result in severe pulmonary hypertension. The consequent marked increase in right ventricular workload may, in turn, produce right ventricular failure. In other words, the clinical condition of a patient with a primary pulmonary problem associated with significant hypoxia, hypercapnia, and/or acidosis may become complicated by right ventricular failure and significant hemodynamic deterioration.

Atelectasis. *Atelectasis* is defined as the collapse of part or all of the lung. Loss of lung air volume is most commonly due to partially or completely obstructed airways (mucous plug, bronchogenic tumor) or may occur with persistently shallow breathing. Atelectasis develops because pulmonary capillary blood rapidly absorbs air from the poorly ventilated alveoli. Atelectasis also may occur when air or fluid enters the pleural space because of loss of the pleural seal (pneumothorax, hydrothorax), or if air, over time, is squeezed from the lung tissue by constrictive scar tissue (pulmonary fibrosis). In addition, diffuse microatelectasis, due to a surfactant deficiency and diffuse small airway disease, is a common pathologic feature of ARDS.

When the lung loses air volume and shrinks, not only are pulmonary capillaries compressed but also pulmonary arteries and veins become kinked and narrowed. Thus, in atelectasis, there are two possible mechanisms that regionally increase pulmonary vascular resistance: (1) hypoxic vasoconstriction in the poorly aerated area of lung and (2) physical distortion and narrowing of the pulmonary vessels.

Increased Pulmonary Blood Flow or Volume. Although pulmonary vascular resistance is normally very low, it may fall further in response to increasing cardiac output or elevations in pulmonary intravascular pressures. For example, if cardiac output increases from 5 to 15 L/min in response to exercise or stress, as pulmonary blood flow and vascular pressures increase, the normally underperfused vessels in zone II open fully and continuously conduct blood flow. This is termed *vascular recruitment.* All of the pulmonary vessels distend to facilitate passage of the increased blood volume from the pulmonary artery to the left atrium. In fact, during strenuous exercise, blood flow through the lungs increases about four to seven times. The overall decrease in pulmonary vascular resistance has a damping effect on pulmonary artery systolic and diastolic pressures, despite the increase in pulmonary blood flow.

This same pulmonary vascular dynamic may occur if left atrial pressure increases owing to left ventricular dysfunction or mitral valve disease. As the elevated left atrial pressure is transmitted to the pulmonary circulation, the vasculature of the lung dilates to damp the pressure effect. This can be noted on chest radiographs as dilation and distention of the vessels near the mediastinum and visualization of the normally nearly collapsed and invisible vessels in the zone II area (upper one third of the lung in an upright chest film). This pattern of redistribution of pulmonary blood flow is termed *cephalization of blood flow.* Once all vessels have been fully recruited and maximally distended, no further decreases in pulmonary vascular resistance can occur. In fact, with worsening of left-sided heart failure and development of pulmonary edema, fluid accumulation around the blood vessel walls (perivascular edema) and hypoxemia result in narrowing of the pulmonary vascular

lumina. The consequent increase in pulmonary vascular resistance, in turn, raises pulmonary artery systolic and diastolic pressures.

Effects of the Left Atrial Pressure and Pulmonary Vascular Resistance. If left atrial pressure increases because of disease of the left side of the heart, pulmonary artery pressures passively increase in proportion to left atrial pressure elevations. This is termed *passive pulmonary hypertension.* In these cases (mitral valve disease, left ventricular dysfunction) the pulmonary artery diastolic to wedge pressure gradient remains less than 4 mm Hg. If, however, disease or other vasoconstrictive stimuli increase pulmonary vascular resistance, the pulmonary arterial pressures increase proportionately to the increase in vascular resistance. However, the measured pulmonary artery wedge pressure (PWP) remains unaffected and reflects only left atrial pressure. Therefore there will be an increase in the pulmonary artery diastolic to wedge pressure gradient that is usually proportionate to the increase in pulmonary vascular resistance. This is termed *active pulmonary hypertension.*

Calculation of Pulmonary Vascular Resistance. Knowledge of changes in pulmonary vascular resistance is diagnostically useful and important to evaluating critically ill or injured patients' hemodynamic and therapeutic responses. No clinical situation requires a therapeutic increase in pulmonary vascular resistance (PVR). However, some clinical situations require lowering of PVR, such as primary pulmonary hypertension and ARDS.[9,10] Intravenous adenosine, inhaled nitric oxide, and intravenous prostacyclin (epoprostenol [Flolan]) all appear to have similar effects in acutely reducing PVR with little effect on the systemic vascular bed. Some patients may benefit from oral calcium channel blockers.[9,10] Other medications may produce systemic hypotension (sodium nitroprusside, phentolamine) or have other cardiovascular effects (isoproterenol) that are undesirable. In selective conditions, removal of the underlying cause is the therapy of choice. These include the lysis or surgical removal of a massive pulmonary embolism and correction of hypoxemia and acidemia in patients with acute or chronic respiratory failure.

Pulmonary vascular resistance cannot be directly measured but may be calculated. There are two calculations:

1. *Total pulmonary resistance.* This calculated value expresses the total resistance to blood flow from the pulmonary artery to the left ventricle in diastole. Total pulmonary resistance is calculated by dividing mean pulmonary artery pressure by cardiac output; normal values are 150 to 250 dynes/sec/cm^{-5}. Because this formula does not take into account left atrial pressure

(which may be very low, normal, or very elevated, and certainly has an impact on blood flow through the lungs), the calculated value will not provide consistent or particularly useful information about the pulmonary vasculature. This formula was widely used more than 25 years ago before it became possible to easily measure left atrial pressure as pulmonary artery wedge pressure, and it is rarely used in clinical practice today.

2. *Pulmonary vascular resistance (pulmonary arteriolar resistance).* This calculated value expresses the resistance to blood flow between the precapillary arterioles (the pulmonary resistance vessels) and the pulmonary capillary bed. This calculated value is more useful in assessing the presence and severity of pulmonary vascular change or disease. Pulmonary arteriolar resistance is calculated by dividing the pressure gradient across the pulmonary circulation (mean pulmonary artery pressure minus left atrial pressure) by pulmonary blood flow (cardiac output). Normal values are 20 to 120 dynes/sec/cm^{-5}.

As PVR increases, concomitant increases occur in pulmonary artery systolic and diastolic pressures accompanied by a widening of the pulmonary artery diastolic to wedge pressure gradient. Normally, the pulmonary artery diastolic pressure is no greater than 4 mm Hg above pulmonary artery wedge pressure. Increases in this gradient correlate with increases in pulmonary vascular resistance.

An important caveat for the clinician to remember is that the calculated pulmonary vascular resistance "number" provides only a general indication of the pressure/flow properties of the lungs. This is because of the normal regional distribution of pulmonary blood volume and pressure (greater at the bottom, least at the top of the lung), as well as the numerous possibilities for local lesions or disturbances that are not reflected in the average of all the regional resistances or global "number." However, this calculated value allows comparisons of an individual patient's values against those known to be standard in health and allows evaluation of the same patient's pulmonary circulatory dynamics over time.

PHYSICAL FACTORS THAT AFFECT DISTRIBUTION OF LUNG BLOOD VOLUME

Up to this point, we have reviewed the anatomic features of the pulmonary circulation and factors that affect PVR. We will now review the physical factors that determine the distribution of lung blood volume and, as a result, affect regional pulmonary vascular pressures. How these physical factors interrelate with alveolar ventilation to determine overall lung gas exchange is also discussed.

Pressures Surrounding the Pulmonary Vessels

The pressures surrounding the pulmonary arteries and veins differ from pressure surrounding the pulmonary capillaries. The perivascular pressure difference between these vessels is due to the fact that the arteries and veins are surrounded by elastic lung tissue, whereas capillaries, which are exceedingly thin and receive little support, are surrounded by alveolar air. For this reason, blood vessels within the lung have been termed *extraalveolar* and *alveolar* pulmonary vessels, respectively. The differences in surrounding pressure profoundly affect the caliber of the blood vessels relative to the phases of breathing.

Extraalveolar vessels (arteries and veins) increase their caliber during inhalation because of the expanding pull of the surrounding lung tissue on their walls.

Alveolar vessels (capillaries) are exposed to and are affected by alveolar pressure. Alveolar pressure is close to atmospheric pressure at end-expiration and fluctuates minimally with quiet breathing. Therefore alveolar pressure does not strongly affect the patency of most of the pulmonary capillaries. However, during normal exhalation when intraalveolar pressure rises to drive out air, the poorly perfused capillaries near the top of the lung may be compressed and flattened by the slight increase in alveolar pressure. This is described more fully in the following section. In patients with labored breathing, the intraalveolar pressures may widely fluctuate and cause the pulmonary capillaries to cyclically collapse or distend.

Effect of Gravity on Lung Blood Volume

In the preceding section, the forces acting on the outside of pulmonary blood vessels and the relationship of alveolar pressure to capillary patency are described. There are also considerable differences in vascular pressures and regional capillary blood flow within the lung because the pulmonary circulation is a low-resistance system and blood flow is highly subject to the effects of gravity. Pulmonary intravascular blood volume affects intravascular pressure, and, in turn, regional pulmonary vascular pressures interrelate with alveolar pressures and affect regional patency of the pulmonary capillaries. The proportion of patent versus collapsed capillaries may affect adequacy of gas exchange and blood flow through the lungs. Collapse of pulmonary capillaries is particularly likely to occur in critically ill patients in whom intraalveolar pressures are frequently increased with mechanical ventilatory support (positive pressure breathing) or in patients who become hypovolemic, which causes a decrease in pulmonary artery pressures. In general, low-pressure blood vessels are more likely to collapse. These induced changes in regional capillary blood flow also may produce inaccurate hemodynamic measurements (see Chapter 10). The effects of gravity on pulmonary blood flow, vascular pressures, and capillary patency are subsequently described.

In the average-size, upright adult, the highest point in the lung (the apex) is about 30 cm above the lowest point (the lung base). Because gravity strongly affects the distribution of lung blood flow, blood flows are greatest at the lung bases and progressively decline toward the apices. Likewise, pulmonary artery, capillary, and venous pressures are greatest at the bases and then progressively decrease upward. Alveolar pressures, however, are not as much affected by gravity and, although slightly greater at the dependent portions of the lung, are fairly consistent throughout the lungs.

The distribution of pulmonary blood flow and pressure is altered by posture changes. When a person lies flat, the distribution of blood flow and pressure from lung apex to base becomes uniform. However, when supine, blood flows toward the person's back (the dependent regions of the lung) and exceeds flow toward the anterior chest (least dependent regions). Overall, the lungs are more evenly perfused when a person is in the recumbent position because of the decrease in the vertical dimension of the lungs.

The pressure/flow differences within the lungs result from the effect of gravity on intravascular hydrostatic pressure—the pressure per unit area imposed by the weight of blood within the vascular structures. Hydrostatic pressure increases in a downward direction and decreases in an upward direction. For example, the hydrostatic pressure difference (mean pulmonary artery pressure difference) between the top and bottom of an upright 30 cm lung is approximately 23 mm Hg, that is, about 0 mm Hg at the apex and 23 mm Hg at the base. At heart level, mean pulmonary artery pressure is about 15 mm Hg.

The local effects on pulmonary artery and venous pressures in relation to alveolar pressure and patency of pulmonary capillaries were originally described by pulmonary physiologist John West and colleagues.[11] The West zone model of the lung is discussed next and is illustrated in Figure 2-12. West's concepts have important clinical significance in evaluating and caring for critically ill or injured patients and also are discussed later in this chapter under ventilation/perfusion mismatch (see also Chapter 10).

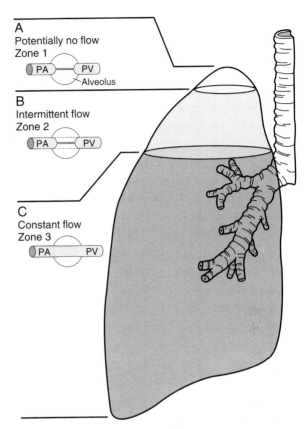

FIGURE 2-12 West's zone model. The effects of gravitational forces of the relationship of alveolar pressure to pulmonary vascular pressures and capillary blood flow. **A,** Zone 1. The least gravity-dependent area of the lung where there may be no blood flow because pulmonary artery and venous pressures are less than alveolar pressure. **B,** Zone 2. Pulmonary artery systolic pressure is greater than alveolar pressure, but alveolar pressure is greater than pulmonary artery diastolic (venous) pressure; as a result flow occurs only during systole because the capillary is obliterated in diastole. **C,** Zone 3. The gravity-dependent area of lung where, under normal circumstances, pulmonary artery pressures always exceed alveolar pressures and capillary blood flow is constant. (NOTE: These are not anatomically fixed zones but rather are functional zones. Any anatomic part of the lung may take on the characteristics of zone 1, 2, or 3 depending on changes in hemodynamic [increased or decreased pulmonary blood volume and pressures] and ventilatory status [PEEP, CPAP, alveolar air trapping]). (Modified from Guyton AC: *Textbook of medical physiology,* ed 10, Philadelphia, 2000, W.B. Saunders.)

Zone I—Pulmonary Capillaries Continuously Compressed (Area of No Blood Flow)

This is the uppermost part of the lungs where pulmonary artery systolic (inflow) and pulmonary venous (outflow) pressures may be less than alveolar pressures.

The capillaries (alveolar vessels) are therefore compressed and obliterated by the higher-pressure alveoli during all phases of the breathing cycle, and no blood flow occurs (see Figure 2-12, *A*). Physiologically, this ventilated but nonperfused region of lung is unavailable for gas exchange (alveolar dead space). Zone I does not occur under normal conditions because pulmonary artery pressures at the top of the lung are normally just high enough to exceed alveolar pressure and force systolic flow through the capillaries. If the pulmonary artery pressures are reduced (hypovolemia), or if alveolar pressures are increased (positive pressure ventilation, PEEP), the zone I area develops.

Zone II—Pulmonary Capillaries Intermittently Compressed (Area of Intermittent Blood Flow)

Farther down the lung, the cyclic pulmonary vascular pressures increase. Pulmonary artery systolic (inflow) pressure now exceeds alveolar pressure, thus allowing systolic blood flow. However, the pulmonary venous (outflow) pressure is less than alveolar pressure and the capillary is therefore compressed and obliterated by the adjacent alveolus in diastole. In this section of lung, which normally begins 7 to 10 cm above the level of the heart and extends up to the apex, there is only intermittent flow. Consequently, the alveoli of this section of the lungs are relatively underperfused (see Figure 2-12, *B*). This flow phenomenon has been variously termed *waterfall, sluice,* or *Starling resistor* effect because similarity has been drawn to a waterfall or sluice where rate of flow at the inflow side (top of waterfall) is not affected by what is happening at the bottom of the waterfall. Applied to the lungs, pulmonary artery systolic pressure is analogous to the top of the waterfall, which determines blood flow, and is not affected by pulmonary venous pressure, which represents the bottom of the waterfall. Instead, blood flow is determined by the relationship of pulmonary artery systolic pressure and alveolar pressure. Zone II conditions can enlarge in a downward direction and involve a larger lung area in patients with hypovolemia or by any factor that increases intraalveolar pressure (PEEP, continuous positive airway pressure [CPAP], intraalveolar air trapping). Alternatively, intravascular volume loading, through its effect on increasing pulmonary intravascular volume and pressures, diminishes the zone II area.

Zone III—Pulmonary Capillaries Constantly Patent (Area of Continous Blood Flow)

Farther down the lungs, pulmonary artery and venous pressures constantly exceed alveolar pressure and the pulmonary vascular channel is continuously open to blood flow. The progressive increase in blood flow downward in zone III is due to the progressively increasing hydrostatic pressures that cause dilation and distention of the capillaries. In this zone there is good matching of ventilated alveoli to perfused capillaries. In health, two thirds of the lung is a zone III area. Hypovolemia or factors that increase intraalveolar pressure shrink zone III. On the other hand, volume loading increases zone III (see Figure 2-12, *C*). Accurate pulmonary artery pressure monitoring requires the catheter tip to be in a gravity-dependent (zone III) area of lung. The pulmonary artery catheter tip flows to a zone III area of lung the greater percent of the time. However, the catheter may float to a zone I or II area. In these cases, obtained pulmonary artery pressures will not correlate with the true intravascular pressures (see Chapter 10).

Increases in zone I or II lung area result in an increase in the area of lung that is overventilated relative to perfusion (wasted ventilation). If significant, this has deleterious effects on blood oxygenation and carbon dioxide removal. Increases in zone I and II areas may also present problems in obtaining accurate pulmonary artery pressure measurements (see Chapter 10).

Matching of Alveolar Ventilation to Pulmonary Capillary Perfusion

The primary functions of the lungs are to remove carbon dioxide and to oxygenate the venous blood delivered to the lungs by the pulmonary arteries. Two physiologic requirements are critical to attainment of these vital endpoints: (1) the alveoli must be adequately ventilated, and (2) the pulmonary capillaries must be adequately perfused. In a perfect world, all alveoli would be perfectly ventilated and all pulmonary capillaries would be perfectly perfused. We live, however, in an imperfect world, and even in healthy persons there is some mismatch of alveolar ventilation to capillary perfusion, as discussed in the preceding section. In patients with cardiopulmonary disease, increased mismatch of ventilation to perfusion frequently results in serious blood gas abnormalities. The concept of the ventilation/perfusion (V/Q) ratio has been developed to help us understand the magnitude of imbalances in patients with abnormalities in alveolar ventilation or pulmonary blood flow (V = alveolar ventilation and Q = blood flow).

Ventilation/Perfusion Ratio (V/Q Ratio)

In health, the total volume of inhaled air that reaches the alveoli (alveolar ventilation) and the total volume of deoxygenated venous blood presented to the lung (cardiac output) per minute fluctuate but remain nearly equal. Resting minute alveolar ventilation averages about 4 to

6 L/min, and resting pulmonary blood flow is about the same. Therefore the normal V/Q ratio is 0.8 to 1.2. For example, a person with a V/Q ratio of 0.8 (4:5) may have 4 L/min alveolar ventilation and pulmonary blood flow of 5 L/min. In this person, at this moment in time, there is slightly less flow of alveolar gas than pulmonary blood. If, at any point in time, a person's alveolar ventilation and lung perfusion were coincidentally perfectly matched, the V/Q ratio would be 1. (These are typical values and may vary in health relative to stress, physical activity, and so forth.)

We now examine the possible extremes of V/Q ratios that may occur with disease. A lung that is nonventilated (apnea, total airway obstruction) but perfused has a V/Q ratio of zero because there is zero ventilation. At the other extreme, a lung that is adequately ventilated but not perfused (massive saddle pulmonary embolism) has an infinite V/Q ratio because ventilation is infinite when matched against no pulmonary blood flow. Obviously, neither of these situations is compatible with life.

The arterial PO_2 and PCO_2 are determined by ventilation and perfusion of all alveoli. This is because of the balance that is set between (1) the rate at which alveolar oxygen is taken up by the pulmonary capillary blood and the rate at which carbon dioxide is yielded from the pulmonary capillary blood, and (2) the rate at which fresh air is inhaled and replenishes alveolar oxygen and the rate at which carbon dioxide is washed out and exhaled.

If a person hyperventilates and, as a result, alveolar ventilation increases, the alveolar PO_2 increases and alveolar PCO_2 decreases. Assuming that pulmonary capillary blood flow remains constant, the arterial PO_2 then increases and the arterial PCO_2 decreases. Conversely, if a person hypoventilates, the alveolar PO_2 decreases and the alveolar PCO_2 increases. Assuming again that pulmonary capillary blood flow remains constant, the arterial PO_2 decreases and the arterial PCO_2 rises. Overall, the effect of alveolar ventilation on arterial PCO_2 is straightforward; if alveolar ventilation is doubled, the arterial PCO_2 is approximately halved, whereas if alveolar ventilation is reduced to one half normal levels, the arterial PCO_2 approximately doubles.

Regional Matching of Ventilation to Perfusion in Normal Lungs

As stated previously, the distribution of pulmonary ventilation and perfusion shows variations relating to gravitational forces dependent on body position. Both increase progressively downward from the apices to the bases when the person is in an upright position, although the volume of blood flow increases about three times more

rapidly than does ventilation. Mean pulmonary artery pressure is about 13 to 15 mm Hg at heart level, and alveolar pressures are about equal throughout the lung, minus 3 to plus 3 cm H_2O with normal, quiet breathing. At the apex, mean pulmonary artery pressure is about 3 mm Hg; therefore the V/Q ratio is higher at the apices (ventilation in excess of perfusion). At the bases, mean pulmonary artery pressure is about 23 mm Hg; therefore blood flow is greater there than at heart level and, in these dependent areas of lung, perfusion is in excess of ventilation (V/Q ratios are lower). Clearly, ventilation is not perfectly matched to perfusion in all areas of the normal lung because gravity prevents the lung from attaining perfect function. The overall effect in healthy persons, however, is that arterial blood is adequately oxygenated and carbon dioxide is adequately removed.

Ventilation/Perfusion Mismatches Induced by Disease

Although some degree of V/Q mismatch always occurs in normal lungs, many diseases result in increased regional or global abnormalities in the matching of ventilation to perfusion. These V/Q imbalances potentially render the lungs less efficient exchangers of both oxygen and carbon dioxide. The greater the number and magnitude of alveolar-capillary units deviating from the idealized V/Q ratio of 1, the less efficient respiratory gas exchange becomes. Unless the problem is hypoventilation, however, patients rarely have an acutely elevated $PaCO_2$. This is because chemoreceptor excitation by the acutely rising $PaCO_2$ immediately triggers an increase in the ventilatory drive, and compensatory hyperventilation returns the arterial PCO_2 to normal levels. Compensatory hyperventilation, however, increases the work of breathing and has a minimal effect on improving arterial oxygenation.

Hypoxemia, defined as a PaO_2 less than 60 mm Hg at sea level, is the blood gas abnormality most frequently observed in patients, and V/Q mismatches are the most common cause. The means by which V/Q imbalances may acutely or chronically lead to respiratory failure covers a broad pathophysiologic spectrum. At one end of the spectrum, absent or decreased alveolar ventilation relative to adequate capillary perfusion predisposes the patient to varying degrees of inadequate gas exchange because blood flow in the diseased area (atelectasis, pneumonia) passes through lung and does not contact and exchange with alveolar air. This is termed *shunting*. At the other end of the spectrum, absent or decreased capillary perfusion relative to ventilation leads to wasted ventilation; alveolar air does not contact and exchange with flowing capillary blood. This is termed *alveolar dead space*. The causes of

V/Q mismatch are discussed separately, although the many causes may coexist regionally or globally in patients with severe lung disease.

Circumstances in Which Pulmonary Capillary Blood Does Not "See" Alveolar Air–Shunt Units

The severity of alveolar dysfunction and hence the severity of the shunt are variable. The alveolus may be completely nonventilated (absolute shunt) or simply inadequately ventilated (shunt effect).

Absolute Shunt (True Shunt). As mentioned earlier, a very small percent of cardiac output normally flows from the venous to the arterial circulation through anatomic shunts, never having exchanged with air. With the development of pulmonary disease, diffusely scattered or local regions of alveoli may be completely nonventilated and nonfunctional because they are filled with fluid or exudate (pulmonary edema, pneumonia, lung abscess, pooled secretions) or are collapsed (atelectasis), while their adjacent capillaries maintain some blood flow. This is an extreme V/Q mismatch in which pulmonary capillary blood "sees" no alveolar air with which to equilibrate. Therefore venous blood flows from the right side of the pulmonary circulation (pulmonary arteries) through the diseased "shunt units" to the left side of the pulmonary circulation (pulmonary veins) without undergoing gas exchange. Here the shunted blood mixes with the oxygenated blood returning from the normal lung units. The PaO₂ composition of the arterial blood pumped into the systemic circulation depends on the percent of deoxygenated "shunted" blood contaminating the mixture. With severe disease, such as diffuse, bilateral pneumonia, arterial oxygenation may be so minimal as to be incapable of supporting the patient's life without aggressive oxygen therapy and ventilatory support.

In Figure 2-13, mixed venous blood enters both alveolar units with a PO₂ of 40 mm Hg and saturation of 75%. Blood perfusing the fully ventilated alveolus reaches ideal oxygen equilibrium—PaO₂ 104 mm Hg, saturation 98%. Blood perfusing the nonventilated alveolus returns to the pulmonary veins unchanged with blood gas values equal to those of mixed venous blood. Assuming 50% distribution of all blood flow through each unit, the combined effect will be an arterial PO₂ of about 55 mm Hg with a saturation of approximately 86%.

A classic feature of *absolute shunt* is that the patient's hypoxemia is very poorly responsive to oxygen administration; increasing the FiO₂ by 20% is met with a PaO₂ increase less than 10 mm Hg. This is termed *refractory*

hypoxemia. For example, if a patient's PaO₂ is 45 mm Hg while breathing room air (FiO₂ 21%), increasing the FiO₂ to 40% with supplemental oxygen will be associated with a PaO₂ increase to less than 55 mm Hg. The oxygenation deficit persists because the shunted blood remains unaffected by the higher alveolar PO₂ that is going only to normal, ventilated alveolar units. The "true shunt" units remain nonfunctional regardless of the amount of oxygen inhaled. Therefore the shunted blood continues to depress the arterial PO₂ with mixed venous blood. However, a minimal elevation in PaO₂ occurs because of the oxygen added to the capillary blood from the normal lung units. (The clinical means of calculating the percent of shunt is discussed in Chapter 10.)

Relative Shunt (Shunt Effect). In this situation, there are areas of subnormally ventilated alveoli relative to the amount of perfusion of the adjacent capillaries. This occurs in persons with airways that are diffusely diseased (severe bronchitis, pulmonary emphysema, status asthmaticus) or

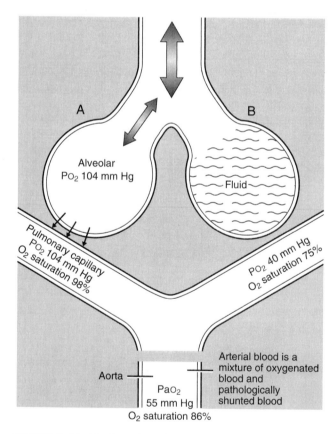

FIGURE 2-13 Absolute shunt (true shunt). *Arrows* indicate the direction of gas flow. **A,** Fully ventilated alveolus. **B,** Nonventilated alveolus.

persons with retained airway secretions. At the involved alveolar-capillary units, pulmonary capillary blood achieves a PaO_2 that is less than ideal. At the pulmonary veins, the less than ideally oxygenated blood mixes with the fully oxygenated blood that has equilibrated at normal alveolar-capillary units.

In Figure 2-14, mixed venous blood enters both alveolar units with a PO_2 of 40 mm Hg, arterial saturation of 75%, and PCO_2 of 45 mm Hg. Alveolus A has normal matching of alveolar ventilation to capillary blood flow and normal equilibration values across the respiratory membrane—PaO_2 of 104 mm Hg and saturation of 99%. Alveolus B is hypoventilated due to bronchial mucus, swelling, or spasm; blood flow across this poorly ventilated unit may achieve equilibration values of PaO_2 of 50 mm Hg and saturation of 80%. Assuming one half of blood flow through each unit, blood gas values derived from both these units as they mix and flow into the arterial circuit will be the average of the two: a PaO_2 of approximately 59 mm Hg and saturation of 89%.

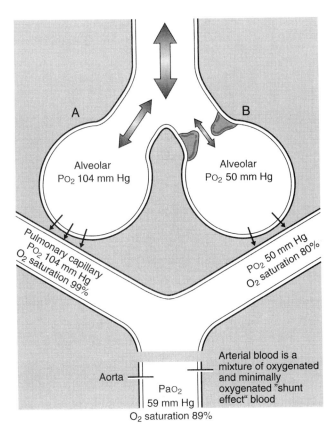

FIGURE 2-14 Relative shunt (shunt effect). *Arrows* indicate direction and magnitude (size of arrows) of gas flow. **A,** Normal alveolus. **B,** Hypoventilated alveolus.

The amount and magnitude of *relative shunt* units may be highly variable among patients. Relative shunt is clinically distinguished from absolute shunt in that it is dramatically responsive to oxygen therapy. This is because as the concentration of oxygen carried to these functional alveoli increases, the arterial PO_2 increases correspondingly.

Critically ill patients typically have both absolute shunt and relative shunt areas of lung. For example, in ARDS, diffuse microatelectasis, in which there is no gas exchange, coexists with poorly ventilated alveoli secondary to diffuse small airway disease and mucous plugs.

Hypoventilation. In patients with pure hypoventilation, the lungs are normal but the volume of air inhaled through the nose or mouth (minute ventilation) and fresh incoming alveolar air are reduced. In other words, there is uniform but decreased total alveolar ventilation relative to normal pulmonary capillary blood flow. Consequently there is an inadequate supply of alveolar oxygen molecules to replenish and maintain the alveolar PO_2 at normal levels and to wash out the alveolar CO_2. The resulting below-normal alveolar PO_2 and above-normal alveolar PCO_2 equilibrate across the alveolar-capillary membrane. On blood gas analysis, hypoventilation is manifest as a decreased PaO_2, a $PaCO_2$ greater than 45 mm Hg, and a decreased pH (respiratory acidosis).

Causes of hypoventilation include depression of the respiratory centers in the brainstem by drugs or anesthesia, disease or trauma to the cerebral medulla, neuromuscular diseases that alter respiratory muscle function, chest or upper abdominal trauma or surgery, upper airway obstruction, respiratory muscle fatigue, or abnormal chest wall loads such as those from extreme obesity.

The hypoxemia associated with hypoventilation responds dramatically to oxygen administration because the increased concentration of oxygen inhaled per breath quickly makes up for the reduced flow of inspired gas. In Figure 2-15, mixed venous blood enters both alveolar units with a PO_2 of 40 mm Hg, saturation of 75%, and PCO_2 of 45 mm Hg. Uniform but globally decreased total ventilation interferes with the elimination of carbon dioxide and the replenishment and uptake of oxygen; therefore the arterial blood gas values reflect decreased arterial PO_2 of 70 mm Hg and increased PCO_2 of 55 mm Hg.

Alveolar Dead Space (Wasted Ventilation). This term applies to an alveolus that is ventilated but not perfused, and therefore not a molecule of oxygen can be exchanged between alveolar gas and the pulmonary circulation. As a result, the alveolar gas in the nonperfused lung region has the same composition as the inspired air. The consequence to the patient is that a portion of the alveolar-capillary surface area is lost for diffusion of gases and a portion of the patient's energy is consumed in moving air in and out of the dead space portions of lung where there is absolutely no gas exchange benefit. The most common cause of alveolar dead space is low cardiac output; however, pulmonary embolism and hyperinflation of alveoli with PEEP, CPAP, or alveolar air trapping also result in dead space units.

In Figure 2-16, although both alveoli are being ventilated, only alveolus A is participating in gas exchange.

As stated earlier, healthy humans have a dead space to tidal volume ratio of approximately 0.3, which means that one third of inhaled air fills the conducting airways and does not participate in gas exchange. With pulmonary vascular occlusive disease, alveolar dead space volume may greatly increase this percent. For example, values as high as 0.85 may occur in patients with massive pulmonary embolism.

Silent Unit. In this circumstance, alveolar-capillary units have neither ventilation nor perfusion and therefore have no effect on gas exchange or expenditure of energy for ventilation. However, the silent unit constitutes a loss of functional surface area for gas exchange and, if significantly large, may severely affect arterial oxygenation. This defect occurs in the context of ARDS wherein diffuse microatelectasis coexists with microthrombotic occlusion of the pulmonary capillaries. This occurs also with pulmonary embolism wherein, over a period of days, the alveoli in the involved ischemic lung area become atelectatic (Figure 2-17).

Critically ill and injured patients may have any combination of regional or global mismatches of ventilation to perfusion due to the complexity of specific pulmonary diseases (ARDS) and the likelihood of complicating, coexisting pathologies such as bilateral pulmonary contusion complicated by pneumonia and pulmonary embolism. The human body also reflexly compensates for V/Q mismatches in order to minimize the energy cost or oxygenation deficit to the patient. For example, poorly

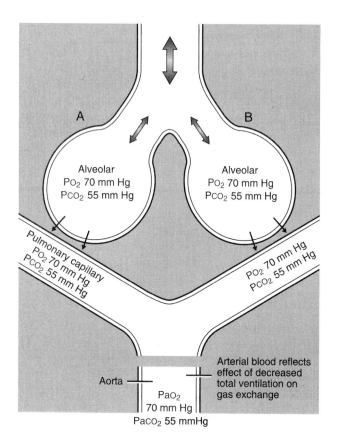

FIGURE 2-15 Hypoventilation. *Arrows* indicate direction and magnitude (size of arrows) of gas flow.

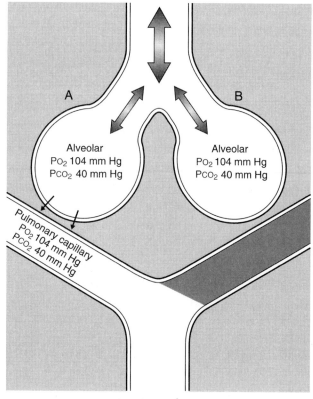

FIGURE 2-16 Alveolar dead space (wasted ventilation). The *shaded area* indicates an area of no blood flow.

ventilated alveoli tend to be underperfused (reflex hypoxic vasoconstriction), thus favoring the delivery of cardiac output to "healthy" lung areas. Poorly perfused areas of lung tend to be underventilated.

TRANSPORT

Oxygenated Blood to Body Tissue

Oxygen that diffuses from the alveoli to the pulmonary capillary blood is transported to the tissues in two forms: physically dissolved in plasma and physically bound to hemoglobin (Figure 2-18) (see also Chapter 12).

Physically Dissolved in Plasma

Oxygen moving across the alveolar capillary membrane immediately becomes dissolved in plasma. Clinically, this component of oxygen is measured as the partial pressure of oxygen in arterial blood (PaO_2). The normal PaO_2 is 90 to 100 mm Hg at sea level when the person is breathing environmental air. At this value, the actual amount of oxygen dissolved in plasma is 0.3 ml per 100 ml and accounts for less than 2% of the total amount of oxygen. Although the actual amount of oxygen in solution is small, this dissolved form is important because oxygen

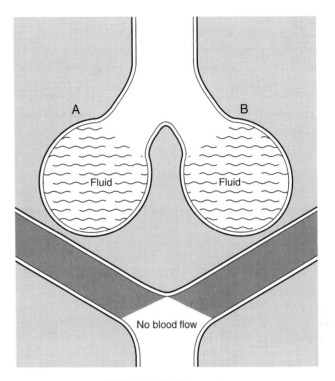

FIGURE 2-17 Silent unit.

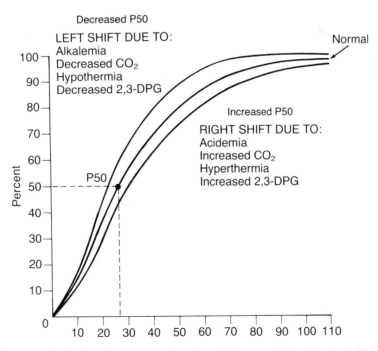

FIGURE 2-18 Oxyhemoglobin dissociation curve. Graphically illustrated is the changing affinity of hemoglobin for oxygen related to the PO_2 of plasma. Binding with oxygen is increased when the PO_2 is high, as at the pulmonary capillary. Conversely, hemoglobin readily dissociates from oxygen when the PO_2 is low, as at the systemic capillaries.

first must be dissolved in plasma before binding chemically with the hemoglobin molecule (the major vehicle for oxygen transport). Factors that influence the PaO_2 level include the gas volume of the lung, the adequacy of alveolar ventilation, the percent of inspired oxygen (FiO_2), the physical characteristics of the lung tissue, the patient's age, and the affinity of hemoglobin for oxygen. The variables that affect the affinity (attraction) of hemoglobin for oxygen are discussed later in this chapter.

Physically Bound to Hemoglobin

Oxygen is transported in reversible combination with the heme (an iron compound) portion of the hemoglobin molecule. Oxygenation transforms hemoglobin to oxyhemoglobin. Deoxygenated hemoglobin is purple in color, which is why low arterial hemoglobin saturation usually results in cyanosis. Oxyhemoglobin is bright red, which is why the mucous membranes of healthy humans are pink and why cyanotic patients who are effectively treated with oxygen therapy "pink up." Oxyhemoglobin accounts for approximately 97% to 98% of the oxygen that is transported to the tissues and about 17 to 20 ml of oxygen in 100 ml of blood.

The affinity of hemoglobin for oxygen directly relates to the PaO_2. This means that when the PaO_2 is elevated, as in the pulmonary capillaries, hemoglobin binds readily with oxygen (increased affinity). Conversely, when the PaO_2 is low, as in the systemic capillaries, oxygen becomes easily dissociated from the hemoglobin molecule (decreased affinity). Oxygen then dissolves in plasma from where it diffuses into the body cells.

Oxygen saturation (SO_2) is a measurement, expressed in percent, of the amount of oxyhemoglobin over the total amount of hemoglobin; normal arterial oxygen saturation values are in the range of 96% to 98%. In other words, of the total amount of hemoglobin in arterial blood, 96% to 98% is fully saturated with oxygen and 2% to 4% of hemoglobin is deoxygenated. If hemoglobin was chemically pure, each gram could maximally bind with 1.39 ml of oxygen, but it is normally contaminated with small amounts of methemoglobin and carboxyhemoglobin. Consequently, each gram of hemoglobin normally binds with 1.34 ml of oxygen. The amount of oxyhemoglobin decreases in patients with methemoglobinemia and carbon monoxide poisoning and, in severe cases, threatens hypoxic death.

In summary, as the PO_2 increases, the percent of fully saturated hemoglobin in blood increases. Conversely, the oxygen saturation (SO_2) falls with decreasing plasma PO_2. The increased affinity of hemoglobin for oxygen at a higher PO_2 and the decreased affinity of hemoglobin for oxygen at a low PO_2 has important physiologic implications with respect to oxygen uptake at the pulmonary capillary level and oxygen unloading at the tissue level.

The *oxyhemoglobin dissociation curve* graphically illustrates the relationship between hemoglobin oxygen saturation and the amount of oxygen dissolved in plasma (see Figure 2-18). The changing affinity of hemoglobin for oxygen (expressed as percent saturation) related to PO_2 gives a characteristic S shape to the curve. The physiologic implications at each point of the curve are described next.

Plateau (see Figure 2-18). At normal arterial PO_2 of 90 to 100 mm Hg, hemoglobin avidly binds with oxygen and becomes nearly completely saturated—96% to 98%. The tendency for hemoglobin to take up and bind oxygen at a high PO_2 facilitates oxygen uptake at the pulmonary capillary level and subsequent transport to tissues. Increasing the PO_2 above 100 mm Hg by the administration of oxygen has a negligible effect of increasing blood oxygen content (the total amount of oxygen in 100 ml of whole blood) because the addition of 1% to 4% oxygenated hemoglobin is trivial. The plateau continues to PO_2 levels of approximately 60 mm Hg and graphically illustrates hemoglobin's continued affinity for oxygen despite a large decrease in PO_2.

The persistently high affinity of hemoglobin for oxygen over a PaO_2 range of 60 to 100 mm Hg is a physiologic safeguard—even if a low alveolar PO_2 (high altitude, hypoventilation) or lung disease (pulmonary edema, fibrosis) causes the arterial PO_2 to drop by more than one third to 60 mm Hg, hemoglobin will continue to readily bind with oxygen. As a result, oxygen saturation undergoes only a minimal decrease from 96% to 99% (PaO_2 90 to 100 mm Hg) to a range of 91% to 92% (PaO_2 60 mm Hg). Thus blood oxygen content is preserved and the body is protected from hypoxia.

Steep Descent (see Figure 2-18). As the PO_2 drops below 60 mm Hg, the affinity of hemoglobin for oxygen progressively decreases. As illustrated in the descending portion of the curve, smaller drops in PO_2 produce greater decreases in oxygen saturation. Given a PO_2 of 40 mm Hg, a normal venous value, one can expect an oxygen saturation of 75%. The progressive tendency for hemoglobin to release its oxygen and become desaturated at a progressively lower PO_2 is important to facilitate tissue oxygen availability at the systemic capillary level. As stated previously, the tendency for hemoglobin to grab and bind oxygen at a high PO_2 facilitates uptake at the pulmonary capillary level and subsequent transport to tissues. However, a pulmonary capillary PaO_2 less than 60 mm Hg, which may be due to severe lung disease or hypoventilation, has unfavorable physiologic implications because the union of hemoglobin to oxygen within the lungs decreases relative to the severity of hypoxemia.

The resulting decreased blood oxygen content may then threaten major organ function and the patient's life.

Other Factors That Affect the Affinity of Hemoglobin for Oxygen. The environment of the red blood cell also affects the affinity of hemoglobin for oxygen, and hence the oxyhemoglobin dissociation curve may be shifted to the right or left. Another way of describing the affinity of hemoglobin for oxygen under differing environmental conditions is a numeric measure termed the *P50*. The P50 is the estimated PO_2 level when the oxygen saturation is 50%. Stated another way, the P50 answers the question "What is the expected PO_2 level in a patient with acidemia, alkalemia, fever, and so forth when the oxygen saturation is 50%?" Any percentage value serves the same purpose; 50% was chosen arbitrarily and in itself has no significance. For example, given normal body temperature, normal arterial pH, and normal levels of 2,3-diphosphoglycerate (2,3-DPG), at a hemoglobin oxygen satura-tion of 50%, the expected PO_2 is 26.6 mm Hg. The P50 may be increased or decreased, or, stated another way, the oxyhemoglobin dissociation curve may be shifted to the right or left because of changes in the affinity of hemoglobin for oxygen, in the following conditions.

Changes in Body Temperature. Increased body temperature decreases the affinity of the hemoglobin molecule for oxygen (increases the P50 and shifts the curve to the right). For example, in a febrile patient, an oxygen saturation of 50% is associated with a PO_2 greater than 26.6 mm Hg (or for any oxygen saturation the PO_2 is greater than what would be expected). The enhanced oxygen unloading means more oxygen is dissolved in plasma, which, in turn, produces a wider plasma-cell oxygen diffusion gradient for uptake and utilization by the tissues. This is advantageous because increases in body temperature are met with proportionate increases in cellular metabolic rate and oxygen demand. Conversely, marked decreases in body temperature are associated with increases in affinity of hemoglobin for oxygen (decreases in the P50 and a shift of the curve to the left). The decreased tendency for oxygen unloading means less oxygen is dissolved in plasma; therefore, at an oxygen saturation of 50%, the PO_2 is less than 26.6 mm Hg. Severe hypothermia is associated with decreased metabolic activity, and less oxygen is demanded by body tissue. Overall, with each 1°C elevation in body temperature, the PaO_2 rises approximately 5%; with hypothermia, the opposite occurs.

Changes in the Quantity of 2,3-diphosphoglycerate. This compound, present in red blood cells, also affects the affinity of the hemoglobin molecule for oxygen. Increased levels of 2,3-DPG, which occur as an adaptation to high al-

titude, in chronic hypoxic conditions, or during strenuous exercise, facilitate oxygen unloading (shifts the curve to the right, increases the P50). Conversely, the concentration of 2,3-DPG falls in banked blood (it may take up to 24 hours for the 2,3-DPG level of transfused, viable red blood cells to return to normal) or in the blood of septic patients and retards the dissociation of oxyhemoglobin (shifts the oxyhemoglobin dissociation curve to the left, decreases the P50). The important clinical point is that patients who have received large quantities of banked blood or septic patients may have acceptable hemoglobin and oxygen saturation "numbers," but because oxygen remains bound to hemoglobin, oxygen availability to the tissues is reduced. The problem is that septic patients and critically injured patients who require multiple blood transfusions commonly have vastly increased tissue oxygen requirements. Hence these patients may be suffering significant oxygen deprivation at the cellular level despite adequate hemoglobin and oxygen saturation measurements.

Changes in pH. If the patient's blood is acidemic, which may also occur locally around rapidly metabolizing tissue (skeletal muscle during exercise), hemoglobin readily dissociates from oxygen (the curve shifts to the right and the P50 is increased). The same principles hold true for increases in CO_2, which create an acid environment. Alkalemia and decreased CO_2 have the opposite effect and have adverse physiologic consequences. Alkalemia reduces oxygen availability at the tissue level by narrowing the oxygen diffusion pressure gradient from plasma to cell. All other factors being normal, an alkalemic patient with a pH of 7.60 will have a PaO_2 of 80, whereas an acidemic patient with a pH of 7.20 will have a PaO_2 of 120 mm Hg.

To summarize, acidemia, increased CO_2, hyperthermia, and increased 2,3-DPG are associated with a decreased affinity of hemoglobin for oxygen, a rightward shift in the oxyhemoglobin dissociation curve, and an increased P50. Thus the PO_2 is greater than normal for any given oxygen saturation (SO_2), allowing a larger plasma-cell oxygen diffusion gradient, which facilitates cellular oxygen uptake. Alkalemia, decreased CO_2, hypothermia, and decreased 2,3-DPG are associated with an increased affinity of hemoglobin for oxygen, a leftward shift in the oxyhemoglobin dissociation curve, and a decreased P50. Because hemoglobin becomes "stingy" and less readily yields up its oxygen, the PO_2 is less than normal for any given oxygen saturation, thus limiting cellular uptake of oxygen.

Other Calculations for Assessing Oxygenation Transport and Consumption

Blood Oxygen Content (CaO_2). Oxygen content defines the amount of oxygen in whole blood and is expressed in milliliters of oxygen in 100 ml of blood or as volume percent (vol%). Because the P_{O_2} defines only the partial pressure of oxygen physically dissolved in plasma and oxygen saturation defines only the percent of oxyhemoglobin as compared with the total amount of hemoglobin, the CaO_2 value has a greater clinical application because it defines exactly how much oxygen is present in the blood (Figure 2-19).

Oxygen content is calculated by multiplying the amount of hemoglobin (in grams) by the known oxygen saturation (SaO_2) by 1.36 (the amount of oxygen a *fully* saturated gram of hemoglobin can carry). Normal blood oxygen content for arterial blood is in the range of 17 to 20 ml per 100 ml of whole blood (17 to 20 vol%). Because only a minuscule amount of oxygen is physically dissolved in plasma (the P_{O_2}), this factor may be eliminated from the calculation. For example, given a patient with a hemoglobin of 14 grams, a PaO_2 of 100 mm Hg, and an oxygen saturation of 98% (the normal value when the PaO_2 is 100 mm Hg):

Hgb $\times$ SaO_2 $\times$ 1.36 = oxygen content expressed in
vol% (ml O_2 in 100 ml of blood)

14 g $\times$ 0.98 $\times$ 1.36 = 18.7 ml in 100 ml blood
or vol%

Progressive drops in P_{O_2} below 60 mm Hg result in progressive and more dramatic drops in oxygen saturation and blood oxygen content. These calculations are based on an assumed pH of 7.40, temperature of 98.6°F (37°C),

and a hemoglobin of 13 g/dl. Values have been rounded off to the nearest whole number.

It is very important for the clinician to understand the distinctions and be clinically mindful of the relationships between P_{O_2}, O_2 saturation, and blood oxygen content. For example, oxygen content can be decreased if the PaO_2 and therefore the oxygen saturation falls or if the hemoglobin level is decreased (Tables 2-6 and 2-7).

It is also clinically significant to note that increasing the PaO_2 above 100 mm Hg through the administration of supplemental oxygen has minimal effect on oxygen content because oxygen saturation cannot exceed 100%. Oxygen saturation is nearly 100% (96% to 98%) at an arterial P_{O_2} of 90 to 100 mm Hg. In fact, a PaO_2 chronically greater than 100 mm Hg places the patient at risk of oxygen toxicity.

Oxygen transport and oxygen consumption are additional valuable calculations in assessing the tissue oxygenation status of patients in whom cardiopulmonary instability or metabolic abnormalities threaten oxidative metabolism.

Calculating Oxygen Transport. Oxygen transport, also termed *oxygen delivery* or *oxygen supply,* defines how much oxygen is pumped out by the heart to body tissue per minute. Remember that the cardiopulmonary unit has as its end-point tissue oxygenation. Consequently, oxygen transport is calculated by multiplying the cardiac output (in liters per minute) by arterial oxygen content in milliliters per 100 ml of blood by 10 (this factor adjusts the

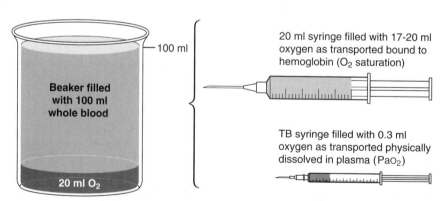

Blood oxygen content equals portion
of oxygen transported as oxyhemoglobin and
that fraction physically dissolved in plasma

FIGURE 2-19 Blood oxygen content equals that portion of oxygen transported as oxyhemoglobin and that fraction of oxygen that is physically dissolved in plasma. The *shaded areas* represent the amount of oxygen contained within the syringes and the beaker. Though oxygen is shown to be separated from the remainder of the blood within the beaker for illustrative purposes, in reality oxygen is evenly distributed throughout any blood sample.

two factors in the formula to the same scale so that the product will be in milliliters). Oxygen transport is normally in the range of 900 to 1100 ml/min and may increase to 5000 ml/min in persons with severe physical stress such as shivering, seizure activity, or exercise.

Given a patient with a cardiac output of 5 L/min and an oxygen content of 18.4 ml O_2 per 100 ml of blood:

Cardiac output $\times$ CaO_2 $\times$ 10 = oxygen transport in ml O_2/min

5 L/min $\times$ 18.4 vol% $\times$ 10 = 920 ml O_2 transported/min

Oxygen transport may be indexed to body surface area. Indexed values normalize (for differing body sizes) any calculations using cardiac output as a factor. Calculation of indexed oxygen transport or oxygen consumption is done simply by dividing the CaO_2 by the patient's body surface area. Resting normal indexed values are 550 to 650 ml O_2/min/m^2.

Oxygen consumption defines the total amount of oxygen consumed by the body per minute. Oxygen consumption is calculated by multiplying the cardiac output (in liters per minute) by the amount of hemoglobin in grams by 1.36 (the amount of oxygen in a fully saturated gram of hemoglobin) by 10 (the conversion factor that unifies the scale to milliliters) by the arteriovenous oxygen difference. The rationale is that by taking arterial oxygen transport (total amount of oxygen carried to the tissues) and subtracting from it venous oxygen transport (total amount of oxygen carried from the tissues), one can determine the amount of oxygen consumed by the body per minute. For example, given a cardiac output of 5 L/min, a hemoglobin of 14 grams, an arterial saturation of 99%, and a mixed venous saturation of 75%:

Cardiac output $\times$ 10 $\times$ Hgb $\times$ 1.36 $\times$ (SaO_2 − SvO_2)
= O_2 consumption in ml O_2/min

5 L/min $\times$ 10 $\times$ 14 $\times$ 1.36 $\times$ (0.99 − 0.75)
= 228.5 ml O_2 consumed by the body per minute

The oxygen consumption for a normal resting adult is approximately 200 to 290 ml/min (115 to 160 ml O_2/min/m^2 indexed values). Factors that affect oxygen consumption include physical activity, body temperature, nervous or endocrine system function, and disease. For example, seizure activity, which is analogous to strenuous exercise, may increase oxygen consumption to 4000 ml/min, whereas hypothermia decreases oxygen consumption proportionate to cold-induced decreases in metabolic activity. Generally, if the patient is not hypothermic, oxygen consumption values less than 100 ml/min/m^2 require immediate intervention because marked decreases in oxygen consumption suggest a severe defect in oxidative metabolism.

Because of the increased metabolic rate and oxygen consumption associated with critical illness or injury, attempts should be made to carefully protect oxygen transport or consider bringing it into a "supernormal" range with inotropic agents, fluid challenges, or administration of packed red blood cells. However, an important clinical point to consider is that the calculated oxygen transport or oxygen consumption (or any of the aforementioned measurements) does not indicate whether body oxygen demands have or have not been met. All merely give global, not organ-specific, information about how much oxygen is available and how much has been used. For example, the measured mixed venous oxygen saturation (SvO_2) is representative of the average of all systems' venous saturation and is not sensitive or specific to oxygenation deficiencies in individually stressed organs. Arterial desaturation (and therefore venous reserve) for each organ system varies depending on differences in functional metabolic need. At rest, the myocardium extracts approximately 70% of the oxygen from its arterial blood, the brain 25%, the liver

TABLE 2-6
Changes in Blood Oxygen Content Related to Changes in Oxygen Saturation

Pao_2 (mm Hg)	O_2 Saturation (%)	Oxygen Content (vol%)
100	98	18
70	94	17
60	90	16
50	85	15
40	75	13
27	50	9

TABLE 2-7
Changes in Blood Oxygen Content Related to Changes in Hemoglobin

Pao_2 (mm Hg)	Oxygen Saturation (%)	Hemoglobin (g/dl)	Content (vol%)
100	98	14	18.7
100	98	12	15.9
100	98	10	13.3
100	98	8	10.7
100	98	6	7.9

20%, and the kidneys 10%. The most vital organs of the body have the greatest resting oxygen requirements and, as an unfortunate consequence, the least oxygen reserve. Furthermore, metabolic needs for oxygen may increase significantly if the specific organ is stressed. For example, seizures pose a threat of cerebral hypoxia because brain oxygen requirements become four to five times greater than normal due to the tremendously increased metabolic activity associated with seizure activity. The cerebral hypoxic threat may be compounded if the amount of oxygen available in arterial blood is drastically reduced because of obstruction of patients' upper airways by the tongue and secretions or absent or spastic ventilatory movements.

Physiologic Consequences of Hypoxia

Normal cell function and therefore major organ function require that oxygen supply (blood oxygen content and cardiovascular performance) is adequate for the amount of oxygen required or demanded by the particular organ system at that moment. With a balanced supply/demand relationship, the amount of oxygen demanded by all organs is met by the supply system; therefore tissue oxygen consumption is equal to tissue oxygen demand. When the body's oxygen transport system fails, the amount of oxygen consumed by the tissues must fall short of tissue demand (what is not supplied cannot be consumed) and cells are forced to metabolize without oxygen. This alternate metabolic pathway results in a twentyfold decrease in energy production and also in lactic acidosis (see Figure 16-2.)

The resulting metabolic acidosis, evidenced on blood gas analysis, predicts physiologic disaster. The acid cellular environment further compromises cell function and consequently major organ function. Failure of major organ systems may then culminate in death.

Complete assessment of critically ill or injured patients entails consideration of the probability of an oxygen supply/demand imbalance, evaluation of the aforementioned oxygen transport and consumption measurements, blood lactate levels, serial blood gases, serial evaluation of major systems' function at bedside, and a consideration of "what the patient looks like," which may be coupled with a "gut sense" for how the patient is doing.

Factors That May Precipitate Hypoxic Injury and Compensatory Mechanisms. The following defects in the oxygen supply system may threaten tissue oxygenation:

1. *Pathologic decreases in cardiac output.* In these cases, tissue hypoxia is due to failure of the heart to pump out oxygenated blood at a rate demanded by normal metabolism. This occurs in patients with severe heart failure or shock.

2. *Fall in hemoglobin saturation.* In affected patients, hypoxia is due to inadequate loading of hemoglobin with oxygen. A decrease in SaO_2 occurs in hypoxemic patients or in patients with carbon monoxide poisoning because hemoglobin preferentially binds with carbon monoxide (producing carboxyhemoglobin, which is physiologically useless) rather than binding with oxygen to produce oxyhemoglobin. Likewise, patients receiving therapy with nitrates or nitrites such as nitroglycerin or silver nitrate (burn therapy), anesthetics such as lidocaine, and sulfonamides may have abnormally high levels of an abnormal hemoglobin called methemoglobin that cannot transport oxygen and may be at hypoxic threat.

3. *Severe anemia.* Severe deficits in blood oxygen content and oxygen transport are due to inadequate amounts of the primary vehicle for oxygen tranport—hemoglobin.

4. *Excessive tissue oxygen requirements.* This form of hypoxia typically occurs in patients with thyroid storm, malignant hyperthermia, extreme prolonged exercise, delirium tremens, or status seizure activity.

5. *An inability of the cells to take up or use the oxygen brought to them.* Common causes of this form of tissue hypoxia include sepsis, cyanide toxicity, and ethanol toxicity.

The body typically attempts to compensate for these defects in one or more of the following ways so that tissue oxygenation and cellular metabolism remain normal:

1. *Increase cardiac output.* The healthy heart can increase cardiac output from normal resting values of 4.5 to 8 L/min to 15 to 25 L/min, thus delivering "the goods" faster. This mechanism is utilized in patients who have excessive oxygen requirements and in those who are anemic or hypoxemic. Many critically ill patients cannot increase cardiac output sufficiently to compensate for any hypoxic threat because of cardiovascular disease and a low or fixed cardiac output.

2. *Increase the arteriovenous oxygen saturation difference.* This compensatory mechanism involves extracting more oxygen from the systemic capillaries, thus drawing on the "oxygen reserve." Normally, hemoglobin in mixed venous blood has an oxygen saturation of 75%, which leaves considerable reserve for additional extraction. This is analogous to having a surplus of money saved from which to draw in times of financial stress. In patients with conditions associated with

increased oxygen requirements, decreased amount of hemoglobin, decreased cardiac output, or hypoxemia, venous saturation can be decreased to levels as low as 31%. Below this critical level, cells are forced into anaerobic metabolism. Because drawing on the venous oxygen reserve is a means of protecting the body tissue from hypoxia, evaluation of mixed venous oxygen saturation can be an important parameter in evaluating the critically ill patient whose oxygen supply/demand relationship is frequently threatened (see Chapter 12). Although extracting more oxygen from the capillary blood is another major safety factor designed to protect the body cells from hypoxic insult, many critically ill patients have serious arterial oxygenation deficits such as refractory hypoxemia that reduce the oxygen reserve.

3. *Increase the amount of hemoglobin.* In chronic hypoxemia, as seen in patients with chronic lung disease or persons living at high altitude, hemoglobin and red blood cell mass increase to maintain oxygen transport and oxidative metabolism. However, this is a slowly developing compensatory mechanism and therefore is of no benefit to acutely ill patients.

These compensatory measures illustrate that the body has excellent adaptive mechanisms designed to protect the various tissue beds from hypoxia. The maintenance of oxidative metabolism is fundamental to preserving the specialized function of various organ systems and life itself. In critically ill or injured patients, one or all of the aforementioned compensatory mechanisms may be compromised.

Clearly, the critically ill patient walks an oxygenation tightrope. It is the responsibility of the clinician to vigilantly monitor all aspects of the oxygen supply/demand system while correlating these serial laboratory measurements with the patient's underlying disease, physical assessment findings, and other laboratory results. It also is of paramount importance to make immediate corrections in oxygenation deficits as they occur.

REFERENCES

1. Genesis 2:7, The Holy Bible, Authorized (King James) Version.
2. Harvey W: *De Motu cordis et Sanguinis in Animalibus (On the motion of the heart and blood in animals)*, 1628.
3. Cournand A, Riley RL, Bradley SE, et al: Studies of the circulation in clinical shock, *Surgery* 13:964, 1943.
4. Shoemaker WC, Montgomery ES, Kaplan E, et al: Physiologic patterns in surviving and nonsurviving shock patients, *Arch Surg* 106:630, 1973.
5. Shoemaker WC, Appel PL, Kram HB: Comparison of two monitoring methods (central venous pressure vs pulmonary artery catheter) and two protocols as therapeutic goals (normal values vs values of survival) in a prospective randomized clinical trial of critically ill surgical patients, *Crit Care Med* 13:304, 1985 (abstract).
6. Finch CA, Lenfant C: Oxygen transport in man, *N Engl J Med* 286:407, 1972.
7. West J: Mechanics of breathing. In West J: *Respiratory physiology — the essentials*, ed 4, Baltimore, 1990, Williams & Wilkins.
8. Bolder PM, Healy TE, Bolder AR: The extra work of breathing through adult endotracheal tubes, *Anesth Analg* 65:853, 1986.
9. Rich S: Primary pulmonary hypertension. In Braunwald E, editor: *Heart disease: a textbook of cardiovascular medicine*, ed 5, Philadelphia, 1997, W.B. Saunders.
10. Rubin LJ et al: Primary pulmonary hypertension, *N Engl J Med* 336:111, 1997.
11. West JB, Dollery CT, Naimark A: Distribution of blood flow in isolated lung: relation to vascular and alveolar pressures, *J Appl Physiol* 19:713, 1964.

SUGGESTED READINGS

Edwards JD, Shoemaker WC, Vincent JL: *Oxygen transport: principles and practice,* Philadelphia, 1993, W.B. Saunders.

Ganong WF: Respiration. In *Review of medical physiology*, ed 19, Stamford, CT, 1999, Appleton & Lange.

George RB, Light RW, Matthay RA, editors: Pulmonary structure and function. In *Chest medicine*, New York, 1983, Churchill Livingstone.

Grossman W: Clinical measurement of vascular resistance and assessment of vasodilator drugs. In *Cardiac catheterization, angiography and intervention*, ed 4, Philadelphia, 1991, Lea & Febiger.

Grossman W, Braunwald E: Pulmonary hypertension. In Braunwald E, editor: *Heart disease: a textbook of cardiovascular medicine*, Philadelphia, 1992, W.B. Saunders.

Guyton A, Hall JE: Respiration. In *Textbook of medical physiology*, ed 9, Philadelphia, 1996, W.B. Saunders.

Leff AR, Schumacker PT: *Respiratory physiology: basics and applications,* Philadelphia, 1993, W.B. Saunders.

Levitsky MG, Cairo JM, Hall SM, editors: Pulmonary anatomy and physiology. In *Introduction to respiratory care*, Philadelphia, 1990, W.B. Saunders.

Malley WJ: Basic physiology and clinical oxygenation. In *Clinical blood gases, application and noninvasive alternatives,* Philadelphia, 1990, W.B. Saunders.

Murray JF: *The normal lung, the basis for diagnosis and treatment of pulmonary disease,* ed 2, Philadelphia, 1986, W.B. Saunders.

Murray JF et al: Scientific principles of respiratory medicine. In Murray JF et al, editors: *Textbook of respiratory medicine,* ed 3, Philadelphia, 2000, W.B. Saunders.

Schlant RC, Sonnenblick EH: Normal physiology of the cardiovascular system. In Hurst JW et al, editors: *The heart*, ed 7, New York, 1990, McGraw-Hill.

Shapiro M, Wilson R, Casar G, et al: Work of breathing through different sized endotracheal tubes, *Crit Care Med* 14:12, 1986.

West JB: *Respiratory physiology—the essentials*, ed 4, Baltimore, 1990, Williams & Wilkins.

West JB: *Ventilation/blood flow and gas exchange*, ed 5, New York, 1990, Blackwell Scientific.

Wilson RF: Pulmonary physiology. In *Critical care manual: applied physiology and principles of therapy*, ed 2, Philadelphia, 1992, Davis.

3

GLORIA OBLOUK DAROVIC

Physical Assessment of the Pulmonary System

This text concerns the acutely ill patient who is a candidate for or is receiving invasive hemodynamic monitoring. Therefore the chapters on physical assessment are limited to the frequent and serial evaluations of the pulmonary and cardiovascular systems as performed in the acute care setting.

OVERVIEW OF PHYSICAL ASSESSMENT

Those who have been involved in critical care longer than 30 years can appreciate the tremendous technologic advances in bedside care and the increased use of invasive and noninvasive monitoring equipment. However, the role of technology in patient care must be kept in perspective. Although the monitors give "beat-by-beat" information of the patient's hemodynamic status, *monitors must be considered an adjunct to patient evaluation and should never replace frequent bedside physical assessment.*

Serial, careful physical assessment, monitoring, and laboratory data must be cross-checked for consistency and appropriateness to the patient's condition. The variability among critical care practitioners to understand and use monitoring equipment correctly, as well as the uncertainty surrounding the accuracy of monitoring data in all patient situations, makes this essential. Frequent close contact between the clinician and patient also allows integration of laboratory and hemodynamic measurements with the so-called gut sense of the experienced clinician for how the patient is doing. *Overall, the tendency to minimize the time spent for the physical assessment or to minimize the*

validity of assessment findings in deference to the enormous amount of invasive and noninvasive monitoring information must be overcome.

Conditions for Accurate Physical Assessment

Adequate lighting, equipment, patient position, time, and complete objectivity are necessary for accurate assessment. However, in the time-pressured intensive care unit (ICU), the tendency to incorporate preconceived ideas and feelings into assessment findings is more likely to occur. In other words, when under stress, we are more likely to perceive largely what we expect or want to perceive. This creates the potential for serious errors in judgment. A careful, nonhurried attitude in assessment is important so that (1) we see and evaluate the patient realistically and not according to our own expectations, and (2) the approach is satisfactory to the patient. The patient who is acutely ill, and who may be feeling like an alien in a strange land, becomes more anxious if the examiner is indifferent, unsympathetic, or rushed. Such an approach may create barriers to effective communication and assessment, as well as produce or heighten the stress "fight-or-flight" response, which may complicate the underlying illness.

Assessment Difficulties Inherent to the Intensive Care Unit

The critical care environment typically is not an optimal setting for examination. Nevertheless, every attempt should be made to provide privacy and a reassuring and comfortable milieu. This is especially important on admission to the unit because the patient's and the family members' first impressions may strongly influence their attitude for the entire hospital stay.

During an emergency admission, the patient may be in too much distress to give a coherent or thorough account of the illness for the clinician to establish the baseline functional state. On these occasions, a family member or close friend may have to be consulted for information to establish what is "normal" or "usual." Patients who are nonresponsive should always be spoken to as if conscious and offered brief, simple explanations about what is going to happen and what is being done.

Physical assessment is made particularly challenging to the examiner because critically ill patients are difficult to examine (Table 3-1). However, the basic principles of physical assessment are the same as those for any other patients.

Although assessment of critically ill or injured patients typically focuses on those systems in which abnormalities have been identified, serial assessment should include a rapid examination of all organ systems. This is particularly important in sedated, unconscious, or intubated patients who are unable to complain.

Transcultural Considerations

Cultural diversity is common to life in North America and some other parts of the world. Health care providers, particularly in large cities, may encounter patients from hundreds of cultures and subcultures. Language or dialect differences may require enlistment of an interpreter. Effective relating to patients and families of varied ethnic/racial backgrounds, socioeconomic status, and sexual orientation necessitates knowledge, understanding, and sensitivity to the cultural values and religious beliefs that relate to health, illness, disability, and other major life events, such as birth and death. For example, although pain and death are universal phenomena, each patient's and family's attitudes, beliefs, and means of coping with pain and death may vary considerably. It is impossible for health care providers to become familiar with all of the details of cultural systems as they relate to health, illness, and death of even the cultures that predominate in one's geographic area. See references 1 through 3 for descriptions of various cultural belief systems, as well as discussion of differences in specific genetic traits and disorders such as sickle cell disease in Africans.

It is essential that each clinician overcome any *ethnocentrism,* which is the tendency to believe that one's own way of life is the most desirable and acceptable. Linked to ethnocentrism is the tendency to try to impose one's own beliefs and values on persons of a different socioeconomic system or culture. Because both can impose serious barriers to a sensitive, healing-based approach to the patient, it is important that we be introspective and aware of our biases

TABLE 3-1
Difficulties in the Physical Assessment of Critically Ill Patients

Difficulty	Cause
Patient unable to cooperate with examination	Comatose (drug or disease effects)
	Combative, restless, confused
	Extreme distress (e.g., dyspnea, pain)
	Metabolic or drug toxicities; substance withdrawal (e.g., drugs, ethanol); blood gas abnormalities; psychiatric problems
Difficult to position the patient for examination of specific part	Orthopedic traction or casts
	Recommended fixed position relative to patient problem, such as supine for shock, sitting for orthopnea
	Burns
Critical care environment	Lack of privacy
	Crowded environment
	Ambient noise
Presence of obstructive devices that obscure visualization, palpation, auscultation	Dressings, orthopedic casts, splints
	Drains, monitoring catheters, equipment
Obscuring of physical signs by severity of disease or support devices	Gross tissue edema
	Massive trauma
	Loud adventitious lung sounds obscure heart sounds
	Peritoneal dialysis
	Gross ascites
	Intraaortic balloon pump
	Ventilators

Adapted from Dobbs GJ, Coombs LJ: Clinical examination of patients in the intensive care unit, *Br J Hosp Med* 38(2):102, 1987.

and prejudices and work to overcome them. This is important to our professional relationships, as well as our own personal and spiritual growth.

SYMPTOMS AND SIGNS OF PULMONARY DISEASE
Symptoms of Pulmonary Disease

Symptoms are patients' subjective accounts of changes in body function or indications of disease. Many of the following symptoms of primary pulmonary disease may be indicative of other conditions as well.

Cough

A sensation of irritation in the pulmonary system, or *cough,* is the most frequent symptom of pulmonary disease. It may be caused by stimuli arising in any part of the airways from the pharynx to the terminal bronchi. The cough may or may not be productive of sputum.

Evaluation of Sputum. Because the character of the sputum, if present, may give important clues to the underlying disorder, sputum should be observed for volume, color, consistency, and odor. It is important that the specimen come from the lungs and not be postnasal secretions or saliva, which are clear, colorless, and watery. In the ICU patient, sputum is frequently collected via suctioning through an endotracheal or tracheostomy tube.

Copious, thick, mucoid, grayish-white, translucent sputum is commonly seen in cigarette smokers and in patients with chronic obstructive pulmonary disease (COPD). Purulent-looking and foul-smelling yellow, brown, or green mucoid sputum is indicative of all bronchopulmonary bacterial infections. Rusty, golden-yellow sputum is seen in pneumococcal pneumonia. Clear or white mucoid sputum is characteristic of asthma; however, eosinophils in the sputum of patients with allergic asthma may cause the sputum to appear purulent.

Hemoptysis. *Hemoptysis* is sputum that is grossly bloody, blood streaked, or pink or that contains small clots. Tumors of the lung or airways and chronic bronchitis are the most frequent causes of hemoptysis in the United States. Patients with pulmonary embolism have blood-tinged sputum when their condition is associated with pulmonary infarction. In acute cardiogenic pulmonary edema, the odorless, frothy, colorless, or peach-colored sputum also may be conspicuously blood streaked due to high-pressure rupture of some pulmonary capillaries. Recurrent bloody sputum is also a common finding in patients with severe pulmonary hypertension due to conditions such as critical mitral stenosis. Trauma to the airways incurred during intubation or tracheostomy or during suctioning may be associated with bright red streaks in the aspirated secretions that resolve quickly unless trauma is recurrent. Hemoptysis also may indicate rupture of a pulmonary artery segment associated with flotation or wedging of the pulmonary artery catheter (see Chapter 10).

Tracheoinnominate Fistula

Tracheoinnominate fistula is a potentially fatal complication of tracheostomy. The inadvertent positioning of the tracheostomy tube against the tracheal wall close to the innominate artery results in the pulsatile movement of the tracheostomy tube. *A pulsatile tracheostomy tube should be quickly repositioned because the throbbing movement eventually results in tracheal erosion.* Subsequent erosion of the adjacent innominate artery segment results in sudden, massive arterial bleeding. Blood may literally spurt across the room. Exsanguination can occur within minutes.

Dyspnea

Dyspnea implies that the act of breathing has become a difficult, conscious effort. Despite the lack of a consistent correlation of the patient's sensation of breathing to the observed respiratory effort, the patient who complains of dyspnea typically appears to have shortness of breath. Theories to explain dyspnea include the following:

1. Excitation of intrapulmonary receptors by irritant substances or abnormalities within the structures of the lung, such as bronchoconstriction or pulmonary edema.
2. Central nervous system mechanisms that relate to the perception of a disparity between work of breathing and adequacy of muscle contraction.
3. Emotional factors, such as hysterical hyperventilation.
4. Circumstances in which minute ventilation (normally approximately 6 L/min) approaches the maximal breathing capacity (normally approximately 200 L/min). This may occur when minute ventilatory requirements are excessively high, such as in extreme exercise; when the maximal breathing capacity is extremely low, such as in COPD; or when respiratory muscle weakness results in diminished ventilatory reserve, such as in weaning from mechanical ventilation.
5. Abnormalities in blood gases, such as hypoxemia or hypercarbia, both of which are associated with compensatory increases in minute ventilation.

Dyspnea related to pulmonary disease is caused by (1) airflow limitations due to obstructive lesions of the airways, such as asthma; (2) conditions that reduce pulmonary compliance, such as atelectasis or adult respiratory distress syndrome (ARDS); (3) conditions that resist lung expansion, such as pneumothorax, pleural effusion, pleural thickening, or inflammation; (4) increases in physiologic dead space, such as pulmonary embolism; and (5) respiratory muscle fatigue, which may occur when the underlying disease, such as airway obstruction, increases the work of breathing beyond the work capacity of the normal ventilatory muscles or when the ventilatory muscles become so weak that they cannot maintain even quiet, normal breathing. Although not related to pulmonary disease, patients with chest wall trauma, such as fractured ribs or flail chest, also may complain of dyspnea.

The clinician should ask patients to compare the present level of dyspnea with that usually experienced, as well as any known precipitating or alleviating factors. Dyspneic patients typically breathe with the mouth open and usually appear distressed and anxious. Flaring of the nostrils and use of the accessory muscles of respiration indicate severe respiratory distress. The rhythm of the patient's speech also may be used to assess the severity of dyspnea. The ability to speak at a normal pace and rhythm indicates the absence of shortness of breath; a gasp between each syllable indicates a potentially life-threatening problem. To test more specifically, the patient is asked to breathe in and then count aloud on exhalation. The inability to count beyond 5 or 10 before exhalation is complete indicates that the patient is at extreme risk of respiratory collapse and should be monitored closely with an intubation tray at the bedside. If the patient cannot reach 5, prophylactic intubation with mechanical ventilatory support is immediately indicated.

Chest Pain

Chest pain due to abnormalities of the pulmonary system includes the following:
1. Upper retrosternal pain as seen in acute tracheitis.
2. Retrosternal pain associated with lesions of the mediastinum, such as acute mediastinitis or pneumomediastinum. This pain has a character similar to that of myocardial ischemic pain. Pain may radiate to the arms and neck but is not related to exertion. Exclusion of myocardial ischemic pain is made by electrocardiogram and serial cardiac enzyme studies.
3. Pleural pain, produced by stretching of an inflamed parietal pleura, is due to pleurisy or pleuritic involvement as a result of pulmonary embolism. Pleuritic pain is typically sharp and stabbing, is aggravated by exertion, and may be present only at the end of a deep inspiration or during a cough.
4. Musculoskeletal pain, which is related to underlying chest wall deformities or injuries.

Signs of Pulmonary Disease

Signs are indicators of disease that are observed by the examiner. Several signs are indicative of pulmonary disease, but, as with symptoms, they also may characterize other pathology.

Level of Mentation

Several conditions, such as blood gas abnormalities, drug effects, perfusion failure, increased intracranial pressure, and circulating toxins, can alter the patient's cerebral function. This discussion focuses on abnormalities in blood gases that result from pulmonary disease or dysfunction.

Hypoxemia (PaO_2 less than 55 to 60 mm Hg) and *acute hypercarbia* ($PaCO_2$ greater than 60 mm Hg) produce changes in affect, perception of reality, and level of consciousness. Accurate assessment may require detailed questioning because a patient who superficially appears alert and lucid may be found to have significantly disturbed mental function on careful interrogation. Blood gas studies are required to accurately evaluate both the PaO_2 and $PaCO_2$.

Hypoxemia/Hypoxia. The term *hypoxia* means a reduction in the oxygen supply to the tissue below physiologic levels. Tissue hypoxia may be due to a variety of factors (see Chapter 2). Hypoxia usually coexists with hypoxemia in persons who are physiologically compromised. Patients cannot perceive hypoxia or hypoxemia. The clinician must therefore be vigilant for the indications of oxygenation failure. Mental signs of *cerebral hypoxia* are nearly identical to those of ethanol intoxication. Initially, there is a loss of higher mental functioning, such as the inability to perform complex mental tasks or think abstractly. Just as drunkenness manifests differently among different people, cerebral hypoxia may variably manifest with restlessness, agitation, confusion, an inappropriate sense of well-being, euphoria, outbursts of hilarity, paranoia, irritability, combativeness, or uncooperativeness. A generalized progressive loss of muscular coordination and visual acuity also occurs. With further decreases in cerebral oxygenation, descending central nervous system depression may ultimately end in stupor, coma, or seizures. *In any restless patient, cerebral hypoxia should be ruled out before giving pain or sedative medications.*

Other generalized signs of hypoxemia include tachycardia, tachypnea, and possibly dyspnea. Ectopic cardiac arrhythmias also may occur with significant decreases in arterial PO_2', but they may develop in patients with cardiac disease or anemia with PaO_2 values in the high 50s. Bradycardia is a late and ominous sign of hypoxemia; cardiopulmonary arrest usually follows within minutes. Consequently, any patient who has any possible cause of hypoxemia who suddenly becomes bradycardic should be immediately and aggressively treated with 100% oxygen and airway management as needed.

Hypercarbia. *Hypercarbia* is defined as a $PaCO_2$ greater than 45 mm Hg. The symptoms of hypercarbia resemble those of central nervous system depression due to anesthetic agents. The patient's behavior may be characterized by lethargy, confusion, slurred speech, and poor coordination-progressing to somnolence, stupor, and coma. The patient also may complain of a headache that results from hypercarbia-induced cerebral vasodilation. Other indications of hypercarbia are tachypnea, tachycardia, respiratory acidosis, and systemic vasodilation, which may be overridden by vasoconstrictive stimulation via the sympathetic nervous system. However, when hypercarbia is severe, systemic vasodilation predominates and the patient may become hypotensive.

Both hypoxemia and hypercarbia have a potent constrictor effect on the pulmonary vasculature. Pulmonary vasoconstriction increases pulmonary vascular resistance and pulmonary artery systolic and diastolic pressures. If mean pulmonary artery pressures acutely exceed 35 to 45 mm Hg, the increased right ventricular workload will produce right-sided heart failure.

Unless the patient is receiving supplemental oxygen, hypercarbia is always associated with some degree of hypoxemia. The clinical picture therefore may be a mixture of the effects of hypercarbia and hypoxemia. In fact, with severe blood gas disturbances, severe mental disturbances such as hallucinations, paranoid or combative behavior, or schizoid behavior may make it appear that the patient has a psychiatric disorder.

Respirations

Patients with pulmonary disease typically have changes in the rate, rhythm, and character of breathing. Patients in intensive care units should be observed for changes in the following.

Frequency of Respirations. The normal respiratory rate for a healthy, nonstressed adult is 10 to 18 breaths per minute. The respiratory rate increases with fever, sepsis, hypercarbia, hypoxemia, acidemia, strong emotional stimuli, agitation, central nervous system lesions, pain, shock, pulmonary embolism, or any condition that produces a sudden increase in the work of breathing, such as bronchospasm or pulmonary edema. Dyspnea does not always correlate with tachypnea; a patient may be breathing slowly but may complain of dyspnea, whereas another patient with rapid breathing may deny dyspnea.

Tachypnea with rates greater than 28 breaths per minute usually indicates significant respiratory distress. If sustained, tachypnea is poorly tolerated because the increased energy expenditure may culminate in patient exhaustion and respiratory collapse. A labored respiratory rate greater than 28 to 34 breaths per minute is usually an indication for intubation with ventilatory assistance.

Warnings of Impending Cardiopulmonary Arrest. Several studies reviewed the clinical events within 6 hours before cardiac arrest in hospitalized patients on the general wards.[4,5] Breathing rates greater than 30 breaths per minute or neurologic deterioration manifested as restlessness, lethargy, or confusion was noted in approximately 70% of all patients. The impression is that cardiac arrest is frequently related to noncardiac disorders. The death event represents the final common pathway of numerous pulmonary or metabolic problems. Efforts to adequately identify high-risk tachypneic patients or patients with mental status changes and immediately institute appropriate therapy, such as bronchodilators or mechanical ventilatory assistance, may prevent cardiopulmonary arrest.

A study done at the Cook County Hospital in Chicago reviewed 150 cases of cardiac arrest on the medical wards.[6] In 99 of a total of 150 cases, a nurse or physician documented deterioration in the patient's condition, primarily neurologic or pulmonary changes, within 6 hours of cardiac arrest. Common staff errors were (1) failure of the nurse to notify a physician of deterioration in a patient's mental status, (2) failure of the physician to obtain or interpret arterial blood gas measurements in patients with mental changes or respiratory distress, and (3) failure of the ICU triage physician to stabilize the patient's condition before transferring the patient to the ICU. The results of this study lend credence to Dr. Stephen Ayres' statement, "The weakest link in patient care is the tendency of the clinician to convince himself or herself that somehow everything will be all right."

Abnormally slow rates of breathing (less than eight breaths per minute) or respiratory rates that are inappropriately slow for the underlying condition (sepsis, pulmonary edema, pulmonary embolism, shock) may also be warnings of impending cardiopulmonary collapse. Because $Paco_2$ also relates proportionally to minute ventilation, inappropriately slow rates of breathing directly result in respiratory acidosis. For example, if a patient with a respiratory rate of 16 and a tidal volume of 500 ml is maintaining a $Paco_2$ of 40 mm Hg, a drop in respiratory rate to eight breaths per minute while maintaining the same tidal volume (50% reduction in minute volume) would result in a 50% increase in $Paco_2$ to 60 mm Hg.

Technique for Counting Respirations. The respiratory rate is counted by auscultating each breath. Counting breaths by visualization or by placing a hand over the abdomen and counting the abdominal efforts may reflect only the respiratory effort and may not correlate with inhaled gas volume and passage of air into the lungs. The number digitally displayed on the mechanical ventilator should never be regarded as indicative of true respiratory rate and pulmonary airflow. The machine may significantly underestimate the number of breaths and lung airflow in

TABLE 3-2
Abnormal Breathing Patterns

Pattern	Cause
Rapid with low tidal volume	Increased sympathetic nervous stimulation
	Decreased chest compliance
	Increased airway resistance
	Pleuritic chest pain or trauma
	Elevated diaphragm
	Residual muscle relaxants
Rapid and deep (Kussmaul respirations)	Metabolic acidosis
	Hysterical hyperventilation
	In the comatose patient, possible infarction of midbrain or pons
Periodic increases and decreases in rate and depth of breathing punctuated by periods of apnea (Cheyne-Stokes respiration)	Brain damage (usually at the brainstem)
	Severe cardiogenic shock
	Uremia
	Drug-induced respiratory depression
Irregular respirations with long periods of apnea (Biot respiration)	Brainstem dysfunction
Slow breathing	Drug-induced respiratory depression
	Increased intracranial pressure
	End-stage respiratory muscle fatigue heralding cardiopulmonary arrest
Apnea punctuated by irregular, gasping breaths (agonal)	Occurs just before death

patients with low spontaneous tidal volumes (intermittent mandatory ventilation breaths) and high spontaneous respiratory rates. *Never accept the digital display on any monitoring or assistive device as absolute truth without physical assessment verification.*

Regularity of Breathing. Changes from regular, rhythmic breathing should be noted and investigated (Table 3-2). Patients also must be observed for changes in the depth and symmetry of ventilatory movements, as well as synchronous movement between chest and abdomen, predominance of thoracic or abdominal breathing, and disturbances specific to the phase of the respiratory cycle.

Depth of Respirations. Depth of breathing is difficult to determine because chest and diaphragmatic movements cannot be accurately measured in the clinical setting; how-

ever, normal breathing is barely visible. Clearly visible ventilatory movements signal a need for immediate investigation and indicate that the minute volume has approximately doubled. Excessively deep breathing also may be observed in severely brain-damaged patients who are victims of head injury or stroke.

Symmetry of Respirations. In health, the two sides of the chest move symmetrically with each breath. To assess chest wall symmetry, the patient should be in the supine position with the chest exposed. From the foot of the bed, the clinician can observe ventilatory movements in the infraclavicular regions, midchest, and lower ribs and abdomen. In obese or grossly edematous patients or patients with thoracic or abdominal dressings, observations may be difficult and assessment may require palpation. The sides of the patient's chest are grasped with the examiner's fingers. The outstretched thumbs should nearly approximate the area of the xiphoid process for anterior palpation and the tenth thoracic vertebra for posterior palpation. If possible, a loose fold of skin should be present between the thumbs as the patient takes a few deep breaths. The excursions of the thumbs are observed, and the range and symmetry of ventilatory movements are felt. Any lag or absence or incomplete expansion should be observed (Figure 3-1).

Asymmetry of chest movement may be due to pleural effusion, obstruction of a major bronchus, or neuromuscular abnormalities. Patients with fractured ribs, flail chest, pleurisy, or area surgery may "splint" one side of the chest to reduce pain. Splinting is making the regional muscles rigid in order to avoid or minimize movement in the involved, painful area of the chest. *Right main bronchus intubation,* or progressive downward slippage of the endotracheal tube into the right main bronchus, may be associated with asymmetric chest movements and diminished breath sounds over the left side of the chest. Auscultation at both axillae may be helpful in determining diminished breath sounds within the left thorax. However, these clinical signs may be absent or difficult to evaluate in some patients, and right main bronchus intubation may be detected only on chest radiograph. As a general rule, in an average-sized male adult it is unlikely to have a right mainstem intubation if the patient's head is neither flexed nor extended and the tube is taped at the 23 cm mark at the teeth. In an average-sized female adult, 21 cm at the teeth is considered correct depth of the tube.

Chest/Abdominal Synchrony and Respiratory Muscle Fatigue. With normal breathing, the chest and abdomen rise and fall smoothly and synchronously with inspiration and expiration. In the supine position, the movement of the abdomen normally is slightly greater than that of the

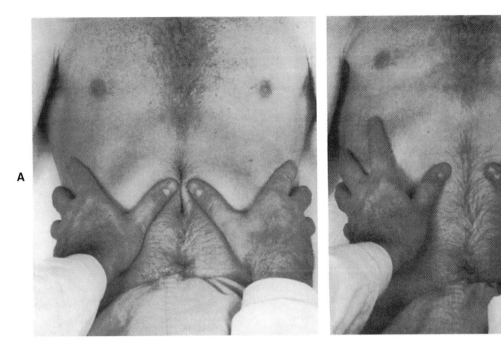

FIGURE 3-1 Technique for evaluating anterior chest excursion. **A,** Placement of examiner's hands at end-expiration. **B,** Location of hands after normal inspiration; note symmetric lateral displacement of examiner's hands. (From Swartz MH: *Textbook of physical diagnosis, history and examination,* ed 3, Philadelphia, 1998, W.B. Saunders.)

rib cage. Ventilatory movement may be felt by the examiner by placing one hand on the abdomen and the other hand on the sternum.

With the onset of respiratory muscle fatigue, the ventilatory movements become rapid and jerky. The abdomen is sucked in on inspiration and balloons out on expiration, producing a paradoxic movement of chest and abdomen. Respiratory paradox imparts a rocking appearance to the act of breathing (Figure 3-2).

Patients who are able to talk typically complain of dyspnea. Because asynchrony between chest and abdomen may herald acute ventilatory failure or arrest, it is important to watch for it in spontaneously breathing patients who have any respiratory distress; patients being weaned from a ventilator; or patients being maintained on intermittent mandatory ventilation. With progression of respiratory muscle fatigue, life-threatening respiratory collapse and apnea usually occur abruptly.

Thoracic versus Abdominal Breathing. As stated earlier, both chest and abdomen move with normal breathing because both intercostal and diaphragmatic muscles are used. Respiratory movements that are entirely thoracic may indicate that diaphragmatic movement is restricted by increased intraabdominal pressure, diaphragmatic paralysis,

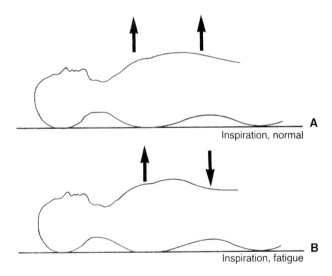

FIGURE 3-2 Respiratory paradox. **A,** With inspiration and descent of the diaphragm, the abdomen rises synchronously with the chest. Both fall smoothly on expiration as the diaphragm ascends. **B,** With respiratory muscle fatigue, as the chest rises during inspiration, the abdomen is sucked in. During expiration, the abdomen moves out as the chest falls. These rapid, uncoordinated respiratory movements may additionally be accompanied by carbon dioxide retention and hypoxemia.

or pain. Respiratory movements that are entirely abdominal may be caused by paralytic involvement of the intercostal muscles. In patients with asthma, emphysema, or diffuse pulmonary fibrosis, or in those having an asthmatic attack, movements of the chest wall may be equally reduced bilaterally. In these patients, breathing appears to be largely abdominal, assisted by the accessory muscles of respiration.

Disturbances Relative to the Phases of the Respiratory Cycle. *Labored inspiration* occurs when adequate intake of air cannot be achieved with normal breathing. The accessory cervical muscles are used to lift the thoracic cage off the diaphragm. The increased negative intrathoracic pressure produces suprasternal, supraclavicular, intercostal, and substernal retractions. The nares are usually flared. This type of breathing occurs when the lungs become stiff, as in severe fibrotic disease, diffuse atelectasis, or pulmonary edema; when there is gross overdistention of the lungs, as in pulmonary emphysema or status asthmaticus; and when there is obstruction or narrowing of the bronchi, trachea, or larynx, or obstruction of an artificial airway, as with a kinked endotracheal tube.

Labored expiration occurs when a disease process interferes with the passive outflow of air. This type of breathing is seen in patients with COPD or ARDS or during an asthmatic attack. To expel air, the accessory muscles of the cervical area, intercostal area, back, and abdomen are enlisted to increase intrathoracic expiratory pressure. Expiratory time also is prolonged. Patients usually prefer to sit upright and may purse their lips or grunt with expiration. These actions keep intra-airway pressures above that of the surrounding tissue and prevent small airway collapse.

The exaggerated intrathoracic pressure fluctuations associated with labored inspiration or expiration are transmitted to the catheter tip in the pulmonary artery and pulmonary artery wedge tracing. This may make the determination of accurate hemodynamic measurements extremely difficult or impossible (see Chapter 10).

Effects of Airway Obstruction on the Character of Breathing. Patients who are not intubated may develop upper airway obstruction if the upper airway or neck has been subjected to trauma, such as cervical spine injury; hematoma formation, such as occurs with inadvertent puncture of a carotid artery during internal or external jugular catheterization; or an inflammatory condition, such as smoke inhalation or epiglottitis. Partial obstruction precedes complete obstruction and usually is accompanied by gurgling or a "crowing" sound, termed *stridor,* along with use of the accessory muscles of respiration.

Respiratory paradox develops as the obstruction becomes more severe. *Stridor suggests greater than 70% obstruction of the upper airway and is an indication for emergency placement of an endotracheal tube or tracheostomy.*

However, endotracheal intubation or tracheostomy does not guarantee an open airway. Airway obstruction in patients with an artificial airway may be due to an intraluminal mucous plug or blood clot or to kinking or torsion of the artificial airway or ventilator tubing. In the spontaneously breathing patient with an artificial airway, the signs of airway obstruction are similar to those previously described. Airway obstruction in the narcotized or paralyzed mechanically ventilated patient is indicated by activation of the ventilator high airway pressure alarm, a diminution or absence of chest movement and breath sounds, and a decrease in continuously monitored oxygen saturations.

Other Signs of Pulmonary Disease

Cyanosis. As the amount of oxygen dissolved in plasma decreases, the binding capacity of the hemoglobin molecule with oxygen likewise decreases. *Deoxygenated hemoglobin* (also termed *reduced or desaturated hemoglobin*) imparts a bluish color to blood. Cyanosis—a diffuse, bluish discoloration of the skin and mucous membranes—becomes perceptible when greater than 5 g per 100 ml of hemoglobin becomes desaturated in the systemic capillaries. This usually occurs when the PaO_2 is approximately 50 mm Hg and arterial saturation is approximately 80%. However, this point is patient variable and relates, in part, to the amount of hemoglobin in the blood. For example, in an anemic patient with a hemoglobin of 8 g per 100 ml, cyanosis is a late sign and may not appear until the patient is severely hypoxemic. Cyanosis cannot occur in a patient who has a hemoglobin less than 5 g per 100 ml and a hematocrit less than 15% because severely anemic patients do not have 5 g of hemoglobin. They can never desaturate the 5 g of hemoglobin necessary to produce cyanosis. On the other hand, the higher the hemoglobin, the greater the likelihood of cyanosis because the amount of desaturated hemoglobin in 100 ml of capillary blood will be greater for any given PaO_2. In patients with an abnormally high hemoglobin, cyanosis may occur before the actual oxygen-carrying capacity (blood oxygen content) is affected. For example, a polycythemic patient with a hemoglobin of 21 g per 100 ml appears chronically cyanotic although the PaO_2 is in an acceptable range and there is no hypoxic threat.

Cyanosis appears first and is most conspicuous at the nail beds, in the mucous membranes, and where skin is thin, such as the tip of the nose and the earlobes. Cyanosis commonly occurs in the absence of disease when the arterioles of the skin, particularly in the hands and feet, constrict in response to cold or anxiety. Vasoconstriction slows blood in these superficial, peripheral capillaries so that increased arterial desaturation occurs in the distal extremities and possibly the nose and earlobes. This has no metabolic consequence to the person.

There are two types of cyanosis

1. In *central cyanosis,* blood leaving the left ventricle is poorly oxygenated. When associated with pulmonary disease, blood fails to become adequately oxygenated by the lungs. This may be due to massive pneumothorax or hemothorax, tension pneumothorax, pulmonary malignancies, severe chronic bronchitis, flail chest, pneumonia, or ARDS. Central cyanosis also may occur in patients with right-to-left intracardiac shunts. Clinically, central cyanosis is evident at the nail beds and earlobes, as well as centrally in the conjunctiva or under the tongue. The skin over the entire body is usually warm.

2. In *peripheral cyanosis,* blood leaving the left ventricle is adequately oxygenated but becomes desaturated in the peripheral systemic circulation. This typically occurs when blood stagnates in vasoconstricted peripheral arterioles because of a cold environment, or from excessive sympathetic nervous system stimulation due to anxiety or circulatory failure. Cyanosis is clinically apparent at the usual peripheral sites; however, the conjunctiva and mucous membranes under the tongue remain pink because these vascular beds never vasoconstrict. The skin is typically cold, and cyanosis disappears as the area is warmed.

Generalized, Dependent Edema. Generalized edema may occur as a consequence of renal, hepatic, endocrine, metabolic, and pure cardiac disease, as well as right ventricular failure due to pulmonary disease termed *cor pulmonale.* The latter most commonly occurs in patients with COPD. The increased venous pressure associated with right-sided heart failure reflects back to the systemic capillaries and increases capillary hydrostatic pressure. High capillary pressures, in turn, result in a transudation of plasma water into body tissue. Swelling is most marked at the dependent parts of the body—the feet when the patient is maintained upright and the back when supine. Visible distention of the superficial veins reflects the increased venous pressure.

Subcutaneous Emphysema. Air in the subcutaneous tissue indicates a pulmonary air leak such as may occur from alveolar rupture in patients receiving positive pressure ventilation. Subcutaneous emphysema is usually evidenced as swelling in the area of the thorax, but air may dissect along fibrous musculoskeletal tissue bands to areas remote from the lungs, such as the scrotum. Palpation of the involved tissue produces a characteristic crackling sensation. Pain may be produced by palpating the areas of swelling, because subcutaneous air tears through the surrounding tissue under the pressure of the examiner's hand. Subcutaneous emphysema does not pose a threat to the patient unless it is significant enough around the throat to compress and occlude the airway and blood vessels. It is, however, a warning that an air leak is present and that the patient is at risk of developing a pneumothorax or already has a pneumothorax.

Posturing as a Sign of Respiratory Failure. The patient's position of comfort relates to the work of breathing. Patients with respiratory difficulty prefer to sit upright while grasping or resting their arms on a stationary object such as the back of a chair. This position enables the patient to stabilize the shoulders and enlist the accessory muscles to augment the respiratory effort. The upright position also increases tidal volume because it allows for greater diaphragmatic descent. Moreover, when sitting, the weight of the anterior chest wall (which can be a significant load in the morbidly obese) does not have to be overcome with inspiration. When dyspneic patients cannot spontaneously assume the upright position because of weakness or the presence of restraints, it is the responsibility of the clinician to assist patients to their position of comfort.

SPECIFIC TECHNIQUES OF PHYSICAL ASSESSMENT

In addition to symptoms and signs of pulmonary disease, the following specific assessment techniques may detect abnormalities in the structures of the pulmonary system.

Percussion

Percussion is a technique used to determine the density or consistency of the underlying lung by evaluating the sounds produced when the chest wall is tapped. When possible, percussion should be performed with the patient sitting upright. The distal part of the examiner's middle finger is pressed firmly against the chest wall, palm side down, with the fingers slightly separated. The middle finger of the other hand, held at a right angle, is used to tap the finger on the chest wall. The entire action must come from the wrist, producing a sharp, hammerlike effect (Figure 3-3).

Percussion begins at the apices and progresses downward. As each site is struck with equal force, symmetric points on the thorax are compared. When percussing the back, patients should have their arms folded across their chest. Percussion over the healthy lung produces a characteristic resonant tone; however, the quality varies depending on the amount of muscle and fat present. Table 3-3 lists the various pulmonary percussion sounds.

Tracheal Position

This assessment technique is used when shift of the mediastinal structures is suspected. The tip of the examiner's index finger is gently pushed into the patient's suprasternal notch. The trachea is located, and deviation of the trachea to either side can then be detected. An increase in volume or pressure on one side of the thorax (as in tension pneumothroax or massive hemothorax) shifts the trachea and mediastinal structures to the opposite side. A decrease in lung volume, as in atelectasis, shifts the trachea and mediastinum to the affected side.

Auscultation of Breath Sounds

Auscultation is the assessment technique, using a stethoscope, of listening for sounds produced by airflow through the tracheobronchial tree. The stethoscope usually has two heads: the bell is used to detect low-pitched sounds, and the diaphragm is used to detect high-pitched sounds. Either may be used to auscultate the lung fields; however, the entire bell or diaphragm must always be in contact with the skin (Figure 3-4). In very thin people, the bell is preferable because complete skin contact with the diaphrahgm is difficult due to protrusion of their ribs. *Auscultation through the patient's gown is not acceptable because fidelity of sounds is significantly compromised by the interposing cloth.* Alternate auscultation of both sides of the chest is essential for comparing the quality of breath sounds. When possible, the patient is asked to sit upright and is asked to breathe deeply with his or her mouth open. The chest is auscultated anteriorly, laterally, and posteriorly. When the back is auscultated, the patient is instructed to cross the arms across the chest so that more of the lung fields are exposed by the separated scapulae. *The patient also should be instructed to breathe slowly with frequent pauses.* Prolonged hyperventilation may produce light-headedness, central nervous system excitability, and cerebral and coronary vasoconstriction.

Patients with gross irregularities in breathing or on intermittent mandatory ventilation are difficult to auscultate because of the effect of variations in the tidal volume on the quality of breath sounds. Nonetheless, decreased breath sounds and abnormal breath sounds have their usual signifi-

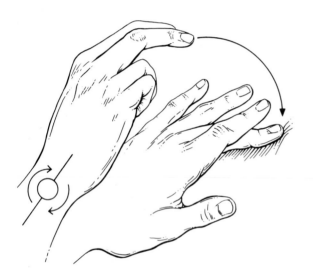

FIGURE 3-3 Technique of percussion. (From Swartz MH: *Textbook of physical diagnosis, history and examination,* ed 3, Philadelphia, 1998, W.B. Saunders.)

TABLE 3-3
Pulmonary Percussion Sounds

Sound	Quality	Clinical Correlates
Resonance	Loud, low in pitch	Sound heard over healthy, aerated lung
Hyperresonance	Very loud, lower in pitch than resonance	Occurs when the amount of air in the thorax is increased, as in emphysema or pneumothorax
Tympany	Musical, clear hollow tone; pitch is usually high	Tension pneumothorax; increased air under pressure
Dullness	Soft intensity, medium in pitch, short duration, damped quality	Occurs when lung is airless as in consolidation, collapse, fibrosis, tumor; or when lung is separated from the chest wall by pleural fluid or thickened pleura

cance. Clamping a nasogastric tube or discontinuing gastric suction eliminates the suction sounds that may obscure or distract from breath sounds.

Breath sounds are produced by turbulent airflow through the airways during inspiration and expiration. The sounds produced are transmitted along the trachea and bronchi and then through the lungs to the chest wall. In passing through the lungs, the intensity and frequency pattern of sounds are altered relative to the interplay of three factors: (1) the volume of airflow, (2) the presence or absence of pleural air or fluid, and (3) the consistency of the underlying lung tissue.

Background sounds can be confused with lung sounds. Consider and rule out these possibilities before making diagnostic judgments. Background sounds include the sound of the examiner's breathing on the stethoscope tubing or the tubing bumping together, patient shivering, or patient hair under the diaphragm of the stethoscope (hairy patient), which may produce sounds likened to crackles.

Types of Breath Sounds

There are two varieties of breath sounds, both of which are normally audible at specific parts of the chest. The first is termed *bronchial breath sounds,* and the second is termed *vesicular breath sounds.* These respiratory sounds are diagrammatically represented in Figure 3-5.

Bronchial breath sounds, also termed *tracheal sounds,* are normally heard only over the trachea. They are high pitched and blowing and have a definite tubular quality. The expiratory sound is as loud and lasts as long as the inspiratory sound. There is a brief pause at peak inspiration. These characteristics are important to remember because bronchial breath sounds heard over lung tissue always indicate pulmonary disease characterized by consolidation or fibrosis.

Vesicular breath sounds are heard over normal lung tissue and have a characteristic low-pitched rustling or "breezy" quality. These sounds resemble the quality of sound created by wind moving through trees. The intensity of the sound increases steadily during inspiration and fades

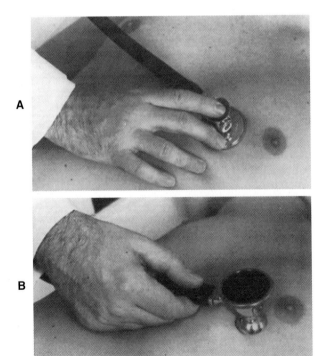

FIGURE 3-4 A, Placement of the diaphragm; the head is applied tightly to the skin. **B,** The bell piece is simply placed on the skin. The application of pressure stretches the underlying skin, which acts as a diaphragm and filters out low-intensity sounds. (From Swartz MH: *Textbook of physical diagnosis, history and examination,* ed 3, Philadelphia, 1998, W.B. Saunders.)

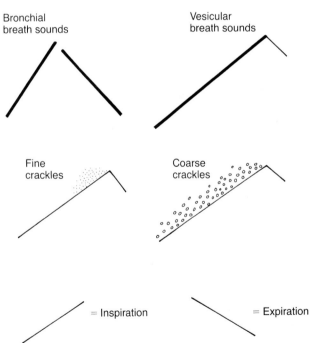

FIGURE 3-5 Breath sounds. The upstroke represents inspiration and the downstroke expiration; the length of each line represents the duration of the sound, and the thickness represents the intensity of the sound. Both sounds are more audible in thin and poorly muscled people, and the sounds are somewhat louder in normal children. Because of differences in patient body build, the standard for normal vesicular breathing is particularly difficult to establish for all people. Instead, individual patient evaluation is based on comparison of symmetric areas.

completely during the first one third of expiration. Vesicular sounds are normally not heard with equal intensity throughout the chest. They are most distinct anteriorly over the upper chest, in the axillae, and posteriorly from the scapular tips downward. Because the audibility of vesicular sounds varies, both sides of the chest should be alternately auscultated so the examiner can compare the regional quality of breath sounds. Auscultation is best begun at the apices and symmetrically auscultated downward to the bases. The midaxillary areas are included in the examination.

Causes of Altered Vesicular Sounds. If there is *airflow limitation,* sounds at the chest wall are diminished or absent. This may be characteristic of status asthmaticus, atelectasis, obstruction of a large bronchus, or pneumothorax. Patients with stage 3 or 4 ARDS, which is characterized by diffuse microatelectasis, also have diminished breath sounds. Vesicular sounds are also diminished in *pulmonary emphysema* because of the decreased force of inspiratory air flow, as well as the fact that the abnormally large volume of air in the hyperinflated lungs damps the transmission of sound. *Pleural thickening* or *effusion* also interferes with the passage of sound to the chest wall. If the lung tissue becomes *consolidated* as in pneumonia, tumor, or fibrotic pulmonary disease, the sounds resemble, but are quieter and more harsh than, bronchial sounds. See Box 3-1 for causes of diminished breath sounds.

Bronchovesicular sounds are a combination of bronchial and vesicular sounds; the inspiratory and expiratory components are of equal length. This type of sound may be heard in patients with diffuse pulmonary fibrosis and COPD.

Abnormal (Adventitious) Breath Sounds. Adventitious sounds are *additional* sounds that, in health, are never heard anywhere in the thorax. These sounds are the result of vibrations produced by pathologic conditions within the airways and lungs.

Crackles, previously called *rales,* are sounds made by the sudden opening of small airways and alveoli previously stuck together; often by fluid or exudate or by movement of air through secretions in the airways. They may be numerous or rare, loud or faint, coarse or fine, bubbly or gurgling. Fine crackles resemble the sound made by rubbing several strands of hair between the thumb and index finger in front of the ear, or the sound made when Velcro is opened. Crackles may occur early or late in inspiration, expiration, or both phases of ventilation. Fine crackles are heard near the peak of inspiration and are due to the explosive reopening of the peripheral airways and alveoli that have closed during expiration. These are heard in patients with restrictive lung disease, pneumonia, pulmonary edema, and intersterstitial fibrosis. Fine crackles that occur early in inspiration are common in patients with COPD and asthma. Both of the previously described fine crackles typically do not clear following coughing or suctioning However, in elderly or bedridden patients, particularly if just aroused from sleep, fine crackles that are heard near the peak of inspiration (atelectatic crackles) are not pathogenic if they disappear after a few deep breaths. Coarse inspiratory or expiratory crackles are bubbly or gurgling in quality, are produced by movement of air through secretions in the larger bronchi, and may or may not clear following coughing or suctioning.

Wheezes, previously called *rhonchi,* are sounds with a wide range of pitch, which may vary from musical and high pitched (sibilant wheezes) to a snoring, moaning, low-pitched sound (sonorous wheezes). Both are produced by the movement of air through diffusely narrowed (sibilant) or obstructed (sonorous) bronchi. Because bronchi normally become shortened and narrowed during expiration, wheezes are most frequently heard during expiration, which also becomes prolonged and labored. Wheezing can occur during both inspiration and expiration in cases of severe bronchial narrowing or when the airways become rigid and do not expand normally during inspiration. Wheezes are commonly associated with asthmatic attacks, ARDS, COPD, pulmonary edema, anaphylactic reactions, irritating inhalants, and pulmonary embolism. If the endotracheal tube tip is near the patient's carina, it may produce a transmitted wheeze. Wheezing may be a normal finding during maximal forced expiration.

Use of terms such as *rales* or *rhonchi* commonly results in misunderstanding among clinicians reporting patient status because there is inconsistency in defining these esoteric terms both in the literature and in clinical settings. The likelihood of accurate communication and

---

BOX 3-1
Causes of Diminished Breath Sounds

Airflow limitation
Status asthmaticus
Atelectasis
Obstruction of a large bronchus
Pneumothorax
ARDS
Pulmonary emphysema
Pleural thickening or effusion
Pneumonia
Tumor
Fibrotic lung disease

clear understanding is increased if clinicians use common adjectives when describing lung sounds or other physical assessment findings.

Stridor is a high-pitched, crowing inspiratory sound due to upper airway obstruction. Stridor is easily audible at a distance from the patient and may quickly result in death. Unless the patient is very obese or edematous, retractions are always visible over the sternal notch, above the clavicles, in the intercostal spaces, and below the sternum. Stridor may be due to laryngeal spasm or swelling, epiglottitis, tracheal stenosis, aspiration of a foreign object, or vocal cord edema. The presence of stridor is an absolute medical emergency, indicating at least a 70% obstruction of the upper airway, and mandates insertion of an artificial airway.

A pleural friction rub is a creaking, leathery sound produced when the surface of the pleura is roughened by inflammation (pleurisy) due to viral or bacterial infection or by pulmonary infarction. The rub occurs toward the peak of inspiration and the early part of expiration. Because the greatest movement of the lungs occurs over the lower lobes, pleural rubs are most commonly heard over the lower thorax. The sound may vary in intensity and disappears when patients hold their breath. In a healthy person, no pleural sound is produced with breathing because the pleural membranes are smooth and moist.

In summary, errors in physical assessment may be minimized if we remain constantly aware of human and monitoring limitations. Judgments based on physical assessment should be tested against laboratory and monitoring data to see if all pieces of patient information fit into a consistent clinical mosaic.

REFERENCES

1. Lipson LG, Dibble SL, Minarik PA: *Culture and nursing care: a pocket guide,* University of California, 1996, The Regents.
2. Jarvis C: Transcultural considerations. In *Assessment in physical examination and health assessment,* ed 3, Philadelphia, 2000, W.B. Saunders.
3. Krieger N, Rowley D, Herman A, et al: Racism, sexism and social class: implications for studies of health, disease, and well-being, *Am J Prev Med* 9(suppl 6):82, 1993.
4. Sax FL, Charlson ME: Medical patients at high risk for catastrophic deterioration, *Crit Care Med* 15(5):510, 1987.
5. Schein RMH, Halday N, Pena M, et al: Clinical antecedent to in-hospital cardiopulmonary arrest, *Chest* 98(6): 1990.
6. Franklin C, Mathew J: Developing strategies to prevent in-hospital cardiac arrest: Analyzing responses of physicians and nurses in the hours before the event, *Crit Care Med* 22(2):244, 1994.

SUGGESTED READINGS

Bates B: The thorax and lungs. In *A guide to physical examination and history taking,* ed 8, Philadelphia, 1995, Lippincott.

Carrieri VK, Janson-Bjerklie S, Jacobs S: The sensation of dyspnea: a review, *Heart Lung* 3:436, 1984.

Crompton GK: The respiratory system. In Munro J, Edwards C, editors: *Macleod's clinical examination,* ed 8, Edinburgh, 1990, Churchill Livingstone.

Ditchey RV: Cyanosis. In Horwitz LD, Groves BM, editors: *Signs and symptoms in cardiology,* Philadelphia, 1985, Lippincott.

Dobbs GJ, Coombs LJ: Clinical examination of patients in the intensive care unit, *Br J Hosp Med* 38(2):102, 1987.

Irwin RS, Widdicome GF: Cough. In Murray JF, Nadel JA, editors: *Textbook of respiratory medicine,* ed 3, Philadelphia, 2000, W.B. Saunders.

Jarvis C: Thorax and lungs. In *Physical examination and health assessment,* ed 3, Philadelphia, 2000, W.B. Saunders.

Lumb PD: Clinical assessment in the intensive care unit. In Civetta JM, Taylor RW, Kirby RR, editors: *Critical care,* ed 2, Philadelphia, 1992, Lippincott.

Malley WJ: *Clinical blood gases, application and noninvasive alternatives,* Philadelphia, 1990, W.B. Saunders.

Murray JF: History and physical examination. In Murray JF, Nadel JA, editors: *Textbook of respiratory medicine,* ed 3, Philadelphia, 2000, W.B. Saunders.

Murray JF, Gebhart GF: Chest pain. In Murray JF, Nadel JA, editors: *Textbook of respiratory medicine,* ed 3, Philadelphia, 2000, W.B. Saunders.

Seidel AM, Ball JW, Dains JE, et al: Chest and lungs. In *Mosby's guide to physical examination,* ed 3, Philadelphia, 1995, Mosby.

Wilson RF: Pulmonary physiology. In *Critical care manual: applied physiology and principles of therapy,* Philadelphia, 1992, Davis.

Weil JV: Dyspnea. In Horwitz LD, Groves BM, editors: *Signs and symptoms in cardiology,* Philadelphia, 1985, Lippincott.

GLORIA OBLOUK DAROVIC

4

Cardiovascular Anatomy and Physiology

OVERVIEW OF THE CARDIOVASCULAR SYSTEM

The function of the cardiovascular system is to transport oxygen, nutrients, and endocrine and exocrine hormones to the tissue and to carry away metabolic waste at a rate proportionate to body needs.

The cardiovascular system is a continuous, closed, fluid-filled, elastic circuit equipped with a pump (Figure 4-1). The component parts include the following:

- *Heart.* The cardiac pump provides the force that drives blood through the vascular system.
- *Arteries.* The arterial vessels serve as a delivery system that distributes cardiac output throughout the body and regulates the volume of flow delivered to each organ system on a moment-to-moment basis, depending on regional metabolic need.
- *Capillaries.* The capillaries are microscopic vessels where the actual exchange of respiratory gases, nutrients, and metabolites occurs between plasma and body cells. They are therefore sometimes referred to as the *nutrient bed.*
- *Veins.* The veins serve as the return system that brings deoxygenated blood back to the cardiopulmonary unit. Veins also act as a reservoir and accommodate approximately 70% of circulating blood volume. Through venoconstriction or venodilation, venous blood volume may be increased or decreased according to the needs of the cardiovascular system.
- *Blood.* Plasma is the liquid medium in which respiratory gases, nutrients, metabolic waste, and hormones

are dissolved, and formed elements of blood (red blood cells, white blood cells, and platelets) are carried.

Normally, with each beat of the heart, equal amounts of blood move through all divisions of the cardiovascular circuit. Because of the continuity of the cardiovascular system, disturbances in flow in one portion of the circulation, such as that which occurs in patients with ventricular septal defect or massive pulmonary embolism, will eventually be reflected as disturbances in flow in all portions of the circulation.

This chapter discusses the anatomic and physiologic features of the specific components of the cardiovascular system, with the exception of blood. It is beyond the scope of this chapter to detail the complex characteristics of blood.

HEART

The heart is a four-chambered muscular organ whose only function is to propel blood forward in an amount that meets the metabolic requirements of the body. The heart is formed of predominantly muscular tissue and some dense fibrous tissue that forms the "skeleton" of the heart. The atria, ventricles, valves, and roots of the great arteries are firmly attached to this connective tissue skeleton. The normal heart is approximately the size of the individual's fist and weighs approximately 2 g per 1 lb of ideal body weight. Therefore an average (150 lb) man's heart weighs approximately 300 g, and the heart of an average (125 lb) woman weighs approximately 250 g.

57

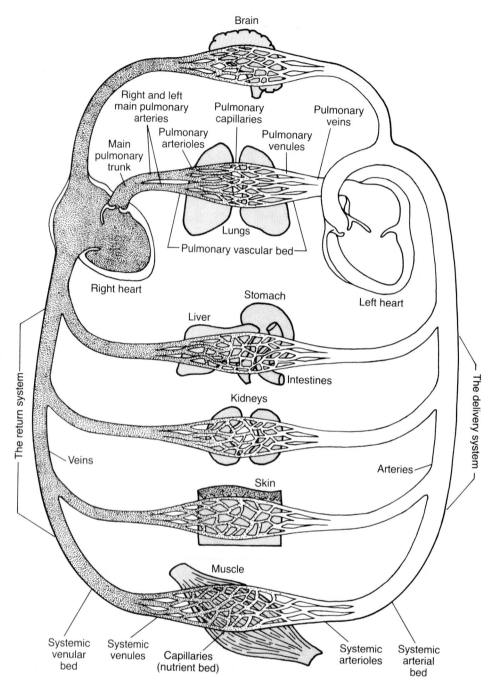

FIGURE 4-1 Cardiovascular circuit.

Structure of the Heart Wall

The cardiac wall is composed of the pericardium, myocardium, and endocardium.

The *pericardium* is a two-layered sac that encases the heart and attaches to the roots of the great vessels. The fibrous, nondistensible, parietal pericardium is the outermost layer. The parietal pericardium then doubles back to form the serous visceral pericardium (also termed *epicardium*), which directly adheres to the myocardial surface. A potential space, which contains 20 to 30 ml of fluid, lies between the parietal and visceral pericardium. Pericardial fluid acts as a lubricant that provides a friction-free surface for the beating heart.

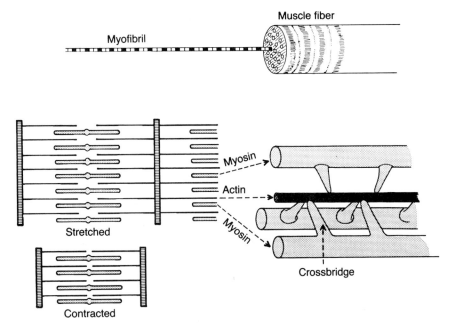

FIGURE 4-2 The myofibrils are composed of overlapping thick myosin and thin actin filaments. The amount of overlap is reduced during muscle stretching and increased during muscle contraction. Crossbridges are noted at regular intervals between the actin and myosin filaments. These crossbridges form linkages on the actin fibers and draw the actin past the myosin during the contractile process. (Adapted from Rushmer RF: *Cardiovascular dynamics,* ed 4, Philadelphia, 1976, W.B. Saunders.)

The *myocardium,* the muscular middle layer of the heart, has contractile properties, as well as the capacity to conduct electrical stimuli for muscle contraction.

The *endocardium* is a serous membrane that lines the inner surface of the heart and extends out to form the heart valves. Rheumatic or infectious endocarditis is frequently associated with scarring and damage of the valve leaflets.

How Heart Muscle Contracts

The myocardium is composed of bundles of microscopic muscle fibers, termed *myofibrils,* that intertwine and form a latticework configuration. The myofibrils, in turn, are made up of two types of filaments; myosin, the first type, is almost twice as thick as actin, the second type. These thick and thin filaments are linked together by crossbridges (Figure 4-2) that project from the myosin fibers at frequent intervals. The dynamics by which actin and myosin produce muscle contraction comprise a process wherein the crossbridges from the myosin filament link to sites on the actin and swivel to a position that causes the two sets of filaments to slide past each other and overlap. This action is termed *interdigitation* and results in the development of muscle tension and shortening. The force of myocardial contraction is related, in part, to the amount of end-diastolic stretch of

cardiac muscle, which is determined by the volume of blood within the heart at end-diastole. Increased stretch of the myofibrils results in an increased force of contraction, just as increased stretch of a rubber band results in forceful shortening on release. Conversely, decreased stretch results in decreased contractile force.[1]

The interdigitation of the actin and myosin fibrils is triggered and controlled by the entrance of calcium ions (Ca^{++}) into a protein called *troponin* located on the actin filament. The calcium comes from outside the cells and also from storage sites that are distributed within the cell. The exit of calcium from the troponin molecules uncouples the crossbridges, and the filaments relax and lengthen. The uptake and removal of ionized calcium from the contractile elements occur within a fraction of a second and repeat with each heartbeat.

The strength of contraction of the cardiac muscle is related, in part, to the concentration of ionized calcium in the extracellular fluid, which increases or decreases calcium availability to the contractile elements. Hypercalcemia excites the cardiac contractile process, whereas hypocalcemia decreases contractility and may result in heart failure. Calcium channel blocking agents, by reducing calcium influx into the myofibrils, also have negative inotropic effects.

The energy required to produce the contractile work of the heart is supplied by the high-energy molecule adenosine triphosphate (ATP) (see Figure 16-2).

Structural Changes in the Myocardium in Health and Disease

Several changes may occur in the structure and function of the myocardium as a result of chronic stress or as a compensatory mechanism or adaptation to heart disease. Changes include hypertrophy of the heart and ventricular dilation.

Hypertrophy of the Heart

When an increased workload is chronically imposed on a muscle, it increases in mass and contractile strength. For example, skeletal and myocardial muscle mass and strength increase in trained athletes to meet the demands of strenuous exercise. Adaptive hypertrophy has no untoward effects in the healthy heart.

Ventricular hypertrophy also develops as a compensatory mechanism in persons with diseases that produce either pressure or volume overload (or both) of the heart. There are two types of hypertrophy. The effects of hypertrophy on the left ventricle are discussed, but the same principles apply to both ventricles.

Concentric hypertrophy develops when the left ventricle chronically contracts against increased pressure (aortic stenosis, hypertension). Myocardial cells adaptively thicken and there is a substantial increase in wall thickness, but the ventricular chamber does not significantly increase in diameter. Consequently, cardiomegaly will not be noted on the chest radiograph and the apex beat can be palpated in the normal, midclavicular position. Instead of growing outward, the expanding ventricular wall encroaches on and diminishes the size of the intraventricular cavity. Therefore ventricular end-diastolic pressure (pulmonary artery wedge pressure [PWP]) will be disproportionately high relative to end-diastolic volume. Hypertrophic hearts may achieve weights of 700 to 750 g (normal 300 g).

Eccentric hypertrophy of the left ventricle adaptively develops in patients with chronic aortic regurgitation or mitral regurgitation. Because there is chronic and progressive volume overload of the left ventricular chamber, myocytes lengthen and may thicken. These changes initially allow ejection of a greater stroke volume, as well as the accommodation of increased intraventricular volume without increases in end-diastolic pressure. Overall, ventricular wall thickness and the internal and external diameters of the heart increase proportionate to the volume load.

Whereas systolic wall tension, heart work, and myocardial oxygen consumption remain normal in patients with adequate compensatory concentric or eccentric hypertrophy, the diastolic distensibility (compliance) and rate of relaxation may be impaired. The penetrating branches of the coronary arteries also elongate relative to the increase in wall thickness. Unfortunately, systolic compression of the elongated penetrating branches compromises systolic blood flow, from endocardium to epicardium. This predisposes to myocardial ischemia even in persons without coronary artery disease.

Whatever the cause of hypertrophy, the enlarging muscle mass eventually reaches a limit beyond which it can no longer compensate for the increased pressure/volume burden. Degenerative myocardial changes, such as lysis, fibrosis, and loss of myofibrillar contractile elements, occur in tandem with the development of heart failure.

Ventricular Dilation

Ventricular dilation may develop as an adaptive process whenever the ventricle cannot empty adequately in systole (heart failure) or in a volume-overloaded ventricle (aortic or mitral regurgitation, intracardiac shunts). As the radius of the ventricle increases, systolic tension, myocardial work, and oxygen requirements proportionately increase. Also, the greater the systolic tension a failing ventricle must develop, the greater the decrease in rate of muscle fiber shortening and velocity of ejection. Consequent to ventricular dilation, the patient becomes more vulnerable to myocardial ischemia, and the development of ectopic arrhythmias further worsens the risk of heart failure and sudden death. Degenerative myocardial changes also develop.

Ventricular Remodeling. This term describes a condition in which the left ventricle is altered in shape and structure. Remodeling was initially used to describe the structural changes that occur after myocardial infarction but has now been extended to include the myocardial effects of chronic pressure and volume overload, chronic valvular disease, and familial hypertrophic and dilated cardiomyopathy. Overall, ventricular mass (hypertrophy) or chamber volume (dilation) or both are increased. The changes in the molecular structure of the myocardium are extremely complex and involve adaptive processes to the underlying problem, as well as degenerative changes that occur at the cellular level. Microscopically, changes involve both myocardial cells and the interspaces (interstitium) of myocardial cells. Myocytes increase in thickness and length, and there may also be fragmentation and loss of myocytes, due to apoptosis. *Apoptosis* is a term generally used to describe cell breakdown and death that is under genetic control. In other words, it is a form of "cell suicide" in that the cell's own genes play a role in its death.

It is a normal process of the cells of various organ systems during development and adulthood. However, abnormal apoptosis may occur in other organs and within the myocardium as a result of hypertrophy and heart failure. An increase in collagen (fibrosis) within the interstitium may account for decreased contractility (systolic dysfunction) and reduced ventricular compliance (diastolic dysfunction). It is probably a combination of hemodynamic, sympathetic nervous system, and hormonal alterations that accounts for the initiation and progression of the remodeling process.

For example, in patients having had a myocardial infarction, the remodeling process begins in the acute period and continues though the late convalescent period. The degree of remodeling depends on infarct size, rate of infarct healing, and left ventricular wall stress. The greater the size of the infarct, the slower the rate of healing or extension of the infarction, and the greater the ventricular wall stress, the greater the extent of remodeling. Once begun, a vicious cycle leads to progressive cardiac dilation and heart failure. Medical management is directed at aborting or slowing the process. Whether this process, once established, is reversible is still unknown.

Endocrine Function of the Heart

The heart can produce angiotensin II, aldosterone, and catecholamines. Various other hormones, termed *natriuretic peptides,* have been discovered.[2] These include the following:

- *Atrial natriuretic peptide* (ANP), which is produced and stored mainly in the right atrium. Release is stimulated by an increase in atrial distending pressure. This peptide causes vasodilation and excretion of increased amounts of sodium in the urine (natriuresis), and it opposes water retention via the renin-angiotensin-aldosterone system.
- *Brain natriuretic peptide (BNP)* is stored in the ventricular myocardium. Release is stimulated by increased ventricular filling pressures. BNP release results in vasodilation and increased urinary losses of sodium.
- *Vasoactive intestinal peptide (VIP)* is present in vagal nerve fibers located in the heart. In response to vagal nerve stimulation, VIP directly dilates the coronary arteries and increases right atrial and ventricular contractility and heart rate.[3,4]

Circulating levels of ANP and BNP are elevated in patients in heart failure proportionate to the severity of heart failure. Also, their natriuretic effect seems to be inhibited in these patients. Serum BNP levels appear to be excellent markers of cardiac status in patients with heart failure. Recent studies have shown that pharmacologic treatment of heart failure guided by serum BNP levels results in reduced total cardiac events and reduced mortality rates.[5,6]

How Electrical Stimuli for Myocardial Contraction Traverse the Heart

Myocardial cells connect in a series at points called *intercalated disks.* These cell boundaries have tight junctions that offer low electrical impedance that, in turn, allows electrical stimuli to pass with ease from cell to cell throughout the latticework interconnections. Stimulation of any muscle fiber therefore results in stimulation of the entire myocardial mass.

The dynamics of excitation of myocardial cells, as well as the sequence of cardiac excitation (depolarization), is described in Chapter 14.

Nervous System Control of the Heart

Heart rate, electrical conductivity velocity, and myocardial contractility are regulated by the sympathetic and parasympathetic nervous systems.

The *sympathetic nervous system* innervates the heart through nerve fibers arising from the upper thoracic spinal cord. Sympathetic nervous system stimulation results in the systemic release of epinephrine and norepinephrine. The cardioexcitatory and vasoactive effects of these hormones are mediated by stimulation of beta- and alpha-adrenergic nerve receptors located within the cardiovascular tissue.

Beta-Adrenergic Receptors

Beta-adrenergic receptors are located within the myocardium and within vascular and bronchial smooth muscle. Stimulation of beta-adrenergic receptors increases the rate of sinus nodal discharge; increases automaticity of all portions of the heart, as well as atrial and ventricular contractility; and promotes a mild dilator effect on arteriolar and venular smooth muscle. Potent sympathetic nervous system discharge, which results in beta-receptor excitation, may raise the resting cardiac output twofold or threefold by increasing heart rate to greater than 200 beats per minute and increasing contractility. Conversely, by decreasing heart rate and contractility, sympathetic nervous system depression may reduce resting cardiac output as much as 30% below normal.[7]

Alpha-Adrenergic Receptors

Alpha-adrenergic receptors are located within vascular smooth muscle; there are no important alpha receptors within the myocardium. Consequently, stimulation of the alpha-adrenergic receptors has no direct effect on the myocardium but produces vasoconstriction in all but coronary and cerebral vascular beds.

The *parasympathetic nervous system* innervates the heart via vagal fibers to both atria and, to a lesser extent, to both ventricles. Vagal stimulation (Valsalva maneuver, gag reflex, carotid sinus massage) results in inhibitory cardiovascular effects, which, in turn, decrease the rate of sinus nodal discharge, decrease contractility, and reduce conduction through the atrioventricular (AV) junction. In fact, potent vagal stimulation can stop the heart for a few seconds. If the vagal effect is sustained, a ventricular escape focus generally begins to drive the heart at a rate of approximately 15 to 35 beats per minute. Strong vagal stimulation also decreases myocardial contractility by as much as 20% to 30%. Overall, parasympathetic nervous system stimulation can decrease cardiac output more than 50%.[7]

Neuronal Transmission of Cardiac Pain and Patterns of Pain

Painful impulses originating within the heart begin in nerve endings located within the coronary vessels and the myocardium. The cell bodies of these sensory nerve fibers are located in the dorsal roots of the thoracic spine, segments T1 through T5. Cardiac pain tends to be referred to skin or skeletal muscles that share nerve supplies from the same or neighboring spinal segments. Therefore cardiac pain is commonly referred to areas innervated by thoracic segments T1 through T5, such as the anterior chest wall; the sternum; the jaw; portions of the abdomen; the scapula; the medial aspects of the forearm, wrist, and hand; and the shoulders and anterior neck. *Chronic or acute unexplained pain in these areas, especially if it occurs in persons with a high-risk profile for coronary artery disease, should be considered the result of angina or myocardial infarction and should be immediately investigated.*

Heart Valves

Four heart valves normally permit only forward blood flow. They are divided into two types according to their structure: semilunar and atrioventricular valves.

Semilunar Valves

Semilunar valves are composed of three delicate half-moon-shaped leaflets attached to a fibrous ring located at the base of the aorta (aortic valve) and pulmonary artery (pulmonic valve). Rising ventricular systolic pressure forces the pliant aortic and pulmonic valve leaflets open, and they are smoothed against the vessel walls (Figure 4-3, *B*). Early in

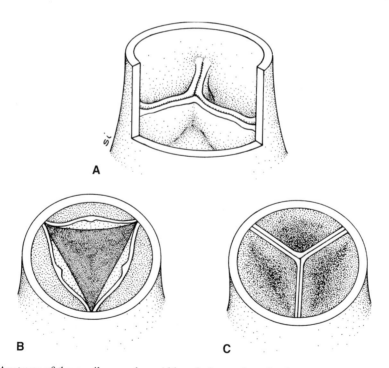

FIGURE 4-3 Anatomy of the semilunar valves. Although the aortic and pulmonic valves are identical in structure, the leaflets of the aortic valve are normally heavier than those of the pulmonic valve. This is because the aortic valve closing pressure (80 mm Hg) is greater than the closing pressure for the pulmonic valve (8 to 15 mm Hg). Thus a structurally stronger valve leaflet is required for the root of the aorta. **A,** Valve closed (diastole) viewed from the side with portion of the arterial wall resected. **B,** Open valve (systole viewed from above). **C,** Closed valve (diastole viewed from above).

ventricular diastole, reversal of blood flow fills and distends the valve cusps. The approximated valve edges then seal off the roots of the great arteries and prevent backflow of blood into the ventricles throughout the remainder of diastole (Figure 4-3, *C*).

Atrioventricular Valves

Atrioventricular valves are so named because they are located between the atria and the ventricles. The right AV valve (tricuspid valve) has three leaflets. The left AV valve (mitral valve) has two leaflets—a larger anteromedial leaflet and a smaller posterior leaflet. Fibrous cords *(chordae tendineae)* connect the edges of the valve leaflets to muscular projections *(papillary muscles)* that arise from

the inner surface of the ventricles. During *diastole,* the leaflets passively open into the ventricles and form a funnel-like shape (Figure 4-4, *A* and *C*). During *systole,* the leaflets spread out like an open parachute and are pushed upward by rising intraventricular pressure. The leaflet edges then approximate and occlude the valve orifice (Figure 4-4, *B*). Contraction of the papillary muscles during systole applies tension to the chordae tendineae, which, in turn, prevent prolapse of the valve leaflets. Valve prolapse would result in regurgitant blood flow into the atria. *All components of the valve apparatus—valve leaflets, chordae, papillary muscles, and supporting myocardium—must be intact for the AV valves to function normally.*

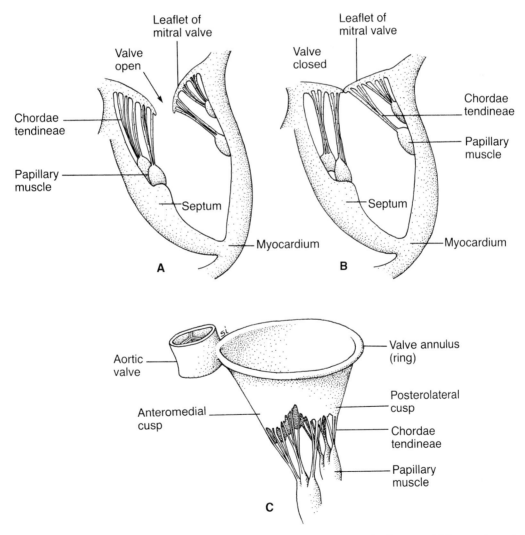

FIGURE 4-4 The atrioventricular valve structure (mitral valve). **A,** The valve leaflets are widely open in ventricular diastole, thus allowing ventricular filling. **B,** Closure of the valve leaflets in ventricular systole seals off the atria from the ventricles as ventricular contraction forces blood into the arterial circulation. **C,** The mitral valve annulus and the funnel-like structure of the valve apparatus.

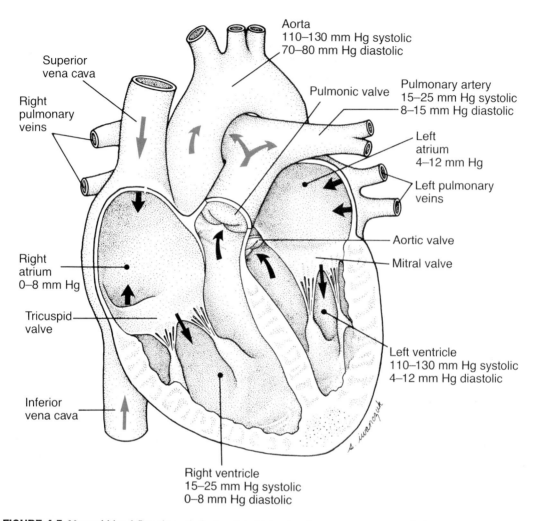

Superior
vena cava

Right
pulmonary
veins

Aorta
110–130 mm Hg systolic
70–80 mm Hg diastolic

Pulmonic valve

Pulmonary artery
15–25 mm Hg systolic
8–15 mm Hg diastolic

Left
atrium
4–12 mm Hg

Left pulmonary
veins

Aortic valve

Mitral valve

Right
atrium
0–8 mm Hg

Tricuspid
valve

Inferior
vena cava

Left ventricle
110–130 mm Hg systolic
4–12 mm Hg diastolic

Right ventricle
15–25 mm Hg systolic
0–8 mm Hg diastolic

FIGURE 4-5 Normal blood flow through the heart and intrachamber pressures; *arrows* indicate normal direction of blood flow. This schematic representation of the heart shows all four chambers and valves visible in the anterior view to facilitate conceptualization of blood flow. (For the correct anatomic position of the heart within the thorax, see Figure 4-6).

Blood Flow and Intrachamber Pressures

The factors responsible for the forward movement of blood through the heart are cyclic, transchamber pressure gradients—in other words, higher pressures in the delivering cardiac chambers and lower pressures in the receiving chambers. The greater the pressure differences between chambers, the greater the rate of blood flow. As pressures approach equilibrium, flow rates decrease. The normal direction of blood flow is represented schematically in Figure 4-5. For an anatomically correct view of the heart as it lies in the chest, see Figure 4-6.

Anatomically the heart is one organ. However, functionally it is two pumps in a series with each side serving a separate and physiologically distinct circulation. The

dynamics of blood flow and intrachamber pressures are presented separately for each side of the heart.

Right Heart

The right atrium and right ventricle receive deoxygenated venous blood from the systemic venous circulation and propel it through the low-pressure, low-resistance pulmonary circulation. Venous blood streams into the thin-walled right atrium (RA) from the superior vena cava, inferior vena cava, and coronary sinus. Right atrial pressure is low, measuring 0 to 8 mm Hg. During *diastole,* as blood flows into the right ventricle, the tricuspid valve is open and the right atrium and ventricle openly communicate. Therefore pressures between the two chambers

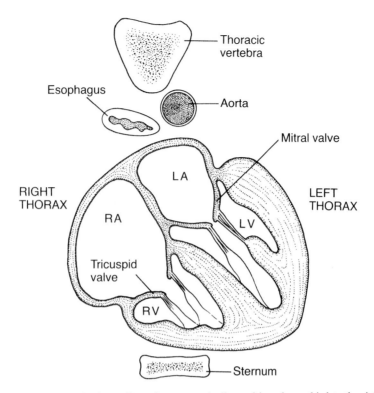

FIGURE 4-6 In situ, the heart is horizontally and asymmetrically positioned one third to the right and two thirds to the left of the sternum. The heart is suspended at the base by its great vessels; the apex is directed anteriorly, inferiorly, and to the left. The right ventricle is the most anterior structure of the heart and lies beneath the sternum. The right atrium lies superior and posterior to the right ventricle. The left ventricle is a posterolateral structure with only approximately one fourth of the total mass visible in the anterior view. The left atrium is an entirely posterior structure lying in front of the aorta, esophagus, and thoracic vertebrae.

equilibrate by end-diastole. This means that *mean right atrial pressure is a hemodynamic correlate of right ventricular end-diastolic pressure.*

At the onset of right ventricular (RV) *systole,* the tricuspid valve closes at the moment when rising right intraventricular pressure exceeds right atrial pressure. A few milliseconds later, the pulmonic valve is opened when right ventricular pressure exceeds the pressure in the pulmonary artery. As right ventricular pressure continues to increase to a systolic peak of 15 to 25 mm Hg, blood flows into the pulmonary circulation. During this time the right ventricle and the pulmonary artery openly communicate, and, as a result, *right ventricular and pulmonary artery systolic pressures correlate.*

As the right ventricle begins to relax at the onset of diastole, right ventricular pressure falls below pulmonary artery diastolic pressure (8 to 15 mm Hg), and the pulmonic valve closes. Blood continues to flow forward through the pulmonary circulation because a pressure gradient of approximately 4 to 8 mm Hg (pulmonary artery

diastolic pressure, 15 mm Hg, and left atrial pressure, 7 mm Hg) facilitates flow through the pulmonary capillaries and veins into the left atrium.

Left Heart

The left atrium and left ventricle pump the newly oxygenated blood through the high-resistance, high-pressure systemic circulation.

The thin-walled left atrium (LA) receives this oxygenated blood from the four pulmonary veins. Mean LA pressure is in the range of 4 to 12 mm Hg. During *diastole,* the mitral valve is open as blood flows into the left ventricle, and, as a result, the left atrium and ventricle openly communicate. Pressure equilibration occurs at end-diastole; therefore *mean left atrial and left ventricular end-diastolic pressures are normally equal (4 to 12 mm Hg).* Because the thick left ventricular wall is less distensible than the thin right ventricular wall, left ventricular end-diastolic (filling) pressure is normally higher than RV end-diastolic pressure despite the fact that right

TABLE 4-1

Normal Intracardiac Pressure and Factors Affecting Means of Bedside Measurement

Means of Bedside Measurement	Normal Pressure Range (mm Hg)	Factors Affecting Pressure Measurements and Means of Bedside Measurement
Right atrial pressure	0–8	Intravascular volume, directly reflects RVEDP in absence of tricuspid valve disease; indirectly reflects pulmonary vascular resistance, left heart function, venous capacitance. CVP line placed in SVC; proximal port of PA catheter
Right ventricular systolic pressure	15–25	Force of RV ejection, which relates to RV preload, afterload, and the contractile state of RV myocardium. PA systolic as measured with a pulmonary artery catheter; RV port of selected PA catheters
Right ventricular diastolic pressure	0–8	Intravascular volume; functional state of RV. CVP line; proximal port of PA catheter; RV port of selected PA catheters
Pulmonary artery systolic pressure	15–25	Pulmonary vascular volume; pulmonary vascular resistance (the resistance to flow through the pulmonary vascular channel). Pulmonary artery catheter, distal port
Pulmonary artery diastolic pressure	8–15	Pulmonary intravascular volume; pulmonary vascular resistance. PA catheter, distal port
Left atrial pressure	4–12*	Intravascular volume, directly reflects LVEDP in the absence of mitral valve disease. LA line; PA catheter in wedge position
Left ventricular systolic pressure	100–130	Force of LV ejection, which relates to preload, afterload, and the contractile state of LV myocardium. Arterial line; arterial systolic pressure
Left ventricular diastolic pressure	4–12	Intravascular volume; functional state of LV. PWP correlates well in absence of mitral valve disease or PWP greater than 20 mm Hg

*Normally the measured pulmonary artery wedge pressure (PWP) is 1 to 4 mm Hg less than the measured PA diastolic pressure (PAd) (termed *PAd-PWP gradient*).

CVP, central venous pressure; *LA,* left atrium; *LVEDP,* left ventricular end-diastolic pressure; *PA,* pulmonary artery; *RV,* right ventricle; *RVEDP,* right ventricular end-diastolic pressure; *SVC,* superior vena cava.

and left ventricular end-diastolic volumes are normally equal—approximately 120 ml.

With the onset of left ventricular *systole,* the mitral valve closes. As intraventricular pressure rises and exceeds pressure in the aortic root, the aortic valve opens. Left ventricular pressure continues to rise to a peak of approximately 110 to 130 mm Hg. This provides the force for movement of blood through the large-volume, high-resistance systemic circulation. During systole, the left ventricle and aorta openly communicate, and, as a result, left ventricular systolic and arterial systolic pressures (as measured in the aortic root) are normally equal. Table 4-1 lists normal intracardiac pressures, the factors affecting them, and the means of obtaining bedside pressure measurements.

Phases of the Cardiac Cycle

The thin-walled atria are entrance and reservoir chambers for the ventricles and contract to augment ventricular filling. The more muscular ventricles supply the power that moves blood through the pulmonary and systemic circulations. The mechanics of ventricular filling (diastole) and ejection (systole) are phasic and applicable to both ventri-

cles. Figure 4-7 illustrates the correlation of the diastolic and systolic events with pressure changes in the cardiac chambers.

Ventricular Diastole

Ventricular diastole is divided into four phases.

Phase I—Protodiastole. This is the very early, brief phase of diastole during which there is reversal of blood flow in the pulmonary artery and aorta as ventricular pressures fall below pressures within the roots of the pulmonary artery and aorta. Retrograde blood flow results in distention and closure of the pulmonic and aortic valves. To open the mitral and tricuspid valves, the pressure within the atria must exceed the pressure within the ventricles. However, at this point in the cycle, ventricular pressures are still higher than atrial pressures, and the AV valves are closed. During this very brief period, all four valves are closed and no blood is flowing.

Phase II—Isometric Relaxation. This is also termed *isovolumic relaxation.* As the ventricles continue

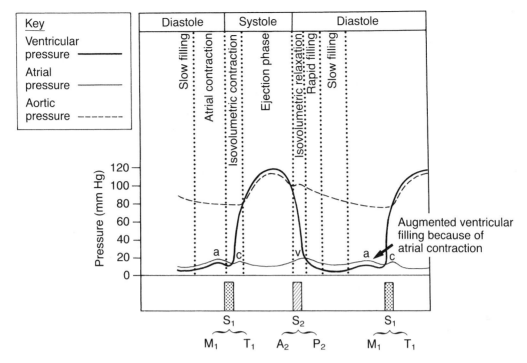

FIGURE 4-7 Cardiac cycle illustrating the pressure changes in the left atrium, left ventricle, and aorta, as well as the relationship of these events to the production of heart sounds. S_1 is the the first heart sound, which occurs synchronously with closure of the mitral and tricuspid valves. S_2 is the second heart sound, which occurs synchronously with closure of the aortic and pulmonic valves. Note the relationship of the waveform with the phases of diastole and systole.

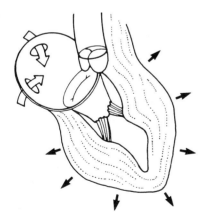

FIGURE 4-8 Isovolumetric relaxation.

to relax, intraventricular pressures decrease and blood continues to flow from the systemic and pulmonary venous systems into the atria. Consequently, intraatrial pressures rise. In Figure 4-8, the solid, outwardly directed arrows indicate ventricular relaxation and the open arrows indicate direction of blood flow.

Phase III—Passive Filling. When pressure within the ventricles falls below atrial pressures, the AV valves passively open and blood rushes into the ventricles. This is termed the *period of rapid filling* during which as much as 60% of ventricular filling may occur. In mid to late diastole, filling of the ventricles becomes progressively slower as atrial and ventricular pressures reach near equilibrium. This is termed the *period of slowed filling,* or *diastasis.* The duration of slowed ventricular filling depends on the heart rate and becomes progressively shorter with rapid heart rates (allowing less time for ventricular filling) and longer with slow heart rates (allowing more time for ventricular filling).

Approximately 70% to 90% of ventricular filling occurs throughout the combined rapid and slowed filling phases. Blood continues to flow into the atrial chambers (Figure 4-9).

Phase IV—Atrial Systole (Atrial Kick). The atrial contribution to ventricular filling is known as the *atrial systole* or the *atrial kick.* Upon atrial contraction, blood flow into the ventricles is again increased. The additional blood volume pumped into the ventricles by the atria contributes approximately 10% to 30% to ventricular end-diastolic volume. Augmented end-diastolic filling, in turn, increases the end-diastolic myocardial fiber length, the force of the subsequent ventricular contraction, stroke volume, and cardiac output. In Figure 4-10, the larger, solid, inwardly directed arrows represent atrial contraction.

Loss of atrial contraction, as may occur in atrial fibrillation, AV dissociation, and some junctional rhythms, has minimal effect on ventricular performance if the patient has a relatively healthy heart. If, however, the patient has an obstruction to ventricular filling (mitral stenosis, left atrial thrombus, or myxoma), has a stiff ventricular muscle (hypertrophy, ischemia), or has heart failure, optimal cardiac function is highly dependent on atrial contraction. In vulnerable patients, hypotension may result from the loss of atrial contraction.

Ventricular Systole
Ejection of the ventricles occurs in three phases.

Phase I—Isometric Contraction. This is also termed *isovolumic contraction.* When applied to muscle, the word "isometric" means muscle contraction occurring without changes in muscle fiber length. During the phase of isometric ventricular contraction, the ventricular walls tense and press toward the center of the ventricular cavities (as represented by the inwardly directed arrows in Figure 4-11), but there is no actual muscle fiber shortening and no blood flow.

This action increases pressure within the ventricular cavities. When ventricular pressures exceed pressures within the atria, the AV valves snap shut. When intraventricular pressures increase to levels greater than the diastolic pressures in the pulmonary artery and aorta (8 mm Hg and 80 mm Hg, respectively), the pulmonic and aortic valves open.

One of the fundamental laws of physics states that an object at rest tends to remain at rest, and an object in motion tends to remain in motion. Just as the greatest work and energy consumption are associated with the muscle tension generated to set a heavy object, such as a large cart, in motion, so too the greatest myocardial energy expenditure and oxygen consumption are associated with isometric contraction.

Phases II and III—Rapid and Slowed Ventricular Ejection. Upon opening of the semilunar valves, the ventricles continue to contract (as represented by the solid, inwardly directed arrows in Figure 4-12) and blood rushes out of the ventricles into the great arteries. Left ventricular pressure continues to build to 120 mm Hg. Within the right ventricle pressure increases to 20 to 25 mm Hg. These respective systolic pressures drive blood into the systemic and pulmonary circulations. This is followed by reduced rates of ejection during which the remaining 40% of ventricular emptying occurs.

Waveforms
Systolic and diastolic hemodynamic events can be correlated with heart sounds and specific components of

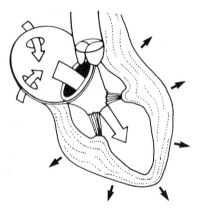

FIGURE 4-9 Passive filling.

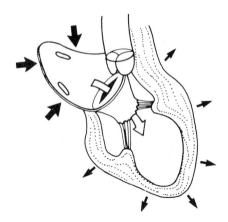

FIGURE 4-10 Atrial systole.

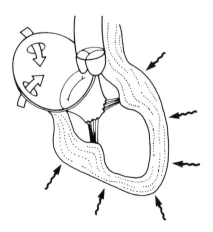

FIGURE 4-11 Isometric contraction.

the atrial, ventricular, and arterial waveforms (see Figure 4-7).

Atrial Pressure Waveform

The shape of the atrial waveform reflects the pressure changes within the atria during the cardiac cycle. In patients with intact atrial contraction, two atrial crests and troughs (which are nearly equal in amplitude) are associated with each heartbeat (Figures 4-13 and 4-14). Right atrial, left atrial, and wedged waveform morphology are fundamentally the same except for minor differences in *a* and *v* wave amplitude.

The a Wave. The first crest is the result of the small pressure rise that accompanies atrial contraction and is preceded by the P wave on a simultaneously recorded electrocardiogram (ECG). A sloped descent, termed the *x descent,* immediately follows the *a* wave and reflects the fall in intraatrial pressure that occurs with atrial relaxation. Occasionally the *x* descent is distorted by a small crest, termed the *c* wave. Inscription of the *c* wave is thought to result partially from upward bulging of the AV valves early in ventricular systole and partially from pressure waves transmitted to the atria from large nearby arteries. When a *c* wave is inscribed, the continued decline in pressure following the *c* wave is termed *x prime,* often written as *x′*.

The v Wave. The second crest occurs as blood flows into and fills the atrial chambers. The continuous vena caval and pulmonary venous inflow occurs against closed, upwardly bulging AV valves throughout systole. The upstroke of the *v* wave (which correlates with atrial filling) follows the QRS complex on a simultaneously recorded ECG. The crest of the *v* wave coincides with opening of the atrioventricular valves. The downstroke, termed the *y descent,* correlates with atrial emptying during the passive filling phase of ventricular diastole.

The a wave is diastolic in timing because it is produced by atrial contraction at the end of ventricular diastole. *The v wave is a systolic event* because it is inscribed as the atria fill during ventricular systole.

However, the *a* wave may not always be present and the *c* waves may not be clearly inscribed. For example, atrial contraction must be present for production of an *a* wave. In patients in atrial fibrillation or flutter, the *a* waves are replaced by continuous fibrillatory or flutter waves that are variably or regularly punctuated by *c* and *v* waves. The sensitivity of the pressure monitoring system also affects the visibility of all components of the atrial waveform. For example, the *c* wave is rarely visible in a pulmonary artery wedge pressure (PWP)

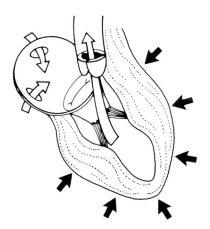

FIGURE 4-12 Rapid and slowed ventricular ejection.

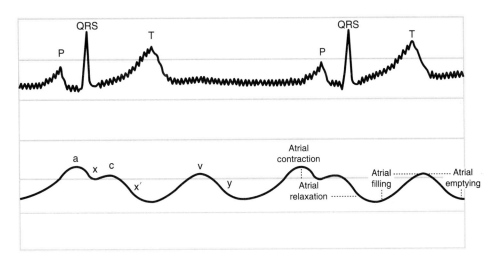

FIGURE 4-13 Components of the atrial pressure waveform correlated with phases of the cardiac cycle.

tracing. The detail of this small wave is attenuated during retrograde transmission through the pulmonary vasculature. The fidelity of bedside monitoring systems is usually inadequate to clearly reproduce it.

Accurate identification of *a* and *v* waves from bedside tracings requires that the atrial waveform be recorded with a simultaneously obtained ECG strip. It is difficult to distinguish *a* waves from *v* waves for two reasons: (1) The *c* wave (which helps identify the *a* wave) may not be clearly inscribed, and (2) both waves are nearly identical in amplitude and shape. If the patient has a slow to normal heart rate, identification of *a* and *v* waves may be possible without a simultaneously recorded ECG strip because the waves are coupled and have noticeable pauses between beats. In such patients, the *a* wave is easily identified as the first wave and *v* as the second wave. However, critically ill and injured patients typically have rapid heart rates. In patients with tachycardia, the cardiac cycles may be so close together that the waves appear to run in continuous succession.

The electrocardiographic components (PQRST sequence) of the cardiac cycle provide a landmark by which *a* and *v* waves may be identified. Just as flicking a light switch to the on position precedes illumination of the light bulb, an electrical stimulus (electrical depolarization of the atrial and ventricular myocardium) precedes mechanical contraction of the atrial and ventricular chambers. The P wave (electrical stimulation of the atria) precedes the *a* wave (the pressure wave produced by atrial contraction). Similarly, depolarization of the ventricles (inscribed on the ECG as the QRS complex) precedes contraction (noted on the pressure tracing as the *v* wave). Increased length of the fluid-filled connecting tubing proportionately increases separation of the P wave from the recorded *a* wave and QRS complex from the recorded *v* wave. This is because the pressure changes within the atrial chambers must transverse a greater distance before striking the transducer diaphragm.

Generally, identification of atrial *a* and *v* waves may be impossible in hospitals or specific intensive care units where the available monitoring equipment does not provide a means of obtaining a simultaneously recorded ECG strip with the atrial waveform.

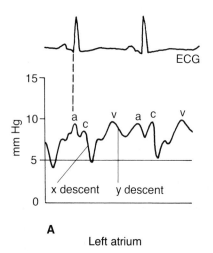

A Left atrium

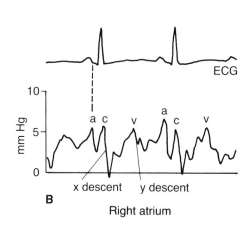

B Right atrium

FIGURE 4-14 Atrial pressure waveform. **A,** Left. **B,** Right. The mechanical events of the cardiac cycle as represented by the pressure waveforms follow the recorded electrical events represented by the ECG. In the recorded atrial pressure tracing, the *a* wave, which relates to atrial contraction, immediately follows atrial depolarization as represented by the P wave. Upward bulging of the AV valves during early ventricular systole produces a *c* wave, which may be seen immediately following the QRS complex (ventricular depolarization). The *v* wave occurs during ventricular systole and represents filling of the atrial chambers. Inscription of the *v* wave follows electrical systole as represented by the QRS complex. The apparent relationship between the electrical and mechanical events may be prolonged if, for example, long tubing connects the transducer to the catheter sensing tip or if there is distance between the catheter sensing tip and the cardiac chamber in which pressure is being measured. For example, the *a* wave usually occurs within the QRS complex, with the left atrial waveform. The catheter tip (in the pulmonary artery) is a distance from the left atrium. In comparison, the right atrial *a* wave usually occurs within the PR interval, with the right atrial waveform. The pressure-sensing port is within the right atrium *(broken lines).*

Ventricular Pressure Waveform

The pressure waveform of both ventricles has the same form but vastly different amplitudes (Figures 4-15 and 4-16).

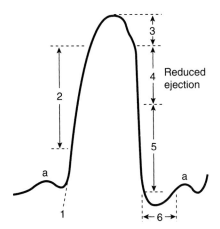

FIGURE 4-15 Components of the ventricular pressure waveform correlated with phases of the cardiac cycle. *a,* atrial contraction (active ventricular filling); *1,* end-diastolic pressure; *2,* isovolumetric contraction; *3,* rapid ejection; *4,* reduced ejection; *5,* protodiastole plus isovolumetric relaxation; *6,* passive filling.

The ventricles begin to contract approximately 6 ms (one and one-half little squares) following the QRS on the simultaneously recorded ECG. This recorded time interval is prolonged if excessive connecting tubing increases the distance from the pressure transducer to the in situ catheter tip and hemodynamic event. The smooth, nearly vertical upstroke coincides with isovolumic contraction and the associated abrupt intraventricular pressure rise to the systolic peak. Opening of the semilunar valves cannot be identified on the recorded waveform. The peak systolic pressure is approximately five times greater for the left ventricle than for the right. At the point of onset of the phase of rapid ventricular ejection, the pressure wave turns downward and forms a brief shelf. It then pursues a more vertical course that is related to the phases of reduced rate of ejection and the isovolumic relaxation phase of diastole. The lowest pressure recorded on the ventricular pressure waveform correlates in time with the onset of passive ventricular filling. Atrial contraction then occurs, and the recorded *a* wave produces a brief increase in pressure. The interval following the *a* wave (immediately before the next systolic upstroke) correlates with ventricular end-diastolic pressure.

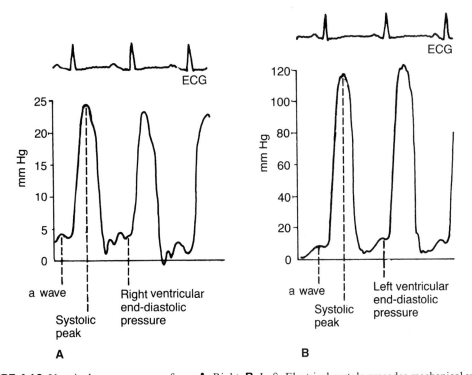

FIGURE 4-16 Ventricular pressure waveform. **A,** Right. **B,** Left. Electrical systole precedes mechanical ventricular systole. The ventricular pressure waveform is usually seen in an area relating to the QT interval of the ECG. However, excessive tubing length may widen the recorded relationship.

Arterial Pressure Waveform
(see also Chapter 7)

The pulmonary arterial and aortic waveforms are similar in contour. The peak systolic pressure for the aorta, however, is approximately five times that of the pulmonary artery (Figure 4-17).

The arterial pressure waveform begins with the opening of the semilunar valves and immediately ascends to the systolic peak. The slope and rate of rise of the upstroke (termed the *inotropic component*) are related to the velocity of blood ejected from the ventricle. The upstroke is steep and rapid as a result of the rapid ejection of a relatively large stroke volume into the arterial circulation in patients with hyperdynamic circulations or decreased systemic vascular resistance secondary to anemia, fever, hyperthyroidism, or mild to moderate aortic regurgitation. The upstroke is slowed and sloped in those with obstruction to ventricular outflow, such as patients with aortic stenosis or those with decreased velocity of ventricular ejection due to systolic (contractile) failure.

Following ejection, pressure in the pulmonary and systemic arteries falls as blood runs through the capillaries and veins. This finding correlates with the descent of the arterial waveform. When intraventricular pressures fall below pressures in the great arteries, the semilunar valves snap shut and a slight distortion in the waveform, the dicrotic notch, is inscribed. This is followed by continued runoff of blood and a steady decrease in pressure that is terminated by the next systole.

The form and numeric values of the systemic arterial pressure waves undergo changes depending on the anatomic site of pressure measurement. The farther the sampling site is from the heart, the higher will be the systolic pressure measurement (10 mm Hg radial artery and 30 mm Hg dorsalis pedis artery). However, the diastolic pressure is approximately 10 mm Hg lower, so the mean arterial pressure remains fairly constant. This change may be observed in patients with intraarterial catheters because differing sampling sites may be used simultaneously, such as a central aortic site (i.e., intraaortic balloon pump catheter that is pressure transduced) and a radial artery site. Also, with intraarterial catheter placement in the distal arteries, the waveform becomes narrower and has a steeper rise, and the dicrotic notch is delayed and lower (Figure 4-18). However, pressure differences are usually not noted by indirect blood pressure measurement techniques because the cuff almost invariably is placed over the brachial artery.

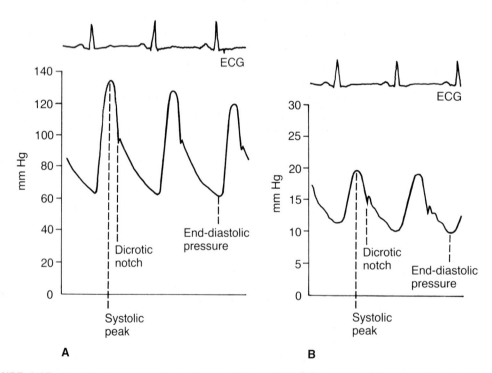

FIGURE 4-17 Arterial pressure waveform. The systolic rise in arterial pressure follows ventricular depolarization represented by the QRS complex. **A,** Aortic pressure. **B,** Pulmonary artery pressure.

FACTORS AFFECTING CARDIAC OUTPUT

Cardiac output is the amount of blood ejected by the heart measured in liters per minute. It is the product of stroke volume (the amount of blood ejected by the heart per beat) and heart rate. This is expressed in Figure 4-19.

Factors that determine stroke volume and cardiac output are also shown in Figure 4-19.

Preload, afterload, myocardial contractility, muscular synchrony, and heart rate, as they relate to cardiac output, are discussed at length in Chapters 10 and 20.

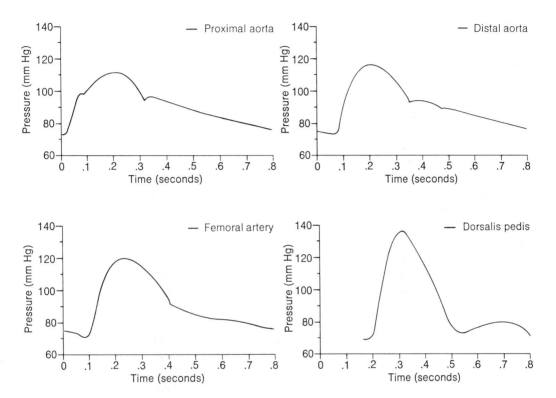

FIGURE 4-18 Contour of the arterial pressure waveform relative to the site used for pressure measurement. Systolic values increase while diastolic values decrease as the pulse moves away from the heart. Note that the mean arterial pressure tends to remain nearly constant (see also Figure 4-24). (From Wilson RF: Cardiovascular physiology. In *Critical care manual,* Philadelphia, 1992, Davis.)

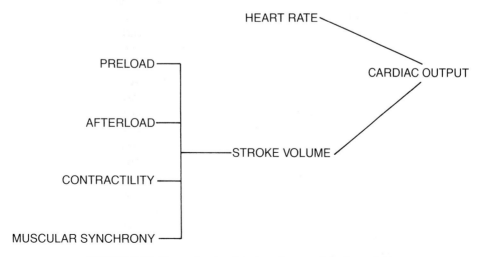

FIGURE 4-19 Determinants of stroke volume and cardiac output.

CORONARY CIRCULATION

Coronary Anatomy

The anatomy of the coronary circulation is illustrated in Figure 4-20. The main coronary arteries extend over the epicardial surface of the heart and surround it like a crown. It is from these arteries and their small penetrating branches that the heart receives all of its blood supply. Only a tissue paper–thin area of the endocardium can obtain oxygen from blood within the cardiac chambers. The two coronary arteries arise from the region of the sinus of Valsalva at the level of the free edges of the aortic valve cusps.

The *right coronary artery (RCA)* originates behind the right aortic valve cusp and runs in a groove between the right atrium and ventricle until it reaches the crux (top of the ventricular septum posteriorly). Here it becomes the

posterior descending branch that runs parallel to the ventricular septum. In 55% to 60% of people, the RCA supplies blood to the sinus node. In 85% to 90% of people, the right coronary artery sends a penetrating branch (at the level of the crux) to nourish the AV node and the initial portion of the bundle of His. The penetrating branches of the posterior descending branch of the RCA also perfuse the posterior one third of the ventricular septum.

The *left main coronary artery* originates in a small opening behind the left aortic valve cusp. It averages approximately 14 mm in length and usually divides into two main branches. The *left anterior descending (LAD) branch* runs anteriorly and downward, parallel to the ventricular septum and, in its course, forms two curves. The first curve is around the base of the pulmonary artery; the second curve is around the apex, where it then ascends 2 to

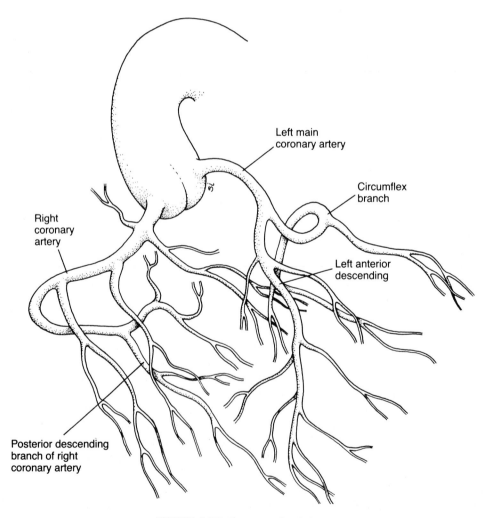

Left main
coronary artery

Circumflex
branch

Right
coronary
artery

Left anterior
descending

Posterior descending
branch of right
coronary artery

FIGURE 4-20 Coronary circulation.

5 cm in the posterior intraventricular groove. The LAD sends some branches to the free wall of the right ventricle (which also usually has anastomosis with branches of the right coronary artery). Some branches also course over the free wall of the left ventricle and include branches to the anterior papillary muscle. Several branches also penetrate the septum to nourish the anterior two thirds of the septum. These branches perfuse conduction tissue such as the bundle of His and right and left bundle branches. In some people, a septal branch also supplies the anterior papillary muscle of the right ventricle.

The *circumflex branch* runs in a groove between the left atrium and ventricle and then descends on the posterior surface of the left ventricle to supply blood to the lateral and posterior portions of the left ventricle. In approximately 8% to 10% of people, it reaches the crux and sends a penetrating branch to the AV node. A *sinus nodal branch* is provided by the circumflex artery in approximately 40% to 45% of people. This discussion describes the most commonly encountered distribution of coronary arteries.

The epicardial coronary arteries and their major branches contribute only approximately 5% to total coronary vascular resistance; no metabolic exchanges occur at these larger-diameter vessels. The majority of coronary vascular resistance is imposed by the very small diameter, penetrating, intramural coronary arterioles that supply oxygen and nutrients to the myocardium.

Individual Variability in Coronary Anatomy

Coronary anatomy varies considerably among people in size, number, and position of arteries. Some people have abundant coronary vessels. For example, the left main coronary artery may send a lavish shower of vessels over the anterolateral surface of the heart. Other people are less fortunate in number or position of vessels and may, for example, have one point of origin to a coronary circulation that perfuses the entire heart. The anatomic distribution of the coronary circulation has no physiologic implications for people with a normal heart and healthy coronary arteries but may become of major significance in the outcome of patients with coronary artery or cardiac disease. For example, sudden thrombotic occlusion or spasm at the origin of a coronary artery that perfuses the majority of the heart is frequently fatal.

The terms *right* or *left dominant circulation* are commonly used but do not imply which circulation supplies the most blood to the heart. The left coronary circulation always provides flow to the greatest portion of the myocardium. The coronary circulation, which perfuses the AV node and supplies the posterior descending artery, is designated as the dominant circulation. A right dominant circulation is present in more than 80% of the population; therefore the right coronary circulation reaches the crux and perfuses the AV node and the inferior aspect of the interventricular septum via the posterior descending branch. A *left dominant circulation* is present in less than 20% of people; therefore the circumflex artery reaches the crux and supplies the posterolateral left ventricular, posterior descending, and AV nodal arteries. In approximately 25% of people in whom both the right coronary and circumflex arteries reach the crux and supply a posterior descending branch, the term *balanced circulation* is appropriate.

FACTORS THAT DETERMINE CORONARY BLOOD FLOW

In health, metabolic and physical factors jointly contribute to regulating the adequacy of coronary blood flow. Disturbances in any factor that is typically associated with disease may profoundly affect myocardial blood flow.

Metabolic Determinants of Coronary Blood Flow

The volume of coronary blood flow is determined primarily by the diameter of the coronary arteries; vessel diameter, in turn, is *autoregulated* by the metabolic requirements of the myocardium. Whenever heart work and oxygen consumption increase, the coronary arteries dilate and coronary blood flow simultaneously increases. When heart work decreases, the coronary arteries narrow. The relationship between myocardial oxygen demand and coronary blood flow is linear. The demand-dependent rate of coronary blood flow ranges from 10 to approximately 600 ml/min/100 g of myocardial tissue.[8]

The coronary circulation is unique because it supplies an organ whose energy expenditure and oxygen consumption are consistently extremely high. Even at rest, the left ventricle extracts approximately 70% of the oxygen from coronary arterial blood. As a result, the normal oxygen content of blood in the coronary sinus is approximately 5 ml per 100 ml of blood, which corresponds to a Po_2 of approximately 20 mm Hg and a saturation of approximately 30% (normal mixed venous Po_2 40 mm Hg, saturation 75%).

The fact that the heart, even at rest, consumes tremendous amounts of oxygen and extracts most of the oxygen in the coronary arterial blood has two important physiologic implications.

The left ventricle is highly dependent on constant delivery of large volumes of oxygen for normal function. *There is no oxygen reserve for additional extraction in times of increased myocardial oxygen need.* Therefore the myocardium is highly flow dependent and normally receives very high flow volumes. Increased metabolic needs, such as occurs with physical or emotional stress, can be met only by increased coronary blood flow.

The term *autoregulation* refers to the inherent capacity of myocardial tissue to maintain constant blood flow proportionate to its need for oxygen and nutrients over a wide range of coronary perfusion pressures by regulating the diameter of the coronary arteries. In times of stress, such as exercise, the normal coronary circulation dilates to increase blood flow four to five times resting values. In health, autoregulation maintains coronary perfusion when mean aortic pressures are as low as 45 mm Hg and as high as 150 mm Hg. If coronary perfusions exceed or are less than these values, coronary blood flow becomes directly dependent on the perfusion pressure (i.e., increasing coronary perfusion pressure increases blood flow, and blood coronary blood flow decreases as perfusion pressures decrease). People with coronary artery disease have impaired autoregulatory mechanisms and may suffer myocardial ischemia with mean aortic pressures considerable higher than 45 to 55 mm Hg. For example, a patient with coronary artery disease and a history of hypertension may develop signs of myocardial ischemia with a mean arterial pressure of 90 mm Hg.

Locally increased carbon dioxide tensions or locally decreased myocardial oxygen tensions (which are associated with increased heart work or obstructive coronary lesions) seem to be the most potent stimuli to coronary vasodilation.

A number of vasoactive substances and physiologic stimuli are also important means by which myocardial blood supply is matched to oxygen demand. Table 4-2 lists these substances, their sources, and their effects on the coronary musculature.

The capacity of the coronary circulation to adapt blood flow to myocardial oxygen requirements is essential to maintain effective cardiac pumping function. *Myocardial contractility relates directly to oxygen availability and therefore to myocardial oxygen consumption.*

The term *coronary reserve* refers to the maximal capacity of the coronary circulation to dilate to increase blood flow to the myocardium. In people with normal coronary vessels, the maximal coronary capacity is a 400% to 500% increase in flow over resting values. Expanding atheromatous plaques, coronary artery constriction or spasm,

TABLE 4-2
Vasoactive Agents and Stimuli That Regulate Coronary Blood Flow in Normal Coronary Arteries

Vasoactive Substance	Source	Vascular Effect
Adenosine	Breakdown of adenosine triphosphate (ATP)	Coronary dilation
Angiotensin	Systemic circulation	Coronary constriction
Bradykinin	Vascular endothelium	Coronary dilation
Dopamine	Adrenergic nerve fibers	Coronary dilation
Endothelin-1*	Coronary endothelium	Coronary constriction
Epinephrine	Adrenal gland and sympathetic nerve fibers	Coronary constriction (elevated blood levels) or dilation (low blood levels)
Histamine	Mast cells and basophils	Coronary constriction (H_1 receptors) or dilation (H_2 receptors)
Magnesium (Mg^{++})	Plasma	Coronary dilator
Nitric oxide (NO)	Vascular endothelium	Coronary vasodilation
Norepinephrine	Adrenergic nerve fibers	Coronary dilation (beta effects) or constriction (alpha effects)
Prostacyclin	Vascular endothelium	Coronary dilation
Respiratory alkalosis	Inappropriate increased minute ventilation	Coronary constriction
Serotonin	Aggregating platelets	Coronary constriction
Thromboxane A_2	Vascular endothelium and platelets	Coronary constriction
Vasopressin	Posterior pituitary gland or intravenous administration	Coronary constriction
Vasoactive intestinal peptide (VIP)	Vagal and intrinsic nerve fibers of the heart	Coronary dilation

Reprinted from *Clinical Cardiology* (1999, vol 22, pp 775–776) with permission from Clinical Cardiology Publishing Company, Inc. and the authors, L. Feliciano and R. J. Henning.

*Endothelin-1 release is stimulated by thrombin, angiotensin II, epinephrine, vasopressin, and cytokines.

or coronary thrombus formation may seriously narrow the lumen of the coronary artery, thereby increasing the resistance to blood flow past the obstructed site. This process simultaneously decreases coronary reserve. In chronically affected people, the coronary reserve may be reduced to levels that render them chronically disabled.

Factors That Determine Myocardial Oxygen Consumption

The major determinants of myocardial oxygen consumption (MVO_2) are ventricular wall tension, myocardial contractility, and heart rate. All of these factors can be manipulated pharmacologically in an attempt to keep myocardial oxygen supply and demand balanced in patients prone to myocardial ischemia. Two minor determinants of myocardial oxygen consumption are electrical depolarization and maintenance of cellular activity; these cannot be therapeutically controlled.

Major Determinants of Myocardial Oxygen Consumption. **Ventricular Wall Tension.** Myocardial oxygen consumption increases proportionately with changes in ventricular wall tension. Wall tension, in turn, is determined by two factors:

1. *Pressure work of the heart.* Increases in afterload are met with linear increases in myocardial oxygen consumption.
2. *Ventricular size.* The ventricular muscle tension required to eject against any pressure load increases proportionately with the diameter of the heart. For example, if the cardiac diameter doubles due to heart failure, and all other variables of oxygen consumption are kept constant, myocardial oxygen consumption doubles.

Contractility—The Inotropic State of the Myocardium. The positive inotropic effects of stress hormones, such as adrenaline and norepinephrine, and the administration of positive inotropic drugs, such as digitalis, dopamine (Intropin), amrinone (Inocor), or calcium ions, increase the metabolic activity of the myocardium and result in a proportionate elevation in myocardial oxygen demand.

Heart Rate. The relationship of heart rate to myocardial oxygen consumption is straightforward. Increases in heart rate are met with proportionate increases in myocardial oxygen demand and consumption. Conversely, myocardial oxygen demand and consumption proportionately decrease with reductions in heart rate.

Minor Determinants of Oxygen Consumption. **Electrical Depolarization.** Excitation of the myocardium accounts for only 0.5% of total myocardial oxygen consumption.

Maintenance of Cellular Activity. Normal myocardial cellular metabolic activity, such as maintenance of the sodium-potassium pump, accounts for 10% to 15% of total myocardial oxygen consumption.

In a person with a healthy coronary circulation, increased demand is met with proportionate increased coronary blood flow and myocardial oxygen consumption. In people with severe coronary artery obstruction, compensatory autoregulatory mechanisms are no longer effective (because coronary dilation is maximized). Such patients are predisposed to myocardial ischemic episodes as a result of even minor stress or drug-induced increases in heart work and oxygen demand. In such patients, drug therapies (beta blockade, etc.) and measures to reduce physical and emotional stress are typically undertaken until definitive therapies (coronary angioplasty, surgical revascularization) are completed.

Physical Factors That Determine Coronary Blood Flow

Blood flow through the coronary circulation is determined primarily by (1) interplay of the pressure gradient across the coronary circulation during diastole and (2) the resistance to coronary blood flow. Resistance to blood flow, in turn, is affected by the diameter of the arteries, which in health is determined solely by autoregulation. However, in people with coronary artery disease, thrombus formation, plaque, and vascular spasm also affect resistance to blood flow.

Coronary perfusion for both ventricles is phasic because aortic pressure is phasic. However, aortic diastolic pressure is the primary determinant of left ventricular blood flow because almost all myocardial perfusion occurs during diastole. Systolic compression of the penetrating coronary artery branches by the thick, strongly contractile left ventricle progressively increases resistance to flow from epicardium to subendocardium. For this reason, the subendocardium (inner one third to one fourth of the ventricular wall) receives no blood flow during systole, whereas the epicardial layer experiences some systolic perfusion. The thinner-walled right ventricle develops less wall tension with systole. Therefore right ventricular penetrating branches undergo less systolic compression, and phasic changes in coronary blood flow are less marked.

In healthy people, the pressure that drives blood across both coronary circulations is approximately 90 to 100 mm Hg; this pressure delivers 90 to 180 ml of blood per minute through the coronary vessels.[8] However, *in people with severely diseased coronary arteries, a normal coronary perfusion pressure of 90 mm Hg may be inadequate to drive the required blood flow beyond the diseased coronary artery segments.* This explains why some chronically hypertensive patients who are effectively treated with antihypertensive drugs may suddenly develop angina when the blood pressure is "normalized." An episode of hypotension in these people may have disastrous ischemic consequences for the myocardium.

Because all blood vessels are somewhat distensible, increasing the pressure within the coronary lumina increases the diameter of the vessels and, as a result, reduces the resistance to blood flow. Although in healthy people coronary blood flow is maintained rather well over a wide range of perfusion pressures, there may be a coronary perfusion pressure below which tension caused by surrounding muscle would close intramyocardial vessels. In normal persons, this *critical closing pressure* is thought to be approximately 20 mm Hg and, when reached, blood flow stops completely.

Factors That May Diffusely or Locally Decrease Coronary Blood Flow

Several factors may occur singly or together to cause mild to profound reductions in coronary blood flow. These include physical obstruction of the coronary artery lumen, reduction of the coronary perfusion pressure, and elevation of the left ventricular end-diastolic pressures.

Physical obstruction or narrowing of the coronary artery lumen by spasm, atherosclerotic plaque, or thrombus formation may reduce coronary blood flow by increasing resistance to blood flow. However, the level of obstruction typically must be advanced before even stress-induced symptoms appear. For example, coronary artery obstruction reducing the lumen diameter by about 70% (equal to 90% cross-sectional area) is necessary to significantly limit the coronary flow required by extreme physical or emotional stress.[9] In affected patients, adequacy of coronary blood flow may be maintained at rest or during moderate activity despite advanced obstruction because compensatory dilation (autoregulatory effects) of the coronary arteries distal to the obstructive lesion helps decrease resistance to flow through the involved vessel.

If, however, compensatory dilation is maximized, further obstruction is met with inadequate coronary blood flow. Initially, the fixed, limited coronary flow may be inadequate to meet increased myocardial oxygen demands imposed by heavy exertion. Then, with progression of obstruction, myocardial ischemia may occur with lesser levels of exertion and then even at rest.

A decrease in aortic diastolic pressure or an increase in right atrial pressure, into which the coronary sinus drains, narrows the transcoronary pressure gradient and

therefore has the potential to reduce coronary blood flow. Patients with coronary artery disease are particularly vulnerable to coronary hypoperfusion even with relatively mild hypotension or increase in right atrial pressure (see Figure 20-3).

Elevated left ventricular end-diastolic pressures also may decrease flow through the coronary microcirculation that drains into the left ventricular chamber (see Figure 20-3).

Overall, the individual patient's *margin of safety* (as it relates to abnormalities in the aforementioned variables) becomes progressively narrower and the individual patient's *critical closing pressure* becomes progressively higher, depending on the severity of the patient's coronary artery disease.

Other Coronary Vasoactive Stimuli

Although coronary blood flow is autoregulated primarily by the moment-to-moment oxygen demands of the myocardium, coronary autoregulation may be pharmacologically or metabolically overridden.

In people with coronary artery disease, the response to pharmacologic or metabolic stimuli is variable. For example, endogenous or exogenous norepinephrine and vasopressin produce direct coronary vasoconstriction, but, in people with a normal heart, these catecholamines indirectly produce coronary vasodilation because of the increased oxygen demand resulting from increases in heart rate and ventricular contractility. However, the vasoconstrictor effects of these hormones may be potentiated in areas of coronary atherosclerosis and may produce a net reduction in coronary blood flow. Acetylcholine normally causes coronary dilation, but it may produce paradoxic vasoconstriction in patients with diseased coronary arteries.

Thromboxane A_2, a prostaglandin released from activated platelets, is a potent coronary vasoconstrictor. If platelets aggregate over a diseased coronary artery segment, the local release of thromboxane A_2 results in localized vasoconstriction that increases intraluminal obstruction. Also, studies have found that although nitric oxide is normally a coronary vasodilator at rest and during stress, when the coronary vascular endothelium becomes atherosclerotic, it becomes dysfunctional and nitric oxide production is significantly reduced and rate of breakdown is increased.[10,11] Consequently, coronary blood flow does not appropriately increase during stress, coronary reserve is reduced, and the patient is at risk of myocardial ischemia. Hypertension also results in coronary endothelial dysfunction and decreased availability of nitric oxide.[12] Ergonovine, a nonspecific vasoconstrictor, has been used diagnostically to induce coronary artery spasm in patients with Prinzmetal's (variant) angina.

However, the response to the drug in patients with normal coronary artery reactivity is minimal.

It has been shown that a sympathetic nervous system–mediated reflex stimulated by ice applied to the skin (so-called cold pressor test) results in significant increases in coronary vascular resistance in patients with coronary artery disease, but in normal people this response is negligible. In some patients, there seems to be a relationship between emotional stress and coronary artery spasm. In addition, it has been demonstrated that respiratory alkalosis due to hyperventilation variably but significantly reduces coronary blood flow and may reduce the angina threshold in susceptible people.[13-15] The myocardial hypoxic insult may be augmented because alkalemia increases bonding of oxygen to hemoglobin (SO_2). The finding that monitored coronary sinus blood oxygen tension (PO_2) is decreased in hyperventilating people validates the alkalemic vasoconstrictor hypothesis.

These potential coronary vasoconstrictor stimuli have several important implications as they relate to patient care. The first is that in mechanically ventilated patients, blood gases and serum pH should be carefully monitored and mechanical ventilator settings adjusted to avoid respiratory alkalosis (particularly in patients with known coronary artery disease). Intubated, paralyzed, or heavily sedated patients are generally unable to notify staff members of the onset of anginal pain if it develops. Furthermore, the ECG monitoring leads may not be oriented to the acutely ischemic area and ST-T wave changes may go undetected. Consequently, the inadvertently induced myocardial ischemic episode may be prolonged and clinically undetected.

The second important implication is that cold stimuli and emotional stress should be avoided whenever possible in patients with coronary artery disease, as should the use of preparations such as ergotamine drugs that are commonly used to treat migraine headache. In addition, when norepinephrine or vasopressin is absolutely indicated in patients with coronary artery disease, the drug should be carefully titrated to achieve a beneficial clinical response without inducing myocardial ischemia.

CIRCUIT (VASCULAR SYSTEM)

Blood flow through the systemic and pulmonary circulations depends on the maintenance of an adequate force within the circulation that drives flow. The distribution of blood flow through the systemic circulation is determined by regional differences in resistance to blood flow—mediated by changes in the diameter of the precapillary arterioles.

Pressure Dynamic (Force) That Drives Blood Flow Through the Systemic and Pulmonary Circulations

The systemic vascular circuit is the conduit that carries blood to and from the cardiopulmonary unit and body tissues. The circuit is composed of arteries, capillaries, and veins. The pulmonary vascular circuit is the conduit that transports blood from the right ventricle to the left atrium. This circuit also is composed of arteries, capillaries, and veins. Resting flow rates through both circulations in resting adults are about 5 to 8 L/min.

Factors Determining Rate and Volume of Blood Flow

The rate and volume of blood flow are determined by two physical factors—the pressure gradient between both ends of each circulation and the resistance to flow through each circulation.

Inflow versus Outflow Pressure Gradient. Blood flow through either circulation can occur only if there is a pressure gradient (difference) between the two ends of the circulation. In the systemic circulation, mean central aortic pressure is approximately 90 mm Hg, whereas central venous pressure is approximately 0 mm Hg. This difference produces a pressure gradient of 90 mm Hg from the central arteries to the central veins. In the pulmonary circulation, mean pulmonary artery pressure is approximately 15 mm Hg and pulmonary venous pressure is approximately 7 mm Hg. This difference produces a pressure gradient of approximately 8 mm Hg across the pulmonary circulation. *These pressure gradients are the force that drives blood through the two circulations.* The rate of flow is partly determined by the magnitude of the pressure gradient between the beginning and end of the vascular bed, not by an absolute inflow or outflow pressure (Figures 4-21 and 4-22).

The pressure gradient across both circulations can be determined with measurements obtained with an intraarterial monitoring system (mean arterial pressure) and a pulmonary artery catheter (right atrial pressure, mean pulmonary artery pressure, and pulmonary artery wedge pressure).

Resistance to Blood Flow. As blood flows through a circulation, several physical factors contribute to resistance or opposition to flow. These include viscosity of the blood, length of the vascular bed, and diameter of the blood vessel.

Viscosity of the Blood. Thick fluid is more resistant to flow than thin fluid. Blood is a viscous fluid, and the

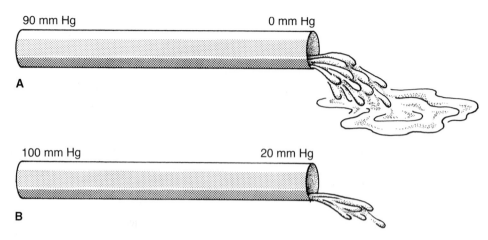

FIGURE 4-21 Rate of blood flow. **A,** A pressure gradient of 90 mm Hg drives fluid through the tube. **B,** Despite a 10 mm Hg increase in pressure at the beginning of the tube, fluid flow rates will be decreased because pressure at the end of the tube is increased to 20 mm Hg. This decreases the pressure gradient, or fluid driving force, to 80 mm Hg.

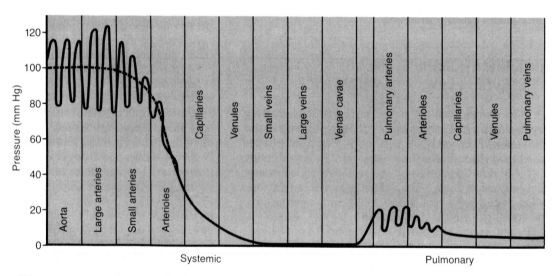

FIGURE 4-22 Blood pressures in the different portions of the systemic and pulmonary circulations. (From Guyton A: *Textbook of medical physiology,* ed 10, Philadelphia, 2000, W.B. Saunders.)

viscous drag of blood in the vasculature contributes significantly to systemic and pulmonary vascular resistance. As the hematocrit value decreases, blood viscosity and resistance to flow decrease, and as the hematocrit increases, blood viscosity and resistance to flow increase. For example, when the hematocrit value is below 40%, vascular resistance decreases by approximately 0.5% for each 1% drop in hematocrit. On the other hand, for hematocrit values greater than 40%, increases in resistance per unit change of hematocrit are much greater (approximately 4% for each 1% of hematocrit change). This becomes clinically significant when the hematocrit exceeds 55% (poly-cythemia or overtransfusion), particularly if the patient has a failing heart. The hematocrit and consequently blood viscosity usually remain constant; therefore this factor is not taken into account when clinically calculating resistance to blood flow.

Length of the Vascular Bed. As the length of a vascular bed increases, flow rates decrease because of the greater friction imposed by the greater length of the vessel walls. The length of either circulation does not change once adult growth has been reached; therefore this factor is not considered when calculating vascular resistance.

Blood Vessel Diameter. The diameter of blood vessels is in a state of constant flux. Vessel diameter profoundly affects resistance to blood flow. The rate of blood flow through a vessel decreases in direct proportion to the fourth power of its diameter. For example, if the diameter is decreased to one half by vasoconstriction, resistance to blood flow is increased 16 times. Therefore *the diameter of the vascular lumen is the most important factor in determining vascular resistance.* The strongly muscled arterioles and precapillary sphincters are the principal sites of changes in vessel diameter. Consequently, they determine resistance and distribution of blood flow and are sometimes referred to as the *resistance vessels.*

Vascular resistance cannot be measured directly; however, calculations of both pulmonary and systemic vascular resistance are used clinically to assess the patient's need for vasodilator or vasoconstrictor therapy (see Chapter 10).

Components of the Vascular Circuit

The vascular system is divided into component parts based on the direction of blood flow relative to the heart, as well as the physical characteristics of each vascular bed. The components of the vascular system include the arteries, capillaries, and veins. Of the total blood volume within the body, approximately 7% is in the heart, 9% is in the pulmonary circulation, 13% is within the arteries, 7% is within the arterioles and systemic capillaries, and 65% to 70% is in the systemic veins and venules.

The anatomic and physiologic characteristics of the systemic and pulmonary vasculature are quite different. The discussion of the vascular circuit is related to that of the systemic circulation (see Chapter 2 for discussion of the pulmonary circulation).

Systemic Arteries

Arteries are vessels that carry blood *away* from the heart. Large arteries branch off the aorta and progressively divide, becoming smaller and smaller in diameter. The small arteries branch into arterioles, which have a strong muscular wall and are the major area of resistance in the systemic circulation. The arterioles divide into metarterioles before merging with the capillary bed. At the level of the metarterioles, a smooth muscle fiber, known as the precapillary sphincter, further regulates regional flow to body tissue.

Arteriolar and metarteriole tone is adjusted by local and systemic chemical, physical, and neural factors. However, local tissue oxygen need is the primary determinant of arteriolar tone; this need profoundly affects capillary blood flow (autoregulation). For example, decreased tissue oxygen tension results in arteriolar dilation (which decreases resistance to flow) and increased capillary blood flow; arteriolar constriction (which increases resistance to flow) results in decreased capillary blood flow.

Overall, the distribution of cardiac output through the various organ systems is controlled chiefly by changes in arteriolar tone. The diameter of the precapillary vessels and the volume of blood flow to any organ system at any point in time are determined primarily by local metabolic need. For example, following a meal, the precapillary sphincters of the abdominal viscera dilate, thereby decreasing resistance to flow and increasing blood flow to the metabolically active digestive tract. At the same time, the precapillary sphincters of skeletal muscle constrict and shunt blood away from the resting, nonmetabolically active musculoskeletal system. There is not enough blood in the cardiovascular system to fill all blood vessels at any single moment. Therefore, by regionally constricting or dilating, the systemic arterioles determine how cardiac output will be distributed.

In summary, the arterial bed is a high-pressure, low-volume, high-resistance portion of the circulation with the purpose of delivering oxygenated blood in required amounts to the capillary network.

Arterial Pressure. Arterial pressure is a measure of the pressure, expressed in millimeters of mercury (mm Hg), exerted by blood per unit area on the arterial wall. This pressure is the same at all points at the same vertical level; the pressure is affected by the influence of gravity on hydrostatic pressure. Hydrostatic pressure results from the weight of blood within the column of the vascular structures and progressively increases downward from heart level and progressively decreases above heart level (Figure 4-23).

To eliminate the influence of gravity on hydrostatic pressure and obtain accurate blood pressure measurements, the limb (usually the arm) used to obtain the blood pressure reading should be supported at heart level. Falsely high blood pressure measurements are obtained when a patient's limb is held in a dependent position, and falsely low measurements are obtained when the limb is held above heart level.

How the Systemic Arterial Pressure Is Controlled. Regulating mechanisms adjust blood pressure by influencing vascular tone and cardiac output over widely varying blood flow requirements determined by body position, physical activity, or emotion. For example, the blood pressure required to meet the flow and oxygen requirements of a stressed person are considerably greater than those of a sleeping person.

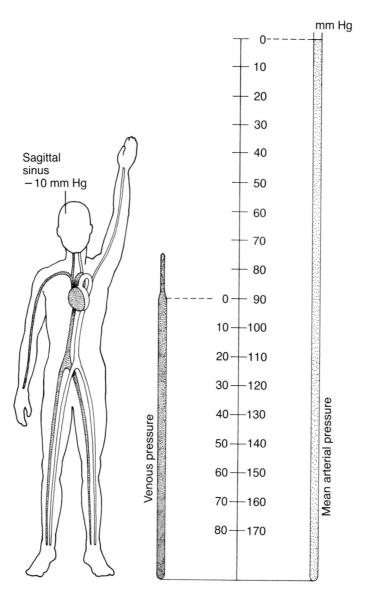

FIGURE 4-23 Effect of hydrostatic pressure on arterial and venous pressure. In the *upright* position, the mean arterial and venous pressures progressively increase from heart level to ankle. With the arm held vertically above the head, the arterial pressure progressively drops in the arm held above heart level. The venous pressure is 0 mm Hg at heart level and becomes progressively more negative in the vascular structures above that level.

Overall, the importance of blood pressure control is that it maintains an adequate and a suitable pressure to drive blood to all areas of the body, despite changes in position and local or systemic tissue oxygen requirements. Generally, a mean arterial pressure of 90 to 100 mm Hg is required to drive blood up the vertical vascular structures of an upright human and to adequately perfuse the structures of the head and neck.

Blood pressure is regulated by arterial baroreceptors, chemoreceptors, and pathways from the central nervous system. These regulatory mechanisms are very potent; they begin to act within seconds of postural or other physiologic changes.

Arterial Baroreceptors. Baroreceptors (also termed *pressoreceptors*) are multiple branching nerve endings located within the walls of the arteries. Baroreceptors are immediately responsive to pressure changes on the vessel wall in which they lie, and therefore they serve as sensors that respond rapidly to changes in blood pressure.

Baroreceptors are present at many arterial sites within the thoracic and neck regions, but they are particularly abundant at the bifurcation of the common carotid artery (carotid sinus) and at the wall of the aortic arch. The nerve endings from the baroreceptors terminate in the cardiovascular regulatory centers in the medulla. An *increase in blood pressure* raises tension on the arterial wall. This increase, in turn, accelerates the rate of discharge from the baroreceptors. These stimuli then enter the medulla, which sends excitatory signals to the vagus nerve. Vagal (parasympathetic) stimulation results in slowing of heart rate and dilation of veins and arteries throughout the systemic circulation. The net effect is a decrease in blood pressure. By a similar mechanism, *carotid sinus massage* produces a reflex slowing of the heart rate in a patient with supraventricular tachycardia.

A *decrease in blood pressure* reduces tension in the arterial walls and has a physiologic effect opposite that of hypertension. The sympathetic nervous system becomes excited by the medulla and increases heart rate and causes systemic vasoconstriction. These effects elevate the arterial pressure toward normal.

Arterial Chemoreceptors. The chemoreceptors are located in the same areas as the baroreceptors and are termed *carotid bodies* and *aortic bodies.* These cells are constantly sampling blood. The cells are extremely sensitive to changes in blood chemistry, such as oxygen lack (hypoxemia), carbon dioxide excess (hypercarbia), and hydrogen ion excess (acidemia). When the blood pressure falls below a critical level, available oxygen to the carotid and aortic bodies likewise falls. At the same time, carbon dioxide and hydrogen ion levels increase in the area of the chemoreceptors because they are not removed by the slow blood flow. Stimulation of the chemoreceptors, in turn, leads to excitation of the vasomotor centers of the brainstem. The systemic vasoconstriction and increased heart rate that result increase the blood pressure.

Pathways from Higher Centers in the Nervous System. Powerful, varied cardiovascular changes are immediately associated with rage, fear, pain, embarrassment, or any intense emotional experience. For example, at the onset of sudden, intense fear, the blood pressure may rise to twice normal levels, owing to selective sympathetic nervous system–mediated increases in arteriolar tone and heart rate. This alarm response provides an increased arterial pressure and cardiac output, which immediately supplies blood to all skeletal muscle so that the person may "fight" or "take flight" from danger, thus favoring short-term survival. However, in current industrialized societies, combat or fleeing from stressful situations is not behaviorally appropriate. Furthermore, today's stressful stimuli, such as work-related conflict, tend to be sustained, with no immediate resolution in situational outcome. Chronic activation of the stress response may predispose to cardiac arrhythmias, sudden cardiac death, hypertension, and other chronic diseases common to industrialized societies.

Blood Pressure Regulation by Hormones. A complex interrelationship of many circulating hormones affects the caliber of arterioles and consequently the blood pressure. Discovery of specific hormones and awareness of the interrelationship of these humoral agents continues to unfold. The interrelationship of these humoral agents is far more complex than previously imagined.

Locally released vasoconstrictor hormones include endothelin-1, serotonin, and thromboxane A_2, which are released from locally aggregated platelets. Local vasodilator hormones include nitric oxide (NO), prostacyclin, and kinins (bradykinin and kallidin). Circulating vasoconstrictor hormones include epinephrine, norepinephrine, angiotensin II, circulating sodium-potassium ATPase inhibitor, and neuropeptide Y. Circulating vasodilator hormones include epinephrine in skeletal muscle and liver, substance P, histamine, VIP, and ANP.

Intravascular fluid balance also affects blood pressure. Various hormones affect fluid balance by enhancing sodium or water retention (antidiuretic hormone, aldosterone).

Overall, blood pressure is not controlled by a single pressure-regulating mechanism but by many interrelated short- and long-term pressure control mechanisms.

Arterial Pressure Pulses. The arterial system receives the pulsatile jets of blood ejected by the heart. The physical arrangement and elastic properties of the arterial walls convey blood down the arterial channels with a minimal loss of pressure but with a damping of the intense pressure fluctuations by the time the blood reaches the capillaries.

At the onset of left ventricular ejection, blood enters the proximal aorta faster than it leaves the distal arterioles. This disparity in flow rates is the result of the inertia of blood in the long, tubular arteries that oppose acceleration. Consequently, blood ejected from the left ventricle accumulates in the first portion of the aorta and stretches and increases tension in the involved arterial walls (Figure 4-24). The increased wall tension in the proximal aorta forces blood into the next aortic segment, which, in turn, is stretched and develops tension. In this manner, a pressure pulse moves quickly down the aorta at a speed that is determined by the elasticity of the patient's arterial walls and blood pressure. The elasticity of the arterial system also facilitates blood flow during diastole.

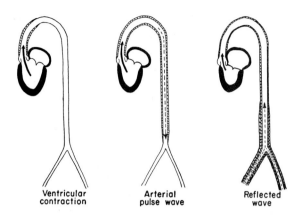

Ventricular   Arterial   Reflected
contraction   pulse wave   wave

FIGURE 4-24 Arterial pressure pulse is a wave of pressure that passes quickly along the arterial system. Blood suddenly ejected into the ascending aorta at the onset of systole has insufficient energy to overcome the inertia of the long columns of blood in the arteries. Consequently, blood tends to pile up and distend the ascending aorta, causing a sudden local increase in pressure. Blood is then forced into the next portion of the aorta, extending the region of distention and initiating a pulse of pressure that travels rapidly along the arteries toward the periphery. These waves of pressure, reflected retrogradely by smaller peripheral vessels, travel back toward the heart and become superimposed on the advancing pulse wave. This results in progressively higher systolic pressures and lower diastolic pressures progressively outward from the heart. The pressure pulse precedes blood flow because the pulse wave velocity is much faster than the velocity of blood flow (see also Figure 4-18). (From Rushmer RF: *Cardiovascular dynamics,* ed 4, Philadelphia, 1976, W.B. Saunders.)

Different components of the pulse wave are transmitted at different rates of speed. The initial more rapid waves of pressure reflect back from the distal arterioles toward the aortic root and become superimposed on the advancing slower pulse waves. This physical phenomenon results in progressively higher systolic pressures, slurring of the dicrotic notch, and lower diastolic pressures progressively down the arterial tree (see Figure 4-18).

Components of the Arterial Pressure (Systole and Diastole). Because of the pulsatile quality of blood flow through the arterial system, arterial pressure has two components. *Systolic pressure* represents the higher pressure and relates to contraction of the ventricles and ejection of a bolus of blood into the arterial system. *Diastolic pressure* is the lower pressure and is related to relaxation of the ventricles and runoff of blood through the vascular system.

The primary factors that influence systolic and diastolic pressure are cardiac output and systemic vascular resistance. However, heart rate, elasticity of the arteries, and intravascular volume also affect the absolute systolic and diastolic pressure measurements.

Vascular Resistance. The arterial diastolic pressure is primarily determined by systemic and pulmonary vascular resistance as influenced by arteriolar tone. Generalized systemic arteriolar constriction increases systemic diastolic pressure. Conversely, decreased systemic vascular resistance reduces diastolic pressure. The same holds true for the pulmonary circulation.

Heart Rate. The level to which the diastolic pressure falls is partially determined by the duration of diastole because the diastolic pressure continues to fall until the next systole. For example, if, in a normal person, the next systole is delayed for 4 seconds (this is equal to a heart rate of 15 beats per minute), the diastolic pressure falls to approximately 10 mm Hg.

Stroke Volume. As the volume of blood ejected with each heartbeat increases, the pulse pressure (difference between systolic and diastolic pressures) increases. As stroke volume falls, the pulse pressure becomes narrower. A narrow pulse pressure is a classic hemodynamic finding in patients in shock with low cardiac output (such as in cardiogenic and hypovolemic shock).

Elasticity of the Aorta and Its Large Tributaries. The walls of the arteries are far less distensible than those of the veins; however, arteries normally do yield somewhat to the bolus of blood delivered from the ventricle. The less elastic the arterial system receiving pulsatile flow, the greater the pulse pressure. With increasing age, the arterial system becomes progressively less distensible and accounts for the wide pulse pressure (pure systolic hypertension) that occurs in some elderly people.

Intravascular Volume. Because the systemic arteries are relatively noncompliant, circulatory volume increases are met with pressure increases. Clinically, fluid overload is usually associated with hypertension, whereas fluid depletion is associated with hypotension.

The *systolic pressure* is determined by a combination of all the aforementioned factors, including systemic vascular resistance, stroke volume, arterial system elasticity, and intravascular volume. All but elasticity can change acutely.

The way in which these factors are interrelated has important clinical implications. For example, a significant decrease in intravascular volume or stroke volume may occur in a patient without a significant decrease in systolic or diastolic pressure, because compensatory vasoconstriction may increase or maintain these pressures within a numerically acceptable range. However, there may be areas of hypoperfusion to organ systems (gut, skeletal muscle, kidneys) that are clinically undetectable.

Pulse pressure is the most important arterial pressure measurement in acute care settings because it reflects acute increases or decreases in stroke volume. If pulse pressure is narrowed by approximately 50%, it can be assumed that stroke volume is decreased by about that much.

In summary, the systolic pressure is determined chiefly by the volume of ventricular ejection in relation to distensibility of the arterial system; the diastolic pressure is determined by the vascular resistance and the duration of diastole as influenced by heart rate.

Mean Arterial Pressure. It is preferable to use mean arterial pressure rather than absolute systolic or diastolic pressure to assess the patient's circulatory status and titrate vasoactive drugs for the following reasons:

1. Mean arterial pressure represents the average pressure driving blood to the body tissue throughout one cardiac cycle.
2. Mean arterial pressure does not change relative to the sampling site. In the supine position, the arterial pressure measurement that is recorded from a site in the thoracic aorta (such as an intraaortic balloon pump catheter) may be 130/88 mm Hg, whereas the pressure measurement recorded from a catheter placed in the posterior tibial artery may be 170/70. The mean pressures, however, are nearly the same. Evaluation of a systolic pressure recorded from a posterior tibial artery (when there are no other sampling sites available) may lead the unwary clinician to believe that the patient has systolic hypertension when in fact the systolic pressure within the central circulation (sensed by the heart and brain) is normal.
3. Mean arterial pressure is less affected by motion artifact and poor fidelity of the fluid-filled monitoring system than the displayed systolic or diastolic pressure measurement.

Calculation of Mean Arterial Pressure. Because at normal heart rates diastole is approximately two thirds of the cardiac cycle, the mean arterial pressure is closer to the diastolic value. The mean arterial pressure may be manually calculated using the following formula:

$$\text{Mean arterial pressure (MAP)} = \frac{\text{systolic} + (\text{diastolic} \times 2)}{3}$$

For a blood pressure of 120/80:

$$\text{MAP 93 mm Hg} = \frac{120 + (80 \times 2)}{3}$$

The formula, however, assumes a resting heart rate of approximately 60 beats per minute during which diastole occupies two thirds of the cardiac cycle. The heart rate of normal humans is not fixed, and the duration of diastole fluctuates with minute-to-minute changes in heart rate. Critically ill and injured patients also typically have sinus tachycardia. At heart rates greater than 100 beats per minute, diastole may be less than one half the cardiac cycle, rendering this calculation grossly inaccurate.

Electrical monitoring systems calculate mean arterial pressure, taking into consideration the area under the arterial pressure curves (which shortens with tachyarrhythmias and lengthens with bradyarrhythmias). These systems precisely calculate and display mean arterial pressure in tandem with changes in the patient's heart rate. For this reason, *the digitally displayed MAP measurement is best used for hemodynamic evaluation of the patient.*

Capillaries

Capillaries are microscopic vessels that branch off the arterioles and ultimately connect with venules. Capillaries are a network of delicate vascular "lace." The total capillary surface area for an average adult is approximately equal to that of a football field (Figure 4-25).

Capillaries are composed of a single layer of endothelial cells that are selectively permeable to water, sugars, electrolytes, respiratory gases, and by-products of cellular metabolism. The extensive capillary network is the sole site of metabolic exchange between circulating blood and tissues. No exchange occurs in the larger blood vessels. Arteries and veins serve only as conduits.

Diffusion is the most important means by which substances are transferred between the intravascular and extravascular spaces. The slitlike gaps between capillary endothelial cells and the diffusion capabilities of endothelial cells themselves allow varying degrees of diffusion for different substances. For example, the capillary membrane is freely permeable to low-molecular-weight substances (e.g., urea, glucose, ions such as sodium and potassium, and water), but the membrane is relatively impermeable to high-molecular-weight substances (e.g., plasma proteins). The large plasma proteins are therefore restricted to and retained within the vascular space.

The permeability of the capillaries of each organ system is specific to the functional requirements of that organ. For example, the capillaries of the liver and kidney are highly permeable because large volumes of plasma water and solutes must filter through these organs. On the other hand, the capillaries of the lungs are relatively impermeable because the lungs must remain relatively dry and air filled to function normally. It is not clinically possible to measure capillary permeability, but assumptions can be made based on the progression and amount of edema

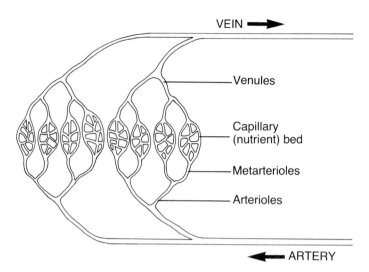

FIGURE 4-25 Capillary (nutrient) bed.

present in patients with conditions that threaten capillary integrity (massive trauma, extensive burn injury, sepsis).

The rate of diffusion is normally determined by the concentration gradient on either side of the capillary membrane. Water diffuses back and forth freely; it is estimated that 3000 ml of water exits and enters the capillary space each minute in a 70 kg adult. Although tremendous two-way movement of fluid occurs across the capillary membrane, the fluid volumes on either side of the vascular membrane must be maintained in delicate balance by an interplay of several forces.

Factors Governing Fluid Movement across the Capillary Membrane

Factors governing fluid movement across the capillary membrane determine intravascular and interstitial fluid volumes. These factors include capillary permeability and the opposite-directed forces of hydrostatic and oncotic pressures.

Hydrostatic Pressure. Hydrostatic pressure is that pressure exerted by a volume of fluid within a given space. The hydrostatic pressure within capillaries is positive and tends to force fluid out of the vascular space into the interstitium (tissue space). *Pulmonary capillary hydrostatic pressure* is estimated at the bedside with a flow-directed pulmonary artery catheter. Pulmonary artery diastolic pressure and wedge pressure closely correlate with the hydrostatic pressure within the pulmonary capillaries. *Interstitial hydrostatic pressures* are estimated to be subatmospheric and act as a vacuum that draws fluid out of the capillaries and into the tissue space. Interstitial hy-

drostatic pressure cannot be measured clinically. In fact, only assumptions of these pressures have been made from research work. It is also not possible to clinically measure systemic capillary hydrostatic pressure.

Oncotic Pressure. Oncotic pressure, also called *colloid osmotic pressure,* is the force generated by the attraction of protein macromolecules for water across the semipermeable capillary membrane. Colloid osmotic pressure is proportional to the number of protein molecules in solution on two sides of the capillary membrane. Fluid moves from the area of lower protein concentration to the area of higher protein concentration. Because capillaries are relatively impermeable to protein, plasma proteins are restricted to the vascular space. This results in a protein concentration gradient between the plasma and interstitium. The protein concentration gradient, in turn, helps maintain plasma water within the blood vessels and protects the body tissue from edema formation.

Plasma oncotic pressure attracts and retains fluid within the vascular space at a force of approximately 24 to 28 mm Hg in a healthy, ambulatory adult. Plasma oncotic pressure decreases in proportion to the severity of illness or prolonged bed rest.

Albumin contributes approximately 75% to the total plasma oncotic pressure; the remainder is contributed by the various globulin fractions, and a very small amount is contributed by fibrinogen. Plasma oncotic pressure is measured with a simple electronic device called an *oncometer.* However, few critical care units or hospital laboratories have the equipment necessary to do this measurement.

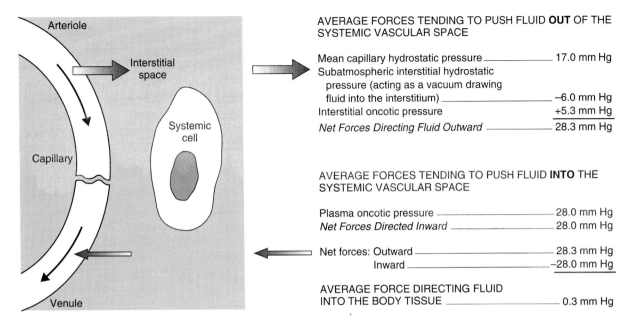

FIGURE 4-26 Systemic capillary fluid dynamics. (Adapted from Wilson RF: Cardiovascular physiology. In *Critical care manual,* ed 2, Philadelphia, 1992, Davis.)

Because albumin contributes nearly three fourths of plasma oncotic pressure, the serum albumin concentration provides a clinical estimate of the patient's plasma oncotic status. For example, a severely hypoalbuminemic patient can be assumed to have a significantly reduced plasma oncotic pressure. The effects are typically expressed clinically as generalized edema that correlates with increased movement of plasma water from the vascular to the tissue space. The threshold for the development of pulmonary edema also is lowered. For example, patients with chronic renal failure (albumin wasting in urine) usually develop acute pulmonary edema with PWPs of only 10 to 12 mm Hg. The PWP threshold level for developing pulmonary edema in a person with a normal plasma protein concentration is greater than 18 to 20 mm Hg.

Interstitial oncotic pressure draws fluid out of the vascular space into the interstitium. This force is the result of the osmotic attraction for water imposed by the small amounts of protein that do escape from plasma across the capillary membrane into the interstitium. Interstitial oncotic pressure cannot be measured clinically, and only preliminary assumptions have been made from related laboratory work.

Hydrostatic and oncotic forces differ in the systemic and pulmonary circulations because the tissue of the lung and the other tissues of the body require slightly different fluid dynamics for normal function. In both circulations, however, the amount of fluid moving out of the capillaries is at near equilibrium to the amount of fluid moving into the capillaries. This state of near equilibrium is produced by the cumulative effects of the opposite-directed forces of net hydrostatic and oncotic pressures at the arterial and venular ends of the capillary bed.

Systemic Capillary Fluid Dynamics

The hydrostatic pressures at either end of the systemic capillaries differ. At the arteriolar end of the capillaries, hydrostatic pressures are approximately 25 to 30 mm Hg, and at the venular end of the capillaries the hydrostatic pressures are about 15 mm Hg less (pressure gradient of approximately 10 to 15 mm Hg). This pressure difference across the capillary bed provides the impetus for blood flow. Because of the large cross-sectional area of the capillary bed, blood flow rates are slow enough to provide suitable time for the reciprocal diffusion of substances from blood vessels to cells. Figure 4-26 illustrates the normal average forces acting at the capillary membrane in a person with an average systemic capillary hydrostatic pressure of 17 mm Hg.

Pulmonary Capillary Fluid Dynamics

At the arteriolar end of the pulmonary capillaries, the hydrostatic pressures are approximately 11 mm Hg and at the venular end approximately 7 mm Hg. Therefore hydrostatic forces at either end of the pulmonary capillary favor a driving pressure through the capillary bed of approximately 4 mm Hg. The normal average forces acting at the pulmonary capillary membrane are illustrated in Figure 4-27.

Although the stated pressure measurements are not absolute and may vary within normal limits, neither systemic nor pulmonary capillary beds maintain a perfect balance between outward- and inward-directed forces. In both circulations there is slightly more fluid exiting than entering the vascular space via the capillaries. In the systemic circulation, this amounts to approximately 1.7 to 3.5 ml/min; in the pulmonary circulation, this amounts to an estimated 10 to 20 ml/hr fluid leak into the lung tissue. This watery extract of plasma that flows into the systemic and pulmonary tissue spaces is drawn up by the systemic and pulmonary lymphatics, which act as a skimming pump, and ultimately is returned to the central veins. In either circulation, if lymphatic drainage is impaired by scarring or compression, the involved area is prone to edema. For example, following radical mastectomy, impaired lymphatic drainage in the same-side arm is expressed as edema in that arm.

Veins

Veins are vessels that collect blood from the capillaries and return it to the heart. *Venules,* which are tiny veins that join with capillaries, merge into larger veins that finally merge into the large central veins (venae cavae). Because veins are subjected to lower pressures than arteries, vein walls are thinner and more distensible. These characteristics allow them to expand and accommodate large volumes of fluids with small changes in intravascular pressure.

At any moment, approximately 65% to 70% of circulating volume is in the veins. For this reason, the venous system is also known as the capacitance bed. The veins are capable of changing capacitance in response to neural, chemical, and hormonal factors. Through venoconstriction, the collective volume of the venous system shrinks by as much as 1 to 1.5 L, and more blood is returned to the central circulation. This, in turn, increases ventricular filling (preload) and pulmonary capillary hydrostatic pressure. Conditions that increase venous tone (decrease venous capacitance) are hypovolemia, acidemia, hypoxemia, hypothermia, and severe pain. Venodilator drugs such as nitroglycerin, sodium nitroprusside (Nipride), and furosemide (Lasix) may increase venous capacity by 1 to 2 L or more. Increased venous capacitance, in turn, decreases ventricular filling and pulmonary capillary hydrostatic pressure. By decreasing the rate and volume of fluid movement into the lungs, this effect is physiologically beneficial in patients with cardiogenic pulmonary edema.

Venous pressures are low, but, like arterial pressures, they are strongly influenced by gravity. That is, venous

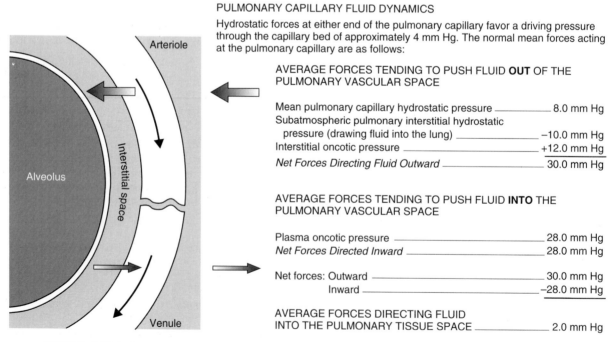

PULMONARY CAPILLARY FLUID DYNAMICS

Hydrostatic forces at either end of the pulmonary capillary favor a driving pressure through the capillary bed of approximately 4 mm Hg. The normal mean forces acting at the pulmonary capillary are as follows:

AVERAGE FORCES TENDING TO PUSH FLUID **OUT** OF THE PULMONARY VASCULAR SPACE

Mean pulmonary capillary hydrostatic pressure	8.0 mm Hg
Subatmospheric pulmonary interstitial hydrostatic pressure (drawing fluid into the lung)	−10.0 mm Hg
Interstitial oncotic pressure	+12.0 mm Hg
Net Forces Directing Fluid Outward	30.0 mm Hg

AVERAGE FORCES TENDING TO PUSH FLUID **INTO** THE PULMONARY VASCULAR SPACE

Plasma oncotic pressure	28.0 mm Hg
Net Forces Directed Inward	28.0 mm Hg
Net forces: Outward	30.0 mm Hg
Inward	−28.0 mm Hg

AVERAGE FORCES DIRECTING FLUID INTO THE PULMONARY TISSUE SPACE _____ 2.0 mm Hg

FIGURE 4-27 Pulmonary capillary fluid dynamics. (Adapted from Wilson RF: Cardiovascular physiology. In *Critical care manual,* ed 2, Philadelphia, 1992, Davis.)

pressure is the same at all points of the same vertical level but changes with height. For example, venous pressures at the feet in an *upright* person may be as high as 90 mm Hg, but venous pressures in the dural sinuses of the head may be in the negative range (see Figure 4-23).

The supine pressure measurement obtained at heart level from the superior vena cava or right atrium is termed *central venous pressure (CVP),* and it averages approximately 0 to 8 mm Hg. Pressure in the peripheral veins is usually 4 to 9 mm Hg higher than central venous pressure. Central venous pressure is influenced by the heart's ability to pump out the blood returned to it, by the volume of venous return (which relates to circulating volume), and by systemic vascular tone. Venous return is augmented by the milking action of the contracting skeletal muscles on veins in the legs, as well as alterations in intrathoracic pressure associated with breathing (the intrathoracic pump mechanism).

In summary, the systemic venous bed is a low-pressure, high-volume, low-resistance system that functions to return deoxygenated blood from the tissues of the body back to the cardiopulmonary unit, to provide a reservoir for the circulation, and to regulate the amount of blood returning to the heart at any moment in time.

The pulmonary and cardiovascular systems are discussed separately in Chapters 2 and 4, although functionally and anatomically the two systems are joined to serve the single life-giving purpose—moment-to-moment oxygenation and removal of metabolic waste from metabolizing tissue over a broad range of changing metabolic activity. The complexity, precision, and balance of the two systems functioning in concert are awe inspiring. Truly, we are "fearfully and wonderfully made."[16]

REFERENCES

1. Starling EH: *The Linacre lecture on the law of the heart,* London, 1918, Longmans, Green.
2. Struthers AD: Ten years of natriuretic peptide research: a new dawn for their diagnostic and therapeutic use, *BMJ* 308:1615, 1994.
3. Feliciano L, Henning RJ: Vagal nerve stimulation during muscarinic and beta-adrenergic blockade causes significant coronary artery dilation, *J Auton Nerv Syst* 68:78, 1998.
4. Feliciano L, Henning RH: Vagal nerve stimulation releases vasoactive intenstinal peptide which significantly increases coronary blood flow, *Cardiovasc Res* 40:45, 1998.
5. Richards AM, Doughty R, Nicholls MD, et al: Neurohumoral prediction of benefit from carvedilol in ischemic left ventricular dysfunction, *Circulation*:786, 1999.
6. Troughton RW, Framption CM, Yandle TG, et al: Treatment of heart failure guided by plasma aminoterminal brain natriuretic peptide (N-BMP) concentrations, *Lancet* 355:1126, 2000.
7. Guyton A: Heart muscle, the heart as a pump. In *Textbook of medical physiology,* ed 8, Philadelphia, 1991, W.B. Saunders.
8. Marcus ML: The coronary circulation in health and disease, New York, 1983, McGraw-Hill.
9. Grossman W, Baim DS: *Cardiac catheterization, angiography and intervention,* ed 4, Philadelphia, 1991, Lea & Febiger.
10. Quyyumi AA, Dakak N, Mulcahy D, et al: Nitric oxide activity in atherosclerotic human coronary circulation, *J Am Coll Cardiol* 29(2):308, 1997.
11. Chester AH, O'Neil GS, Moncada S, et al: Low basal and stimulated release of nitric oxide in atherosclerotic epicardial vessels, *Lancet* 336:897, 1990.
12. Liao JK: Nitric oxide and vascular disease, *Cardiol Rounds* 2(5):1, 1998.
13. Mudge GH et al: Comparison of metabolic and vasoconstrictor stimuli on coronary vascular resistance in man, *Circulation* 59(3):544, 1979.
14. Neill WA et al: Respiratory alkalemia during exercise reduces angina threshold, *Chest* 80(2):149, 1981.
15. Rowe GG et al: Effects of hyperventilation on systemic and coronary hemodynamics, *Am Heart J* 63:67, 1962.
16. Psalms 139:14, The Holy Bible, Authorized (King James) Version.

SUGGESTED READINGS

Bache RJ: Regulation of coronary blood flow. In Willerson JT, Cohn JN, editors: *Cardiovascular medicine,* ed 2, New York, 2000, Churchill Livingstone.

Baroldi G, Scomazzoni G: *Coronary circulation in the normal and pathologic heart,* Washington, DC, 1967, Office of the Surgeon General, Department of the Army.

Braunwald E: Coronary blood flow and myocardial ischemia. In Braunwald E, editor: *Heart disease: a textbook of cardiovascular medicine,* Philadelphia, 1992, W.B. Saunders.

Cohn PF: *Clinical cardiovascular physiology,* Philadelphia, 1985, W.B. Saunders.

Colucci WS, Braunwald E: Pathophysiology of heart failure. In *Heart disease: a textbook of cardiovascular medicine,* ed 5, Philadelphia, 1997, W.B. Saunders.

Dor V, DiDonato M: Ventricular remodeling. In *Coronary artery disease,* New York, 1997, Rapid Science Publishers.

Feliciano L, Henning RJ: Coronary artery blood flow: physiology and pathophysiologic regulation, *Clin Cardiol* 22:775, 1999.

Ganong WF: Circulation. In *Review of medical physiology,* ed 19, Stamford, CT, 1999, Appleton & Lange.

Ganz P, Braunwald E: Coronary blood flow and myocardial ischemia. In *Heart disease: a textbook of cardiovascular medicine,* ed 5, Philadelphia, 1997, W.B. Saunders.

Guyton A, Hall E: The heart. In *Textbook of medical physiology,* ed 9, Philadelphia, 1996, W.B. Saunders.

Hoffman BB, Lefkowitz RJ: Adrenergic receptors in the heart, *Annu Rev Physiol* 44:475, 1982.

Kern MJ et al: Interpretation of cardiac pathophysiology from pressure waveform analysis: coronary hemodynamics, part III. Coronary hyperemia, *Cathet Cardiovasc Diagn* 26:204, 1992.

Marcus ML: *The coronary circulation in health and disease,* New York, 1983, McGraw-Hill.

Rushmer RF: *Cardiovascular dynamics,* ed 4, Philadelphia, 1976, W.B. Saunders.

Sarnoff SJ: Myocardial contractility as described by ventricular function curves, *Physiol Rev* 35:107, 1955.

Schriner DK: Using hemodynamic waveform to assess cardiopulmonary pathologies, *Crit Care Nurs Clin North Am* 1(3):563, 1989.

Swynghedauw B, Caraboeuf E: Cardiac hypertrophy and failure. In Willerson JT, Cohn JN, editors: *Basic aspects in cardiovascular medicine,* ed 2, New York, 2000, Churchill Livingstone.

Wilson RF: Cardiovascular physiology. In *Critical care manual: applied physiology and principles of therapy,* ed 2, Philadelphia, 1992, Davis.

Wilson RF et al: Transluminal, subselective measurement of coronary artery blood flow velocity and vasodilator reserve in man, *Circulation* 72(1):82, 1985.

5

GLORIA OBLOUK DAROVIC and HENRY J.L. MARRIOTT

Physical Assessment of the Cardiovascular System

The only function of the cardiovascular system is to deliver oxygenated blood and nutrients to the body at a rate equal to body need and remove metabolic waste at the tissue level. In the critical care setting, a mere glance at the patient may reveal the present hemodynamic status. For example, an ashen, restless, confused, or obtunded appearance is characteristic of severe perfusion failure. The patient's underlying illness or injury and level of hemodynamic stability determine the frequency and rapidity of assessment, as well as the sequence in which the assessment procedure is done. For example, in a crisis, physical assessment is brief and focuses on parameters that are key to perfusion—heart rate and rhythm, presence and quality of pulses, capillary refill, color of skin and mucous membranes, level of consciousness, and urine flow rates.

This chapter focuses on the serial physical assessment techniques applicable to critically ill and injured patients. For that reason, a detailed discussion of history taking and psychosocial considerations is not included in this chapter, although this by no means minimizes their importance in routine patient evaluation.

SYMPTOMS AND SIGNS OF CARDIOVASCULAR DISEASE

In assessing the symptoms and signs of cardiovascular disease, the influence of environmental or emotional factors or body position should be noted because such information may be pertinent in prevention or management of disease manifestations.

Symptoms

Symptoms are the patient's subjective perception of changes in body function or indications of disease. The following are common symptoms of cardiovascular disease.

Chest Pain

Chest pain of cardiac origin is most commonly the result of myocardial ischemia due to coronary artery disease. The areas of pain are variable and may involve the chest, back, neck, teeth, shoulder, arms (usually the left), and epigastrium. Rarely, the pain may be in the kidney region, groin, rectum, legs, or any "weak" spot, such as a surgical scar. The pain is commonly described as a "discomfort" characterized by a great pressure, burning, or crushing sensation. In some people only a sensation of heaviness or tightness is perceived. Most patients remain quiet during the painful episode; this may reduce the severity of pain by reducing heart work. Others become very restless and agitated. Myocardial ischemic pain may be made worse by lying down because the augmented preload increases heart size, ventricular wall tension, and therefore myocardial oxygen demand. Because of the variability in the site, character, and patient response to ischemic myocardial pain, atypical pain or discomfort should not be dismissed as noncardiac in origin. This is especially important in patients whose age and history suggest risk of coronary artery disease, particularly if pain is associated with weakness, indigestion, or irregularities in the pulse.

In the postinfarction period or following heart surgery, chest pain may indicate *pericarditis.* Pericardial pain is sharp and stabbing and may radiate to the neck, back, and left shoulder. The severity of the pain is increased or appears abruptly from activities that usually do not affect myocardial ischemic pain, such as lying supine, deep inspiration, rotation of the trunk, or coughing, because these activities stretch the inflamed pericardium.

Noncardiac causes of chest pain that must be ruled out include musculoskeletal problems, pulmonary or pleural disease, aortic dissection, and referred pain from the abdomen.

Cultural and gender differences, as well as individual personality characteristics, such as stoicism or the need to deny disease or pain, may influence the pain threshold or may produce distorted information on patient questioning. Patients also may try to please the examiner, and care must be taken not to ask leading questions such as "You don't appear to be having any pain; are you?" An inclusive question such as "Are you having any *discomfort,* pain, pressure sensations, or unusual sensations in your chest, neck, face, teeth, arms, back, or abdomen?" may help the patient disclose valuable information. If pain is acknowledged, a scale of 0 through 10 (0 being complete freedom from pain, 10 being intolerable pain) helps the clinician objectively assess the severity of pain and the efficacy of analgesics. Precipitating or aggravating factors, the activity threshold at which pain occurs, and measures that reduce the severity of pain also should be determined. Visceral pain may be distinguished from musculoskeletal pain by asking patients to indicate with their hands the location of pain. Patients usually use a finger to point to the pain of musculoskeletal disorders, whereas they commonly place a clenched fist over areas of visceral pain.

Dyspnea

In the cardiac patient, dyspnea usually reflects *pulmonary edema* due to left heart failure. Generally, a pulmonary artery wedge pressure (PWP) greater than 18 to 20 mm Hg is associated with greater than normal movement of fluid into the lung. Factors that may produce cardiac dyspnea include the following.

Increased Venous Return. A normal right ventricle easily transports a normal or an increased venous return through the pulmonary circulation. An impaired left ventricle, however, functions on a depressed preload/stroke volume relationship so that a disproportionately high preload is required to generate the same output for the left ventricle.

For example, with an end-diastolic volume that produces an end-diastolic pressure of 0 mm Hg, the right

ventricle delivers 70 ml of blood into the pulmonary circulation (Figure 5-1). In order to match the right ventricular stroke volume, an impaired left ventricle may require an increased end-diastolic volume, which produces an end-diastolic pressure of 15 mm Hg. These values may be the patient's steady state when upright and at rest. At such a time, the lungs would be clear to auscultation and there would be no complaint of dyspnea.

If, however, venous return increases (volume loading, exercise, lying down), right ventricular end-diastolic volume increases to produce an end-diastolic pressure of, perhaps, 3 mm Hg. Note that in Figure 5-1 the small increase in right ventricular preload raises the normal right ventricular stroke volume from 70 to 85 ml. An impaired left ventricle may be able to match the increased right ventricular stroke volume with an increased filling volume associated with an end-diastolic pressure (measured as PWP) of 30 mm Hg. The grossly elevated left ventricular end-diastolic pressure is transmitted back to the pulmonary capillary bed. An acute elevation in pulmonary

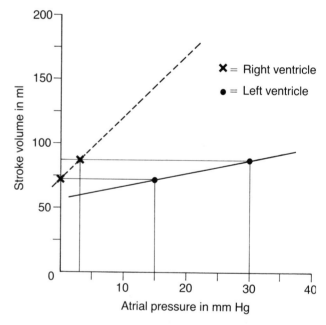

FIGURE 5-1 The relationship between atrial pressure (a correlate of ventricular end-diastolic pressure) for the right heart is plotted by the broken line and for the left heart is plotted by the solid line. The left ventricular filling volume required to establish the new dynamic equilibrium in stroke volume between the two ventricles may be associated with a left ventricular end-diastolic pressure sufficiently high to produce pulmonary edema. (Adapted from Bradley RD: *Studies in acute heart failure,* London, 1977, Edward Arnold Publishers. Reproduced by permission of Edward Arnold, Limited.)

capillary hydrostatic pressure to 30 mm Hg produces overwhelming extravasation of fluid into the lung. Acute pulmonary edema and its clinical hallmarks, tachypnea and dyspnea, result.[1]

Sudden Myocardial Ischemic Event. The sudden reduction in left ventricular distensibility associated with acute myocardial ischemia may be associated with elevations in left ventricular end-diastolic pressure (diastolic failure) that, if significant, may lead to pulmonary edema. Acute ischemic cardiac events also produce variable degrees of regional abnormalities in left ventricular wall motion that may significantly compromise pump function (systolic failure). Therefore, through two pathophysiologic mechanisms, acute ischemic myocardial dysfunction may lead to increased left ventricular end-diastolic pressures and the potential for pulmonary edema. Indeed, in some patients, dyspnea or cough may be the only symptom of an acute myocardial ischemic event.

Some noncardiac causes of dyspnea that must be differentiated from dyspnea induced by cardiac disease, or those that may coexist with cardiac disease, include disease of the lung tissue or vasculature, hysterical hyperventilation, and musculoskeletal problems such as extreme obesity.

Weakness and Fatigue

The sudden onset of ventricular dysfunction precipitated by an acute ischemic event may produce sudden-onset perfusion failure with its associated symptoms of acute weakness or fatigue. Chronic congestive heart failure is typically associated with chronic feelings of weakness, tiredness, and exercise intolerance proportional to the severity of heart failure.

Signs

Signs represent objective indications of changes in body function or illness. The clinician caring for acutely ill patients observes for the following.

Level of Mentation

Because of its immediate need for steady-state oxygenated blood flow, the brain is a sensitive indicator of the patient's perfusion status. Very early signs of cerebral underperfusion include any one or all of the following: the inability to think abstractly or perform complex mental tasks, restlessness, apprehension, uncooperativeness, and irritability. Short-term memory also may be impaired. A friend or family member of the patient may be needed for documentation of the patient's normal personality and intellectual status.

Studies have noted that a relatively consistent finding in hospitalized patients (approximately 70% of those studied) during the hours before cardiac arrest was deterioration of respiratory or mental function (see also Chapter 3).[2-4] Consequently, deviations from the patient's normal mental status should be immediately reported to and aggressively investigated by the physician in charge of the patient.

Skin Color and Temperature

In patients with circulatory failure, blood is shunted from skin and skeletal muscle to central organs necessary for survival in an amount roughly proportionate to the severity of perfusion failure. Therefore cool, pale skin may indicate circulatory failure. The patient's hands and feet should be touched and observed periodically and each time there appears to be a change in the patient's condition. With a progression in cardiovascular deterioration, cool, cyanosed, mottled, or pale skin changes begin at the distal extremities and move centrally toward the trunk. The anatomic site of color and temperature change should be noted, such as cool and clammy lower extremities and warm and dry trunk and upper extremities. These sites should be checked serially as a means of tracking remission or worsening cardiovascular dysfunction. The skin overlying bony prominences such as knees may also appear blanched in patients with severe circulatory failure.

Cool extremities, pallor, and perhaps peripheral cyanosis also may be found in patients with peripheral vascular disease, in those exposed to a cool environment, and in patients receiving potent vasoconstrictor agents such as epinephrine (Adrenalin), norepinephrine (Levophed), and phenylephrine (Neo-Synephrine). In these patients, skin color and temperature changes do not have the critical diagnostic or prognostic significance that they do in patients with circulatory failure not on vasoconstrictor drugs.

Cyanosis

Central cyanosis may be due to right-to-left intracardiac shunts such as that in tetralogy of Fallot. Peripheral cyanosis is apparent in patients with severe perfusion failure such as cardiogenic shock (see Chapter 3).

Urine Output

Low urine output in a patient known to be adequately hydrated may indicate hypoperfusion secondary to acute left ventricular systolic dysfunction. For example, a 10% to 20% drop in cardiac output may produce minimal blood pressure changes, but because renal vascular resistance increases immediately and disproportionately to the drop in cardiac output, renal blood flow and glomerular filtration rate may fall by as much as 20%.[5] Consequently, urine output may fall long before other signs of impaired tissue perfusion become clinically evident. The scanty urine produced in sudden-onset perfusion failure is typically concentrated (specific gravity greater than 1.025) and has a low urine sodium. Even if the perfusion deficit is slower in onset and urine output does not fall noticeably, the urine produced is more concentrated and the urine sodium is low. Generally, a progressive decrease in mean arterial pressure from the normal values of approximately 90 to 100 mm Hg is associated with a progressive decrease in urine output. When mean arterial pressure is approximately 50 mm Hg there is usually a nearly complete cessation in urine flow.[6] *Any recent diuretic therapy invalidates urine output as an indicator of acute circulatory changes and renal perfusion or function.*

Nutritional Status

Fragile, slack skin and muscle wasting, especially in the small muscles of the patient's hands, suggest protein-calorie malnutrition and impaired resistance to infection. The nutritional deficiency may be the result of poor absorption of foodstuffs or anorexia in patients with severe chronic heart failure or may be secondary to the hypermetabolic state characteristic of critical illness or injury (see also Chapter 17).

SPECIFIC TECHNIQUES OF PHYSICAL ASSESSMENT

The following techniques are used to obtain and expand information about the cardiovascular function. Included are considerations specific to evaluation of critically ill or injured patients.

Evaluation of Heart Rate

When the patient is hemodynamically unstable, the accuracy of the heart rate should be determined by auscultating heart sounds rather than noting the digital display on the monitoring console. Changes in the quality of heart sounds and the appearance of murmurs and gallop rhythms then may be detected earlier on. Although rare, *pulseless electrical activity* (formerly termed *electrical-mechanical dissociation*) also may be detected in patients with profound hypovolemia and advanced cardiac tamponade. Pulseless electrical activity is, in essence, cardiac arrest and is clinically noted in an unresponsive patient as the absence of heart sounds and palpable carotid pulses despite electrocardiographic evidence of any type of cardiac rhythm, including normal sinus rhythm.

Tachycardia is defined as a heart rate greater than 100 beats per minute, and *bradycardia* is defined as a heart rate less than 60 beats per minute. In the clinical setting, the appropriateness of the heart rate and its hemodynamic consequences are far more significant than the absolute values. The medications the patient is receiving (digitalis, beta-adrenergic and calcium channel blocking agents, or beta agonists) also must be considered when evaluating heart rate.

Evaluation of Cardiac Rhythm

A variety of factors may cause disturbances in cardiac rhythm in critically ill or injured patients. An electrocardiogram (ECG) rhythm strip should be analyzed at least once each 8-hour shift and again each time there is a change in the patient's condition. As with heart rate, the hemodynamic and clinical tolerance of the patient to the cardiac rhythm is more significant than the specific arrhythmia, such as atrial fibrillation or second-degree atrioventricular block, type I. The patient's hemodynamic tolerance to the arrhythmia determines the urgency with which corrective therapy is instituted (or whether corrective therapy is necessary at all).

Evaluation of the Arterial Pulses

Several factors determine the quality of the arterial pulse. These include stroke volume and ejection velocity, systemic vascular resistance, and pressure waves that reflect back from the peripheral arterioles. In the critical care setting, the upper and lower extremity arterial pulses are routinely checked for rate, rhythm, and volume. Bilateral comparisons of pulse volumes are made.

Pulse Rate and Rhythm

If the pulse is irregular, the pattern of the irregularity is noted. Comparisons also are made between the heart rate counted at the apex and the peripheral pulse rate.

Pulse Volume

The volume of the arterial pulse reflects left ventricular stroke volume. The closer to the heart the vessel is palpated, the less influence the characteristics of the vessel wall have on the quality of the pulse. Therefore the carotid or brachial pulses are more reliable in assessing stroke volume than the distally located radial or pedal pulses.

Extrasystolic beats, whether atrial, junctional, or ventricular, are weak beats because of the decreased ventricular filling time. If they occur early enough in diastole and are associated with abnormal systolic contractile dynamics, such as occurs with ventricular premature beats, extrasystolic beats may not be palpable at all (nonperfus-

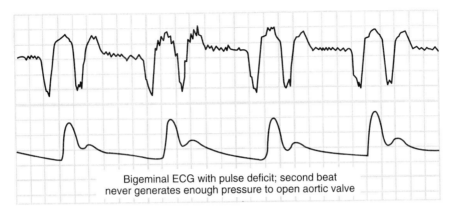

Bigeminal ECG with pulse deficit; second beat
never generates enough pressure to open aortic valve

FIGURE 5-2 Surface electrocardiogram (ECG) demonstrates a bigeminal rhythm. The simultaneously obtained systemic arterial waveform graphically illustrates that only the beat following the longer cycle is a "perfusing" beat. The premature beat never generates enough pressure to open the aortic valve; heart rate counted by ECG is 100 beats per minute, hemodynamically significant pulses are 50 per minute.

ing beats) (Figure 5-2). Usually the beat following the premature beat is stronger than normal because the compensatory pause allows more time for ventricular filling. As a general rule, a shorter cycle ends with a weaker beat and a longer cycle ends with a stronger beat. This rule also applies to the variably spaced beats in patients with atrial fibrillation.

Palpating a peripheral pulse while auscultating at the apex discloses the number of *perfusing beats.* For example, in ventricular bigeminy, a total of 76 beats (38 sinus and 38 ventricular premature beats) are counted at the apex and visualized on the ECG oscilloscope. Because of the shortened ventricular filling time, absence of the atrial contribution to ventricular filling, and distorted ventricular contractile dynamics, the ventricular beats may be so weak that they do not eject blood out of the semilunar valves and are, in essence, nonperfusing beats. Therefore only the 38 perfusing sinus beats are palpated at the wrist. Functionally, the patient has significant bradycardia (see Figure 5-2).

The volume of all pulses is increased in patients with hyperdynamic circulations such as those that occur with fever, anemia, emotional excitement, pregnancy, compensated aortic regurgitation, or systemic inflammatory response syndrome (SIRS). Pulse volume is decreased in patients with significant tachyarrhythmias or in those with hypodynamic circulations, for example, with left ventricular failure or hypovolemia.

When evaluating patients with profound circulatory failure and hypotension, if the radial pulse can be palpated, the systolic pressure is at least 80 mm Hg; if the femoral pulse can be palpated, the systolic pressure is at least 70 mm Hg; and if the carotid pulse can be palpated, the systolic pressure is at least 60 mm Hg.

Pulsus alternans

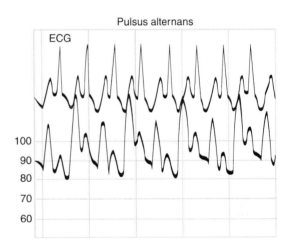

FIGURE 5-3 Pulsus alternans. Arterial pressure tracing from a 37-year-old man with severe congestive cardiomyopathy who died the next day. Note the regular alternation in amplitude in the arterial pulse waveforms. This patient's left ventricular end-diastolic pressure was 50 mm Hg. The simultaneously obtained ECG demonstrates left bundle branch block. (Courtesy of Dr. William P. Nelson.)

Assessment of Beat-by-Beat Variability in Pulse Volume

Alterations in cardiovascular function may be associated with characteristic beat-by-beat changes in the volume of the arterial pulses.

Pulsus alternans manifests as a regular alternation in the force of beats, so that a weak pulse regularly follows a strong pulse (Figure 5-3). The underlying cardiac rhythm is usually regular. The alternating pulse volume is produced because stroke volume increases and then decreases from beat to beat. In some patients this variability is attributed to alterations in ventricular end-diastolic pressure (due to

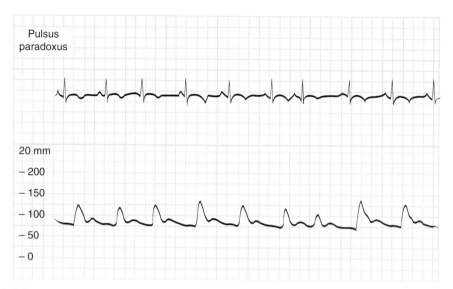

FIGURE 5-4 Pulsus paradoxus. Note the phasic variability in the systolic pressures; systolic pressures decrease on inspiration and increase during exhalation. If the patient does not have an intraarterial line and the pulsus paradoxus cannot be graphically documented, the sphygmomanometer technique may be employed (see Figure 5-5).

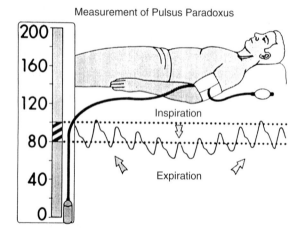

FIGURE 5-5 Sphygmomanometer technique for determination of pulsus paradoxus. Although patients may be tachypneic and perhaps dyspneic, they should be instructed to breathe as regularly and continuously as possible. The arm cuff is then inflated. While auscultating over the brachial artery, the arm cuff is deflated gradually until the Korotkoff sounds are heard phasically. The intermittent appearance of sounds corresponds with expiration. The cuff is then slowly deflated until all sounds are auscultated throughout the entire breathing cycle. The pressure difference between the phasic and the consistent sounds is a measure of the pulsus paradoxus. A pressure difference greater than 10 mm Hg is abnormal. However, in a hypotensive patient with a pulse pressure of 10 mm Hg, an inspiratory decrease in pressure of 5 mm Hg is considered a significant pulsus paradoxus. (From Stein L, Shubin H, Weil MH: Recognition and management of pericardial tamponade, *JAMA* 225:503, 1973. Copyright 1973, American Medical Association.)

changing myocardial compliance) that, in turn, affect ventricular filling. In other patients, there seems to be a primary alteration in contractility without changes in end-diastolic volume. Pulsus alternans may be noted in patients with severe heart failure, particularly when there is increased resistance to left ventricular ejection such as occurs with systemic hypertension or critical aortic stenosis. Pulsus alternans also may occur in patients with heart failure due to cardiomyopathies and also has been noted for a few beats following severe tachycardia in patients with normal hearts.

Pulsus paradoxus is an exaggerated decrease in pulse volume during inspiration and increase in pulse volume during exhalation. Normally, there is an approximately 3 to 4 mm Hg fall in systolic pressure with inspiration, which produces no discernible change in the quality of the pulse. When detectable, a systolic pressure reduction greater than 20 mm Hg is usually present. Rarely, the weak pulse may be imperceptible. The cyclic changes in systolic pressure of pulsus paradoxus can be visually appreciated by continuous intraarterial pressure monitoring (Figure 5-4.) When intraarterial pressure monitoring is not available, a sphygmomanometer may be used for documentation of pulsus paradoxus (Figure 5-5). Pulsus paradoxus is commonly seen in patients with cardiac tamponade; severe obstructive airway disease, such as asthma or chronic obstructive pulmonary disease (COPD); severe hypovolemia; and pulmonary embolism (see also Figure 23-21). See Table 5-1 for common causes of an abnormal pulse in critically ill patients.

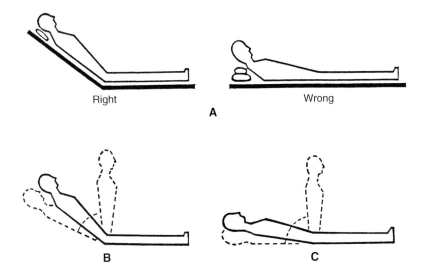

FIGURE 5-6 Positions of patients for venous viewing. **A,** Correct position: head and trunk are in line, the neck is not flexed. Wrong position: the neck is flexed by pillows. **B,** Range of possible positions for assessing jugular venous pressure/distention. **C,** Range of possible positions for studying internal jugular venous pulsations. (From Marriott HJL: *Bedside cardiac diagnosis,* Philadelphia, 1993, Lippincott.)

Evaluation of Venous Pressure and Right Heart Function

Venous pressure may be noninvasively estimated by examining the patient's jugular veins or the veins at the dorsum of the hands. Venous pressure, in turn, is a reflection of the filling pressure and function of the right ventricle due to the close diastolic correlation between right atrial and right ventricular end-diastolic pressure.

Examination of the Jugular Veins

The jugular veins, particularly the right internal jugular vein, are direct vascular conduits to the right atrium. In the absence of a catheter for direct monitoring of right atrial or central venous pressure, inspection of the external or internal jugular veins may give information about venous pressure. Certain clinical situations, however, present pitfalls to neck vein examination. These include patients with (1) short, thick necks, which may make visualization of these veins impossible; (2) surgery, trauma, tracheostomy tape, or dressings about the neck area; (3) obstruction in the superior vena cava as may occur with intrathoracic tumors or hematoma; (4) increased intrathoracic pressures secondary to positive pressure mechanical ventilation (particularly with positive end-expiratory pressure or continuous positive airway pressure) or expiratory difficulty as is common with COPD or asthma; or (5) circulatory failure or hypovolemia due to the associated sympathetic nervous system–induced venoconstriction.

For examination of the jugular veins, the patient should be relaxed and breathing normally with the head in a neutral position on a small pillow (Figure 5-6). A source of light, such as a pocket flashlight, that strikes the neck at an angle may be used to cast shadows and enhance visualization of the neck veins and venous pulsations.

TABLE 5-1

Common Causes of an Abnormal Pulse in Intensive Care Patients

Type of Pulse	Cause
Thready, low-volume pulse	Severe heart failure
	Hypovolemic shock
	Severe aortic stenosis
	Hypodynamic sepsis
Bounding pulse	Hyperdynamic sepsis
	Fever
	Anemia
	Aortic regurgitation
Pulsus paradoxus	Cardiac tamponade
	Mechanical ventilation, particularly if the patient is hypovolemic or if high peak airway pressures are used; severe chronic obstructive airway disease (COPD)
	Status asthmaticus
Pulsus alternans	Very low cardiac output, severe left ventricular dysfunction

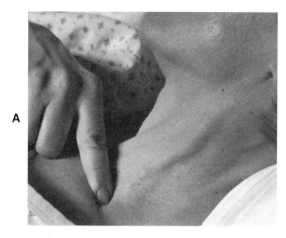
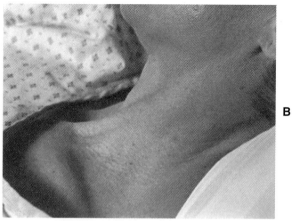

A

B

FIGURE 5-7 A, Compression of the superior border of the midclavicle allows filling and identification of the external jugular vein. **B,** On removal of compression, the vein column briskly collapses. The level of the crest of the fallen vein column is noted; normally it hovers just above the superior border of the midclavicle.

External Jugular Veins. The nonpulsatile external jugular veins are easily visualized because they lie superficially in the neck. Normally, at a 30-degree angle the crest of the vein column is just above the superior border of the midclavicle. Gentle compression of that site with the examiner's thumb or forefinger allows the vein to fill from above, become distended, and thus be identified. When the finger is removed and the vein column falls to its previous level, the height of the crest is then noted (Figure 5-7, *A* and *B*).

Normally, the full length of the partially distended external jugular vein is visible with the patient in the supine position; nonvisibility (venous collapse) suggests hypovolemia in supine patients (Figure 5-8).

Internal Jugular Veins. The right internal jugular vein most accurately reflects right atrial pressure because it lacks valves and extends in an almost straight line toward the head from the superior vena cava.

The internal jugular veins lie lateral to the carotid arteries deep within the neck. As a result of their deep anatomic location, the vein column is not visible. However, the crest of the venous column pulsates with each heartbeat and imparts flicking movements, which correlate with a and v waves, on the overlying skin. Visible carotid and jugular cutaneous pulsations may be confused by the examiner. The guidelines in Box 5-1 help distinguish one from the other.

For examination of the internal jugular veins, the patient is positioned as illustrated in Figure 5-6. The examiner begins with a 30-degree elevation of the patient's trunk and then elevates or lowers the bed appropriately. Internal jugular pulsations are normally observed just above the superior border of the clavicle in normovolemic

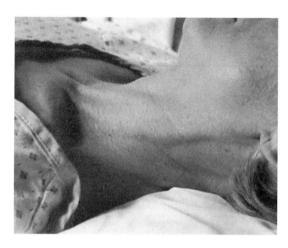

FIGURE 5-8 With the patient supine, note the normal slight distention of the full length of the external jugular vein column (clavicle to level of jaw).

persons with normal right heart function. Therefore a low venous pressure may require a nearly supine position to visualize the venous pulsation above the clavicle. On the other hand, an extremely high pressure may be missed if the flickering crest is very high; in fact, visualization of the crest of the vein column may be possible only if the patient is seated in an upright position.

Noninvasive Technique for Estimation of Central Venous Pressure. The anatomic reference level against which central venous pressure is estimated is the sternal angle of Louis. This reference point is used because of the assumption that the relationship between the center of the right atrium and the sternal angle remains constant regardless of the person's position. Normally, the sternal angle is 5 cm above the center of the right atrium and is located by running the forefinger centrally down the sternum. Very early the sternal ridge will be noted. The sternal angulation is formed by the junction of the manubrium and the body of the sternum and its union with the second ribs.

The jugular veins may be thought of as a central venous pressure (CVP) water manometer attached to the right atrium; CVP measurement correlates with the level of the venous pulsations. Normal CVP measurements using this technique are 3 to 11 cm H_2O, which correlates with 0 to 8 mm Hg. First, a centimeter ruler is vertically placed on the sternal angle. The straight edge of another ruler or tongue blade is then aligned, like a T-square, to the top of the pulsating vein column (Figure 5-9).

Central venous pressure is calculated to be the height of the blood column plus the 5 cm from the right atrium to the sternal angle. Thus, if the vertical height of the pulsation is 10 cm above the sternal angle, 10 cm + 5 cm = CVP of 15 cm H_2O. The normal vertical distance from the crest of the pulsating vein column to the level of the sternal angle is less than 6 cm, or a central venous pressure less than 11 cm H_2O.

This cost-effective and noninvasive technique has some drawbacks. This technique is difficult because the pulsating vein crest may be difficult to see, and assessment results among practitioners are variable. Also, due to the number of clinical variables other than right heart function and volume status that affect the height of the vein column (such as positive pressure ventilation, expiratory difficulty), the measurements obtained by this technique may be misleading.

Examination of the Veins at the Dorsum of the Hand

The patient is positioned with the trunk elevated 30 degrees or higher and the right arm (when possible) extended in a dependent position. The veins at the dorsum of the hand then immediately distend. The extended arm is slowly raised by the examiner. When venous pressure is normal, the veins collapse when the dorsum of the hand reaches the level of the sternal angle (heart level). Early collapse suggests a low venous pressure because of dehydration or hypovolemia; venous distention beyond that point suggests an elevated venous pressure.

Causes of Elevated Venous Pressure

Cardiac causes of elevated venous pressure include (1) right ventricular failure secondary to left heart failure (left ventricular ischemia, mitral valve disease, aortic valve disease, dilated cardiomyopathy); (2) primary right ventricular failure (right ventricular infarction, right ventricular contusion, cardiomyopathies); (3) cor pulmonale; (4) tricuspid or pulmonic stenosis; (5) pericardial effusion or tamponade; (6) restrictive cardiomyopathy or constrictive pericarditis; or (7) space-occupying lesions of the right heart (right atrial thrombosis or tumor).

Noncardiac causes of elevated venous pressure include (1) superior vena caval obstruction (thoracic tumor, hematoma, scarring, intravascular thrombus formation); (2) increased blood volume; (3) increased intrathoracic pressure due to positive pressure mechanical ventilation, Valsalva maneuver, obstructive airway disease, or tension pneumothorax; and (4) increased intraabdominal pressure due to pregnancy, obesity, or ascites.

Hepatojugular Reflux for Evaluation of Right Ventricular Function

In early right heart failure, venous blood volume may be increased but the elastic, distensible venous system may initially be able to accommodate the increased volume without increased venous pressure. A more sensitive indicator of right heart failure is the hepatojugular reflux.

First the patient is positioned comfortably at a 20- to 30-degree trunk elevation and asked to breathe quietly through an open mouth. Then firm, sustained gentle pressure is applied over the patient's abdomen just below the rib cage or right upper quadrant for 30 to 60 seconds. This pressure empties venous blood out of the liver sinusoids and increases venous return. The jugular veins are observed throughout. In patients with normal cardiovascular function, the initial jugular venous distention is followed quickly by collapse of the jugular veins because the right

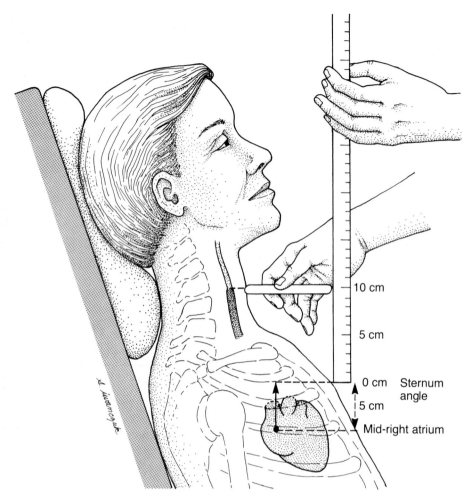

FIGURE 5-9 Estimation of central venous pressure using the vertical distance from the sternal angle to the pulsating crest of the internal jugular vein.

ventricle quickly adjusts its output to the increasing venous return. In patients with right heart failure or restrictive pericardial or myocardial disease, jugular venous distention continues during the 30 to 60 seconds of abdominal compression because the failing or constrained heart cannot accommodate the transient increase in venous return. A positive hepatojugular reflux test, however, may be observed in patients with intravascular volume overload and normal hearts.

Palpation of the Anterior Chest

Abnormally palpable heart sounds are termed *shocks,* abnormally pronounced precordial movements are termed *thrusts,* and palpable murmurs are termed *thrills.* The fingertips are best for feeling arterial pulsations, the apex beat, and the right ventricular thrust, whereas the palm, at the base of the fingers, is best for analyzing

shocks and thrills. It is best to palpate the anterior chest with the patient supine; elevation of the patient's trunk to greater than 45 degrees may alter the position of the heart in the chest. However, some patients with cardiac or pulmonary disease or increases in intracranial pressure may not tolerate the supine position. Nonetheless, it must be remembered that no assessment procedure, no laboratory test, and no hemodynamic measurement justifies placing the patient in a position that will not be clinically tolerated. In unstable patients, assessment trends are evaluated with the body position remaining as consistent as possible, such as at a consistent 45-degree backrest elevation.

The patient's body build will affect the examiner's perception of cardiac movements and sounds. Weak or undetectable impulses or sounds occur in patients with obese, muscular, swollen, or bruised chests; pulmonary or subcutaneous emphysema; pericardial tamponade; or effusion. In these patients, forceful pressure with the examiner's hand may be necessary for perception of precordial movements, and even then they may be imperceptible. Also, asking the patient to exhale and then "hold it" may help in locating or hearing cardiac activity. Conversely, cardiac movements or sounds may seem exaggerated in patients with thin, small chest walls.

Assessment of the Apex Beat

The *apex beat* or *impulse* is the most lateral and inferior point at which examiners can see or feel the cardiac impulse and is an excellent indicator of heart size and cardiac activity. It often, but not necessarily, coincides with the *point of maximal impulse (PMI)*. The apex beat is produced early in ventricular systole when the hardened, contracted left ventricle rotates anteriorly and to the right, causing the apex to tap the anterior chest wall. The apex beat occurs synchronously with the carotid impulse and is only briefly sustained. The apex beat is examined for location, duration, and character.

Location. In people with a normal heart and average build, the apex beat is in the fifth left intercostal space at or just medial to the midclavicular line (Figures 5-10, *A,* and 5-11). However, in short, obese adults, or in those with distended abdomens, the apex beat of the horizontally displaced heart may be in the fourth left intercostal space. In tall, thin people, the apex of the more vertical heart may be closer to the lower left sternal border. As a consequence of individual variance in body build and cardiac position, changes in the position of the apex beat over time are more important than absolute standards.

As the left ventricle enlarges with failure, the apex beat is displaced downward and left of the midclavicular line, for example at the anterior axillary line in the sixth intercostal space (Figures 5-10, *B,* and 5-11, *B*). With left ventricular hypertrophy, as may be seen in patients with chronic hypertension, the thickening myocardium tends to grow inward, encroaching on the ventricular cavity, and the apex beat usually occupies its normal position (Figure 5-11, *A*). In hypertensive patients, leftward deviation of the apex beat usually indicates hypertrophy complicated by ventricular failure and dilation.

Duration. Normally, perception of the apex beat ends within the first two thirds of systole. In patients with left ventricular failure and dilation, the apex beat extends into systole, sometimes lasting to the second heart sound. A prolonged impulse also is typical of hypertrophy due to increased left ventricular afterload (hypertension, aortic stenosis). Generally, the more severe the hypertrophy and increased afterload, the more sustained the apex beat.

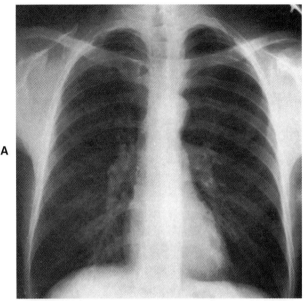

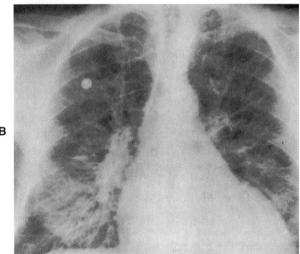

FIGURE 5-10 A, Normal upright chest radiograph, posteroanterior projection of an asymptomatic 26-year-old man. Note the position of the cardiac apex just medial to the left midclavicular line. **B,** Posteroanterior radiograph of a patient with left ventricular failure. The apex of the dilated left ventricle is shifted leftward and appears to be drooping below the level of the diaphragm. There are multiple linear densities scattered throughout both lung fields indicative of interstitial pulmonary edema. (From Frazer RC, Pare JAP: *Diagnosis of diseases of the chest,* vols 1 and 2, ed 4, Philadelphia, 1999, W.B. Saunders.)

Character. The normal apical beat is light and tapping and is felt over an area of the chest wall no larger than a nickel. Any condition associated with a hyperdynamic circulation will produce a more forceful impulse that is not sustained. This occurs in patients with anxiety,

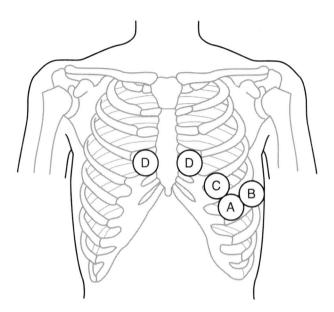

FIGURE 5-11 Areas of palpable precordial impulses. **A,** Normal apex beat. **B,** Position of apex beat in a patient with left ventricular enlargement. **C,** Position of ectopic impulse in a patient with anterior wall infarction. **D,** Positions of possible right ventricular activity (thrusts) in patients with pressure or flow overload of the right ventricle.

catecholamine administration or excess, fever, sepsis, anemia, or hyperthyroidism. Decreased force with increased duration and size occurs in patients with ventricular dilation resulting from damage to the ventricle, such as the failure due to ischemic heart disease. The apex beat is typically very weak or imperceptible in hypotensive patients.

The apical beat may not be detectable in some normal people (particularly men over age 50 years) while in the supine position. Turning such patients to the left lateral position brings the heart closer to the anterior chest wall and may make the apex beat palpable, especially at end-expiration. However, the left lateral position shifts the heart, and in turn the apex beat, leftward. This must be taken into consideration when evaluating the location of precordial pulsations.

Evaluation of Ectopic Precordial Impulses

The appearance of an *ectopic impulse* is an important finding in patients with ischemic heart disease. The acutely ischemic area of myocardium fails to contract in systole (ischemic paralysis) and may paradoxically bulge outward. Functional loss of a portion of the myocardial mass and paradoxic ventricular wall motion compromise heart function. If significant, this may result in heart failure. The systolic bulge may be visualized over the midpre-

cordial or apical area, and when palpated it feels like a distinct double impulse separated by a few centimeters. The ischemic ectopic impulse may occur in early, mid, or late systole and may be present only during an anginal attack or may be persistent in patients with myocardial infarction or ventricular aneurysm. A further indication of acute myocardial infarction sometimes may be obtained by simple inspection to see if a systolic bulge is visible within the midprecordium (Figure 5-11, *C*).

Right Ventricular Impulse (Right Ventricular Thrusts)

Although the right ventricle lies closer to the anterior chest wall than does the left ventricle, a palpable right ventricular impulse is normal only in some children and in slender adults. Abnormal left parasternal activity may be associated with central circulatory pressure or flow changes.

Increased Pulmonary Artery Pressures. In patients with elevations in pulmonary artery systolic and diastolic pressures, forceful right ventricular activity may be visualized and felt at the left or right lower sternal border. This may be noted in patients with chronic mitral valve disease, COPD, or primary pulmonary hypertension. A right ventricular thrust also may present acutely in patients with massive pulmonary embolism; it reflects the sudden systolic pressure overload and dilation of the acutely failing right ventricle (Figure 5-11, *D*). A chronic right ventricular thrust also may be observed in patients with pulmonic stenosis.

Right Ventricular Flow Overload. Atrial septal defect and acute or chronic tricuspid regurgitation both produce right ventricular diastolic flow overload that, if significant, may be associated with a brisk, left parasternal thrust. A right ventricular thrust also is a finding in patients with tetralogy of Fallot (pulmonic stenosis and systolic flow overload due to ventricular septal defect).

Auscultation of the Heart
Heart Sounds

Opinions differ as to the precise mechanism producing heart sounds—whether they are produced by actual valve closure or the acceleration/deceleration of blood associated with valve closure. Because the issue is not yet resolved, we will simply state that the first heart sound occurs simultaneously with closure of the atrioventricular (mitral and tricuspid) valves, and the second heart sound occurs synchronously with semilunar (aortic and pulmonic) valve closure. Because most heart sounds are near the lower end of the range of human hearing, the clinician must optimize conditions for auscultation.

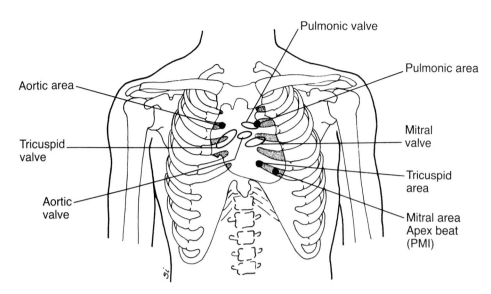

FIGURE 5-12 Areas of auscultation of heart valves. *Aortic area*—second intercostal space to the right of the sternum. *Pulmonic area*—second intercostal space to the left of the sternum. *Tricuspid area*—fifth intercostal space to the left of the sternum. *Mitral area*—over the apex beat (normally in the fifth intercostal space in the midclavicular line).

The *environment* should be as quiet as possible, requiring, for example, silencing of a bubbling chest tube drainage system by temporarily discontinuing wall suction or nasogastric tube suction.

The *stethoscope* design should maximize transmission of heart sounds. Earpieces should fit tightly enough to produce slight discomfort when in place, and the total length of the stethoscope tubing should be about 12 inches. The *diaphragm* chest piece is used for auscultating high-frequency sounds, such as the sounds associated with pulmonic or aortic valve closure or the ejection sounds associated with full opening of the semilunar valves. The *bell* chest piece is used to detect low-frequency sounds such as third and fourth heart sounds or the diastolic rumble of mitral stenosis. If the bell is applied with too much pressure, the underlying stretched skin acts as a diaphragm and filters out the low-pitched sounds. As a result, diagnostically significant low-intensity heart sounds may be missed.

If cooperative, the patient may assist with auscultation by breath holding to eliminate the noise of breath sounds. Breath holding at end-expiration also brings the chest wall (and stethoscope head) closer to the heart and thus increases audibility of heart sounds. A sustained hand grasp also may bring out a sound by increasing left ventricular filling, cardiac output, and arterial pressure. Turning the patient to the left shifts the heart against the anterior chest wall and amplifies many left-sided events. For example, the opening snap and diastolic rumble of mitral stenosis, as well as left ventricular third and fourth

heart sounds, may be audible only with the patient in this position. The left breast of large-breasted women will need to be lifted up and away from the intended area of auscultation, such as the apical area, with the examiner's nondominant hand (the dominant hand controls the stethoscope).

Cardiac auscultation is a difficult art and science requiring time, practice, and patience for the practitioner to become clinically adept. The critical care practitioner is particularly challenged with cardiac auscultation because heart sounds may be swamped or obscured by unavoidable factors such as the sounds made by mechanical ventilator breaths, the action of the intraaortic balloon pump, the adventitious lung sounds, or the sound-damping effects of generalized edema. Extra time and effort are frequently required to detect heart sounds. However, it is possible to hear only that which is humanly possible to hear. Sometimes effective cardiac auscultation is impossible for even the most experienced practitioner, and inaudibility of heart sounds should be noted on the chart.

Three concepts help convey the principles of auscultation:

1. Heart sounds normally occur synchronously with valve closure. Normal valves do not generate sounds on opening.
2. Heart sounds are heard best "downstream" from the source of the sound (Figure 5-12). However, auscultation should not be limited to just these areas because valve sounds may be heard all over the precordium.

Therefore the stethoscope head should inched from area to area over the entire precordium.

3. The intensity (loudness) of the sound depends partially on the pressure at which the cardiac event occurs. For example, the aortic closure sound is louder than the pulmonic closure sound.

First and Second Heart Sounds. The first heart sound (S_1) signals the onset of ventricular systole. It has two components: M_1 coincides with mitral valve closure, and T_1 coincides with tricuspid valve closure (Figure 5-13, *B*). Normally these two events occur so close together that the human ear is usually unable to separate them. However, when tricuspid valve closure is delayed, as in right bundle branch block, both components may be heard separately. This is termed *splitting of the first heart sound* and is best heard over the left lower sternal border in the fifth intercostal space (tricuspid area).

The *second heart sound* (S_2) coincides with closure of the aortic (A_2) and pulmonic (P_2) valves and signals the onset of ventricular diastole (Figure 5-13, *D*). During expiration, the two components are nearly inseparable. However, during inspiration, P_2 is delayed because right ventricular systole is slightly prolonged because of increased venous return. The normal physiologic splitting of the second heart sound is best heard at the left sternal border in the second intercostal space (pulmonic area) with the diaphragm of the stethoscope. The intensity of the second heart sound depends on two factors: (1) aortic and pulmonic diastolic pressures—the audibility of A_2 and P_2 is increased in systemic arterial and pulmonary hypertension, respectively, and is decreased in hypotension; and (2) the mobility of the valve leaflets and their ability to close. For example, the intensity of A_2 is decreased in aortic stenosis or regurgitation because of the abnormal dynamics of aortic valve closure.

Identification of S_1 and S_2. The first step in cardiac auscultation is identification of the S_1 and S_2 sounds. S_1 coincides with the onset of systole and S_2 with the onset of diastole. Identification of each sound establishes a sonic landmark relative to the cardiac cycle against which other sounds can be identified. For example, any other sounds occurring after S_1 are systolic in timing, whereas sounds occurring after S_2 are diastolic in timing. These sounds can then be further identified as early, mid, or late systolic or diastolic.

At normal heart rates, diastole is longer than systole, and it is easy to isolate and identify the first and second heart sounds. At faster heart rates the two sounds run in uninterrupted cadence and it may become difficult to differentiate S_1 from S_2. A hemodynamic landmark may be identified by placing a finger over the carotid pulse or apical beat while listening to the heart. The pulsation felt will be synchronous with the first heart sound (S_1). S_1 ("lubb") is also lower in pitch and more prolonged than S_2, which has a higher-pitched, abrupt closing sound ("dupp"). This difference in the character of the sounds may help the examiner differentiate S_1 from S_2.

Third and Fourth Heart Sounds. When the atrial contraction is intact, as in sinus rhythm and some atrial rhythms, three filling phases—rapid, slow, and active—occur during diastole. The rapid and active filling phases may be associated with audible sounds—a third and fourth heart sound, respectively.

Rapid Filling Phase. Early in diastole, the mitral and tricuspid valves open followed by rapid flow of blood into the ventricle, which may generate a third heart sound. If audible, the third heart sound occurs shortly after S_2 (early diastole) (Figure 5-13, *F*).

Slow Filling Phase. Rapid ventricular filling is followed by a slow filling phase during which ventricular diastolic pressures are normally low. At this time, 70% to 90% of ventricular filling has occurred.

Active Filling Phase. Atrial contraction augments ventricular filling late in diastole. Through volume loading of the ventricle, atrial contraction normally increases end-diastolic pressure a few mm Hg and generates a fourth heart sound. If audible, the fourth heart sound will occur just before S_1 (late diastole) (Figure 5-13, *A*).

Accentuated and possibly palpable third (S_3) or fourth (S_4) heart sounds result from large intraventricular diastolic pressure changes (ventricular failure), increased ventricular distending forces (hyperdynamic circulation producing increased blood flow), or decreased ventricular compliance due to myocardial ischemia, ventricular hypertrophy, or pericardial constriction.

Because third and fourth heart sounds are of very low intensity, the sudden appearance of the majority may go undetected, and the first subtle clue to the presence of heart disease may be missed. Therefore the examiner must optimize conditions to detect them. The patient's room should be as quiet as possible. S_3 or S_4 sounds from the left ventricle are best heard with the patient in the left lateral position with the bell of the stethoscope *lightly* applied over the apical beat. S_3 or S_4 sounds from the right ventricle are best heard with the bell of the stethoscope over the left lower sternal border with the patient recumbent. S_3 or S_4 becomes more audible when intracardiac blood flows are increased. Therefore having the patient cough a few times or maintain a sustained hand grasp increases blood flow and may bring the sound into the range of the examiner's hearing.

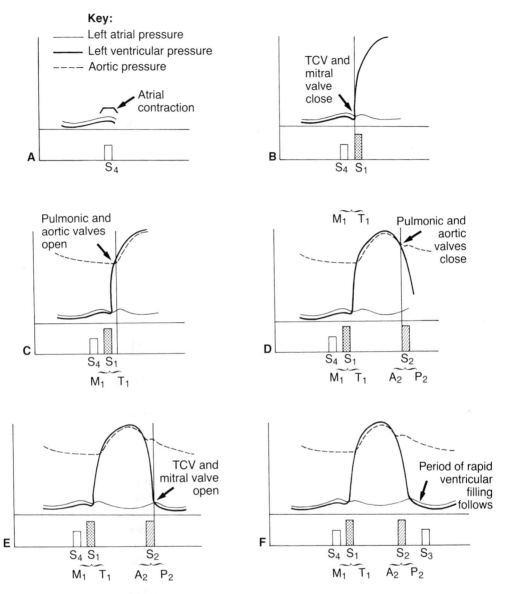

Key:
⎯⎯ Left atrial pressure
⎯⎯ Left ventricular pressure
- - - - Aortic pressure

FIGURE 5-13 Relationship of cardiac events to the production of heart sounds. S_4, fourth heart sound; S_1, first heart sound; M_1, mitral component of the first heart sound; T_1, tricuspid component of the first heart sound; S_2, second heart sound; A_2, aortic component of the second heart sound; P_2, pulmonic component of the second heart sound; S_3, third heart sound.

Clinical Significance of the Third Heart Sound

This low-intensity sound, which is audible shortly after S_2, is produced by sudden distention of the ventricular wall due to rapid early diastolic filling. When audible, a distinct triple rhythm is produced. The first two components are the normal S_1 and S_2 sounds, and the low-intensity third component is the S_3 sound. The auscultated cardiac cycle sounds like "lubb-dupp-up," in which "lubb-dupp" represents S_1 and S_2 and the softer "up" is the third heart sound (Figure 5-14).

A third heart sound can be heard in most children, but, with maturity, it gradually diminishes and becomes inaudible in adults. It may be a normal finding beyond age 30 years in thin-chested adults, particularly women, but is rarely audible after 40 years of age. S_3 becomes louder when cardiac output and flow rates are increased, as occurs in anemia, hyperthyroidism, exercise, anxiety, and so on. When present in a healthy, young person, the term *physiologic S₃* or *third heart sound* is used.

With advancing age, an audible third sound is abnormal and is termed *S₃ gallop* or *ventricular gallop*. Its presence implies an enlarged failing ventricle with an elevated end-diastolic pressure. The pathophysiologic S_3 sound is produced when atrial blood rushes into a ventricle incompletely emptied from the previous beat and unable to yield to the incoming blood. The audibility of S_3 becomes fainter with improvement or louder with worsening of failure. A ventricular gallop also may be palpable in patients with major elevations in left ventricular filling volume and pressure. Constrictive pericarditis also may produce a ventricular gallop (pericardial knock) because diastolic distention of the ventricles is limited by the constraining pericardium.

Clinical Significance of the Fourth Heart Sound

This sonic event is produced when ventricular filling is augmented by atrial contraction; therefore a fourth heart sound can be produced only when effective atrial activity is present. This low-intensity sound occurs shortly before S_1, and the triple cadence, which sounds like "la-lubb-dupp," may rarely be audible in people with healthy hearts, especially in older people (Figure 5-15).

The following features help distinguish a pathologic S_4 sound from a physiologic S_4. An S_4 is pathologic if it appears suddenly when it was not previously audible; if a previously audible S_4 becomes particularly prominent; or if it becomes palpable at the apex when there is decrease in ventricular compliance.

Overall, when the sound appears acutely or increases in loudness, is palpable, and occurs in the context of heart disease, the terms *atrial gallop* and *S₄ gallop* are applied.

An atrial gallop is associated with a decreased ventricular compliance and an increased ventricular end-diastolic pressure, although pressure in early diastole may be normal. Clinically, this is seen in patients with ventricular hypertrophy (particularly with outflow obstruction), ischemic heart disease, or acute mitral regurgitation. When present in patients with ischemic heart disease, the atrial gallop may become more intense or audible only during an ischemic attack.

The term *gallop* was chosen to distinguish physiologic S_3 and S_4 sounds from those heart sounds resulting from heart disease. Although the cadence of gallop rhythms is suggestive of the sounds made by a galloping horse, the auscultatory characteristics or cadence of sounds do not characterize normal from abnormal. Rather, the clinical setting in which the sounds appear helps distinguish normal from abnormal. For example, an S_3 sound in a teenage trauma patient is likely to be physiologic, but an S_3 sound in an adult with acute ischemic heart disease is always a ventricular gallop.

Quadruple Rhythm

In patients with established ventricular failure, two gallop sounds may be present in addition to the two normal heart sounds. If the heart rate is sufficiently slow, all four sounds are separate and distinct and produce a quadruple rhythm that sounds like "la-lubb-dupp-up" (Figure 5-16).

Summation Gallop

At heart rates that typically accompany heart failure, the atrial and ventricular gallop sounds are nearly synchronous and produce a loud sound termed a *summation gallop*. The summation sound is typically louder than the first and second heart sounds (Figure 5-17).

Heart Murmurs

A cardiac murmur is an auscultatory sound that arises when (1) rapid rate of flow occurs across a normal cardiac structure, as with innocent heart murmurs; (2) flow occurs across a constricted area, as in aortic stenosis; (3) flow occurs across an abnormal structure without obstruction, as in congenital bicuspid aortic valve; (4) regurgitant flow occurs through an incompetent valve, as in mitral regurgitation; (5) flow occurs into a dilated structure, as in the aortic root or pulmonary trunk in patients with systemic or pulmonary hypertension; or (6) blood is shunted from a high- to a low-pressure area through an abnormal opening such as a ventricular septal defect. Overall, the loudness

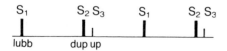

FIGURE 5-14 Auscultated cadence of the third heart sound.

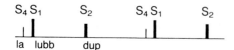

FIGURE 5-15 Auscultated cadence of the fourth heart sound.

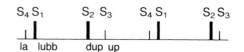

FIGURE 5-16 Auscultated cadence of quadruple rhythm.

of a murmur increases as cardiac output increases, and, conversely, it may be difficult to hear a murmur in patients with low cardiac output or hypotension.

Systolic Murmurs. Systolic murmurs are evident following S_1 because this sound is a sonic landmark that heralds the onset of ventricular systole. Innocent murmurs are always systolic in timing, and many types of valvular defects, as well as congenital and acquired heart defects, are characterized by systolic murmurs. Innocent murmurs, aortic stenosis, acute and chronic mitral regurgitation, and ventricular septal defect are described next.

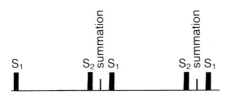

FIGURE 5-17 Auscultated cadence of summation gallop.

Innocent (Functional) Murmurs. The presence of a murmur does not necessarily indicate heart disease. Innocent (functional) murmurs are common and systolic in timing and may be consistent or intermittent. People with innocent murmurs demonstrate no clinical, electrographic, echocardiographic, or radiographic evidence of heart disease. These murmurs have many causes, such as episodic vibrations of the pulmonary valve leaflets at their attachments to the pulmonary trunk or exaggerations of normal ejection vibrations within the pulmonary trunk. An innocent systolic flow murmur may be heard at the base of the heart (aortic or pulmonic areas) in patients with hyperdynamic circulations resulting from pregnancy, sepsis, anemia, hyperthyroidism, or SIRS. In these patients, the murmur usually disappears when cardiac output returns to normal.

Aortic Stenosis

Aortic stenosis is a chronic valve disease characterized by progressive narrowing of the valve opening and obstruction to left ventricular outflow. Clinical features include systemic underperfusion, a predisposition to pulmonary

---

Murmurs are described according to the following characteristics:

1. Pitch—high or low.
2. Quality—musical, harsh, blowing, machinelike, and so forth.
3. Shape:
   a. Crescendo—increasing in intensity.

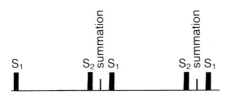

   b. Decrescendo—decreasing in intensity.

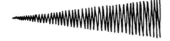

   c. Crescendo-decrescendo, diamond shaped—increasing in intensity to a peak, then decreasing in intensity.

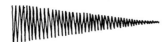

   d. Plateau—consistent intensity throughout.

   e. Variable—intensity waxes and wanes variably.

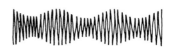

4. Location—where the murmur is maximally heard, as well as its direction of radiation, if applicable.
5. Timing—early, mid, or late systolic or diastolic. If the murmur occurs throughout systole, it is termed *holosystolic* or *pansystolic*. If the murmur occurs throughout diastole, it is termed *holodiastolic* or *pandiastolic*.
6. Intensity (loudness)—the intensity of a murmur may be graded from I to VI:
   a. Grade I—the murmur is barely audible in a quiet room. Detection may require breath holding on the part of the patient (because normal breath sounds may obscure the sound of the murmur) and a "warm-up" period on the part of the listener. It is often astonishing what can be seen, felt, and heard after 15 to 20 seconds of warm-up that could not be appreciated in the initial 5 or 10 seconds of auscultation.
   b. Grade II—the murmur is faint but immediately audible.
   c. Grade III—the murmur is audible but not loud.
   d. Grade IV—the murmur is loud and is usually accompanied by a thrill.
   e. Grade V—the murmur is very loud, is always accompanied by a thrill, and can be heard with only one edge of the stethoscope in contact with the chest wall.
   f. Grade VI—the murmur is very loud, is accompanied by a thrill, and may be heard with the stethoscope close to but not touching the chest wall.

edema, and potential for myocardial ischemia even in the absence of coronary artery disease. Common causes include rheumatic fever and fibrotic or calcific valve changes that occur in some people as a function of aging and are termed *senile aortic stenosis.*

The murmur of aortic stenosis is usually most audible in the second intercostal space to the right of the sternum (aortic area) and radiates to the neck. The murmur is harsh in quality, and the sound is similar to that of a whispered R. Beginning after S_1, the murmur crescendos to a systolic peak and then decrescendos and ends before S_2. The intensity of the murmur coincides with the rise and fall in blood flow in systole across the aortic valve and creates the characteristic crescendo-decrescendo. The more severe the aortic outflow obstruction, the later in systole the summit of the murmur. Patients with aortic stenosis develop compensatory hypertrophy of the left ventricle. Therefore, as an associated finding, the apex beat is prolonged and forceful.

Mitral Regurgitation

All components of the mitral valve apparatus (leaflets, chordae tendineae, papillary muscles, adjoining structures) must be normal and intact for normal valve function. Mitral regurgitation, which may be acute or chronic, occurs when damage or distortion of the structures of the valve apparatus prevents complete valve closure. Incomplete valve closure, in turn, allows retrograde blood flow into the left atrium during ventricular systole, which is associated with a murmur. The clinical, hemodynamic, and auscultatory findings differ dramatically between chronic and acute mitral regurgitation.

Chronic Mitral Regurgitation. Chronic mitral regurgitation is due most commonly to mitral valve prolapse but may also result from rheumatic distortion of the mitral valve leaflets or chordae tendineae. The rheumatic form is typically associated with compensatory left atrial dilation, which protects the pulmonary circulation from high pressures induced by the regurgitant flow. This valve disorder is generally well tolerated for decades.

The large, compliant atrium accommodates the regurgitant flow throughout systole; consequently, a pansystolic murmur ends with the aortic component of the second heart sound. The murmur, which is best heard over the apex, is typically high pitched and blowing.

Acute Mitral Regurgitation. This potentially life-threatening condition may be the result of damage or dysfunction of a papillary muscle, rupture of the chordae tendineae, disruption or distortion of valve leaflets, or dilation of the mitral valve annulus because of severe left ventricular failure. Acute mitral regurgitation may occur in the clinical context of infective endocarditis, acute myocardial infarction, or blunt anterior chest trauma.

Acute mitral regurgitation is frequently accompanied by sudden hemodynamic deterioration, which may rapidly result in death. Early recognition and aggressive, appropriate patient management are therefore critical determinants of patient outcome.

The regurgitant blood streams into the normal, small, relatively noncompliant left atrium and produces significant increases in left atrial pressure, which predispose patients to pulmonary edema and may be noted as large v waves in the PWP tracing. With severe mitral regurgitation, the v waves may approach left ventricular pressures in late systole. Near equilibration of left atrial and left ventricular systolic pressure suppresses the regurgitant flow; therefore the murmur is decrescendo in character (regurgitant flow is maximal in early systole and minimal in late systole) and may end before the second heart sound. The quality of the murmur is low pitched and blowing. It may be as loud as grade V to VI but diminishes in intensity if the patient becomes hypotensive.

Acute Ventricular Septal Defect

The majority of septal ruptures occur within the first week and affect 1% to 3% of patients with anterior or inferior wall myocardial infarction. Rapidly progressive systemic underperfusion and development of pulmonary edema characterize this potentially lethal defect. The murmur is pansystolic because left ventricular pressures are higher than right ventricular pressures throughout systole. Consequently, ventricular blood is shunted from left to right. The murmur may sometimes occur only in midsystole. This is the period when the left ventricle reaches its peak pressure. The source of the murmur is produced within the right ventricle by the turbulence of shunted blood. The murmur may cover a large area but is typically loudest at the left sternal border at the third, fourth, and fifth intercostal spaces. It is high pitched and harsh in quality, sometimes accompanied by a thrill, and is usually associated with progressive hemodynamic deterioration.

Diastolic Murmurs

Diastolic murmurs are evident following S_2 because this sound signals the onset of ventricular diastole. Diastolic murmurs always indicate the presence of heart disease. The murmurs of mitral stenosis and aortic regurgitation are discussed next.

Mitral Stenosis. Mitral stenosis is a chronic, progressive valve disease in which impairment of valve function and narrowing of the mitral valve orifice restrict the free flow of blood from the left atrium to the left ventricle. The most common cause of mitral stenosis is rheumatic fever. Clinical features in patients with severe disease include chronic fatigue and predisposition to pulmonary edema and manifest as dyspnea occurring with very little provocation.

Blood passing across a stenosed mitral valve produces a jet stream that makes an impact on the endocardial surface of the left ventricle at the apex and produces a low-pitched, rumbling diastolic murmur. Generally, the more advanced the stenosis, the longer the murmur, and thus in less severe disease the murmur may be middiastolic or presystolic. With severe disease the murmur may occupy all but the first moments of diastole. Other auscultatory findings include an accentuated S_1, with a tapping, metallic quality, and S_2 may be followed by an opening snap.

The murmur is best heard with the bell of the stethoscope lightly applied to the apical area with the patient lying in the left lateral position. This position brings the apex closer to the chest wall and overlying stethoscope, which increases the audibility of the characteristically low-intensity murmur.

Aortic Regurgitation. Aortic regurgitation is an acute or chronic valve disease in which incompetence of the aortic valve results in reflux of blood from the aorta into the left ventricle in diastole.

Chronic aortic regurgitation is commonly due to rheumatic heart disease or hypertension with dilation of the aortic root. This valve defect is associated with a hyperdynamic circulation and is usually well tolerated for decades or a lifetime.

Acute aortic regurgitation may result from infective endocarditis, proximal dissection of the aorta, and valve damage due to blunt thoracic trauma. With high levels of retrograde flow, patients with acute aortic regurgitation generally develop circulatory shock. If the valve defect is not aggressively corrected, the patient's condition rapidly deteriorates to death. Consequently, a high level of suspicion for the possibility of valve dysfunction is necessary in high-risk patients. Careful auscultation, early detection, and surgical correction (valve replacement) may be lifesaving.

When the aortic valve fails to close completely, backflow of blood into the left ventricle produces a high-pitched, blowing murmur. The murmur begins with the aortic component of the second heart sound and is decrescendo in character, which reflects the progressive reduction in the rate of retrograde flow throughout diastole. Murmurs of aortic regurgitation may be of all grades of intensity. When very soft, the murmur resembles a breath sound and may be heard only when patients lean forward and hold their breath at expiration. For detection, the diaphragm of the stethoscope should be applied with firm pressure at the left sternal border.

Other Cardiac Sounds and Clinical Caveats

Infective Endocarditis

A sudden-onset diastolic or pansystolic murmur in a critically ill or injured patient should always raise the suspicion of infective endocarditis with cardiac valve involvement. Multiple invasive catheters and support devices predispose these often immune-compromised patients to this potentially lethal disease. Patients known to be intravenous drug abusers also are at risk of infective endocarditis. Associated possible signs include fever, heart failure, pericardial rub, eyelid petechiae, neurologic changes, hypertensive crisis, proteinuria, and hematuria.

Pericardial Friction/Rub

Inflammation of the pericardium may be associated with "to-and-fro" noises synchronous with ventricular contraction and relaxation. These noises sound like friction between two rough surfaces and may be described as leathery, scratching, creaking, or squeaky. The rub is best heard with the patient leaning forward with breath held in full expiration with the stethoscope diaphragm held firmly over the left midprecordium. The audibility of pericardial friction is usually maximal at the left of the lower sternum. In sinus rhythm, the rub may have three components—midsystolic, middiastolic, and late diastolic (atrial contraction). Pericardial rubs may be mistaken for murmurs; however, the relationship of a rub to a heart sound, such as S_1 or S_2, is less fixed than that of a murmur. A pericardial rub also may be palpable all over the precordium.

All types of pericarditis (viral, bacterial, acute myocardial infarction, acute rheumatic fever, uremia, drug sensitivity) may be associated with a rub. The rub may disappear if a pericardial effusion develops. The most common in-hospital situation in which pericardial rubs are heard is in patients immediately following open heart surgery. In the rare patient, the rub may be so loud as to swamp the normal heart sounds. Alternatively, a crunching noise that occurs synchronously with the beating heart, audible over the apex, may be detected and is caused by air in the mediastinum (Hamman's sign). Mediastinal air has no clinical or hemodynamic consequence in the immediate postoperative period in patients who have had cardiac surgery.

Prosthetic Heart Valves

The sounds made by prosthetic heart valves differ from those made by normal, human valves. The sounds vary with the type of valve. For example, the majority of bioprosthetic valves have an audible opening mechanical-sounding click. Tilting and bivalve mitral prostheses typically are silent on opening. A soft, short diastolic rumble may occasionally be heard in porcine mitral valves. Auscultatory caveats relative to prosthetic valves include the following: (1) any diastolic murmur is abnormal and should be promptly investigated; (2) holosystolic mitral regurgitant murmurs in any prosthetic mitral valve are abnormal; and (3) decrease or disappearance of a prosthetic valve closing sound may be related to the development of a valve thrombus or valve fibrosis.

The importance of careful, serial physical assessments in critically ill or injured patients cannot be overstated. The condition of these patients is one of either potential or actual hemodynamic and physiologic instability. Dramatic changes in the patient's condition may occur within seconds to minutes. The potential or actual instability of the patient's physical condition mandates the expert vigilance of critical care clinicians.

REFERENCES

1. Bradley RD: *Studies in acute heart failure,* London, 1977, Edward Arnold Press.
2. Sax FL, Charlson ME: Medical patients at high risk for catastrophic deterioration, *Crit Care Med* 15(5):510, 1987.
3. Schein RM, Hazday N, Pena M, et al: Clinical antecedents in in-hospital cardiopulmonary arrest, *Chest* 98(6):1388, 1990.
4. Franklin C, Mathew J: Developing strategies to prevent in-hospital cardiac arrest: analyzing response of physicians and nurses in the hours before the event. Unpublished manuscript.
5. Wilson RF: *Critical care manual: applied physiology and principles of therapy,* ed 2, Philadelphia, 1992, Davis.
6. Guyton A: *Textbook of medical physiology,* ed 8, Philadelphia, 1991, W.B. Saunders.

SUGGESTED READINGS

Chatterjee K: Physical examination. In Topol EJ, editor: *Textbook of cardiovascular medicine,* Philadelphia, 1998, Lippincott-Raven.

Dobb GJ, Coombs LJ: Clinical examination of patients in the intensive care unit, *Br J Hosp Med* 38(2):102, 1987.

Horwitz LD, Groves BM: *Signs and symptoms in cardiology,* Philadelphia, 1985, Lippincott.

Lumb PD: Clinical assessment in the intensive care unit. In Civetta JM, Taylor RW, Kirby RR, editors: *Critical care,* ed 2, Philadelphia, 1992, Lippincott.

Marriott HJL: *Bedside cardiac diagnosis,* Philadelphia, 1993, Lippincott.

Munro J, Edwards C: The cardiovascular system. In Munro J, Edwards C, editors: *Macleod's clinical examination,* ed 8, Edinburgh, 1990, Churchill Livingstone.

O'Rourke RA, Shauer JA, Salerni R, et al: History, physical examination and cardiac auscultation. In Alexander RW, Schlant RC, Fuster V, editors: *Hurst's the heart,* ed 9, New York, 1998, McGraw-Hill.

Perloff JK: *Physical examination of the heart and circulation,* ed 2, Philadelphia, 1990, W.B. Saunders.

Perloff JK, Braunwald E: Physical examination of the heart and circulation. In Braunwald E, editor: *Heart disease: a textbook of cardiovascular medicine,* ed 5, Philadelphia, 1997, W.B. Saunders.

Topol EJ: The history. In Topol EJ, editor: *Textbook of cardiovascular medicine,* Philadelphia, 1998, Lippincott-Raven.

Willerson JT, Smitherman T: The history and physical examination. In Willerson JT, Cohn JN, editors: *Cardiovascular medicine,* ed 2, New York, 2000, Churchill Livingstone.

Unit Two

MONITORING TECHNIQUES

6

GLORIA OBLOUK DAROVIC and JOSEPH P. ZBILUT

Fluid-Filled Monitoring Systems

From the time of the first cannulated artery to the electronics revolution of the 1960s, various techniques of direct cardiovascular pressure monitoring were available for laboratory use. These methods were quite cumbersome and, from a clinical standpoint, impractical. The electronics revolution brought about the development and introduction into clinical medicine of methods to monitor patient hemodynamics in a relatively simple yet relatively accurate manner. Refinements continue today as computerized systems and advanced microcircuits are added to improve the efficiency, reliability, and accuracy of these systems.

It is imperative that clinical practitioners become familiar with the physical characteristics of fluid-filled pressure monitoring systems because (1) hemodynamic monitoring using fluid-filled catheter/transducer systems is routine in critical care units, (2) characteristics of these monitoring systems are unique, and (3) errors in many controllable factors may result in waveform distortion and inaccurate pressure measurements.

This chapter begins with a brief discussion of the types of currently available pressure monitoring systems and the components of these systems. This discussion is followed by a description of the sources of pressure waveform distortion and inaccurate pressure measurements, as well as techniques of monitoring system preparation, zeroing, and calibration that optimize the fidelity of the monitoring system. The terminology specific to physical properties of a fluid-filled system is included in the glossary at the end of the chapter.

FLUID-FILLED MONITORING SYSTEMS

Bedside monitors display pressures in various compartments of the cardiovascular system for assessment of cardiovascular function. The physical principle underlying current methods of invasive monitoring is that a change in pressure at any point in an unobstructed fluid-filled system results in similar pressure changes at all other points of the system. A fluid medium is not very compressible and therefore allows accurate transmission of pressure from the catheter tip located within the patient's body to an appropriately zeroed and calibrated water manometer or a transducer/amplifier/monitor. This principle is elaborated on later in this chapter, taking into account the inherent shortcomings of fluid-filled pressure monitoring systems.

TYPES OF MONITORING SYSTEMS

Fluid System Attached to a Water Manometer

In this first type of monitoring system, an in situ catheter is attached to fluid-filled connecting tubing, which, in turn, is attached to a calibrated water manometer. This simple technique was originally used for central venous pressure (CVP) monitoring and was later extended for use in intracranial pressure monitoring. Drawbacks included the following:

1. Values were available only intermittently and had to be obtained manually.
2. System contamination due to accidental overflow of fluid from the manometer tip with possible backflow

of contaminated fluid into the system was a major risk factor.

This technique is nearly obsolete today and has been largely replaced by fluid systems attached to a transducer/amplifier/monitor system.

Fiberoptic Monitoring Systems

The miniaturization of electronics and the advancement of fiberoptic technology have allowed for monitoring systems that do not depend on principles of fluid dynamics. Instead, probes with transducers at the tip are inserted into the areas to be monitored; such as the ventricles of the brain. The signal can then be sent to a monitor by means of the fiberoptics. Compared with fluid-filled systems, they are simpler to maintain. However, their cost is higher, they cannot be passed through a catheter smaller than 18 gauge, they cannot be recalibrated once inserted, and they are very fragile. Their usage, originally in laboratory settings, is increasing for intracranial pressure monitoring.

However, with refinements in this technology, fiberoptics may eventually be used for monitoring cardiovascular pressures.

Fluid System Coupled with a Transducer/ Amplifier/Monitor

The most commonly used method for bedside measurement of cardiovascular pressures involves a fluid-filled intravascular catheter, fluid-filled connecting pressure tubing, a pressure transducer, and an electronic amplifier/monitor. The pulsatile pressures at the catheter tip are transmitted through the fluid-filled connecting tubing to the transducer diaphragm, which then converts pressure-induced motion of the transducer diaphragm into low-voltage electrical signals. These low-level signals are then amplified and conditioned by the amplifier/monitor for continuous, real-time waveform display on an oscilloscope. Pressure measurements are also continuously digitally displayed in mm Hg or torr (1 mm Hg = 1 torr) (Figure 6-1).

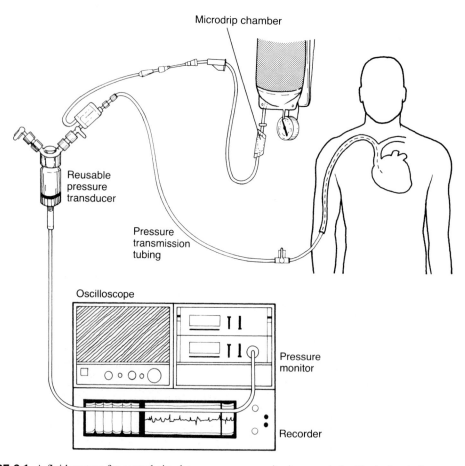

FIGURE 6-1 A fluid system for central circulatory pressure monitoring coupled with electronic instrumentation.

For the electronic fluid-filled electronic system to measure pressures accurately, the pressure signal from the patient must be transmitted through an unobstructed fluid system, and the transducer must be zeroed, leveled, and calibrated. The frequency response and damping characteristics of the system must also be optimized. These factors are discussed later in this chapter.

COMPONENTS OF THE FLUID-FILLED ELECTRONIC MONITORING SYSTEM

The basic components required for invasive pressure monitoring include the in situ catheter coupled with low-compliance extension tubing, the pressure transducer, and the amplifier/monitor. A strip chart recorder also may be used to obtain hard-copy recordings. When monitoring cardiovascular pressures, the fluid-filled components of the system are connected to an automatic flush device and inflatable pressure bag for continuous, low-volume catheter irrigation (see Figure 6-1). Each of these components is briefly explained.

Catheter and Low-Compliance Extension Tubing

A fluid-filled semirigid catheter is introduced into the body compartment to be monitored. The external end of the catheter is connected to fluid-filled semirigid connecting tubing. The enclosed fluid transfers the pressures from the in situ catheter tip to the pressure transducer. Several commercially available preassembled kits for invasive pressure monitoring contain all the necessary tubing, stopcocks, connectors, and transducer. Preassembled kits

significantly reduce setup time, reduce the margin for monitoring error by maintaining consistency of this portion of the setup, and reduce the risk of system contamination during assembly.

Pressure Transducer

A *pressure transducer* is an electromechanical device that converts applied pressure into an electrical signal.

Several types of pressure transducers are used in clinical practice. *Reusable transducers* (such as the one depicted in Figure 6-1) were the clinical rule in the past. They usually used the strain gauge and Wheatstone bridge for determination of pressures applied to the diaphragm. These transducers were easily damaged, and some were relatively large. Pretested, precalibrated, and presterilized *disposable transducers* (Figure 6-2) allow electrical isolation from the patient and are used most commonly at the present time because of their small size, durability, accuracy, and relatively low cost.

Miniaturized in situ *catheter-tip transducers* eliminate the problems of waveform and pressure distortion inherent to coupling an external transducer to the vascular or intracranial compartment via fluid-filled tubing. However, catheter-tip transducers are very expensive, and they develop baseline drift over time, which makes long-term clinical use impractical. Currently, catheter-tip transducer use is limited to research laboratories.

All transducers have a pressure-sensitive diaphragm enclosed by a fluid-filled dome. As the patient's pressure pulsations, transmitted by the fluid, physically strike the diaphragm, mechanical movement of the diaphragm is converted into an electrical signal that can then be processed and intelligibly displayed by the amplifier/monitor.

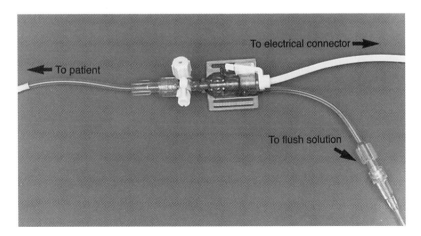

FIGURE 6-2 Disposable transducer with continuous flush device.

A final word about pressure transducers: the word "transducer" comes from the Latin *trans,* which means across, and *ducere,* which means to lead, calculate, or draw along. An alternative meaning of *ducere* is to charm, influence, or mislead. This secondary meaning should remind the clinician that all invasive monitoring information should be viewed within the context of the complete clinical situation, also taking into account the patient's history, physical assessment, and laboratory findings.

Amplifier/Monitor

The purpose of the amplifier/monitor is to take the very small electrical signal generated by the transducer and increase it to a form and an amplitude that is clinically useful, filter out unwanted signals, and then accurately reproduce and display the pressure waveform on the oscilloscope. The monitor also digitally displays the pressure measurements.

An amplifier must possess the quality of *linear response,* which means that a 1 mV signal is reproduced by the amplifier in such a way that it will consistently be 10 times the amplitude of the original signal. This is an important requirement because it ensures that, using arterial monitoring as an example, a systolic pressure of 200 mm Hg is accurately represented by a waveform that is twice the height of one that is 100 mm Hg. Thus visual trending (observed changes in waveform height) and numeric readouts can be relied on to be both accurate and reproducible. However, if the fluid-filled portion of the monitoring system is poorly set up or improperly zeroed and calibrated, the quality of linear response and accuracy of displayed measurements is limited by flaws within the system.

The amplifier/monitor also must respond rapidly and precisely to changes in pressure. Certainly, a pressure monitoring system is of little value if it takes a full minute to accurately represent a change in applied pressure from 120 mm Hg to 60 mm Hg. The shorter the time it takes for the monitoring system to respond to physiologic changes, the greater the fidelity in timing to the actual event. The monitoring systems in use today are capable of responding to pressure changes within milliseconds. This quick response characteristic means that wide and rapid changes in pressure, such as occurs with arterial pressure monitoring, are received by the system and visually displayed as a rapid rise (systole) followed by a relatively rapid decline (diastole). This nearly instantaneous response time also allows for accurate timing with other displayed physiologic events, such as myocardial depolarization and repolarization (the electrocardiogram [ECG]).

Oscilloscope and Strip Chart Recorder

The oscilloscope provides continuous, real-time viewing of the amplified pulse pressure wave. Strip chart recorders document the waveform on paper for analysis and accurate pressure measurement when there is significant movement of the baseline. Such baseline irregularities commonly occur in mechanically ventilated or dyspneic patients. Strip chart recorders vary in sophistication and versatility. Single-channel recorders are limited for waveform analysis because the pressure pulse cannot be obtained with a simultaneously recorded ECG tracing. Consequently, specific waves, such as right or left atrial *a* and *v* waves, may be impossible to identify, particularly if the patient has a rapid heart rate. Multiple-channel recorders simultaneously record ECG activity with pressure waveforms from one or multiple invasive lines so that specific components of the pressure waveforms may be identified by their relationship to PQRS and T waves (see Chapter 4).

Flush System

The flush system consists of a bag of normal saline (to which heparin may or may not be added), which is connected to the monitoring catheter via stopcocks and noncompliant (semirigid) extension tubing. The flush solution is surrounded by an inflatable pressure bag that is maintained at 300 mm Hg. Housed within the tubing, which leads from the patient to the transducer, is a continuous flush device that, if maintained at a constant pressure of 300 mm Hg, ensures a continuous flow (usually 3 to 5 ml/hr) of flush solution via a minidrip/air filter chamber through the monitoring system. Flush devices prevent clotting and backflow of blood through the vascular catheter, provide a means of intermittent and rapid manual flushing of the system, and provide a method of dynamic response (square wave) testing described later.

Although the continuous flush devices are carefully industry tested, the remote but possible chance exists that a defective flush device may allow rapid administration of intravenous (IV) fluid. Microdrip chambers provide a measure of safety against accidental patient fluid overload. However, if the flush device totally fails to limit fluid flow, the flow of flush solution will be greatly augmented by the surrounding pressure bag under 300 mm Hg pressure. Consequently, patients may receive a rapid bolus of fluid despite the use of the microdrip chamber. *Smaller bags of flush solution (150 ml or 50 ml) are recommended for some adult patients (those with oliguric renal failure, heart failure) in whom fluid overload may precipitate a hemodynamic crisis.*

PHYSICAL PRINCIPLES INVOLVED IN PRESSURE MONITORING SYSTEMS

Several important considerations related to the physical properties of fluid-filled monitoring system profoundly affect the fidelity of pressure measurement and waveform morphology. Failure of the clinician to take these considerations into account when setting up and maintaining the monitoring system may result in significant distortion of waveforms and inaccurately displayed pressure measurements. The following considerations are interrelated; however, they are explained point by point for organization and clarity. Clinically appropriate comments are included in the discussion.

Measurement of Hydrodynamic Pressure

Fluid in motion exerts *hydrodynamic pressure.* Monitored cardiovascular pressures are hydrodynamic because of the pulsatile forces initiated by ventricular systole, as well as diastolic runoff of blood.

Effect of Inertia on Hydrodynamic Pressure Monitoring

Ideally, pressure changes within the cardiovascular and central nervous systems and pressure changes within the monitoring system should be transmitted simultaneously and with equal force. However, because of inertia, the fluid column within the monitoring system cannot respond precisely in tandem with the physiologic events. As a result, the action of the fluid column lags behind and cannot respond with perfect fidelity to the pulsatile intravascular waves. This explains why, as the length of the connecting tubing is increased, the recorded hemodynamic waveforms lag farther behind the simultaneously recorded ECG on a multichannel strip chart recorder. As the patient's heart rate and associated pulsatile pressure swings increase in frequency, the fluid column becomes even less able to precisely track pressure changes. Because of the physical properties and limitations of fluid-filled monitoring systems, this lag period cannot be modified. However, by keeping the tubing length as short as possible, the lag is minimized. When properly set up, modern monitoring systems are acceptably pressure accurate. Cyclic pressures are also displayed with rapidity, and continuous realtime oscilloscope displays allow tracking of hemodynamic trends.

Effect of Natural Frequency and Frequency Response Characteristics of Biologic and Electronic Monitoring Systems

Many systems, when stimulated, oscillate (vibrate) at a characteristic frequency that is determined by their individual mass and compliance (stiffness). Examples include waves on the surface of water, string instruments, cymbals, and tuning forks. The structures of the cardiovascular system and components of the electronic monitoring system such as the pressure transducer, connecting tubing, and electronic amplifier also oscillate when stimulated. The frequency at which any structure oscillates is termed its *natural frequency.* This also is referred to as the *fundamental* or *resonant frequency.* The natural frequency (the rate of vibrations per second) decreases with increased mass and decreased stiffness. In other words, the greater the mass of an object or the more compliant (flabby) the object, the lower the natural frequency. For example, the low notes of a harp (low frequency sounds) are generated when the longer, heavier, relatively more compliant strings are plucked and vibrate at a low natural frequency. Conversely, the high notes (high-frequency sounds) are generated by plucking the shorter, thinner, more tightly stretched strings, which vibrate at a high natural frequency.

The number of oscillations is described in terms of number of cycles per second or hertz (Hz). One hertz is equal to one cycle per second. A system that oscillates 120 times per minute is equal to 2 Hz (2 cycles per second). A patient with a heart rate of 90 beats per minute can alternatively be described as having a heart rate of 1.5 Hz. Heart rate is never described in this manner in clinical practice.

Complex pulsatile waves, such as blood pressure pulses (waveforms), are composed of multiple oscillating waves of differing amplitude and frequency whose sum yields the observed waveform. The oscillating frequency of the individual component waves is termed *harmonics,* and each harmonic is a multiple of the fundamental frequency (Figure 6-3). For example, the fundamental frequency of arterial pressure waves occurring at a rate of 120 beats per minute is 2 Hz (two cycles per second), and the first five harmonics of the composite oscillating waves are 2, 4, 6, 8, and 10 Hz.

An optimal monitoring system should be able to respond equally to the varying frequency components (harmonics) contained within each pressure pulse wave and display the summated waveform accurately in shape and amplitude (Figure 6-4, *A*).

For this reason, the natural frequency of all components of the monitoring system must be greater than that of

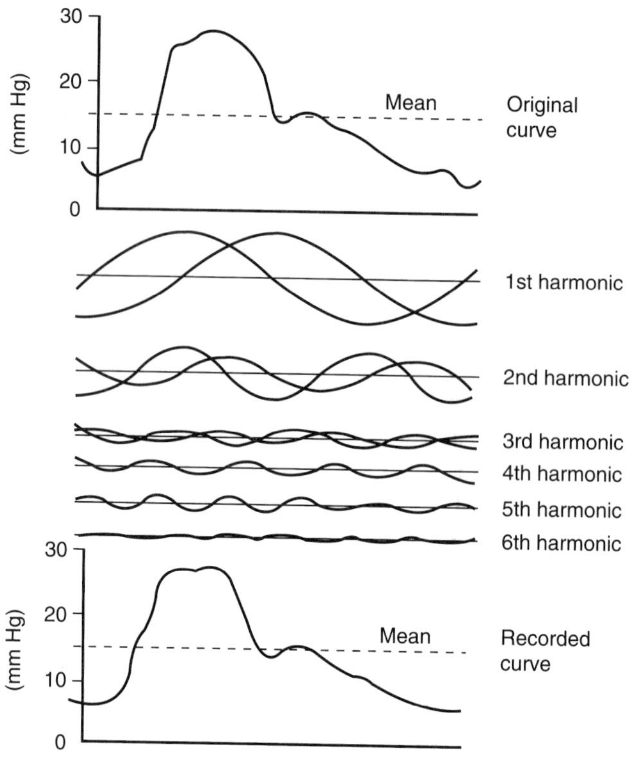

FIGURE 6-3 Frequency components of pressure waveforms. (From Waltham MA: *Guide to physiologic pressure monitoring,* 1977, Hewlett-Packard Company. Courtesy of Hewlett-Packard Company.)

the highest oscillating component (harmonic) of the pulsatile signal. Otherwise, components of the pressure wave will be either exaggerated or blunted. The following two examples illustrate the possible monitoring consequences.

Underdamping (Exaggerated Response). If the extension tubing is compliant ("flabby") and long—both of which decrease the natural frequency of the system—and the pressure waves being transmitted contain a harmonic whose frequency is *identical* to the natural frequency of the extension tubing, the tubing will vibrate more intensely. This vibration will produce an *overshoot* spike that extends over the upstroke of the pressure waveform followed by multiple, small spikes termed *ringing* on the downstroke (Figure 6-4, *B*). If the ringing is severe, negative spikes also appear on the diastolic portion of the monitored waveform and are termed *undershoot.* In the clinical setting, overshoot, undershoot, and ringing are commonly referred to as *artifacts.* The cumulative effect of these artifacts may result in an overestimation of the true systolic pressure and an underestimation of the true diastolic pressure. The presence of these artifacts may also make waveform analysis impossible.

Overdamping (Blunted Response). If the frequency response of components of a monitoring system are *less than* the specific components' frequencies of the pulsatile waveform, the amplitude of that portion of the waveform will be blunted. For example, the dicrotic notch of the aortic pressure wave contains frequencies greater than 10 Hz. If the monitoring system cannot respond to frequencies greater than 10 Hz, the dicrotic notch will be blunted and obscured (Figure 6-4, *C*).

Overall, a monitoring system with frequency response characteristics that are inadequate for those of the pressure pulses being monitored is analogous to a high-quality symphonic recording being played on an inexpensive audio system. Because of the system's inability to reproduce the highest- and lowest-frequency sounds of the recording (inadequate dynamic response range), the music lacks depth and sounds tinny. On the other hand, an audio system with a very wide dynamic frequency response range may reproduce the symphonic sound so faithfully that the depth and tonal quali' of the music is almost equal to that heard in a conc hall.

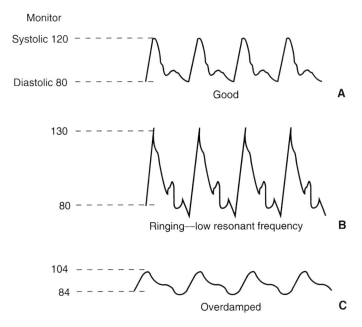

FIGURE 6-4 Normal and distorted systemic arterial waveforms. **A,** Dynamic response characteristics of the monitoring system provide good reproduction of the arterial waveform. **B,** Effects of exaggerated response because of decreased natural frequency of the fluid-filled system. Overshoot artifact results in overestimation of the true systolic pressure, and ringing artifact obscures the true waveform morphology. **C,** Damped waveform (blunted response) results in underestimation of the systolic pressure, overestimation of the diastolic pressure, and total obscuration of the dicrotic notch.

Patient and Monitoring System Factors That Affect Frequency Response

Many monitoring system characteristics and patient variables may occur in isolation or interrelate to produce inaccuracies in displayed pressures and reduce the fidelity of waveform reproduction. Monitoring system–related factors include the following:

- *The length of the pressure connecting tubing.* Excessively long tubing may reduce the natural frequency to as low as 7 Hz; this is never clinically acceptable. Under no circumstances should the length of the connecting tubing exceed 3 to 4 feet.
- *The method of application of the transducer dome (reusable transducers).* Lower frequency responses of the system result when the dome is applied without water between the diaphragm and transducer dome.
- *The presence of air bubbles in the fluid system.* Small, pinpoint air bubbles may cause a decrease in the monitoring system's natural frequency.
- *Stiffness of the extension tubing.* Soft, low-compliance tubing results in a decrease in the natural frequency of the monitoring system.
- *The intraluminal size of the vascular catheter and extension tubing.* Small-diameter intravascular catheters have a lower natural frequency than large-bore catheters.

Patient-related factors may increase the natural frequency of the pulsatile signals and thereby require higher frequency responses of the monitoring system:

- *Patients with a hyperdynamic circulation* (sepsis, aortic regurgitation, stress response) require a higher frequency response of the monitoring system, as do elderly patients with atherosclerosis and hypertension. In these patients, the high-frequency arterial pressure waves generated have a rapid rate of rise and a steep upstroke that also may appear serrated. An overshoot spike also may be noted on the arterial waveform, which will result in false-high systolic pressure measurements.
- *Tachycardia.* Increases in heart rate generate more pressure signals per minute. For example, if the patient's heart rate increases from 60 beats per minute (1 Hz or pressure signal per second) to 180 beats per minute (3 Hz or 3 pressure signals per second), the monitoring system must be capable of reproducing a minimum natural frequency of 30 Hz. If there are coexisting factors that increase the biologic signal's natural frequency, such as hypertension, frequencies up to 60 Hz may be required by the monitoring system to faithfully reproduce a tachycardic, hypertensive patient's pressure pulses.

Faithful transmission and reproduction of the pulsatile cardiovascular and intracranial pressure signals require that the components of the monitoring system have a natural frequency of *at least* 20 Hz. However, patient-related circulatory changes may increase the frequency response requirement of the monitoring system. The components of the transducer/tubing systems currently available for *clinical* use have frequency responses of approximately 40 to 50 Hz, which still may not be adequate for all clinical situations.

A higher-frequency response system may be achieved by using a short, stiff, wide-bore, in situ catheter connected to a transducer without pressure extension tubing and filled with saline. Air will not be dissolved in a boiled solution; this excludes air bubble formation and consequent decreased natural frequency following setup. Clearly, such a system is highly impractical for clinical use and also is grossly underdamped. The conclusion is that it is impossible to design and set up a "perfect" system to meet all monitoring needs. However, available monitoring systems are adequate for most clinical applications. Fiberoptic intracranial pressure monitoring systems avoid the problem of waveform distortion inherent to currently used fluid-filled systems.

In summary, a decreased natural frequency of the monitoring system or an increased natural frequency of the patient's pressure pulse may be associated with overshoot and ringing artifact in the recorded waveforms, as well as overestimation of systolic pressure and underestimation of diastolic pressure or distortion of components of pressure waveforms. The objective in assembling and maintaining the catheter-to-transducer system is to maintain the natural frequency as high as possible so that it is well removed from the natural frequency of any pulsatile signals transmitted regardless of rate or amplitude.

Effect of Damping of the Monitoring System

If a cymbal were to be struck in the absence of friction and wind resistance, it would continue to oscillate indefinitely at its natural frequency. Likewise, if the fluid-filled monitoring system were to be excited by the pressure pulse, in the absence of resistance and friction, it would forever oscillate at its natural frequency. *Damping* represents loss of the vibrating energy of the physiologic signal through frictional resistance to movement of the fluid and distortion of the plastic components of the monitoring system until the physiologic signal ultimately comes to rest. When applied to invasive pressure monitoring, damping is a function of the frictional resistance to movement of the fluid and absorption of pulsatile energy by the monitoring system's plastic components or by air bubbles.

Mechanical systems may be optimally damped, underdamped, or overdamped. To illustrate *underdamping,* banging a hammer against a noncompliant, underdamped

surface such as a metal bell transmits energy from the hammer to the bell and converts it to an amplified, high-intensity sound, which gradually diminishes over several seconds. An example of *overdamping* is placing a pillow over the bell and striking it with the hammer. This time, a brief, flat, low-intensity sound is produced because the pillow absorbs (damps) much of the energy.

Applied clinically, an *underdamped* system exaggerates systolic pressures and may display artifact. In an *overdamped* system, some of the oscillating energy of the pulsatile signal is lost through friction or buffering before having an impact on the transducer diaphragm. As a consequence, the systolic pressure measurement is underestimated, the diastolic pressure is overestimated, and the waveform appears less distinct. Components of the waveform, such as the dicrotic notch, may be obscured. An *optimally damped* system faithfully transmits the pulsatile signal in a clearly defined waveform and an accurate pressure display.

The effect of damping is especially significant in pulmonary artery pressure monitoring because these pressures are much lower than systemic arterial pressures, and there are many high-frequency components to the pressure signal. If the monitoring system is *overdamped,* the high-frequency components (such as the dicrotic notch) are not visible and the magnitude of the waveform is reduced. In such a system, the transition from pulmonary arterial to wedge waveforms may be imperceptible, digitally displayed pulmonary arterial systolic measurements may be falsely low, and accurate waveform interpretation may be difficult or impossible.

Factors That Produce Overdamping. Overdamping may be produced by several factors:

- *Distensible (compliant)* or *excessively long extension tubing* causes some of the pulsatile energy to be lost in distending the tubing with each systole.
- *Air bubbles in the circuit.* Liquids are slightly compressible, whereas air is highly compressible. If air bubbles are in the connecting tubing, stopcocks, or transducer dome, part of the energy of the pressure pulse is absorbed by the bubbles and is lost before exciting the transducer diaphragm. In other words, there is more motion at the fluid column on the patient's side of the air bubbles and less motion at the transducer side of the air bubbles. The extent of damping effect is proportional to the size, number, and location of air bubbles present. For example, large air bubbles near the transducer diaphragm cause significant overdamping. Air bubbles may result in air emboli during flushing of an arterial line.
- *Catheter diameter, length, and stiffness.* Monitoring catheters with small intraluminal diameters and long

catheters increase frictional resistance to fluid movement. Soft, compliant catheters "stretch" with each heartbeat and absorb pulsatile energy. As a result, energy of the pressure pulse being transmitted is diminished.

Factors That Produce Underdamping. Underdamping occurs when the pressure wave being transmitted contains a harmonic whose frequency is identical to the natural frequency of components of the monitoring system. In this circumstance, the high-frequency components of the patient's pulsatile waveform are transmitted with a

---

BOX 6-1
Guidelines for the Setup and Maintenance of a Reliable Monitoring System

Use as simple a system as possible. Extra stopcocks and manifolds decrease the fidelity of the monitoring system, increase the risk of fluid leak and bacterial line contamination, and are the source of air bubble collection.

Monitoring catheters should have large bores, no smaller than 18 gauge or 7 French. Monitoring catheters for pediatric use should be as large bore as possible.

All connecting tubing between the transducer and patient catheter should be of low compliance and no longer than 3 to 4 feet. IV connecting tubing is too soft and absorbs pulsatile energy. Low-compliance tubing is identified on packaging as "monitoring tubing" and is clear, difficult to compress, and stiff. The shorter tubing length needed for a patient-mounted transducer versus a pole-mounted transducer increases the fidelity of the system by increasing the natural frequency. Therefore the likelihood of overshoot and undershoot artifacts is reduced.

Use tight tubing connectors and inspect frequently for fluid leaks. Luer-Lok connections safeguard against accidental disconnection. Plastic stopcocks are preferred over metal ones because they are electrically safe and less likely to leak.

Use a continuous flush device for cardiovascular pressure monitoring. Because the pressure bags surrounding the flush solution often lose pressure, frequently check to ensure that the recommended 300 mm Hg pressure is maintained. Routine "fast flush" of the monitoring catheter may be necessary to keep the monitoring catheter patent in hypercoagulable patients such as those with acute myocardial infarction.

Carefully inspect the fluid-filled components of the system for air bubbles following setup and periodically thereafter. Air may come out of the flush solution just as dissolved air comes out of solution in a standing glass of water. Even pinpoint air bubbles affect the fidelity of the monitoring system.

Keep the connecting tubing away from areas of patient movement such as the shoulder and chest. Movement of the tubing results in movement of the fluid within the system and produces an externally induced whip artifact.

---

magnified amplitude and ringing artifact. In other words, underdamping is noted in monitoring systems with a frequency response that is inadequate for the patient's pulsatile signals. (See earlier section on monitoring and patient variables that affect frequency response.)

Guidelines for Reliable Pressure Monitoring

From the preceding discussion of the elements of frequency response and damping effects, we can appreciate that attention to detail in system setup and an understanding of the monitoring pitfalls inherent to fluid-filled systems are necessary to avoid distorted waveforms and inaccurate hemodynamic measurements.

The potential for monitoring system inaccuracies directly correlates with the complexity of the fluid-filled system. A simple system is far more likely to provide accurate information than a complex system fitted with multiple stopcocks, extension tubing, and other pieces of hardware such as adapters.

The highest natural frequency and the least amount of damping is obtained by using short, stiff catheters with an intraluminal size no smaller than 7 French or 18 gauge in adult patients. The largest possible catheters should be placed in infants and children.

Overall, the catheter-to-transducer system should be as short, simple, and direct as possible; the pressure extension tubing should be stiff, with as large an internal diameter as possible; the monitoring catheter intraluminal size should be large; air bubbles should be removed from the system at the time of setup; and the fluid-filled components of the system should be assessed for air bubbles periodically thereafter. See Box 6-1 for guidelines for the setup and maintenance of a reliable monitoring system.

DYNAMIC RESPONSE TESTING

The term *dynamic response* refers to the ability of the fluid-filled monitoring system to faithfully reproduce the patient's pressure pulse on the amplifier/monitor. Dynamic response is related to the interplay of the natural frequencies of the monitoring system and the pulsatile pressure signals, as well as the amount of damping present in the monitoring system.

The fidelity of the monitoring system and dynamic response characteristics may be tested using the *square wave test* (also termed *fast flush test* or *snap test*). This procedure, done with low-compliance, continuous flush devices, determines if the natural frequency and damping characteristics of the system faithfully represent the pressure waveform and produce accurate digital displays. The rapidly closing valve in the continuous flush device generates a response of the pressure measuring system on the oscilloscope or hard copy, which is then evaluated (Box 6-2).

BOX 6-2

Dynamic Response Testing (Square Wave, Frequency Response Testing) Using the Fast Flush System

There is an extensive literature explaining how systems may be painstakingly evaluated for their dynamic responses. In point of fact, most of these tests are really "static" in that they look at the response of the monitoring system to some laboratory-induced stimulus, in a relatively controlled research setting. Use of such tests in the clinical setting must be considered in the context of a constantly changing patient physiologic status. Exact, complex measurements of the monitoring system behavior are of questionable use in clinical situations. We recommend the following simple dynamic response testing procedure for bedside practitioners.

Optimally Damped System

When the fast flush of the continuous flush system is activated and quickly released, a sharp upstroke terminates in a flat line at the maximal indicator on the monitor and hard copy. This is then followed by an immediate rapid downstroke extending below baseline with just one or two oscillations within 0.12 second (minimal ringing) and a quick return to baseline. The patient's pressure waveform is also clearly defined with all components of the waveform, such as the dicrotic notch on an arterial waveform, clearly visible.

Square wave test configuration

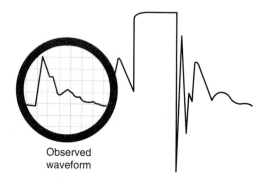

Observed waveform

Intervention

No adjustment is required in the monitoring system.

Overdamped System

The upstroke of the square wave appears somewhat slurred, the waveform does not extend below the baseline after the fast flush, and there is no ringing after the flush. The patient's waveform displays a falsely decreased systolic pressure and false-high diastolic pressure, as well as poorly defined components of the pressure tracing such as a diminished or absent dicrotic notch on arterial waveforms.

Square wave test configuration

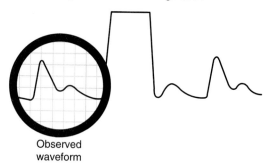

Observed waveform

Intervention

To correct for the problem:
1. Check for the presence of blood clots, blood left in the catheter following blood sampling, or air bubbles at any point from the catheter tip to the transducer diaphragm, and eliminate these as necessary.
2. Use low-compliance (rigid), short (less than 3 to 4 feet) monitoring tubing.
3. Connect all line components securely.
4. Check for kinks in the line.

Underdamped System

The waveform is characterized by numerous amplified oscillations above and below the baseline following the fast flush. The monitored pressure wave displays false-high systolic pressures (overshoot), possibly false-low diastolic pressures, and ringing artifacts on the waveform.

Square wave test configuration

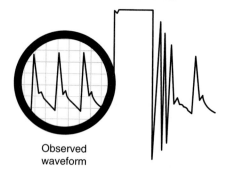

Observed waveform

Intervention

To correct the problem, remove all air bubbles (particularly pinpoint air bubbles) from the fluid system; use large-bore, shorter tubing; or use a damping device.

ORIENTATION OF THE INTRAVASCULAR CATHETER RELATIVE TO THE FLOW OF BLOOD AND CATHETER WHIP ARTIFACT

The position of an intravascular catheter tip relative to the flow of blood and pulsatile movement also affect hemodynamic pressure measurements.

Orientation of the Catheter Tip

A catheter-sensing tip that is facing into the flow of blood provides a more accurate representation of the hemodynamic pressure being generated within the vessel than one whose sensing tip is directed in the same direction as blood flow. Hemodynamic pressures measured from a catheter tip that is perpendicular to blood flow are invalid; this circumstance never occurs clinically. However, shifts in catheter-tip position or catheter movement may alter waveform morphology and obtained hemodynamic measurements.

Arterial catheters are placed with the catheter tip directed into the flow of blood (toward the patient's heart) to maximize fidelity of arterial pressure reproduction. However, an arterial catheter that is too short or too compliant may move around within the vessel (not face directly into the flow of blood), and the recorded pressure pulses will be less than the maximal amplitude. In such patients, variances in measured arterial pressure and sporadic damping of the waveform are said to be "positional." The catheter tip also may rest against the vessel wall. Repositioning of the catheter within the vessel so that the long axis of the catheter is in line with the long axis of the artery is generally associated with a return to a well-defined, well-amplified waveform.

Catheter Whip Artifact

Because of anatomic limitations, the tip of *pulmonary artery catheters* cannot be directed into the flow of blood. Rather, they are placed in the same direction as flowing pulmonary arterial blood. A problem encountered with pulmonary artery catheters (not systemic arterial catheters) is *catheter whip artifact.* This also is commonly referred to as *catheter fling* or *noise.* Because the pulmonary artery catheter tip rests in the central circulation, the force of contraction of the right ventricle, particularly in a patient with a hyperdynamic heart (sepsis, anemia, excessive circulating catecholamines) may impart pulsatile motion to the catheter. The resulting whip artifact may produce positive and negative waves superimposed on the pulmonary artery waveform in amplitudes of as high as plus or minus 10 mm Hg (Figure 6-5). This is a high-frequency artifact

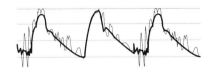

FIGURE 6-5 Pulmonary arterial waveform reproduced with fidelity *(heavy dark lines)* with whip artifact drawn superimposed on the original waveform. The digitally displayed values reflect the highest and lowest waveform excursions and consequently overestimate systolic pressure and underestimate the diastolic pressure.

and may be eliminated by incorporating a high-frequency filter or damping device into the monitoring system.

Some clinicians introduce air bubbles into the transducer system to "damp out" the whip artifact. We do *not* recommend this approach because air bubble–induced damping reduces the frequency response, distorts the waveform, and renders systolic and diastolic measurements inaccurate. More important, particularly in pediatric patients, air in the monitoring line risks accidental air embolization that may be associated with significant patient morbidity.

When confronted with the problem of whip artifact, we recommend tracking changes in *mean* pulmonary artery pressures, which are not significantly affected by the bobbing catheter.

ASSEMBLY OF THE MONITORING SYSTEM

Different institutions have slightly different protocols for monitoring system assembly. The generic procedure outlined below applies to most of the commercially available monitoring kits. However, *the manufacturer's guidelines should be reviewed before the assembly of any newly purchased system and carefully followed during assembly.* Meticulous aseptic technique should be used for all components in contact with the fluid column. If contamination or defect in any portion of the system is a possibility, that portion of the system should be replaced by a new, sterile unit.

Because use of disposable transducers predominates in clinical practice, the following description relates to the setup of a disposable transducer/flush system assembly. All the components of the pressure transducer/flush system, including the microdrip chamber with air filter, usually come packaged as a single unit.

Collect the material needed for the setup, including (a) a bag of sterile saline IV flush solution with or without heparin (dextrose is not recommended because it supports growth of gram-negative bacteria), (b) a transducer/flush system assembly with a microdrip chamber, (c) dead-ended caps, (d) an intravenous standard with a pressure transducer mount device (if institutionally used), and (e) an inflatable flush solution pressure bag.

Heparinize the saline IV bag according to institutional protocol. Heparin-induced thrombocytopenia, from even the very-low-dose heparin used in flush solutions or heparin-bonded catheters, may lead to thromboembolic events in patients who are immunologically sensitive to heparin. Concern about the risks of heparin-induced thrombocytopenia versus the risks of intravascular catheter thrombosis prompted a large-scale (5139 patients from 198 participating institutions), randomized, clinical trial that evaluated the effects of heparinized versus nonheparinized flush solutions on the patency of intraarterial pressure monitoring sites.[1] The results of the study showed that the probability for catheter patency is significantly greater over time in arterial pressure lines maintained with heparinized flush solution. Other factors known to prolong line patency include an arterial catheter longer than 2 inches, placement of the catheter in the femoral artery, and concomitant systemic administration of anticoagulant or thrombolytic agents. Female patients are suspected to be more prone to line thrombosis than male patients. Clinicians are required to weigh the risks of heparin-induced thrombocytopenia against the risk of thrombotic arterial line occlusion (which also may result in embolization to a downstream vascular site). However, *nonheparinized flush solutions should be used in patients with known heparin sensitivity.*

Open the IV bag and squeeze all of the air out of the bag. Spike the bag and gravity fill the transducer/flush system until it is completely free of air. Rapid flushing with the saline solution pressurized by the inflatable bag is associated with turbulent flow that may result in the entry of excessive air bubbles into the system; these can be difficult and time consuming to remove. All components of the transducer/flush system should be carefully inspected to ensure that all air bubbles are cleared from the system before zeroing, calibration, and connection to the patient. Air bubbles clinging to the walls of the transducer or tubing may be mobilized by tapping the involved area. Because air rises, the mobilized bubbles are then cleared with the flush solution by holding the exit port at a level higher than any other part of the flush/transducer system.

Place the bag of flush saline solution in the inflatable pressure bag and pump the pressure bag up to 300 mm Hg. Place the transducer on its mount and position the venting port level with the patient's midchest.

After the monitoring system has had sufficient warm-up time (5 to 15 minutes), zero and calibrate the transducer/ amplifier/monitor assembly according to the manufacturer's monitoring system protocol.

Close the system and double check that all connections are secure and that no air bubbles are present. Sterility of all ports must be protected by sterile deadheads.

Connect the fluid-filled system to the patient's in situ catheter. At the time of setup, count and confirm that the flush rate is 3 to 6 minidrops per minute and periodically check that the inflatable bag is pressurized at 300 mm Hg. A rate greater than 3 to 6 minidrops per minute indicates that the flow system may be defective and the patient may be accidentally volume loaded. On the other hand, less than 3 to 6 minidrops per minute may result in catheter thrombosis.

PATIENT POSITION FOR ZERO REFERENCING AND PRESSURE MONITORING

The hemodynamic values that we regard as "normal," against which patients' measurements are judged, were obtained from supine, healthy humans. Therefore the supine position is considered the standard position for pressure measurement. Raising or lowering the patient's head and thorax affects measured pressures because of the effects of gravity on blood flow and intravascular pressure. However, head and thorax elevations up to 30 to 40 degrees are generally not associated with a change from supine measurements.

Many patients cannot tolerate the supine or 40-degree elevated position for even the few minutes it takes to record central circulatory pressures. Such patients (those with severe congestive heart failure, acute respiratory failure) should not be lowered to the supine position to obtain hemodynamic pressure measurements. In these special circumstances, consideration that head or trunk elevated measurements may be less than those recorded from the supine position is important when making clinical judgments. The important point, however, is that evaluating *trends* in measured pressures over time as they relate to the patient's clinical presentation is the focus of meaningful clinical and hemodynamic evaluation. If the patient's condition requires a change in position from that in which hemodynamic pressures were previously measured, the time and degree of positional change should be noted on the flow sheet and also should be mentioned when verbally communicating pressure measurements. The difference between hemodynamic measurements obtained in the supine versus backrest elevated position should also be noted and recorded on the flow sheet at the time of the position change.

ZERO REFERENCING

The transducer/monitor system must be given a zero reference point to establish a standard, neutral level for all measured pressures. This procedure eliminates the effects of atmospheric and hydrostatic pressure from the measured pressure readings. *The establishment of a zero reference point is an extremely important monitoring technique that should be performed at the time of setup, during each shift, or at any time that the validity of the monitored values is in question.* Errors in zero referencing may make clinically significant differences in all measured pressures. This is particularly true of central circulatory pressures (right atrium [RA] pressure, pulmonary artery [PA] pressure, pulmonary artery wedge pressure) and intracranial pressures because the normal range of these pressures is very narrow. Zero referencing *must always* be done by opening the stopcock that is aligned with the patient's reference level appropriate to the specific type of monitoring (see Leveling, later in this chapter).

Eliminating the Effects of Atmospheric Pressure

The ocean of air that surrounds our planet has a weight that exerts its force (pressure) on any object on the earth's surface. This is termed *atmospheric pressure* and is equal to 760 mm Hg (torr) at sea level. In obtaining physiologic pressure measurements, the values are not affected by atmospheric pressure because the monitor's display is set to read "zero" while the transducer diaphragm is exposed to atmosphere. In other words, by programming the monitoring system to read "zero" when opening the system to air, the effects of atmospheric pressure are eliminated from the patient's physiologic pressures.

Eliminating the Effects of Hydrostatic Pressure

The liquid that fills the connecting tubing and monitoring catheter also has weight. If the force of the liquid's weight is applied to the transducer diaphragm or water manometer, a pressure that is proportional to the height of the fluid column is added to the hemodynamic measurement. The term *hydrostatic pressure head* is the pressure exerted on the transducer diaphragm due to its position relative to the catheter tip (see also Leveling). For example, if a transducer is positioned *below* the catheter tip, gravity-directed flow and the pressure head will be transmitted from the monitored site to the transducer diaphragm. For every inch the transducer is below the catheter tip, the *positive* hydrostatic pressure head produces a measured value approximately 2 mm Hg greater than the true physiologic value. In Figure 6-6, *A*, the true pressure is assumed to be zero.

If, on the other hand, a transducer is positioned *above* the reference level of the catheter tip, gravity-directed flow and the pressure head will be directed from the transducer diaphragm to the catheter. For every inch that the transducer is above the catheter tip, the *negative* hydrostatic pressure head produces a measured value approximately 2 mm Hg less than the true physiologic pressure (Figure 6-6, *B*).

When the zero reference point and catheter tip are at the same vertical level, the physiologic measurements will not be contaminated by positive or negative hydrostatic pressure heads (Figure 6-6, *C*).

In clinical practice, this principle is illustrated when lowering a bag of IV solution to check intravenous catheter patency. With the bag lowered, the negative pressure head at the dependent IV bag means that fluid will flow from the patient to the solution bag (from higher to lower pressure) and the characteristic streak of blood backing up into the tubing will be observed. When the IV solution is placed back on the IV pole, above the level of the IV catheter, the positive pressure head at the IV bag ensures that solution will flow into the patient.

When the transducer is leveled (see below) to the proposed catheter-tip site, the effects of the positive or negative pressure head are essentially eliminated. The transducer still must be zeroed to atmosphere, however.

When setting up a monitoring system using method 2 (see Leveling a Pressure Transducer for Hemodynamic Pressure Measurements, later in this chapter), the effect of the positive or negative pressure head and atmosphere pressure is eliminated by zero referencing.

LEVELING

Because the catheter tip to pressure measurement device is fluid filled, the vertical distance from the midchest to the measuring device exerts a hydrostatic pressure against the transducer diaphragm or water manometer that may add to or subtract from the actual cardiovascular pressure. All circulatory pressure measurements are referenced to the midchest position, also termed the *phlebostatic axis* (one half of the patient's anteroposterior diameter), below the sternal angle[2,3] (Figure 6-7). The midchest position was chosen because fluoroscopic examination using a cross-table lateral projection has shown that the left ventricle and aorta are usually located midway between the sternum and the top of the mattress (with the patient supine).[2] In most cases the tips of the catheters placed for pressure monitoring of the central circulation are approximately at this level. A study has also radiographically documented that in the majority of patients, the pulmonary artery catheter tip is located at the midchest area.[4]

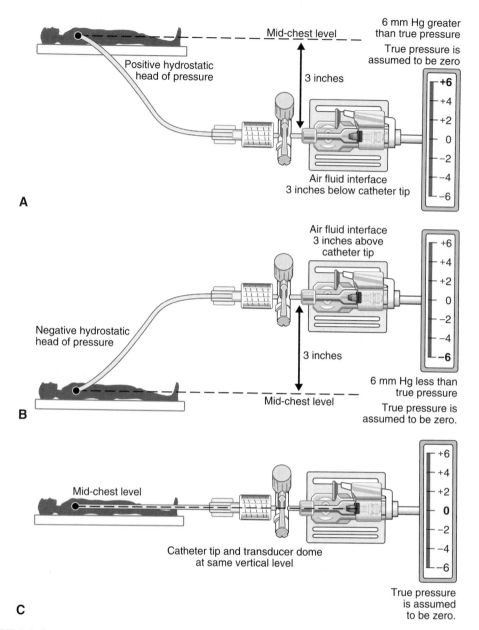

FIGURE 6-6 A, Pressure transducer positioned 3 inches below the in situ catheter tip. **B,** Pressure transducer positioned 3 inches above the in situ catheter tip. **C,** Pressure transducer positioned at the same vertical level as the in situ catheter tip.

Once the midchest point is identified, it should be marked with an ink pen or felt-tipped marker so that all clinicians have the same external reference. Precise location of the catheter tip correlated with an area on the patient's chest wall is impossible. However, the midchest area constitutes a "leap of faith" based on the probability that the catheter tip is at that level. *The important clinical point is that absolute consistency in all aspects of pressure measurement, such as the midchest reference point, be maintained from shift to shift and from clinician to clinician.* This allows meaningful tracking of *changes* in the patient's condition without distortion introduced by shift-to-shift and clinician-to-clinician variability in pressure measurement technique.

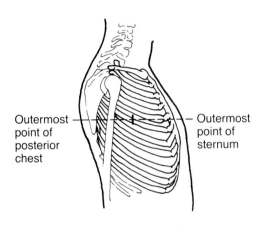

FIGURE 6-7 Midchest reference point for monitoring circulatory pressures. This is a point midway between the outermost portion of the anterior and posterior surfaces of the chest and under the sternal angle of Louis.

Leveling a Pressure Transducer for Hemodynamic Pressure Measurements

There are two methods for zeroing a pressure transducer to eliminate the hydrostatic pressure effect induced by the vertical difference in catheter tip to transducer diaphragm position.

Method One

In the first method, the transducer stopcock, which is connected to the extension tubing, is leveled to the midchest level with the transducer diaphragm closed to the patient and open to the atmosphere. The monitor display is then zeroed (Figure 6-8, *A*).

In the case of a small, disposable transducer, the transducer may be taped to the patient's thorax at the midchest level as long as pressures are recorded with the patient lying on his or her back. The pressure transducer also may be secured to an IV standard at the midchest level using a yardstick to which a carpenter's level has been taped. One end of the yardstick is placed at the inked-in area on the patient's midchest and the other end of the yardstick at the appropriate transducer stopcock. The transducer also may be placed on the mattress and elevated to the midchest position by rolled towels or an inverted basin.

Method Two

In the second method, the transducer may be placed at any vertical level relative to the patient's chest (Figure 6-8, *B*). However, a stopcock located between the in situ catheter and the transducer is leveled and fixed at the patient's midchest and is closed to the patient and opened to the atmosphere. By then adjusting the monitor to register zero pressure, any positive or negative hydrostatic pressure difference between the transducer diaphragm and the open stopcock is compensated for electrically.

Choice of Method

With either method, the vertical transducer level relative to the midchest zero reference point cannot be changed without rezeroing the transducer. However, it is our *strong* recommendation that the first method be used consistently throughout all critical care units for the following reasons:

1. The increased length of tubing and the addition of a stopcock to the fluid-filled system (required for the second method) may impair the dynamic response characteristics and decrease the natural frequency response of the monitoring system.
2. In the second method, changes in the height of the patient's bed (or short clinician versus tall clinician) relative to a transducer fixed to an IV standard may not be easy to spot. For example, if the patient's bed is raised 15 cm so that a tall technician can obtain an ECG, the measured pressures will increase by 10 mm Hg. The patient then may receive inappropriate therapy for a monitoring system change. It is much easier to "eyeball" and spot changes in transducer position if the vertical relationship is always fixed at the midchest level.
3. The concept of the first method is easier to understand than the concept of the second. Where confusion reigns, errors in system setup and pressure measurements are much more likely to occur.

Either method chosen for zeroing the pressure transducer should be followed in all critical care areas of the hospital to avoid errors in monitoring system setups or measurements of hemodynamic values when critical care personnel are rotated or when they "float."

Procedure for Zero Referencing

1. Allow the monitoring system and transducer sufficient time to warm up (approximately 5 to 15 minutes).
2. Check to see that the fluid-filled components of the system are free of air.
3. Arrange the stopcocks so that pressure from the patient is turned off and the fluid in the transducer is exposed to atmosphere. The digital and monitor displays should both read 0 mm Hg. If they do not, follow the manufacturer's instructions and adjust the zeroing mechanism to achieve a measurement of 0 mm Hg. Failure to zero also may be due to a defect in the transducer, monitoring cable, or monitor console.
4. When properly zeroed, close the stopcock that exposes the transducer to air and open the line to the patient. Check again to see that the system is air free.

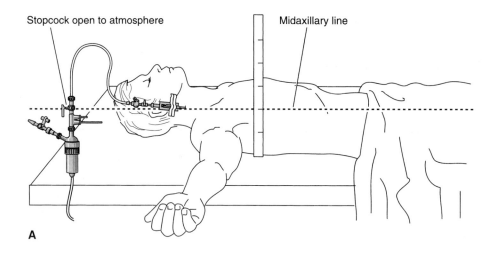

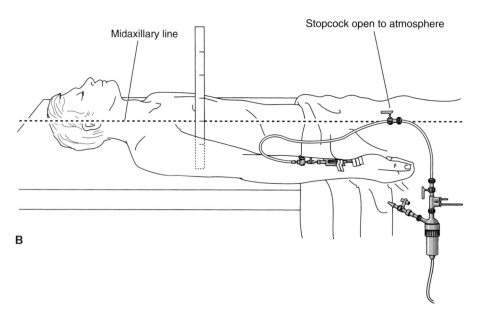

FIGURE 6-8 A, The air-fluid interface in the pressure transducer stopcock is placed at the midchest level and the transducer is then zeroed. Note that changes in the transducer-midchest vertical relationship are easy to spot. **B,** The stopcock at the end of the indwelling catheter is opened to air for zeroing and placed at the midchest level. The transducer may be placed at any level because the effects of hydrostatic pressure on the transducer diaphragm are eliminated when the monitor is zero balanced. (From Gardner RM, Hollingsworth KW: Optimizing the electrocardiogram and pressure monitoring, *Crit Care Med* 14:651, 1986.)

Problem of Drift from the Zero Reference Point

The monitoring system should be rezeroed periodically (every 8 hours, whenever pressure measurements are in question) during use because transducer drift from the zero reference point occurs over time. The main factors causing transducer drift are (1) temperature effects on the transducer (temperature changes of 10° C usually change the monitored pressure by about 1 mm Hg)[5] and (2) the effects of transducer domes that contain diaphragms. Drifts of 15 mm Hg over 3 hours have been reported.[6] Loosening of the transducer dome may cause 80 mm Hg negative drift.[7]

Because drift may cause significant inaccuracy of values, which may lead to inappropriate therapies (especially when low pressures such as central circulatory pressures are being measured), systems should be rezeroed at frequent intervals.

Overall, when zeroing the monitoring system, and at all times while hemodynamic pressure monitoring is in process, the appropriate transducer or extension tubing stopcock *must* be leveled to the midchest. Furthermore, the PA waveform should be continuously transduced for early identification of spontaneous wedging or backward slippage of the PA catheter into the right ventricle. An exception is the few minutes required to obtain right atrial pressure if a single transducer is used for PA and RA pressure monitoring.

MONITOR AND TRANSDUCER CALIBRATION

Monitor Calibration

The need and technique for monitor calibration varies by manufacturer and model. Manufacturer recommendations should be meticulously followed. Some monitoring systems have a calibration button that, when activated, feeds a known electrical signal into the amplifier just as though that signal had come from the transducer. By observing the output display and the numeric readout on the monitor, the clinician is able to tell if the signal rises to the appropriate pressure level and then falls back to zero at the end of the test. When monitoring pressures in the 0 to 300 mm Hg range (systemic arterial pressure monitoring), set the sensitivity control to 200; when monitoring pressure in the 0 to 60 mm Hg range (PA pressure, CVP), set the sensitivity control to 40. Set the sensitivity control to 60 if the patient has pulmonary hypertension. Performing this test indicates only that the electronics of the system are functioning as designed, but performance does *not* correct for any disturbances in the remainder of the system.

Transducer Calibration

Reusable pressure transducers are industry tested and standardized to a fixed sensitivity. Although they are usually reliable, reusable transducers may lose pressure sensitivity and accuracy over time, usually because of damage of the pressure-sensitive diaphragm or cable. Therefore, if there is question regarding the reliability of the transducer (after performing appropriate checks), it should be replaced.

CONCLUSION

"User beware" of blind faith in expensive, high-technology monitors. Relative accuracy of displayed data is not ensured unless the entire system is meticulously set up, zero balanced, leveled, and calibrated (Table 6-1). The least accurate measurement tends to be systolic pressure (systemic and pulmonary arterial) because it is most affected

---

TABLE 6-1
Troubleshooting Pressure Monitoring Systems

Problems	Possible Causes/Solutions
No waveform	Check power supply.
	Check the pressure range setting on the monitoring equipment.
	Check zero reference and calibration of the equipment.
	Check for loose connection in the pressure-monitoring line.
	Check to be certain that stopcocks are not turned off to the patient.
	Be certain that the connecting tubing is not kinked or compressed. It is possible that the catheter is occluded or has moved out of the vessel. If this is suspected, try to aspirate blood from the line.
	NOTE: Fast flushing the line may dislodge a loose clot and cause distal embolization.
	Never use a syringe to aggressively flush any hemodynamic monitoring line.
Artifact	Check for electrical interference.
	Check for patient movement.
	Catheter whip may be the problem (pulmonary artery catheters).
	Do dynamic response test to determine underdamping.
	Use alternative method of measurement when possible, such as cuff arterial blood pressure monitoring.
Waveform drifting	Temperature change of IV solution (new flush bag hung) or environmental temperature change.
	Rezero the system.

Continued

TABLE 6-1

Troubleshooting Pressure Monitoring Systems—cont'd

Problems	Possible Causes/Solutions
Unable to flush line with the continuous flush system	Check stopcocks and tubing for kinks.
	Check to see that the pressure bag is inflated to the appropriate level.
	Reposition catheter to move it away from vessel walls or to remove catheter kinks.
	Aspirate with a syringe (do not apply excessive force to aspirate).
Reading too high	Check zero and calibration.
	Check to see if the transducer is located at the midchest level.
	Check stopcocks and make certain they are open to the patient.
	Check flow rate of the automatic flush device (flow too fast). The standard flush device delivers 3 microdrops/min.
	Check for underdamping of the system. If due to overshoot or undershoot artifact, track mean pressures.
Reading too low	Check to see if the transducer is located at the midchest level.
	Check for loose connections and leaks.
	Check for air bubbles.
	Rezero and calibrate.
Overdamped waveform	Check for air bubbles in the system.
	Check for kinks in the tubing.
	Check for blood in the system.
	Suspect possible occlusion at the catheter tip (i.e., thrombus), or the catheter tip may be resting against the vessel wall. NOTE: A term sometimes used for this phenomenon is *high-pressure damping.* This refers to a baseline that elevates and remains elevated—usually at the upper limit of the pressure monitoring range. This is invariably caused by either an electrical failure of the monitor/amplifier or by total occlusion at some point in the fluid-filled line. Check stopcocks, tubing, and catheter patency.

by electronic filters that manufacturers add to equipment and it is the measured value most subject to artifact.

Technical and patient factors also must be investigated when waveforms or digitally displayed data are suspect. Even the most scrupulously set up monitoring system may give grossly inaccurate information, for example, if the pressure transducer monitoring blood pressure accidentally falls off the bed or if the transducer holder slips down the IV pole. In these cases, vasodilator therapy initiated to treat a "hypertensive crisis" without first investigating all possible patient and nonpatient causes may lead to a therapeutic tragedy. On the other hand, grossly damped arterial waveforms noted on patients showing clinical evidence of shock indicate an emergent situation, rather than a monitoring problem.

GLOSSARY

Physics Terminology for Fluid-Filled Systems

Artifact (noise)—False signals superimposed on the true signal. Artifacts may be due to inadequate dynamic response characteristics of the monitoring system or movement of the monitoring extension tubing or in situ catheter.

Calibration—The introduction of a selected pressure to the amplifier/monitor or transducer to verify faithful reproduction of the pressure signal.

Catheter whip (noise, fling, artifact)—Movement of the catheter tip within the circulation in response to pulsatile blood flow. As a consequence of this whipping movement, artifact is superimposed on the pressure waveform.

Damping—Loss of the energy and vibrations within the monitoring system due to frictional resistance to movement of the pressure signal line obstruction by air bubbles or clots and/or absorption of the pulsatile energy by the monitoring system plastics.

Dynamic response—The monitoring system's ability to measure physiologic pressure changes. Dynamic response relates to the natural frequency and damping characteristics of the in situ catheter/extension tubing/transducer system.

Fidelity—An indication of the pressure monitoring system's capacity to faithfully reproduce the pressure signal. For example, a high-fidelity system faithfully reproduces the original pressure wave/measurement, whereas a poor-fidelity system fails to accurately reproduce the pressure wave and hemodynamic measurements.

Hydrodynamic pressure—The pressure produced by fluid in motion.

Hydrostatic pressure—The pressure exerted by a stationary fluid column.

Natural frequency (resonant frequency, fundamental frequency)—The frequency at which the in situ catheter and monitoring "plumbing" vibrate when stimulated by pulsatile signals. This is measured in cycles per second, or hertz; one hertz is equal to one cycle per second. For example, when a tuning fork is struck, it resonates (vibrates, oscillates) at a particular frequency determined by its material, size, and shape.

Overshoot/undershoot—Monitoring system vibration that occurs when the patient's pressure wave contains a component frequency equal to the monitoring system's natural frequency. The upstroke of the pressure waveform is exaggerated and appears "spiked," and the downstroke is likewise exaggerated and spiked.

Ringing—Multiple, small spikes on the pressure waveform due to an inadequate dynamic response characteristic of a component of the "plumbing" system. This artifact usually results in false-high systolic pressure measurements and low diastolic pressure measurements.

Zeroing—A procedure performed to eliminate the effects of atmospheric and hydrostatic pressure from the measured physiologic reading. The zero reference point is taken at midchest level for cardiovascular pressure measurements.

REFERENCES

1. Evaluation of the effects of heparinized and non-heparinized flush solutions on the patency of arterial pressure monitoring lines: the AACN Thunder Project, *Am J Crit Care* 2(1):3, 1993.

2. Lambert CR, Pepine CJ, Nichols WW: Pressure measurement. In Pepine CJ, Hill JA, Lambert CR, editors: *Diagnostic and therapeutic cardiac catheterization,* Baltimore, 1989, Williams & Wilkins.

3. Grossman W: Pressure measurement. In Grossman W, Baim DS, editors: *Cardiac catheterization, angiography and intervention,* ed 4, Philadelphia, 1991, Lea & Febiger.

4. Kronberg GM, Quan SF, Schlobohm RM, et al: Anatomic location of the tips of pulmonary artery catheters in supine patients, *Anesthesiology* 51:467, 1979.

5. Disposable pressure transducers—evaluation, *Health Devices* 13:268, 1984.

6. Gordon VL, Welch JP, Carley D, et al: Zero stability of disposable and reusable pressure transducers, *Med Instrum* 21:87, 1987.

7. Sisko F, Hagerdal M, Neufeld GR: Artifactual hypotension without damping, a hazard of disposable diaphragm domes, *Anesthesiology* 51:263, 1979.

SUGGESTED READINGS

Carroll GC: Blood pressure monitoring, *Crit Care Clin* 4(3):411, 1988.

Geddes LA, Bourland JD: Technical note: estimation of the damping coefficient of fluid-filled, catheter-transducer pressure-measuring systems, *J Clin Engineer* 13(1), 1988.

Kiyoshi M, Koepchen HP, Polosa C: *Mechanisms of blood pressure waves,* Tokyo, 1984, Japan Scientific Societies Press.

Loeb R: Intravascular pressure monitoring systems. In Lake CL, editor: *Clinical monitoring,* Philadelphia, 1994, W.B. Saunders.

Marini JJ, Wheeler AP: Hemodynamic monitoring. In *Critical care medicine—the essentials,* Baltimore, 1989, Williams & Wilkins.

Milnor W: *Hemodynamics,* ed 2, Baltimore, 1989, Williams & Wilkins.

7

GLORIA OBLOUK DAROVIC

Arterial Pressure Monitoring

Reverend Stephen Hales performed the first measurement of arterial pressure when he cannulated a mare's artery with a goose quill connected to a length of goose trachea. This, in turn, was connected to an 8-foot glass column manometer. Performed in 1731, this creative although awkward technique clearly had no practical clinical application. In 1896, Riva-Rocci proposed using a sphygmomanometer along with palpation for noninvasive blood pressure measurement. In 1905 Korotkoff proposed the auscultatory method. Although these techniques were simple, safe, and reasonably accurate, the medical community was initially reluctant to adopt routine blood pressure monitoring. However, by 1930, measurement of blood pressure became a clinical standard for evaluation of the cardiovascular system.

The electronics revolution in the late 1960s ushered in a new era of sophisticated monitoring technology. Electromechanical devices, developed for clinical practice, allowed application of continuous intraarterial pressure monitoring for hemodynamic assessment and management of critically ill and injured patients. Today, the goose quill has been replaced by intraarterial catheters, the goose trachea has been replaced by low-compliance plastic tubing, and the glass column manometer has been replaced by electromechanical pressure transducers connected to electronic amplifiers and display systems.

This chapter first defines systemic arterial pressure and the factors affecting measured values at various points within the arterial circulation. The underlying principles, measurement techniques, and advantages and drawbacks for both indirect and direct blood pressure measurements are then discussed. The components of the pulse-pressure (arterial) wave are described, as are anticipated changes in waveform morphology with hemodynamic abnormalities. Insertion protocol, catheter maintenance, and the hazards and complications of direct arterial pressure measurement are then discussed. Finally, comparisons are made between direct and indirect monitoring techniques, and the settings in which each technique is best applied are defined.

DEFINITION OF ARTERIAL PRESSURE

Blood flows through the arteries under tremendous force. Blood pressure is a measure of this force as it is exerted on the arterial walls by the blood contained within the arterial system. Blood pressure is the result of the pressure generated by the beating heart and resistance to blood flow through the arteries (see Chapter 4). Blood flow and pressure are pulsatile in character, representing systolic and diastolic activity. Normal pressure values for an adult range from 100 to 130 mm Hg systolic and 60 to 90 mm Hg diastolic when recorded at heart level. These figures represent the height that a column of mercury is pushed by the pressure of blood at the point in the arterial system where pressure is being measured. Arterial pressure measurements in the critical care setting are useful for screening and assessment of trends as they relate to cardiovascular function. For this reason, *it is important to know the patient's preillness blood pressure to properly assess and manage the individual whose baseline blood pressure is not within the "normal" range.*

Blood pressure is not the same at all points in the arterial system. There are two reasons for these differences:

1. *Arterial* pressure progressively increases downward from heart level and progressively decreases upward from heart level because of the effects of gravity on blood flow. Differences are most pronounced when a person is standing up (see Chapter 4, Figure 4-23), and arterial pressures are most homogeneous throughout the body when a person is supine. Blood pressure is, however, the same at all points at the same vertical level such as at both feet, the hips, and the shoulders in an upright person. This remains true whether the blood pressure is obtained by indirect or direct blood pressure monitoring techniques. Consequently, a standard reference level must be used for blood pressure measurements. *The standard reference level, for all anatomic sites used to obtain blood pressure measurements using any technique, is heart level.*

2. The *systolic* blood pressure becomes progressively higher toward the distal peripheral arteries as compared with pressure measured in the thoracic aorta. The left ventricle ejects blood and a pressure wave precedes the actual flow of blood and is reflected back from the small, tapering, distal arterioles to produce a wave that is added to the oncoming original wave in the peripheral vessels. This is described in greater detail later in this chapter under characteristics of the arterial waveform.

The important clinical point is that central circulatory aortic pressures are the most significant in the critical care setting because aortic root pressures determine the force at which blood is driven through the cerebral and coronary circulations and determine left ventricular afterload. Unfortunately, true aortic root systolic and diastolic pressures cannot be estimated using measurements obtained from a cannulated or "cuffed" peripheral artery. Generally, the only available clinical option is to track mean arterial pressure or, when indicated and available, to use the transduced tip of an intraaortic balloon catheter for central aortic systolic, diastolic, and mean pressure measurements.

Mean Arterial Pressure

This measurement indicates the average driving force in the arterial system throughout the cardiac cycle. However, the arithmetic mean (midpoint between systolic and diastolic pressure) is not a valid means of determining mean arterial pressure. It is common to approximate the mean pressure by the formula illustrated in Chapter 4. This formula also is usually invalid because it assumes diastole is two thirds of the cardiac cycle, which occurs at a heart rate of 60 beats per minute. A fixed heart rate of 60 beats per minute is not a clinical reality, and most intensive care unit (ICU) patients maintain heart rates greater than 100 beats per minute.

There is no quick, easy, and accurate means of determining mean arterial pressure when monitoring blood pressure by manual cuff technique. However, currently manufactured noninvasive automated systems display systolic, diastolic, and mean values. When blood pressure is monitored invasively, computer circuits in pressure monitoring systems make precise running calculations of mean arterial pressure by taking into account the systolic and diastolic pressures and the area under the arterial pressure curve (Figure 7-1). The digitally displayed value is derived from data averaged over several cardiac cycles.

When available, the mean arterial pressure should be used in hemodynamic assessment and therapeutic decision making for four reasons: (1) mean pressures are essentially the same in all parts of the arterial tree; (2) pulmonary and systemic vascular resistances are derived from mean pressure; (3) mean pressure is not significantly affected by overshoot artifact (ringing), due to poor damping and frequency response characteristics of the monitoring system; and (4) mean arterial pressures approximate the pressure within the vital systemic and cerebral capillary beds.

CLINICAL CAVEATS FOR ALL TYPES OF ARTERIAL PRESSURE MEASUREMENTS

1. Any time blood pressure measurements are suspicious (suddenly too high, too low, or inappropriate to the patient's condition), first evaluate the patient to be sure there is not a sudden change in his or her condition.

2. After it has been determined that the patient is stable, readjust the cuff and attempt pressure measurements on different limbs and different instruments. Remember that cuffs and hoses may develop leaks and that pressure release mechanisms, aneroid gauges, and automated systems may become defective and display errors in pressure measurement.

3. Never become so preoccupied with equipment setup or problems that the patient is ignored.

4. In both indirect and direct techniques, the limb used for pressure measurement must be at heart level. Higher than true pressure is recorded if the arm is lower than heart level (a common occurrence when blood pressures are taken with the patient sitting with the arm relaxed at his or her side). Values are falsely low if the arm is held above heart level.

INDIRECT METHODS OF MEASURING BLOOD PRESSURE

Indirect blood pressure measurement techniques are *noninvasive* and depend on blood *flow* within the body part used for pressure measurement. When compression on an extremity is gradually released and return to blood flow is detected by a return to pulses or Korotkoff sounds, a correlation of intraarterial pressure with the externally applied cuff pressure is assumed.

Two basic methods are used for noninvasive blood pressure monitoring: manual and automated methods. *Manual techniques* include auscultation, palpation, auscultation assisted with a handheld Doppler device, manometer oscillation observation, and photoelectric devices. *Automatic systems* include oscillometry, infrasonde, ultrasonic (Doppler) determination of axial flow, and arterial tonometry.

Manual Methods

Generally, indirect "cuff" measurements obtained by various techniques coincide, but *systolic* values may be up to 20 mm Hg *lower* than the directly measured "arterial line" pressures. Conversely, *diastolic* pressures measured by cuff are generally *higher* than arterial line pressures.

Auscultation

The most common method of measuring blood pressure is the auscultatory (Riva-Rocci) method employing a sphygmomanometer and a stethoscope.

Principle. Pulsatile blood flow through major, unobstructed arteries is largely streamline. Therefore the sound of blood flow is inaudible by a stethoscope. However, the pulsatile, turbulent flow through an externally com-pressed artery creates vibrations and low-frequency sounds (termed *Korotkoff sounds*) between systole and diastole that are audible with a stethoscope. This method depends on adequate pulsatile flow to produce vascular vibrations associated with sounds within the range of human hearing.

Technique. All air should be removed from the cuff before it is applied. Instruct the patient to remain quiet and not move his or her arm or hand during the procedure. The cuff is then wrapped snugly around an extremity; for an adult, "snug" means tight enough to allow only one finger to slip under the cuff. The cuff should be applied so that an inflatable bladder, located within the cuff, lies directly over a superficial artery. If the systolic pressure is unknown, the pulse immediately distal to the cuff is then palpated. This is usually the brachial artery, but in extremely obese or edematous patients the radial artery may have to be used. The cuff is then inflated to a pressure approximately 30 mm Hg greater than that in which the palpated pulse is noted to disappear or that of the expected systolic pressure if blood pressure measurements have recently been taken. The bell or diaphragm of a stethoscope is then placed over the artery. When properly positioned, inflation of the cuff air bladder compresses the underlying artery against bone, and there is no blood flow and no sound (Figure 7-2).

The cuff is slowly deflated at approximately 3 mm Hg per second. Too-rapid cuff deflation tends to underestimate systolic pressure and either overestimates or

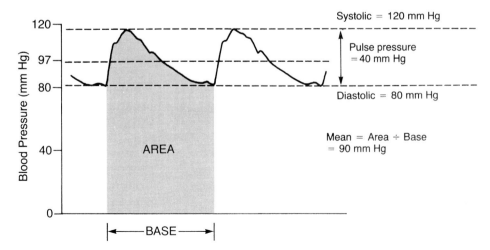

FIGURE 7-1 Determination of mean arterial pressure. If the arterial waveform were perfectly symmetric, the arithmetic mean pressure would represent the average perfusion pressure. However, the waveform is not symmetric; systole and diastole occupy variable percentages of the cardiac cycle relative to heart rate. Mean pressure is computer derived by dividing the vertical area by the horizontal base.

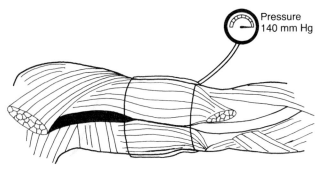

FIGURE 7-2 Artery is occluded by cuff pressure.

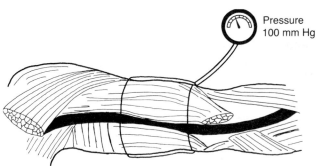

FIGURE 7-4 Vascular compression continues; vascular vibrations are louder.

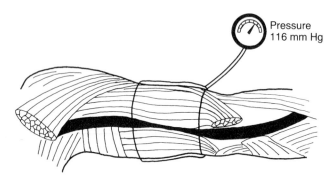

FIGURE 7-3 Beginning turbulent blood flow in the partially occluded artery is associated with audible vascular vibrations (systole).

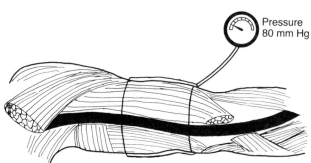

FIGURE 7-5 The artery is fully open. Streamlined blood flow is inaudible.

underestimates diastolic pressure because the onset of the Korotkoff sounds is difficult to correlate with the level of a rapidly falling mercury column or aneroid pressure gauge needle. This margin of error is increased in patients with bradycardia or irregular heart rhythms. On the other hand, too-slow deflation or reinflation before the cuff is fully deflated (to double-check the systolic reading) results in venous congestion and muffling of the Korotkoff sounds near the diastolic level.

The gradual reduction in externally applied pressure eventually permits the first spurts of turbulent blood flow through the mechanically deformed vessel under the cuff. If stroke volume and vascular tone are normal, the associated vascular vibrations are detected as clear, tapping Korotkoff sounds that correlate with systolic pressure (Figure 7-3).

As the external pressure on the artery is progressively decreased, more flow occurs and audible Korotkoff sounds continue within the deformed vessel. During this progressive decompression phase, the character of the sounds progresses to louder "popping" noises (Figure 7-4). As the pressure immediately approaches the diastolic value, Korotkoff sounds become muffled. When the vessel fully

opens, blood flow once again is streamlined and the Korotkoff sounds disappear (Figure 7-5).

Controversy still exists about whether to measure the diastolic value at the muffling or disappearance of sound. Muffled Korotkoff sounds may occur at very low diastolic levels in people with hyperdynamic circulations (high stroke volume and low systemic vascular resistance). This phenomenon may be noted in children, healthy young adults, patients with systemic arteriovenous shunts (as in the case of cirrhosis), severe anemia, and patients with compensated severe aortic regurgitation. In patients in whom prolonged muffling of sounds occurs before total disappearance, the blood pressure should be recorded using the three-component format. All three values (onset of Korotkoff sounds, muffling, and cessation of sound) are recorded (e.g., 120/66/20). In some patients, Korotkoff sounds may still be heard over the brachial artery even when the cuff has been completely deflated. Because a diastolic pressure of zero is a hemodynamic impossibility, the point of sudden muffling of sounds probably correlates with true diastolic pressure in patients who exhibit the three-component phenomenon.

TABLE 7-1
Commonly Available Blood Pressure Cuff Sizes

Size	Arm Circumference (cm)	Bladder Size (cm)
Newborn	6–11	2.5 × 5
Infant	10–19	6 × 12
Child	18–26	9 × 18
Adult	25–35	12 × 23
Large arm	33–47	15 × 33
Thigh	46–66	18 × 36

Courtesy of W.A. Baum Co., Inc., Copiague, NY.

When initially measuring arterial pressure of any patient, the pressure should be taken in both arms and then compared. A 15 mm Hg systolic pressure difference between arms indicates obstructive lesions in the aorta or subclavian arteries on the side with the lower pressure measurement. The extremity with the higher pressure should therefore be consistently used for pressure measurement.

If the arms are not available or suitable for cuff pressure measurements (amputation, heavy dressings), blood pressure may be measured using the popliteal or posterior tibial artery. However, appropriately sized thigh cuffs must be used.

Advantages. Equipment is minimal and readily available in all areas of the hospital and outpatient facilities. The technique is relatively simple, and there is no risk to patients.

Disadvantages. The following caveats and weaknesses must be considered with use of the auscultatory technique despite the common use and familiarity of this method.
1. The examiner must have normal hearing acuity and background noise should be kept to a minimum, otherwise it may override Korotkoff sounds. To maximize audibility through the sound-sensing instrument, the total length of the stethoscope should not exceed 16 inches.
2. The mercury column must be vertical, unbroken, and resting at the zero point. Aneroid gauges must be periodically calibrated against mercury by biomedical engineering department personnel to ensure accuracy.
3. Appropriate cuff size is essential to obtain accurate pressure measurements, residual air must be squeezed from the cuff, and the cuff must be properly applied. It should also fit snugly around the arm, should be cen-

tered over the monitored artery, and should be of appropriate bladder length and cuff size. Bladder length should be at least 80% of arm circumference, and cuff width should be equal to 40% of arm circumference (Table 7-1). If the cuff is too small or is applied loosely or if air remains trapped in the cuff, the pressure measurements will be falsely elevated (Figure 7-6). If the cuff is too large for the patient, the measurement may be inaccurately low; the margin of error is not as great as for a cuff that is too small.
4. Obese people or those with cone-shaped (muttonlike) arms present difficulties in obtaining accurate auscultatory pressure measurements because of inadequate or uneven compression of the underlying tissue and artery. In these patients, accuracy may be increased if the clinician applies the cuff to the forearm and determines the point at which the auscultated or palpated radial pulse returns during cuff deflation. If this site is to be used in ICU patients, this site will be more comfortable than the upper arm for frequent, repeated measurements, but the effects of vasoconstriction in "shocky" patients will be more pronounced and readings may be very inaccurate or impossible to obtain.
5. False-low systolic pressure measurements may be obtained because of an auscultatory gap. This phenomenon usually occurs in a small percentage of hypertensive patients and is characterized by the appearance of Korotkoff sounds at a hypertensive value followed by their disappearance and subsequent reappearance at a lower level. Erroneously low systolic pressure measurements are prevented when the clinician is certain that cuff pressure is 30 mm Hg above the point at which the palpated pulse is lost or the cuff is initially inflated to 300 mm Hg.
6. In "shocky" patients with severe vasoconstriction and reduced stroke volume, Korotkoff sounds may be damped, variable in audibility, or even inaudible with a standard stethoscope. This may result in inaccurately low or unobtainable blood pressure values. A classic study by Cohn[1] documented that directly measured (intraarterial) systolic pressures were significantly higher and diastolic pressures were lower than those pressures obtained by auscultation or palpation in patients with cool, clammy skin; oliguria; dulled sensorium; or vasopressor therapy. Pulse pressure also was significantly underestimated by the auscultatory method (Figure 7-7).

Generally, a fall in blood pressure is associated with a shifting of the Korotkoff sound spectrum to lower frequencies that may be out of the range of human hearing.

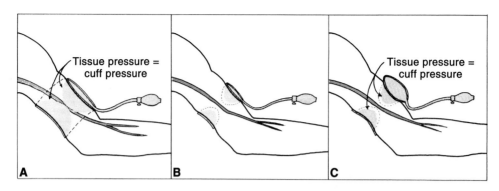

FIGURE 7-6 Transmission of cuff pressures to tissues of the arm. **A,** When a sphygmomanometer cuff of sufficient width in relation to the diameter of the arm is properly applied, the tissue pressure around deep arteries under the cuff equals cuff pressure. However, pressure under the edge of the cuff does not penetrate as deeply as that under the center of the cuff. **B,** A cuff that is too narrow in relation to the diameter of the limb does not transmit its pressure to the center of the limb. Under these conditions, the cuff pressure must greatly exceed arterial pressure to produce complete occlusion of the artery, and erroneously high systolic and diastolic pressures will be read from the mercury manometer. **C,** If a cuff of sufficient width is applied too loosely, it becomes rounded before exerting pressure on the tissues and produces the same sort of error as a narrow cuff. (From Rushmer RF: *Cardio-vascular dynamics,* ed 4, Philadelphia, 1976, W.B. Saunders.)

There are two interrelated reasons for this:

1. *Insufficient pulsatile flow* (low stroke volume) occurs through the compressed vessel and lowers the natural frequency and audibility of sound.
2. *Vasoconstriction* causes the vascular wall to be less likely to produce palpable pulses and audible vibrations.

These have profound clinical implications. Blind faith in cuff pressures that significantly underestimate the true blood pressure may lead the clinician to order inappropriate vasopressor therapy. Complications of such therapy include severe hypertension, hemorrhagic stroke, heart failure, and increased capillary oozing in patients with recent trauma or surgery.

Warning! If there is no intraarterial pressure for comparison and the character and indirectly obtained numeric values have *changed,* this indicates that the patient's *hemodynamic status may have changed.* This requires immediate patient assessment and possible management with therapy such as inotropic agents or fluid loading. When possible, an arterial line should be placed for more accurate evaluation of blood pressure trends. (See Table 7-2 for pitfalls in measuring auscultatory blood pressure.)

Other Special Considerations. Each patient's clinical circumstance determines the frequency of blood pressure measurements. If it appears that the period for frequent blood pressure monitoring (every few minutes to every half hour) is going to be long and an arterial line

will not be placed, the cuff should be moved to alternate sites at least once each shift. This will help prevent injury, edema, or petechiae from repeated cuff compressions. Also, if there is excess skin that might be pinched by the cuff or the patient's skin is friable, the portion of the arm or leg over which the cuff is to be placed should first be covered with thin stockinet. This soft material between cuff and skin will not alter blood pressure measurements but will reduce the likelihood of skin injury or discomfort.

Palpation

This method is simple and requires a blood pressure cuff, an aneroid gauge or a mercury manometer, and palpable brachial or radial pulses. This method is highly subjective and is of limited value for serial measurements that involve numerous examiners.

Principle. During slow cuff deflation, the point of return to the palpable pulse of an artery distal to the cuff is taken as the initial return to blood flow. The simultaneously measured pressure value is then assumed to be the systolic pressure.

Technique. The radial or brachial artery is palpated, and the cuff is inflated 20 to 30 mm Hg above the point where the loss of the pulse is noted. The cuff is then slowly deflated. The point at which the pulse returns is

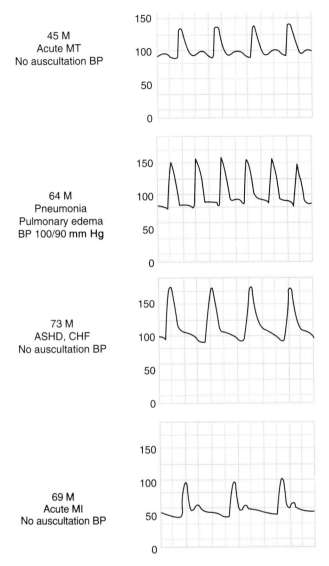

45 M
Acute MT
No auscultation BP

64 M
Pneumonia
Pulmonary edema
BP 100/90 mm Hg

73 M
ASHD, CHF
No auscultation BP

69 M
Acute MI
No auscultation BP

FIGURE 7-7 Examples of the discrepancy between arm cuff pressure and simultaneously measured femoral arterial pressure in four patients in shock. No pressure could be obtained by auscultation or palpation of the brachial artery in three patients despite normal or high arterial pressure. In the other patient, low systolic and pulse pressure measured by cuff were factitious. (From Cohn JM: Blood pressure measurement in shock, *JAMA* 199(13):972, 1967. Copyright 1967, American Medical Association.)

applied to the popliteal or posterior tibial arteries, although it may be somewhat more difficult to palpate these pulses.

Advantages and Disadvantages. The advantages of this technique are that it is not dependent on the hearing acuity of the examiner, the equipment is not complex, and there is no risk to the patient. The numerous and significant disadvantages are (1) the diastolic pressure cannot be measured; (2) in severely hypotensive patients, the pulses may be nonpalpable; (3) if two systoles are close together, as in premature beats and atrial fibrillation, the examiner may miss a beat and interpret the systolic pressure as lower than it actually is; and (4) the palpation method may *underestimate* systolic pressure in patients who are bradycardic, have low cardiac output, or are receiving vasopressor agents. This is because the amplitude of the peripheral pulses depends on stroke volume, as well as the ability of the examiner to compress the vessel and perceive vascular expansion with each pulse wave. As stroke volume falls, the amplitude of each pulse diminishes, and the vasoconstricted smaller arteries may be less compressible and may expand less with each pulse wave. Overall, systolic measurements by palpation are lower than those determined by Korotkoff sounds.

Auscultation Assisted with Doppler Flow Detectors

This technique requires a sphygmomanometer and a handheld Doppler device. When Korotkoff sounds are faint or absent (low flow state) and the patient has no arterial line, a handheld flow detector placed over a brachial or radial artery during cuff deflation may be helpful in detecting the return to blood flow, allowing an estimate of systolic pressure. This technique may be useful in the evaluation of systolic pressure trends in response to therapy in "shocky" patients.

Principle. Because there is no blood flow or movement of the arterial wall when the artery is closed, no Doppler signal is detected above systolic pressure. The appearance of a Doppler signal is detected at systolic pressure due to resumption of blood flow and arterial wall motion. Diastole cannot be detected clinically.

Technique. The pulse detector is placed over the brachial or radial artery distal to the cuff. The cuff is then inflated to a pressure above the expected arterial pressure. As the cuff pressure is reduced, the appearance of the characteristic shushing sound (shhhh, shhhh, shhhh) signifies

recorded as the systolic pressure. This method is applicable in situations in which a stethoscope may not be available, ambient noise may obscure Korotkoff sounds, and a primary check for the systolic pressure is done using the auscultatory method. The same technique also can be

TABLE 7-2

Pitfalls in Measuring Auscultatory Blood Pressure

Problem	Cause	Rationale
False-high reading	Cuff too small	Small cuff does not adequately disperse the pressure over the arterial surface
	Cuff not centered over the brachial artery	More external pressure is needed to compress the artery
	Cuff not applied snugly	Uneven and slow inflation results in varying tissue compression
	Arm below heart level	Hydrostatic pressure imposed by weight of intraarterial blood column above site of auscultation additive to arterial pressure; reposition arm to heart level
	Very obese arm	Cuff too small for large arm will cause too little compression of the artery at the suitable pressure level; apply a large thigh cuff to the upper arm if necessary
	Cone-shaped arm	Uneven pressure with a circular cuff transmitted to the underlying artery within a conical arm; employ forearm blood pressure measurements
False-low reading	Cuff too large	Pressure is spread over too large an area and produces a damping effect on the Korotkoff sounds
	Arm located above heart level	Hydrostatic pressure in the elevated arm causes resistance to pressure and flow generated by the heart
	Failure to correctly determine the onset of the first Korotkoff sound	Difficult to correlate sounds with rapidly falling mercury column; cuff deflation should not exceed 1–3 mm Hg/sec

blood flow and vascular motion. The pressure at which the first shushing sound is heard is recorded as the systolic pressure. The shushing sounds continue as long as the device is held over the open artery.

Advantages and Disadvantages. This small device is easy to use but may be unavailable "in the unit" when needed. Also, only systolic pressures are available. Doppler device estimates of systolic pressure are higher than those obtained with palpation but are somewhat lower than those obtained with an intraarterial line. However, the relationship to arterial line systolic pressures remains good over a wide pressure range (both rise and fall proportionately).

Mercury Manometer or Aneroid Pressure Gauge Oscillation Observation

Only a cuff and mercury or aneroid manometer are required for this simple technique.

Principle. During slow cuff deflation, systolic pressure may be estimated by observation for the appearance of fluctuations of the top of the mercury column or "flicking" of an aneroid gauge needle. These oscillations are synchronous with the heartbeat.

Technique. The cuff is pressurized until no oscillations are observed at the mercury column meniscus or pressure gauge needle. The cuff pressure is then slowly decreased until oscillations are observed, which allows for an estimate of systolic pressure. The pressure is then allowed to fall farther until oscillations become maximal and then begin to decrease. The maximal point of oscillation provides an estimate of mean arterial pressure.

Advantages and Disadvantages. The advantages of this technique are that little equipment is required and it may be done by examiners with hearing impairment. Conversely, this technique is highly subjective as to the precise point of systolic and mean pressure measurement. Further doubt as to the accuracy of this method is based on the fact that the arteries proximal to the cuff may be able to pulsate under the upper edge of the cuff while the vessel underlying the cuff is still occluded; this is particularly pronounced in patients with a hyperdynamic circulation. These pulsations may be detected as oscillations and therefore interpreted as falsely high systolic values. Other disadvantages are lack of means of determining diastolic pressure and possibly minimal oscillations in hypotensive patients.

Systolic Pressure Measurement by Photoelectric Devices

Pulse oximeters that are currently used for monitoring arterial oxygen saturation also serve as pulse detectors for estimating systolic pressure by pulse reappearance during cuff deflation.

Principle. This technology involves the measurement of light absorption from the photoelectric device placed against the skin on a finger. Changes in absorption of infrared light are produced by phasic changes in blood volume associated with pulsatile blood flow. A pulse wave identical in appearance to an intraarterial waveform is displayed.

Technique. An arm cuff, placed in the same limb as the digit used for placement of the light source, is inflated above systolic pressure. The displayed pulse wave flattens to an isoelectric line. The cuff is then slowly deflated. The initial, sudden oscillation correlates with resumption of blood flow in the involved digit and is recorded as the systolic pressure. Following the initial systolic "blip," the amplitude of the pulse wave progressively returns to normal as the cuff deflates.

Advantages and Disadvantages. This technique is easy to use, but motion of the detector (due to finger movement) is associated with errors. The technique also is unreliable if the blood vessels of the finger become constricted because of a cold environment, anxiety, perfusion failure, or peripheral vascular disease.

Automated Monitoring Instruments

Automated indirect blood pressure devices provide measurements of systolic, diastolic, and mean arterial pressures without a stethoscope, without manual inflation and deflation of the sphygmomanometer cuff, and without patient contact because the systems can be programmed to measure blood pressure at specified time intervals. In ICUs, automated blood pressure systems are built into recently manufactured bedside monitoring consoles. Freestanding models are also available for ICU, step-down, emergency department, outpatient, or research purposes. Some models intended for step-down, research, or emergency settings also variously display electrocardiogram, SpO_2, heart and respiratory rates, capnometry, and core temperature, along with intermittent or continuous blood pressure measurements (manufacturer dependent). In instruments intended for hospital use, built-in alarm systems alert clinicians of hemodynamic change.

These devices are all dependent on adequate pulsatile blood flow to the extremities for accurate measurement. Under ideal conditions and when applied to normal, healthy individuals who are hemodynamically stable, studies indicate that these devices are generally accurate to plus or minus 5 mm Hg compared with a centrally placed arterial catheter.[2,3]

Reliability and accuracy are questionable in patients with rapid variations in blood pressure and heart rate; subclavian artery compression due to patient positioning; calcific vascular disease; hypotension with low pulse pressure and vasoconstriction; or patient movement (shivering, seizure activity, restlessness). Paradoxically, the patients who require the most accurate and reliable blood pressure measurements are those most likely to have inaccurate blood pressure measurements recorded.

Clinical Application

Automatic devices release clinicians from frequent, routine blood pressure measurements in patients who are hemodynamically stable but who require frequent measurements. Applications include patient monitoring during or following operative or diagnostic procedures or patients in whom arterial lines cannot be immediately placed (emergency transport situations) or are contraindicated. Patients who are also good candidates for automated devices are those in hypertensive crisis (malignant hypertension, acute pulmonary edema) or patients in whom cardiovascular deterioration in the immediate future is possible (trauma, suspected gastrointestinal bleeding, acute myocardial infarction). *These devices are useful in following trends but should be avoided in patients who become hypotensive or patients who are receiving potent vasoactive drug titration.*

Principles

Automated indirect blood pressure devices estimate blood pressure by one of five technologies:
1. *Oscillometric* detection of pulsatile arterial wall vibrations by an automatically inflating/deflating cuff coupled to electronic instrumentation (Dinamap; Critikon, Tampa, FL).
2. *Infrasonde* detection, by microphone, of the pulsatile vibrations of the arterial wall underlying the automatically deflating cuff (Puriton Bennett Corp., Carlsbad, CA).
3. *Ultrasonic* detection (using the Doppler principle) of the speed and direction of blood flow by determination of the change in pitch in the sound of flowing blood as it gets nearer to and then suddenly "downshifts" as it passes a sensing device housed within the encircling

cuff (Arteriosonde 1216, Roche Medical Electronics Division, Cranbury, NJ).

4. *Arterial tonometry,* which uses a pressor sensor, positioned over and partly flattening the radial artery against the underlying bone. The pressor sensor detects the pulsatile forces exerted by the artery. The beat-to-beat forces are then converted to an electrical signal, which is computer analyzed and continuously displayed (Pilot Model 7000, Colin Medical Instruments Corp, San Antonio, TX, and Vasotrac Model AMP205A, Medwave, Inc., St. Paul, MN).

It is beyond the scope of this textbook to more extensively list and describe the physical principles and mechanics of all commercially available automated devices. It is the clinician's responsibility to obtain, carefully read, and understand manufacturers' recommendations for operation; possible sources of inaccuracy in systolic, diastolic, and mean pressures; and troubleshooting techniques for each manufacturer's instrument.

Currently, the oscillometric method is the most commonly used. Two hoses on the cuff connect the cuff to the instrumentation. Through one hose, a pneumatic inflation system pressurizes the cuff until no vascular vibrations (oscillations) are detected. This is usually approximately 160 mm Hg for the first blood pressure measurement or approximately 30 mm Hg above the previously obtained systolic pressure. If the patient's systolic pressure exceeds the cuff pressure (oscillations are still detectable), the cuff will immediately pressurize to approximately 200 mm Hg. If cuff pressure is still less than systolic pressure, the instrument will measure only mean arterial pressure. The cuff will then completely deflate to restore circulation and will then reinflate to a maximum of 250 mm Hg.

A second hose connects the cuff to the pressure sensor within the electronics enclosure. As the cuff is microcomputer deflated, vascular oscillations cause cuff-detectable expansion within the patient's arm during each systole. The time of each decrement in cuff pressure is determined by the time it takes for two consecutive heartbeats to produce two roughly equal pressure oscillations. Throughout the deflation cycle, the averaged pairs of oscillations and corresponding cuff pressures are computer analyzed to determine systolic, diastolic, and mean arterial pressures. Normally, the entire time period from onset of measurement to display is 20 to 45 seconds.

Mean arterial pressure is easier for the oscillometric device to read than systolic and diastolic pressures because they are more affected by hypotension and rapid variations in blood pressure. Consequently, displayed mean arterial pressure is measured reliably even in shock patients, even though systolic and diastolic pressures may not be displayed.

Possible causes of difficulty relating to oscillometric blood pressure measurement technique include the following:

1. If there is muscular activity in the cuffed arm, the instrument may not be able to differentiate between muscle and vascular motion. In this case, the device stops the cuff deflation and waits for a period of time before continuing.

2. The cyclic tourniquet effect may be disturbing to some patients.

3. The cuff should not be applied to a limb with an intravenous infusion distal to the cuff to avoid venous distention, clotting of the vascular catheter, or extravasation of fluids.

4. Measurements taken each minute may result in artificially high pressure measurements. The process of inflating and deflating the cuff may produce an increase in blood volume in the involved arm that can last for several minutes. Generally, a delay of 3 minutes between pressure measurements allows time for complete resumption of the steady state.

5. Failure to squeeze all the air from the cuff before application to the patient's arm may result in inaccurate pressure measurements.

6. Arm cuffs may abrade the skin or result in cutaneous pressure injuries, particularly when ridges or wrinkles are present in the cuff. Application of stockinet to the area under the cuff, periodic removal of the cuff, and inspection and cleansing of the underlying skin should prevent this problem.

Overall, automated blood pressure devices have a role in tracking blood pressure *trends* and are generally reliable in stable patients. Unfortunately, their accuracy is questionable in hypotensive patients or in circumstances in which blood pressure is likely to rapidly fluctuate. An additional problem is that clinicians may develop an inappropriate sense of security that the patient is "being monitored" and that the device will sound the alarm when necessary. Unfortunately, mechanisms fail and alarms may become defective, or alarm limits may not be set specific to the individual patient's condition or may not be set at all. *Comprehensive, safe patient care requires that the clinician evaluate patient, monitor, and alarm status on a regular basis.*

DIRECT ARTERIAL PRESSURE MEASUREMENT

Intraarterial pressure of a catheterized vessel can be converted to an electrical signal by a pressure transducer. The signal is then amplified and continuously displayed as an oscilloscopic waveform and digital numeric value. The physical setup involves direct connection of a fluid-filled intraarterial catheter and extension tubing to a pressure transducer that, in turn, connects to an electronic amplifier/monitor.

The indirect methods of blood pressure measurement described previously depend on the detection of blood *flow* beneath the pressurized cuff. The direct (intraarterial) method actually measures pressures within the cannulated artery, which do not necessarily correlate with volume of blood flow. The shape of the displayed arterial pressure waveform also reflects changes in cardiovascular function such as stroke volume, ventricular performance, and systemic vascular resistance (see conditions that affect waveform morphology later in this chapter).

Continuous Intraarterial Pressure Monitoring

This is the most reliable method of continuously monitoring real-time systemic arterial systolic, diastolic, and mean pressures. It also offers the advantage of relatively pain-free, simple, and low-risk access for arterial blood sampling.

Indications and Contraindications

There are two main indications for arterial cannulation, several relative contraindications, and no absolute contraindications (Box 7-1).

Physiology of the Arterial Pressure-Pulse Wave (Arterial Waveform)

Left ventricular ejection results in the creation of a pressure wave and blood flow into the arterial system. The pressure wave is transmitted to the peripheral arteries more rapidly and precedes blood flow; the pressure wave moves at a rate of 10 meters per second, whereas blood flows at a rate of 0.5 meters per second.[4] This phenomenon is illustrated by the following example. When an examiner places a finger on a patient's radial pulse, the pulse felt does not correspond with the passage of blood ejected by the ventricle during that cardiac cycle. Rather, the examiner is feeling the pressure wave, which travels much faster than the actual flow of blood. The ejected blood reaches the same point several heartbeats later.

Understanding the morphology of the arterial waveform is based on the two-component nature of the pressure-pulse wave forms: (1) transmission of a pressure wave and (2) the pulsatile displacement of stroke volume through the arterial circulation. These are described relative to the phases of the cardiac cycle (Figure 7-8).

BOX 7-1
Indications and Contraindications for Arterial Cannulation

Indications*
1. Continuous arterial pressure monitoring—critically ill or injured patients or patients undergoing major surgical procedures so that sudden changes in pressure are immediately detected, trends in pressure change may be evaluated, and the effects of therapy may be assessed
   a. Surgical procedures requiring cardiopulmonary bypass
   b. Major vascular, thoracic, abdominal, or neurologic procedures
   c. All hemodynamically unstable patients
   d. Patients receiving potent vasopressor or vasodilator drugs
   e. Patients supported on the intraaortic balloon pump (IABP)
   f. Patients receiving intracranial pressure monitoring
   g. Hypertensive crisis such as overdissecting aortic aneurysm
2. Serial blood gas measurements
   a. Patients in respiratory failure
   b. Patients being maintained on or being weaned from mechanical ventilatory support
   c. Patients with severe acid/base abnormalities
   d. If, for any reason, more than three to four arterial blood samples are required on a daily basis

Relative Contraindications*
1. Patients with peripheral vascular disease
2. Patients with hemorrhagic disorders
3. Patients on anticoagulants or patients receiving thrombolytic agents
4. Arterial puncture is relatively contraindicated in areas of infection, where skin is weeping, at sites of previous vascular surgery (particularly cutdown), or through synthetic vascular graft material

*Whether an arterial catheter is or is not placed in these situations depends on the severity of the patient's illness.

Phase I, the Inotropic Component

This occurs during early systole when opening of the aortic valve transfers the tremendous energy generated by the contracting left ventricle to the aorta. This creates the pressure wave that moves rapidly down the arterial tree. At the same time, the first portion of stroke volume is delivered into the aortic root. The initial steep upstroke, termed the *anacrotic rise* (*ana*—up, *krotos*—beat [Greek]), normally ascends to a systolic peak of approximately 100 to 140 mm Hg. Because the steepness, rate, and height of the

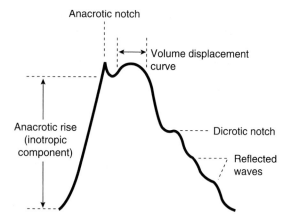

FIGURE 7-8 Pressure-pulse wave. Creation of the arterial pressure wave and acceleration of blood flow correlate with the inotropic upstroke. The rounded shoulder represents blood volume displacement and distention of the arterial walls. Normally, the peak of both the inotropic and volume displacement phases are equal in amplitude. The descending limb represents diastolic runoff of blood; the dicrotic notch separates systole from diastole. Additional humps on the downslope relate to pulse waves reflected from the periphery.

anacrotic rise are related to the rate of acceleration of blood, these waveform characteristics are indicators of left ventricular contractility. For example, the inotropic component is typically decreased in amplitude and becomes sloped in patients with contractility failure (ischemic disease, cardiomyopathy, certain drug therapies) or in those with hypovolemia because an underfilled ventricle empties with little force. On the other hand, the inotropic component is nearly vertical and is of increased amplitude in patients with hyperdynamic circulations (anemia, thyroid toxicosis, compensated moderate to severe aortic regurgitation).

Phase II, the Volume Displacement Curve

This fills out and sustains the pressure pulse. The rounded appearance is produced by continued ejection of stroke volume from the left ventricle, displacement of blood, and distention of the arterial walls. The volume displacement curve is narrow and of low amplitude in patients with low stroke volume. An "anacrotic notch" may be noted and is thought to mark the change from the inotropic component (initial generation of the pressure pulse) to the volume displacement curve.

Phase III, Late Systole and Diastole

This is associated with a sloping decline as rate of peripheral runoff of blood exceeds volume input into the arterial circulation. Aortic valve closure heralds the onset of diastole and is evident by inscription of the

dicrotic notch (*di*—twice, *krotos*—beat [Greek]). Following the dicrotic notch, as blood continues to run off into the capillaries, there is a continuous decline until the next systole. Undulations may be noted on the diastolic decline and are due to reflections of pressure waves from the distal arterioles.

Changes in the Arterial Pressure-Pulse Wave as it Moves from the Aorta toward the Periphery

As the pressure-pulse wave moves from the aorta toward the periphery, changes normally occur. These include the following:

1. Delays in transmission occur, so that pressures measured simultaneously in an upper and a lower extremity are out of phase.
2. The anacrotic and dicrotic notches become less conspicuous and eventually disappear.
3. The systolic portion becomes more peaked, of greater amplitude, and narrower so that a lower extremity systolic pressure is considerably higher than the systolic pressure of an upper extremity (see Figure 4-18). The pressures recorded from the catheter tip are the *actual pressures* at that *point* in the arterial circulation. Mean arterial pressure, however, is essentially the same at all points within the arterial circulation.

The changes in the shape of the arterial waveform, particularly the systolic portion, account for the differences between intraarterial pressures measured at different anatomic sites. Also, systolic pressures may differ at the same site between those measured by intraarterial versus various indirect "cuff" measurement techniques. This is why Brunner[5] stated that "blood pressure is a function of the way it is measured." Anatomic site, as well as technique of blood pressure measurement, must be considered when interpreting data, particularly when vasopressor or vasodilator drugs are being titrated. For example, the systolic pressure measured from an arterial line placed in the dorsalis pedis artery will be different from that measured by an automated system with the cuff placed over the brachial artery, which will be different from that measured from the tip of an intraaortic balloon catheter tip located just distal to the aortic arch. However, mean arterial pressure measured with various technologies and different anatomic sites should be nearly equal.

Cause of Waveform Morphology Changes from the Aorta to the Periphery

The major factor responsible for the changes in waveform amplitude and configuration is the reflection of pressure waves from the periphery. This concept is illustrated by the following analogy. When an object is dropped into a dish of water, waves are produced that move concentrically outward. When these waves hit the edge of the dish, they are reflected back and add to and amplify the oncoming waves. This effect is greatest near the edge of the dish. Similarly, in the arterial tree, as the leading pressure wave hits the small, abruptly tapering arterioles, much of it is reflected backward. The amplitude of the reflected waves, also termed *echo waves,* is added to the oncoming waves. The summation of waves is greatest at the periphery and is most noted in radial and dorsalis pedis arterial waveforms. Reflected waves also may be observed as undulations in the descending limb of the arterial waveform.

Changes in vascular tone also affect the shape and amplitude of the arterial waveform:

- *Vasodilation* (decreased systemic vascular resistance) reduces the effects of reflected waves because the energy of the pressure-pulse wave passes through the arterioles without much reflection. This causes the peripheral arterial waveform contour to be more like that of the central aorta.

- *Vasoconstriction* (increased systemic vascular resistance) results in a greater contribution of reflected waves and an exaggeration of the systolic pressure value at radial or dorsalis pedis sites. This is because the site of greatest reflection is at the catheter tip located nearest the arterioles. Vasoconstriction also results in a generalized increase in arterial pressure.

Difficulty Determining True Systolic Pressure When Two Systolic Peaks Are Present on the Arterial Waveform

Normally, the amplitudes of the inotropic spike (anacrotic notch) and the volume displacement curve are essentially the same, and measurement of the systolic pressure is uncomplicated. However, under various circumstances, two distinct systolic peaks may be observed in the pressure waveform when blood pressure is measured at peripheral sites: the first is the inotropic spike and the second is the volume displacement curve. Either peak may be taller and may determine peak systolic pressure. The monitor interprets and digitally displays the taller peak as systolic pressure. Increases in the inotropic spike may be due to (1) increased rate of left ventricular pressure generation and increased acceleration of aortic blood flow (Figure 7-9, *A*), (2) increased reflection of pressure waves from the periphery, or (3) overshoot artifact. Decreased amplitude of the inotropic spike may be the result of (1) myocardial depression, (2) hypovolemia, or (3) decreased systemic vascular resistance (vasodilation), which reduces the generation of reflected waves.

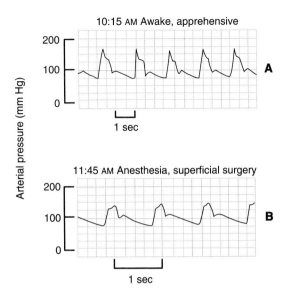

FIGURE 7-9 Two systolic peaks are commonly observed in the pressure pulse; either peak may determine systolic pressure. After induction of anesthesia, note decline of peak 1 (or inotropic component), while peak 2 remains unchanged. Radial artery cannula. (From Bruner JMR, Krenis LJ, Kunsman JM, Sherman AP: Comparison of direct and indirect methods of measuring arterial blood pressure. *Med Instrum* 15(1):14, 1981. Reprinted with permission of AAMI, Arlington, VA.)

It is important to note that various "word of mouth" techniques have been applied to determine "true" systolic pressure in circumstances in which two peaks are clearly visible and one peak significantly dominates the other. *None of these techniques is valid because either peak can be systolic pressure depending on the patient's hemodynamic status* (see Figure 7-9). Furthermore, dominance of the inotropic spike or volume displacement curve may change over a short period of time, depending on systemic vascular resistance and left ventricular contractility.

Warning! Overshoot of systolic pressure due to catheter/transducer system underdamping or inadequate frequency response relative to that of the pulsatile pressure signal may produce a falsely high systolic pressure display (see Chapter 6 for further discussion). In fact, systolic overshoot artifact is one of the most common artifacts of the arterial waveform in clinical practice. The important clinical point is that the possibility of this artifact must be investigated by dynamic response (snap, square root) testing (see Chapter 6, Box 6-2) and ruled out before beginning what could be inappropriate antihypertensive therapy. The overshoot artifact may occur briefly or may come and go transiently when the patient's pressure-pulse signal contains high-frequency components that approximate those of the monitoring system. This occurs in patients who develop hyperdynamic circulations or rapid heart rates.

The solution to the problem of dominance of one wave over the other, or overshoot artifact, is simple and straightforward. Mean arterial pressure remains unaffected because inotropic spikes contribute little to the area under the arterial waveform in spite of their height. *Consequently, in all the aforementioned situations, patient evaluation and therapy should be based on mean arterial pressure rather than digitally displayed or calculated systolic pressure.*

Arterial Waveform Analysis to Determine Other Indices of Circulatory Function

There has been some interest in determining hemodynamic variables such as stroke volume and cardiac output by evaluating the area under the systolic ejection portion of the arterial pressure curve, as well as the systemic vascular resistance by the height of the dicrotic notch. Because of the relatively poor fidelity of recording systems in clinical use, as well as the numerous pitfalls inherent in fluid-filled systems, there is currently no clinical application for these techniques. However, it has been suggested that left ventricular ejection time (LVET), or *dP/dT,* an index of the speed and force of ventricular ejection, can be estimated using the arterial waveform.[6]

The beginning of the systolic upstroke and peak of the systolic pressure are identified. Then a vertical line is drawn from the systolic peak to the level of diastolic pressure. LVET is estimated, in milliseconds, from the beginning of the systolic upstroke to the peak identified by the vertical line. The shorter the time interval from the upstroke to the peak systolic pressure, the greater the force and velocity of ventricular ejection. Conversely, the greater the time interval, the weaker the force and velocity of ejection. Changes in ventricular function can thus be easily and noninvasively assessed over time if the waveform is artifact free and optimally damped (Figure 7-10).

Changes in Arterial Waveform Morphology Specific to Certain Clinical Conditions

The commonly encountered conditions that affect waveform morphology are subsequently described.

Arrhythmias

Premature supraventricular and ventricular contractions are associated with decreased ventricular contractile dynamics, decreased rate of acceleration of blood flow, and decreased stroke volume because of the shortened ventricular filling time. The corresponding arterial pressure wave will show a sloped anacrotic rise with a lower peak pressure. Multiple, consecutive extrasystoles or sustained tachycardia may lower systolic pressure significantly.

The sinus beat following the compensatory pause generally displays a rapid, steep anacrotic rise and increased peak pressure because of increased ventricular filling time and, as a result, increased ejection velocity and stroke volume (Figure 7-11). In tachyarrhythmias in which the R-to-R intervals are variable, such as during atrial fibrillation, the arterial waveform will show variable peak systolic pressures (Figure 7-12).

Hypertension and Hypotension

Hypertension and hypotension are common occurrences in critically ill patients. In *hypertension,* a rapid anacrotic rise reaches an initial peak pressure of greater

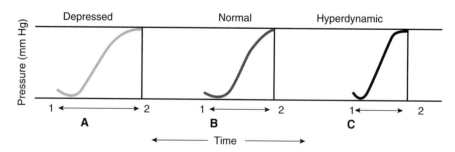

FIGURE 7-10 Three examples of estimating left ventricular ejection time *(dP/dT)* using the arterial waveform. **A,** Depressed left ventricular junction. Note the sloped upstroke and increased time interval from point 1 to point 2. **B,** Normal left ventricular function. **C,** Hyperdynamic left ventricular function. Note the steep upstroke and decreased time interval from point 1 to point 2. (Adapted from Hanlon-Pena P, Pitner J: Updated clinical management of the IABP patient: pharmacological considerations, *Canadian Perfusion* 10:18, 2000.)

than 140 mm Hg, and the end-diastolic pressure may be 90 mm Hg or higher. Each phase of the waveform is clearly visible and may be significantly enlarged. Reflectance waves may be noted in the descending limb of the waveform (late systole and diastole) (Figure 7-13).

In *hypotension,* the peak of the inotropic component and the dicrotic notch disappear. The rate, slope, and amplitude of the anacrotic rise decrease, and maximal peak

systolic pressures are 90 mm Hg or less. Overall, the waveform appears damped (Figure 7-14).

Aging

With aging, the difference between central aortic and distal systolic pressures decreases because the pressure-pulse wave does not change significantly as it progresses distally. The inotropic component of the waveform also

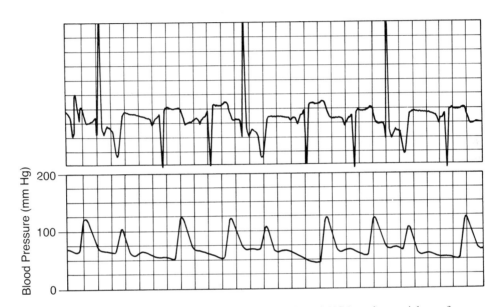

FIGURE 7-11 Effect of premature ventricular contractions (PVCs) on the arterial waveform.

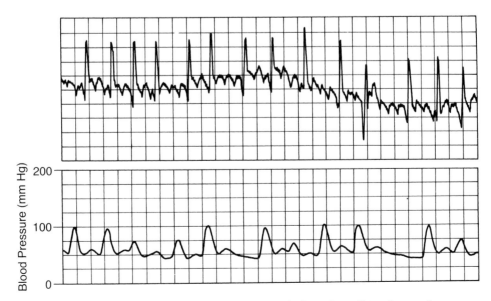

FIGURE 7-12 Effect of rapid, irregular supraventricular tachycardia on the waveform.

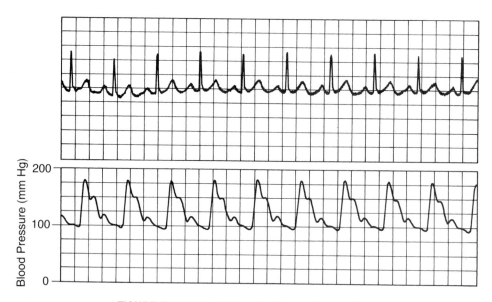

FIGURE 7-13 Effect of hypertension on the waveform.

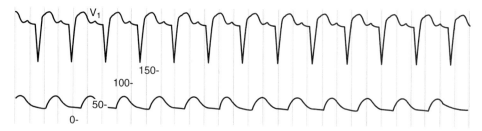

FIGURE 7-14 Effect of hypotension on the waveform.

tends to be dominant. In other words, in elderly patients, systolic pressure and waveform morphology recorded in the radial artery are not significantly different from those recorded in the aortic root. This is thought to be caused by the loss of compliance of the arteries with advancing years. Alternatively, in children, the dicrotic notch in the peripheral arterial waveforms is augmented, and the difference in aortic and peripheral waveform morphology is generally marked.

Initial Postoperative Period following Major Vascular or Cardiac Surgery

Significant overshoot of the inotropic component (20 to 40 mm Hg) may be noted within the initial 48 hours of surgery. Postoperative hemodynamic changes are associated with the production of high-frequency components of the arterial pressure-pulse wave that are equal to the resonant frequency of the fluid-filled system. In other words, the overshoot is probably largely due to an artifact of the fluid-filled system. Cuff pressure usually corresponds with

the peak of the volume displacement curve. In this situation, clinical decision making should be based on mean arterial pressure.

Hypovolemia or Vasoconstriction in Patients with Normal Left Ventricular Function

A tall, spiking inotropic component relates to increased systemic vascular resistance in patients with anxiety, hypovolemia, or chilling, or those receiving vasopressor medications. The reduced amplitude and narrow width of the volume displacement component directly reflect the low stroke volume in hypovolemic patients (Figure 7-15).

In summary, the shape of the recorded pulse-pressure wave is variable and depends on the interplay of factors such as the site of arterial pressure measurement, the hemodynamic status of the patient, and the fidelity of the monitoring system to accurately reproduce the pressure-pulse wave. *Measurement of mean arterial pressure generally remains accurate and relatively consistent despite the cause of the altered waveform except in the*

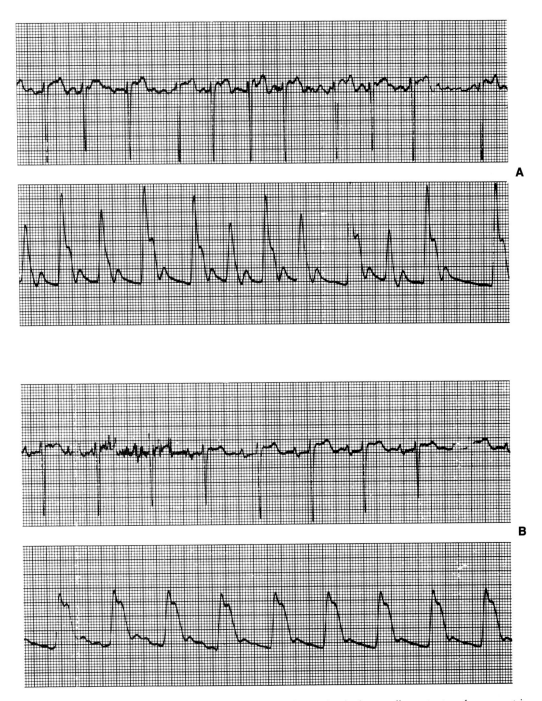

FIGURE 7-15 Arterial pressure tracing from a patient with hypovolemia, low cardiac output, and vasoconstriction. Blood pressure by digital readout is 210/49; mean arterial pressure is 79 mm Hg **(A).** Systolic pressure at the shoulder of the waveform averages approximately 148 mm Hg. After the addition of volume and restoration of normal sinus rhythm **(B),** cardiac output is improved, and the waveform has much less systolic overshoot. The volume displacement wave is unchanged. Arterial pressure now reads 144/45; mean arterial pressure is 71 mm Hg. (From Kirkland LL, Veremakis C: Arterial pressure monitoring. In Carlson RW, Geheb MA, editors: *Principles and practice of medical intensive care,* Philadelphia, 1993, W.B. Saunders.)

case of arrhythmias. In patients with varying R-to-R intervals, stroke volume and mean arterial pressures can vary significantly from beat to beat.

Checking Systolic Pressure by the Monitored Occlusion Technique

This method utilizes a sphygmomanometer and the observation of the arterial waveform from an indwelling arterial catheter.

Principle

Externally applied cuff pressure compresses the underlying artery. The absence of flow is associated with an "isoelectric line" on the arterial pressure channel. As cuff pressure is decreased, the return to flow is noted as the first deflection ("blip") in the isoelectric line and is interpreted and recorded as the systolic pressure.

Technique

Two observers are required. The first observer inflates the cuff to levels 20 to 30 mm Hg greater than the point after which the arterial waveform becomes a flat line. He or she then slowly deflates the cuff while watching the manometer. The second observer, watching the arterial pressure channel on the oscilloscope screen, signals when the first deflection, or blip, appears on the isoelectric line. The pressure value that is noted simultaneously on the manometer is taken to represent the systolic pressure.

Advantages and Disadvantages

The systolic pressure estimated by this method correlates fairly well with the volume displacement curve of the continuously displayed arterial pressure waveform because that portion correlates with actual blood flow. The clinician should recall that the peak systolic pressure may be determined by either of the two systolic peaks in the waveform, whichever is higher. The first peak (the inotropic component) is related to the inotropic state of the heart and may not be associated with flow. There also is a reasonable correlation between systolic pressure as estimated by the indirect auscultation (Riva-Rocci) method and the monitored occlusion technique. Diastolic and mean pressure cannot be determined by this technique. Its clinical application is to "see" the return to blood flow and correlate this with the simultaneously measured systolic pressure on the mercury manometer.

Clinical Caveats of Intraarterial Pressure Measurements

Several important considerations are related to the clinical use of directly obtained arterial pressure measurements.

1. *Pressure values obtained by direct intraarterial pressure measurement do not necessarily correlate with peripheral blood flow.* From the applied laws of physics, one may deduce that the higher the arterial pressure (the higher the driving force behind the flow of arterial blood), the greater the flow through the systemic capillaries. This principle would hold true if systemic vascular resistance were constant. However, vascular tone and systemic vascular resistance frequently change dramatically and may profoundly affect flow. Vasoconstriction tends to increase blood pressure but also increases vascular resistance, which, in turn, decreases systemic blood flow. If, for example, an incision is made in the arm of a patient receiving a potent vasopressor supporting a "normal" blood pressure, the incisional site is likely to be nearly bloodless. The bloodless wound indicates that the intensely vasoconstricted peripheral tissues are severely underperfused. In such patients, the normal blood pressure maintains the delivery of cardiac output only to the vital heart and brain while increased systemic vascular resistance sacrifices blood flow to all other body tissue.

   On the other hand, vasodilation decreases systemic vascular resistance. There are several effects on blood pressure and flow. Systolic pressure may actually increase as a result of increased stroke volume. In some significantly vasodilated patients, a subnormal blood pressure may still be associated with normal blood flow. However, if vasodilation is profound (neurogenic shock, anaphylactic shock), both blood pressure and flow decrease.

   The clinical point of this discussion is that measured intraarterial blood pressure and peripheral blood flow do not necessarily correlate, and the clinician must not be lulled into a false sense of security because the "blood pressure numbers" are normal. Clinical assessment findings provide the backdrop against which hemodynamic "numbers" and perfusion status are evaluated.

2. *The measured systolic pressure increases progressively from the ascending aorta to the peripheral arteries.* Mean arterial pressure provides a more stable and reliable estimate of central circulatory pressures because it is unchanged from the thoracic aorta to the periphery and therefore does not vary with arterial pressure sampling sites (brachial versus dorsalis pedis artery).

3. *The arterial line insertion site and transducer air-fluid interface should ideally all be referenced to*

heart level. If the patient is being maintained in the supine position, there is no problem. But if the patient is placed in a sitting position and the arm is allowed to be dependent or the dorsalis pedis site is used, both pressure sampling sites will be below heart level and the weight of the column of blood in the arteries from heart to sampling site will result in a deceptive increase in systolic, diastolic, and mean pressure values. In this common circumstance, the pressure transducer should be releveled to the wrist or foot to avoid greater errors in blood pressure measurement and the pressure differences between supine and sitting values noted.

Worse yet, if the transducer is placed on rolled towels, the transducer may fall off the bed and hang at any point from mattress to floor. For every 15 cm (6 inches) the transducer is placed below sampling site level, the blood pressure increases approximately 10 mm Hg. Failure to reference the catheter insertion site and the transducer to the same level can result in large differences in measured pressures due to gravity effects on the fluid in the connecting tubing. Poor catheter site–to–transducer leveling may result in serious therapeutic misadventures if the patient is being maintained on vasopressor or vasodilator drugs. The most accurate pressures recorded are those in which both the catheter insertion site and pressure transducer are leveled to heart level. In one particular situation, due to the pressure transducer hanging off the bed several feet below heart level, a newly admitted patient with malignant hypertension was receiving sodium nitroprusside (Nipride) titrated to the blood pressures that were displayed. When the transducer was brought up to the radial artery catheter level, the blood pressure measurements changed from 150/96 to 108/54, a level too low for a patient who was just admitted for hypertensive crisis.

4. *The capacity of the monitoring system to faithfully represent intravascular pressures profoundly affects measured values* (see Chapter 6). The resonant frequency, dynamic response, and damping characteristics of the monitoring system most profoundly affect systolic pressure measurement. Mean arterial pressure is not much affected by monitoring system physics imbalances.

Arterial Catheter Placement
Technique
Informed consent must be obtained before arterial cannulation except in emergency situations. The sites are selected based on the patient's underlying condition and anticipated time of arterial cannulation. See Table 7-3 for strong

---

TABLE 7-3
Strong and Weak Points for Arterial Cannulation Sites

Advantages	Disadvantages
Radial Artery Site	
The artery is superficial and easy to identify and cannulate	Complication rate is high with prolonged use, such as thrombus formation
The site is accessible during most types of surgery	Possible injury to the adjacent nerves by hematoma or insertion trauma
Dual arterial circulation to the hand is easy to document and risk of distal vascular insufficiency is low	Considerable augmentation of systolic pressure makes hemodynamic evaluation of central circulatory systolic pressure difficult
Ease of immobilizing the site, comfortable for the patient	Small intraluminal arterial size requires a small-gauge catheter with a lower natural frequency, which predisposes to overshoot artifact; small bore also predisposes to thrombus formation and vascular occlusion by catheter
	Site of pulse wave reflection may be directly at site of catheter; high-frequency pressure wave harmonics may result in overshoot artifact and require a higher natural frequency than is available in most monitoring systems

Continued

TABLE 7-3

Strong and Weak Points for Arterial Cannulation Sites—cont'd

Advantages	Disadvantages
Brachial Artery Site	
Artery is larger than radial artery, is easy to cannulate, and can accommodate a large-gauge catheter with a higher natural frequency	Difficulty in immobilizing the elbow; restriction of arm movement is uncomfortable for the patient
Less subject to systolic pressure augmentation due to reflected waves	Possibility of median nerve damage from hematoma formation or traumatic arterial puncture
Collateral vessels at the elbow joint reduce likelihood of vascular insufficiency	Thrombus formation occurring in a patient with poor collateral circulation may compromise blood flow to the ulnar and radial arteries
Femoral Artery Site	
Less likely to become nonfunctional and has fewer complications with prolonged use	Atherosclerotic plaque may make catheter passage difficult or plaque may break off and embolize distally
Useful site in shock when other peripheral pulses are nonpalpable	Possibility of massive, retroperitoneal hematoma formation
May accommodate a large-gauge catheter with a high-frequency response, thus minimizing overshoot artifact	Discontinuation required if an intraaortic balloon must be placed in the same artery
	Difficult to immobilize the site, particularly in restless patients
	Comment: Systolic, diastolic, and mean pressures are usually the same in the brachial and femoral arteries, although waveform morphology differs
Axillary Artery Site	
Large size results in fewer complications with prolonged use and allows use of large-gauge catheters with higher natural frequencies (less likelihood of overshoot artifact)	Possibility of cerebral air or clot embolism during flushing of the catheter or blood sampling (use of the left axillary artery versus the right reduces this possibility)
Useful option in patients with severe peripheral vascular disease such as Raynaud disease	Location within the neurovascular sheath predisposes to neurologic complications with hematoma formation
Proximity to the aortic arch gives a pulse-pressure wave similar in morphology to that of the aortic root	Cannulation is technically difficult and requires prolonged extension, hyperabduction, and rotation of the arm at the level of the shoulder
Minimal systolic augmentation due to reflectance waves; systolic and diastolic pressures most closely approximate central circulatory pressures	*Comment:* Systolic and diastolic pressures most closely correlate with central aortic pressures
Considerable collateral flow reduces the likelihood of vascular insufficiency	
Useful in shock when other peripheral pulses may be nonpalpable	
Dorsalis Pedis Artery Site	
Useful option in situations when arteries in the upper extremities are unavailable such as trauma or previous arterial catheterization	Generally a poor site for hemodynamic evaluation; subject to the greatest systolic pressure augmentation; mean arterial pressure may be inaccurate in patientswith regional flow deficits or alterations in vascular tone
Dual circulation minimizes risk of vascular insufficiency	Small vessel size predisposes to thrombotic occlusion
	Small-gauge catheter with low natural frequency required for cannulation
	Difficult to immobilize the site, uncomfortable for the patient, and impossible to stand or walk the patient
	Comment: The systolic peak is as much as 20 mm Hg higher than radial artery pressure; generally indicated when the arterial line is placed primarily for serial blood gas analysis

and weak points for each site. Physicians should be experienced with catheterization of all sites, although radial and femoral artery sites are used in approximately 90% of all arterial cannulations. The radial artery is usually the first site attempted unless the radial pulses are not palpable.

In the case of brachial, femoral, and axillary artery cannulation, the adequacy of the distal pulses should be assessed, before and after arterial cannulation, to rule out vascular insufficiency. Testing the collateral circulation before placement of a radial and dorsalis pedis artery catheter is essential to determine that blood supply to the hand or foot would not be eliminated if the radial or dorsalis pedis arteries became occluded by a thrombus, vascular spasm, or obstruction by the catheter (large vessel, small catheter). Such tests are described next. The operator must have a thorough understanding of normal arterial anatomy and common anatomic variants in order to safely insert the catheter and also effectively manage unexpected findings. For a comprehensive review of arterial anatomy for arterial access, see reference 7; for more detailed descriptions of arterial line placement for radial, dorsalis pedis, brachial, femoral, and axillary artery cannulation, see reference 8.

Radial Artery Placement

The hand is perfused via the radial and ulnar arteries, which unite to form a branching circulation in the hand. The *Allen test* evaluates the adequacy of the ulnar circulation and patency of the deep palmar arch (Figure 7-16). When possible, cannulation of the radial artery of the nondominant hand allows patient use of the more dexterous hand and also minimizes the risk of severe permanent disability in the event that distal ischemia occurs.

Dorsalis Pedis Placement

The foot is perfused by the dorsalis pedis and posterior tibial arteries. The collateral flow is provided via the posterior tibial artery. Both the posterior tibial and dorsalis pedis arteries are manually compressed and occluded with one hand while compressing and blanching the great toenail bed with the other hand. After 15 seconds, compression of the toenail and posterial artery is relieved while observing the return to color of the nail bed. The significance of the findings is evaluated by applying the same time frames as those used when performing the Allen test before radial artery cannulation.

If an abnormality of the hand or foot circulation is detected, a Doppler test should be performed to assess the state of the circulation, or a different site should be selected for arterial cannulation.

Adherence to surgical sterile technique is mandatory in all but emergency situations. The intended site is surgically

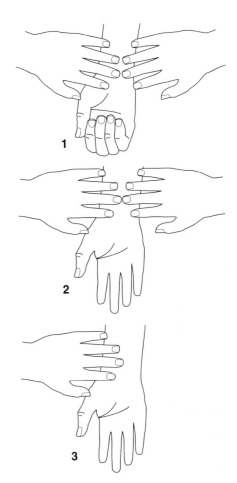

FIGURE 7-16 The Allen test is performed before cannulation of the radial artery to ensure adequacy of the ulnar and radial arteries and patency of the deep palmar arch. *1,* The examiner compresses both arteries while the patient repeatedly makes a tight fist to squeeze blood out of the hand. *2,* After the patient relaxes the fingers, the examiner observes the waxen hand. The patient should be instructed not to hyperextend the fingers and wrist because this may result in a false-positive test. *3,* Compression of the ulnar artery is released and the hand is observed for a blush or hyperemia. If color does not return within 5 to 10 seconds, radial artery cannulation should not be done. If brisk filling occurs, the test is repeated with the radial artery to test radial artery competency. If both vessels are competent, the radial artery may be used for puncture. (From Schwartz GR, editor: *Principles and practice of emergency medicine,* Philadelphia, 1978, W.B. Saunders.)

prepared and draped to provide an adequate sterile field around the exposed site. The operator and assistants should wear sterile gowns, gloves, caps, masks, and protective eyeshields.

Percutaneous puncture is the preferred method for arterial cannulation and may be performed using catheter-over-needle devices or the Seldinger method. (For a detailed description of these techniques, see Chapter 8.) The cutdown technique is rarely used; cannulation is performed under direct visualization of the artery.

Following arterial cannulation, the procedure is documented in the medical and nursing records to include date and time of catheter insertion, anatomic site, operator's name, description of the procedure, and any difficulties or complications encountered.

Hazards and Complications of Arterial Pressure Monitoring

Although arterial pressure monitoring is a relatively low-risk procedure, a number of hazards and complications are associated with its use. Complications such as hematomas, vascular insufficiency, infection, arterial or cerebral embolism, hemorrhage, accidental injection of medication, and disconnection are applicable to all sites. Frequent patient and site assessment is essential for early identification of complications. Factors that predispose to complications are listed in Box 7-2.

Arterial Embolization Resulting in Localized Tissue Ischemia or Necrosis

Embolization into the vascular bed beyond the catheter tip may result in ischemia or necrosis in the distal tissue. For example, with radial arterial catheterization, this may lead to necrosis of the digits. Retrograde flow with embolization can result in cerebral

---

BOX 7-2
Factors that Predispose to Complications of Arterial Catheterization

Large catheters (greater than 20 gauge except for the femoral and axillary arteries)
Septicemia
Burns or other inflammatory problems at insertion site
Cutdown placement
Vasopressor therapy
Hypercoagulable or hypocoagulable states
Low cardiac output
Multiple puncture attempts
Atherosclerosis
Frequent "cuff" blood pressure determinations on arm with arterial catheter
Poorly functioning flushing system
Frequent patient movement (restless, seizures, ethanol withdrawal)

---

ischemia secondary to embolization. *Fibrin emboli* are usually seeded from a primary thrombus that forms at the end of the indwelling catheter. *Particulate matter emboli* may result from pieces of dried blood or clots that formed when the stopcock and connecting tubing were improperly cleared following arterial sampling. *Air emboli* may be introduced into the system through improper line setup, as a result of blood sampling procedures, or through vigorous flushing of the catheter. *The practice of manual irrigation of an intraarterial line with a syringe is absolutely discouraged.*

Meticulous technique during catheter and system setup and manipulation, avoidance of vigorous flushing, and infusion of irrigation solution with a continuous flush device help prevent clot and air-bubble formation within the monitoring lines. The pressure bag must be pumped up to a level higher than systolic pressure to prevent reverse blood flow into the catheter and extension tubing. A pressure of 300 mm Hg, when used with the intraflow system, ensures a continuous irrigation of 3 ml/hr. Patients with hypercoagulable states (myocardial infarction, fever, cancer, pregnancy) may require occasional "fast flushes" with the continuous flush device lasting no longer than 2 to 3 seconds. *Whenever particles or air bubbles appear in the line, they should be aspirated and cleared before using the fast flush device.*

Cerebral Embolism

Vigorous manual flushing with a syringe or opening the fast flush valve for more than 2 to 3 seconds (which allows overaggressive manual flushing of the line) may result in cerebral ischemia due to retrograde flow of irrigation solution, particulate matter, or air bubbles into the cerebral circulation. From the radial artery, flush volumes as little as 3 to 12 ml may result in retrograde flow. Generally, the amount of irrigation solution required to reach the central circulation correlates with the patient's height.[9] If the patient is sitting or standing, air is more likely to travel into the cerebral arteries because air travels up.

Vascular Insufficiency

The risk of vascular insufficiency seems to be greater with smaller (radial) than larger (femoral) vessels. Factors that tend to predispose a patient to ischemic complications include low cardiac output, multiple arterial punctures, vasoconstriction (particularly with the administration of vasopressors), large catheter size, severe atherosclerosis, peripheral vascular insufficiency (e.g., Raynaud disease), diabetes, extended duration of arterial cannulation, and brachial or radial artery catheter placement.

Vascular occlusion may be due to occupation of the vascular lumen by the catheter (large catheter, small vessel), thrombus formation, embolization of air or debris, dislodgement of atherosclerotic plaque (femoral catheterization), or arterial spasm. Arterial spasm usually occurs shortly after catheter insertion or removal and is of short duration. Some clinicians use lidocaine (Xylocaine) or phentolamine (Regitine) to minimize the likelihood of spasm.

The portion of the cannulated extremity distal to the catheter site should be frequently assessed for skin temperature and color, tactile stimulation, and motor responses. When possible, the patient should be questioned to determine whether pain or altered sensation is present. In a patient with evidence of ischemia, prompt removal of the catheter diminishes the risk of significant sequelae. Ischemic injury also may persist or may not develop for hours after removal of the catheter.

Ischemic Necrosis of the Overlying Skin

This complication is associated with radial artery cannulation and is the result of thrombosis of the small, cutaneous branches of the radial artery. Patients at risk of this complication may be identified by intense blanching of the skin over the intraarterial catheter when the line is fast flushed. Smaller catheters for arterial catheterization and continuous catheter irrigation help minimize the likelihood of thrombus formation.

Infection

This hazard is related to local as well as systemic infection (see Chapter 13). The risk of arterial catheter infection is greater for patients in medical and burn ICUs because of the chronic, debilitating nature of the illness and the likelihood of ongoing infection from other sources. Generally, the risk of infection increases with the duration of catheter indwelling time. Catheter-related infection may manifest locally as redness, tenderness, and drainage at the insertion site or systemically as hyperthermia or hypothermia, chills, leukocytosis or leukopenia, and tachycardia and tachypnea without apparent cause. If infection is suspected, the catheter should be removed immediately and cultured using the semiquantitative technique described in Chapter 13.

Hemorrhage

This is the most common hazard and is more likely to occur in elderly, restless, or very obese patients; in patients with hemorrhagic disorders (thrombocytopenia, disseminated intravascular coagulation); in patients receiving anticoagulants; and in patients who have recently been or are being given thrombolytic agents.

External oozing around the insertion site may occur. Occult bleeding may result from a puncture wound in the posterior wall of the artery, from catheter dislodgment, or from catheter removal with insufficient pressure or time allowed for arterial compression. In such a situation, the bleeding will take the path of least resistance, which may be in surrounding soft tissue or a body cavity. Hemorrhage into the soft tissue surrounding a radial or brachial artery catheter is not likely to be associated with significant blood loss, but large hematomas may compromise blood supply and neurologic function to nearby tissues. For example, median nerve compression by a spreading hematoma in the area of the radial or brachial artery may result in neuropathy (pain, weakness, hand wasting). A puncture leak of the axillary artery may be associated with filling of the axillary sheath around the neurovascular bundle. The forming hematoma compresses the cords and branches of the brachial plexus, leading to clinical evidence of neurologic dysfunction of the involved arm.

Bleeding from the femoral artery into the retroperitoneal space may be difficult to detect, and the patient may lose 1000 to 1500 ml of blood before significant clinical and hemodynamic signs of hemorrhage become evident. Because unexplained swelling or bruising at the insertion site may be the only clue to bleeding, inspect for bruising or firmness on palpation in the lower abdominal quadrant, particularly following catheter insertion and removal.

Accidental disconnection of an 18-gauge arterial catheter could result in 500 ml blood loss per minute, if cardiac output is normal,[10] resulting in rapid exsanguination. Because all nonlocking connectors are subject to "creep of the plastics," only Luer-Lok connectors (Becton-Dickinson Company, Rutherford, NJ) should be used in pressure monitoring systems. Accidental malposition of a stopcock also may result in massive, rapid blood loss. The arterial cannulation site and all points in the catheter-to-transducer system should be exposed and visible to everyone involved in patient care. Arterial pressure monitor alarm limits *must* be set to ensure that accidental blood loss through the monitoring system is immediately detected and corrected.

Accidental Intraarterial Drug Injection

Accidental injection of pharmacologic agents through an arterial line may result in serious ischemic or necrotic complications of the involved extremity. Arterial pressure tubing should be clearly labeled to eliminate the possibility that it will be confused with adjacent intravenous lines, particularly in resuscitation situations.

Diagnostic Blood Loss

A cavalier attitude about the number of diagnostic blood samples obtained may result, over time, in significant blood loss for the patient. Blood sampling should be reduced to that needed for essential laboratory tests, and the volume for each withdrawal should be kept to a minimum, using pediatric collection tubes. Closed-sampling tubing systems may help prevent line contamination and prevents additional blood loss because there is no need to discard the initially withdrawn saline/blood samples necessary with open systems.

Less common complications include pseudoaneurysm formation, heparin-associated thrombocytopenia (see Chapter 6), bowel perforation (femoral artery catheterization), and arteriovenous fistula.

Overall, arterial catheters should be inserted only when they are absolutely necessary and removed when they are no longer needed. Too often, they are left in place for convenience in blood sampling or "just in case something happens." Because the likelihood of complications increases with length of indwelling time, the possibility of "something happening" also increases.

Care of Arterial Catheters

Dressings over the insertion site are changed according to institution protocol. The catheter insertion site is carefully inspected for redness, drainage, and bruising and blanching of the overlying skin on fast flush of the catheter. The presence of dressing does not preclude frequent inspection of the area for unusual firmness or swelling.

The joint used for arterial cannulation should be immobilized to prevent joint flexion or extension and kinking or dislodgement of the arterial catheter. When the *radial artery* is cannulated, the patient's hand is fixed in a neutral position to an armboard. Care is taken *not* to hyperextend the wrist because, over time, this position may result in neuromuscular injury to the hand. The hand is positioned with the palm on the armboard, and a small gauze square or folded washcloth may be placed behind the wrist for a cushion effect only. Alternatively, the armboard may be secured to the lateral instead of dorsal aspect of the hand.

Other sites are stabilized in such a manner that the joint or limb is in a neutral position and the patient is comfortable. If the patient is unconscious or paralyzed, this is usually not a problem; however, joints such as the elbow (brachial cannulation) become a challenge to clinicians caring for restless patients.

Obtaining Blood Samples from an Arterial Catheter

An indwelling arterial catheter provides simple and ready access for blood sampling for any purpose. Even prothrombin time (PT) and partial thromboplastin time (PTT) assays, withdrawn via the arterial catheter, have been shown to be accurate in patients not receiving medical-dose heparin.

When using the open system for blood collection, samples should be drawn from the stopcock closest to the insertion site. When obtaining blood samples, the sterile cap covering the port is removed and protected from contamination by placing it on a sterile gauze square or in the gauze packaging. A sterile syringe is attached in its place. The stopcock is then turned off to the flush system. Approximately 3 to 5 ml of flush-blood solution (to be discarded) must be withdrawn. This ensures that the specimen is undiluted with saline solution so that blood gas, hematology, or chemistry results are reliable. Each institution should determine its optimal discard volume based on the institution-specific, fluid-filled system used.

The stopcock is turned off to the patient and sample port, and the discard syringe is removed. The anticoagulated blood gas syringe (typically prepackaged) is then attached in its place. When prepackaged syringes are not available, heparinization of the syringe is accomplished by aseptically drawing up approximately 0.5 ml of 1:1000 sodium heparin, pulling back on the plunger to coat the inside of the syringe and needle and then expelling *all* of the heparin. The stopcock is then again turned off to the flush system and the desired amount of blood is drawn *gently* and *slowly* into the syringe. Rapid, forced withdrawal may injure the arterial segment. Next, the stopcock is turned off to the sample port, the syringe is removed and set aside, and the system is flushed for 1 to 3 seconds using the mechanism on the continuous flush device (pigtail or squeeze clamp) in order to rapidly infuse irrigation solution back through the catheter lumen.

The next step is the one most often forgotten but perhaps is the most important for preventing catheter thrombus formation and in-line bacterial growth. The stopcock is turned off to the patient and the intraarterial catheter, extension tubing, and sample stopcock are flushed (using the pressurized continuous flush system) with the irrigation solution to clear the sample port. Holding a piece of sterile gauze over the port to collect the expelled solution prevents spillage onto the bed. The stopcock is turned off to the sample port, so that monitoring can continue, and a sterile cap is reapplied. *When obtaining samples for tests other than blood gas analysis, the sampling syringe should not be heparinized.*

The newer closed systems allow collection of arterial blood samples without the need to open the system to air or discard the initial saline/blood aspirate withdrawn before obtaining the laboratory sample.

Sources of Inaccuracy in Blood Gas Determinations

Air bubbles trapped in the syringe cause time-related changes in blood gas results. These changes occur more rapidly if entrapped air is "foamed" because of the larger surface area per unit volume. If air is present in the arterial sample, significant changes in blood gases may occur within 2 to 3 minutes. To avoid inaccurate blood gas results, air should be immediately expelled and the syringe should be tightly capped. If the blood sample is at room temperature, specimen analysis should occur within 10 minutes of collection. If the sample is iced, specimen analysis may be extended to 30 minutes.

An excess of heparin in the sample syringe also may result in inaccurate blood gas results. These errors are avoided by expelling *all* the heparin and obtaining at least 3 ml of blood. Pre-anticoagulated syringes are commercially available for blood gas analysis and reduce the likelihood of inaccurate laboratory results.

Indwelling blood gas electrodes placed through the intraarterial catheter are being researched for clinical use. At this time, there are no known manufacturers for these devices. The capability of continuously monitoring PaO_2, $PaCO_2$, and arterial pH would be an exciting, major advancement for assessment and management of patients with cardiopulmonary disease. These devices would require use of at least a 20-gauge catheter. This will preclude placement in radial or dorsalis pedis sites.

Technique for Removal of Intraarterial Catheters

Arterial catheters should be discontinued when they are no longer needed. Frequently, they are left in place as a convenience to clinicians or "just in case something happens." This is not justifiable on a risk-benefit basis. Usually, however, they become nonfunctional after 3 to 4 days because of thrombus accumulation.

Sutures, if any, are removed, and the site and surrounding tissue are inspected. The technique recommended by Bedford[11] includes application of firm pressure proximal and distal to the catheter insertion site while the catheter is removed with continuous suction applied with a syringe. This technique facilitates aspiration of thrombi (Figure 7-17).

Following catheter removal, firm *manual* pressure is maintained over the insertion site for 10 minutes. Patients with coagulopathies may require the application of manual pressure for a greater length of time. Following the period of manual compression, a small pressure dressing is applied. For the first few hours thereafter, the site is routinely inspected for signs of external or internal bleeding.

Following catheter removal, a note should be made in the medical or nursing record concerning the appearance of the arterial site, motor and sensory integrity of the involved limb, and any difficulties encountered during the procedure.

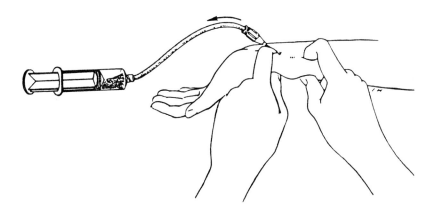

FIGURE 7-17 Technique for removal of arterial catheters—compression of the artery distal and proximal to the catheter site while the catheter is removed during continuous aspiration. This method allows aspiration of clots surrounding and within the catheter. (From Lake CL: Monitoring of arterial pressure. In Lake CL, editor: *Clinical monitoring,* Philadelphia, 1990, W.B. Saunders.)

COMPARISON OF DIRECT AND INDIRECT BLOOD PRESSURE MEASUREMENTS

Once an arterial catheter has been placed, the pressure measurements are generally found to conflict with auscultatory cuff measurements. Much controversy and debate are usually then generated around the use of "cuff" versus "art line" pressures for patient assessment and management. Although intraarterial pressures are the research "gold standard" against which the accuracy of noninvasive techniques are judged, some clinicians have greater faith in the older, more traditional auscultatory method that uses the examiner's "eyes and ears." At other times, the pressure values that are most acceptable for the patient's condition (i.e., most comforting for the clinician to believe they are) or "normal" are honored and recorded as arterial pressure. This is the worst of both possible worlds and results in an illogical and inconsistent acceptance of one technique and pressure measurement over the other. Selected therapies may consequently be inconsistent and inappropriate to the patient's clinical and hemodynamic status.

Unfortunately, we live in an imperfect world, and clinical interpretation of arterial pressure measurements obtained by neither pressure measurement technique (indirect versus direct) is ideal, simple, and straightforward. Pressure measurements with the two techniques are also based on different variables (pressure versus flow). Table 7-4 lists the differences and weaknesses of indirect and direct monitoring systems.

The problem inherent to both indirect and direct techniques is the potential for clinicians to unquestionably accept measured pressures. The practitioner must remain ever mindful that simple as well as complex blood pressure

---

TABLE 7-4

Comparison of Indirect versus Direct Arterial Pressure Monitoring

Indirect	Direct
Pressure estimate relies on blood *flow* under the compressing cuff	Directly measures actual *pressure* at the anatomic site of catheter insertion
Provides only "spot" estimates of arterial pressure; generally requires that a clinician be available for measurement	Provides continuous, real-time estimates of systolic, diastolic, and mean arterial pressure; does not require a clinician for pressure measurements
Vasoconstriction and decreasing stroke volume (shock, severe heart failure) may make Korotkoff sounds difficult or impossible to hear; generally, obtained pressures significantly underestimate true systolic pressure in vasoconstricted patients with low stroke volume	In patients with hemodynamic instability, blood pressure may not correlate with blood flow in the cannulated vessel or throughout the aterial tree, therefore adequacy of tissue perfusion is difficult to evaluate based on direct blood pressure measurements
Oscillometry, palpation, and auscultation show close agreement over high and low pressure ranges; however, these indirectly measured blood pressures tend to *underestimate* systolic blood pressure and *overestimate* diastolic pressure when compared with simultaneously obtained direct readings, particularly in patients with vasoconstriction and low stroke volume	Systolic and diastolic pressures are site variable; systolic pressure increases with increasing distance from the aortic root; mean arterial pressures are consistent throughout the arterial circulation
Defects in the aneroid gauge or mercury manometer, poor operator technique, or patient factors such as extreme obesity may result in inaccurate pressure measurements	Pressure distortion may occur as a result of underdamping or overdamping; also, a natural frequency close to the natural frequency of the pressure-pulse signal results in overshoot and a digitally displayed overestimation of the systolic pressure
The noninvasive technique has a lower patient risk profile; however, the devices may serve as an electrical current route, and "runaway" automated systems may result in compression nerve injury, venous congestion, IV infiltration, and skin-pressure lesions by prolonged or repetitive cuff inflations	Invasion of the arterial circulation is associated with several potential hazards and complications (see section on hazards and complications in text)

Comment: When a systolic pressure measured by an intraarterial catheter (arterial line) is less than that measured by an indirect method, errors in indirect technique or monitoring equipment should be suspected.

monitoring systems are predisposed to mechanical failure and the misleading effects of artifact. In today's age of high technology, the most effective monitoring and alarm system for any patient remains a vigilant bedside clinician.

REFERENCES

1. Cohn JN: Blood pressure measurement in shock: mechanism of inaccuracy in auscultatory and palpatory methods, *JAMA* 199(13):118, 1967.
2. Borow KM, Newburger JW: Noninvasive estimation of central aortic pressure during the oscillometric method: a comparative study of brachial artery pressure with simultaneous central aortic pressure measurements, *Am Heart J* 103:879, 1982.
3. Nystrom E, Keod KH, Bennett R, et al: A comparison of two automated indirect arterial blood pressure meters: with recordings from a radial arterial catheter in anesthetized surgical patients, *Anesthesiology* 62:526, 1985.
4. Remington JW: Contour changes of the aortic pulse during propagation, *Am J Physiol* 199:331, 1960.
5. Brunner JMR: *Handbook of blood pressure monitoring,* Littleton, MA, 1978, PSG.
6. Hanlon-Pena P, Pitner J: Updated clinical management of the IABP patient, *Pharmacological Considerations in Canadian Perfusion* 10(2):18, 2000.
7. Mathers LH Jr: Anatomical considerations in obtaining arterial access, *J Intensive Care Med* 5:110, 1990.
8. Seneff MG: Arterial line placement and care. In Irwin RS et al, editors: *Procedures and techniques in intensive care medicine,* ed 2, Philadelphia, 1999, Lippincott Williams & Wilkins.
9. Lowenstein E, Little JW, Lo HH: Prevention of cerebral embolization from flushing radial artery cannulas, *N Engl J Med* 285:1414, 1971.
10. Lantiegne KC, Civetta JM: A system for maintaining invasive pressure monitoring, *Heart Lung* 7:610, 1978.
11. Bedford RF: Removal of radial artery thrombi following percutaneous cannulation for monitoring, *Anesthesiology* 46:430, 1977.

SUGGESTED READINGS

Ahrens TA, Taylor LA: Normal arterial waveforms, and technical considerations in obtaining hemodynamic waveform values. In *Hemodynamic waveform analysis,* Philadelphia, 1992, W.B. Saunders.

American Association of Critical Care Nurses: Evaluation of the effects of heparinized and nonheparinized flush solutions on the patency of arterial pressure monitoring lines: the AACN Thunder Project, *Am J Crit Care* 2(1):3, 1993.

Bruner J et al: Comparison of direct and indirect methods of measuring arterial blood pressure, *Med Instrum* 15(1):11, 1981.

Byra-Cook C, Dracup K, Lazik A: Direct and indirect blood pressure in critical care patients, *Nurs Res* 39(5):285, 1990.

Campbell B: Arterial waveforms: monitoring changes in configuration, *Heart Lung* 26:204, 1997.

Carroll GC: Blood pressure monitoring, *Crit Care Clin Intensive Care Monitoring* 4(3):411, 1988.

Chyun DA: A comparison of intra-arterial and auscultatory blood pressure readings, *Heart Lung* 14(3):223, 1985

Cohn P, Brown E, Vlay S: *Clinical cardiovascular physiology,* Philadelphia, 1985, W.B. Saunders.

Gingsary Y, Pizour R, Sprung CL: Arterial and pulmonary artery catheters. In Parrillo JE, None RC, editors: *Critical care medicine: principles of diagnosis and management,* St Louis, 1995, Mosby.

Hand H: Direct or indirect blood pressure measurement for open heart surgery patients: an algorithm, *Crit Care Nurse* 12(6): 52-4, 1992.

Henneman E, Henneman P: Intricacies of blood pressure measurement: reexamining the rituals, *Heart Lung* 18(3): 263, 1989.

Hines RL, Barash PG: Hemodynamic monitoring in the intensive care unit. In Scharf SM, Cassidy SS, editors: *Heartlung interactions in health and disease,* New York, 1989, Marcel Dekker.

Imperial-Perez F, McRae M: Arterial pressure monitoring in hemodynamic monitoring series: protocols for practice, *AACN Crit Care,* 1997.

Kaye W: Invasive monitoring techniques: arterial cannulation, bedside pulmonary artery catheterization, and arterial puncture, *Heart Lung* 12(4):395, 1983.

Keckeisen M, Monsein S: Techniques for measuring arterial pressure in the postoperative cardiac surgery patient, *Crit Care Nurs Clin North Am* 3(4):699, 1991.

Kirkland LL, Veremakis C: Arterial pressure monitoring. In Carlson RW, Geheb MA, editors: *Principles and practice of medical intensive care,* Philadelphia, 1993, W.B. Saunders.

Lake C: *Monitoring of arterial pressure,* Philadelphia, 1990, W.B. Saunders.

Maltby A, Wiggers CJ: Studies on human blood pressure criteria and methods. I. The effects of partial and complete occlusion on actual pressures in compressed arteries, *Am J Physiol* 100, 1932.

Mark JB: *Atlas of cardiovascular monitoring,* New York, 1998, Churchill Livingstone.

Nelson W, Egbert A: How to measure blood pressure accurately, *Primary Cardiology,* Sept 1984, p 14.

O'Rourke MF: The arterial pulse in health and disease, *Am Heart J* 82(5):687, 1971.

Pascarelli EF, Bertrand CA: Comparison of blood pressures in the arms and legs, *N Engl J Med* 270(14), 1964.

Pierson D, Hudson L: Monitoring hemodynamics in the critically ill, *Med Clin North Am,* Nov 1983, p 1343.

Pursley P: Arterial catheters: nursing management to decrease complications, *Crit Care Nurse,* July, Aug, 1981.

Ramsey M: Blood pressure monitoring: automated oscillometric devices, *J Clin Monitor* 7(1):28, 1991.

Rebenson-Piano M et al: An evaluation of two indirect methods of blood pressure measurement in ill patients, *Nurs Res* 38(1):42, 1989.

Rebenson-Piano M, Holm K: Evaluation of automatic blood pressure devices for clinical practice, *Dimens Crit Care Nurs* 7(4):228, 1988.

Rushmer RF: Systemic arterial pressure. In *Cardiovascular dynamics,* ed 4, Philadelphia, 1976, W.B. Saunders.

Seneff MG: Arterial line placement and care. In Irwin RS et al, editors: *Procedures and techniques in intensive care medicine,* ed 2, Philadelphia, 1999, Lippincott Williams & Wilkins.

Shah N, Bedford RF: Invasive and noninvasive blood pressure monitoring. In Lake CL, Hines RL, Blitt CD, editors: *Clinical monitoring: practical applications for anesthesia and critical care,* Philadelphia, 2001, W.B. Saunders.

Sladen A: Complications of invasive hemodynamic monitoring in the intensive care unit, *Curr Probl Surg* 25(2):69, 1988.

Taylor RA, Piwinshi SE: Invasive and noninvasive measurement of blood pressure. In Levine RL, Fromm RD, editors: *Critical care monitoring from pre-hospital to the ICU,* St Louis, 1995, Mosby.

Urbina LR, Kruse JA: Blood gas analysis and related techniques. In Carlson RW, Geheb MA, editors: *Principles and practice of medical intensive care,* Philadelphia, 1993, W.B. Saunders.

Venus B, Smith RA: Direct versus indirect blood pressure measurements in critically ill patients, *Heart Lung* 14(3):228, 1985.

Yamakoshi K, Rolfe P, Murphy C: Current developments in noninvasive measurement of arterial blood pressure, *J Biomed Eng* 10(2):130, 1988.

ANAND KUMAR and GLORIA OBLOUK DAROVIC

Establishment of Central Venous Access

Central venous access with catheterization of the beating human heart was first performed in a small German hospital in 1928. Dr. Werner Forssmann, then a recent medical school graduate, conceived the idea of passing a catheter through the venous system into the right atrium for the purpose of injecting medications for life-threatening conditions or cardiac resuscitation. Up to that time, it was believed that the living human heart could not be catheterized without danger. In spite of his supervisor's refusal of permission, Forssmann secretly went to an operating room and performed antecubital venisection on himself and then courageously advanced a urethral catheter 1 foot into his venous circulation. Minutes later, in the nearby x-ray room, the catheter tip was seen to be in the right side of his heart.

Forssmann subsequently repeated the experiment on himself and in 1929 published his reports of safe catheterization of the living, human heart.[1] However, acceptance of human cardiac catheterization was slow until Cournand applied the procedure to clinical medicine while working with traumatic shock patients.[2] This 1941 publication, "Catheterization of the Right Auricle in Man,"[3] drew attention to the clinical application of this procedure. In the following two decades, diagnostic right and then left heart catheterization, pioneered by Brannon and colleagues[4] and Zimmerman and colleagues,[5] ultimately led to the development of cardiac angiography, central circulatory blood oxygen determinants, and pressure recordings.

As valuable as these techniques were diagnostically, they allowed only one hemodynamic "picture" to be obtained in the cardiac catheterization laboratory. Mean-while, at the bedside, diagnosis of and therapy for changes in the patient's condition were based on assessment and speculation derived from physical and laboratory evaluation. A continuous, real-time means of bedside hemodynamic monitoring was needed for management of physiologically labile critically ill patients.

In 1962, Wilson and co-workers[6] described the technique, management, and clinical utility of continuous central venous pressure (CVP) monitoring in the acutely ill. This first step in bedside invasive cardiac monitoring allowed direct determination of right heart function and assessment of intravascular volume status; however, correlation with the left heart function was found to be unpredictable and therefore unreliable in the critically ill (see Chapter 9, section on assessment of cardiac function).

The introduction into clinical medicine of the balloon-tipped, flow-directed pulmonary artery catheter by Swan, Ganz, and colleagues[7] in 1970 had an enormous impact on bedside management of the critically ill because the pulmonary artery "wedge" measurement normally correlates well with left atrial and left ventricular end-diastolic pressures. These catheters have since been further developed to allow measurements of right and left heart pressures, cardiac output, and right ventricular ejection fraction and end-diastolic volume, as well as a means of calculating pulmonary and systemic vascular resistances and oxygen transport and consumption.

Before direct pressure and flow monitoring of the central circulation, all of the normal and pathophysiologic cardiovascular principles described by the great innovators and pioneers (Harvey, Laënnec, Starling, Frank, Wood)

TABLE 8-1
Sites for Central Venous and Pulmonary Artery Catheter Insertion

Advantages	Disadvantages*
Central Venous Access—Subclavian Vein	
Easily accessible	Risk of air embolism
Ease in maintaining a sterile, intact dressing	Possible puncture or laceration of subclavian artery
Unrestricted neck and arm movement	Possibility of disastrous blood loss (hemothorax, hemomedi-astinum) because pressure cannot be applied to bleeding subclavian anterior tear
Less likely displacement of the catheter once in place	
Reduced incidence of thrombotic complications because of rapid venous flow rates	Risk of pneumothorax
	Phrenic nerve injury or brachial nerve injury
	Possible tracheal perforation
	Possible endotracheal tube cuff perforation
	Risk of major complications increased in patients with prior surgery in the subclavian area, emphysema, mechanical ventilation (especially PEEP)
Central Venous Access—Internal Jugular Vein	
Relatively short and direct pathway to superior vena cava or right atrium	Risk of air embolism
Reliable site for correct catheter placement	Possible puncture or laceration of the common carotid artery
Catheter displacement not likely	Possible puncture of the trachea or endotracheal tube cuff
Rapid venous flow rates decrease thrombotic complications	Risk of pneumothorax (more common in the left than in the right internal jugular vein)
Lower incidence of arterial laceration or puncture and pneumothorax than with subclavian site	Thoracic duct injury (left internal jugular only)
Central Venous Access—Femoral Vein	
Readily accessible	Presence of local smaller veins that may be cannulated inadvertently with subsequent inability to pass catheter
Familiarity with site; used by clinicians for central venous access longer than other approaches	Possible increased risk of infection due to proximity to groin
Greater ease in insertion in elderly patients with tortuous subclavian and jugular veins	Difficult in maintaining an intact, sterile dressing
	Difficult to locate in obese patients
No risk of pneumothorax; minimal risk of air embolism	Thrombosis of femoral vein is high risk factor for pulmonary embolism (risk increased in hypercoagulable states)
	Difficulty in immobilizing leg; increased risk of catheter displacement, particularly if the patient is restless

were based on astute observations derived from clinical work and animal and cadaver dissection, hypothesis, experimental demonstration, and logical deduction. Dating from the general availability of laboratory and bedside cardiac catheterization, as well as continuous hemodynamic monitoring, the expansion of understanding of the human circulation in health and disease has been explosive in growth and staggering in magnitude within the past three decades.

This chapter discusses techniques of intravenous access that ultimately allow central venous cannulation and right heart catheterization for hemodynamic monitoring, hyperalimentation, or administration of fluids, medications, and electrolytes (Box 8-1).

INSERTION SITES

Access to the central circulation may be accomplished with the initial insertion of a catheter into either a central or peripheral vein. Central venous access is defined by the location of the catheter tip rather than the site of insertion. Central venous access devices have the distal catheter tip positioned at the proximal superior vena cava/right atrial juncture.[8]

There is no ideal insertion site for cannulation of the central venous circulation. The site chosen frequently relates to the experience of the physician, but patient-related factors, such as body build; trauma areas; and specific clinical circumstances, such as coagulation abnormalities, hyperinflated lungs (positive end-expiratory

TABLE 8-1
Sites for Central Venous and Pulmonary Artery Catheter Insertion—cont'd

Advantages	Disadvantages*
Peripheral Venous Access—External Jugular Vein	
Easily accessible, especially in children, because of superficial location of the vein	Successful passage of catheter less likely than with internal jugular vein; J wire guide may be necessary to facilitate passage through junction to central veins
Minimal risk of carotid artery puncture or pneumothorax	Risk of carotid anterior puncture or laceration
	Possibility of malposition into axillary or azygos vein
	Venous flow rates less than central veins, increasing risk of thrombosis
	Risk of pneumothorax
	Difficulty in maintaining a sterile dressing, especially if patient has tracheostomy
	Increased risk of vessel thrombosis
Peripheral Venous Access—Antecubital Sites (Cephalic or Basilic Sites)	
No risk of pneumothorax or major hemorrhage	Difficult to locate in obese or edematous patients
Bleeding from site more easily controlled in patients with coagulopathies or anticoagulation	Advancement of catheter to central veins may be difficult
	Vein may not be large enough to accept a large-lumen catheter
	Access may be limited because of previous venous cutdown or venipuncture
	Venous spasm may prohibit catheter passage
	Catheter displacement is more common
	Increased risk of vessel thrombosis

*The most common disadvantage to all central venous line insertion sites is catheter-related infection, which may occur in up to 25% of cases (see Chapter 13). The importance of scrupulous sterile insertion technique cannot be overstated.

BOX 8-1
Indications and Contraindications for Central Venous Cannulation

Indications	**Relative Contraindications**
Administration of fluids and electrolytes	Coagulopathy
Drug therapy	Thrombolytic therapy
Venous access for monitoring central venous pressure	Anticoagulation
Venous access for insertion of a pulmonary artery catheter	Infection at proposed site
Parenteral nutrition	High risk of pneumothorax (PEEP, CPAP, emphysema)
Insertion of transvenous pacemaker	Severe vascular disease at proposed site
Administration of blood and blood components	Distorted vascular anatomy
Lack of accessible peripheral veins; trauma, plaster casts; chemically sclerosed, thrombosed, or inflamed peripheral veins	Suspected vena caval injury
	Combative patient
	Unsupervised, inexperienced operator

---

pressure [PEEP], continuous positive airway pressure [CPAP], pulmonary emphysema), tracheostomy, and anticoagulation should receive strong consideration. Table 8-1 lists the advantages and disadvantages of the variously used sites, which are illustrated in Figure 8-1.

In this chapter, techniques of vascular access of the internal jugular, subclavian, and femoral veins are discussed, because these are the most common vascular insertion sites. The reader is referred to other sources for techniques in cannulating other venous sites.[9-13]

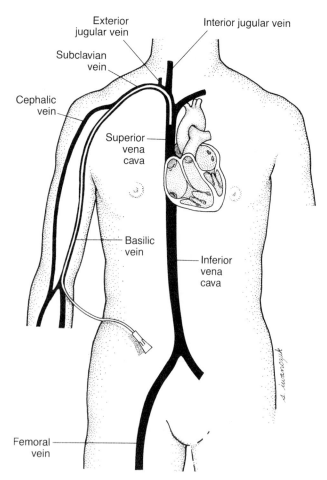

FIGURE 8-1 Sites for central venous or pulmonary artery catheter insertion. In the illustration, a CVP monitoring catheter is inserted at the antecubital fossa into the basilic vein. The catheter tip rests in the superior vena cava.

EQUIPMENT FOR CANNULATION OF THE CENTRAL VEINS

Many brands of prepackaged kits are now on the market, and they vary with the manufacturer. Bedside caregivers should be familiar with the equipment available in their institution. Box 8-2 provides a checklist for the equipment required for access and placement of a catheter in the central circulation.

PREINSERTION PROTOCOL AND CONSIDERATIONS

Patient and Family Teaching

An explanation of the purpose and technique of the procedure and expected outcome in simple language, with careful avoidance of technical terms, is an essential first step.

It is important that the patient and family members clearly understand the nature and purpose of the procedure so that they can believe that they are giving a truly informed consent. Having a confused or comatose patient does not eliminate the need to talk to the patient and explain what is being done during the procedure. Whenever possible, touching the patient for purposes of reassurance and nurturing (handholding, stroking of the brow) may contribute much to relieving the patient's anxiety and sense of alienation.

Preparation of Equipment

The appropriate equipment is assembled and set up, and the monitoring equipment and central venous pressure or pulmonary artery catheter are appropriately prepared (see Chapter 10, section on testing and preparation of the pulmonary artery catheter).

Central Venous Catheters

Three types of central venous catheters are commonly used. Each of these types serves a different clinical purpose.

Large-Gauge, Single-Lumen Catheter

The large-gauge, single-lumen catheter is used for rapid administration of fluid. To maximize flow rate, the catheter diameter should be as large as possible and the length as short as possible. In critical care units, physicians commonly insert a pulmonary artery catheter sidearm introducer (8.5 French) for present or anticipated rapid fluid administration (flow rates of approximately 1 L/min). Such large catheters are ideal for resuscitation of patients in hemorrhagic or traumatic shock using packed red blood cells and other blood components.

Multilumen Central Venous Catheters

Multilumen central venous catheters are used for the administration of multiple infusions. These are commonly used in critical care units. The multiple lumina of these catheters enable simultaneous fluid and drug administration, as well as continuous CVP monitoring. One port opens to a 16-gauge lumen, and the remaining ports open to 18-gauge lumina. Through either the 18- or 16-gauge lumen, approximately 1 L of colloid solution may be given in 60 minutes with a volumetric infusion pump. Before inserting the multilumen central venous catheters, the proximal lumina are flushed with saline solution (the use or the amount of heparin in the flush solution is institution variable) and capped to prevent intraluminal clotting and air entrainment into the circulation during the insertion procedure. The distal port is threaded over a guide wire. Once the catheter is inserted and the tip is in the proper position within the vessel lumen, aspiration of blood from all ports should be possible.

Peripherally Inserted Central Venous Catheters

A resurgence of percutaneous catheters used for extended intravenous therapy has been observed with the reintroduction of the peripherally inserted central venous catheter. These subcutaneously tunneled and totally implanted catheters are inserted for a variety of purposes (chronic administration of intravenous medications, chemotherapy, hyperalimentation, etc.) by trained nurses and physicians. They are commonly inserted using an antecubital approach.

Patient Preparation and Evaluation

Physical assessment and vital signs are obtained before and serially throughout the procedure by someone other than the operator and scrubbed assistants. Typically, during central line placement, the focus of clinicians is on the surgical site, while the often critically ill patient is in a therapeutic "limbo." Extreme vigilance at this time is necessary. Simply placing the patient in the Trendelenburg position, for the purpose of line placement, may predispose the patient to cardiovascular or respiratory distress. The patient's status should be continuously monitored and any changes promptly investigated.

Immediate life-threatening complications may occur as a consequence of the procedure, particularly subclavian or internal jugular catheterization. These complications include tension pneumothorax and venous air embolus. Both can result in profound respiratory and circulatory compromise. Consequently, a working intravenous access site and emergency resuscitation equipment should be available.

Surgical aseptic technique *must* be followed to reduce the risk of infection associated with central venous catheter insertion. The patient's face is draped and hair should be isolated with a cap before preparation and draping of the site begin. The patient's head should be turned in the direction opposite the insertion site, with the chin pointed slightly upward. The operating physician and assistants must perform a full surgical scrub and wear sterile gowns and gloves, as well as masks and caps. If the patient is in a private or semiprivate room, the door to the room should be closed and anyone circulating or entering the room for any reason must also wear a mask and cap. The area for catheter insertion is considered a surgical site and is prepared and appropriately isolated with sterile drapes. The preparation includes shaving, antiseptic scrub for 2 to 3 minutes, antiseptic paint, and a sterile drape large enough to cover the patient from head to toe while providing room

---

BOX 8-2

Equipment Required for Insertion of Catheter for Central Hemodynamic Monitoring

Central venous pressure catheter kit
Stopcocks
Suture material, needle holder
Sterile drapes
Infusion solution with administration set
Caps, masks, and sterile gowns
Local anesthetic agent (lidocaine 1% to 2% without epinephrine)
10 ml syringes
25-gauge, 1.5-inch needle for local anesthetic
21-gauge, 1.5-inch needle for exploration
18-gauge, 1.5-inch needle to aspirate lidocaine
18-gauge, 2.75-inch needle (Cook needle)
Scalpel and number 11 blade; number 15 blade if cutdown technique used
Non-Luer-Lok 10 ml syringe for exploring needle
4 × 4-inch gauze pads (10)
Transparent surgical dressing (optional)
Iodine antiseptic solution
Nonallergic tape
Dilator-sheath-sidearm assembly
Extension tubing
Intravenous atropine and lidocaine in case of cardiac arrhythmias
Suture scissors
Tincture of benzoin
Antibiotic ointment
Small straight hemostat (mosquito)
Pressure transducer
Electronic monitor/amplifier system
Pressure bag
Flush saline solution (use of heparin is variable with institution)
Flush system
Pressure tubing

Emergency Equipment

Electrocardiogram and noninvasive blood pressure monitors
Oxygen and airway management equipment
Defibrillator unit
Pulse oximeter

Surgical Dress

Cap and mask for all persons in the room
Surgical gowns and gloves for operator and assistant(s)

for two operators to perform the procedure without contaminating the equipment. A half-body drape is acceptable. Many consider a full-body drape ideal.[14]

Nasogastric feedings should be turned off approximately 10 minutes before the procedure to allow gastric emptying, and the nasogastric tube should be connected to suction for the duration of the procedure. This measure reduces the risk of aspiration of gastric contents while the patient is maintained in the Trendelenburg position.

The skin and subcutaneous tissue at the insertion site and along the expected "track" of the needle used to cannulate the vein are anesthetized with 1% to 2% lidocaine (Xylocaine) *without epinephrine.*

For cannulation of the central veins, the patient is positioned in a head- and trunk-down, supine (Trendelenburg) position of 15 to 30 degrees. If the external jugular veins are distended when the patient is in a trunk-elevated position or if the patient is orthopneic, the patient should not be lowered below the position of comfort or tolerance. The Trendelenburg position promotes distention of the veins of the chest, head, and neck; makes venous cannulation easier; and reduces the risk of air embolism. A small percentage of patients, such as the massively obese, nonetheless do not have easily identifiable anatomic landmarks or veins. Awake and cooperative patients may be instructed to perform a Valsalva maneuver during exploration and cannulation. This helps enhance venous distention and further reduces the risk of air embolism. Abdominal compression, by an assistant, may help distend the veins of unconscious or paralyzed patients or patients with pulmonary edema or other respiratory distress in whom the Trendelenburg position is absolutely contraindicated. Preprocedure sedation should be considered in restless or uncooperative patients.

Overall, the success and complication rates associated with insertion of percutaneous catheters into nonvisible veins (internal jugular, subclavian) are related to the experience of the operator. Experience should be gained under the close supervision of an expert; lack of experience is a contraindication to unsupervised placement of a central venous catheter (see Box 8-1).

TECHNIQUES FOR GAINING VENOUS ACCESS

Preprocedure preparation and positioning of equipment is crucial to performance of a low-risk, successful procedure. The procedure tray should be rearranged to suit the operator. Ideally, the equipment should be prepared so that the operator requires only one hand for handling of the equipment at all times. This may include attaching needles to syringes and removing the guards, loading syringes with lidocaine anes-

thetic or saline, and advancing the wire out of its sheath. All needles should point away from the operator. The catheter should be readied for insertion by flushing and locking secondary lumina (those not accepting the guide wire). All connection ports should be prepared. This frees the other hand of the operator to apply hemostasis in case of emergency.

Venous access for catheter insertion may be accomplished via the cutdown or percutaneous techniques. In all techniques, the preinsertion protocol previously described precedes vascular cannulation.

Cutdown Technique

Surgical cutdown is performed when venous access is not possible because veins are undetectable visually or by palpation (profoundly hypovolemic patients) or when anatomic landmarks are difficult to identify (grossly obese or edematous patients). Cutdown is occasionally necessary in infants because their very small veins are difficult to cannulate. Antecubital cutdown may have to be used when central venous catheterization is attempted from the cephalic or basilic venous sites and venous access cannot be gained by the percutaneous technique.

For the procedure, an incision is made directly over the desired vein. Once the vein is isolated, the catheter is inserted by a direct needle puncture, or a small incision is made in the vein through which the catheter is threaded. The venotomy is then closed snugly around the catheter by a fine vascular suture. Surgical cutdown significantly increases the likelihood of catheter-related sepsis (see Chapter 13). Overall, in today's clinical practice, cutdown is rarely indicated for adults.

Percutaneous Catheter Insertion

The vessel is initially located using a 21-gauge, 1.5-inch "exploring" needle attached to a 10 ml non-Luer-Lok syringe. After the needle penetrates the skin, a constant, gentle negative pressure is applied to the syringe as the needle is advanced. When the needle enters the vein, dark blood appears in the syringe. The syringe is not filled with fluid, so that the dark color of venous blood aspirated on cannulation of the vein may be accurately evaluated. Blood diluted with fluid may appear bright red, which could be mistakenly attributed to arterial puncture. Following venipuncture, the syringe is carefully removed to avoid movement of the needle tip, which may result in vascular injury or dislodgement of the needle from the vein lumen. A small hemostat may help stabilize the needle hub to prevent motion during disconnection of the syringe.

The exploring needle may then be connected to the pressure transducer if the operator is uncertain whether the needle is in a vein or an artery. The introducing needle, used with any of the anatomic approaches mentioned in the following sections, is then carefully inserted immediately adjacent to the exploring needle. The exploring needle is used as a guide and removed following entry into the vein by the introducer needle.

Deep veins may collapse against the pressure of the exploring or introducing needle tip, and the needle may pass through the vein without yielding blood (Figure 8-2, *A*). After the needle passes through the vein, the vessel reexpands (Figure 8-2, *B*), but no blood can be aspirated. If a gentle, negative pressure is applied with the syringe as the needle is slowly withdrawn, blood may be freely aspirated when the needle tip again enters the lumen of the vein (Figure 8-2, *C*).

A

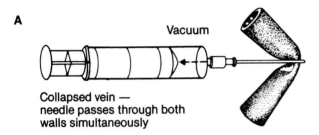

Vacuum

Collapsed vein —
needle passes through both
walls simultaneously

B

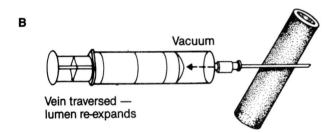

Vacuum

Vein traversed —
lumen re-expands

C

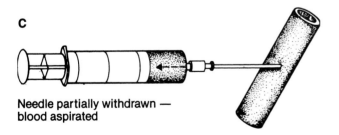

Needle partially withdrawn —
blood aspirated

FIGURE 8-2 The exploring or introducing needle may penetrate both vein walls as it is advanced. Location of the needle tip within the vein lumen, recognized by aspiration of blood, may occur if the needle is slowly withdrawn while gently pulling back on the plunger of the syringe. **A,** Needle passes through the vein without yielding blood. **B,** Vessel reexpands. **C,** Gentle, negative pressure is applied and the blood may be freely aspirated. (From Parsa MH, Tobora F, Al-Sawwaf M: Vascular access techniques. In Shoemaker WC et al, editors: *Textbook of critical care,* ed 4, Philadelphia, 2000, W.B. Saunders.)

PERCUTANEOUS ACCESS SYSTEMS AND TECHNIQUES

Most vascular catheters are inserted using one of the following percutaneous approaches: the Seldinger technique or the catheter-over-the-needle technique.

Seldinger Technique

The Seldinger technique is the preferred and most commonly used percutaneous technique for intravenous access. It employs a guide wire over which the catheter is advanced into the vessel. This method is thought to minimize trauma to the cannulated vessel and adjacent structures.

SELDINGER TECHNIQUE

1. The selected vein is cannulated. The vein lumen is known to be cannulated when free-flowing venous blood is easily aspirated.

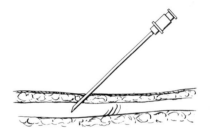

2. The syringe is carefully removed, and the hub of the introducing needle is obstructed by the operator's gloved finger to prevent accidental entry of air into the patient's venous circulation. Spontaneously breathing patients are asked to hold their breath at peak expiration at the moment of vascular insertion and whenever the catheter or needle is open to air. This maneuver increases intrathoracic pressure and prevents accidental entry of air into the patient's bloodstream. A flexible-tipped guide wire (called a J wire) is then smoothly advanced through the needle. The guide wire should be threaded until approximately 5 to 10 cm (2 to 4 inches) of the wire is in the vein. The greater portion of the guide wire should still be exposed.

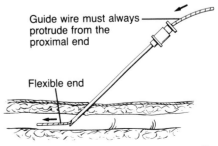

Guide wire must always
protrude from the
proximal end

Flexible end

Continued

3. Because guide wires are delicate and may bend, break, or kink, no pressure should be applied. A force of greater than 4 pounds may rupture the wire. If obstruction is met, the guide wire should be pulled back into the needle, turned, then readvanced. If further obstruction is met, the wire should be removed and free flow of venous blood reconfirmed. On reconfirmation of venous cannulation, advancement of the guide wire may again be attempted. When the guide wire has been successfully advanced, the needle is removed over the wire. At this point only the guide wire is in the vessel.

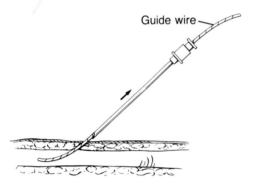

4. The insertion site is then enlarged by making a small incision in the skin with a number 11 scalpel. For best results, the blade is held parallel to the guide wire. The incision should be approximately the size of the desired intravascular catheter to prevent buckling of the sheath introducer.

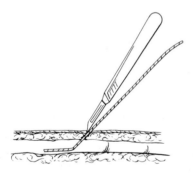

5. The dilator (and sheath assembly in the case of catheters designed for use with pulmonary artery catheters) is advanced over the guide wire to the skin. The guide wire must at all times be visible through the hub of the dilator or sheath to prevent inadvertent progression of the wire into the right side of the heart. If the guide wire is lost at the catheter hub, it is pulled back from the skin through the dilator until it is again visible at the hub. The wire must then be manually controlled by the second operator or clamped with a small hemostat.

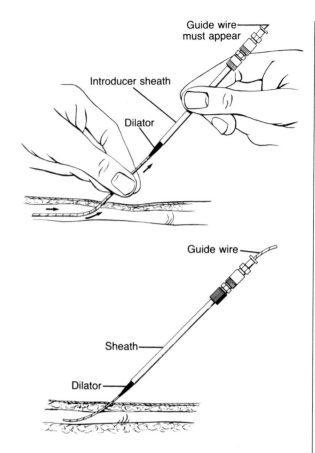

6. While grasping the dilator sheath close to the insertion site, the assembly is advanced over the guide wire using firm, gentle pressure and a rotating motion. Attempting to hold the hub or any proximal portion of the dilator sheath during advancement results in buckling of the assembly and splaying of the tip of the sheath.

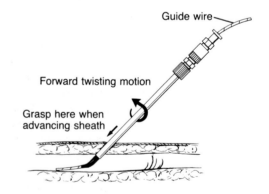

7. The dilator is advanced only a few inches into the vessel. For central access devices designed for subsequent placement of pulmonary artery catheters, the sheath assembly can then slide over the dilator into the vessel.

Once this is accomplished, the guide wire and dilator are removed. Sheath assemblies designed for pulmonary artery catheters are designed to be inserted to the hub. In the case of most single-lumen and multilumen catheters, the catheter is directly threaded over the wire once the dilator is removed. Ideal insertion distance can be determined by mapping against external landmarks. The tip of the catheter should be positioned above the right atrium in the superior vena cava. An insertion distance of 5 to 6 inches is typical for right subclavian or internal jugular access points.

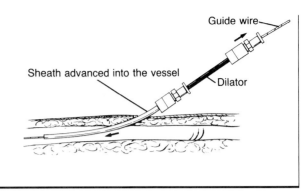

Illustrations from Sacchetti A: Large-bore infusion catheters (Seldinger technique of vascular access). In Roberts JR, Hedges JR, editors: *Clinical procedures in emergency medicine,* ed 3, Philadelphia, 1998, W.B. Saunders.

Following placement, most central venous access devices require aspiration of blood followed by a saline or heparinized saline flush to ensure that no air is inadvertently introduced. The introducer sheath may be topped by a hemostasis valve that prevents the backflow of blood. It also has a sidearm that may be used for aspiration of blood samples or as a port for infusion of fluids.

Insertion of the Catheter over the Needle

Once the needle tip is located within the lumen of the vein, the catheter is advanced over the needle and in through the puncture site of the vessel wall (Figure 8-3). The most common length is 5.5 to 6 inches, which allows the catheter tip to reach the superior vena cava from the right internal jugular or subclavian vein. The catheter occupies the entire skin and vascular puncture wound, minimizing bleeding. The major disadvantage to this

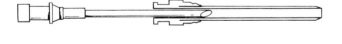

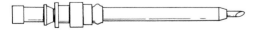

FIGURE 8-3 Insertion of catheter over needle. (From Sacchetti A: Large-bore infusion catheters [Seldinger technique of vascular access]. In Roberts JR, Hedges JR, editors: *Clinical procedures in emergency medicine,* ed 3, Philadelphia, 1998, W.B. Saunders.)

system is that the needle tip may be in the vein lumen while the leading edge of the catheter may fail to enter the vein.

SITES OF CENTRAL VENOUS CATHETER INSERTION

Right Internal Jugular Vein

The highest success rate of advancing the catheter tip into the superior vena cava or into the right heart with a pulmonary artery or central venous catheter is achieved via the right internal jugular vein. The right internal jugular vein is preferred over the left because it forms an almost straight, unobstructed route into the superior vena cava; is larger than the left internal jugular vein; and is farther from the common carotid artery at the base of the neck.

Anatomy

The internal jugular vein runs obliquely down the neck under the sternocleidomastoid (SCM) muscle. With the patient's head turned to the side, the vein follows a straight line down from the ear to the point where the clavicle joins the sternum. The only structure that maintains a fixed anatomic relationship with the internal jugular vein is the carotid artery; the vein lies slightly anterior and lateral to the carotid artery. Consequently, the major risk to this approach is carotid artery puncture or laceration. For this reason, the internal jugular approach should be used with great caution if the patient has impaired hemostatic function. Fortunately, the carotid is accessible for direct pressure (unlike the subclavian) in case of actual laceration and hemorrhage.

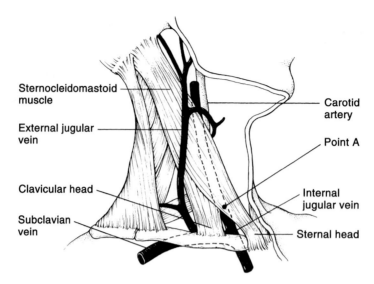

FIGURE 8-4 Superficial and deep veins of the neck and shoulder. (Redrawn from Bone RC, George RB, Hudson LH, editors: *Acute respiratory failure,* New York, 1987, Churchill Livingstone.)

Insertion Technique

The internal jugular vein may be entered from a central, a posterior, or an anterior approach. A pillow placed under the patient's shoulders to extend the neck may be useful in a very muscular or obese patient or in one with a short neck.

Central Approach. The triangle created by the two heads of the SCM is identified. The intended skin puncture site is at the apex of the triangle (point A, Figures 8-4 and 8-5). The patient's head is turned to face away from the intended insertion side.

Before venipuncture, the carotid artery is palpated to ensure that it is medial to the puncture site. A 21-gauge "exploring" needle mounted on a non-Luer-Lok syringe, which has been purged with the flush solution, is advanced with the bevel facing up and the needle at a 45-degree angle with the skin surface while negative pressure is maintained on the syringe. If the vessel lumen is not located by a depth of approximately 5 cm, the needle tip is withdrawn to the skin and reinserted more laterally. When the vein is located, the needle is carefully detached from the syringe and covered with the operator's gloved thumb. If arterial-appearing blood is withdrawn from the syringe, the needle is removed and pressure is applied manually to the area for 5 to 10 minutes. If the carotid artery is punctured, attempts at cannulation of the internal jugular veins on either side should be resisted or made with great caution because bilateral carotid hematomas may have serious consequences. As stated earlier, when in doubt, the small-gauge "exploring needle" is best connected to

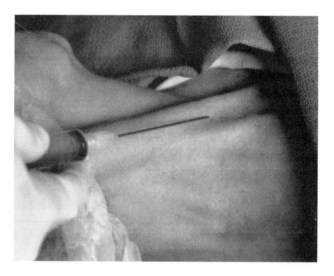

FIGURE 8-5 Venipuncture site for the central approach to internal jugular vein cannulation.

a pressure transducer to rule out arterial cannulation because critically ill patients may have poorly saturated arterial blood that may look deceptively dark and venous in origin.

If the needle is in the jugular vein, the detached exploring needle is left in the vein as a locator. Immediately superior to the locator needle, the introducer needle is inserted for introduction of the guide wire and catheter using the Seldinger technique. Alternatively, the needle-through-the-catheter technique may be done.

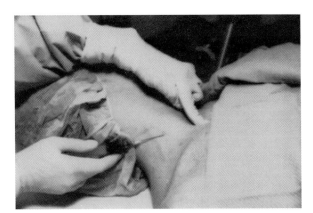

FIGURE 8-6 Venipuncture site for the posterior approach to the internal jugular vein. Note the position of the needle relative to the horizontal plane.

Posterior/Lateral Approach. The posterior approach may seem more awkward than the central approach, and there is a slightly higher risk of carotid artery puncture, but there is less risk for pneumothorax. The head is turned slightly away from the insertion side. The external jugular vein is identified on the surface of the SCM (see Figure 8-4). This is at the junction of the middle and lower third of the lateral border of the SCM muscle (approximately 2 to 3 finger breadths above the clavicle). The "exploring" 21-gauge needle is advanced from just under the belly of the SCM and is directed toward the suprasternal notch at an upward angulation of 30 to 45 degrees from the horizontal plane (Figure 8-6). The vein usually can be cannulated by the time the tip of the needle has been advanced 3 to 5 cm from the skin surface. Once the position of the internal jugular vein is determined by the small exploring needle, the introducing needle is inserted immediately superior to the exploring needle. Venous catheterization is completed using the Seldinger or needle-through-the-catheter technique.

Medial/Anterior Approach. The medial/anterior approach may be preferred in obese patients in whom landmarks for the central or posterior approach are difficult to determine. The head is midline or directed slightly contralaterally to the insertion site. Slight extension of the neck is helpful. The carotid is palpated between the trachea and the medial head of the SCM. For right internal jugular vein access, the SCM muscle and common carotid artery are separated with the index and middle fingers of the left hand. The arterial pulsation should be directly below the middle and other fingers. The needle should enter at a 45-degree angle to the skin just to the right of the palpated carotid artery and left of the SCM muscle at the

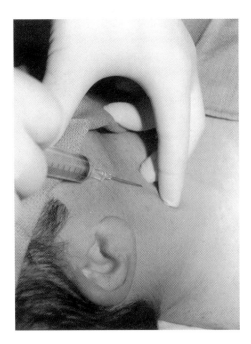

FIGURE 8-7 Venipuncture site for the medial/anterior approach to the internal jugular vein. Note the use of the index and middle fingers to separate the common carotid artery and the body of the sternocleidomastoid muscle.

midpoint of the SCM (between the level of the cricoid and thyroid cartilages). The direction of insertion should be parallel to the carotid artery and toward the junction of the medial and middle thirds of the ipsilateral clavicle (Figure 8-7). The vessel is typically entered 3 to 6 cm from the skin surface; however, in obese patients, a much greater depth may be required. For these patients, the finder needle (if used) may need to be several inches long. The internal needle portion of an angiocatheter may be effective. In experienced hands, the risk of pneumothorax or carotid artery injury is very low.

Subclavian Vein

The subclavian vein may be the site chosen because it is the method of venous access most familiar to the operator; it is easier to secure the catheter to the chest wall and maintain an intact dressing; the catheter has minimal movement with changes in the patient's head position; the surrounding tissue helps keep the vein from collapsing; and the insertion wound is away from neck wounds, such as tracheostomies. The disadvantage is that it has a higher complication rate (pneumothorax, hemothorax due to subclavian artery puncture). In fact, in patients with hyperinflated lungs (PEEP, CPAP, pulmonary emphysema) or impaired hemostatic function, this approach should be avoided or used only with great caution. Further, it should be completely avoided whenever possible in patients with severe coagulopathy or thrombocytopenia due to the total inability to provide direct compression in the event of arterial laceration.

Anatomy

The vein begins at the outer border of the first rib and runs under the clavicle. Behind the junction of the sternum and clavicle, it meets the internal jugular vein, where these vessels unite to form the innominate vein (see Figure 8-4). Then, behind the manubrium of the sternum, the innominate vein forms the inferior vena cava.

Important anatomic landmarks for the approach to subclavian vein cannulation are the anterior scalene muscle behind the clavicle and the head of the SCM as it inserts at the clavicle. The subclavian vein lies on the anterior scalene muscle, and the subclavian artery lies beneath the muscle.

Insertion Technique

In most cases the right side is favored as the cannulation site because the dome of the pleura is lower on the right (reducing the risk of pneumothorax) and the risk of thoracic duct puncture is eliminated. When the purpose of cannulation is the introduction of a pulmonary artery catheter, the left side may be preferred. This is because the venous anatomy favors balloon-tip flotation into the right ventricle from this access site more so than it does from the right subclavian site. The initial preparation proceeds as described earlier.

A small, rolled towel placed vertically between the scapulae brings the shoulders back, raises the medial portion of the clavicle, and separates the subclavian vein from the apex of the lung when the patient is lying on a soft surface such as a bed. However, care must be taken not to bring the shoulders too far back. See Figure 8-8 for the desired shoulder position.

The clavicular head of the SCM, as it inserts on the clavicle, is identified. This point is at the junction of the middle and inner thirds of the clavicle; the muscle and the clavicle form an angle where they meet. The skin puncture is done just under the clavicle. The index finger of the free hand is placed on the suprasternal notch for use as a reference point for needle direction during insertion. While gently aspirating, the advancing needle is directed just above the top of the needle puncture site. This provides a horizontal approach to the vein (Figure 8-9).

The vein should be entered at a distance of approximately 1 to 2 cm below the skin surface. If the vein is not entered, the needle is withdrawn slowly with gentle aspira-

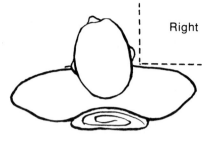
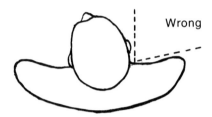

FIGURE 8-8 Correct position of the patient for insertion of a subclavian catheter. The patient's arms are at the side and a rolled towel is placed vertically along the thoracic spine. (From Grant JP: *Handbook of total parenteral nutrition,* Philadelphia, 1980, W.B. Saunders.)

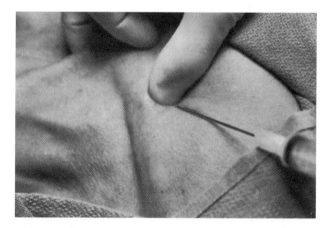

FIGURE 8-9 Hand and needle position for venipuncture of the subclavian vein. Note that the operator's left index finger is placed on the suprasternal notch and the left thumb is positioned at the outer junction of the middle and inner thirds of the clavicle.

tion. The landmarks are reevaluated, and reentry is directed slightly more upward and medially. The needle should not be directly posteriorly because the vein does not lie behind the anterior scalene muscle but the subclavian artery and lung do. Once the position of the subclavian vein is determined by the exploring needle, the introducing needle is

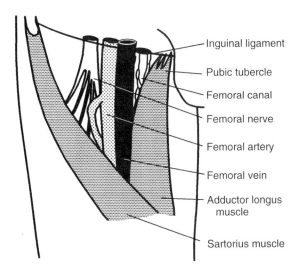

- Inguinal ligament
- Pubic tubercle
- Femoral canal
- Femoral nerve
- Femoral artery
- Femoral vein
- Adductor longus muscle
- Sartorius muscle

FIGURE 8-10 Anatomy of the femoral triangle. (From Rosen M, Latto P, Ng S: *Handbook of percutaneous central venous catheterisation,* ed 2, Philadelphia, 1992, W.B. Saunders.)

inserted immediately next to the exploring needle. Venous catheterization is then completed using the Seldinger or needle-through-the-catheter technique.

Femoral Vein

Cannulation of the femoral vein is an option in patients with severe coagulopathy or thrombocytopenia because like the internal jugular site, the femoral site allows for direct compression of the adjacent artery if lacerated. The risk of catheter-related sepsis is higher than with a subclavian site for insertion (although it may be comparable with the internal jugular site). The site can also be used for pulmonary artery catheterization, albeit with some difficulty (fluoroscopy may be required).

Anatomy

Anatomy in the area of catheter insertion into the femoral vein is shown in Figure 8-10. The femoral triangle, delineated by the inguinal ligament superiorly, the sartorius muscle laterally, and the adductor longus muscle medially, contains the major anatomic structures in the area. These structures include, in order lateral to medial, the femoral nerve, artery, vein, and canal (lymphatics). Several significant branches of the femoral vein including the great saphenous vein enter the vessel within this triangle.

Insertion Technique

A Trendelenburg position is not required for catheterization of the femoral vein. The femoral artery is pal-

pated below the inguinal ligament. Insertion of the needle at a 45-degree incline is directed toward the head just medial to the femoral artery pulsation 2 inches below the inguinal ligament. The vein should be entered within 2 to 4 cm depending on the body habitus. Several smaller branches of the femoral vein exist in this area. If blood return is sluggish or the guide wire fails to advance easily, a subsidiary vein may have been entered. In this circumstance, a repeat cannulation attempt may be necessary to enter the femoral vein. It is crucial to ensure that needle entry into the vein occurs below the inguinal ligament. Entry of the needle into the vein above the ligament impairs the ability to apply direct pressure in case of arterial laceration and may lead to retroperitoneal blood accumulation.

IMMEDIATE LIFE-THREATENING COMPLICATIONS

Complications of central venous cannulation are described in Chapter 9. However, a brief description of tension pneumothorax and venous air embolism is presented here because it may develop during catheter insertion, may be rapidly fatal, and is preventable.

Pneumothorax may occur as a result of inadvertent puncture of the pleura and perforation of the lung during the procedure. Pneumothorax is a well-recognized complication of both subclavian and internal jugular vein approaches; the overall incidence is approximately 1% to 2%. In patients receiving mechanical ventilation or patients with respiratory distress, a simple pneumothorax (produced by needle puncture) may suddenly convert to a tension pneumothorax. This complication can result in life-threatening respiratory and circulatory compromise.

The risk of pneumothorax can be minimized by using a no-risk (femoral rather than either internal jugular or subclavian) or low-risk (posterior internal jugular rather than subclavian) approach in high-risk patients (emphysema, lung hyperinflation, high airway pressures). Use of an exploring needle may also be helpful. Signs of a tension pneumothorax include hypotension in association with diminished breath sounds and hyperresonance on the side of the catheterization attempt; tracheal shift away from the side of the attempt; and a marked increase in respiratory distress in spontaneously breathing patients or marked increase in airway pressures in mechanically ventilated patients. Hypoxemia may also occur but is not universal.

If a significant suspicion exists, immediate therapy is warranted. A percutaneous needle thoracostomy (midclavicular line in the second intercostal space) should be placed. This should be followed by tube thoracotomy (chest tube insertion).

Venous air embolism may occur when the intrathoracic pressure is negative (during spontaneous inspiration) and the introducing needle, intravenous line, or monitoring system is open to air. The negative intrathoracic pressure then brings venous pressure below that of the atmosphere. This allows air to flow through the disconnected needle, intravenous line, or monitoring system and enter the circulation. This is particularly likely to occur if central venous pressures are low (hypovolemia) or the patient has inspiratory difficulty because labored inspiration is associated with marked drops in intrathoracic pressure. However, a pressure gradient of even 4 mm Hg across a 14-gauge catheter may draw approximately 90 ml of air per second into the venous circulation and produce a sudden, fatal air embolism.

The air that enters the central veins passes through the right heart chambers and embolizes into the pulmonary circulation. This occurrence may be associated with a mortality rate of at least 50%. The patient typically develops sudden dyspnea, tachypnea, chest pain, hypotension, or cardiac arrest.

Several precautionary measures may be taken to prevent this potentially fatal complication. Central venous pressure is elevated by placing the patient in the Trendelenburg position during catheter insertion. During the time when the vein and catheter system are "open to air," asking conscious, cooperative patients to perform a Valsalva maneuver, or abdominal compression applied by an assistant, transiently raises central venous pressure, thereby reducing the risk of venous entry of air. Covering the open hub of the needle with the operator's thumb prevents entry of air into the circulation. Likewise, caution must be used when removing a large-bore catheter that has been in place for a prolonged period of time, especially if the patient is thin. An occlusive dressing must be applied over the insertion site.

If air embolism is suspected, the patient is immediately placed in the left lateral decubitis position with the head down, and attempts are made to aspirate the air out of the circulation from the venous catheter.

POSTINSERTION PROTOCOL AND SITE MAINTENANCE

Once the catheter has been successfully inserted, it should be sutured in place with 3-0 to 4-0 silk suture and covered with a sterile dressing. A transparent surgical dressing or sterile gauze may be applied according to individual hospital policy for centrally placed lines. Venous placement is

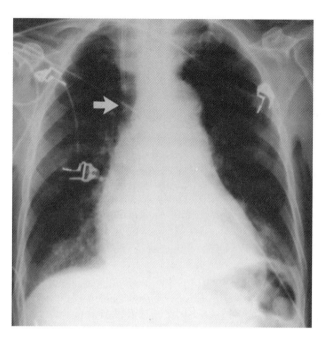

FIGURE 8-11 Proper position of the central venous catheter tip within the superior vena cava.

verified initially at the bedside by aspirating blood following cannulation or by lowering the intravenous fluid bag (when this is applicable) below the patient's body level. Certainty that the catheter tip is in the correct location and position is affirmed by a postinsertion chest radiograph. Central venous catheters should be located with the catheter tip positioned at the proximal superior vena cava/right atrial junction well away from the vena caval wall (Figure 8-11). The tip also should be kept away from the right atrium to avoid perforation of the thin right atrial wall or spontaneous migration into the right ventricle. The latter may cause life-threatening ventricular arrhythmias secondary to catheter irritation of the septal area. Chest radiographs also can rule out the presence of pneumothorax and hemothorax (see Chapter 9, section on complications). The dressing is changed according to hospital policy.

CENTRAL VENOUS CATHETER REMOVAL

Correct technique during removal of central venous catheters is crucial. Technique is especially important during removal of catheters whose sites are located close to or within the thoracic cavity (subclavian, internal jugular). The generation of negative intrathoracic pressure can result in air embolus during catheter removal.

The patient should be recumbent or in a slight Trendelenburg position. All catheter ports should be securely clamped or closed. The dressing should be removed and the site cleaned with povidone-iodine. Once the povidone-iodine is dry, any sutures should be cut.

Cooperative patients should be asked to perform the Valsalva maneuver while the catheter is steadily withdrawn over 1 to 3 seconds. Removal in patients who cannot perform the Valsalva maneuver should be timed to coincide with expiration. Removal should be timed to mid-inspiration in mechanically ventilated patients. These maneuvers ensure that a positive intrathoracic pressure exists during line removal. The positive intrathoracic pressure minimizes the risk of air embolus.

During catheter removal, resistance should be minimal. If significant resistance is met, the catheter position may need to be assessed by x-ray (catheter knot or other problem). Immediately following removal, firm pressure should be placed on the catheter exit site. The pressure should be continued for 5 to 15 minutes until venous stasis is obvious (total duration depends on the patient's coagulation status/platelet function, the catheter diameter, and duration catheter was in place). Following establishment of hemostasis, a pre-prepared occlusive dressing (two twice-folded 4 × 4-inch gauze pads covered by pressure dressing tape or vaseline occlusive dressing) should be applied. The patient should remain in bed for 15 minutes following removal of smaller catheters (e.g., triple-lumen catheter, pulmonary artery catheter) and 30 minutes following removal of larger catheters (apheresis catheters, dialysis catheters).

REFERENCES

1. Forssmann W: The catheterization of the right side of the heart, *Klin Wochenschr* 8:2085, 1929.
2. Cournand A: Cardiac catheterization: development of the technique, its contribution to experimental medicine, and its initial applications in man, *Acta Med Scand* 579(suppl):7, 1975.
3. Cournand A, Ranges HA: Catheterization of the right auricle in man, *Proc Soc Exp Biol Med* 46:462, 1941.
4. Brannon ES, Weens HS, Warren JV: Atrial septal defect. Study of hemodynamics by the technique of right heart catheterization, *Am J Med Sci* 210:480, 1945.
5. Zimmerman HA, Scott RW, Becker NO: Catheterization of the left side of the heart in man, *Circulation* 1:357, 1950.
6. Wilson JN, Grow JB, Demong CV, et al: Central venous pressure in optimal blood volume maintenance, *Arch Surg* 85:55, 1962.
7. Swan HJC, Ganz W, Forrester JS, et al: Catheterization of the heart in man with use of flow-directed balloon tipped catheter, *N Engl J Med* 283:447, 1970.
8. Whitman ED: Complications associated with the use of central venous access devices, *Curr Probl Surg* 33:331, 1996.
9. Seneff M: Central venous catheters. In Rippe JM et al, editors: *Intensive care medicine,* ed 2, Boston, 1991, Little, Brown.
10. Venous B, Mallory DL: Vascular cannulation. In Civetta JM, Taylor RW, Kirby RR, editors: *Critical care,* ed 2, Philadelphia, 1992, Lippincott.
11. Butterworth JF: Central venous cannulation. In *Atlas of procedures in anesthesia and critical care,* Philadelphia, 1992, W.B. Saunders.
12. Grauer K, Cavallara D, Gourid J, et al: Intravenous access. In *ACLS certification preparation,* vol 1, ed 3, St Louis, 1993, Mosby.
13. Parsa MH, Tobora F, Al-Sawwaf M: Vascular access techniques. In Shoemaker WC et al, editors: *Textbook of critical care,* ed 2, Philadelphia, 1989, W.B. Saunders.
14. Raad II, Hohn DC, Gibbreath BJ, et al: Prevention of central catheter related infections by using maximal sterile barrier precautions during insertion, *Infect Control Hosp Epidemiol* 15:231, 1994.

SUGGESTED READINGS

Amin D, Shah PK, Swan HJC: The Swan-Ganz catheter, insertion and technique, *J Crit Care Illness*, 1986.

Doren SC: Subclavian venipuncture. In Roberts JR, Hedges JR, editors: *Clinical procedures in emergency medicine,* Philadelphia, 1985, W.B. Saunders.

Lemen RJ, Quan SF: Intravascular line placement in critical care patients. In Fallot RJ, Luce JM, editors: *Cardiopulmonary critical care management,* New York, 1988, Churchill Livingstone.

Marino PL: Central venous access. In *The ICU book,* Philadelphia, 1991, Lea & Febiger.

Otto CW: Central venous pressure monitoring. In Blitt CD, editor: *Monitoring in anesthesia and critical care,* ed 2, New York, 1990, Churchill Livingstone.

Schwenzer KJ: Venous and pulmonary pressures. In Lake CL, editor: *Clinical monitoring,* Philadelphia, 1990, W.B. Saunders.

Seldinger SI: Catheter replacement of the needle in percutaneous arteriography: a new technique, *Acta Radiol* 39:369, 1953.

Seneff MG: Central venous catheters. In Irwin RS et al, editors: *Procedures and techniques in intensive care medicine,* ed 2, Philadelphia, 1999, Lippincott Williams & Wilkins.

Swan HJC, Shah PK: Bedside hemodynamic monitoring in critically ill patients. In Parrillo PL, editor: *Current therapy in critical care medicine,* St Louis, 1986, Mosby.

Walsh J, Dull R: Hemodynamic monitoring. In Hurford WE, editor: *Critical care handbook of the Massachusetts General Hospital,* ed 3, Philadelphia, 2000, Lippincott Williams & Wilkins.

GLORIA OBLOUK DAROVIC and ANAND KUMAR

Monitoring Central Venous Pressure

The 1962 introduction of bedside central venous pressure (CVP) monitoring was the first important step in invasive clinical assessment of cardiac function and intravascular volume status. To measure CVP, a single-lumen or multilumen catheter is advanced from a peripheral or central vein until the catheter tip rests in the proximal superior vena cava (Figure 9-1). Because the superior vena cava openly communicates with the right atrium, central venous and right atrial pressure can then be measured continuously or intermittently. *The normal range of CVP measurements is 0 to 8 mm Hg.*

CLINICAL APPLICATION OF CENTRAL VENOUS PRESSURE MEASUREMENTS

The CVP directly measures the pressure in the great thoracic veins as deoxygenated blood returns to the heart. Generally, as venous return decreases, central venous pressures decrease, and as venous return increases, central venous pressures increase. Serial or continuous measurement of CVP also provides a direct means of assessing right heart function and an indirect means of assessing left heart function and intravascular volume status. The central venous catheter also provides central intravenous access that can be used as a route to administer medications, fluids, and electrolyte solutions, as well as to withdraw blood samples. The catheter also may serve as an emergency route for temporary pacemaker insertion.

Assessment of Cardiac Function

The CVP measurement allows direct measurement of right atrial (RA) pressure and right ventricular end-diastolic pressure. In patients with a normal cardiac structures and normal lungs, the CVP also correlates with left ventricular end-diastolic pressure.

Assessment of Right Ventricular Function

The right atrium is a thin-walled, low-pressure chamber that receives venous blood. *Mean* pressure in the right atrium is normally 0 to 8 mm Hg and normally correlates with the end-diastolic (filling) pressure of the right ventricle. This correlation is possible because when the tricuspid valve is open, the right atrium and right ventricle openly communicate, and pressures equilibrate at end-diastole. If right ventricular compliance remains constant, an elevated right atrial pressure suggests right ventricular failure or intravascular volume overload. Both conditions will probably be accompanied by peripheral and jugular venous distention. The patient in *right heart failure* is likely to have a right ventricular gallop (S3), increased heart rate, a narrow pulse pressure and possibly weakened pulses, restlessness, and decreasing urine output. Dependent edema and an enlarged, tender liver also develop over time. The *volume-overloaded* patient is likely to have bounding pulses, no gallop rhythm, and an increase in blood pressure and urine output with a low urine specific gravity. In patients being treated for heart failure, a decreasing CVP indicates an improvement in cardiac performance.

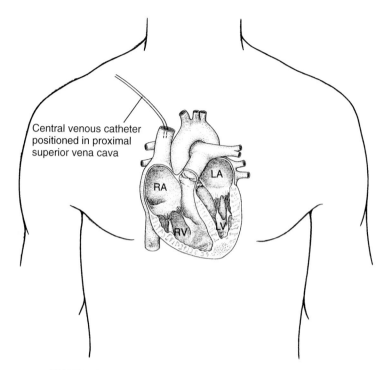

FIGURE 9-1 Anatomic position of a central venous catheter.

A low CVP in patients with signs and symptoms of low cardiac output indicates hypovolemia.

Assessment of Left Ventricular Function

Ordinarily, right ventricular end-diastolic pressure and left ventricular end-diastolic pressure correlate reasonably well in healthy persons. In the normal heart, left ventricular end-diastolic pressure can be estimated to be twice that of right ventricular end-diastolic pressure plus 2. For example, given a right ventricular end-diastolic pressure of 3 mm Hg, left ventricular end-diastolic pressure is 8 mm Hg (3 mm Hg $\times$ 2 + 2 = 8 mm Hg). Therefore, if the patient is young and without cardiopulmonary dysfunction, the CVP may be used as a guide for fluid therapy. However, in patients with differences in right and left heart function, the CVP may not correlate with left ventricular end-diastolic pressure.

In fact, there is no correlation in patients with right heart dysfunction due to tricuspid, pulmonic, or mitral valve defects; right ventricular myocardial disease or injury; or right heart failure secondary to pulmonary hypertension (chronic obstructive pulmonary disease, massive pulmonary embolism, primary pulmonary hypertension).

If the left ventricle fails in patients without pulmonary vascular or right heart disease, the CVP may be within normal limits and may not reflect the hemodynamic changes that are occurring or have occurred in the left ventricle for the following reason. When the left ventricle fails, stroke volume decreases and left ventricular end-diastolic volume and pressure increase. This volume/pressure overload is then reflected to the cardiac and vascular structures in back of the failing left ventricular chamber as elevated left atrial, pulmonary venous, pulmonary capillary, and pulmonary arterial pressures. However, as long as the right ventricle is able to eject adequately against the increased afterload, CVP remains normal. Only if the right ventricle ultimately fails are elevated pressures measured from the central veins. By this time, pulmonary edema, the consequence of left heart congestive failure, is well established and clinically evident (Figure 9-2).

After the introduction of the pulmonary artery catheter (PAC), evaluation of cardiopulmonary function in the intensive care unit (ICU) focused on the measurements obtained with the PAC. For a period of time, use of isolated CVP monitoring in most ICUs had been nearly abandoned. However, there is renewed interest in and strong arguments for increased use of CVP monitoring, rather than pulmonary artery catheterization, in patients with normal cardiopulmonary anatomy and ventricular function. Passage of a catheter through the right heart into the pulmonary circulation and maintenance is associated with risks and complications not found with simple CVP monitoring. Highly emergent situations do not allow the time for pulmonary

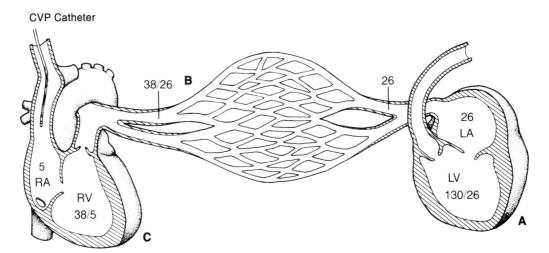

FIGURE 9-2 The left ventricle **(A)** is failing and the elevated left ventricular end-diastolic pressure is reflected back to the level of the pulmonary arterial circulation **(B).** However, the right ventricle **(C)** is able to mount a systolic pressure commensurate with the increased impedance to ejection and is not in failure. Therefore right atrial or central venous pressure does not reflect left ventricular failure.

artery catheterization. Furthermore, central venous catheters are commonly placed as a route for fluids, medications, and nutrition. Attachment of one port of a multilumen central catheter to a pressure transducer is a simple means of assessing hemodynamic change or a means of guiding fluid therapy in low-risk surgical patients. One recent study compared the use of pulmonary artery pressure versus CVP monitoring in low-risk patients undergoing coronary artery bypass grafting (CABG).[1] The patients in the pulmonary artery catheterization group experienced greater weight gain, increased total hospital charges, and longer intubation and ICU stay time than the CVP group. The use of only CVP monitoring in low-risk CABG patients is not without precedent. Other studies dating back as far as 1983 reported similar findings.[2-4] Possible explanations for these findings include chance differences in patient outcome between the two groups; bias when the surgeon or anesthesiologist selected a pulmonary artery rather than CVP catheter in terms of patient age; left ventricular ejection fraction (all were greater than 0.40); and history of congestive heart failure and the difference in the volume of postoperative fluid therapy between the two patient groups.

Assessment and Management of Intravascular Volume Status

Central venous pressure measurements can be used to assess and manage intravascular volume status because pressure in the great thoracic veins generally correlates with the volume of venous return. Also, because the volume of blood that returns to the heart is normally ejected by the heart, in patients with severe hypovolemia, subnormal CVP measurements are usually associated with a decreased cardiac output. Patients with significant volume overload typically have elevated CVP measurements and cardiac output. However, CVP measurements that are within a normal range do not necessarily indicate normal intravascular volume and cardiovascular dynamics. This is because the venous system is able (within physiologic limits) to adjust to changes in circulatory volume by compensatory constriction or dilation in order to maintain venous return and cardiac output at normal levels. For example, a rapid, small-to-moderate decrease in vascular volume immediately results in a decrease in venous return, as well as decreased right atrial pressure. However, the venous system quickly constricts to increase venous return, and right atrial pressure and cardiac output return toward normal. The reverse happens with volume overload.

Therefore, when evaluating intravascular fluid losses or gains and monitored responses to fluid therapy, isolated CVP measurements are not as meaningful as are clinical and CVP responses to fluid challenges. A rapid infusion of 300 to 500 ml of fluid in a normovolemic, healthy adult results in a CVP increase of approximately 2 to 4 mm Hg with a return to near baseline within 10 to 15 minutes. Rapid increases in CVP that do not decrease toward normal values within 10 minutes suggest either an increased intravascular volume, a noncompliant right ventricle, or both. On the other hand, if the CVP fails to increase or increases and then returns to baseline within 5 minutes, a reduced intravascular volume is suggested.

Overall, CVP reflects the interrelationship among intravascular volume, venous tone, and right ventricular function and is a means of indirectly assessing left heart function in persons without cardiopulmonary disease.

Administration of Fluids or Drugs

Peripheral venous administration of hypertonic or caustic fluids, such as potassium chloride at concentrations greater than 40 mEq/L, causes vein irritation, pain, and phlebitis due to the relatively slow peripheral venous flow rate and consequent delayed wash-out of intravenous (IV) solutions. However, blood flow in the great veins of the thorax is rapid and dilutes the IV solution immediately on entry into the circulation.

Peripheral venous catheters also tend to be less stable than centrally placed catheters. Subcutaneous infiltration of irritating or vasoactive drugs, such as norepinephrine (Levophed), may result in regional tissue necrosis. Overall, central venous catheters are recommended for administration of such vasoactive and caustic medications, as well as concentrated electrolyte solutions such as potassium.

LIMITATIONS OF CENTRAL VENOUS PRESSURE MONITORING

Several factors, if present, may affect central venous pressure measurements and prevent them from being a dependable index of circulating volume or cardiac function.

Patient-Related Factors

A single, isolated CVP measurement is of little value unless it is very high or low. Evaluation of CVP trends, along with other hemodynamic and assessment data, is essential to effective patient evaluation.

Systemic Venoconstriction

If the patient has systemic veins that are constricted (hypovolemia, low-cardiac-output states, administration of norepinephrine and dopamine), the measured CVP may be greater than that appropriate for the circulating blood volume. In other words, a normal or near-normal CVP measurement may not betray the underlying hypovolemia.

Decreased Right Ventricular Compliance

Acute or chronic decreases in right ventricular compliance due to ischemia, hypertrophy, restrictive or constrictive cardiomyopathy, cardiac tamponade, acidosis, or myocardial fibrosis may render the right ventricular chamber less distensible. As a result, the measured CVP value may be disproportionately and deceptively high for any given intravascular or intraventricular blood volume.

Venous Patency

The accuracy of the CVP measurement depends on the patency of the venous system. If, for example, there is a tumor mass or hematoma compressing the vena cava or any problem with the patency of the veins or structure of vein valves, central venous flow and pressure are affected. Venous pressure will be higher proximal to the venous obstruction and lower distal to the obstruction. As a result of the obstructed venous flow, measured CVP does not accurately reflect intravascular volume status or right ventricular filling.

Tricuspid Valve Disease

Mean CVP does not correlate with right or left ventricular end-diastolic pressure in patients with significant tricuspid regurgitation or stenosis.

Tricuspid Regurgitation. This is associated with recirculation of blood within the right heart chambers. The regurgitant systolic v waves produce elevations in mean CVP that are out of proportion to blood volume changes and right ventricular end-diastolic pressure. The v waves also may be noted in the central venous waveform (see Chapter 22, Fig. 22-23).

Tricuspid Stenosis. This defect impedes blood flow to the right ventricle and prevents end-diastolic equilibration across the stenotic valve. Consequently, measurement of right ventricular end-diastolic pressure is impossible. In patients with significant tricuspid stenosis, the measured CVP correlates only with right atrial and central venous pressures. However, judgments about circulating blood volume are difficult because this valve defect is characterized by elevated right atrial and central venous pressures.

Other cardiac abnormalities, such as those producing left-to-right intracardiac shunts (acute ventricular septal defect), also make isolated or trend interpretation of CVP measurements difficult if not impossible.

Mechanical Ventilator–Induced Factors

If the patient is receiving positive-pressure ventilatory support, the mean CVP may be falsely elevated because of the cyclic positive pressure ventilator breaths. Positive pressure ventilator breaths applied to the patient's airway are transmitted to the intrathoracic cardiovascular structures and increase right atrial and measured central venous pressures. At the same time, the externally applied positive intrathoracic pressure impedes venous return and consequently decreases cardiac output.

The problem of ventilator-induced artifact is compounded by the addition of *positive end-expiratory pressure* (PEEP; *continuous positive airway pressure* [CPAP]). At levels greater than approximately 10 to 15 cm H_2O, there is an unpredictable disparity between CVP measurements and cardiac output measured on and off the ventilator. This makes interpretation of CVP measurements and cardiac function difficult. However, removing a patient from the mechanical ventilator, particularly with PEEP, to obtain CVP measurements is not recommended. The clinician should be aware that the CVP may be overestimated in patients with ventilatory support and that decreases in cardiac output also may be ventilator induced (Figure 9-3).

Generally, evaluation of the direction of change in consistently obtained CVP measurements over time is more clinically sound than basing diagnostic or therapeutic judgments on isolated measurements. Because the accuracy of obtained measurements may be temporarily or consistently distorted by patient, mechanical ventilator, and monitoring artifacts, it is important that clinicians consider the *probability* of inaccuracy of CVP measurements. This is particularly true if the CVP does not correlate with serially obtained physical assessment findings and other laboratory and monitored data.

CENTRAL VENOUS PRESSURE MEASUREMENTS OBTAINED BY A PRESSURE TRANSDUCER VERSUS A CALIBRATED WATER MANOMETER

Before the widespread use of electronic pressure monitoring, CVP measurements were typically obtained using a calibrated water manometer. With the zero point of the water manometer held at midchest (right atrial) level, the CVP is equal to the height of the water column as it reaches pressure equilibrium with blood within the central vein invaded by the central venous catheter. Measurements obtained using a water manometer are recorded in cm H_2O. The main advantage of this system is simplicity, as well as rapid setup time. Disadvantages include (1) the need to convert CVP measurements from cm H_2O to mm Hg for comparative evaluation of other cardiovascular pressure measurements; (2) the unavailability of the RA waveform for analysis; (3) the slow response time of the water column to equilibrate to RA pressure; (4) respiratory-induced fluctuations in the water column that may make CVP interpretation difficult; (5) intermittent "snapshot" rather than continuous CVP measurements; and (6) risk of system contamination if the water manometer is filled for pressure readings and water spills over the top of the plastic manometer.

In current clinical practice, CVP is typically measured with an electronic monitoring console and a pressure transducer connected to the in situ central venous catheter or proximal (right atrial) port of a pulmonary artery

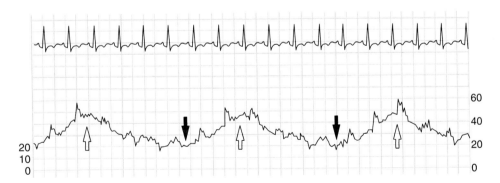

FIGURE 9-3 Right atrial waveform, from a pulmonary artery catheter, with simultaneously recorded ECG from a head-injured male with neurogenic pulmonary edema. The patient is being maintained on controlled mechanical ventilation with 30 cm H_2O PEEP. Peak inspiratory pressures are 100 cm H_2O. The *open arrows* indicate the positive pressure (ventilator) breaths, and the *solid arrows* indicate end-expiration. It is at this point that right atrial pressure is recorded. Note that the end-expiratory pressure measurement is approximately 20 mm Hg. This grossly elevated value should not be considered to be a "true" indication of intravascular volume or right ventricular function. Rather, the pressure measurement is spuriously elevated as a result of the excessively high intrathoracic pressures surrounding the heart and blood vessels. In this circumstance, patient evaluation and management is based on "trend analysis" of central circulatory pressures.

catheter. Measurements by the electronic monitoring unit are recorded in mm Hg. Only this technique will be discussed because the water manometer technique is rarely, if ever, used in current practice. The reader is referred to manufacturer's instructions for use (enclosed in manometer and tubing packaging) on the rare occasions when this technique is chosen.

CENTRAL VENOUS INSERTION SITES AND PROTOCOL FOR CATHETER INSERTION

Sites and surgical technique for central venous access are discussed in Chapter 8.

Catheter tip location is an extremely important consideration. The ideal location of the catheter tip, confirmed by chest radiograph, is the distal innominate or proximal superior vena cava, 3 to 5 cm proximal to the caval-atrial junction (see Figure 9-1). The caval-atrial junction is approximately 13 to 17 cm from right-sided subclavian vein or right internal jugular venous insertion sites and 15 to 20 cm from left-sided insertions.[5]

The importance that the catheter tip *not* lie within the right atrium cannot be overstated; a right atrial catheter tip may also migrate into the right ventricle. Perforation of the thin atrial wall may result from the action of the beating heart against the stiff catheter tip, as well as patient arm and neck movements; two thirds of patients with secondary tamponade die[6] (see Perforation of the Cardiac Chambers, later in this chapter). Atrial and ventricular arrhythmias may also develop from mechanical irritation or infusion of caustic fluids or drugs.

TYPES OF CATHETERS USED FOR CENTRAL VENOUS PRESSURE MEASUREMENT

Various types of catheters may be used to measure central venous pressure. The pulmonary artery catheter is discussed in detail in Chapter 10. Central venous catheters are made of various materials and may have a single lumen or multiple lumina.

Catheter Material

Catheters for central venous insertion are made of various materials, none of which is ideal for all clinical uses. See Table 9-1 for comparison of central venous catheter materials.

The potential for catheter-related complications is related, in part, to the level of *catheter inertness*. For example, polyvinyl chloride (PVC), polypropylene, and polyethylene catheters are the least inert (most reactive) and most likely to be associated with development of phlebitis and catheter-related thrombosis, whereas Silastic catheters are the most inert.

Flexibility also characterizes catheter material. A rigid catheter is more easily passed through the skin and subcutaneous tissue but, unfortunately, is more likely to perforate a blood vessel or the right atrial wall. Teflon is the most rigid of the catheter materials, whereas Silastic is the most flexible (similar to cooked noodles). Highly flexible catheters make venous access difficult without a stylet or guide wire.

The decision for a type of catheter material is based on the use intended. For example, catheters for long-term hyperalimentation should be the most inert and flexible (Silastic catheters). Clinicians choose catheters that are

---

TABLE 9-1
Comparison of Central Venous Catheter Materials

Type of Material	Chemical Inertness	Thrombogenicity	Flexibility	Transparent?
Polyvinyl chloride (PVC)	− − −	+ + +	+ +	Yes
Siliconized PVC	−	+ +	+ +	Yes
Polyethylene	− −	+ + +	+ +	Yes
Polypropylene	− −	+ + +	+ +	Yes
Siliconized polypropylene	0	+	+ +	Yes or no
Teflon	−	+	+	No
Silastic	0	0	+ + + +	No
Polyurethane	− −	+	+ + +	No

From Blitt CD, editor: *Monitoring in anesthesia and critical care medicine,* New York, 1985, Churchill Livingstone, by permission.

0, None; +, minimal; + +, moderate; + + + and + + + +, large; −, less; − −, much less; − − −, markedly less.

stiff (Teflon, polyethylene) and easy to insert for emergency fluid resuscitation.

Number of Catheter Lumina

A single-lumen or multilumen catheter may be used for CVP monitoring purposes. The disadvantage of the single-lumen catheter is that any continuous fluid or drug infusion must be temporarily interrupted to obtain the CVP reading. The multilumen catheters provide more therapeutic options and have gained wide acceptance in the operating room and intensive care units. The multilumen catheter has three distinct infusion ports that terminate 2.2 cm apart at the distal end (Figure 9-4, *A* and *B*).

With a percutaneous sheath introducer with a sidearm infusion port, four lumina are available for use. The multilumen catheter is not recommended when insertion will be via a peripheral vein because of its large outside diameter (7 French).

Central venous multilumen catheters can be used to (1) withdraw venous blood samples; (2) administer different or incompatible drugs simultaneously; (3) administer hyperalimentation solutions; (4) administer blood, blood products, or fluids; (5) phlebotomize the patient as necessary; and (6) obtain CVP measurements.

PROTOCOLS FOR OBTAINING CENTRAL VENOUS PRESSURE MEASUREMENTS USING A PRESSURE TRANSDUCER/ ELECTRONIC MONITOR

This system may be used for obtaining intermittent or continuous CVP measurements. Patient position and the point at which the transducer is zeroed are important factors in accurate CVP measurement.

Patient Position

Ideally, the patient is supine without a pillow. However, if the patient's condition does not permit the supine position, the reading may be performed with the head of the bed elevated to 30 degrees without changing the measured

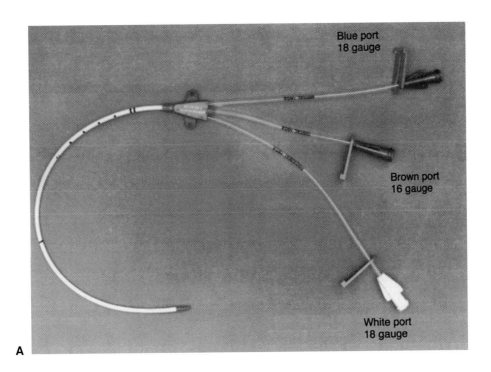

A

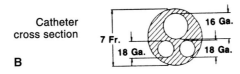

Catheter cross section

B

FIGURE 9-4 A, A multilumen central venous catheter. **B,** Catheter cross section illustrating intraluminal size. (From Arrow International, Inc., Reading, PA 19605.)

values. If, however, the patient is orthopneic, even a 30-degree trunk elevation may not be clinically and hemodynamically tolerated. In this case, the patient should be allowed to remain in his or her position of comfort, and the CVP should be measured consistently from the trunk-elevated position until the orthopnea is resolved. The central venous pressures measured from the upright position are lower than values in the supine position because of the gravity-induced changes in intrathoracic blood volume. However, as stated earlier, therapeutic judgments and decisions are best based on monitoring and clinically observed changes over time and *not* on an isolated measurement. Any variation in the measurement procedure (upright versus supine patient position), as well as any observed difference between upright versus supine measurements, should be documented in the chart and bedside flow sheet and taken into consideration when interpreting measurements or relating them to others.

Leveling the Zero Reference Point to Midchest

The transducer is leveled to the midchest position, regardless of patient's backrest position. This provides a zero reference point at the right atrium (see Chapter 6, Fig. 6-7).

Equipment and Setup

Several possible setups may be used, many of which involve commercially available kits. Equipment and kits may be adapted to meet the individual unit's needs.

CVP measurements may be recorded from the proximal port of a pulmonary artery catheter or from a separate single-lumen or multilumen central venous catheter. Two methods of setup for central circulatory pressure measurement are possible. One uses two separate transducers—one for the proximal (right atrial) pulmonary artery catheter port or a separate central venous catheter and one transducer for the distal (pulmonary artery) port. The advantage to the double-transducer system is that both right atrial and pulmonary artery pressures and waveforms are continuously displayed. This method, however, is chosen less frequently than the single-transducer technique, which conserves equipment and is therefore more cost effective. When the single-transducer method is used, the monitor should record and continuously display the pulmonary artery pressures rather than right atrial pressure. The reason is to observe for spontaneous pulmonary artery catheter migration into the wedge position, which is indicated by gradual damping of the pulmonary artery

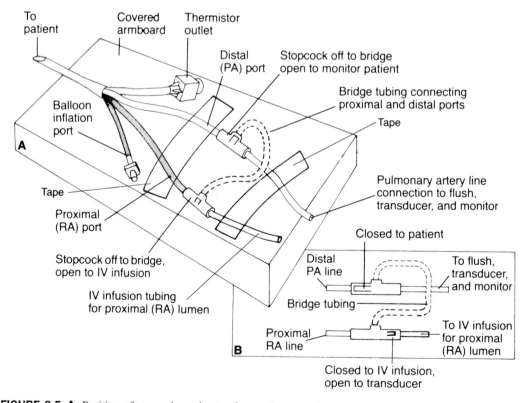

FIGURE 9-5 A, Position of stopcocks and setup for continuous pulmonary artery pressure monitoring with intermittent right atrial pressure measurements. **B,** Position of stopcocks for right atrial pressure measurements.

waveform. Another reason is that the pulmonary artery diastolic pressure normally correlates well to left ventricular end-diastolic pressure. The filling pressure of the left ventricle is a far more important hemodynamic measurement to continuously assess in critically ill or injured patients.

One possible single-transducer setup has an extra bridge tubing (Figure 9-5). In this setup, the end of the pulmonary artery catheter, with its infusion ports, is secured to a short armboard covered with clear, nonallergenic tape. This setup provides stabilization and easy identification of all pulmonary artery catheter ports. A right atrial waveform (Figure 9-6) and pressure measurement may be quickly obtained with a turn of two stopcocks.

COMPLICATIONS OF CENTRAL VENOUS PRESSURE MONITORING

Complications associated with CVP monitoring are essentially the same as those associated with access to a central vein for any purpose. Complications include, but are not limited to, hemorrhage, vascular erosion, arrhythmia, local and systemic infection, fluid overload, thromboembolic problems, electrical microshocks, air emboli, perforation of the cardiac chambers, and pneumothorax.

Hemorrhage

Hemorrhage may occur overtly, as in the case of bleeding from the insertion site. Bleeding also may be occult, such as hematoma formation deep in body tissue or oozing into a body cavity due to laceration or through-and-through perforation of the involved vessel. The risk of hemorrhage is increased in patients receiving anticoagulant therapy, having deficient clotting factors, having coagulopathy, or having undergone multiple catheter insertion attempts. It is the responsibility of the clinician to check for both visible and occult bleeding by signs such as bruising or swelling. Oozing into a body cavity may be manifest only as signs and symptoms of hypovolemia, such as restlessness, apprehension, pallor, cool distal extremities, tachycardia, or thirst. Attempted central venous access into the femoral vein carries with it the risk of bleeding into areas that can accommodate large volumes of blood before overt local evidence of hemorrhage is apparent. If the catheter is correctly placed below the inguinal ligament, significant bleeding (a liter or more) may occur into the thigh with little local evidence of hemorrhage. If puncture of the vein is inadvertently superior to the inguinal vein, any hemorrhage will track posteriorly into the retroperitoneum. Extremely large amounts of blood can collect at this site without overt local evidence of hemorrhage. Similarly, subclavian or internal jugular venous catheterization may be complicated by substantial bleeding into the

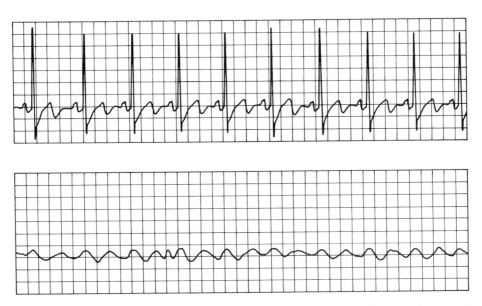

FIGURE 9-6 Right atrial waveform compared with a surface ECG tracing. The oscillations relate to right atrial *a* and *v* waves; absence of oscillations suggests catheter occlusion or an overdamped monitoring system. Right atrial pressures are monitored on the lowest available scale, usually 0 to 30 mm Hg.

mediastinum (hemomediastinum) or the pleural space (hemothorax) with little evidence of a problem at the insertion site. Of course, inadvertent penetration of the local artery with either an exploring or introducer needle or with the catheter itself substantially increases the risk of hemorrhage. If undetected and untreated hemorrhage does occur, decompensated shock (hypotension) eventually results.

Hemorrhage that cannot be stopped by applied pressure may require removal of the catheter, as well as surgical cutdown at the site of the bleeding for exploration and possible repair of the damaged vessel. The rate of bleeding from the jugular or subclavian veins may be reduced by elevating the patient's head and thorax because this position decreases the pressure in the veins by gravity effect.

Vascular Erosions

Vessel erosion typically occurs 1 to 7 days following catheter insertion. Erosion may be due to repeated irritation of the vessel wall by a stiff catheter or by the infusion of caustic or hypertonic solutions. This complication is more common with central venous catheters placed via the left internal or external jugular vein because the catheter tip is more likely to be up against the superior vena caval wall (Figure 9-7).

Extravascular catheter tips may result in the accumulation of IV solution or blood in the pleural space or medi-

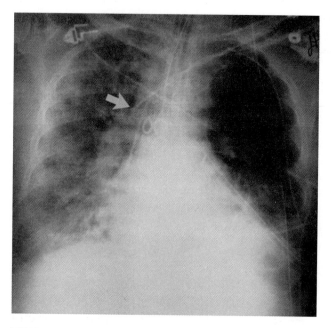

FIGURE 9-7 Chest radiograph illustrating a central venous catheter tip resting against the superior vena caval wall (*arrow*). The catheter was inserted via the left subclavian vein.

astinum. Therefore a new pleural effusion or widening of the mediastinum may be noted on the chest radiograph. The patient also may have sudden-onset dyspnea, tachypnea, and tachycardia. Proper positioning of the catheter tip (parallel to the vessel wall) should be confirmed on the catheter postinsertion chest radiograph and any routine films obtained thereafter. Free aspiration of blood from the catheter does not rule out vascular perforation.

Arrhythmias

Irritation of the right atrial or right ventricular endocardium by a CVP catheter tip that has migrated from the SVC may precipitate a variety of arrhythmias. Ventricular arrhythmias (ventricular premature beats, ventricular tachycardia) are most common and are associated with spontaneous catheter advancement into the right ventricle. The arrhythmia may also be precipitated by turning the patient (more likely to the left) because position change may cause the catheter tip to fall against and irritate the ventricular endocardium. If this occurs, the patient should be immediately brought back to the original position. This simple maneuver may terminate the arrhythmia until the catheter is pulled back to the superior vena cava by a physician.

Right ventricular migration is easily and immediately documented by the appearance of a right ventricular waveform if the central venous port is transduced. When in doubt, a chest radiograph documents catheter location. As stated earlier, to ensure safe distance from the right ventricle, the catheter tip should be located in the proximal superior vena cava.

Infectious Complications

All central venous lines are potential sources of nosocomial infections and septicemia. Insertion site or catheter contamination can occur as a result of poor sterile technique during insertion, downward migration of normal skin flora following catheter placement, catheter colonization from distant infected foci or contaminated tubing, pressure transducers, or IV and flush solutions. Once the catheter has become colonized, it may become the source of systemic infection. Polyurethane CVP catheters combined with silver compounds are now commercially available. The release of silver ions from the catheter kills colonizing bacteria and may afford some protection from catheter-related infection.

All patients with invasive lines must be carefully monitored for signs or symptoms associated with infections, such as fever or hypothermia; chills; localized redness; swelling; heat; purulent discharge or pain at or above the insertion site; or the development of an unexplained, elevated, or abnormally decreased white blood cell count. It is imperative that signs of a local inflammatory response or systemic infection be considered to be potentially infusion-related sepsis, investigated, and appropriately treated (see Chapter 13).

Staphylococcus aureus, S. epidermidis, and entero-cocci are the most common bacterial infectious agents associated with contaminated invasive lines. *Candida* species are also becoming major pathogens in catheter-related infections. Peripheral insertion sites for central venous catheters are at increased risk of sepsis. Pinella and co-workers[7] reported an increased infection rate of 20% when the antecubital route was used for insertion versus 7% when the subclavian route was chosen. Specific catheter characteristics and duration of catheterization also affect risk of infection (see Chapter 13).

The risk of infection increases in the case of improperly capped stopcocks, frequent catheter repositionings, and contaminated infusates caused by poor admixture technique when adding medications or electrolyte solutions. Immunosuppressed patients (major trauma, major surgery, major burn injury, congenital or acquired immunodeficiency diseases) are especially susceptible to the development of infections. Clinical signs of infection in such patients may be blunted. Patients with infectious sites such as tracheostomies may also be at greater risk of catheter-related sepsis.[8]

Sterile technique is mandatory during catheter insertion, during subsequent dressing changes, and whenever interruption of the fluid-filled system is necessary. The dressing should be changed every 48 to 72 hours and when dressings are soiled, moist with perspiration, or the edges are not intact. As with all invasive lines, the catheter should be left in place no longer than is absolutely necessary to minimize the septic potential. If catheter-related infection occurs, the catheter must be removed and the catheter tip sent to the laboratory for culture and sensitivity studies. The specificity of catheter culture improved when Maki and colleagues[9] introduced a solid agar technique that differentiates colonized from contaminated catheters. When removing the catheter for the purpose of microbial study, meticulous care must be taken to prevent accidental contamination of the tip as it is prepared for the laboratory. Simultaneous peripheral blood cultures should be obtained to document the presence of the same bacterial or fungal contaminant as that found to be colonizing the suspected intravascular catheter.

Fluid Overload and Hypothermia

Fluid overload may be caused by unregulated infusion of IV solution owing to a defective or an improperly adjusted flow device, or failure to manually adjust the solution flow rate with the standard IV tubing roller clamp. Even relatively small amounts of accidentally infused fluids are hazardous, particularly to patients sensitive to alterations in fluid balance, such as those with congestive heart failure and oliguric renal failure. The symptoms of acute fluid overload are most often present shortly after the accidental volume bolus; tachypnea, dyspnea, hypertension, and adventitious lung sounds are related to the severe volume overload causing pulmonary edema. The CVP is elevated in proportion to the severity of hypervolemia. Forced diuresis, with potent medications such as furosemide (Lasix), may be lifesaving.

In situations where aggressive resuscitation is called for, infusion of appropriate amounts of room-temperature resuscitative fluids may result in marked hypothermia. This may result in coagulopathy and platelet dysfunction, as well as cardiac dysrhythmias. When large amounts of resuscitative fluids are being infused, an in-line heater device or prewarming of infusates to body temperature is indicated.

Thromboembolic Complications

Catheter kinking or poor fluid flow through the catheter can predispose the patient to occlusion of the catheter lumen by a blood clot. Catheter design and composition (thrombogenicity) are also related to the predisposition to formation of a fibrin clot that may surround the catheter (regionally or entirely) from its point of entry into the vein to its distal tip. Patient-related factors that increase the thrombogenic risk include diseases or conditions associated with hypercoagulability, such as polycythemia, fever, myocardial infarction, cancer, estrogen therapy, antithrombin deficiency, and others. Trauma sustained by the vessel wall during or after insertion also predisposes the patient to clot formation on the wall of the vein. Most of these intravascular thrombi are clinically silent. Significant or total occlusion of the vein occurs in a small percentage of patients and may be clinically evidenced as edema of the involved arm, the neck, and the face. Unexplained sepsis may be the presenting sign of a catheter thrombus that has become infected with bacteria or fungi (septic thrombus). Fragmentation or complete migration of the central venous thrombus clot may result in pulmonary embolization and infarction of lung tissue.

Forceful flushing of the central venous line should be avoided to prevent the possibility of dislodging a clot that may have formed around the catheter tip. If blood cannot be easily aspirated or free flow of IV solution does not occur, the presence of a clot on the catheter tip should be suspected. When a port of a multilumen catheter is not used for continuous IV infusion, intermittent saline flushes may help prevent thrombus formation. An infusion control device is recommended to ensure an adequate and a consistent flow rate for continuous infusions.

Treatment of a central venous thrombus requires removal of the catheter, culture of the catheter tip, and initiation of medical dose heparin therapy. Local symptoms should resolve in several days.

Electrical Microshocks

An invasive pathway directly to the heart exists whenever a patient has a central venous catheter in place. Heart muscle is particularly sensitive to electrical stimulation. *Microshocks,* or electrical currents of less than 1 ampere, can travel via the central venous catheter to the myocardium and produce life-threatening arrhythmias such as ventricular fibrillation. Normally microshocks are imperceptible and do not affect the person because of the natural defense afforded by intact skin. The skin also serves as a barrier against a low level of electrical current found on all electrical equipment, termed *leakage current.* The presence of IV lines, moist skin, gel for attaching electrocardiogram (ECG) electrodes, and any break in the skin surface decreases the natural resistance to electrical complications.

General electrical safety guidelines must be enforced in order to decrease the potential for electrical complications. These guidelines include the following:

1. Keep the external portion of the catheter dry.
2. Use only properly grounded electrical equipment in the patient environment. This includes only three-pronged plugs and wall outlets. All patient monitoring equipment must be either grounded or double-insulated per federal regulations.
3. Provide for routine, qualified inspection of permanent electrical equipment, as well as portable devices such as infusion pumps, automated blood pressure units, and the like. All equipment should be identified as having been inspected and dated by biomedical engineering personnel.
4. Inspect all cords and plugs for signs of wear such as fraying, cracking, or cuts.
5. Use extreme care when handling liquids, such as intravenous fluids, near electrical equipment. Never store liquids on top of electrical devices.
6. Use only dry hands to plug in or disconnect electrical equipment.
7. Remove a plug from a socket by firmly grasping the plug, not the cord.
8. Turn the power off before disconnecting electrical devices.
9. Keep the patient as dry as possible; this may require frequent linen changes for the patient who is diaphoretic or incontinent.
10. Do not use electrical extension cords.
11. Remove all unnecessary electrical equipment from the patient's room, such as electric cooling blankets that are not being used. Limit the patient's personal electrical equipment, including radios, portable televisions, hair dryers, and similar items. If used, those pieces of equipment should pass a safety inspection by the biomedical engineer.
12. Accidentally spilled fluids on the floor should be *immediately* wiped dry to reduce the risk of electrical injury to hospital staff and patients, as well as the risk of injury due to slippage.

Venous Air Embolism

The potential for pulmonary air emboli exists whenever air enters the systemic venous circulation (usually via a central catheter inserted into an intrathoracic location). Intravascular entrance of air may occur at the time of catheter insertion or any time the catheter or tubing become disconnected. Entrained air may then travel through the vena cava, travel through the right side of the heart, and enter the pulmonary circulation. The risk is substantially increased if the catheter is open to atmosphere while the patient is generating significantly negative intrapleural pressures (labored or forced inspiration) or is volume depleted. A pulmonary air embolism should be suspected if the patient suddenly develops cyanosis, tachypnea, dyspnea, coughing, tachycardia, and hypotension, especially during central venous catheter manipulation (either insertion or removal) or when connections to a central venous line have been interrupted. Cardiovascular collapse may quickly result in death.

The diagnosis is supported by the presence of a classic "mill wheel" murmur over the precordium. Monitored patients may demonstrate peaked T waves and ST depression in the inferior leads. If an echocardiogram can be obtained expeditiously, air in the right heart chambers may be apparent. (Figure 9-8 shows an air embolism that has traversed an intracardiac shunt to completely opacify the left atrium and ventricle.) Aspiration of air from the central venous catheter may serve as a definitive diagnostic maneuver.

Preventive measures include asking the conscious, cooperative patient to perform a Valsalva maneuver whenever the catheter hub or monitoring tube is disconnected. If the patient is on controlled mechanical ventilation or cannot cooperate, gentle abdominal compression, applied by an assistant, transiently raises central venous pressure. Elevation of central venous pressure reduces the likelihood that air will be drawn into the venous circulation. Additional precautions that

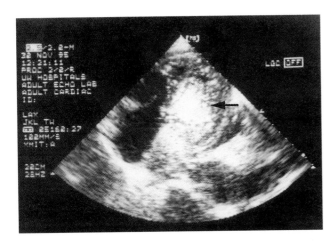

FIGURE 9-8 Modified apical four-chamber view of heart demonstrating complete opacification of left ventricle and atria with air bubbles. Performed approximately 15 minutes after clinical event in which patient suffered cardiac arrest during line insertion.

prevent venous air embolism include ensuring that all connections are secured using Luer-Lok equipment and clamping the central venous line during necessary interruptions of the system.

Immediate therapy for venous air embolism involves positioning the patient on the left side; this maneuver may prevent the air embolism from entering the pulmonary circulation and minimize obstruction to flow. The patient should also be tilted with the head down (Trendelenberg position) for the same reason and also in order to protect the cerebral circulation for the small but significant number of patients who may have an unrecognized right-to-left shunt (e.g., atrial septal defect). Initiation of 100% oxygen, in addition to treating hypoxemia, has been shown to enhance reabsorption of air from the circulation. This occurs because air in the circulation consists primarily of nitrogen that will diffuse easily into alveoli if alveolar gases contain only oxygen. For direct therapy, the central venous catheter can be used to aspirate air from the right ventricle. This ideally requires fluoroscopy (see Chapter 8).

Perforation of the Cardiac Chambers

Perforation of the right atrium or right ventricle can occur from improper catheter placement during insertion or from spontaneous catheter migration facilitated by blood flow or patient movement. Radiographic documentation of the catheter tip in the superior vena cava following insertion, and inspection of subsequent chest films, assesses for intracardiac catheter location. Cardiac perforation associated with hemorrhage or collection of infused

IV fluids into the pericardium (cardiac tamponade) is more likely to occur in patients with elevated right atrial or right ventricular pressures. Any patient with a central venous catheter who suddenly develops distended neck veins, venous hypertension, narrowed pulse pressure, hypotension, distant heart sounds, and pulsus paradoxus should be suspected of having cardiac tamponade secondary to catheter perforation of the heart wall. The ECG may show decreased PQRST voltage and electrical alternans. Treatment is directed at relieving the tamponade through pericardiocentesis or surgical evacuation of the accumulated pericardial blood or fluid and repair of the perforation.

Pneumothorax

The occurrence of pneumothorax, as a complication of central venous pressure catheter insertion, is increased when the subclavian veins (as opposed to the internal jugular veins) are used for venous access, particularly if the patient has hyperinflated lungs due to PEEP, CPAP, or pulmonary emphysema. The overall incidence of pneumothorax due to central line placement is 1% to 2%. A portion of a lung or an entire lung may collapse. Signs and symptoms of a pneumothorax are usually abrupt in onset and include dyspnea, cough, and sharp chest pain. In patients with massive pneumothorax, chest wall movements may be abnormal or absent on the affected side. In patients being mechanically ventilated or patients with respiratory distress, a simple pneumothorax may progress to a tension pneumothorax and result in life-threatening respiratory and circulatory collapse. This is usually associated with a marked increase in peak airway pressures (in mechanically ventilated patients) and hypoxemia. Diagnosis of pneumothorax is confirmed by chest radiograph.

Treatment is evacuation of air from the pleural cavity. Eventually this is followed by reinflation of the affected lung, using closed chest drainage. If, in tension pneumothorax, the patient's condition does not allow time for radiographic confirmation and chest tube insertion, a diagnostic and therapeutic tap with a large-bore needle should be performed. The needle is slipped over the *top* of the rib in the second intercostal space in the midclavicular line. This needle insertion position avoids laceration of the intercostal vessels that lie along the underside of each rib and laceration of the internal mammary artery that lies closer to the mediastinum.

CATHETER REMOVAL

See Chapter 8 for discussion of proper technique for catheter removal.

REFERENCES

1. Stewart RD, Psyhojos T, Lahey SJ, et al: Central venous catheter use in low-risk coronary artery bypass grafting, *Ann Thorac Surg* 66:1306, 1998.
2. Loop FD, Christiansen EK, Cosgrove DM, et al: A strategy for cost containment in coronary surgery, *JAMA* 250:63, 1983.
3. Bashein G, Johnson PW, Davis KB, et al: Elective coronary bypass surgery without pulmonary artery catheter monitoring, *Anesthesiology* 63:451, 1985.
4. Pearson KS, Gomez SK, Moyers JR, et al: A cost/benefit analysis of randomized invasive monitoring for patients undergoing cardiac surgery, *Anesth Analg* 69:336, 1989.
5. Long R, Kassman D, Donen N, et al: Cardiac tamponade complicating central venous catheterization for total parenteral nutrition: a review, *J Crit Care* 2:39, 1987.
6. Czepiak CA, O'Callaghan JM, Venus B: Evaluation of formulas for optimal positioning of central venous catheters, *Chest* 107:1662, 1995.
7. Pinella JC, Ross DF, Martin T, et al: Study of the incidence of intravascular catheter infections and associated septicemia in critically ill patients, *Crit Care Med* 11:21, 1983.
8. Schoemaker WC, Ayres S, Grenvik A, et al: *Textbook of critical care,* ed 2, Philadelphia, 1989, W.B. Saunders, p 856.
9. Maki DG, Wise CE, Sarafin HW: A semiquantitative culture method for identifying intravenous catheter related infection, *N Engl J Med* 296:1305, 1977.

SUGGESTED READINGS

Aldridge HE, Jay AWL: Central venous catheters and heart perforation, *Can Med Assoc J* 135:1082, 1986.
Banasid J, Broderson M: The effect of lateral positions on CVP, *Heart Lung* 20:296, 1991.
Cook DJ: Clinical assessment of central venous pressure in the critically ill, *Am J Med Sci* 299:175, 1990.
Davis CL: Upper extremity venous thrombosis and central venous catheters, *Crit Care Nurse* 11:16, 1991.
Garcia-Rodriguez CR, Hilton AK, Mark JB: Intra-operative hemodynamic monitoring. In Willerson JT, Cohn JN, editors: *Cardiovascular medicine,* ed 2, Philadelphia, 2000, Churchill Livingstone.
Halck S, Walther-Larsen S, Sanchez R: Measurement of central venous pressure after open heart surgery and effect of positive end-expiratory pressure, *Danish Med Bull* 38:181, 1991.
Haywood GA: Influence of posture and reference point on central venous pressure measurement, *Br J Med* 303:626, 1991.
Otto CW: Central venous pressure monitoring. In Blitt CD, editor: *Monitoring in anesthesia critical care medicine,* New York, 1990, Churchill Livingstone.
Rajacich N et al: Central venous pressure and pulmonary capillary wedge pressure as estimates of left atrial pressure: effects of positive end-expiratory pressure and catheter tip malposition, *Crit Care Med* 17:7, 1989.
Schwenzer KJ: Venous and pulmonary pressures. In Lake C, editor: *Clinical monitoring,* Philadelphia, 1990, W.B. Saunders.
Seneff M: Central venous catheters. In Rippe JM et al, editors: *Procedures and techniques in intensive care medicine,* ed 2, Boston, 1999, Little, Brown.
Sladen A: Complications of invasive hemodynamic monitoring in the intensive care unit, *Curr Probl Surg* 25:73, 1988.
Sprung CL, Ginosar Y: Central venous and pulmonary artery catheter monitoring. In Levine RL, Fromm RE, editors: *Critical care monitoring from pre-hospital to ICU,* St Louis, 1995, Mosby.
Tocino IM, Watanabe A: Impending catheter perforation of superior vena cava: radiographic recognition, *Am J Radiol* 146:487, 1986.

GLORIA OBLOUK DAROVIC

Pulmonary Artery Pressure Monitoring

Before the availability of invasive hemodynamic monitoring devices for bedside use, the clinician had only physical signs and symptoms to assess cardiac function and guide therapy. However, physical assessment findings are expressions of pathophysiologic changes that occur secondary to the primary problem. As such, they are neither early nor specific indicators of deterioration in cardiopulmonary function and may be diagnostically misleading. For example, dyspnea, tachypnea, cough, and adventitious lung sounds suggest either a primary cardiac *or* pulmonary problem. A significant decrease in cardiac output (hypovolemic or cardiogenic shock) may not be accompanied by a corresponding drop in blood pressure because of compensatory vasoconstriction.

Furthermore, a lag time of several hours may occur between correction of a cardiac problem and resolution of the associated clinical findings. For example, auscultatory and radiographic evidence of cardiogenic (high-pressure) pulmonary edema may persist for several hours following reduction of left atrial pressure to normal values. The delay between the onset or resolution of the pathologic event and the appearance or disappearance of clinical signs and symptoms is particularly clinically relevant for intensive care unit (ICU) patients, who commonly have rapid changes in cardiopulmonary function. Coexisting multisystem disease further complicates clinical assessment in these patients. It would be an obvious diagnostic and therapeutic advantage to have a bedside means of real-time, continuous, accurate cardiac monitoring.

The 1962 introduction of central venous pressure (CVP) monitoring was the first step in direct, bedside

hemodynamic monitoring. In the absence of tricuspid valve disease, the CVP correlates with right ventricular end-diastolic pressure (RVEDP). Consequently, estimates of intravascular volume status and right ventricular function can be serially evaluated through intermittent or continuous CVP measurements. The initial assumption was made that left ventricular end-diastolic pressure (LVEDP), also termed *filling pressure,* could likewise be tracked with CVP measurements because a close relationship between the filling pressures of the two ventricles had been demonstrated in normal humans. In the normal heart, LVEDP can be estimated to be twice that of RVEDP plus 2. For example, given an RVEDP of 3 mm Hg, LVEDP is estimated to be 8 mm Hg: (3 mm Hg $\times$ 2) + 2 = 8 mm Hg. However, it was later found that the CVP correlated poorly with LVEDP in patients with any abnormalities in the cardiac or vascular structures for function between the CVP catheter tip and left ventricle. The CVP may be considerably higher and may bear no predictable relationship to left ventricular filling pressure in these patients or in mechanically ventilated patients with high levels of positive end-expiratory pressure (PEEP). Even in a patient with a normal vascular channel from the right atrium to the left ventricle, correlation between right and left ventricular filling pressure may be poor because CVP changes are relatively late indicators of left ventricular dysfunction (see Chapter 9, Fig. 9-2).

Because the left ventricle pumps blood to all the vital organs, an immediate and accurate means of tracking left ventricular filling and performance is essential in managing many ICU patients.

The development and clinical application of the double-lumen, balloon-tipped, flow-directed *pulmonary artery catheter* by Swan and Ganz in 1970 provided a relatively simple, safe, rapid, and accurate means of bedside estimate of LVEDP (as estimated by the pulmonary artery wedge pressure [PWP]), as well as pulmonary artery systolic and diastolic pressures (PWP is variously termed *pulmonary artery capillary wedge pressure* [PCWP] or *pulmonary artery occlusion pressure* [PCOP]). Abnormalities affecting the right heart or pulmonary circulation did not prohibit evaluation of left ventricular filling pressure and function. Indeed, the pulmonary artery catheter made it clinically possible to distinguish cardiogenic from noncardiogenic pulmonary edema and establish hemodynamic profiles that could differentiate among multiple causes of perfusion failure.

Several refinements and modifications of the original double-lumen catheter have been developed. With the more complex and sophisticated catheters, it is now possible to intermittently or continuously monitor cardiac output, determine right ventricular ejection fraction and end-diastolic volume, continuously monitor right atrial pressure and mixed venous oxygen saturation, and pace the atrium or ventricle. Important calculations, such as pulmonary and systemic vascular resistance, oxygen transport and consumption, arteriovenous oxygen difference, and intrapulmonary shunt fraction, also can be obtained from hemodynamic and blood gas measurements. However, the potential clinical benefit of these sophisticated monitoring devices is only as good as the ability of the clinician to (1) safely insert and maintain the in situ catheter, (2) accurately obtain and interpret the hemodynamic measurements, (3) correlate the monitored information with clinical and laboratory data, and (4) integrate all the information to form an effective therapeutic plan.

INDICATIONS FOR PULMONARY ARTERY CATHETERIZATION

Despite the numerous functions now available, the pulmonary artery catheter is essentially a *diagnostic tool* that may also be used to assess and guide management of critically ill and injured patients. The anticipated benefits of any diagnostic, therapeutic, or monitoring technique must clearly outweigh anticipated risks and justify expense. There is no absolute rule defining the need for the pulmonary artery catheter. Each individual patient circumstance must be carefully considered.

Generally, the pulmonary artery catheter is indicated in patients in whom cardiopulmonary pressures and flows require precise, intensive management. Therapeutic goals guided by information obtained from these devices are to (1) maximize cardiac output and oxygenation delivery and (2) prevent or target therapy of pulmonary edema. Besides the conventional diagnostic and therapeutic uses for the pulmonary artery catheter, newer, more innovative applications include the detection and treatment of air embolism in patients positioned upright during neurosurgery and the withdrawal of pulmonary arterial blood to recover diagnostic cells and debris in patients with amniotic fluid embolism, fat embolism, and lymphangitic carcinomatosis (Box 10-1).

CONTRAINDICATIONS AND SPECIAL CONSIDERATIONS OF PULMONARY ARTERY CATHETERIZATION

There are no absolute contraindications to pulmonary artery pressure monitoring. However, *invasive hemodynamic monitoring is not justified if the patient's disease or injury cannot be modified or corrected by therapy.* Patients with relative contraindications include the following:

1. *Patients with a severe coagulation defects.* Overt or occult hemorrhage during and after venous access may be problematic.
2. *Patients with a prosthetic right heart valve.* The catheter may knot or loop around the valve and cause valve malfunction.
3. *Patients with an endocardial pacemaker.* The monitoring catheter may dislodge or knot around the intracardiac pacing electrode.
4. *Patients with a severe vascular disease.* The catheter may coil or take an abnormal path within the tortuous, diseased blood vessels. Abnormal systemic venular or pulmonary arterial walls also increase the risk of inadvertent vascular puncture or injury. For these reasons, if pulmonary artery catheterization is essential, insertion should be aided by fluoroscopy.
5. *Patients with pulmonary hypertension.* The incidence of pulmonary arterial rupture is greatest in the distended, friable vessels of those with elevated pulmonary artery pressures.
6. *Patients in locations with an unavailability of physicians trained and skilled in insertion and flotation of the catheter or trained in the principles of blood flow, measurement of intravascular pressures, and interpretation of hemodynamic data.* Likewise, the absence of a nursing staff trained in the principles of pulmonary arterial catheterization, catheter maintenance, and acquisition and interpretation of data renders safe and effective use of this highly invasive and sophisticated monitoring device impossible.

Pulmonary artery catheter flotation and placement is difficult in patients with severe systemic hypotension or low cardiac output due to decreased rates of blood flow through the right heart and pulmonary artery. Circulatory improvement with therapies based on the suspected underlying cause should be attempted before passage of the pulmonary artery catheter. In some cases, fluoroscopy may be required to successfully advance the catheter from the right atrium to the pulmonary artery.

Another important consideration is the financial cost of pulmonary artery pressure monitoring. One study estimated that the patient cost of uncomplicated pulmonary artery catheterization and maintenance is approximately $6,000 per week[1] (Table 10-1). This cost constitutes a significant addition to the patient's hospital bill when the absolute benefits of invasive hemodynamic monitoring are not yet well established. Overall, the decision to use invasive monitoring must involve careful assessment of the existing risks and predicted benefits for each patient.

EFFECTS OF PULMONARY ARTERY CATHETERIZATION ON PATIENT OUTCOME

Although the pulmonary artery catheter provided a quantum leap in physiologic measurements available for diagnosis and management of critically ill and injured patients, unresolved questions related to its use include the following:

1. Does invasive monitoring reduce length of hospital stay?
2. Does invasive monitoring reduce the cost of patient care?
3. Most important, does invasive monitoring reduce patient morbidity and mortality?

Despite the fact that more than 1 million pulmonary artery catheters are inserted in the United States annually, concern has been voiced relating to its frequent use, and research continues to be variable in documenting a benefit in patient outcome.[2-17] Several considerations may, in part, shed light on the causes of the differing study results and may also give insights into improving patient outcomes with diagnosis and management guided by the pulmonary artery catheter.

The first consideration is that physician and nurse knowledge and understanding of the basic principles and use of the pulmonary artery catheter are highly variable and significantly inadequate in all aspects.[18-21] The conclusion is that the *pulmonary artery catheter is not likely to have a positive effect on patient outcome if it is not used properly and if obtained data are contaminated by artifact*

BOX 10-1
General Indications for Pulmonary Artery Pressure Monitoring

Assessment of Cardiovascular Function and Response to Therapy in Patients with:

Complicated myocardial infarction
Cardiogenic shock
Severe congestive heart failure (cardiomyopathy, constrictive pericarditis)
Structural defects, such as acute ventricular septal defect or papillary muscle rupture
Acute right ventricular dysfunction
Cardiac tamponade
Perioperative monitoring of the cardiac surgical patient

Perioperative Monitoring of Surgical Patients with Major Systems Dysfunction Undergoing Extensive Operative Procedures

Shock of All Types

If severe or prolonged
Shock of unknown cause

Assessment of Pulmonary Status and Response to Therapy in Patients with

Cardiogenic vs. noncardiogenic pulmonary edema (ARDS)
Acute respiratory failure (COPD in crisis, pulmonary embolism, etc.)
Pulmonary hypertension: diagnosis and evaluation during acute drug therapy

Assessment of Fluid Requirements in Patients with

Severe, multisystem trauma
Large-area, deep-partial, or full-thickness burns
Severe sepsis

Assessment of Obstetric Patients with Severe Eclampsia Complicated by Refractory Hypertension, Oliguria, or Pulmonary Edema

Therapeutic Indications

Aspiration of air emboli in neurosurgical patients in the upright position during operation
Ventricular pacing using the pacemaker thermodilution pulmonary artery catheter

Diagnostic Indications

Aspiration of pulmonary arterial blood for cytologic diagnosis of amniotic fluid embolism, fat embolism, and lymphangitic carcinomatosis
Right heart catheterization in the cardiac catheterization lab

TABLE 10-1
1989 Costs of Pulmonary Artery Catheter*

	Cost to Hospital	Cost to Patient
Materials		
Catheter introducer kit, transducer, IV fluids, gowns, etc.	$127.23	$497.30
Initial Care		
Insertion, arterial blood gases, cardiac profile, chest radiograph, radiograph interpretation, nursing time		$667.50
Total charge to the patient		$1164.80
Total Daily Charges		
Daily radiograph, interpretations (not essential based on pulmonary artery catheter alone), IV fluids, cardiac profiles, syringes, arterial blood gases, nursing time		$745.00
Weekly Charges		
Initial charges		$1164.80
Daily charges × 7		+$5215.00
Total charge/week		$6379.80

Adapted from Pesce RR: The Swan-Ganz catheter: it goes through your pulmonary artery and you pay through the nose, *Respir Care* 34:785, 1989.

*Current charges may differ and are institutionally variable. Prices have not been adjusted for inflation.

or are misinterpreted. This finding emphasizes the need for expert training and proficiency testing of physicians and nurses in pulmonary artery catheter use.

A second consideration is the hemodynamic end-points of therapies for different patient problems. Since the introduction of the pulmonary artery catheter into clinical practice 20 years ago, critically ill patients who were hemodynamically monitored had their measurements adjusted to the "normal" range. The standardized "normal" hemodynamic values, against which patients' measurements were judged and therapy was directed, were derived from *healthy* humans in the supine position. In 1988 a prospective study demonstrated that patients therapeutically adjusted to or spontaneously maintaining greater than normal values (cardiac output, oxygen transport, oxygen consumption), while recovering from major surgery, experienced improved survival rates, whereas patients therapeutically adjusted to or spontaneously maintaining "normal" values had significantly lower survival rates.[22] The importance of these findings is that traditional therapy has been directed at maintaining the patient's hemodynamic values within the "normal" range. However, normal values may be suboptimal therapeutic end-points to support the "supernormal" physiologic needs imposed by the hypermetabolism associated with critical illness or injury. Although much interest has been generated over the ensuing years, the specific goal for attaining adequate oxygen delivery continues to be a topic of debate and controversy.[23,24] Optimized end-points for specific diseases or conditions have yet to be uniformly defined and accepted. It is likely that they will be complex and varied.

The third consideration is the distant location of the catheter tip from the left ventricle. As a consequence, accuracy of measurement may be affected by disease, distortion, or obstruction of the anatomic structures from the catheter tip to the left atrium or ventricle (chronic obstructive pulmonary disease [COPD], pulmonary venous disorders, massive pulmonary embolism, mitral valve disease).

A fourth consideration is staff members' delay in decision making and preparation to use the pulmonary artery catheter. Such delays may prolong the initiation of appropriate therapeutic actions. One university hospital study looked at the time elapsed before deciding to use a pulmonary artery catheter in 104 critically ill patients.[25] The study showed that the time interval to decide to use the pulmonary artery catheter is never less than 45 minutes and that it is greater than 120 minutes in half of the patients.

Fifth, patients selected for pulmonary artery catheterization are typically gravely ill with complex conditions (severe sepsis, cardiogenic shock, multiple-system organ dysfunction, severe trauma). All are associated with complex biochemical abnormalities that profoundly affect metabolism and hemodynamics. The resolution of these problems depends on elimination of the underlying problem, modulation of the biochemical alterations, prevention of complications, and hemodynamic support. In other words, hemodynamic support is a small part of a very complex whole. Currently, there are no "quick fix" or known effective therapies for many conditions common to ICU patients.

Most likely, the problem of inconsistent study results examining the benefit of the pulmonary artery catheter is not in the design of the pulmonary arterial monitoring system but, rather, in how it is used. Certain assumptions are implicit in its use. The clinicians using the device must do the following:

1. Understand and follow the indications for pulmonary artery catheter use.
2. Rapidly make the decision to insert the pulmonary artery catheter, and quickly initiate appropriate therapies.
3. Practice meticulous technique in setting up the fluid-filled monitoring system and catheter insertion.
4. Be able to interpret the hemodynamic waveforms and understand the physiologic data and their relationship to the underlying clinical problem.
5. Be aware of the potential for patient-related and monitoring system–induced artifacts and error.
6. Understand the need for vigilant, continuous evaluation of obtained measurements, as well as the need to readjust therapy appropriate to changes in the underlying problems.
7. Be competent in prevention and treatment of potential complications.

CATHETER DESIGN AND TYPES

Pulmonary artery catheters are available in a number of sizes suitable for adult and pediatric patients. They range from 60 to 110 cm in length and 4.0 to 8.0 French in caliber. Balloon inflation volumes range from 0.5 to 1.5 ml; balloon diameters range from 8 to 13 mm. The catheter material is polyvinyl chloride, which is pliable at room temperature and softens further at body temperature. The shaft of the catheter is marked at 10 cm increments by black bands; these aid in determining the location of the catheter tip within the central circulation. For example, when the catheter is inserted via the right internal jugular vein, advancement of the catheter tip to the level of the pulmonary artery is usually achieved at the 40 to 45 cm mark (Box 10-2).

There are 10 types of pulmonary artery catheters (differing capabilities) and three manufacturers. Manufacturer-specific catheter models offer a wide range of clinical applications. Apart from the various models of catheters, there are also many pulmonary artery catheter options available (e.g., heparin versus nonheparin coating, differing catheter body firmness, encased in sterile protection guard). Product information specific to each model is also included within the packaging. *It is the responsibility of the caregiver to familiarize himself or herself with each manufacturer's guidelines for specific catheter model insertion and use.* The pulmonary artery catheter manufacturers (and their toll-free technical support telephone numbers) are Edwards Lifesciences LLC (formerly Baxter Healthcare

---

BOX 10-2
Distances to Right Atrium, Pulmonary Artery, and Wedged (PWP) Position

Right Atrium
Right internal jugular vein: 15 cm
Left internal jugular vein: 20 cm
Right antecubital vein: 45 cm
Left antecubital vein: 50 cm
Subclavian vein: 10 cm (R), 15 cm (L)

Right Ventricle
Right internal jugular vein: 25 cm
Left internal jugular vein: 30 cm
Right antecubital vein: 60 cm
Left antecubital vein: 65 cm
Subclavian vein: 20 cm (R), 25 cm (L)

Pulmonary Artery
Right internal jugular vein: 40 cm to PWP 45 cm
Left internal jugular vein: 45 cm to PWP 50 cm
Right antecubital vein: 75 cm to PWP 80 cm
Left antecubital vein: 80 cm to PWP 85 cm
Subclavian vein: 35 cm to PWP 40 cm (R), 45 to 50 cm (L)

Distances are approximations based on the average-sized adult. Appropriate adjustments must be considered in patients whose height is less or greater than average.

Corporation), Irvine, California, 1-800-822-9837; Abbott Laboratories, Abbott Critical Care Systems, North Chicago, Illinois, 1-800-241-4002 option 5; and Arrow International, Reading, Pennsylvania, 1-800-447-4227.

Double-Lumen Pulmonary Artery Catheter

In its original and simplest form, the 5-French catheter contains two lumina; one is for transmission of pressures from the catheter tip in the pulmonary artery to the pressure transducer/monitoring system, and the other is for balloon inflation.

Quadruple-Lumen Thermodilution Catheter

The most commonly used catheter for adults is the quadruple-lumen thermodilution catheter (Figure 10-1). This catheter is available in 5- and 7-French sizes. The distal (pulmonary artery) port *(A)* opens to a lumen that runs the length of the catheter and terminates at the catheter tip. The distal port measures pulmonary artery pressures and PWP. Mixed venous blood samples may also be drawn from the distal port when the catheter tip lies within the pulmonary artery. Drugs and caustic or hyperosmotic solutions should

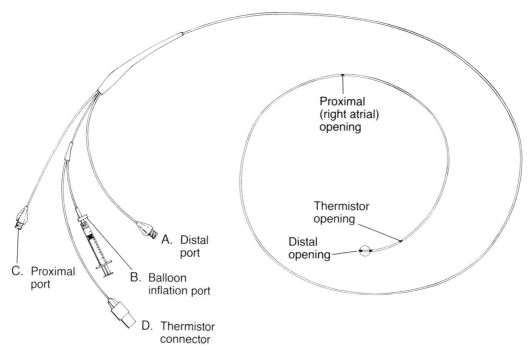

FIGURE 10-1 Number 7 French quadruple-lumen, thermodilution pulmonary artery catheter.

not be administered through the pulmonary artery port because a concentrated infusion into a small pulmonary artery segment may result in an untoward local vascular or tissue reaction. The balloon inflation port *(B)* opens to a lumen that terminates within the balloon. The proximal (right atrial [RA]) port *(C)* opens to a lumen that terminates 30 cm from the tip of the catheter. This opening lies within the right atrium when the catheter tip is in the pulmonary artery. The RA port may be employed to monitor RA pressure; administer intravenous [IV] fluids, electrolytes, or medications; sample right atrial blood; and receive the injectate solution for cardiac output studies.

The RA port should not be used for infusion of vasoactive or inotropic drugs if cardiac output studies are being considered because the patients will receive miniboluses of the highly active cardiovascular medications with each cold indicator injection. The thermistor port *(D)* incorporates a temperature-sensitive wire that terminates approximately 4 to 6 cm proximal to the tip of the catheter. The terminal portion of the wire, termed the *thermistor bead,* lies in one of the main pulmonary arteries when the catheter tip is properly positioned. Connection of the thermistor port to a cardiac output computer allows determination of a "spot" cardiac output measurement following injection of a cold indicator solution by measuring the magnitude of blood temperature change over time (see Chapter 11).

Thermodilution Pulmonary Artery Catheter with Additional Right Atrial (Proximal) Port

This 7.5-French thermodilution pulmonary artery catheter has an additional right atrial (proximal) port for fluid, electrolyte, and drug infusion. The catheter design permits cardiac output measurements via the proximal injectate port without interruption of continuous drug infusions via the proximal fluid-administration port.

A second generation of this catheter type offers an additional third lumen that empties into the right ventricle. The V.I.P. + TriLumen Infusion Thermodilution catheter (Edwards Lifesciences LLC, Irvine, California) increases the capability to infuse a variety of drugs without risk of incompatibility and also allows continuous right atrial and right ventricular (RV) pressure monitoring.

"Position Monitoring" Thermodilution Pulmonary Artery Catheter

The original thermodilution pulmonary artery catheter has been modified by moving the proximal infusion port, located 30 cm from the catheter tip, to 10 cm from the tip. This places the opening of the proximal lumen within the right ventricle just proximal to the pulmonic valve. Guided by the RV port pressure waveform, distal migration of the catheter can be detected by a change from a right ventricular waveform and pressures to a pulmonary artery waveform and pressures. The clinician may then withdraw the catheter to a position that restores the right ventricular waveform and pressure readings.

This "position monitoring catheter" adds a margin of safety to pulmonary artery pressure monitoring by preventing catheter-associated pulmonary artery rupture due to distal migration of the catheter tip into the small, peripheral pulmonary arteries. Proper catheter tip position also enables accurate cardiac output measurement and central circulatory pressure monitoring. The overall cost of pulmonary artery pressure monitoring is lowered with this catheter by eliminating the need for chest radiographs to assess proximal versus distal catheter tip location.

Fiberoptic Thermodilution Pulmonary Artery Catheter

The fiberoptic thermodilution pulmonary artery catheter allows continuous in vivo monitoring of mixed venous oxygen saturation. This standard thermodilution catheter has an additional lumen that contains two fiberoptic bundles, which are exposed near the catheter tip, for light transmission. Red light is transmitted from one fiberoptic bundle and strikes the red blood cells. The amount of light that is reflected toward the receiving (second) fiberoptic bundle depends on the amount of oxygenated versus deoxygenated hemoglobin in the mixed venous blood. A photodetector in the attached computer module calculates the fraction of saturated hemoglobin (oxyhemoglobin) and continuously displays and records it in real time.

Knowledge of mixed venous oxygen saturation has practical diagnostic, prognostic, monitoring, and therapeutic implications and is valuable in calculating parameters used in evaluating the patient's oxygenation status (see Chapter 12).

Pacemaker Thermodilution Pulmonary Artery Catheters

Pulmonary artery catheters are available that offer pacemaking capabilities in addition to the standard means of obtaining hemodynamic measurements. One pacing-thermodilution catheter has five electrodes: two intraventricular electrodes located 18.5 and 19.5 cm from the catheter tip and three intraatrial electrodes located 28.5, 31.0, and 33.5 cm farther back from the catheter tip. This catheter may be used for atrial, ventricular, and atrioventricular (AV) sequential pacing. It also has the capability to record an intracardiac rhythm strip.

Another pacing model has a right ventricular port that opens 19 cm from the catheter tip. This port allows the introduction of a pacing wire (Chandler Transluminal V-pacing Probe) for emergency ventricular pacing (Figure 10-2). Another modification of a pacemaker pulmonary artery

catheter provides a right atrial port, in addition to the right ventricular port, for AV sequential pacing.

Indications for pacing pulmonary artery catheters include (1) second- or third-degree heart block, (2) bifascicular or trifascicular block, (3) digitalis toxicity, (4) severe bradycardias, (5) intracardiac electrocardiogram (ECG) for diagnosis of complex arrhythmias, and (6) overdrive suppression of tachyarrhythmias.

Thermodilution Ejection Fraction Pulmonary Artery Catheter

A recently introduced 7.5-French thermodilution ejection fraction catheter also allows the calculation of right ventricular end-systolic and end-diastolic volumes. Knowledge of right ventricular function in a variety of critical care situations may provide new insights into ventricular interdependence and overall cardiac function in patients with cardiopulmonary disease.

The catheter has three unique characteristics:
1. Two intracardiac electrodes (one of which lies in the right ventricle and the other in the pulmonary artery) that sense ventricular depolarization.
2. A specialized multihole injectate opening that creates a spray of cold solution into the right atrium. The spray ensures a rapid intraatrial mixing of the iced thermal indicator solution.
3. A rapid thermistor response time of 50 ms (thermal response time with a standard thermodilution catheter is 300 to 1000 ms) that is rapid enough to sense beat-by-beat temperature variation. Each cardiac cycle is sensed by the intracardiac electrodes.

Bedside computer calculation of right ventricular ejection fraction is derived from a thermal wash-out curve. The normal right ventricular ejection fraction using the thermodilution technique is approximately 40%. Right ventricular stroke volume and end-systolic and end-diastolic volumes may be calculated using the following formulas:

Right ventricular (RV) stroke = Cardiac output ÷ Heart rate

RV end-diastolic volume (preload) = RV stroke volume ÷ Ejection fraction

RV end-systolic volume = RV end-diastolic volume − RV stroke volume

Additional information is available with the ejection fraction catheter. Changes in right ventricular compliance are reflected in changes in the relationship of right ventricular end-diastolic volume to end-diastolic pressure. Increases or decreases in right ventricular contractility are reflected in changes in stroke volume relative to

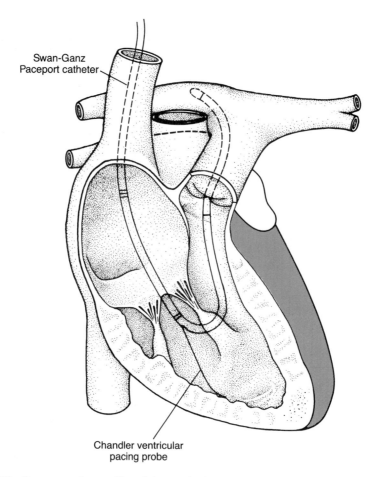

Swan-Ganz
Paceport catheter

Chandler ventricular
pacing probe

FIGURE 10-2 The Paceport catheter with a right ventricular port for passage of a Chandler ventricular pacing probe. A modification of this catheter type also allows passage of a probe for atrial pacing. The Paceport catheter with the atrial port has the capability of atrial, ventricular, and atrioventricular pacing. (Reprinted with permission. © 2001 Edwards Lifesciences LLC. Swan-Ganz® is a trademark of Edwards Lifesciences Corporation, registered in the U.S. Patent and Trademark Office. All rights reserved.)

changes in ejection fraction. Right ventricular function curves may be plotted with stroke volume and cardiac output (see the section on clinical applications later in this chapter).

Thermodilution Pulmonary Artery Catheter for Continuous Cardiac Output Measurements

This pulmonary artery catheter provides continuous thermodilution cardiac output measurements. The 8-French catheter with a built-in thermal filament is powered and controlled by its companion cardiac output computer. The 10 cm thermal filament is located within the right ventricle and transfers 7.5 W of energy to heat the surrounding blood. At all times the filament surface remains below 44°C, which has no harmful effect on the myocardium or blood components. The blood temperature change is detected by a thermistor located in the pulmonary artery near the tip of the catheter and is cross-correlated with the right ventricular thermal input to produce a thermodilution wash-out curve. Cardiac output is calculated by the bedside computer from an equation using the area under the thermodilution curve. Every 30 seconds the displayed cardiac output is updated and reflects the average cardiac output of the preceding 3 to 6 minutes and is graphically displayed to illustrate cardiac output "trends over time." The effects of therapeutic interventions, as well as the effects of routine patient care maneuvers, can then be evaluated and adjusted to optimize the patient's hemodynamic condition (Figure 10-3).

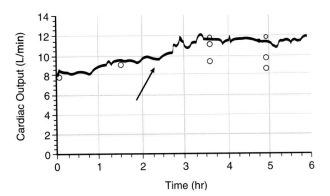

FIGURE 10-3 The patient is changed from controlled ventilation to spontaneous breathing at the *arrow*. Note the increase in cardiac output required by the increased flow demands brought on by the work of spontaneous breathing. The continuous line represents continuous thermodilution, and the open circles represent bolus thermodilution. (From Yelderman ML et al: Continuous thermodilution cardiac output measurement in intensive care unit patients, *J Cardiothorac Vasc Anesth* 6:271, 1992.)

Models are also available that combine continuous cardiac output and Svo_2 monitoring.

CCOmbo V Pulmonary Artery Catheter

The newest addition to the family of pulmonary artery catheters and its companion bedside computer (Edwards Lifesciences, Irvine, California) provides continuous display of cardiac output (derived by the thermodilution technique), right ventricular end-diastolic volume, ejection fraction, stroke volume, and Svo_2. Also available are calculation and cross-calculation of hemodynamic and oxygenation parameters.

The advantages of continuous cardiac output measurements relate to patient safety, clinical efficiency, and possible increased accuracy of measurements. The risk of fluid overload due to multiple injectate boluses is completely eliminated. Continuous display of cardiac output and cardiac index provides immediate information on the patient's responses to care activities and treatments, as well as physiologic changes. Therefore appropriate interventions may be instituted in a timely manner. Continuous measurements save staff time by eliminating the need for intermittent manual bolus measurements. Any errors in cardiac output measurement inherent in the manual, bolus technique (respiratory variation, prolonged or irregular injectate administration, etc.) are eliminated. The catheter is available in sizes 7.5 to 8 French, depending on the number of proximal lumina and flow rates via these lumina.

METHODS AND SITES OF PULMONARY ARTERY CATHETER INSERTION

There is no *ideal* method or site for pulmonary artery catheter insertion. The method and site chosen are frequently determined by the operator's preference and personal expertise. However, patient-related factors, such as age, body build, areas of regional trauma or burns, and anticipated duration of catheterization, and specific clinical circumstances, such as coagulation or perfusion abnormalities, anticoagulation, and severe pulmonary hypertension, should weigh heavily in the decision making.

The three vascular access techniques are as follows:

1. *The percutaneous approach using a large-bore catheter over a needle.* This technique is rarely, if ever, done.
2. *The cutdown approach.* A catheter is directly placed into a surgically isolated, exposed vein. This technique is commonly used when cannulating the relatively small-caliber basilic or cephalic veins of an adult or the very small veins of infants and children.
3. *The percutaneous approach using the modified Seldinger technique.* This is currently the catheter insertion procedure of choice. Following creation of a puncture wound, a sheath introducer inserted over a guide wire provides a conduit for the catheter to pass into the lumen of the vein. This technique is commonly used for catheter insertion into the central veins. Complications related to this technique include cardiac or vascular puncture by the guide wire or vessel dilator and migration of the guide wire into the central circulation (see Chapter 8).

The percutaneous vascular approaches are preferable to the cutdown approach because of the increased risk of infection from cutdown. *When the catheter cannot be easily placed from a specific anatomic site using any of the aforementioned techniques, another vascular insertion site should be considered rather than risking complications from repeated manipulations at the same site.* The insertion sites for pulmonary artery catheterization are the same as those for central venous catheterization (see Chapter 8, Table 8-1 and Figure 8-1).

PREPARATION AND EQUIPMENT SETUP

An important and often overlooked part of the procedure is discussion, with the patient and family, of the intended procedure with focus on the improved diagnostic, assessment, and treatment/response potentials. Informed consent should also be obtained. In the rush and pressure of the critical care environment, attention may focus on the underlying disease, technology, and equipment so that the patient as a person, as well as the family, is forgotten. The patient is generally acutely ill; consequently, the fear of disability and death is felt by both the patient and family members. An invasive procedure that directly involves the heart reinforces the extraordinary nature of the illness. Fears and misconceptions should be identified and discussed. The presence of confusion or coma does not eliminate the need to talk to the patient and explain what is being done. The caregiver's touch and voice may be the patient's only conscious contact with reality.

Premedication with sedative or analgesic medications helps reduce the pain and anxiety that accompany placement of central circulatory catheters and may help limit patient movement throughout the procedure, particularly in restless patients.

Equipment Required

Details related to the pulmonary artery catheter insertion equipment and setup vary among institutions. Generally, as experience is gained with pulmonary arterial catheterization, physicians and hospital staff adopt a protocol that they find most efficient and with which they are most comfortable.

Chapter 8 (Box 8-2) lists the equipment required for entering a central vein. The following equipment also is usually required for pulmonary artery catheter insertion and maintenance:

1. An IV pole and transducer holder (optional). Alternatively, the pressure transducer may be mounted, at the level of the patient's midchest, on a rolled towel or taped to the patient's arm (if not uncooperative, restless, or with tremor disorder).
2. Sterile three-way stopcocks. The number of stopcocks required depends on the number of vascular pressures being monitored (RA, RV, and pulmonary artery). The number of stopcocks and the length of connecting tubing should be kept to a minimum in order to maximize fidelity of the fluid-filled monitoring system.
3. A bag of flush solution attached to low-compliance connecting tubing with a microdrip chamber. Normal saline is preferable to dextrose as a flush solution because growth of microorganisms of the Enterobacteriaceae family is enhanced by sugar.
4. A pressure transducer connected to the fluid-filled tubing and electronic monitoring console. The monitoring console is turned on, allowing 15 minutes for the system to "warm up."
5. A small sterile cup or basin of sterile saline to test balloon integrity.

Figure 10-4 illustrates the components of the pulmonary artery catheter monitoring system.

Preparation for Insertion and Flotation of the Pulmonary Artery Catheter

Typically, the catheter is advanced at the ICU bedside. However, pulmonary artery catheterization may be performed in any area of the hospital where monitoring and cardiopulmonary resuscitation equipment are available. *Familiarity with the catheter manufacturer's directions and specifications is mandatory before beginning the procedure.* This information is included in the catheter packaging.

The patient's physical assessment and vital signs are obtained before catheter insertion and are reevaluated any time during the procedure that a change is suspected in the patient's condition. A pulse oximeter is applied, and, if the patient has no arterial line, an automated blood pressure monitoring device is set to record blood pressure every 5 minutes. If present, nasogastric feedings are turned off and the nasogastric tube is connected to suction. IV tubing used for emergency drug administration should be conspicuously labeled.

Extubated patients should wear surgical masks, if their condition allows, to minimize site contamination from oral and nasal flora. *All personnel participating in catheter insertion must be dressed in full surgical scrub; no circumstance obviates the need for absolute sterile technique.* Personnel circulating in the room should wear caps and masks. There is clearly no risk associated with surgical dress, and the added expense is minimal. The benefit of reducing the risk of catheter-related sepsis in these acutely ill and often immune-compromised patients needs no elaboration.

Catheter testing and preparation are done while the patient is being positioned, prepared, and draped. This minimizes the time the patient must remain motionless, covered with drapes. The patient is positioned so that accessibility to the catheter insertion site and comfort are maximized. Care must be taken to clear the proposed work area of IV or other tubing, ECG leads, and the like. These pieces of equipment are secured so that they will not shift into the sterile field during the catheter insertion procedure.

Testing and Preparation of the Pulmonary Artery Catheter

The sterile catheter is removed from its packaging, and the balloon is inflated with air to the manufacturer's recommended inflation volume, which is indicated on the catheter shaft (0.5 to 1.5 ml). In approximately 3% of

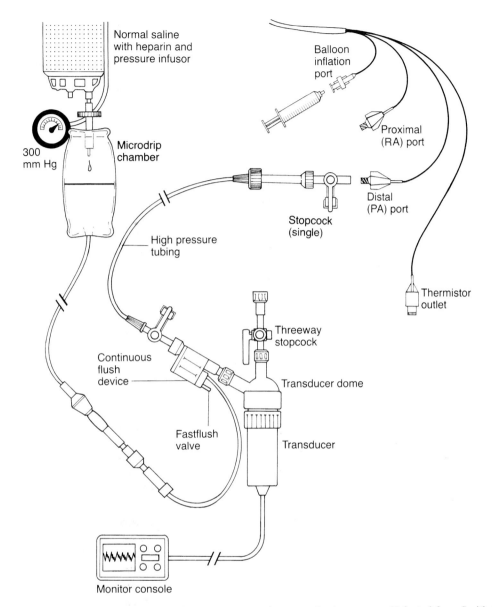

FIGURE 10-4 The components of the pulmonary artery catheter monitoring system. (Adapted from Smith RN: Invasive pressure monitoring, *Am J Nurse* 9:1514, 1978. Copyright 1978 The American Journal of Nursing Company. Used with permission. All rights reserved.)

newly unpackaged pulmonary artery catheters, there is a defect with balloon inflation or integrity. Therefore the balloon must be inspected for integrity, symmetric inflation, and catheter tip protection. The catheter tip should be recessed in the center of the inflated balloon with the sensing tip exposed (Figure 10-5).

Fluids should *never* be used as a balloon inflation medium because fluids may be difficult to retrieve. In addition, the fluid-filled balloon is incompressible and may stress and injure the walls of the pulmonary vessels.

The presence of right-to-left intracardiac shunts, such as septal defects, places the patient at risk for systemic or cerebral air embolization if the inflated balloon ruptures during flotation or wedging. If communications between the right and left sides of the circulation are known to exist, carbon dioxide (rather than air) should be used for balloon inflation because carbon dioxide is rapidly absorbed in blood and minimizes the risk of cerebral or systemic air embolization. Carbon dioxide also diffuses more easily than air through the latex balloon and reduces balloon

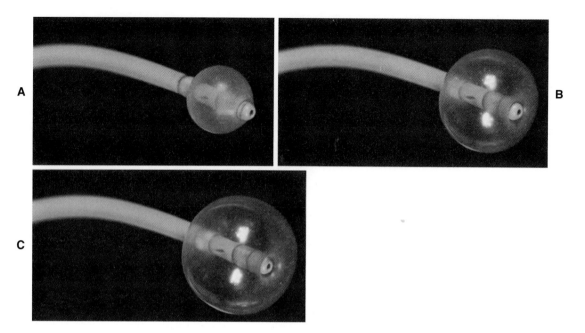

FIGURE 10-5 Number 7 French thermodilution pulmonary artery catheter balloon inflated with 0.5 ml of air **(A)** and 1.0 ml of air **(B).** Note that the hard catheter sensing tip is exposed. Trauma or irritation to the endocardial surface may occur during catheter insertion, and damage to the pulmonary artery may occur on wedging. In **C,** the balloon is inflated to the manufacturer's recommended volume, 1.5 ml. The balloon protrudes over and cushions, but does not cover, the sensing tip.

volume at a rate of approximately 0.5 ml/min. If balloon flotation is significantly prolonged, rapid loss of balloon volume may result in balloon wedging in the smaller, more peripheral pulmonary arteries. When restoration of balloon volume is required during prolonged flotation, the balloon should be completely deflated before reinflation to the recommended volume. This precaution prevents accidental overinflation, pulmonary vascular injury, and possible balloon rupture.

Balloon integrity is further tested by submerging it in a small amount of sterile water or saline and checking for air leaks. The balloon is then passively deflated by removing the syringe from the balloon inflation port. Manual removal of gas with a syringe may pull the latex balloon into the inflation lumen and result in balloon rupture.

Stopcocks are attached to the proximal ports and distal (pulmonary artery) port. The proximal (right atrial or right ventricular) and distal lumina are flushed with saline solution with a syringe attached to one of the stopcock ports. The stopcocks are then closed to keep the flush solution within the catheter lumina. If a pacemaker pulmonary artery catheter is being inserted, air in the pacing wire channel should be flushed out with saline. *Air must be cleared from all catheter channels before insertion.*

The outside of the catheter is then wiped with a gauze pad soaked with sterile water or saline. Wetting the catheter before advancement helps reduce vein irritation. The catheter is then passed through the sterility shield (Figure 10-6). An assistant connects the thermistor port to the cardiac output computer. If the thermistor wires, connecting cable, and computer display are functional, room temperature will be displayed on the cardiac output computer.

The stopcock at the distal (pulmonary artery) port is attached to connecting tubing and flush solution. These are then attached to the properly "air zeroed" transducer/monitor system.

Vascular Insertion

A discussion of techniques of vascular access is presented in Chapter 8. The catheter insertion procedure should be performed or supervised by an experienced physician to minimize insertion time, as well as the risk of complications. When constant observation of the oscilloscope is not possible, the ECG audiosignal is turned on to detect arrhythmias that may occur during balloon flotation. A defibrillator and lidocaine (Xylocaine) are present at the bedside in the event that major or life-threatening arrhythmias occur during the procedure.

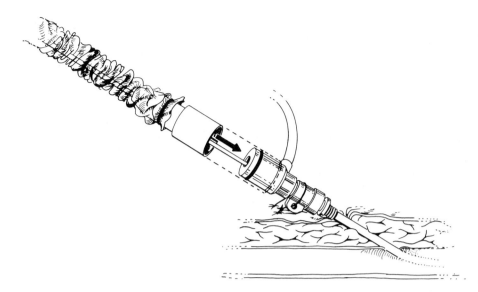

FIGURE 10-6 After the sterile sheath has been secured to the catheter, the "sterile" portion can be distinguished from the "contaminated" portion of the catheter. (From Butterworth JF: Pulmonary artery catheterization. In *Atlas of procedures in anesthesia and critical care,* Philadelphia, 1992, W.B. Saunders.)

During catheter insertion and throughout flotation, the entire length of the catheter is continuously observed to guard against accidental contamination. After establishing vascular access, the operator introduces the catheter, with the balloon deflated, into the vein lumen. The distal (pulmonary artery) lumen is gently aspirated with the attached syringe to ensure free flow of blood and gently flushed with saline solution. The stopcock is then turned to open the pulmonary artery lumen to the pressure monitoring system. The thermistor should register the patient's body temperature.

Peripheral Venous Insertion

The catheter is advanced with the balloon deflated until the catheter tip reaches a central thoracic vein. Upon balloon inflation, the stream of venous blood aids in directing the inflated balloon, which acts as a sail, into the vena cava and right atrium. Catheter tip location within the thoracic veins is documented by respiratory-induced fluctuations in the baseline. If position of the catheter is in question (intrathoracic versus extrathoracic), a patient who is conscious and cooperative is instructed to cough. A sedated, mechanically ventilated patient may be given a few deep, manual breaths with a bag-valve device. Marked deflections in the baseline confirm position of the catheter in the thorax (Figure 10-7).

Central Venous Insertion

The balloon may be inflated as soon as the catheter tip and balloon are introduced into the lumen of the internal jugular, subclavian, or femoral veins. Inflation of the balloon to its *recommended inflation volume* (1.5 ml for the 7-French thermodilution catheter, 0.8 ml for the 5-French double-lumen catheter) ensures that the balloon extends over, but does not cover, the hard sensing tip. This cushions the catheter and protects the endocardial structures and pulmonary vessels from trauma during balloon flotation (see Figure 10-5, *C*). Inflation beyond recommended levels may cause balloon rupture. The bursting volume of the balloon is approximately 3.0 ml.

Flotation of the Pulmonary Artery Catheter

As the catheter passes from the central venous circulation through the heart, waveforms characteristic of the chamber being traversed are encountered. Obtained pressure measurements and waveform morphology, in turn, provide a basis for hemodynamic diagnosis of various cardiopulmonary diseases.

Normally, passage of the pulmonary artery catheter from the right atrium to the pulmonary artery "wedged" position occurs within 10 to 20 seconds. The approximate distance for catheter advancement from various insertion sites to the right atrium, right ventricle, and "wedged" position are listed in Box 10-2.

Catheter passage may take longer than normal or flow-direction of the catheter may be difficult in patients with (1) abnormal blood flow patterns within the heart, such as tricuspid or pulmonic stenotic or regurgitant valve lesions; (2) elevated right ventricular pressures; (3) low flow states, such as heart failure or shock; (4) dilated right heart chambers; or (5) pulmonary hypertension. The use of catheters of small French size may also predispose to coiling within the right ventricle or pulmonary circulation.

In these patients, stiffening the catheter with a cold saline flush or use of a 21-gauge, 120 cm guide wire placed within the distal (pulmonary artery) lumen of the catheter improves catheter stiffness and torque to facilitate catheter passage. In a patient with tricuspid or pulmonic stenosis, less than recommended balloon inflation volume may be necessary to facilitate passage across the narrowed valve orifice. Simple maneuvers such as turning the patient so that the right side is lower than the left or having the patient take deep breaths also may favor flow-direction through the desired cardiovascular channels. Catheter advancement may have to be guided by fluoroscopy in patients in whom difficulty with balloon flotation and catheter passage is anticipated or encountered.

The shapes of the hemodynamic waveform and pressure measurements are noted on entry into each cardiopulmonary chamber. Patients in whom pulmonary artery catheterization is indicated frequently have hemodynamic measurements that are significantly different from those considered "normal." However, if at any time the obtained measurements are in doubt (because they do not fit the clinical picture or are grossly abnormal), the distal catheter lumen should be flushed and the monitoring system rezeroed. Calibration testing may be required for older (non–fixed-calibration) monitoring systems. Otherwise, important therapeutic decisions may be based on incorrect hemodynamic information. Box 10-3 summarizes normal hemodynamic values and causes of abnormal hemodynamic pressure measurements (see also Box 10-4).

Entry into the Right Atrium
On entry into the right atrium, the following waveform and pressures are observed. The waveform is characterized

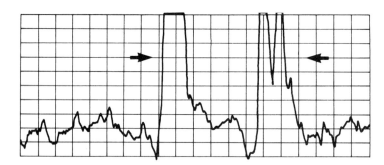

FIGURE 10-7 The catheter tip, now located in the thorax, reflects the marked pressure changes occurring with the patient coughing *(arrows)*.

BOX 10-3
Normal and Abnormal Hemodynamic Values

Right Heart Pressure Profile
Right Atrium
Normal values: 0 to 8 mm Hg
Increased pressure:
- RV failure secondary to left heart failure: mitral stenosis/regurgitation, aortic stenosis/regurgitation, cardiomyopathies, ischemia
- RV failure secondary to factors that increase pulmonary vascular resistance: pulmonary embolism, hypoxemia, COPD, ARDS, sepsis, shock, primary pulmonary hypertension

- RV failure due to intrinsic disease: RV infarction, cardiomyopathies
- Right-sided valve disease (tricuspid regurgitation or pulmonic stenosis/regurgitation)
- Cardiac tamponade/effusion
- Intravascular volume overload
- Obstructive right atrial myxoma
- Restrictive cardiomyopathies
Decreased pressures:
- Hypovolemia

BOX 10-3
Normal and Abnormal Hemodynamic Values—cont'd

Alterations in RA waveform:
- Large *a* waves: RV failure of any cause, decreased RV compliance due to ischemia or hypertrophy; absent *a* waves in atrial flutter (sawtooth waves), atrial fibrillation (undulating baseline, atrial standstill [flat baseline]); tricuspid stenosis (large *a* waves); sporadic appearance in atrioventricular dissociation
- Large *v* waves: tricuspid regurgitation due to valve disease or due to significant right ventricular dilation; AV dissociation

Right Ventricle
Normal values: 15 to 25 mm Hg systolic; 0 to 8 mm Hg diastolic
Increased systolic pressure:
- Factors that increase outflow resistance: COPD, pulmonary embolism, hypoxemia, ARDS, sepsis, pulmonary vascular volume overload due to left heart dysfunction or left-to-right shunts (ventricular septal defect or atrial septal defect), pulmonic stenosis
- Primary pulmonary hypertension
- Significant atrial or ventricular septal defect
Decreased systolic pressure:
- RV failure due to ischemic disease or myopathies
- Hypovolemia, tamponade
Increased diastolic pressure:
- All factors that increase RA pressure
Decreased diastolic pressure:
- Hypovolemia
- Tricuspid stenosis
Alterations in waveform:
- Slurred upstroke with narrow pulse pressure in severe RV failure, hypovolemia; overall, damped-appearing tracing
- Pulse pressure wide in atrial or ventricular septal defect with steep upstroke

Pulmonary Circulation Pressure Profile
Pulmonary Artery Pressures
Normal values: 15 to 25 mm Hg systolic; 6 to 12 mm Hg diastolic
Increased systolic pressure:
- Factors that increase pulmonary vascular resistance: pulmonary embolism, hypoxemia, COPD, ARDS, sepsis, shock, primary pulmonary hypertension, restrictive

cardiomyopathies, significant left-to-right shunt (atrial septal defect, ventricular septal defect)
Increased diastolic pressure:
- All factors that increase pulmonary artery systolic pressure
- Intravascular volume overload
- Left heart dysfunction of any cause; LV failure, mitral stenosis/regurgitation, aortic stenosis/regurgitation, decreased LV compliance (altered volume-pressure relationship)
- Restrictive cardiomyopathies
- Cardiac tamponade/effusion
Pulmonary artery systolic and diastolic pressure decreased:
- Hypovolemia
- Severe tricuspid or pulmonic stenosis
Alterations in waveform:
- Retrograde *v* waves may distort the pulmonary artery pressure waveform in acute or severe mitral regurgitation
- Pulse pressure narrow in tamponade or shock states
- Pulse pressure wide in significant ventricular or atrial septal defect

Pulmonary Artery Wedge Pressure (PWP)
Normal values: 4 to 12 mm Hg
Increased:
- Left heart dysfunction: mitral stenosis/regurgitation, aortic stenosis/regurgitation, left ventricular failure of any cause, decreased left ventricular compliance (ischemia, fibrosis, hypertrophy)
- Intravascular volume overload
- Tamponade/effusion
- Obstructive left atrial myxoma
- Restrictive cardiomyopathies
Decreased:
- Hypovolemia
Alterations in waveform:
- Large *a* waves: mitral stenosis, left ventricular failure of any cause, or decreased left ventricular compliance (ischemia, fibrosis, hypertrophy); absent *a* waves in atrial flutter, fibrillation, or standstill (see above, RA waveform); sporadic appearance in atrioventricular dissociation
- Large *v* waves: mitral regurgitation; severe left ventricular dilation; severe, acute ventricular septal defect

Pulmonary artery wedge pressure does not approximate left ventricular end-diastolic pressure in patients with mitral stenosis; mitral regurgitation with large *v* waves; left atrial myxoma; pulmonary venous occlusive disease (thrombosis, fibrosis, tumor); COPD; decreased LV compliance; increased pleural pressures (PEEP, CPAP); severe left ventricular failure; location of pulmonary artery catheter tip in a nondependent zone of the lung, such as West zone I or II; or tachycardia (greater than 130 beats per minute). See also Box 10-4.

A pulmonary artery diastolic to pulmonary artery wedge pressure gradient greater than 4 mm Hg occurs in patients with acute or chronic pulmonary disease associated with increased pulmonary vascular resistance.

by continuous oscillations in the baseline (*a* and *v* waves), as shown in Figure 10-8.

In the absence of tricuspid valve disease, mean right atrial pressure is equal to RVEDP. This correlation is possible because if the tricuspid valve is open, the right atrium and right ventricle openly communicate and pressures equilibrate at end-diastole. The right atrial *a* wave (which is diastolic in timing) directly reflects RVEDP.

When the tricuspid valve is closed during ventricular systole, the right atrial pressure associated with atrial filling, the *v* wave (which is systolic in timing), normally rises to a level nearly equal to the *a* wave.

When the catheter tip is in position in the pulmonary artery, right atrial pressure may be continuously monitored using the proximal lumen attached to a pressure transducer.

Entry into the Right Ventricle

Directed by the flow of blood, the balloon enters the right ventricle, at which time there is a dramatic change in the waveform morphology and peak pressure. Systolic and diastolic pressures are noted and recorded. The right ventricular waveform (Figure 10-9) is characterized by a steep upstroke ascending to a peak pressure that is normally two to three times higher than the mean right atrial pressure. The sharp downstroke, without a dicrotic notch, dips and then plateaus to reach a baseline that directly records RVEDP. As stated earlier, this is normally equal to mean right atrial pressure. Premature ventricular contractions, ventricular tachycardia, or ventricular fibrillation may occur during balloon passage through the right ventricle due to stimulation of the ventricular septum at the right ventricular outflow tract by the advancing catheter.

Entry into the Pulmonary Artery

As the catheter traverses the pulmonic valve and enters the pulmonary circulation, relatively subtle changes in waveform morphology and pressure are noted (Figure

---

BOX 10-4

Conditions Resulting in a Discrepancy between Pulmonary Artery Wedge Pressure (PWP) and Left Ventricular End-Diastolic Pressure (LVEDP)

Measured PWP Is Less Than True LVEDP

Left ventricular failure with PWP greater than 15 to 20 mm Hg
Decreased left ventricular compliance

Measured PWP Is Greater Than True LVEDP

Use of positive end-expiratory pressure (PEEP, CPAP)
Zone 1 or 2 catheter tip placement
Tachycardia (greater than 130 beats per minute)
Mitral regurgitation
Mitral stensosis
COPD
Pulmonary veno-occlusive disease

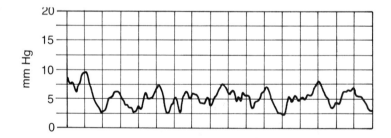

FIGURE 10-8 Right atrial waveform.

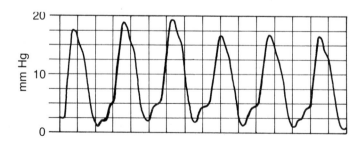

FIGURE 10-9 Right ventricular waveform.

10-10). The shape of the waveform is altered by the presence of a dicrotic notch, which is caused by pulmonic valve closure. The recorded pulmonary artery diastolic pressure does not correlate with right ventricular diastolic pressure because the closed pulmonic valve seals off the pulmonary artery from the right ventricle. The hemodynamic factors that contribute to pulmonary artery diastolic pressure are left atrial pressure and the resistance to diastolic runoff of blood through the pulmonary arteries, capillaries, and veins. Pulmonary artery diastolic pressure is normally only 1 to 4 mm Hg higher than left atrial pressure because the highly distensible pulmonary circulation offers little resistance to blood flow. Pulmonary artery systolic pressure is normally equal to right ventricular systolic pressure because the two chambers are in open communication when the pulmonic valve is open.

In patients with pulmonary hypertension, the catheter tip may reverse direction and reenter the right ventricle, leaving a loop of catheter in the pulmonary artery. The redirected catheter tip may press against the right ventricular wall. The damped tracing that results then may be misinterpreted as a "wedged" position. The sudden appearance of ventricular ectopic arrhythmias also suggests RV malposition of the pulmonary artery catheter tip.

Direction of the Balloon and Catheter Tip into the Wedged Position

Guided by the flow of blood, the inflated balloon continues to act as a sail and floats into the peripheral pulmonary arteries (Figure 10-11). When the inflated balloon lodges *(a)* within a segment of the pulmonary artery that is slightly smaller than the inflated balloon, no blood flows distal to the

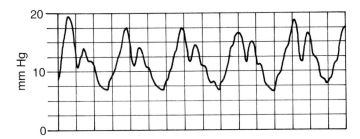

FIGURE 10-10 Pulmonary artery waveform.

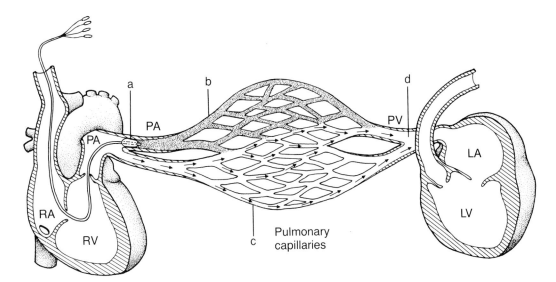

FIGURE 10-11 Schematic representation of the pulmonary artery catheter in the wedged position. From its position in a small occluded segment of the pulmonary circulation, the pulmonary artery catheter in the wedged position allows the electronic monitoring equipment to "look through" a nonactive segment of the pulmonary circulation to the hemodynamically active pulmonary veins and left atrium.

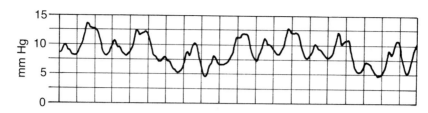

FIGURE 10-12 Pulmonary artery wedged waveform.

balloon-occluded segment of the pulmonary circulation. This creates a nonmoving column of blood within a small portion of the pulmonary circulation *(b)*, which is an extension of the nonmoving fluid column within the pulmonary artery catheter/pressure transducer system. Blood in the nonoccluded portion of the pulmonary circulation *(c)* continues to flow into the pulmonary veins and left heart. The catheter sensing tip records the pressure at the first junction *(d)* where vessels from the occluded and nonoccluded portions of the pulmonary circulation merge. This point is within the pulmonary veins. In other words, hemodynamic activity from the pulmonary veins (which are the next active portion of the pulmonary circulation) will be sensed by the pulmonary artery catheter tip. Hemodynamic activity in the pulmonary veins also reflects left atrial activity. Therefore, as long as there is a nonflowing, patent vascular channel from the catheter tip through to the pulmonary veins and left atrium, clinicians have a means of assessing left atrial activity at the bedside. Wedging of the catheter is associated with a dramatic change from the pulmonary artery waveform to a low-amplitude tracing (Figure 10-12) that relates to left atrial pulsations (phasic *a* and *v* waves).

The wedged catheter tip provides an estimate of left atrial pressure and activity. However, because the lungs lie between the catheter tip and left atrium, transmission of *a* and *v* waves is delayed and the waveform appears somewhat damped. In fact, the *c* wave is rarely visible even in a clear tracing.

Correlation of the Wedged Pressure to Left Ventricular End-Diastolic Pressure

When the mitral valve is open in ventricular diastole, there is an open channel from the catheter tip in the pulmonary artery to the left ventricle. Therefore the *a* wave (diastolic wave) of the wedged waveform correlates with LVEDP. When the mitral valve closes in ventricular systole, the catheter sensing tip records the left atrial *v* wave (systolic wave), which relates to left atrial filling against the closed mitral valve. Because the *a* and *v* waves are normally of equal amplitude, there is no significant systolic to diastolic pressure change. Therefore mean PWP correlates with LVEDP.

In summary, the mean PWP normally reflects mean left atrial pressure, which in turn normally reflects LVEDP (Figure 10-13). The balloon should not be allowed to remain inflated in the wedged (occluded) position beyond 15 seconds or two to three respiratory cycles. Minimum balloon inflation time reduces the vascular wall stress and the risk of pulmonary artery injury or rupture. Reduced wedging time also lessens the risk of ischemia of the lung segment distal to the catheter.

Prolonged wedging may result in falsely elevated pressure measurements for two reasons: (1) The catheter sensing tip may eventually shift position and protrude into the vessel wall. The transducer then records the pressure within the occluded vascular catheter, which is affected by the buildup of pressure delivered from the flush system. (2) The balloon, which is compressed by the surrounding pulmonary artery, may "herniate over" and pressurize the sensing tip of the catheter.

Hyperinflation of the balloon may also result in catheter tip occlusion by the aforementioned mechanisms. In either circumstance (prolonged balloon inflation or hyperinflation), the waveform pattern usually does not display *a* and *v* waves, rises slowly and progressively, and may then abruptly decline only to slowly rise again (Figure 10-14).

On deflation of the balloon, the catheter recoils into the main pulmonary artery (usually right), and the pulmonary artery waveform should immediately reappear.

If a wedged waveform ever continues after balloon deflation, the catheter should be carefully withdrawn until the recommended balloon inflation volume again produces a characteristic left atrial waveform. If, on the other hand, inflation of the balloon fails to produce a wedge waveform, and the balloon is thought to be intact, the catheter may have slipped backward and should be advanced with the balloon inflated. *Never advance the catheter with the balloon deflated and then inflate it later.*

An intact balloon offers a slight resistance to inflation that may be perceived by the examiner. In addition, when thumb pressure is removed from the plunger, it usually spontaneously moves back to the extended position.

Following flotation of the catheter, the sterile protective sheath is advanced over the catheter and attached to

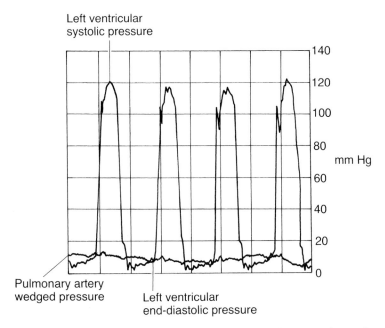

Left ventricular
systolic pressure

mm Hg

Pulmonary artery
wedged pressure

Left ventricular
end-diastolic pressure

FIGURE 10-13 Simultaneously obtained left ventricular pressure waveform superimposed on the pulmonary artery wedged pressure waveform. Note that the left ventricular end-diastolic pressure is equal to mean PWP. Waveforms are from a middle-age woman with a normal heart.

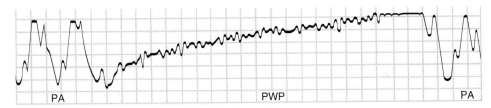

PA   PWP   PA

FIGURE 10-14 The continuously rising pressure associated with "overwedging" is due to the buildup of intra-catheter pressure from the high-pressure flush system. Obtained values are hemodynamically meaningless.

the introducer assembly (see Figure 10-6). The sheath is secured to the catheter with the adhesive strip packaged with the sheath. Once the sheath is secured to the catheter, the enclosed portion of the catheter remains sterile and that portion of the catheter may be advanced if necessary. *The catheter should never be advanced if sterility has not been maintained or if a break has occurred in the plastic sheath.* The skin surrounding the catheter insertion site is cleansed, and a dry sterile dressing is applied while continuing surgical sterile technique.

Techniques to Document a True Wedged Position

Several factors, such as improper catheter tip location and defective balloon inflation, may be associated with inaccuracies in wedge pressure measurements. Following attainment of the wedged pressure position during catheter

insertion, or at any time a wedged pressure measurement is in question, the first two criteria and possibly the third criterion may be used to verify a true wedge position.

1. *The pulmonary artery pressure trace flattens to a characteristic left atrial pressure trace immediately on balloon reinflation* (Figure 10-15). Distinct *a* and *v* waves may not be identifiable. However, an oscillating baseline, which corresponds to *a* and *v* waves, should be visible. The baseline should remain flat or follow respiratory excursions. On balloon deflation, the pulmonary artery pressure waveform should immediately return. A "partial wedge" position is characterized by a waveform that has characteristics of both the pulmonary arterial and left atrial waveforms. The "partial wedge" pressure measurement has no value in hemodynamic assessment.

2. *The mean PWP is lower than the mean pulmonary artery pressure or pulmonary artery diastolic (PAd)*

pressure. A PWP that is higher than the PAd pressure is *never* hemodynamically valid except for the following clinical circumstance. In patients with acute mitral regurgitation with "giant" *v* waves, the mean left atrial pressure, and consequently the measured PWP, is higher than the PAd pressure because of the systolic reflux of blood into the left atrium and pulmonary circulation. In all other clinical circumstances, a PWP measurement that is higher than PAd is an artifact that results from a problem within the catheter-monitoring system. The source of the artifact, such as overwedging, should be sought and corrected.

3. *Blood withdrawn from the wedged catheter tip is highly oxygenated and resembles arterial blood.* Blood gas analysis of "wedged" blood is usually performed only when doubt exists about catheter position because the

first two criteria are generally reliable and because the cost for extra blood gas studies is unnecessary. However, significant doubt about catheter position may occur when giant left atrial *v* waves (acute mitral regurgitation) distort the PWP waveform and thus create the appearance of a pulmonary artery waveform when, in fact, the balloon is truly wedged (Figure 10-16).

The rationale for the third criterion is that the wedged catheter tip has been separated from the mixed venous blood that is proximal to the inflated balloon. As a result of pulmonary artery occlusion, a sample of blood withdrawn from the wedged catheter tip represents oxygenated blood aspirated back from the pulmonary capillaries.

The "wedged" blood sample is obtained in the following manner:

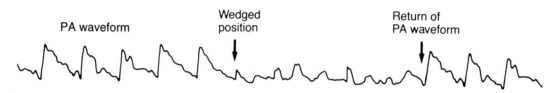

FIGURE 10-15 Balloon inflation stops when the pulmonary artery tracing flattens to a characteristic left atrial pressure trace. On deflation of the balloon, the pulmonary artery waveform reappears.

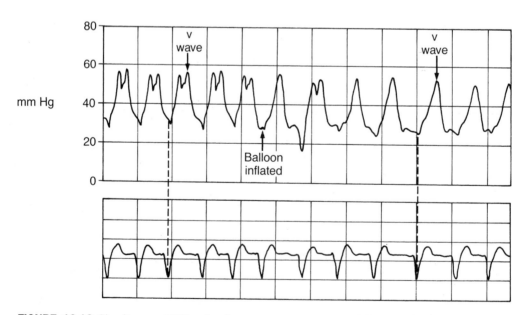

FIGURE 10-16 Simultaneous ECG and pulmonary artery pressure and PWP tracing in a patient with mitral regurgitation. Note the giant *v* wave distorting the pulmonary artery waveform, thus giving it a notched appearance. On inflation of the pulmonary artery catheter balloon, only the giant *v* wave is seen in the wedged waveform, giving it the appearance of a pulmonary artery waveform. The *v* wave is located later in the cardiac cycle than the pulmonary artery systolic peak. (Courtesy of Cedars-Sinai Medical Center, Department of Hemodynamics.)

Step 1. With the balloon inflated, 5 ml of the mixed flush solution and blood is rapidly aspirated and cleared from the distal (pulmonary artery) catheter lumen and then discarded.

Step 2. With the balloon still inflated, a second syringe is filled with 2 ml of blood, labeled *PWP aspirate,* iced, and sent to the laboratory for blood gas analysis. The balloon is deflated and the distal lumen is then flushed with irrigating solution. Blood drawn from the distal lumen with the balloon inflated has a slightly higher Po_2 than systemic arterial blood and should be fully saturated with oxygen.

This test may not be reliable if, in the wedge position, blood is drawn from areas of lung with significant shunting, such as regional atelectasis or pneumonia. In this circumstance, a low oxygen saturation is noted because the capillary blood in shunted areas of lung does not exchange gas with alveolar air.

Analysis of a mixed venous (pulmonary arterial) blood sample is not necessary for this test. However, the oxygen tension and saturation of true mixed venous blood provide diagnostic information and are necessary for calculation of the fraction of intrapulmonary shunt and various oxygen transport indices (see Chapter 12).

Withdrawal of a Pulmonary Arterial Blood Sample for Analysis of Mixed Venous Blood

The balloon is left deflated and the flush solution/pulmonary arterial blood mixture is cleared from the line by withdrawing 2 to 5 ml of blood very slowly (1 ml per 20 seconds). This blood sample is discarded. A second 2 ml sample is then obtained very slowly, labeled *pulmonary artery aspirate,* and iced.

Rapid aspiration of blood may draw arterialized (pulmonary capillary) blood into the syringe and may "contaminate" the mixed venous specimen and produce a false-high oxygen saturation. When in doubt about the purity of the drawn specimen, comparing the mixed venous and arterial carbon dioxide tensions helps identify mixed venous blood that is "contaminated" with arterialized pulmonary capillary blood. A mixed venous CO_2 equal to or lower than a simultaneously drawn arterial CO_2 suggests withdrawal of pulmonary capillary blood.

Evaluation of the PAd-PWP Gradient

The pulmonary artery diastolic pressure and the left atrial pressure (measured as PWP) closely correlate in patients with a normal pulmonary circulation. This correlation is possible because during diastole, the catheter sensing tip located in a main pulmonary artery is able to "see through" the pulmonary circulation, which has no valves, to the left atrium. During systole, no correlation between pulmonary artery pressure and left atrial pressure exists because of the systolic thrust of blood from the right ventricle.

PAd pressure, however, is normally 1 to 4 mm Hg higher than left atrial pressure because of the slight resistance to diastolic runoff imposed by the friction of flowing blood against the highly distensible pulmonary vascular walls. When the catheter is "wedged," there is no blood flow distal to the catheter tip and hence no resistance to flow. Measurements thereby reflect only left atrial pressure.

The correlation between left atrial pressure and the PAd pressure is not close when pulmonary vascular resistance is increased secondary to hypoxemia, acidemia, massive pulmonary embolism, or pulmonary vascular disease. In these cases, the PAd pressure is significantly higher than measured PWP. The greater the increase in pulmonary vascular resistance, the wider the PAd-PWP gradient. Generally, a *PAd-PWP gradient greater than 4 to 5 mm Hg is indicative of increased pulmonary vascular resistance.* The difference between PAd pressure and PWP may be used as an index in assessing pulmonary vascular resistance. For example, a PAd-PWP gradient of 7 mm Hg indicates a slight increase in pulmonary vascular resistance, whereas a PAd-PWP gradient of 50 mm Hg indicates a marked increase in pulmonary vascular resistance.

Rewedging Protocol

The frequency with which PWP measurements are done depends on the acuity of the clinical situation and the patient's hemodynamic status. Generally, if a good correlation is known to exist between the PAd pressure and PWP, the PAd pressure (rather than PWP) may be used to track left atrial pressure. This reduces the number of balloon inflations, which may prolong balloon life, and reduces the risk of ischemic lung injury and pulmonary vascular damage or rupture. If, however, factors known to increase pulmonary vascular resistance are present, the predictable correlation between pulmonary artery diastolic pressure and PWP no longer exists. In such cases, serial PWP measurements should be used to assess left atrial pressure and left ventricular filling. In order to accurately measure the PWP, the balloon must totally occlude the pulmonary artery branch but not be hyperinflated relative to the size of the vessel. Sufficient time (approximately one respiratory cycle) must elapse so that pressures can fully equilibrate across the pulmonary vascular bed.

For rewedging, the balloon is *slowly* inflated while the pulmonary artery waveform is being observed. Inflation is immediately stopped when the pulmonary artery waveform changes to a PWP waveform (see Figure 10-15). This indicates that the inflated balloon has entered and is occluding a pulmonary vessel that is slightly smaller than the balloon. Inflation beyond this point risks damage to the smaller pulmonary artery segment. The compressed balloon also may herniate over and pressurize the catheter sensing tip. This results in a falsely elevated pressure measurement termed *overwedging.*

Postinsertion Protocol

Following completion of the pulmonary artery catheter insertion procedure, any unusual events (arrhythmia or difficulty in passing the catheter) are recorded, along with the type of catheter used for insertion and the balloon volume for flotation and wedging.

If the catheter is advanced under fluoroscopy, the tip of the catheter should be seen to move freely within the left or right pulmonary artery and then advance to a visibly "wedged" position when the balloon is inflated. If performed without fluoroscopy, an *overpenetrated* postinsertion chest radiograph is then inspected to document catheter placement and to rule out pneumothorax. When in proper position, the tip of the catheter should not be evident beyond the silhouette of the mediastinal structures (Figure 10-17). Location beyond the mediastinal border indicates placement of the catheter too far into the distal pulmonary

circulation. Peripheral catheter tip location may have the following adverse monitoring and clinical implications:

1. *Cardiac output measurements may be in error.* The thermistor bead should be located in a large, main pulmonary artery or a major vascular segment to adequately sample the injected fluid bolus and estimate cardiac output. If the catheter has migrated distally to a smaller pulmonary artery branch, the thermistor sensing bead may be against the smaller vessel wall or may receive a less than indicative sample of right ventricular output and pulmonary blood flow.

2. *Damage to the pulmonary vasculature may occur.* The tip of the pulmonary artery catheter normally lies in the right main pulmonary artery. Upon inflation of the balloon, the catheter rapidly moves forward until it wedges. If wedging is accomplished with less than the recommended inflation volume, the hard, unprotected catheter tip may impale and possibly perforate the vessel wall.

3. *The catheter may spontaneously migrate into a wedged position.* Prolonged wedging predisposes the patient to ischemic injury or infarction of the lung tissue located beyond the pulmonary artery segment occluded by the catheter.

4. *Blood drawn from the pulmonary catheter for a mixed venous "specimen" may be contaminated with arterialized blood.* Because of the decreased flow rates in

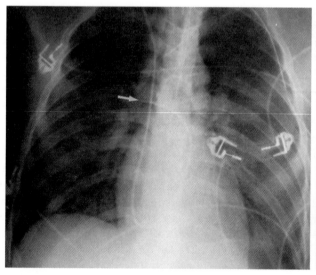 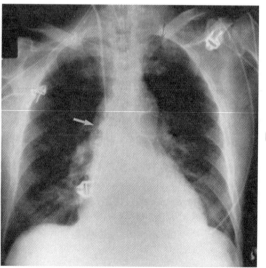

A   B

FIGURE 10-17 A, Overpenetrated portable chest radiograph showing proper pulmonary artery catheter placement. Note that the length of the catheter may be visualized within the cardiovascular structures. The catheter is most commonly positioned in the right main pulmonary artery; however, left main placement may occur and has no monitoring or clinical significance. In this patient, the catheter tip is located near the right mediastinal border *(arrow).* **B,** Standard portable chest radiograph showing proper pulmonary artery catheter position. The catheter tip is just within the right heart border *(arrow).* Note that the catheter is nearly invisible within the cardiac silhouette, which makes determination of catheter coiling or knotting difficult.

the more peripheral pulmonary arteries, even careful aspiration of blood might draw oxygenated blood from the pulmonary capillaries.

On the other hand, *proximal* location of the catheter tip in the main pulmonary trunk may be associated with significant catheter whip artifact. The normally turbulent blood flow just above the pulmonic valve imparts spasmodic motion to the catheter tip. The whip artifact spikes that result may significantly distort the pulmonary artery waveform. Proximal location also risks downward slippage of the catheter tip into the right ventricle and the possible generation of ventricular ectopy.

REMOVAL OF THE PULMONARY ARTERY CATHETER

Removal of the pulmonary artery catheter is done after viewing the most recent chest radiograph. An overpenetrated chest radiograph is preferred over a standard chest radiograph to visualize the catheter within the mediastinal silhouette. Thus a knotted or coiled intracardiac catheter can be identified before attempts at catheter removal (see catheter knotting in the section on complications of pulmonary artery catheterization).

The procedure for catheter removal is explained to the patient, and the patient is instructed in performing a Valsalva maneuver. At least one return demonstration is performed to ensure that the patient clearly understands not to inhale as the catheter is removed. Patients are then placed in a supine position if their condition allows.

The stopcocks at the end of the proximal and distal ports are closed to the patient. Immediately before catheter withdrawal, the patient is asked to repeat the practiced Valsalva maneuver, which is maintained throughout catheter withdrawal. The associated increase in intrathoracic pressure helps prevent accidental entry of air into the circulation. The catheter is then smoothly and gently withdrawn. *The catheter is never "jerked out," nor is withdrawal forced if resistance is encountered. Resistance indicates catheter attachment to a cardiac structure.*

Following removal, sterile dressings are applied to the catheter insertion site and the patient is watched for changes in cardiopulmonary function.

Although the reported incidence of complications encountered with pulmonary artery catheter removal is low, some complications may be associated with significant transient or permanent functional impairment or even with death. In one reported case, a thrombus was apparently stripped off the pulmonary artery catheter during removal and embolized across a ventricular septal defect into the cerebral and coronary circulations.[26]

Because of the low incidence of complications associated with 215 pulmonary artery catheters removed by nurses, Roundtree[27] suggests that removal of pulmonary artery catheters be delegated to critical care nurses if they receive "proper education and training." The American Association of Critical-care Nurses (AACN) also recommends pulmonary artery catheter removal by nurses who have successfully completed a competency-based program following a physician's order and using a written protocol.[28] Unfortunately, in many cases, proper education and training of critical care practitioners may be more the ideal and less the reality. In view of the tremendous variability in critical care education, experience, on-the-job training, and supervision of critical care practitioners, as well as the potential for immediate life-threatening complications, there are reservations about this practice being generally endorsed by state boards of nursing and this liability being readily accepted by nurses. If a major complication occurs during or immediately following catheter removal, such as massive pulmonary embolism or catheter fracture and embolization, a physician may not be readily available for intervention. Although removal of pulmonary artery catheters by nurses is becoming increasingly common, it is recommended that catheter removal be generally performed by an experienced physician and the preparatory setup, patient education, and transfer of pharmacologic drips and IV infusates remain the responsibility of the nurse.

The insertion of a pulmonary artery catheter sometimes is an urgently needed procedure. Catheter removal is not urgent. Waiting a few hours until an experienced physician is available has no clinical significance for the patient.

CLINICAL APPLICATIONS OF THE PULMONARY ARTERY CATHETER

The pulmonary artery catheter is most commonly used in the diagnosis and assessment of patient responses to therapy of circulatory or pulmonary disorders such as pulmonary edema. Safe and effective patient management requires that the clinician has the ability to understand the physiologic variables that determine cardiac output and fluid movement into the lung and the ability to understand and interpret the physiologic data available with the pulmonary artery catheter.

Risk of Observer Error

Because we generally see what we expect or want to see, preconceived ideas may lead to significant clinical mistakes. In one case, an admission white blood cell count that was 700 and a platelet count that was 15,000 were read by both nurses and physicians as 7000 and 150,000, respectively. The error was not detected until the following day when the patient was moribund with severe sepsis. At that time, the white blood cell count was 500 and the platelet count was 9000.

When reviewing a patient's hemodynamic profile on the bedside flow sheet or computer printout, it is of critical importance that the measurements be evaluated as they actually are. To reduce the likelihood of observer misinterpretation or error, rather than mentally scanning the hemodynamic data, silently "talk to yourself," as if communicating measurements to another person. Then formulate your hemodynamic interpretation and "discuss" with yourself the reasons for your conclusions. This more deliberate approach may help minimize significant assessment errors.

This section focuses on the role of the pulmonary artery catheter as an adjunct in evaluating and managing patients with circulatory and pulmonary dysfunction.

Assessment of Variables in Circulatory Function Using the Pulmonary Artery Catheter

The hemodynamic determinants of cardiac output are heart rate and stroke volume.

Heart Rate

Heart rate and rhythm are routinely monitored for all patients in critical care units. Disturbances in heart rate and rhythm may be treated with drugs or cardiac pacing to optimize the patient's hemodynamics.

Stroke Volume

Stroke volume, the volume of blood ejected by the heart with each beat, ranges from 60 to 130 ml. The relationship of stroke volume and heart rate to cardiac output is illustrated in the following formula:

Stroke volume $\times$ Heart rate = Cardiac output

For example,

70 ml per beat $\times$ 70 beats per minute = 4900 ml/min

A reduction in stroke volume is the fundamental defect in systolic (contractile) failure due to ischemic heart disease, cardiomyopathy, or myocardial depressant drugs or factors. Hypovolemia, pericardial disease, and cardiac tamponade are extracardiac causes of a reduced stroke volume.

50 ml per beat $\times$ 70 beats per minute = 3500 ml/min

In patients with mild systolic failure, a compensatory increase in heart rate usually maintains acceptable cardiac output while the patient is at rest and performing mild exercise. However, exercise tolerance is limited because of the limited stroke volume and reduced reserve for increases in heart rate.

50 ml per beat $\times$ 98 beats per minute = 4900 ml/min

Signs and symptoms of heart failure are usually noted by the patient only when compensatory mechanisms are exhausted by the severity of heart failure. At this time, significant decreases in stroke volume are usually present.

Stroke volume, which can be calculated at the bedside, is a more sensitive indicator of subtle changes in ventricular performance than cardiac output. Stroke volume can be calculated by dividing cardiac output, measured in milliliters, by heart rate:

$$\frac{5000 \text{ ml (cardiac output)}}{100 \text{ beats per minute (heart rate)}} = 50 \text{ ml (stroke volume)}$$

Stroke volume is determined by the degree of myocardial fiber shortening and circumferential ventricular size reduction. These factors, in turn, are affected by preload, afterload, and myocardial contractility.

Preload

The term *preload* refers to the amount of end-diastolic stretch on myocardial muscle fibers. This, in turn, is determined by the volume of blood filling the ventricle at end-diastole; the greater the filling volume, the greater the stretch. Increased ventricular muscle fiber stretch results in a more forceful contraction and greater stroke volume up to a physiologic limit. In other words, the larger the ventricular filling volume (cardiac input) and myocardial fiber length, the greater the stroke volume (cardiac output).

A means of measuring myocardial fiber length is not available. One-time "snapshot" estimates of biventricular ventricular filling volume are available with bedside echocardiography. Ventricular filling volume can also be measured by specific new technologies (see Chapter 11). However, these newer technologies are not available in most ICUs.

In the *normal* heart, a close correlation exists between ventricular end-diastolic (filling) volume and ventricular end-diastolic (filling) pressure. The filling pressures of both ventricles, which serve as a gauge to filling volume, can be estimated at the bedside using the pulmonary artery catheter. In the absence of tricuspid valve disease, mean right atrial pressure (measured with the proximal RA port) correlates with right ventricular filling pressure. In the absence of mitral valve disease, PWP (measured with the distal pulmonary artery port) correlates with left ventricular filling pressure. In the absence of pulmonary vascular abnormalities, the pulmonary artery diastolic pressure also correlates with left ventricular filling pressure.

Knowledge of ventricular preload is clinically valuable in evaluating acute changes in ventricular function, circulating blood volume, ventricular compliance, and myocardial oxygen consumption. The ways in which preload measurements can be of clinical value are discussed next.

Preload Measurements as a Means of Evaluating Ventricular Function

Preload measurements provide a bedside means of evaluating acute changes in ventricular performance through the construction of ventricular function curves (VFCs).

Construction of Ventricular Function Curves. The VFC graphically illustrates the relationship between ventricular filling volumes or pressure and stroke volume. Right ventricular preload may be expressed as end-diastolic volume (using the thermodilution ejection fraction pulmonary artery catheter); right and left ventricular preload may be expressed as ventricular filling pressure (RA pressure for the right ventricle and PWP for the left ventricle). Serial assessment of the shape of the VFC gives valuable information regarding the functional characteristics of each ventricle at any period in time. Changes in contractility, ventricular compliance, afterload, and preload can all produce changes in the ventricular function, and therefore VFCs are variable from patient to patient and in the same patient at different points in time due to physiologic changes.

Figure 10-18 shows sample graphs for correlating RV and LV end-diastolic volume or pressure with stroke volume in milliliters. Using this or similar graph paper, align the patient's stroke volume or cardiac output (on the vertical axis) with the patient's filling pressure or end-diastolic volume (on the horizontal axis). The point of intercept indicates ventricular output for that particular level of preload. Then draw a line starting from the lower left corner of the graph to the point of intercept. Note the slope of the curve (steep or depressed) (Figure 10-19). The goal of fluid, unloading, or inotropic therapy is to optimize ventricular output (increase the slope of the curve) while keeping the PWP as close to normal as possible. The shape of the VFC as affected by normal, failing, and hyperdynamic ventricular function is described next.

The *function curve of a person with a normal left ventricle* has a steep upstroke that plateaus (point of intercept) at filling pressures of approximately 8 to 10 mm Hg (see Chapter 20, Figure 20-2, *A*). The *normal right ventricular function curve* has a sloped upstroke and a lower

filling pressure for any given stroke volume and may not possess a plateau.

The effect of the *function curve of a person with systolic (contractile) failure* is elaborated on because many ICU patients have cardiac problems that are related to contractile dysfunction. In the patient with systolic failure, stroke volume decreases. Because the ventricle fails to empty adequately with each beat, the filling volume and pressure of the ventricle increase in proportion to the severity of heart failure. Increases in preload are met with minimal or no increase in stroke volume because the weakened ventricle cannot respond normally to increases in end-diastolic filling. These hemodynamic features produce two characteristic changes on the ventricular function curve.

First, the decreased stroke volume and poor response to increases in ventricular filling volume/pressure are manifest by a flat, depressed function curve. Second, the increase in ventricular filling volume/pressure shifts the point of intercept to the right. In other words, for the left ventricle, the preload measurement at which "optimum" stroke volume is attained is higher—perhaps 16 mm Hg rather than the normal 8 to 10 mm Hg. Beyond that critical limit, ventricular performance may decrease and the patient is likely to develop pulmonary congestion and edema. The upper limit for improving the function of an impaired right ventricle has not been defined.

The *function curve of a hyperdynamic ventricle* (anemia, early sepsis, pregnancy, hepatic cirrhosis) has a steep upward slope and is heightened and shifted to the left. In other words, ventricular output is greater than normal for any level of preload, and the "optimum" ventricular output (point of intercept) is attained at a lower than normal level of preload.

The Effect of Altered Ventricular Compliance on Preload and the Ventricular Function Curve

As stated, in the normal ventricle, an increase or a decrease in end-diastolic volume is associated with predictable increases or decreases in end-diastolic pressure. In patients with heart disease, ventricular filling volume and pressure may not correlate if compliance of the ventricle is altered.

Ventricular compliance is increased (more distensible) in some patients with dilated cardiomyopathy, as well as in patients with anemia or mild-to-moderate aortic regurgitation. In these persons, a large increase in ventricular filling volume may be accompanied by only a small change in filling pressure. In such patients, serial function curves usually show a blunted stroke volume response to fluid challenges.

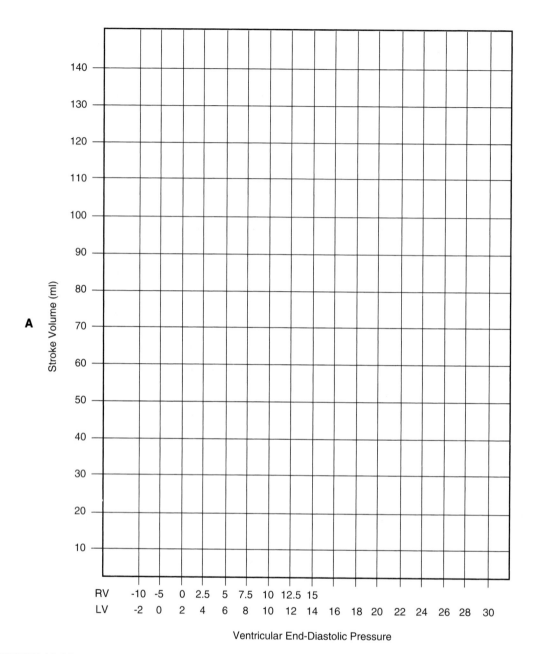

FIGURE 10-18 Sample graphs for plotting left or right ventricular function curves using either right ventricular end-diastolic pressure (standard thermodilution catheter) **(A)** or volume (thermodilution RV ejection fraction catheter) **(B)** against stroke volume. Use of serially constructed ventricular construction curves enables identification of "optimum preload" for either ventricle.

Ventricular compliance is decreased (stiff ventricle) in patients with hypertrophic, ischemic, or fibrotic heart disease. In these patients, the ventricular filling pressure is disproportionately increased relative to ventricular filling volume. In other words, a small fluid challenge may be associated with striking increases in ventricular filling pressures without significantly increasing stroke volume. Serial VFCs usually show a blunted stroke volume response to fluid challenges and abnormally large increases in PWP to any given stroke volume.

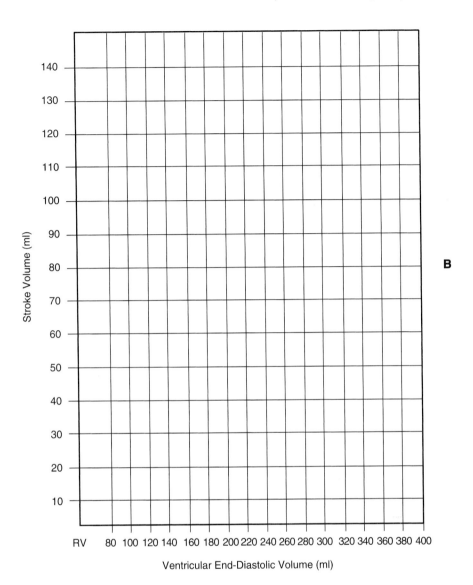

FIGURE 10-18, cont'd

A sudden decrease in myocardial compliance (diastolic failure) is one of the first changes associated with acute myocardial ischemia, and it actually precedes the onset of pain by several minutes. An acute increase in PAd pressure or PWP, which occurs in patients not receiving fluid challenges or vasopressor drugs, is a sensitive indication of early left ventricular ischemia. Unexplainable increases in PWP may be particularly helpful warnings of acute myocardial ischemia in patients who are unable to verbalize their pain (intubated, sedated, incoherent, non–English speaking).

Preload Measurements as a Means of Evaluating Circulatory Volume

In patients with normal ventricular compliances, venous tone, and cardiac function, an increase in central circulatory pressure measurements and cardiac output indicates a proportionate increase in intravascular volume. Conversely, a decrease in these measurements indicates a proportionate decrease in circulating blood volume. In other words, intravascular volume changes are *normally* met with similar changes in intracardiac and pulmonary vascular pressure

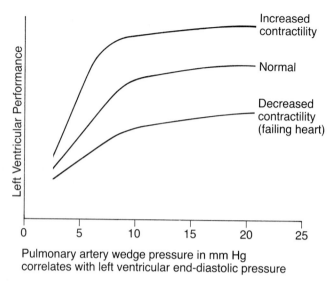

FIGURE 10-19 The ventricular function curve. Note that in the failing heart, increases in intraventricular volume, as reflected by increases in filling pressure, produce disproportionately smaller increases in performance compared with the normal ventricle. Conversely, with increased contractility due to catecholamine stimulation of the normal myocardium, more work is produced for any given filling pressure.

measurements. Stroke volume likewise increases up to a physiologic limit. Because ICU patients frequently have acute or chronic changes in ventricular compliance, cardiac dysfunction, and changes in venous tone, preload measurements may not accurately reflect intravascular volume status unless values are very low.

Influence of Preload on Myocardial Oxygen Consumption

Myocardial oxygen consumption (MVo_2) increases in direct proportion to the diameter of the heart. For example, if heart size doubles, MVo_2 can be expected to double. Therefore increases in ventricular end-diastolic volume, which may be the result of heart failure or hypervolemia, can have disastrous effects on the ischemia-prone heart. On the other hand, if intraventricular volume and heart size are reduced through the use of diuretics or venodilator agents, myocardial oxygen consumption can be expected to decrease. In fact, preload reduction is the primary mechanism of action of nitroglycerin in relieving ischemic myocardial pain (see Chapter 21, Figure 21-4).

In summary, evaluation of ventricular performance, myocardial compliance, and circulating volume is possible by evaluation of right and left ventricular preload and its relationship to cardiac output. Pharmacologic or fluid therapy adjustments in preload allow the clinician to manipulate cardiac performance and myocardial oxygen consumption. Because of the tremendous variability in ventricular function and myocardial compliance in pa-

tients with acute and chronic heart disease, there is no universal "best preload" level that serves as a therapeutic end-point. Overall, the *optimal* preload level for the left ventricle of any patient is that which produces an adequate cardiac output without causing pulmonary edema or worsening myocardial ischemia.

Afterload

The term *afterload* relates to the sum of all the loads (forces) against which the muscle fibers of both ventricles must shorten in order to eject blood into the arterial circulations. Afterload for either ventricle is affected by several factors, the most important of which is vascular resistance. Other factors include the mass of blood and diastolic pressure in the great arteries, the viscosity of blood, and compliance of the arterial walls. As afterload *increases,* stroke volume falls and myocardial oxygen consumption rises proportionate to the increased load placed on the heart. As afterload *decreases,* stroke volume rises and myocardial oxygen consumption falls proportionate to decreasing ventricular workload. Increases in the pressure surrounding the heart, as with the use of PEEP, reduces afterload because the increased extracardiac pressure applied during systole helps the ventricle "lift the load" (see Chapter 20, Figure 20-2).

Afterload cannot be directly measured. However, pulmonary vascular resistance and systemic vascular resistance, as well as pulmonary artery and aortic diastolic pressures, provide a guide to the level of right or left ventricular afterload.

Physical Determinants and Calculation of Vascular Resistance

The resistance to flow through the systemic and pulmonary circulations is the result of friction between flowing blood and the vascular walls. The diameter of the blood vessels is the principal factor determining resistance to blood flow. The resistance to blood flow disproportionately increases by a reduction in the cross-sectional area of the vascular bed. For example, if vasoconstriction decreases the cross-sectional area of the arterial circulation by one half, resistance to flow increases 16 times.

If the arteries of either the systemic or pulmonary circulation constrict, the mean arterial pressure must increase to maintain blood flow through the narrowed vascular channels. Therefore the volume of blood flow distal to a vasoconstricted circulation may fall if:

1. The involved ventricle cannot increase systolic pressure proportionate to the increased vascular resistance. In this case, the patient develops circulatory failure.
2. Vascular resistance is locally increased (coronary artery spasm, cerebral vascular spasm, peripheral vascular spasm) and the blood pressure remains constant. In this case, only the tissue distal to the intensely constricted artery is underperfused and in ischemic jeopardy.

Calculation of Vascular Resistance

Vascular resistance cannot be directly measured. The following formula can be applied to the calculation of systemic and pulmonary vascular resistances:

$$\text{Vascular resistance} = \frac{\overbrace{\substack{\text{Mean inflow} \\ \text{pressure}} - \substack{\text{Mean outflow} \\ \text{pressure}}}^{\substack{\text{Pressure gradient} \\ \text{across circulation}}}}{\substack{\text{Volume of blood flow in} \\ \text{one minute (cardiac output)}}}$$

There are two means of calculation and several terms (for the same method of calculation) that are used to describe the physical units that express vascular resistance. Neither calculation nor any term is superior to the others, and the general lack of consistency has the potential to cause confusion among practitioners. *Resistance units,* expressed in mm Hg/L/min, are used more commonly in laboratories, whereas *metric units,* expressed in dynes/sec/cm^{-5}, are most commonly used in clinical practice and are therefore used throughout this textbook.

Resistance units (R units) are expressed in mm Hg/L/min. Blood flow is expressed in liters per minute and central circulatory pressures are measured in millimeters of mercury (mm Hg). Resistance units are also termed *absolute resistance units* (ARUs), *hybrid units,* or

Wood units, because this unit measure of vascular resistance was first introduced by Dr. Paul Wood, a pioneer cardiologist.

For metric units, pressure in millimeters of mercury is changed to dynes/cm^{-2} and flow in liters per minute is changed to cm^{-3}. The only significant difference between the two units is that calculation of metric resistance units uses the basic vascular resistance formula multiplied by a conversion factor of 80, whereas R units are calculated using only the formula. As a result, the range of values for R units is considerably lower than that of metric resistance units.

Systemic vascular resistance (SVR) represents the average resistance to blood flow throughout the entire systemic circulation. Clinically, it is calculated by subtracting central venous (RA) pressure from mean arterial pressure (the pressure gradient across the systemic vascular bed) and then dividing by cardiac output (the rate of flow through the vascular bed). The result is multiplied by 80, which is the conversion factor for adjusting the value to dynes/sec/cm^{-5}. Newer monitoring systems and cardiac output computers automatically compute SVR from hemodynamic measurements. The formula for calculating SVR manually is

$$\text{SVR dynes/sec/cm}^{-5} = \frac{\text{Mean arterial pressure} - \text{Central venous pressure}}{\text{Cardiac output}} \times 80$$

In a patient with a mean arterial pressure of 90 mm Hg, a right atrial pressure of 5 mm Hg, and a cardiac output of 5 L/min,

$$1360 \text{ dynes/sec/cm}^{-5} = \frac{90 \text{ mm Hg} - 5 \text{ mm}}{5 \text{ L/min Hg}} \times 80$$

Normal SVR values range from 770 to 1500 dynes/sec/cm^{-5} (9.6 to 18.9 R units). Decreased values are due to generalized vasodilation. Increased values relate to generalized vasoconstriction. The SVR measurement has diagnostic importance and may be used as a guide to vasodilator or vasopressor therapy to optimize the patient's hemodynamic status.

Clinical factors that decrease SVR and left ventricular afterload include vasodilator therapy, hyperdynamic septic shock, cirrhosis, compensated aortic regurgitation, anemia, and anaphylactic and neurogenic shock. Clinical factors that increase SVR and left ventricular afterload include hypovolemia, hypothermia, low cardiac output syndromes, and excessive catecholamine secretion (stress response, pheochromocytoma) or administration.

When calculating SVR, it is important for the clinician to remember that this calculated value represents an average of the various resistances of the entire systemic circulation. Thus SVR measurements do not reflect regional differences in vascular resistance and blood flow. For example, as cardiac output begins to fall, significant increases in renal vascular resistance may occur without significant increases in calculated SVR.

Pulmonary vascular resistance (PVR) represents the average resistance to blood flow through the entire pulmonary circulation. It is calculated by subtracting PWP from mean pulmonary artery pressure (the pressure gradient across the pulmonary vascular bed), dividing by cardiac output, and then multiplying by 80.

$$\text{PVR dynes/sec/cm}^{-5} = \frac{\text{Mean pulmonary artery pressure } - \text{ PWP}}{\text{Cardiac output}} \times 80$$

For example, in a patient with a mean pulmonary artery pressure of 15 mm Hg, a PWP of 8 mm Hg, and a cardiac output of 5 L/min,

$$112 \text{ dynes/sec/cm}^{-5} = \frac{15 \text{ mm Hg } - \text{ 8 mm Hg}}{5 \text{ L/min}} \times 80$$

Because the pulmonary circulation is normally a highly compliant, low-resistance circulation, PVR is considerably less than SVR. Normal values range from 20 to 120 dynes/sec/cm^{-5} (0.25 to 1.7 R units).

Factors that may increase pulmonary vascular resistance and, in turn, right ventricular afterload include massive pulmonary embolism, cardiogenic and noncardiogenic pulmonary edema, sepsis, acidemia, hypoxemia, idiopathic primary pulmonary hypertension, and some congenital or valvular heart diseases. Factors that may decrease pulmonary vascular resistance and right ventricular afterload include use of pulmonary vasodilator drugs such as epoprostenol (prostacyclin), as well as correction of hypoxemia or acidemia.

Calculation and Clinical Value of Total Pulmonary Resistance

Total pulmonary resistance relates to the resistance to flow from the pulmonary artery to the left atrium, not taking into account left atrial pressure. It is calculated using the following formula:

$$\text{Total pulmonary resistance} = \frac{\text{Mean pulmonary arterial pressure}}{\text{Cardiac putput}}$$

Values range from 150 to 250 dynes/sec/cm^{-5}. This measurement does *not* provide information that relates *only* to changes in the pulmonary vasculature. For example, changes in left atrial pressure, which commonly occur in critically ill patients, influence this calculation. This calculation and measurement was widely used more than

25 years ago before it became possible and convenient to measure left atrial pressure at the bedside and incorporate it into the vascular resistance formula. However, it is rarely used today.

Contractility

This term describes the inotropic state of the myocardium that relates to the velocity and extent of myocardial fiber shortening regardless of preload and afterload. Changes in ventricular contractility strongly affect the patient's perfusion status and the slope of the ventricular function curve. Positive inotropic stimuli (endogenous or exogenous catecholamines, positive inotropic drugs) produce a steeper function curve and shift it upward and possibly to the left (increased contractility; see Figure 10-19). Negative inotropic stimuli (severe acidemia and hypoxemia, myocardial disease, negative inotropic drugs) produce a flattened, depressed function curve that may be shifted to the right (decreased contractility; see Figure 10-19). Pharmacologic agents affecting contractility also have effects on preload, afterload, or both (see Chapter 14). Contractility cannot be measured at the bedside; however, judgments about contractility are based on the characteristics of the patients' ventricular function curves and perfusion status.

Indexed Measurements Used in Assessing Circulatory Function

Body Size in Relation to Hemodynamic Measurements

A person's body size affects certain hemodynamic measurements. For example, a cardiac output that is suitable to meet the metabolic needs of a small person must be greater to meet the metabolic needs of a large person. The resting cardiac output of a very small adult may be one half or even one third that of a very large adult. As a more precise means of assessing tissue perfusion relative to body size, hemodynamic measurements (such as cardiac output and stroke volume) are related to the amount of blood (in liters per minute) flowing to a standardized area of tissue (square meter of body surface).

As an example, the average male adult weighing 70 kg has a body surface area of approximately 1.7 square meters; a small female adult may have a body surface area of 1.45 square meters; and a large male adult may have a body surface area of 2.4 square meters. Cardiac index standardizes hemodynamic parameters for all these persons to a square meter of body surface.

The body surface area for each patient may be obtained with a nomogram, such as the DuBois Body Surface Chart, which uses height and weight to calculate body surface area. Currently, most institutions are equipped with computerized monitors that automatically calculate cardiac index after the patient's height and weight are programmed in (see Chapter 11 for further discussion of indexed values, and see Figure 11-1).

Cardiac Index

This calculated value provides the means by which cardiac output of people of different sizes can be compared, eliminating differences in body build. The range is 2.5 to 4.2 L/min/m² and is typically higher in youth, normally diminishing with age. Cardiac index (CI) is calculated by dividing cardiac output (CO) by body surface area (BSA):

$$CI = \frac{CO}{BSA}$$

Stroke volume index is determined by dividing cardiac index by heart rate or by dividing stroke volume by body surface area. The range is 30 to 65 ml/min/m².

Vascular Resistance Index

Pulmonary and systemic vascular resistance index is calculated by substituting cardiac index for cardiac output in the aforementioned formulas. The important clinical point related to indexed measurements is that they are not without shortcomings and weaknesses (see Chapter 11). Although indexed values have gained almost universal acceptance over the past 30 years, there has been no documentation that their clinical use has improved patient outcome. *No measured or calculated hemodynamic parameter yields absolute truth, and all must be regarded as hemodynamic "estimates." These "estimates" are then related to each patient's history and physical findings, as well as current laboratory measurements.*

Assessment of Measurements of Pulmonary Function Using the Pulmonary Artery Catheter

Evaluation of Hemodynamic Measurements in Pulmonary Edema

In people with normal cardiopulmonary systems, pulmonary artery diastolic pressure, pulmonary capillary hydrostatic pressure, pulmonary venous pressure, left atrial pressure, and LVEDP are nearly equal. Knowledge of one measurement therefore allows a reasonable estimate of all measurements (see Chapter 18, Figure 18-23).

Pulmonary capillary hydrostatic pressure, as estimated by PWP, is the principal determinant of fluid movement from the pulmonary capillaries into the lung. Therefore this hemodynamic measurement is of major significance in the assessment and management of patients with pulmonary congestion and edema. In people with normal plasma oncotic pressure (which relates to

serum protein levels) and normal pulmonary capillary permeability, PWP values below 18 mm Hg are associated with normal lung fluid content. At values of 20 to 30 mm Hg, fluid movement into the lung typically exceeds the pulmonary lymphatic pumping capacity and the lungs become edematous. Pulmonary edema is classically associated with tachypnea, dyspnea, wheezing, crackles, cough, restlessness, and anxiety. With PWP measurements in excess of 30 to 35 mm Hg, florid pulmonary edema develops and is usually incompatible with survival beyond a few hours.

Patients who are exceptions to the aforementioned critical threshold PWP measurements are commonly encountered in clinical practice. For example, people with chronic elevated left atrial pressures (mitral stenosis or insufficiency) may tolerate elevated left atrial pressures with considerably less fluid shift; therefore they have a higher PWP threshold for developing overt pulmonary edema. On the other hand, patients with the acute respiratory distress syndrome (ARDS) extravasate large volumes of plasma into the lungs with a PWP in the normal range, because the damaged pulmonary capillaries become highly porous.

Patients with chronic, fibrotic pulmonary disease are also vulnerable to pulmonary edema. They have a reduced lymphatic pumping capacity and tend to develop pulmonary edema with less provocation (heart failure, fluid overload) than people with normal pulmonary lymphatic channels.

Calculation of Oxygen Transport and Consumption

The maintenance of adequacy of blood oxygen transport relative to total body oxygen consumption is fundamental to the maintenance of normal organ function and patient viability. Neither parameter can be measured directly but can be calculated taking into account measurements of cardiac output, hemoglobin, and mixed venous and arterial oxygen saturations. Elaboration of the clinical application of oxygen content, transport, and consumption calculations and the formulas necessary for calculation of these parameters are discussed in Chapters 2 and 12.

Estimation of the Fraction of Intrapulmonary Shunt

A common cause of hypoxemia in critically ill or injured patients is increased intrapulmonary shunting of mixed venous blood. The *pulmonary shunt fraction* refers to the percent of right ventricular output that perfuses the pulmonary circulation without going through ventilated areas of lung. In other words, this is the percent of cardiac output that does not come in contact with alveolar air and therefore cannot become oxygenated. The end-capillary

P_{O_2} of shunted pulmonary blood is identical to that of mixed venous blood and is also termed *venous admixture*. When mixed with the oxygenated blood draining into the left heart, venous admixture lowers the arterial P_{O_2}. In healthy people, the fraction of shunted pulmonary blood is approximately 5% to 8% of cardiac output and is the result of normal anatomic vascular shunts. This small volume of venous admixture entering the systemic arterial circulation has minimal effect on arterial P_{O_2} (see Chapter 2).

Pulmonary disease is commonly associated with shunt units (perfused but not ventilated alveoli) that are the result of atelectasis, alveolar edema, or consolidation due to pneumonia. As the percent of shunted pulmonary blood increases, the arterial P_{O_2} decreases. The hypoxemia that results from the intrapulmonary shunt is not significantly affected by oxygen therapy because nonventilated alveoli and the fraction of blood that perfuses the nonventilated alveoli are unaffected by oxygen administration. In patients with significant increases in the fraction of shunted pulmonary blood, hypoxemia is refractory to increases in FiO_2.

A pulmonary shunt fraction in excess of 25% suggests significant lung disease, and the patient should receive mechanical ventilatory support with consideration for the addition of PEEP.

Calculation of the Intrapulmonary Shunt Fraction. The calculated shunt fraction is the most sensitive and accurate indicator of the onset of ARDS. It is also the most accurate index of the amount of pulmonary dysfunction occurring in patients with acute respiratory failure. Calculation of the shunt fraction requires determination of mixed venous (pulmonary arterial) and systemic arterial oxygen contents and a calculation of the pulmonary capillary oxygen content. Because the pulmonary capillary blood is inaccessible for direct measurement, its oxygen content is assumed to be that which the arterial blood would have if it were fully equilibrated with alveolar air. Because the alveolar oxygen tension of patients breathing 100% oxygen is always greater than 150 mm Hg, the blood of the adjacent pulmonary capillaries can be assumed to be fully saturated with oxygen. For this reason, an FiO_2 of 100% was traditionally used for the shunt study because it simplifies the overall calculation. However, inhalation of an excessively high FiO_2, in patients with airway obstruction or disease, can lead to absorption atelectasis and more intrapulmonary shunting. Lesser concentrations of oxygen are often used for the study but require further calculation of the capillary oxygen content with the alveolar gas equation. In this text, the intrapulmonary shunt is calculated assuming that the patient's FiO_2 is 1.00 (100%). The intrapulmonary shunt fraction can be calculated from the following formula:

$$\text{Shunt fraction} = \frac{\begin{array}{c}\text{Pulmonary capillary oxygen content} -\\ \text{Arterial oxygen content}\end{array}}{\begin{array}{c}\text{Pulmonary capillary oxygen content} -\\ \text{Mixed venous oxygen content}\end{array}}$$

If a patient is breathing 100% oxygen for the shunt study, with a hemoglobin of 14 g, a capillary oxygen content of 20 ml/dl, an arterial content of 19 ml/dl, and a mixed venous oxygen content of 14 ml/dl, the shunt formula is calculated in the following manner:

$$\text{Shunt fraction } 17\% = \frac{20 - 19}{20 - 14} = \frac{1}{6} = 17\%$$

Cardiac output also must be taken into account when evaluating the shunt fraction. If, for example, cardiac output becomes very low, the available blood flow selectively perfuses better-ventilated portions of the lung. Therefore, for any given level of pulmonary pathology, the calculated shunt fraction tends to be lower although the actual number of shunt units has not changed. On the other hand, if the patient develops a high cardiac output, increased amounts of blood perfuse the shunted areas of lung and the calculated shunt fraction increases, although, again, the actual number of shunt units is unchanged. Overall, for any level of lung pathology, as cardiac output increases, the calculated shunt fraction increases, and as cardiac output decreases, the calculated shunt fraction decreases (Table 10-2).

Calculation of the PaO_2/FiO_2 Ratio. A noninvasive (but crude) way to evaluate patients with oxygenation deficits, to estimate pulmonary shunt and level of pulmonary dysfunction, is to calculate the PaO_2 to FiO_2 ratio. For example, if a patient has a PaO_2 of 80 mm Hg while breathing 40% oxygen, the PaO_2/FiO_2 ratio is 80/0.4, or 200. A ratio of less than 200 corresponds with a shunt fraction of approximately 20%. The more the PaO_2/FiO_2 ratio is below 200, the worse the degree of pulmonary dysfunction and the greater the need for aggressive ventilatory support with PEEP (Table 10-3). An important caveat to consider when using the PaO_2/FiO_2 ratio in evaluating patients with pulmonary disease is that PaO_2 also is affected by cardiac output. For example, if cardiac output decreases, the PaO_2 decreases, although no change in pulmonary function has occurred.

POTENTIAL PROBLEMS AND PITFALLS IN OBTAINING ACCURATE HEMODYNAMIC MEASUREMENTS

To effectively use the pulmonary artery catheter and maximize the patient's risk/benefit ratio, it is important to understand the potentials for invalid pressure

TABLE 10-2
Relationship between Shunt Fraction, Pao$_2$, and Cardiac Output When Breathing 100% Oxygen*

Arterial Po$_2$ (Pao$_2$)	Shunt Fraction		
	If CO = 2.5L/min; AV Do$_2$	If CO = 5 L/min; AV Do$_2$	If CO = 10 L/min; AV Do$_2$
600	2	4	8
500	5	10	17
400	8	16	25
300	11	19	32
200	13	24	38
150	14	26	42
100	18	31	47
90	20	34	50
80	22	36	53
70	24	39	56
60	28	44	61
50	33	50	67

From Wilson RF: *Critical care manual,* ed 2, Philadelphia, 1992, FA Davis.

AV Do$_2$, Arteriovenous oxygen difference.

*Assuming an oxygen consumption of 250 ml/min and hemoglobin of 10.0 g/dl.

TABLE 10-3
Relationship of Pao$_2$/Fio$_2$ Ratio to Shunt Fraction as It Correlates with the Severity of Pulmonary Disease

Pao$_2$	Fio$_2$	Pao$_2$/Fio$_2$ Ratio	Intrapulmonary Shunt (%)	Abnormality
240	0.4	600	5	None
120	0.4	300	10	Minimal
100	0.4	250	15	Mild
80	0.4	200	20	Moderate
60	0.4	150	30	Severe
40	0.4	100	40	Very severe

From Wilson RF: *Critical care manual,* ed 2, Philadelphia, 1992, FA Davis.

measurements inherent to fluid-filled monitoring systems (see Chapter 6). A number of patient factors or technically related factors also may result in significantly inaccurate pressure measurements. Therefore reliance on digitally displayed pressure measurements increases the likelihood of clinical reliance on flawed hemodynamic profiles. Appreciation of these potential sources of error combined with an understanding of the patient's pathophysiology reduces the risk that the patient's diagnosis and therapy will be based on inaccurate hemodynamic information.

Body Position

Patients are often placed in the supine position for hemodynamic pressure measurement. This protocol is based on the assumption that this position is necessary to obtain the "standard supine" values against which all obtained pressure and flow measurements are judged. However, conditions such as acute pulmonary edema necessitate continuous elevation of the patient's upper body. In these patients, lowering the backrest to the supine position may precipitate a clinical disaster. The repetitive backrest position changes (usually hourly) also may disturb the patient's rest.

Generally, the backrest position may vary within a range of 0 to 60 degrees without significantly affecting a supine patient's pulmonary artery pressure and PWP measurements. If the patient's condition requires upper body elevation beyond this range or if the patient is hypovolemic, obtained hemodynamic measurements may be less than measurements obtained with the patient supine because gravity reduces venous return to the central circulation. However, in clinical practice, directional changes in hemodynamic measurements over time (correlated with the patient's clinical appearance) are more valid indices of the patient's condition than "absolute" measurements. The degree of change from the supine to the trunk-elevated measurements also should be noted at the time of position change so that the pressure differential may be taken into account when evaluating the upright pressure changes.

Accuracy of pulmonary artery pressure measurements of patients positioned in lateral positions less than 90 degrees (90 degrees defined as lying squarely on the right or left side) with the backrest flat have not yet been validated. If the flat bed, 90-degree lateral position is used, the transducer reference point varies with right- or left-side positioning. For both sides, the fourth intercostal space is used. However, when the patient is lying on the right side, the point of intersect is at midsternum. When lying on the left side, the reference point is the left parasternal border. The important points to remember when changing backrest position are as follows:

1. The transducer air-fluid interface must be leveled to the patient's midchest each time the level of the upper body is changed (Figure 10-20).

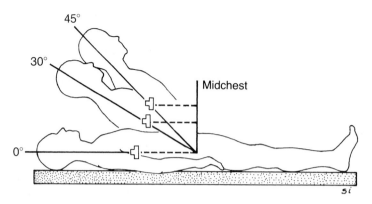

FIGURE 10-20 The transducer must be leveled to the patient's midchest each time the backrest position is changed.

2. The change in position must be indicated on the flow sheet next to recorded hemodynamic measurements or when verbally communicating hemodynamic data to other members of the care team.
3. Allow 5 minutes following patient position change before measuring pulmonary artery pressures.

Generally, technique should be as consistent as possible each time a hemodynamic profile is obtained. However, when changes in the patient's body position are required, appropriate consideration must be given to clinical interpretation of hemodynamic data.

Inadvertent Connection of the Transducer to an Inappropriate Catheter Port

Accidental connection of one of the proximal pulmonary artery catheter ports to the pressure transducer rather than to the distal port can result in misleading pressure measurements and cardiac output studies. This problem may result in serious errors in clinical decision making. Likewise, the inadvertent infusion of medications, concentrated electrolyte solutions, or hypertonic solutions (meant for the RA port) into a pulmonary artery segment may result in regional lung injury.

Cardiac Dysfunction

Interpretation of hemodynamic waveforms and pressure measurements may be difficult, or the close correlation between pulmonary artery wedge pressure, left atrial pressure, and LVEDP may not exist, in the following circumstances.

Mitral Regurgitation

Several problems are present in patients with acute severe mitral regurgitation due to the increased amplitude v wave that is a hemodynamic characteristic of this

valve defect (see Chapter 22, section on acute mitral regurgitation).

First, in affected patients, the PWP is higher than LVEDP because the regurgitant v wave elevates the averaged PWP pressure. Estimates of LVEDP (preload) may be obtained by measuring the crest of the a wave if the patient is in sinus rhythm or the base of the waveform (just before the v wave) if the patient is in atrial fibrillation, flutter, or standstill. However, the mean PWP does correlate with mean pressure in the left atrium and pulmonary veins and is valuable to assess patient risk for pulmonary edema.

Another problem is that in patients with acute, severe mitral regurgitation, the v wave produced by systolic regurgitant flow into the left atrium resembles a pulmonary artery systolic wave. Therefore, if the v waves are large, the PWP waveform may resemble the pulmonary artery waveform and lead the unwary clinician to believe that the catheter has not wedged and is still in the pulmonary artery position. This can result in repeated attempts to wedge the catheter (with the risk of pulmonary artery damage) or may result in prolonged wedging (with the risk of pulmonary infarction).

To differentiate between the pulmonary artery or PWP waveform in patients with severe mitral regurgitation, the simultaneously recorded ECG rhythm strip is correlated with the balloon-deflated and balloon-inflated tracings. The giant v wave of the wedge waveform will be located later in the cardiac cycle than will the pulmonary artery systolic wave (see Figure 10-16).

Left Ventricular Dysfunction

In patients with a noncompliant or failing left ventricle, a forceful left atrial contraction is necessary to maximally fill the ventricle and ensure an optimal stroke

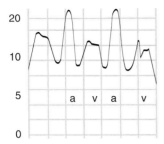

FIGURE 10-21 The increased amplitude *a* wave in this PWP waveform suggests increased resistance to left ventricular end-diastolic filling.

volume. Consequently, left atrial contraction may be associated with an increased amplitude *a* wave of the PWP waveform. Because the amplitude of the *v* wave is unaffected by ventricular dynamics, the "averaged" left atrial (PWP) pressure does not closely correlate with LVEDP. The crest of the *a* wave correlates with LVEDP (Figure 10-21).

The relationship of LVEDP to PWP seems to become less reliable at LVEDPs greater than 15 to 20 mm Hg. For example, at a very high LVEDP of 30 to 35 mm Hg, the averaged PWP may underestimate LVEDP by 5 to 10 mm Hg. Although this effect complicates hemodynamic evaluation, it is physiologically desirable because left atrial contraction can increase LVEDP without a proportionate rise in pulmonary capillary hydrostatic pressure. This situation decreases the patient's risk of pulmonary edema.

In summary, *in patients with either mitral regurgitation or left ventricular dysfunction, the crest of the PWP a wave most closely estimates LVEDP.*

Mitral Stenosis, Left Atrial Myxoma

Obstruction within the left atrial chamber by a tumor mass or stenotic mitral valve prevents diastolic equilibration of pressures between the left atrium and left ventricle. In these cases, measurement of LVEDP is possible only by direct left ventricular cannulation performed in the cardiac catheterization laboratory. However, the measured PWP is clinically valuable because it correlates with pulmonary capillary hydrostatic pressure, which is the primary determinant of fluid movement into the lung.

Miscellaneous Other Patient-Related Factors

Tachycardia

At heart rates greater than 130 beats per minute, diastolic time is shortened and does not allow sufficient time for PWP to equilibrate to LVEDP. In this circumstance, the measured PWP will be greater than true LVEDP relative to the severity of the tachycardia.

Chronic Obstructive Pulmonary Disease

Positive intrathoracic pressure induced by the combination of purse-lip breathing, intrapulmonary air trapping, and forced expiration may elevate PWP to an unpredictable level. Consequently, according to obtained "numbers," it may appear that the patient is developing heart failure or is fluid overloaded when, in fact, this is not the case. Analysis of PWP trends, along with careful physical assessment, is necessary.

Hemodynamic Measurements in Patients with Pulmonary Veno-Occlusive Disease

Pulmonary veno-occlusive disease is characterized by narrowing and occlusion of pulmonary venules and veins by fibroelastic tissue. In afflicted people, pulmonary capillary hydrostatic pressure may be elevated despite normal PWP measurements. In other words, the measured PWP is unpredictably less than with pulmonary capillary hydrostatic pressure.

The difference between the two is explained by the fact that the static column of blood produced by balloon inflation reflects only the normal pressure within the left atrium. When pulmonary blood flow resumes after balloon deflation, pressure in the pulmonary capillaries proximal to the diseased, narrowed venous segments passively increases because of impaired systolic and diastolic runoff of blood. Affected patients have radiographic evidence of interstitial pulmonary edema, dyspnea on exertion, and high pulmonary artery systolic and diastolic pressures. The PWP will be normal if the patient has normal left heart function.

Catheter Whip (Fling, Noise, Artifact)

Motion of the pulmonary artery catheter tip within the central circulation is associated with spikelike artifacts superimposed on the pulmonary artery pressure waveform (see Chapter 6, Figure 6-5). Spikes may be as great as plus or minus 10 mm Hg in amplitude and can make determination of accurate pressure measurements difficult or impossible. The monitor displays high-pressure artifacts as systolic pressures and low-pressure artifacts as diastolic pressures. Both measurements bear no relationship to the patient's true hemodynamic condition. The spike artifacts disappear after balloon inflation because the catheter tip is immobilized in the wedged position. The following are possible causes of and remedies for whip artifact.

Hyperdynamic Heart

In patients with a hyperdynamic circulation (early sepsis, catecholamine administration or excess, systemic inflammatory response syndrome, pregnancy, thyroid toxicosis), the force of right ventricular contraction may cause the catheter to pulsate within the pulmonary artery with each heartbeat. The pulsations, in turn, cause the fluid within the catheter lumen to vibrate and result in a noisy tracing. Devices can be incorporated into the monitoring system to filter out the high-frequency artifact, but they may produce excessive waveform damping. As a consequence, pulmonary artery systolic pressure may be underestimated, diastolic pressures may be overestimated, and the dicrotic notch may be obscured. Because neither option (presence of whip artifact or overdamping) is desirable, mean pulmonary artery pressure should be used for hemodynamic assessment because it is least affected by either problem.

Excessive Catheter Length

An excess of catheter in the right ventricle may be associated with pulsating catheter movement and related disturbances of the waveform. A reduction in the length of catheter within the ventricle may substantially reduce or eliminate the whip artifact.

Location of the Catheter Tip Near the Pulmonic Valve

The high-velocity, turbulent flow in this portion of the central circulation causes a quivering movement of the catheter tip, which may produce a whip artifact. Forward flotation of the catheter by a physician to the right or left main pulmonary artery may eliminate the whip artifact. This also reduces the risk that the catheter will accidentally slip back into the right ventricle.

External Sources of Noise

If a length of catheter or connecting tubing lies across the patient's chest, precordial movements or movement of the patient's chest related to breathing, shivering, and the like may impart movement to fluid within the monitoring system and may create artifact. The catheter and connecting tubing should be placed away from areas of movement.

Generally, *if the whip artifact cannot be eliminated, the recorded pulmonary artery systolic and diastolic pressures are not reliable. Because the mean pressure is the least unreliable, directional changes in mean pressure are recommended for hemodynamic assessment.*

Ventilatory Effects on Pulmonary Artery Pressure Measurements

This section begins with a brief discussion of how the electronic monitoring system processes the pressure transducer input for digital display so that the potential for inaccuracies in displayed hemodynamic measurements can be understood. This is followed by a discussion of the effects of nor-

mal and labored breathing, the effects of pulmonary artery catheter tip location within the lung, and the effects of mechanical ventilation on displayed pressure measurements.

Electronic Monitoring System

Monitors analyze the transducer input for a defined period of time termed the *scanning interval*. This is usually the time required for one screen width of corresponding pressure data. During the scanning interval, the monitor designates the lowest transducer input as the diastolic pressure measurement and the highest pressure input as the systolic measurement. These numeric values are then digitally displayed. The displayed "mean" pressure represents the average pressure over the scanning interval.

The monitor cannot distinguish high- or low-pressure inputs due to artifact (catheter whip or "ringing" due to underdamping), nor can systolic and diastolic pressure measurements obtained from a grossly wandering waveform baseline be distinguished from valid systolic and diastolic pressure measurements that would be obtained from a stable baseline. Therefore, if the highest- or lowest-pressure inputs are artifact ("fiction"), the digitally displayed systolic or diastolic measurements will likewise be nonfactual, and the mean values will be an average of fact and fiction.

Although sophisticated computer algorithms have been developed and incorporated into the monitoring system to deal with positive and negative artifacts, displayed pressure measurements still may not be accurate in patients with complex combinations of artifacts or changes in artifacts. Consequently, analysis of strip-chart recordings of central circulatory waveforms, combined with patient assessment, helps eliminate diagnostic artifact-induced errors in patients with "messy" hemodynamic waveforms.

Hemodynamic waveforms contaminated by a significant whip artifact or a grossly unstable baseline sometimes defy interpretation by even the most experienced clinician and must be acknowledged as "uninterpretable." These "messy" tracings occur when there is significant catheter whip artifact, when there are poor dynamic response characteristics of the fluid-filled system, or when there are wide swings in intrathoracic pressure associated with labored breathing or ventilator breathing with elevated peak inspiratory pressures. In these circumstances, clinical attention is best directed at relief or correction of the underlying patient-related problem (such as airway obstruction). When possible, the cause of the monitoring artifact, such as catheter whip, should be eliminated rather than "guessing" at pressure measurements.

Effects of Intrathoracic Pressure on Central Circulatory Pressure Measurements. If the heart and blood vessels were absolutely rigid (like the metal pipes of a plumbing system), changes in pressure surrounding these structures would not affect central circulatory pressure measurements. However, the walls of the heart and blood vessels are pliable and compressible. Therefore hemodynamic pressures recorded within the thorax are affected by the cyclic respiratory pressure changes exerted on the outer wall of these structures. These cyclic, respiratory pressures can be assumed to be the same as pleural pressure.

The pressure transducer monitoring system is zero referenced to atmospheric pressure. Any pressure at the catheter tip, whether purely intravascular or a combination of intravascular and intrathoracic pressure, is sensed by the catheter/pressure transducer system. The hemodynamic pressure is then compared with atmospheric pressure and graphically represented on the oscilloscope screen and digitally displayed. Consequently, the intrathoracic pressure effects of spontaneous breathing or mechanical ventilation may significantly affect the baseline of the hemodynamic waveform and digitally displayed hemodynamic measurements.

Effects of Quiet, Spontaneous Breathing on Hemodynamic Pressure Measurements. During quiet breathing, inspiration and expansion of the lung require a slight decrease in pleural pressure. On the other hand,

exhalation and deflation of the lung slightly increase pleural pressure. These cyclic changes in intrathoracic pressure are transmitted to the catheter/transducer system and impart a minimally wandering baseline to the hemodynamic pressure waveform. In people with nonlabored breathing, digitally displayed or strip-chart recorded central circulatory pressures are negligibly affected by the slight phasic intrathoracic pressure changes. Therefore either may be used to record and assess hemodynamic pressure measurements (Figure 10-22).

Effects of Labored Breathing on Hemodynamic Pressure Measurements. The effects of labored breathing produce a significantly wandering baseline of the pressure tracings because much greater swings in intrathoracic pressure are required to move air into or out of the lungs. The conspicuous inspiratory troughs or expiratory peaks are related to phases of breathing. The monitor detects pressures only during the expiratory highs and inspiratory lows during the scanning interval and therefore may display pressure measurements that have nothing to do with the patient's circulatory status.

The specific baseline changes are related to the underlying pulmonary problem and associated breathing

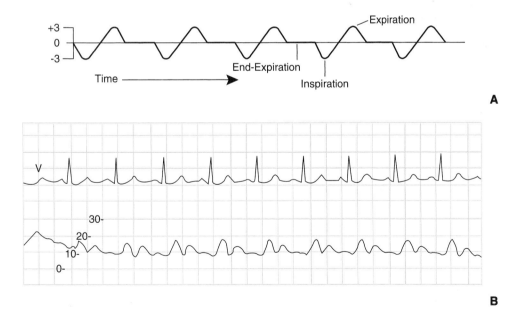

FIGURE 10-22 A, Airway curves during resting, spontaneous breathing. A negative airway pressure draws fresh air into the lungs, whereas a positive airway pressure forces expired air out of the lungs. **B,** The minimal changes in intrathoracic pressure have minimal effect on this pulmonary artery waveform baseline and measured pressures.

difficulty. If *lung compliance is decreased* (ARDS, cardiogenic pulmonary edema, diffuse atelectasis) or if upper airway obstruction is present, large negative waveform excursions may be produced by the extraordinary efforts the patient makes to inhale. The cyclic baseline dips affect the validity of systolic, diastolic, and mean pulmonary artery pressure measurements obtained during the scanning interval.

On the other hand, large positive expiratory-induced waveform excursions may be produced by patients who are "bucking the ventilator" or patients who have *increased airflow resistance* (status asthmaticus, bronchitis).

Most patients have both inspiratory *and* expiratory difficulty, and the waveform swings between inspiration and expiration can be dramatic. The widely changing digitally displayed hemodynamic measurements challenge accurate interpretation of displayed values (Figure 10-23).

To produce a stable baseline, it may seem reasonable to ask the patient to momentarily stop breathing at the end of a breath. In theory, if pressure readings were taken at this point, intravascular pressures would not be contaminated by respiratory-induced pressure changes surrounding the cardiovascular structures. Unfortunately, breath holding is impossible for a dyspneic patient. Even if breath holding were possible, most people

hold their breath against a closed glottis (Valsalva maneuver), which increases intrathoracic pressure and produces falsely elevated central circulatory pressure measurements.

Rationale and Technique for Measuring Hemodynamic Pressures at End-expiration

Intrathoracic pressure at end-expiration is normally equal to that of the atmosphere. At this time, there is minimal airflow and change in pleural pressure to be reflected on the cardiovascular structures and monitoring catheter tip.

Hemodynamic pressure measurements evaluated at end-expiration provide a standard reference point that is uncontaminated by extravascular pressures. Unfortunately, tachypnea typically coexists with dyspnea, and currently available monitors do not display the pressure during the very brief end-expiratory periods. It has been suggested that pulmonary artery pressures, airway pressures, or end tidal volume CO_2 values be simultaneously displayed on the oscilloscope or strip-chart recorder as a means of correlating end-expiration with recorded hemodynamic waveforms. This capability is determined by the technical sophistication of the monitoring equipment available at individual hospitals and is not available to most practitioners.

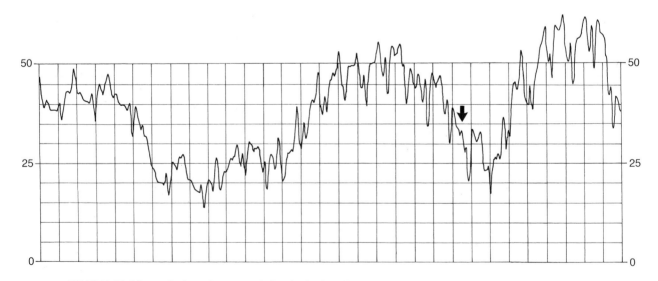

FIGURE 10-23 Marked respiratory variation in the baseline of a PWP tracing in a 64-year-old woman with pulmonary edema secondary to critical mitral stenosis. Note the marked negative deflection associated with labored inspiration (decreased pulmonary compliance) and marked positive deflection associated with labored exhalation (increased airflow resistance). The patient also is tachypneic and an end-expiratory plateau is not apparent. Therefore the PWP is measured at a point where end-exhalation *(arrow)* is estimated to occur.

The most practical and reasonable method of identification of end-expiration for measurement of central circulatory pressures uses a calibrated pressure tracing taken from a strip-chart recorder. When possible, three respiratory cycles should be included in the pressure analysis (Figures 10-24 and 10-25; see also Figures 10-22 and 10-23).

If a calibrated hard copy is not available, end-expiratory pressure measurements may be obtained from a frozen calibrated oscilloscope screen. However, if the point at which end-exhalation occurs cannot be determined with confidence and the true accuracy of measured pressures is in question, this uncertainty should be stated on the chart or flow sheet next to the recorded value so that other members of the health care team take this fact into consideration when making diagnostic judgments or therapeutic decisions.

Other Pulmonary Variables Influencing Hemodynamic Pressure Measurements

The correlation between PWP and left atrial pressure depends on an uninterrupted column of blood between the catheter sensing tip located in the pulmonary artery and the pulmonary veins. Changes in catheter tip location within the vertical plane of the lung or intrapulmonary hemodynamic changes may result in obliteration of the open vascular column, which, in turn, results in inaccurate hemodynamic pressure measurements.

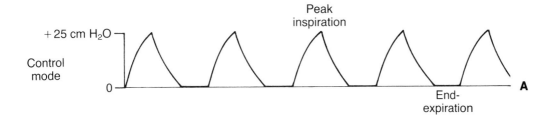

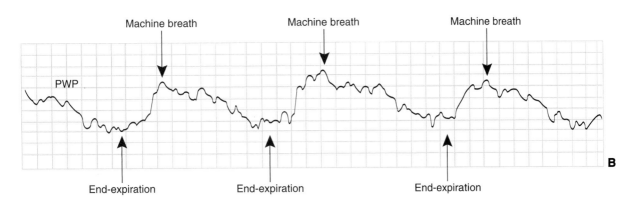

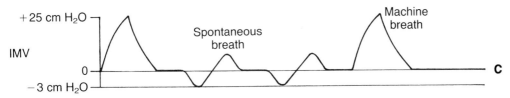

FIGURE 10-24 Airway pressure curve for ventilator (machine) breathing. The control mode **(A)** is used for apneic patients; the ventilator completely determines ventilatory rate and tidal volume. A positive pressure pushes the prescribed tidal volume into the patient's lungs, and the associated pulmonary artery or wedged waveform **(B)** follows the intrathoracic pressure excursions. Hemodynamic measurements are recorded at end-expiration *(arrows)*. **C,** With intermittent mandatory ventilation (IMV), the patient's spontaneous breaths are interspersed with a prescribed number of ventilator breaths. The hemodynamic waveform baselines follow a combination of machine breaths and spontaneous breaths.

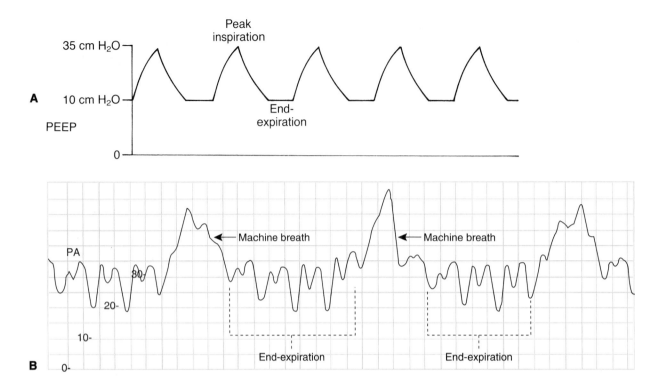

FIGURE 10-25 A, Airway pressure curve for ventilator breathing with positive end-expiratory pressure (PEEP). While machine ventilated, the patient's airway pressure at end-expiration is maintained at a positive value, most commonly in a range of 5 to 15 cm H_2O. The hemodynamic waveform baseline will correspond with pressure fluctuations within the chest. **B,** Pulmonary artery waveform taken from a 36-year-old man with catastrophic head injury and neurogenic pulmonary edema. The patient is receiving mechanical ventilatory support with 30 cm H_2O PEEP; peak airway pressures for the machine-induced breaths *(arrows)* are 100 cm H_2O. End-expiration is indicated by the area within the broken lines. The PAd pressure measurement is estimated at approximately 20 mm Hg, which is not a hemodynamic reality. The elevated recorded pressure is a reflection of the extraordinarily elevated intrathoracic pressures induced by positive pressure breathing with PEEP. Although it is impossible to determine "true" values (which would be less than those recorded) without removing the patient from the ventilator, the clinical objective is to assess changes over time correlated with the patient's clinical condition.

Relationship of Gravity to Lung Blood Flow and the Patency of Pulmonary Vessels

Gravity strongly influences the flow and distribution of blood in the lungs; pulmonary blood volume and pulmonary vascular pressures increase progressively down the lung, whereas alveolar pressures are about equal throughout the lung. (Figure 2-12 illustrates the relationship of alveolar pressures and gravitational forces to pulmonary vascular pressure, lung blood flow, and the patency of pulmonary blood vessels.) This concept was originally described by John West, a pulmonary physiologist.[29] The gravity-dependent zones of lung perfusion have therefore been termed *West zones 1, 2, and 3.*

The uppermost portion of the lung is in zone 1. In an upright person, this is the apex, but in a supine person this area is directly under the anterior chest wall. Zone 1 is a lung area with potentially no blood flow because alveolar pressure exceeds pulmonary artery systolic and diastolic pressures throughout the respiratory cycle. A pulmonary artery catheter wedged in the least dependent (zone 1) portion of the lung does not reflect left atrial pressure because the catheter tip does not have a patent vascular lumen to "look through" to the left atrium. Instead, the catheter tip reflects only alveolar pressures (Figure 10-26, zone 1).

Zone 2 is directly under zone 1. Here alveolar pressure is less than pulmonary artery systolic pressure. During systole, blood flows through the pulmonary circulation. However, alveolar pressure is greater than pulmonary artery diastolic pressure, and the higher alveolar pressure may compress and obliterate the pulmonary capillaries and venules during diastole. If the wedged pulmonary artery catheter tip is located in this intermediate lung zone, only

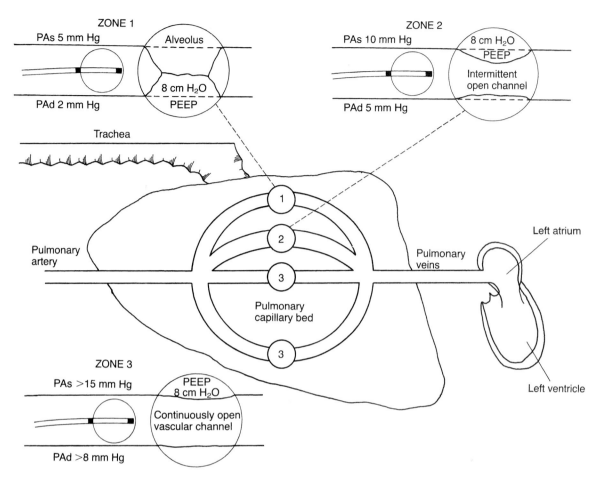

FIGURE 10-26 Schematic representation of a lung while the patient is in the supine position showing the theoretical effects of 8 cm H_2O PEEP on the pulmonary vasculature. *PAs,* pulmonary artery systolic pressure; *PAd,* pulmonary artery diastolic pressure. In *zone 1,* alveolar pressure is greater than pulmonary artery systolic pressure and diastolic pressure. Consequently, the capillary is pinched shut throughout the cardiac cycle and the pulmonary artery catheter tip senses only intraalveolar pressure. In *zone 2,* the pulmonary vascular channel is open during systole but is compressed during diastole. Intermittent closure of the vascular channel renders obtained hemodynamic measurements hemodynamically inaccurate. In *zone 3,* intravascular pressures exceed intraalveolar pressures throughout the cardiac cycle, and the open vascular channel allows accurate measurement of pulmonary artery and "wedged" pressures.

alveolar pressure is measured and displayed in diastole. A PWP measurement obtained from this area of lung is hemodynamically invalid (see Figure 10-26, zone 2).

In the most dependent portion of the lung, zone 3, pulmonary artery systolic and diastolic pressures are consistently higher than alveolar pressure. Therefore a constantly open vascular channel from the pulmonary artery catheter tip in the small pulmonary arteries to the left atrium allows the wedged pulmonary artery catheter to accurately reflect left atrial pressure. In supine patients, most of the lung is a zone 3 area and most wedged pulmonary artery catheters float to zone 3 (see Figure 10-26, zone 3).

However, the balloon may "float" upward, rendering obtained measurements invalid.

Zone 1 and 2 lung areas may increase in size and surround the pulmonary artery catheter tip. As a result, hemodynamic pressure measurements may be invalid. This is likely when (1) pulmonary vascular pressures are generally decreased because of hypovolemia and (2) alveolar pressures are increased owing to air trapping or therapeutically applied positive end-expiratory pressure (PEEP, continuous positive airway pressure [CPAP]). Zone 1 or 2 areas are particularly likely to occupy larger lung areas with PEEP or CPAP levels greater than 10 to 15 cm H_2O

(see the section on effects of mechanical ventilation later in this chapter).

In summary, invalid or inconsistent hemodynamic measurements may be the result of (1) inadvertent rewedging of the catheter tip in the uppermost (zone 1 or 2) areas of lung or (2) increases in the size of zone 1 or 2 areas of the lung secondary to hypovolemia or increases in alveolar pressures.

The following criteria may be used to assess for catheter tip location in a zone 3 lung area:

1. Identification of consistent left atrial *a* and *v* waves should be possible in the PWP waveform. A damped "wedged" tracing suggests zone 1 or 2 conditions if the fluid-filled monitoring equipment is known to be patent.

2. If the pulmonary artery catheter tip is in a zone 1 or 2 position, the PWP can exceed pulmonary artery diastolic pressure, and significant respiratory variations may be noted on the waveform baseline.

3. A cross-table lateral chest film also can determine catheter tip position in the vertical plane. If the catheter tip is below the left atrium, it can be assumed to be in zone 3 in patients with PEEP values less than 15 cm H_2O.

4. An increase or decrease in PEEP results in a proportionate increase or decrease in PWP. For example, a 5 cm H_2O decrease results in a 4 mm Hg decrease in PWP (5 cm H_2O = 4 mm Hg).

Effects of Mechanical Ventilation on Pulmonary Artery Pressure Measurements

As mentioned earlier, the forces (pressures) acting on the outside of cardiovascular structures affect the pressures inside the cardiovascular structures. Mechanical ventilator breaths are positive pressure breaths and may significantly reflect on the heart and vascular structures of the thorax. The more compliant the patient's lungs, the more the positive pressure breaths are reflected on the cardiovascular structures. This phenomenon has the potential to confound accurate interpretation of hemodynamic pressure measurements for three reasons:

1. *Hemodynamic waveform excursions reflect the pressure fluctuations that are related to the ventilator mode for that patient* (see Figure 10-24). When the ventilator delivers a breath, hemodynamic waveform baseline is transiently elevated. The higher the patient's peak airway pressures, the greater the positive deflection of the waveform baseline. Hemodynamic pressures measured during the scanning period may therefore be misleadingly high. However, the pulmonary artery pressures recorded at end-expiration should not be affected (i.e., intrathoracic pressure should be equal to that of atmospheric pressure). Therefore central circulatory pressure measurements should be taken between machine breaths from a calibrated strip-chart recorder or from a frozen, calibrated oscilloscope screen.

2. *Cardiac output tends to decrease as mean airway pressure increases in patients who are being mechanically ventilated.* Venous return, the filling volume of both ventricles, and stroke volume fall because of the effects of increased intrathoracic pressures, as well as loss of the thoracic pump mechanism. The positive pressure surrounding the heart also may produce a tamponade effect on the ventricles that further interferes with diastolic filling. However, despite the decreased ventricular filling volume, the positive pressure surrounding the cardiovascular structures, CVP, mean pulmonary artery pressure, and PWP may actually rise. Intraventricular blood volume, not pressure, determines stroke volume. Therefore the cardiac output of mechanically ventilated patients may fall despite normal or elevated central circulatory pressure measurements. In other words, hemodynamic pressure measurements that appear to be normal or elevated may be inadequate to support cardiac output because the cardiovascular volume/pressure relationships have been distorted by positive pressure ventilation.

3. *Positive alveolar pressure (PEEP, CPAP, alveolar air trapping) may increase the size of zone 1 and 2 lung areas, particularly if pulmonary artery pressures are low.* If a zone 1 or 2 area develops in the region of the pulmonary artery catheter tip, the PWP measured no longer accurately reflects left atrial pressure. Instead, the PWP is entirely or partially distorted by alveolar pressure. Of special consideration are patients with severe airway obstruction (COPD, asthma). These patients are particularly likely to have increased zone 1 or 2 lung areas because they tend to develop alveolar air trapping with hyperinflation (termed *auto-PEEP, occult PEEP*) with or without mechanical ventilatory support.

The intrathoracic pressure effects on hemodynamic measurements are especially pronounced in patients with pulmonary emphysema because the positive pleural pressures are easily transmitted to the cardiovascular structures through the highly compliant lung tissue. In these patients, pulmonary artery pressures may be misleadingly high relative to true intravascular or left ventricular filling volumes. A patient may receive inappropriate diuretic therapy for an elevated PWP measurement when, in fact, the patient may have normal blood volume or normal left ventricular function. On the other hand, patients with hypovolemia may go unrecognized because the artificially elevated high hemodynamic "numbers" indicate normovolemia.

Effects of Positive End-expiratory Pressure or Continuous Positive Airway Pressure on Central Circulatory Pressure Measurements and Cardiac Output

With the application of positive end-expiratory pressure, all of the aforementioned interpretative and hemodynamic problems are increased. Airway pressures remain positive throughout the ventilatory cycle. Elevated airway pressures, in turn, increase both intrathoracic and central circulatory pressure measurements. One would expect hemodynamic measurements recorded at end-expiration to rise nearly proportionate to increases in PEEP. This, however, is not the case. Studies that have investigated the effects of PEEP on left atrial pressure, LVEDP, and PWP measurements have shown variable effects on hemodynamic measurements. The variability in findings may relate to patient-to-patient differences in the particular ventilatory mode (controlled ventilation, intermittent mandatory ventilation, pressure support), circulating blood volume, catheter tip location, or regional or global differences in lung compliance.

Generally, at PEEP levels of 10 cm H_2O or less, the PWP correlates well with left atrial pressure and LVEDP measured with the patient off the ventilator. However, at levels of PEEP greater than 10 to 15 cm H_2O, there is an increasing likelihood of significant differences in hemodynamic measurements recorded with the patient on or off the mechanical ventilator (see Figure 10-25).

The application of continuous positive pressure to the thoracic cavity also increases zone 1 and 2 areas and produces changes in circulatory dynamics. PEEP-induced compression of the pulmonary capillaries increases right ventricular afterload, which, in turn, may reduce right ventricular stroke volume. With the advent of right ventricular failure, RVEDP may increase to levels greater than those of the left ventricle and thus shift the intraventricular septum toward the left ventricular cavity. Septal deviation, in turn, reduces the volume capacity of the left ventricle. This is manifested as a decreased stroke volume and a disproportionately high PWP relative to left ventricular filling volume. In such a patient, the measured PWP appears to be adequate but the cardiac output is low. An errant clinical judgment that left ventricular contractile failure has developed may be made.

Clearly, the cardiopulmonary changes associated with the application of mechanical ventilation, particularly with PEEP, are multifaceted and complex. The following techniques have been suggested to minimize or solve the

problem created by continuous positive intrathoracic pressures. However, each technique has significant drawbacks.

Technique—Calculating Pressure Using a Mathematic Formula

Pressure surrounding the heart and blood vessels can be estimated to be one third to one half of alveolar pressure (1 mm Hg = 1.36 cm H_2O). This calculated pressure is then subtracted from the PWP measurement. For example:

PEEP applied = 15 cm H_2O (11 mm Hg)

Measured PWP = 18 mm Hg

One half of 11 mm Hg PEEP = 5.5 mm Hg pressure surrounding the heart and blood vessels

Therefore

$$\begin{array}{r} 18 \text{ mm Hg measured PWP} \\ - 5.5 \text{ mm Hg PEEP applied perivascular and pericardial pressure} \\ \hline 12.5 \text{ mm Hg true PWP reading} \end{array}$$

Some clinicians simply subtract 1.0 mm Hg from the measured PWP for every 3.0 cm H_2O PEEP above 10 cm H_2O.

Drawbacks. Because lung and chest wall compliance and the effects of PEEP differ from patient to patient and in different areas of the lungs (such as areas of pneumonia, atelectasis) in the same patient, this technique is not uniformly reliable. This technique also does not take into account the possibility of positive pressure–induced changes in circulatory dynamics (zone 1 and 2 conditions).

Technique—Disconnection of Mechanical Ventilation or Positive End-expiratory Pressure

In some hospitals, mechanical ventilation or PEEP is temporarily discontinued for hemodynamic pressure measurements. This technique has two significant drawbacks.

Drawbacks. Because mechanical ventilation, especially with PEEP, produces pressure changes in the thorax that affect blood flow, removing the patient from the ventilator may cause abrupt circulatory changes. Venous return suddenly increases (autotransfusion effect), and PEEP-applied compression of the pulmonary capillaries and cardiac chambers is relieved. Thus more blood flows into the central circulation, and cardiac output increases. The hemodynamic measurements obtained during this time reflect a circulatory condition that exists only when the patient is removed from ventilatory support. Circulatory status should be assessed when patients are being therapeutically supported and not during the period when PEEP is suddenly discontinued.

Second, there is a risk that the patient's condition will deteriorate after the removal of PEEP. Sudden volume overload of the left ventricle and pulmonary circulation may result in a rapid extravasation of fluid into the lung from the autotransfusion effect. When PEEP is removed, loss of alveolar stability and small airway collapse may result in sudden, severe hypoxemia.

Technique—Measuring Serial Changes in Hemodynamic Measurements with Changes in Positive End-expiratory Pressure Levels

The effects of PEEP or CPAP may be judged by measuring the changes in pulmonary artery pressures with each change in PEEP during PEEP therapy.

Drawback. This technique addresses only the effect of applied extravascular pressure on hemodynamic pressure measurements and does not take into account the secondary circulatory changes.

In summary, mechanical ventilation, especially with high alveolar pressures, may affect hemodynamic pressure measurements and confound interpretation of hemodynamic data via three mechanisms: (1) transmission of intrathoracic pressures to the cardiovascular chambers and monitoring catheter tip, (2) intermittent or complete vascular obstruction from the pulmonary arterioles to the pulmonary venules by PEEP-compressed capillaries, and (3) the effects of decreasing venous return and cardiac output. The difficulties and uncertainties in measurement of true central circulatory pressure in patients supported by mechanical ventilation underscore the importance of evaluation of changes in hemodynamic measurements (trend analysis). The relationship of these changes to alterations in clinical and laboratory data rather than reliance on isolated hemodynamic measurements is also important.

IDENTIFICATION AND SOLUTION OF MONITORING PROBLEMS

The absolute accuracy of hemodynamic pressure measurements is difficult to determine. However, if consistency in technique is maintained when obtaining hemodynamic measurements, if dynamic response characteristics of the monitoring system are adequate, if waveform morphology and pressure measurements are appropriate for the clinical setting, and if hemodynamic measurements and waveforms do not change without apparent cause, obtained pressure measurements are accepted as accurate. Distortion of the monitored waveforms, inappropriate pressure measurements, or inability to obtain pressure measurements may occur as a result of many technical problems.

Problem—Marked Changes in Pressure Measurements or Pressure Measurements Inappropriate to the Patient's Condition

Numeric values that have suddenly changed or do not fit the clinical picture should be suspected as inaccurate and investigated. Causes and corrective maneuvers include the following.

Position Changes

If the upper part of the patient's body or the patient's bed has been raised or lowered, but the transducer mounted on an IV pole has not been re-referenced to the midchest, significant errors in pressure measurements may occur. For example, for each inch the pressure transducer is located *below* the pulmonary artery catheter tip, an error of approximately 2 mm Hg *above* the true reading is obtained. Conversely, a falsely *low* 2 mm Hg reading is obtained for each inch the transducer is *above* the midchest level. Leveling and zero referencing the pressure transducer to the midchest is particularly important when measuring pressures in the central circulation because an error of as little as 5 mm Hg may result in significant errors in diagnosis and therapy.

Inaccurate Static Reference Points and Pressure Scales

The zero reference point is established by turning the transducer stopcock off to the patient and open to air (the transducer dome is open to atmospheric pressure). When checking the accuracy of the zero point, the protective cap (sometimes termed *dead-ended cap*) should be removed from the venting port. Otherwise the protective cap may obstruct the port and prevent transducer equilibration to atmospheric pressure.

If non–fixed-calibration monitoring systems are used or any time accuracy of the transducer or monitoring system is in question, the calibration point should be tested by the department of biomedical engineering for accuracy (see Chapter 6).

The monitor pressure scale should be appropriate to the type of pressure monitoring. Typically, a pressure scale and amplifier setting of 40 mm Hg is used for pulmonary artery pressure monitoring; a 60 mm Hg scale is required for patients with pulmonary hypertension. A pressure scale of 200 mm Hg is used for arterial pressure monitoring.

To ensure accurate hemodynamic measurements, an important principle to remember when setting up, zeroing, and calibrating the monitoring system is "garbage in = garbage out."

Problem—Inability to Obtain a Wedged Pressure Measurement

If a wedge waveform does not follow balloon inflation with the proper amount of air, balloon rupture or retrograde slippage of the catheter into the pulmonary trunk or right ventricle should be suspected. A chest radiograph may be required to document backward slippage. Once documented, catheter advancement and redirection of the inflated balloon to the right or left main pulmonary artery branches, by a physician, allow rewedging.

Problem—Damped Pulmonary Artery Waveform

If the amplitude of the waveform decreases (lower systolic pressure), the patient should be immediately assessed for shock. If it is determined that the patient's condition is stable, technical causes of a damped waveform should be investigated. These include the following:

1. Air in the tubing.
2. Clotted blood at the catheter tip or within the catheter lumen. This may have occurred as a result of inadequate line irrigation. A leaky irrigation solution pressure bag (less than 300 mm Hg pressure) is a common cause of this problem.
3. Kinking or knotting of the catheter or tubing.
4. A loose connection with a small leak in the system. Streaks of blood backing up from the pulmonary artery catheter may be present.
5. Spontaneous catheter migration into a near-wedged position.
6. Catheter tip positioned against the vessel wall.
7. Amplifier setting in the wrong pressure range. For example, a pulmonary artery pressure monitored at an arterial pressure scale (200 mm Hg) may appear severely damped.
8. A loose or cracked transducer or air in the dome.

Problem—No Waveform

The complete absence of a pulmonary arterial waveform may be the result of the following:

1. Pulmonary artery transducer improperly engaged in the monitor outlet or engaged in the wrong outlet
2. Defective transducer
3. Large leak in the system (blood will probably back up from the pulmonary artery catheter)

4. Loose or cracked transducer dome or air in the dome
5. Stopcock turned to the wrong position
6. Amplifier on zero or off
7. Catheter lumen or catheter tip is completely clotted
8. Defective cable connecting the pressure transducer to the monitor/amplifier

A Systematic Approach to Problem Solving

After it has been determined that the altered waveform and pressure are not related to changes in the patient's condition, a systematic approach is taken to identify and solve the problem. This begins as simply and noninvasively as possible and with the most common sites of disturbance. If necessary, investigation may then proceed to more complex, manipulative, and time-consuming approaches to troubleshooting.

Problems are most frequently located within the fluid-filled portion of the system. The transducer dome and tubing are first inspected for the presence of blood, kinks (this may require removal of dressings), and air bubbles, as well as a loose fit at connection sites, inappropriate position of stopcocks, or defects such as cracks in the transducer dome. The pressure bag also should be checked for adequate inflation pressure—300 mm Hg. An inadequate bag-inflation pressure should raise suspicion of catheter thrombosis.

If air bubbles or blood is seen in the tubing, the system is gently aspirated with a syringe until blood from the pulmonary artery appears in the aspirating syringe. This ensures that clotted blood or air has been cleared from the line. The line is then gently flushed with irrigating solution. Aspiration or irrigation should not be undertaken if there is a possibility that the catheter has spontaneously wedged because of the risk of damage or rupture to the distal pulmonary artery segment. If blood or air is seen within the transducer dome, the dome is purged of air or blood.

If the problem cannot be visibly identified proximal to the catheter, it may be within the length of the catheter or at the catheter tip. Problems may be related to catheter position. If gentle aspiration followed by flushing does not improve the waveform, the catheter tip may be resting against the vessel wall. Turning the patient to the left or right side, or having the patient cough, may move the catheter tip away from the vessel wall. A completely clotted catheter (i.e., difficulty in withdrawing blood along with inability to flush the line) frequently requires catheter replacement. The catheter should not be force irrigated because the obstructing thrombus may be dislodged and propelled into the distal arterioles and become a pulmonary embolism. Spontaneous wedging, or kinks or knots within the heart or great vessels, may require a chest

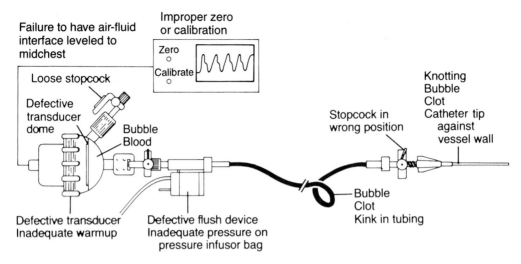

FIGURE 10-27 A step-by-step approach to problem source identification begins noninvasively with the most common sites of disturbance.

radiograph for diagnosis. If spontaneous wedging is verified as the cause of the problem, the catheter is withdrawn carefully until a wedged waveform reappears after balloon reinflation to the recommended volume. If catheter knots are the problem, intracardiac knots may be eliminated using fluoroscopic manipulation of the catheter. Knots may require removal of the catheter via transvenous or surgical routes.

If the fluid-filled components of the monitoring system are found to be free of problems, the monitoring instruments are checked. First, the connecting cable should be changed before performing more time-consuming and costly transducer changes. If the problem persists, the existing transducer is replaced by a new transducer. If the original problem persists, the monitoring consoles are tested and exchanged. Figure 10-27 illustrates possible problem sites encountered with pulmonary artery pressure monitoring.

COMPLICATIONS OF PULMONARY ARTERY CATHETERIZATION

Any procedure that introduces a foreign body into the circulation introduces risks to the patient. The responsibility of the clinician in preventing complications is related not only to the purely moral and ethical issues of "doing no harm," but also to reducing time and cost of the hospital stay. The following guidelines may contribute significantly to reducing the incidence of complications associated with pulmonary artery catheterization.

1. Catheter insertion and flotation should be performed or supervised by an experienced physician.

2. Scrupulous attention should be paid to manufacturer's recommendations for catheter placement and maintenance.

3. The pulmonary artery catheter should be used only as long as the patient's condition requires pulmonary artery pressure monitoring.

4. All complications related to access of central veins and central venous catheter placement may occur with pulmonary artery catheterization (see Chapter 8). The following are additional complications specific to pulmonary artery catheterization.

Cardiac Arrhythmias

Atrial and ventricular arrhythmias are caused by irritation of the endocardium by the pulmonary artery catheter. They may occur any time during catheter flotation and maintenance, as well as when the catheter is pulled back through the right heart for removal. However, the incidence of arrhythmias, particularly ventricular ectopy, is greatest during catheter insertion. This finding underscores the importance of careful ECG monitoring during catheter flotation and the bedside availability of cardiopulmonary resuscitation equipment.

The incidence of arrhythmias is significantly higher in patients with acute myocardial ischemia, shock, hypoxemia, ventricular failure, acidosis, hypocalcemia, hypokalemia, hypomagnesemia, or digitalis toxicity, and during prolonged catheter flotation time. Whenever possible, arrhythmia risk factors should be corrected before catheter insertion. The risk of arrhythmias also may be minimized by inflating the balloon to its recommended volume so that the hard catheter tip is cushioned by the inflated balloon. This practice reduces endocardial stimulating effects. No circumstance, other than tricuspid or pulmonic stenosis, justifies flotation of the balloon with less than the manufacturer's recommended inflation volume. Placing the patient in a 5-degree head-up, right lateral tilt position during catheter insertion may result in a lower incidence of malignant arrhythmias than the traditional supine or Trendelenburg position by facilitating balloon flotation from the right ventricle to pulmonary artery.

Ventricular ectopy may also occur if the catheter tip slips down into the right ventricle after being placed in the pulmonary artery. Backward slippage is associated with the appearance of a right ventricular waveform (dicrotic notch absent and lowered end-diastolic pressure) from the transduced distal (pulmonary artery) port. Temporarily inflating the balloon to its recommended volume may redirect the catheter to the pulmonary artery position. If redirection cannot be accomplished by the physician and the arrhythmia continues despite lidocaine (Xylocaine) therapy, the pulmonary artery catheter should be promptly pulled back to right atrial level.

Right bundle branch block also may complicate pulmonary artery catheterization. Mechanical irritation of the conduction tissue or damage to the bundle of His during catheter passage is believed to be the cause. High-risk patients include those with acute anteroseptal myocardial infarction or pericarditis. Most cases of right bundle branch block are clinically benign and transient. However, patients with a preexisting left bundle branch block may develop complete heart block. In these cases, an external transthoracic pacing device should be immediately available. Alternatively, a pulmonary artery catheter with pacing capabilities, rather than a nonpacing pulmonary artery catheter, should be inserted.

Balloon Rupture

Inflation of the balloon is typically associated with a feeling of resistance. Absence of this resistance, failure to wedge, and the ability to aspirate blood through the inflation port is diagnostic of balloon rupture. The one-time introduction of 0.8 to 1.5 ml of air into the pulmonary circulation is not harmful; however, repeated injections of air may result in pulmonary air embolism. Therefore a piece of tape labeled *balloon rupture* should be applied to the inflation port so that other clinicians will not repeat the wedging attempts.

The latex material of the balloon gradually loses elasticity and weakens as it absorbs lipoproteins from the blood. Balloon life also may be shortened by multiple inflations (the average balloon can withstand approximately 72 inflations), manual removal of air from the inflated balloon via a syringe, and exceeding the recommended balloon inflation volume for flotation or wedging.

A monitoring problem occurs with balloon rupture because the PWP measurement is no longer available. However, if there was a known good correlation between the PAd pressure and the PWP, the pulmonary artery diastolic pressure may be used to track left heart filling and function.

Potential patient risks associated with balloon rupture include embolization of balloon fragments into the distal pulmonary circulation and, in the presence of right-to-left shunts, cerebral or systemic air embolization on injection of air into the ruptured balloon. *If a right-to-left shunt is known to exist, carbon dioxide should be used for balloon inflation instead of air. Fluid should never be employed for balloon inflation because the high balloon wall tension may rupture the pulmonary artery.*

Catheter Knotting

Knotting of the pulmonary artery catheter may occur within the blood vessels and cardiac chambers and around intracardiac structures and other intravascular catheters. Knotting is more likely to occur with a small-caliber pulmonary artery catheter, when the catheter is repeatedly withdrawn and readvanced; when the patient has dilated cardiac chambers; and when an excessive length of catheter has been inserted. The insertion of excessive catheter length is more likely to cause the formation of coils or kinks that may then form knots. Any time an extraordinary length of catheter has been inserted without achievement of the anticipated chamber pressures and waveform, catheter coiling should be suspected (see Box 10-2 for anticipated distances from insertion sites to central circulatory chambers). Other important signs of knotting include the development of ventricular arrhythmias, at a time when the distal (pulmonary artery) port indicates right atrial placement; waveforms appearing damped; and difficulty with aspirating or flushing the catheter.

Knotting also should be suspected when resistance is encountered during withdrawal of the catheter for removal or repositioning. When gentle traction is applied to the catheter, the presence of a pulse-by-pulse tug suggests involvement of the tricuspid valve apparatus. Catheter withdrawal should be *immediately stopped* to prevent traumatic disruption of the tricuspid valve and its supportive structures.

An *overpenetrated* chest radiograph confirms the diagnosis of catheter knotting and defines the location and extent of catheter knotting within the cardiac silhouette. The catheter may be removed transvenously or unknotted by a physician with fluoroscopic manipulation assisted by guide wire placement. In difficult cases, venotomy or thoracotomy and cardiotomy may be required for catheter removal.

Infectious Complications

Several physical characteristics of the pulmonary artery catheter and factors associated with its use increase the potential for local and systemic infections (see Chapter 13). These factors include (1) the intracardiac location of the catheter; (2) the breaks in the closed monitoring system for withdrawal of blood samples; (3) the repeated repositioning of the catheter; (4) the possibility of spontaneous migration of the catheter, with entry of a non-sterile portion of the catheter into the vascular system; and (5) the thrombogenic and adherence characteristics of the polyvinyl chloride catheter for microorganisms. Critically ill patients, many of whom are in an immune-compromised condition, are also more susceptible to these infections.

The threat of infectious disease is subtle because the cause (microorganisms) is invisible to the naked eye. There also is a tendency to believe (consciously or unconsciously) that that which cannot be seen is either not there or is inconsequential. The effects of pulmonary artery catheter or wound contamination also are typically not clinically evident as site infection or septicemia until 24 to 48 hours after the incident that allowed contamination of tissue or blood. Therefore the cause-and-effect relationship of infectious disease is not always well established. The patient is said to have "become septic" as though by some unfortunate twist of fate.

Sepsis is a major and often avoidable cause of morbidity and mortality in the critically ill patient. It is incumbent on clinicians to use meticulous sterile technique during catheter insertion and maintenance; to keep blood withdrawals and catheter repositioning maneuvers to a minimum; to be keenly alert to any signs of infection; and to remove the catheter as soon as it is no longer needed. It has been shown that the incidence of infectious complications, as well as catheter fault (balloon rupture, thermistor malfunctions, luminal obstruction), progressively increases the longer the catheter is in place (Figure 10-28).

Thromboembolic Complications

Any catheter in the vascular system can promote thrombus formation, particularly in patients who have prolonged circulatory failure. The polyvinyl chloride pulmonary artery catheter also is known to initiate a thrombogenic response. The clot can form anywhere along the length of the pulmonary artery catheter, within the catheter lumen, and may also cover the catheter tip. The incidence of

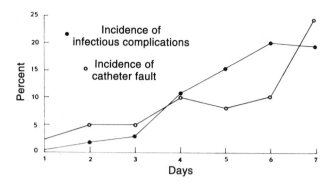

FIGURE 10-28 Incidence of infectious complications and catheter fault as related to pulmonary artery catheter indwelling time. Catheters maintained longer than 72 hours had a significantly higher incidence of both infectious complications and catheter fault. (From Sise MJ et al: Complications of the flow-directed pulmonary artery catheter: a prospective analysis in 219 patients, *Crit Care Med* 9:317, 1981. Copyright Williams & Wilkins.)

clot formation appears to be far greater than what would be indicated by clinical evidence. For example, one study revealed postmortem and venographic evidence of internal jugular vein thrombosis at the catheter insertion site in 22 of the 33 patients entered in the study.[30] No patients had clinical evidence of thrombosis in the area of the catheter. However, patients with catheter-related thrombosis had a significantly lower cardiac output 12 hours following catheter insertion. Nonheparin-bonded pulmonary artery catheters were used in the study. Another study showed that 53% of patients had autopsy evidence of thrombosis along the catheter, five of whom also had evidence of catheter-related pulmonary embolism.[31] The incidence of catheter thrombosis was statistically higher in patients whose catheters were in place longer than 35 hours.

The clinical and monitoring implications of catheter-related thrombosis include the following:
- Extensive clot material in the area of the catheter tip may occlude the pulmonary vessels distal to the catheter tip, resulting in ischemic injury to the lung.
- A thrombus anywhere in the systemic veins, right heart, or pulmonary arterial system can dislodge or fragment and result in pulmonary embolism. The clot also may be stripped from the catheter and may embolize on catheter withdrawal.
- Subclavian venous thrombosis may interfere with venous drainage from the head or same-side upper extremity. This is clinically evidenced as unilateral jugular venous distention, upper extremity edema, dyspnea, facial congestion, and cough.

- The accuracy of pulmonary artery pressure or thermodilution cardiac output measurements may be adversely affected by the presence of a thrombus over the pulmonary artery pressure sensing tip or thermistor bead.

The presence of a clot may be detected by (1) consistently damped waveforms without evidence of peripheral catheter migration; (2) poor infusion of IV fluids or flush solution via the proximal (RA) or distal (pulmonary artery) ports; or (3) increased pulmonary artery systolic and diastolic pressure, with a widening of the PAd-PWP gradient without apparent cause. This hemodynamic finding should raise the suspicion of pulmonary embolism. Signs and symptoms of pulmonary ischemic injury or infarction are discussed later in this chapter.

Prevention of catheter thrombus formation requires consideration of anticoagulation in hypercoagulable patients if pulmonary artery pressure monitoring is prolonged or if catheter insertion is known to have been traumatic. Heparin-bonded catheters also reduce catheter thrombogenicity. Continuous infusion of a saline solution (2 to 3 ml/hr) helps prevent clot formation in the lumen or around the catheter tip. Additional flushes using the in-line flush device also may be required in patients known to be hypercoagulable. If clotting of the proximal or distal sensing port is suspected, gentle aspiration of blood with clots followed by gentle irrigation may clear the line.

Pulmonary Complications

Pulmonary complications include pneumothorax, pulmonary infarction, and damage to or rupture of the pulmonary artery.

Pneumothorax

Although previously discussed in the section on complications of CVP monitoring, pneumothorax is mentioned again in relation to pulmonary artery pressure monitoring because of its relative frequency. For example, in one study of 320 pulmonary artery placements done in 219 patients, 10 major complications occurred.[32] Of these, six were pneumothoraces; five occurred at catheterization of new sites and one at a preexisting CVP access site.

The pulmonary artery catheter postinsertion chest radiograph should be carefully inspected not only for correct catheter tip placement and in situ catheter coiling or knotting but also for the presence of pneumothorax.

Pulmonary Ischemic Injury or Infarction

Mechanical occlusion of the pulmonary artery by clot material or a persistently wedged catheter predisposes the patient to pulmonary ischemic injury. The likelihood of pulmonary infarction is increased in patients with elevated pulmonary venous pressures or inadequacy of the bronchial collateral circulation (fibrotic lung disease, COPD).

Factors that predispose patients to pulmonary artery catheter–related ischemic lung injury include the following:

1. *Persistent wedging due to spontaneous forward migration of the catheter tip into a small peripheral branch of the pulmonary arterial circulation.* Following insertion, the pulmonary artery catheter warms to body temperature and softens. Pulsatile blood flow may then move the more pliant catheter more peripherally until any excessive catheter loop tightens or the uninflated balloon spontaneously wedges in a vessel slightly smaller than the catheter tip. Ischemic lung lesions are usually small and asymptomatic. Some may be diagnosed solely by the sudden appearance of a new unexplained density on the chest radiograph in the area of the peripherally located catheter tip.

2. *Persistent or prolonged inflation of the balloon in the wedged position.* Because a relatively large branch of the pulmonary arterial circulation remains obstructed, a significant area of lung is at risk to ischemic injury.

Ischemic lung injury due to persistent wedging may be prevented by (1) not leaving the catheter in the wedge position longer than 15 seconds or two to three respiratory cycles; (2) ensuring that a clearly defined pulmonary artery waveform returns when the wedged balloon is deflated; and (3) inspecting the postcatheter insertion chest radiograph, and following routine or emergency radiographs to verify correct position of the catheter tip. With the balloon fully deflated, the catheter recoils into a main pulmonary artery. In the correct position, the catheter tip should not be visible beyond the mediastinal silhouette (see Figure 10-17).

If peripheral migration is suspected, the catheter should be withdrawn slowly and carefully until a full or nearly full inflation volume produces a PWP trace.

Damage to or Rupture of a Pulmonary Artery Segment

The spectrum of pulmonary artery injuries may vary from clinically undetectable vascular injury to life-threatening hemorrhage. Possible causes of pulmonary vascular injury include the following:

1. *Spontaneous distal migration of the catheter with damage to the pulmonary vessel by the uncushioned, unprotected catheter tip.* As the catheter advances into the narrower lumen of a more peripherally located vessel, the pulsatile action of blood flow may cause the catheter tip to rhythmically strike against the vessel wall, ultimately resulting in erosion or perforation.

2. *Balloon flotation using less than the manufacturer's recommended inflation volume or rewedging that requires less than recommended inflation volume.* Normally, when in the pulmonary artery position, the catheter lies in a main, usually right, pulmonary artery. With the onset of balloon inflation, the balloon moves rapidly forward. If wedging occurs with a smaller balloon inflation volume, the hard, unprotected catheter tip may spear the distal vessel wall. In addition, asymmetric balloon inflation, which typically occurs in a peripherally located catheter during prolonged balloon inflation, may cause the catheter tip to protrude into and injure or puncture the vessel wall.

3. *Overinflation of the balloon in a vessel too small to accommodate the excessive volume.* This typically occurs when the catheter has migrated to a smaller peripheral vessel and the previously used volume of gas for balloon inflation is injected for rewedging. An inflated balloon that is "too big" for the surrounding vessel may damage or rupture the pulmonary arterial wall.

4. *Irrigation of the distal (pulmonary artery) lumen of the pulmonary artery catheter, particularly if the flush is manual and forceful.* The likelihood of vascular damage or rupture is increased if the catheter is wedged or located in a small, peripheral vessel.

5. *The pressure difference, across an inflated balloon, may be very high in patients with pulmonary hypertension.* The pressure difference may then act as a driving force to push the balloon or exposed catheter tip through the vessel wall.

Any condition that produces chronic pulmonary hypertension (mitral valve disease, COPD) increases the risk of vascular damage or rupture, because the pressure-dilated pulmonary arteries allow the catheter to wedge more peripherally. Pulmonary hypertension also may be associated with degenerative changes in the vessel walls, such as sclerosis or aneurysmal dilation, in which case the vessel walls are noncompliant and friable. Inflation of the balloon in these stiff vessels may alter balloon shape and cause the catheter tip to protrude into the vessel wall. Other risk factors for pulmonary vascular damage include advanced patient age, female gender, excessive catheter manipulation, and stiffening of the catheter with hypothermia. There may be a cumulative risk of pulmonary artery rupture with each balloon inflation. For this reason, it is recommended that if there is a good initial correlation between PAd pressure and PWP, PAd pressure should be tracked instead of PWP. Systemic anticoagulation or blood dyscrasias increase the risk of severe hemorrhage should the vessel perforate or rupture.

Patients may be clinically asymptomatic with only mild damage to the pulmonary artery segment. At one end of the clinical spectrum, patients with vascular rupture may have minimal blood-tinged sputum. At the other end, massive hemoptysis may quickly lead to shock and death. If hemoptysis is scanty, it may be difficult to differentiate pulmonary artery rupture from infarction. However, aspiration of air through the distal (pulmonary artery) lumen indicates pulmonary artery rupture.

If the patient's condition is stable, pulling the catheter back, conservative management, close observation, and reversal of anticoagulation (if relevant) may suffice. With significant, active bleeding, the patient should be placed with the affected side (usually right) down to prevent spillage of blood into the uninvolved lung with pullback of the catheter tip. Control of the airway, ventilatory support, and circulatory support are primary goals. The application of PEEP also may tamponade hemorrhage. Although the simple removal of the pulmonary artery catheter may help in patient stabilization, emergency thoracotomy with resection of the involved lung lobe may be required.

The following guidelines should prevent damage or rupture of the pulmonary artery:

1. Do not advance the catheter with the balloon deflated.

2. Carefully obtain PWP measurements by *slowly* inflating the balloon while continuously observing the pulmonary artery waveform. Inflation is stopped *immediately* when the pulmonary artery trace changes to a wedged pressure trace.

3. Do not inflate the balloon with fluid because the incompressible balloon increases stress on the vessel wall.

4. Keep the wedging time and the number of balloon inflation/deflation cycles to a minimum. If a close pulmonary artery diastolic/wedge pressure relationship exists, pulmonary artery diastolic pressure may be used to assess left atrial pressure.

5. Position the catheter tip in a central pulmonary vessel so that the full or nearly full recommended inflation volume produces the wedge waveform.

6. Avoid excessive catheter manipulation.

7. Avoid irrigating the pulmonary artery lumen under high pressure. This is sometimes attempted when it is assumed that the damped tracing is the result of a clot at the catheter tip. If a clot is indeed present, it may be distally propelled and result in pulmonary embolism. On the other hand, the damped tracing may be due to spontaneous wedging, and forced irrigation may produce rupture of the pulmonary artery.

8. Survivors of short-term hemorrhage should be evaluated for the possibility of pseudoaneurysm formation. Traumatic pulmonary artery pseudoaneurysms may later rupture.

Miscellaneous Complications

Other potential complications include spontaneous catheter fracture and embolization, cerebral air embolism, and embolization of a catheter knot during attempts at pulmonary artery catheter removal.

Although studies have been conducted to determine the incidence of complications associated with pulmonary artery catheterization, the true incidence is unknown and may be underestimated for several reasons. A single-center study indicates the number of complications only at the institution participating in the study, and the number of complications is influenced by protocol for catheter insertion and maintenance. Knowledge that a prospective study examining the incidence of complications is being conducted may influence clinicians to be more fastidious with technique of insertion and maintenance; this may cause a bias in the outcome. Generally, insertion and management techniques may vary widely among institutions and, for that matter, within an institution among different critical care units and practitioners. Another reason that complications may be underestimated is that a minor complication, such as a small pulmonary embolism or infarction, may go unrecognized.

Although pulmonary artery catheterization offers distinct assessment and management advantages, it is not a benign procedure. When considered, the anticipated benefits to the patient should clearly outweigh anticipated risks. Unfortunately, the likelihood of complications tends to increase as the patient becomes more seriously ill. Consequently, pulmonary artery catheterization should be used with extreme caution in patients with bleeding tendencies; hypercoagulable states; immunosuppression, especially granulocytopenia, and recurrent sepsis; and in patients who are on anticoagulants or have hemorrhagic blood disorders.

REFERENCES

1. Pesce RR: The Swan-Ganz catheter: it goes through your pulmonary artery and you pay through the nose, *Respir Care* 34:785, 1989.
2. Robin ED: The cult of the Swan-Ganz catheter, *Ann Intern Med* 103:445, 1985.
3. Robin ED: Death by pulmonary artery flow-directed catheter: time for a maratorium? *Chest* 92(4):727, 1987.
4. Rapoport J, Teres D, Steingrub J, et al: Patient characteristics and ICU organizational factors that influence frequency of pulmonary artery catheterization, *JAMA* 283:2559, 2000.
5. Viellard-Baron A, Girao E, Valente E, et al: Predictors of mortality in acute respiratory distress syndrome, *Am J Crit Care Med* 161:1597, 2000.
6. Connors AF, Speroff T, Dawson NV, et al, for the SUPPORT Investigators: The effectiveness of right heart catheterization in the initial care of critically ill patients, *JAMA* 276:889, 1996.
7. Dalen JE, Bone RC: Is it time to pull the pulmonary artery catheter? *JAMA* 276:916, 1996.
8. Baxter JK, Beilman GJ, Abrams HJ, et al: Effectiveness of right heart catheterization: time for a randomized trial, *JAMA* 277:108, 1997.
9. Tuman KJ, Roizen MF: Outcome assessment and pulmonary artery catheterization: why does the debate continue? *Anesth Analg* 84:1, 1997.
10. Hollenberg SM, Hoyt J: Pulmonary artery catheters in cardiovascular disease, *New Horizons* 5(3):207, 1997.
11. Kirton O, Civetta JM: Do pulmonary artery catheters alter outcome in trauma patients? *New Horizons* 5(3):222, 1997.
12. Ivanov RI et al: Pulmonary artery catheterization: a narrative and systemic critique of randomized controlled trails and recommendations for the future, *New Horizons* 5(3):268, 1997.
13. Ivanov RI et al: Pulmonary artery catheterization: a balanced look at the controversy, *J Crit Illness* 12, 1997.
14. Connors AF: Right heart catheterization: is it effective? *New Horizons* 5:195, 1997.
15. Gore JM et al: A community-wide assessment of the use of pulmonary artery catheters in patients with acute myocardial infarction, *Chest* 92:721, 1987.
16. Cooper AB, Doig GS, Sibband WJ: Pulmonary artery catheters in the critically ill: an overview using the methodology of evidence-based medicine, *Crit Care Clin* 12(4):777, 1996.
17. Brandstetter RD, Grant G, Estilo M, et al: Swan-Ganz catheter: misconceptions, pitfalls, and incomplete user knowledge—an identified trilogy in need of correction, *Heart Lung* 27:218, 1998.
18. Iberti TJ, Fischer EP, Leibowitz AB, et al: A multicenter study of physicians' knowledge of the pulmonary artery catheter, *JAMA* 264:2928, 1990.
19. Iberti TJ, Daily EK, Leibowitz AB, et al: Assessment of critical care nurses' knowledge of the pulmonary artery catheter, *Crit Care Med* 22:1674, 1994.
20. Burns D, Burns D, Shively M: Critical care nurses' knowledge of the pulmonary artery catheter, *Am J Crit Care* 5:49, 1996.
21. Wilson RF et al: Pulmonary artery diastolic and wedge pressure relationship in critically ill and injured patients, *Arch Surg* 123:933, 1988.
22. Shoemaker WC, Appel PL, Dram HB, et al: Prospective trial of supernormal values of survivors as therapeutic goals in high risk surgical patients, *Chest* 94:1176, 1988.
23. Ganninoni L, Brazzi L, Pelosi P, et al: A trial of goal-oriented hemodynamic therapy in critically ill patients, *N Engl J Med* 333:1025, 1995.
24. Hayes MA, Yau EHS, Timmons AC, at al: Response of critically ill patients to treatment aimed at achieving supernormal oxygen delivery and consumption, *Chest* 103:886, 1993.
25. Lefrant JY, Muller L, Pascal B, et al: Insertion time of the pulmonary artery catheter in critically ill patients, *Crit Care Med* 28(2):355, 2000.

A special thank you to R. Phillip Dellinger, MD, FCCP, Professor of Medicine at Rush University and Director of Medical Intensive Care at Rush Presbyterian—St. Luke's Medical Center, Chicago, Illinois, for his review of and suggestions for this chapter.

26. DeVitt JH, Noble WH, Byrick RJ: A Swan-Ganz catheter-related complication in a patient with Eisemenger's syndrome, *Anesthesiology* 57:335, 1982.

27. Roundtree WD: Removal of pulmonary artery catheters by registered nurses: a study in safety and complications, *Focus Crit Care* 18:313, 1991.

28. Keckeisen M: Pulmonary artery pressure monitoring. In *Protocols for practice. Hemodynamic monitoring series,* 1997, AACN Critical Care funded by Abbott Critical Care Systems.

29. West JB, Dollery CT, Naimark A: Distribution of blood flow in isolated lung: relationship to vascular and alveolar pressures, *J Appl Physiol* 19:713, 1964.

30. Chastre J, Cornud F, Bouchama A, et al: Thrombus as a complication of pulmonary artery catheterization via the internal jugular vein, *N Engl J Med* 306:278, 1982.

31. Connors AF et al: Complications of right heart catheterization: a prospective autopsy study, Chest 88:567, 1985.

32. Sise MJ, Hollingsworth P, Brim J, et al: Complications of the flow-directed pulmonary artery catheter: a prospective analysis in 219 patients, *Crit Care Med* 9:315, 1981.

SUGGESTED READINGS

Ahrens TS, Taylor LA: *Hemodynamic waveform analysis,* unit II, Principles of waveform analysis, unit IV, Application of waveform analysis, Philadelphia, 1992, W.B. Saunders.

Bennett D, Boldt J, Brochard L: European Society of Intensive Care Medicine Expert Panel: the use of the pulmonary artery catheter, *Intensive Care Med* 17:1, 1991.

Boscoe MJ, de Lange S: Damage to the tricuspid valve with a Swan-Ganz catheter, *BMJ* 283:346, 1981.

Butterworth JF: Pulmonary artery catheterization. In *Atlas of procedures in anesthesia and critical care,* Philadelphia, 1992, W.B. Saunders.

Chandrakant P et al: Acute complications of pulmonary artery catheter insertion in critically ill patients, *Crit Care Med* 14:195, 1986.

Chastre J et al: Thrombosis as a complication of pulmonary-artery catheterization via the internal jugular vein, *N Engl J Med* 306:278, 1982.

Connors AF et al: Assessing hemodynamic status in critically ill patients: do physicians use clinical information optimally? *J Crit Care* 2:174, 1987.

Connors AF Jr et al: Hemodynamic states in critically ill patients with and without acute heart disease, *Chest* 98:1200, 1990.

Damen J, Bolton D: A prospective analysis of 1400 pulmonary artery catheterizations in patients undergoing cardiac surgery, *Acta Anaesthesiol Scand* 30:386, 1986.

Davidson CJ, Fishman RF, Bonow RO: Cardiac catheterization. In Braunwald E, editor: *Heart disease—a textbook of cardiovascular medicine,* ed 5, Philadelphia, 1997, W.B. Saunders.

Davis RF, Sakuma G: Comparison of semi-continuous thermodilution to intermittent bolus thermodilution cardiac output determinations, *Anesthesiology* 77:A477, 1992.

Dorman BH et al: Use of a combined right ventricular ejection fraction–oximetry catheter system for coronary bypass surgery, *Crit Care Med* 20:1650, 1992.

Eidelman LA, Pizov R, Sprung CL: Pulmonary artery catheterization—at the crossroads? *Crit Care Med* 22:543, 1994.

Eisenkraft JB, Eger EI: Nitrous oxide anesthesia may double the balloon gas volume of Swan-Ganz catheters, *Mt Sinai J Med* 49:430, 1982.

Ermakov S, Hoyt JW: Pulmonary artery catheterization. In *Critical care clinics, procedures in the ICU,* Philadelphia, 1992, W.B. Saunders.

Ewer MS, Ali MK, Gibbs HR: Nodus migrans: the case of the migrating knot, *Am J Crit Care* 1:108, 1992.

Fletcher EC: Pulmonary artery rupture during introduction of the Swan-Ganz catheter: mechanism and prevention of injury, *J Crit Care* 3:116, 1988.

Friesinger GC, Williams SV: Clinical competence in hemodynamic monitoring. A statement for physicians from the ACP/ACC/AHA Task Force on Clinical Privileges in Cardiology, *J Am Coll Cardiol* 15:1460, 1990.

Ganz P, Swan HJC, Ganz W: Balloon-tipped flow-directed catheters. In Grossman W, Baim D, editors: *Cardiac catheterization, angiography and intervention,* ed 4, Philadelphia, 1991, Lea & Febiger.

Gilbert HC et al: Evaluation of continuous cardiac output in patients undergoing coronary artery bypass surgery, *Anesthesiology* 77:A472, 1992.

Gore JM et al: Superior vena cava syndrome, *Arch Intern Med* 144:506, 1984.

Gore JM et al: A community-wide assessment of the use of pulmonary artery catheters in patients with acute myocardial infarction, *Chest* 92:721, 1987.

Iberti TJ et al: A multicenter study of physicians' knowledge of the pulmonary artery catheter, *JAMA* 264:2928, 1990.

Keusch DJ et al: The patient's position influences the incidence of dysarrhythmias during pulmonary artery catheterization, *Anesthesiology* 70:582, 1989.

Kirton OC et al: Flow-directed, pulmonary artery catheter–induced pseudoaneurysm: urgent diagnosis and endovascular obliteration, *Crit Care Med* 20:1178, 1992.

Lake CL: Monitoring ventricular function. In Lake C, editor: *Clinical monitoring for anesthesia and critical care,* ed 2, Philadelphia, 1994, W.B. Saunders.

Lichtenthal PR et al: A safety comparison between a new continuous cardiac output (CCO) monitoring system and a standard pulmonary artery catheter in sheep, *Anesthesiology* 77:A473, 1992.

Marshall WK, Bedford RF: Use of a pulmonary artery catheter for detection and treatment of venous air embolism: a prospective study in man, *Anesthesia* 52:131, 1980.

Masson RG, Ruggieri J: Pulmonary microvascular cytology, a new diagnostic application of the pulmonary artery catheter, *Chest* 88:908, 1985.

Mimoz O, Rauss A, Rekik N, et al: Pulmonary artery catheterization in critically ill patients: a prospective analysis of outcome changes associated with catheter-prompted changes in therapy, *Crit Care Med* 22:573, 1994.

Moore FA et al: Alternatives to Swan-Ganz cardiac output monitoring, *Surg Clin North Am* 71:699, 1991.

Moorthy SS et al: Cerebral air embolism during removal of a pulmonary artery catheter, *Crit Care Med* 19:981, 1991.

Morris AH: Hemodynamic guidelines, *Crit Care Med* 22:1096, 1994.

Morris D, Mulvihill D, Lew WYW: Risk of developing complete heart block during bedside pulmonary artery catheterization in patients with left bundle-branch block, *Arch Intern Med* 147:2005, 1987.

Mullerworth MH, Angelopoulos P, Couyand MA, et al: Recognition and management of catheter-induced pulmonary artery rupture, *Ann Thorac Surg* 66:1242, 1998.

Naylor CD, Sibbald WJ, Sprung CL, et al: Pulmonary artery catheterization. Can there be an integrated strategy for guideline development and research promotion? *JAMA* 269:2407, 1993.

Nolan TE et al: Invasive hemodynamic monitoring in obstetrics, *Chest* 101:1429, 1992.

O'Toole JD et al: Pulmonary-valve injury and insufficiency during pulmonary-artery catheterization, *N Engl J Med* 301:1167, 1979.

Paul M, Heard S, Varon J: Interpretation of the pulmonary artery occlusion pressure: physicians' knowledge versus the experts' knowledge, *Crit Care Med* 26:1761, 1998.

Paulson DM et al: Pulmonary hemorrhage associated with balloon flotation catheters, *J Thorac Cardiovasc Surg* 80:453, 1980.

Perreas KG, Kumar S, Khan A: A knot in the heart—surgical removal of a pulmonary artery catheter entangled in the tricuspid valve chordae, *Eur J Cardiothorac Surg* 15:112, 1999.

Poses RM, Chaput de Saintonge M et al: An international comparison of physicians' judgements of outcome rates of cardiac procedures and attitudes toward risk, uncertainty, justifiability and regret, *Med Decis Making* 18:131, 1998.

Puri VK, Carlson RW, Bander JJ, et al: Complications of vascular catheterization in the critically ill, *Crit Care Med* 8:495, 1980.

Putterman C: The Swan-Ganz catheter: a decade of hemodynamic monitoring, *J Crit Care* 4:127, 1989.

Randolph AG, Cook DJ, Gonzales CA, et al: Benefit of heparin in central venous and pulmonary artery catheters: a meta-analysis of randomized controlled trials, Chest 113:165, 1998.

Ray CE, Kaufman JA, Geller SC, et al: Embolization of pulmonary catheter–induced pulmonary artery pseudoaneurysms, *Chest* 110:1370, 1996.

Robin ED: The cult of the Swan-Ganz catheter, *Ann Intern Med* 103:445, 1985.

Robin ED: Death by pulmonary artery flow-directed catheter, *Chest* 92:727, 1987.

Rowley KM: Right-sided infective endocarditis as a consequence of flow-directed pulmonary-artery catheterization, *N Engl J Med* 311:1152, 1984.

Schmitt EA, Brantigan CO: Common artifacts of pulmonary artery and pulmonary artery wedge pressure: recognition and interpretation, *J Clin Monit* 2:44, 1986.

Schwartz AJ et al: Carotid artery puncture with internal jugular cannulation, *Anesthesiology* 51:S160, 1971.

Schwender KJ: Venous and pulmonary pressures. In Lake C, editor: *Clinical monitoring for anesthesia and critical care,* ed 2, Philadelphia, 1994, W.B. Saunders.

Shoemaker WC et al: The efficacy of central venous and pulmonary artery catheters and therapy based upon them in reducing mortality and morbidity, *Arch Surg* 125:1332, 1990.

Shoemaker WC, Appel PL, Kram HB: Hemodynamic and oxygen transport responses in nonsurvivors of high-risk surgery, *Crit Care Med* 21:977, 1994.

Sise MJ, Hollingsworth P, Brimm JE, et al: Complications of the flow-directed pulmonary artery catheter: a prospective analysis in 219 patients, *Crit Care Med* 9:315, 1981.

Smart FW: Complications of flow-directed balloon-tipped catheters, *Chest* 97:227, 1990.

Sprung CL: *The pulmonary artery catheter: methodology and clinical application,* Closter, NJ, 1993, Critical Care Research Association.

Stancofski ED, Sardi A, Conaway GL: Successful outcome in Swan-Ganz catheter induced rupture of pulmonary artery, *Am Surg* 64:1062, 1998.

Swan HJC, Ganz W: Complications with flow-directed balloon-tipped catheters, *Ann Intern Med* 91:494, 1979.

Swan HJC, Ganz W: The Swan-Ganz catheter: past and present. In Blitt CD, editor: *Monitoring in anesthesia and critical care medicine,* New York, 1985, Churchill Livingstone.

Swan HJC, Ganz W, Forrester J, et al: Catheterization of the heart in man with use of a flow-directed balloon-tipped catheter, *N Engl J Med* 283:447, 1970.

Swan HJC, Prediman KS: The rationale for bedside hemodynamic monitoring, *J Crit Illness* 24, 1986.

Swan-Ganz monitoring systems, Santa Ana, Calif, American Edwards Laboratories.

Tremblay N et al: Successful non-surgical extraction of a knotted pulmonary artery catheter trapped in the right ventricle, *Can J Anaesth* 37:388, 1990.

Tuman KJ, Ivankovich AD: High-cost, high-tech medicine: are we getting our money's worth? *J Clin Anesth* 5:168, 1993.

Understanding hemodynamic measurements made with the Swan-Ganz catheter, Santa Ana, Calif, American Edwards Laboratories.

Urbach DR, Rippe JM: Pulmonary artery catheter placement and care. In Rippe JM, Irwin RS, Alpert JS, et al, editors: *Intensive care medicine,* Boston, 1985, Little, Brown.

Varon AJ: Hemodynamic monitoring: arterial and pulmonary artery catheters. In Civetta JM, Taylor RW, Kirby RR, editors: *Critical care,* ed 2, Philadelphia, 1992, JB Lippincott.

Voyce SJ, Urbach D, Rippe JM: Pulmonary artery catheters. In Rippe JM et al, editors: *Intensive care medicine,* ed 2, Boston, 1991, Little, Brown.

Wadas TM: Pulmonary artery catheter removal, *Crit Care Nurse* 14(3):63, 1994.

Weed HG: Pulmonary "critical" wedge pressure not the pressure in the pulmonary capillaries, *Chest* 100:1138, 1991.

Wilson RF et al: Pulmonary artery diastolic and wedge pressure relationships in critically ill and injured patients, *Arch Surg* 123:933, 1988.

Yelderman ML et al: Continuous thermodilution cardiac output measurement in intensive care unit patients, *J Cardiothorac Vasc Anesth* 6:270, 1992.

11

GLORIA OBLOUK DAROVIC, PATRICIA G. GRAHAM, and MARY ANN F. PRANULIS

Monitoring Cardiac Output

The provision and transport of oxygenated blood to the body and removal of cellular waste is a complex process that involves the integrated actions of the pulmonary and cardiovascular systems. The cardiovascular system fulfills the role as pump and transporter of vital cellular substrates and metabolic waste. *Cardiac output* is the quantity of blood delivered to the systemic circulation. This measured value is represented in both volume and time, resulting in a measurement of liters per minute (L/min). The normal resting range of cardiac output for a range of average adults is 4 to 8 L/min.

Cardiac output is an important measurement in the overall assessment of cardiovascular function. It is essential to the calculation of stroke volume, blood oxygen transport, and intrapulmonary shunt, as well as pulmonary and systemic vascular resistance. Various measurement techniques are available, but all require precision and expertise on the part of the clinician. *The cardiac output measurement procedure should be adequately covered in orientation to critical care practice both in theory and clinical procedure by qualified instructors and experienced personnel.*

The physiologic variables that determine cardiac output, as well as the principles, techniques, and drawbacks that are specific to currently available methods of measuring cardiac output, are discussed in this chapter.

FACTORS AFFECTING CARDIAC OUTPUT

Cardiac output is a product of stroke volume times heart rate. Stroke volume is the amount of blood ejected by the heart with each contraction; the normal range is 60 to 130 ml. The major factors affecting stroke volume include preload, afterload, and contractility. (See Chapter 4, Figure 4-19; Chapter 10; and Chapter 21.)

Variables that affect the cardiac output range for any person, at any point in time, include metabolic rate and oxygen demand, gender, body size, age, and posture.

Metabolic Rate and Oxygen Demand

The most potent determinant of cardiac output is the body's metabolic oxygen demand. As metabolism and oxygen demand increase, cardiac output increases; as oxygen demand decreases, cardiac output decreases. Sepsis, strong emotion, major trauma or surgery, and exercise increase metabolism and therefore cardiac output. Critically ill and injured patients generally require a cardiac index that is approximately 50% greater than normal because of the increased metabolic needs imposed by their underlying conditions (e.g., systemic inflammatory response syndrome [SIRS], sepsis, multisystem organ dysfunction). Body temperature also directly affects metabolism and cardiac output, increasing with fever and decreasing with hypothermia.

Gender

Females tend to have a smaller skeletal muscle mass and more body fat than males. Adipose tissue is far less metabolically active and vascular than skeletal muscle. Consequently, the cardiac output of a female is approximately 10% less than that of a male of equivalent body mass.

Body Size

The larger the person's body size, the greater the cardiac output required to perfuse the tissue mass. For example, the resting cardiac output required for a 250 lb person (approximately 10 L/min) is considerably greater than that required for a 100 lb person (approximately 4.5 L/min). Consequently, the "range" of required cardiac outputs for adults may differ considerably owing to the tremendous range of body sizes. The values of 4 to 8 L/min are those required for a scatter of average adults.

Cardiac Index

Cardiac index adjusts the cardiac output to the individual person's body size by representing blood flow relative to a square meter of body surface area; the normal adult range is 2.5 to 4.2 L/min/m². Cardiac index is calculated by dividing the cardiac output by the person's body surface area because metabolic rate (the predominant determinant of cardiac output) is thought to correlate with body surface area. Body surface area is not measured directly but is calculated from a nomogram, such as the *Dubois Body Surface Chart,* which uses the person's height and weight as factors in the calculation (Figure 11-1). Most free-standing cardiac output computers and computers built into bedside monitoring consoles automatically calculate cardiac index, along with other indexed measurements, such as stroke volume index with each averaged cardiac output measurement after the patient's body weight and height are entered into the console database.

The cardiac index has gained favor over the cardiac output as an assessment parameter because it adjusts cardiac output to a defined measurement of body tissue (square meter of body surface area). This eliminates the effects of differences in body size. Cardiac index, however, does have pitfalls because the relationship of metabolism to body surface area differs among people according to personal build. Obese persons have less metabolically active tissue for their body surface area than a heavily muscled person of the same body height and weight. The type of tissue mass cannot be factored into the cardiac index calculation. The presence or absence of specific diseases, such as hyperthyroidism or hypothyroidism, also profoundly affects metabolism, independent of body surface area. A patient's weight (and therefore calculated body surface area) may change dramatically on a daily basis owing to third-space fluid shifting or diuresis. Edema does not strongly affect metabolism, nor does pooled fluid, such as ascites, but these factors do affect body surface area. Therefore, in these cases, cardiac index should be based on the patient's estimated or known normal or usual weight.

Age

Cardiac index is highest in childhood and progressively diminishes with age. For example, the cardiac index of a neonate is triple that of an adult; an 8-year-old may have a cardiac index of 4.5 L/min/m², whereas a cardiac index of 2.8 L/min/m² is common in healthy persons over 70 years of age.

Posture

A cardiac output measured from a supine position decreases by approximately 20% when the person stands up. Consequently, measured cardiac outputs may vary in patients purely because of postural changes (supine versus high Fowler's position), and obtained measurements must be evaluated in light of these changes.

EFFECT OF ANATOMIC SHUNTING AND REGURGITANT FLOW ON CARDIAC OUTPUT MEASUREMENTS

In the absence of underlying pathology such as anatomic intracardiac shunts, the output for both ventricles and pulmonary and systemic blood flow is the same. If the output of either ventricle increases or decreases for any reason, the output for the other ventricle quickly adjusts its output to match the change, and a new dynamic equilibrium is established. Therefore measurements of blood flow sampled from any portion of the cardiovascular system are representative of blood flow throughout the system.

Anatomic Intracardiac Shunts

Patients with anatomic intracardiac shunts have differences in the volumes of pulmonary and systemic blood flow. Oxygen saturation in the cardiac chambers, pulmonary circulation, and arterial circulation are also variably abnormal. In patients with *left-to-right anatomic shunts,* such as atrial or ventricular septal defects, there is systolic flow overload of the right ventricle. Pulmonary blood flow is greater than systemic blood flow, and mixing of oxygenated and deoxygenated blood in the right heart occurs. As a consequence, the oxygen saturation of blood samples obtained from the right heart or pulmonary artery is greater than that expected for mixed venous blood. *Right-to-left anatomic shunts,* such as in tetralogy of Fallot, are associated with pulmonary blood flow that may be less than that of systemic blood flow. Subnormal arterial oxygen saturation, due to the mixing of venous and arterial blood in the left heart, is clinically evidenced by central cyanosis.

All invasive methods of measuring cardiac output sample flow through the pulmonary circulation, and interpretations are based on the assumption that pulmonary and

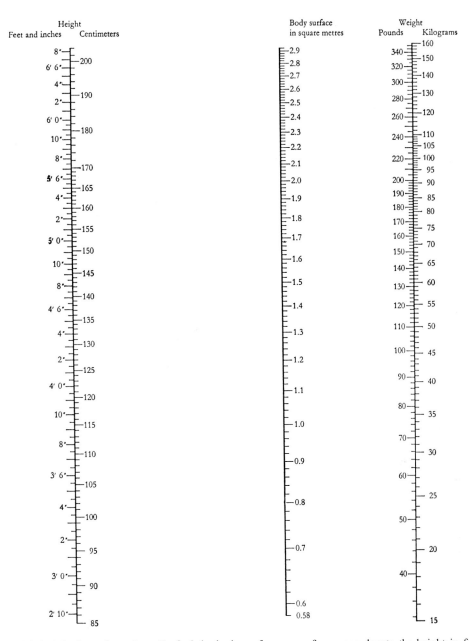

FIGURE 11-1 A body surface chart. To find the body surface area of a person, locate the height in feet and inches or centimeters on scale 1 and the weight in pounds or kilograms on scale 3, and place a ruler between these two points. The ruler intersects on scale 2 at the person's body surface area. (From Meschan I, Ott DJ: *Introduction to diagnostic imaging,* Philadelphia, 1984, W.B. Saunders.)

systemic blood flow are equal. The presence of intracardiac shunts renders all methods of cardiac output measurement invalid because pulmonary and systemic blood flow are unpredictably unequal. Another important consideration is that intact intracardiac chambers are necessary for the test indicator substance (dye, cold injectate) to be adequately mixed within the right ventricle in order to obtain an unspoiled pulmonary arterial blood sample (mixed venous blood) containing all of the indicator solution.

Regurgitant Heart Lesions

Cardiac output measurements may not be representative of flow throughout the cardiovascular system in patients with regurgitant valve lesions. If regurgitant flow goes unmeasured; the greater the volume of regurgitant flow, the greater the ventricular output that goes unmeasured and the less blood that goes into the receiving circulation. Tricuspid and pulmonic regurgitation is associated with such significant recirculation of blood in the right heart chambers (which may vary beat by beat) that measurements made by the dye-dilution and thermodilution methods are completely invalid. In patients with severe mitral regurgitation, the "regurgitant jet" may contaminate blood at the pulmonary artery sampling site and thus render the thermodilution and dye-dilution cardiac output techniques invalid (see Chapter 22).

CLINICAL APPLICATION OF CARDIAC OUTPUT MEASUREMENTS

During the past 20 years, cardiac output measurements have become increasingly used as adjuncts to the management of critically ill patients. Cardiac output is probably the most important hemodynamic measurement to assess the patient's perfusion status because other circulatory measurements may be influenced by other factors or may not be sensitive indicators of hemodynamic deterioration. For example, cardiac output may decrease by one third before there is a significant drop in systolic blood pressure. Because systemic arterial pressure is the product of systemic vascular resistance (SVR) and cardiac output, reflex vasoconstriction may increase SVR and maintain a normal or increased blood pressure despite a decreasing cardiac output. A patient may then "crash" when compensatory vasoconstriction is maximized if cardiac output continues to fall.

Generally, a sudden fall in cardiac index to less than one half normal may be life threatening, and a cardiac index less than 1.0 L/min/m^2 is incompatible with life. However, critically ill or injured patients are commonly hypermetabolic and have supernormal oxygen demands. In hypermetabolic patients, a sudden fall in cardiac index to less than 2.0 to 3.0 L/min/m^2 may be immediately life threatening.

Because isolated pieces of hemodynamic information can be misleading, cardiac output measurements must be considered in relation to other monitoring and assessment data. *The integrated information then helps the clinician to develop and guide a more effective therapeutic program for critically ill or injured patients.*

INVASIVE METHODS OF CALCULATING CARDIAC OUTPUT

Three methods are used to calculate cardiac output: the Fick oxygen consumption method, the indicator-dilution method, and the thermodilution method. All three methods are discussed; major emphasis is given to the thermodilution method because this is the technique used nearly exclusively in clinical practice. Noninvasive measurement of cardiac output using Doppler ultrasonography and thoracic electrical bioimpedance is briefly discussed.

Fick Oxygen Consumption Method

The Fick oxygen consumption method was the first technology available for measuring cardiac output and is sometimes referred to as the "gold standard." This method is based on the principle, described by Adolph Fick in 1870, that the total uptake or release of a substance by an organ is the product of the blood flow through that organ and the arteriovenous difference of that substance.[1]

Principle

The minute volume of blood flow may be calculated if the amount of a tracer substance, such as oxygen, entering or leaving an organ, such as the lungs, and the tracer concentration difference resulting from entry and removal from the organ are known. Applying the Fick principle to measurement of cardiac output, pulmonary blood flow over 1 minute may be determined by measuring the arteriovenous oxygen difference across the lungs and the rate of oxygen uptake by blood from the lungs over 1 minute. In the absence of intracardiac or intrapulmonary shunts, pulmonary blood flow is equal to systemic blood flow. This concept is expressed in the following formula:

$$\text{Cardiac output (L/min)} = \frac{\text{Oxygen consumption (ml/min)}}{\text{Arteriovenous oxygen content difference (ml/dl blood)}}$$

The factors that constitute the Fick formula are explained next.

Oxygen Consumption. The oxygen consumption for a normal, resting adult is approximately 220 to 290 ml/min. Oxygen consumption is calculated by analyzing the oxygen content difference of inspired minus expired air that is collected from the patient over a 3-minute period.

Arteriovenous Oxygen Difference. A quantity of 100 ml of arterial blood contains approximately 19 to 20 ml of oxygen, whereas 100 ml of mixed venous blood contains approximately 15 to 16 ml of oxygen. Therefore, for every 100 ml of blood perfusing the systemic circulation, 4 to 5 ml of oxygen is normally consumed by body tissue. Therefore the normal arteriovenous oxygen difference for every 100 ml of blood is 4 to 5 ml. Applying the Fick principle to the clinical setting, consider a patient with a measured oxygen consumption of 240 ml/min and a measured arteriovenous oxygen difference of 4 ml/dl (4 ml/100 ml of blood):

$$\frac{240 \text{ ml/min}}{19 \text{ ml/dl} - 15 \text{ ml/dl}} = \frac{240 \text{ ml/min}}{4 \text{ ml/dl}} = \text{ or } \frac{6000 \text{ ml/min}}{6 \text{ L/min}}$$

| (arterial oxygen content) | (mixed venous oxygen content) | (arteriovenous oxygen content difference) | (cardiac output) |

Technique

Measurement of cardiac output by the Fick technique requires the simultaneous measurement of oxygen content in arterial and mixed venous blood samples and oxygen uptake by the lungs (measured in terms of oxygen consumption). Each of these measurements must be done precisely while the patient remains in a steady metabolic state. The classic, standard method for determining oxygen consumption requires measurement of the percent of oxygen of the inhaled gas by any oxygen analyzer, as well as oxygen uptake by the lungs as determined by the gaseous mixture the patient exhales. In the past, only a 60 L collection (Douglas) bag was available to analyze the patient's exhaled gases. Currently, direct expired gases and oxygen consumption can be easily measured with a breath-by-breath metabolic monitor (Medgraphics Corp., St. Paul, Minnesota). The patient's oxygen consumption is then displayed on a computer screen.

In many clinical settings, however, the breath-by-breath metabolic rate monitor and the Douglas bag are not available to or easily accessible by bedside clinicians. Therefore many institutions rely on an estimated Fick cardiac output rather than the standard Fick methods described previously. An estimated Fick cardiac output assumes that the average adult patient's resting oxygen consumption is approximately 3.5 ml/kg/min, rather than measuring the patient's actual oxygen consumption.

Although this method does not have as high a degree of reliability as direct measurement of oxygen uptake by the lungs, it does provide useful trending information. It is also more accurate than thermodilution cardiac output measurements in patients with regurgitant tricuspid or pulmonic valves.

A continuous Fick method for determining cardiac output has also been described.[2] In this technique, a gas exchange metabolic monitor (MGM II, Utah Medical, Midvale, Utah) measures inhaled and exhaled gas content and volume and displays the cardiac output every 20 minutes. Pulse oximetry and mixed venous oximetry (using the oximetric pulmonary artery [PA] catheter) numbers are used to determine oxygen content and oxygen extraction

ratio. The correlation with the thermodilution method is 0.86; however, thermodilution outputs are always higher.

A primary advantage of this method over thermodilution is that cardiac output is not viewed alone, but rather with the knowledge of oxygen demand and oxygen extraction ratio. The disadvantage of this method is the expense and time involved. An oximetric PA catheter is considerably more expensive than a standard PA catheter.

Additionally, this method for continuous Fick cardiac output requires the practioner to hand calculate or use a personal computer to calculate the oxygen content and oxygen extraction ratios. This is often too time consuming for the busy critical care practitioner.

Drawbacks

Although the Fick technique is considered the gold standard, a number of potentials for flawed results are inherent in the technical process. These include the following:

1. The patient must maintain a steady hemodynamic and metabolic state during the period of the test, such as unchanging left and right ventricular outputs, oxygen consumption, and arterial and mixed venous oxygen saturations. Shivering, strong emotion, pain, and irregularities in breathing all introduce error into the cardiac output measurement.
2. Incomplete collection and timing of the expired air sample may occur when the Douglas bag method is used.
3. Improper collection of mixed venous and arterial blood samples or errors in the calculation of oxygen consumption and mixed venous and arterial oxygen content can occur.
4. In the presence of intracardiac or intrapulmonary shunts, obtained measurements are invalid.

Other drawbacks are that the Fick method allows only a "one-shot" measurement of cardiac output, is time consuming, requires multiple personnel using meticulous technique, and is cumbersome at the bedside. This technique is occasionally used in cardiac catheterization laboratories and in some intensive care units to measure cardiac output in patients with regurgitant valve lesions such as tricuspid regurgitation secondary to cardiomyopathy. When not performed correctly, this technique carries a greater likelihood of error than the dye or thermodilution techniques. (See Box 11-1 for advantages and disadvantages of the Fick method.)

Overall, the Fick method is most accurate in patients with low cardiac output. Generally, there is an approximately 6% to 10% margin of error in the carefully performed oxygen consumption method.[3,4]

BOX 11-1
Advantages and Disadvantages of Cardiac Output Measurement Systems

Invasive
Fick Oxygen Consumption Method
Advantages
When performed correctly, the most accurate method of measuring cardiac output
Most accurate when cardiac output is low
Disadvantages
Invalid in the presence of intracardiac or intrapulmonary shunts
Patient must be in a steady metabolic state (usually for 3 minutes)
Requires multiple, highly trained personnel to perform (original technique)
Time consuming, requires meticulous technique
Blood withdrawal necessary (original technique)
Risk of infection
Does not provide easily repeatable or continuous cardiac output measurements
Results not readily available for immediate clinical intervention
Least accurate if cardiac output is high
Comments
Usually used in laboratory or research settings

Dye-Dilution Method
Advantages
Most accurate in high-cardiac-output states
Disadvantages
Invalid in patients with intracardiac shunts, valve regurgitation, or shock
Risk of allergic reaction to dye; dye is unstable and must be mixed fresh daily
Requires multiple, trained personnel using meticulous technique
Time consuming
Blood withdrawal necessary
Does not provide easily repeatable or continuous cardiac output measurements
Patient must be in a stable metabolic state for approximately 40 seconds
Least accurate if cardiac output is low
Comments
Currently used only in research settings

Thermodilution Method
Advantages
Blood withdrawal not necessary
Easily and quickly performed and repeated by one trained person or continuous information also available (type of cardiac output computer specific)
Results readily available for immediate clinical intervention

Disadvantages
Not accurate in the presence of tricuspid regurgitation, intracardiac shunts, possibly severe mitral regurgitation
Least accurate if cardiac output is low
Risk of infection
Comments
Most common technique used clinically

Noninvasive
Doppler Ultrasonography
Advantages
Noninvasive, no risk of infection
Potential for use in outpatient setting
Disadvantages
Requires experienced personnel
Time consuming
Difficult to repeat, cannot provide continuous cardiac output monitoring
Not accurate in patients with anemia, tachycardia, subcutaneous emphysema, sternal decisions
Comments
Needs further study and refinement before widespread clinical application

Transthoracic Electrical Bioimpedance—Impedance Cardiography
Advantages
Provides continuous real-time hemodynamic data, as well as thoracic fluid content
Noninvasive—no risk of infection, bleeding, or pneumothorax
Rapid computer processing, analysis, and display of data facilitates immediate assessment of patient responses to treatment
Does not require extensive operator training
Immediately available for hemodynamic profile determination in hospital and outpatient settings
Cost-effective technique
Not affected by mitral or pulmonic regurgitation
Disadvantages
Accuracy affected by high left bundle branch block, left-to-right intracardiac shunts, aortic regurgitation, sepsis
Uncontrolled muscle movement (shivering, seizures) and inability to cooperate produce artifact
Comments
TEB technology is being incorporated into bedside hemodynamic monitoring systems that measure and record other cardiorespiratory parameters. However, further investigation is needed before the full range of clinical application in critical care settings can be achieved.

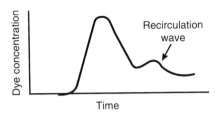

FIGURE 11-2 A normal dye-dilution curve.

Dye-Dilution Method

The difference between the dye-dilution method and the Fick method is that the marker substance is a dye rather than oxygen. This technique is usually restricted to research laboratories.

Principle

A bolus of a marker substance, in this case nontoxic dye, is injected into the right side of the circulation (usually the pulmonary artery). At the same time, a continuous dye/blood sample is withdrawn from a systemic artery at a constant rate. The concentration of sampled dye in the arterial blood is plotted against time by a computer and produces a curve that displays cardiac output.

Technique

A known amount of indocyanine green dye, usually 1 ml, is injected into the pulmonary artery and flows into the left side of the heart where it thoroughly mixes with blood. The injection must be followed by an immediate flush of intravenous solution to ensure that the total amount of indicator dye has been delivered. Failure to do so may allow dye to remain in the injection line or stopcock ports and produce inaccurate measurements. Further downstream, the blood/dye solution is sampled from a systemic artery (brachial, radial, or femoral) at a constant rate via a mechanical device called a *densitometer*. The densitometer measures the concentration of the dye in the blood over time and records a curve on paper until recirculation has occurred (Figure 11-2). Cardiac output equals the amount of indicator injected divided by the area under the dye/concentration time curve.

Drawbacks

Precision of technique and preparation of dye are essential to obtaining accurate cardiac output measurements. Because of all the possible sources of error and clinical disadvantages, this procedure is impractical for bedside practice. Drawbacks and sources of error include the following:

1. The need for the patient to be in a steady hemodynamic/metabolic state for approximately 40 seconds may not be fulfilled.

2. Indocyanine dye is unstable with time and is photosensitive. Dye must be made daily and protected from light until injected.
3. Imprecise measurement or administration of dye is possible.
4. Imprecise rate of arterial sample withdrawal, due to air bubbles entering the system through loose tubing connections, may occur.
5. Invalid in patients with intracardiac shunts because an intact chamber (left ventricle) is necessary for the blood and all of the indicator dye sample to mix before the arterial sample is obtained.
6. Invalid in patients with severe valve regurgitation or shock because the first-pass curve is so prolonged that recirculation begins before the downstroke of the cardiac output curve is fully inscribed. This makes accurate calculation of cardiac output impossible.
7. The dye-dilution technique is cumbersome, requires extreme precision using several highly trained persons, and provides a one-shot estimate of cardiac output. Clearly, this technique is impractical for bedside, serial measurements of cardiac output. See Box 11-1 for advantages and disadvantages of the dye-dilution method.

In contrast to the Fick method, the dye-dilution method is least accurate in a low-cardiac-output state. The dye-dilution method has an error rate of 5% to 10% when performed correctly.[3]

Thermodilution Method

The thermodilution method is currently the most widely used technique to calculate cardiac output. It was first described by Fegler[5] in 1954 but did not gain widespread acceptance until the development, by Ganz and colleagues,[6] of the thermodilution pulmonary artery catheter. In this method of cardiac output measurement, the "indicator" is a cold solution and the "concentration" of indicator is the temperature of the injectate. A cardiac output computer, attached by a cable to the thermistor port of a pulmonary artery catheter, provides a thermal cardiac output curve and an immediate digital readout of cardiac output.

Principle

The principle behind the thermodilution method is similar to the indicator-dilution principle. A specific quantity of known indicator solution, in this case a solution with a temperature less than that of blood, is injected into the proximal injectate port of the thermodilution pulmonary artery catheter (Figure 11-3). The cold injectate solution is introduced rapidly and smoothly as a bolus into the right atrial chamber *(a)*. The thermal bolus passes into the right ventricle *(b)* and is then ejected into the pulmonary artery.

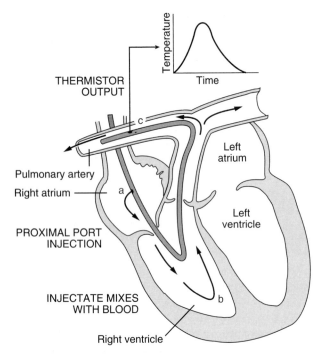

FIGURE 11-3 Schematic illustration of the thermodilution method using the pulmonary artery catheter. The cold injectate is introduced into the right atrium *(a)*, mixes completely with blood within the right ventricular chamber *(b)*, and the cooled blood flows into the pulmonary arterial circulation and past the thermistor bead near the tip of the pulmonary artery catheter *(c)*. (Adapted from Marino PL: Thermodilution cardiac output. In *The ICU book,* Philadelphia, 1991, Lea & Febiger.)

The patient's baseline blood temperature is established and recorded by the cardiac output computer before the injection. During the test, the temperature of the mixed blood (a combination of the cold indicator solution and blood) is recorded farther downstream in the pulmonary artery by a thermistor bead located near the tip of the pulmonary artery catheter *(c)*.

The cardiac output is plotted as the difference in blood temperatures on a time/temperature curve. Time is plotted on the horizontal axis and blood temperature differential on the vertical axis. A normal cardiac output curve is smooth, with a rapid rise to a peak and a slow return to baseline. The top or peak of the curve represents the lowest temperature or greatest temperature differential between the baseline blood temperature and the injectate/blood mixture as it is sensed by the thermistor bead near the tip of the catheter. The curve then drops back to baseline as the cold indicator solution washes out of the pulmonary artery and the temperature of the blood in the pulmonary artery returns to normal. Overall, the thermal curve has a lower peak and a longer tail than the dye-dilution curve.

The volume of cardiac output is inversely proportional to the area observed under the curve. A high cardiac output characteristically has a small area under the curve. The rapid rise of the curve is due to the rapid appearance of the cold indicator, and the small area under the curve is produced by rapid blood flow through the central circulation (Figure 11-4, *A*). In patients with a low cardiac output (Figure 11-4, *B*), the upstroke of the curve may be slurred,

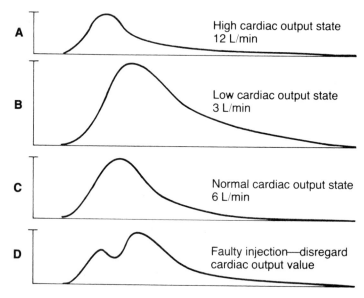

FIGURE 11-4 Variations in cardiac output thermodilution curves. (Copyright Hewlett-Packard Company. Reproduced with permission.)

and the area under the curve is large because wash-out of the cold indicator is prolonged.

The cardiac output curve should be inspected for deviations from the expected normal shape; the computed/calculated readout should never be accepted without question. Faulty technique may cause an artifactual curve variation (Figure 11-4, *D*) in which the peak may be notched or the upstroke may not be well defined and is slow. When this occurs, the measurement results should be discarded and the cardiac output measurement procedure repeated.

The final cardiac output measurement is digitally displayed on the front panel of the cardiac output computer. Thermodilution cardiac output always should be based on the average of at least three individual measurements that are within 10% of each other.

The thermodilution method is least accurate in patients with low cardiac output and most accurate in patients with high cardiac output. The reproducibility of triple measurements is approximately 5%.[4]

Thermodilution cardiac output can be performed easily at the patient's bedside by one person. When performed by a skilled operator, the technique can be done quickly and with a high degree of reproducibility. The capacity to calculate cardiac output and index and related hemodynamic indices is built into most bedside monitoring systems in current clinical use along with the standard electrocardiogram (ECG), systemic and pulmonary artery pressures, and SpO_2. Data such as patient height and weight must be entered only at the time of systems setup. However, pulmonary artery wedge pressure and arterial blood pressure (if not monitored via an intraarterial line) must be entered into the computer at the time of each cardiac output study. The core temperature, obtained from the thermistor at the tip of the PA catheter, is continuously displayed when the catheter is connected to the monitoring console.

PROCEDURAL REVIEW

Initial Preparation

1. *Meticulously follow specific manufacturer's recommendations and institutional protocols for systems setup and the cardiac output procedures.*
2. *Assemble the necessary equipment* (assuming the prior insertion of a thermodilution PA catheter):
   - A free-standing cardiac output computer or computer housed within the bedside monitoring system
   - A closed injectate system setup (if the iced injectate method will be used, a container with ice/slush solution cooled to 0° to 4° C)
   - A 500 or 1000 ml bag of 5% dextrose in water

   Types of injectate systems. Open and closed injectate systems are available for use with the thermodilution catheter. The open injectate system was the only system available when the thermodilution PA catheter was initially introduced into clinical medicine. However, the closed system is currently preferred for the following reasons: reduced likelihood of systems contamination; considerably less labor intensive, more cost effective; reduced risk of accidental injection of air, and reduced likelihood of accidental disconnection of the syringe. Because the closed system is preferred, the procedural review for only the closed delivery system is described.

   Types and temperature of injectate solution. The preferred injectate solution is 5% dextrose; use of saline can produce a 2% artifactual decrease in cardiac output measurements.[7] However, use of saline is acceptable in patients with contraindications to receiving dextrose-containing solutions or in whom saline infusions are recommended (hyponatremia). All other types of fluids, such as Ringer's lactate, have varying specific heats and densities that affect the accuracy of the cardiac output measurement and should never be used. *There is presently no evidence to justify generalized use of iced rather than room-temperature solutions in adults.* Room-temperature injectate offers the advantages of less expense, ease of preparation, and less chance of accidental spills than iced solutions. However, because the signal-to-noise ratio is two to three times greater with iced rather than room-temperature injectate, its use is indicated in some situations. The signal is the amount and temperature of the injectate, and the noise is the patient's PA blood (core) temperature. The patient's core temperature is obtained via the thermistor bead and continuously displayed on the monitor. It is important to have an adequate gradient (greater than 10° C) between the signal and the noise in order to produce a reliable thermodilution wash-out curve. The temperature of the injectate is typically obtained during injection from an in-line temperature probe incorporated into the closed delivery system. (The location is manufacturer specific). See Figure 11-5.

   Use of iced injectate. Use of iced injectate should be considered only when: large fluctuations in pulmonary artery blood temperature are probable. Instances include patients with large tidal volumes who are mechanically ventilated, as well as patients who have deep spontaneous respirations; patients who cannot lie still for the study; and patients who are shivering or panting. Use of iced injectate may also be considered when the temperature of the room (and therefore the room-temperature injectate) is very warm (burn units) to ensure an adequate difference between the injectate temperature and the patient's temperature; when cardiac outputs are less than 3.6 L/min; when a catheter thrombus or fibrin

Continued

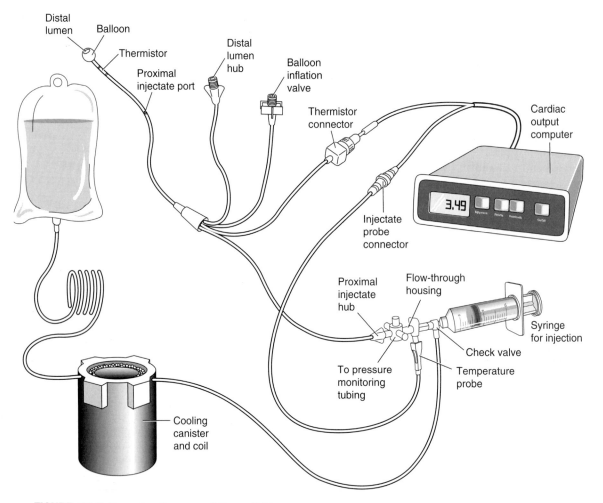

FIGURE 11-5 Example of commercially available closed-iced injectate system. The cooling coil filled with injectate is submerged in an ice-slush. The injectate is withdrawn from the cooling coil through the "check valve" and is injected through the "flow through housing" into the injectate lumen of the thermodilution pulmonary artery catheter. (Modified Co-Set, from Baxter Healthcare Corporation. Edwards Critical Care Division, Santa Ana, CA.)

is thought to be present over the thermistor bead (see the section on drawbacks to the thermodilution technique); or when 5 ml rather than 10 ml of injectate is indicated (patients with fluid restrictions). **Warning!** *To decrease the chance of electrical hazards or equipment damage, do not store iced injectate solution on any instrument.*

3. *Powering the cardiac output computer.* Most cardiac output computers are now incorporated into the bedside monitoring console. Free-standing models, however, must be plugged into an electric outlet and turned on manually. The computer is typically continuously connected to wall current or to battery power for brief periods of time. A line voltage regulator placed on the back of the unit maintains electrical safety when the computer is attached to wall current. Batteries should be left in the recharging mode. Cardiac output computers should be inspected routinely by a biomedical engineering service.

4. *Verify that no vasoactive or inotropic drugs are being infused through the blue cardiac output injection port.* If medications are being infused through the blue port, introduction of the injectate will abruptly push approximately 2 ml of vasoactive medication into the circulation and cause a brief period of hemodynamic instability. If no other lines are available for drug infusion, and titratable drugs are being given via this port, it is imperative that the drug be withdrawn from the line followed by a saline flush before the cardiac output study.

5. *Verify correct position of the PA catheter tip and also verify that the opening of the injectate (RA) port is beyond the end of the introducer to obtain accurate cardiac output measurements and prevent complications.* Types of catheter malpositioning include distal or proximal catheter tip location and location of the proximal (injectate) port within the introducer sheath.

The thermistor bead (near the tip of the PA catheter) must be located in either the left or right main pulmonary artery. Following catheter insertion, catheter tip position is confirmed by chest radiograph. Visibility beyond the left or right mediastinal structures or catheter tip location in the main pulmonary artery or right ventricle requires repositioning by an experienced physician. Thereafter, the routine chest radiographs should be inspected to document continuing acceptable catheter placement (see Chapter 10, Figure 10-17).

Other means of determining that the thermistor is not located too far distally include observing for a clear pulmonary artery waveform and maintaining an appropriate wedging balloon inflation volume of 1.25 to 1.5 ml. Spontaneous distal migration of the catheter tip is suggested by damping of the PA waveform and balloon inflation wedging volumes of less than 1.25 ml. Positioning of the catheter tip within the main pulmonary artery is suggested by the appearance of catheter whip. Right ventricular placement is indicated by the appearance of a right ventricular waveform or development of ventricular ectopic rhythms.

Periodic evaluation of the PA catheter tip position should also be done as an electrical safely measure. Current leakage from the thermistor bead can induce ventricular arrhythmias if the catheter tip lies within the right ventricle. Other reasons for correct catheter tip placement can be found in Chapter 10 in the section on postinsertion protocol for the PA catheter.

A right atrial tracing from the proximal port indicates that the injectate port is properly positioned beyond the end of the introducer sheath. Placement within the introducer sheath is indicated by a damped or flat tracing. Another indication that the injectate port may be within the sheath is the detection of resistance to the fluid bolus during injection. If the injectate port opening lies within the introducer sheath, flow may occur retrogradely or into the sidearm. The loss of the volume of forward injectate flow that results from this type of malpositioning produces errors in cardiac output measurements.

Procedure

1. *Briefly and simply explain the procedure to the patient (if the procedure is to be done for the first time) even if the patient does not seem to be cognitively intact and awake.* Also instruct the patient to lie as still as possible during the procedure. Family members, if present, should be included in the explanation. Each time a full hemodynamic profile is to be done, tell the patient just before beginning.
2. *When possible, place the patient in the standard (supine) position.* When using the thermodilution technique, an elevated backrest position of 20 degrees or less should not differ from supine cardiac output measurements.[8,9] If the patient cannot tolerate lowering of the head of the bed below 30 degrees (orthopnea or increased intracranial pressure), the measured cardiac output will probably be less than that measured from the supine position. The decreased measurement is due to the reduction in cardiac filling as a result of gravity effects. The important clinical point is that *all cardiac output measurement techniques be carried out as consistently as possible.* If the patient's condition requires a position change, a note of this change should be made next to the cardiac output measurement on the chart and should be mentioned when verbally relaying patient information.

3. *If done for the first time, introduce an appropriate computation constant, the patient's height and weight, and any other information specific to manufacturer's recommendations into the computer database.* The computation constant is a number predetermined by the manufacturer to provide accurate results by adjusting for catheter size and injectate volume and temperature. The computation constant varies depending on PA catheter model, the amount of injectate, and the temperature of injectate (iced or room temperature). Computation constants are listed on the PA catheter insert and should be displayed at the bedside for clinical reference. The appropriate computation constant should be reentered whenever the catheter type and size, temperature, or amount of injectate changes. If the incorrect computation constant has been used, the following formula may be used to correct for the inaccurate data entry rather than performing the cardiac output series over again:

$$\text{Incorrect cardiac output} \times \frac{\text{Correct computation constant}}{\text{Incorrect computation constant}}$$
$$= \text{Accurate cardiac output}$$

4. *Select the appropriate volume of injectate for the specific patient. Use of 10 ml of injectate solution is generally recommended for adults.* A recent study, however, concluded that thermodilution cardiac outputs measured with 5 and 10 ml injectates do not differ significantly.[10] This study did, however, identify greater variability of measurement with the 5 ml injectate in patients with low ventricular ejection fractions. Because intensive care unit patients who are candidates for PA catheterization frequently have unstable cardiac function, the use of lower injectate volumes is indicated only in patients with fluid restrictions. In these patients, use of iced injectate is recommended to produce a more powerful thermal signal. Another important point of consideration is that if 3 or 5 ml of injectate is used in adults, relatively small errors in volume of injectate drawn into the syringe (such as 3.4 ml rather than 3 ml) will result in significantly inaccurate cardiac output measurements.

5. *Use the manufacturer's recommendation for injectate port selection.* One type of thermodilution catheter has a proximal injectate port that exits 30 cm from the catheter tip, as well as a proximal infusion lumen that exits 31 cm from the catheter tip. The manufacturer recommends that the proximal (30 cm) injectate lumen be selected for cardiac output measurements. However, if the injectate port becomes occluded, the other proximal port may be used.[11] If there are significant differences between the last measurement obtained with the 30 cm port and the measurement obtained with the 31 cm port and the patient's condition

Continued

appears unchanged, the change in injectate ports must be considered in evaluating the cardiac output measurement.

6. *Note the core temperature recorded from the PA catheter.*

7. *Open the clamp between the bag of injectate solution and syringe.*

8. *Adjust the stopcock for flow between the injectate syringe and solution.*

9. *Press the START button on the cardiac output computer.* Withdraw the exact amount of injectate and open the stopcock for flow between the injectate syringe and PA catheter injection port.

10. *Inspect for air bubbles in the tubing or injectate syringe before injection.* Failure to remove air bubbles before injection could cause pulmonary or systemic air emboli (in patients with right-to-left shunts), as well as interfere with reliable test data. The margin of error increases as the size of the air bubble(s) increases or the injectate volume decreases. Also check for leaks in the cardiac output syringe and stopcocks.

11. *When the computer signals READY, inject the saline within 4 seconds, preferably at end-expiration, holding the syringe by the flange.* Holding the barrel results in injectate warming, if an injectate system does not have an in-line temperature probe that measures injectate temperature as it enters the circulation. In normothermic patients, a 1° C error in iced injectate temperature causes a 2.7% error in measured output (7.7% error with room temperature injectate).[12]

12. *Watch the ECG monitor for the simultaneous appearance of arrhythmias.* Disturbances in cardiac rhythm and sudden, brief changes in heart rate (paroxysmal supraventricular tachycardia, ventricular tachycardia) will produce a wide range of measurements and warrant repeated studies, preferably during periods of regular rhythm (if possible). If the patient has atrial fibrillation, the wide scatter of cardiac output that results is caused by irregular R-R intervals and variable ventricular filling times.

13. *Evaluate the cardiac output curve and note the digitially displayed measurement.* The normal curve should have a smooth baseline, upstroke, and downstroke (see Figure 11-4, *B* and *C*). Assess for abnormal inflections in the contour (faulty injection technique) (see Figure 11-4, *D*); delayed upstroke and low-amplitude peak (slow injectate administration) (Figure 11-4, *A*); irregular curve with oscillating baseline (patient movement, respiratory effects, changes in blood pressure or heart rate, contact of the thermistor with the vessel wall); low-amplitude curve (temperature difference of less than 10° C between injectate and blood); and a broad, low-amplitude curve with increased artifact (recirculation of blood in the right heart such as tricuspid and pulmonic stenosis). If an abnormal-looking curve appears, the measurement should be discarded, possible causes investigated, and the procedure repeated.

14. *Repeat the procedure three times, at least 90 seconds apart, to permit restoration of steady blood temperature.* An average of three injections determines the cardiac output. The readings should fall within a 10% range. If not within this range, technical errors or patient-related problems may have occurred. If there is wide scatter of the results, all three measurements may have to be repeated with careful attention to technique or patient-related issues such as cardiac arrhythmias.

15. *Upon completion of the study, close the clamp leading from the injectate fluid to the syringe hub and open the stopcock to flow between the proximal catheter port and IV fluid.* These steps are easily overlooked and may result in the formation of a thrombus on or within the catheter lumen or inadvertent fluid bolusing.

16. *Enter the patient's currently obtained central circulatory pressures (if not monitored via intraarterial line) into the computer.* The computer will then display and print out the entire hemodynamic profile.

Other Considerations

1. *Periodically replace components of the cardiac output measurement equipment.* The Centers for Disease Control and Prevention (CDC) currently recommends that the PA pressure tubing, flush system, cardiac output tubing, disposable transducer, stopcocks, and cardiac output solution be changed no more frequently than every 72 hours. Because the CDC has no recommendations for the frequency of dressing changes, institutional standards are the clinician's guide for the frequency of change and type of dressings used.

2. *Interpret cardiac output and cardiac index values in context with other hemodynamic measurements, indices of tissue oxygenation, and laboratory and physical assessment findings.* "Normal" cardiac output and cardiac index values may be unacceptably low and should be investigated in patients with sepsis, SIRS, thyroid toxicosis, hyperthermia, or severe anemia. On the other hand, a subnormal cardiac output may be appropriate and acceptable (hypothermia).

Drawbacks to the Thermodilution Technique

The displayed cardiac output measurement is obtained over the several heartbeats it takes the injectate to travel from the right atrium to the pulmonary artery. The displayed measurement is a calculation of what the volume of blood flow would be over a minute if physiologic conditions remained constant. Rapid, phasic physiologic and hemodynamic changes that occur during each isolated cardiac output study result in a wide scatter of thermodilution cardiac output measurements.

Many other possible sources of inconsistency or inaccuracy are possible with the thermodilution technique. Carefully consider that variabilities between cardiac output measurements or values incongruent with the patient's condition may result from patient-related factors or from inconsistencies in the operator's technique. Furthermore, technical factors such as improper constants, inaccurate systems measurement of patient or injectate temperature, or computer or catheter defects also may produce flawed readings. Sources of inaccuracy include the following:

1. *Respiratory variations.* Random measurement of cardiac output with the respiratory cycle may produce variability in results for two reasons. First, pulmonary artery blood temperature decreases during inspiration, particularly during mechanical ventilation, sighing, or labored breathing due to right ventricular cooling by the overlying lung. Second, cardiac output is phasic because venous return and right ventricular output (which is measured with the thermodilution technique) increase during inspiration and decrease during expiration. Study results looking at this issue are variable. Some investigators indicate that respiratory variability in cardiac output measurements is insignificant,[13,14] whereas others indicate that variability can be clinically significant.[15]

   Two solutions to the problem of respiratory-induced variations in cardiac output measurements have been proposed; neither is ideal. The first solution uses a fixed point in the respiratory cycle. End-expiration has been suggested because absence of chest wall movement makes it easy to identify and because of absence of respiratory noise, and it provides a convenient determination for injection time. Some practitioners, however, choose to use peak inspiration as the fixed point. The fixed-point technique may be associated with less variation and more reproducibility. It may, however, be impossible to uniformly time the injection at the same point in the respiratory cycle in a patient with rapid, labored, or irregular breathing.

   In the second solution, average measurements are obtained randomly throughout the respiratory cycle. It has been suggested that a better mean value for cardiac output is achieved by this technique. Regardless of which technique is used, it is important that there be consistency in method between practitioners, whether measurements are obtained at peak inspiration or end-expiration, or average measurements are used.[13] Overall, if there is significant variability in obtained measurements and no other cause can be determined, the possibility of respiratory artifact should be considered when interpreting cardiac output measurements and applying them to diagnosis and management decisions.

2. *Alterations in ventricular performance due to arrhythmias.* The time it takes the cold indicator to arrive at and flow past the thermistor after the bolus injection may vary considerably owing to arrhythmia-induced changes in stroke volume and ejection velocity. In patients with arrhythmias, such as frequent premature beats, atrial fibrillation, or brief runs of tachyarrhythmias or bradyarrhythmias, this problem may be impossible to avoid. Variability in cardiac output due to irregularities in heart rhythm should be considered when diagnostic or therapeutic decisions are being made.

3. *Intracardiac flow abnormalities.* In order to obtain accurate cardiac output measurement and inscribe a normal curve, all of the cold injectate must enter the right ventricle and then pass the thermistor bead located near the catheter tip in the pulmonary artery. When tricuspid regurgitation, pulmonic regurgitation, or intracardiac shunt exists, recirculation and dilution of the cold injectate before the first pass through the pulmonary artery flattens and prolongs the curve. Consequently, cardiac output measurements are completely invalid. In patients with regurgitant valve lesions, use of the Fick method is indicated when available. Inaccurate thermodilution measurements also may be obtained in patients with severe mitral regurgitation due to mixing of pulmonary arterial blood with the regurgitant flow (Figure 11-6).

4. *Low cardiac output.* Loss of cold indicator may occur owing to warming of the indicator/blood mixture by cardiac and vascular walls and surrounding tissue. Investigators in one study found that thermodilution cardiac output overestimated cardiac output consistently in patients with outputs of less than 3.5 L/min, and the margin of error was greatest in patients whose outputs were less than 2.5 L/min.[16]

5. *Injectate factors.* Use of the wrong injectate, wrong temperature, or wrong injectate volume, or prolonged injectate administration, may cause significant error in measured cardiac output (Figure 11-7, *A*).

6. *Thermistor factors.* Three thermistor-related factors may result in significant error in cardiac output measurements: (a) The presence of a thrombus on the catheter delays cooling and rewarming of the thermistor bead with the cold bolus injection. This results in overestimation of the area under the curve and decreased cardiac output measurements proportionate to the size of the thrombus. Likewise, after the thermodilution catheter has been in place for 24 to 48 hours, the deposition of plasma proteins on the thermistor bead may result in a loss

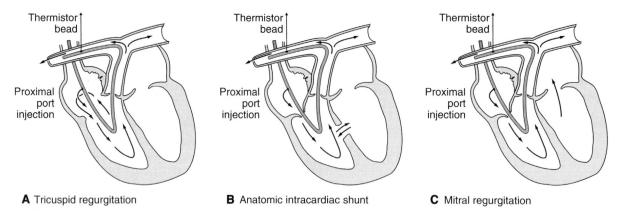

A Tricuspid regurgitation   **B** Anatomic intracardiac shunt   **C** Mitral regurgitation

FIGURE 11-6 The effects of structural cardiac defects on the cold injectate/blood mixture and cardiac output. **A,** Tricuspid regurgitation is associated with significant recirculation of blood and cold injectate in the right side of the heart. This makes accurate thermodilution cardiac output measurement impossible. **B,** Dilution of cold injectate from left-to-right shunts (acute ventricular septal defect) or loss of cold injectate from right-to-left shunts (tetralogy of Fallot) invalidates thermodilution cardiac output results. **C,** Significant systolic regurgitant flow through an incompetent mitral valve may contaminate the injectate/blood mixture at the sampling site in the pulmonary artery. (Adapted from Marino PL: Thermodilution cardiac output. In *The ICU book,* Philadelphia, 1991, Lea & Febiger.)

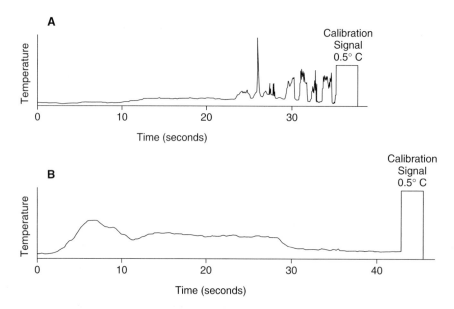

FIGURE 11-7 A, The thermodilution curve is distorted and low, rendering measurements invalid when injectate is administered slowly over 15 seconds. **B,** The pulmonary artery catheter is in the wedge position, placing the thermistor against the vessel wall. The cardiac output curve is irregular and of low amplitude. (From Lake CL: Monitoring of ventricular function. In Lake CL, editor: *Clinical monitoring,* Philadelphia, 1990, W.B. Saunders.)

of sensitivity to temperature change and an underestimation of cardiac output. The reduction in thermistor sensitivity may be minimized by employing iced injectate to maximize the thermal signal. This step, however, does not correct for the thermistor defect, and the possibility of underestimation of true cardiac output should be considered

in hemodynamic evaluation. (b) A defect in the pulmonary artery catheter septum between the proximal and distal lumina artificially decreases cardiac output values. (c) Location of the thermistor in a location other than the center of the right or left main pulmonary artery can occur. Distal migration of the catheter may result in erroneous cardiac output measurements because a smaller, more distal vessel may receive a less than representative sample of cardiac output. A temperature difference also exists between the lateral and central portions of flowing blood; consequently, if the thermistor is in close approximation to the vessel wall, errors in cardiac output values result (Figure 11-7, *B*). As stated earlier, positioning of the injectate port within the introducer rather than the right artery may also produce inaccurate cardiac output measurements.

7. *Rapid intravenous fluid infusions, which act as an additional indicator, during the cardiac output measurement procedure.* The area under the curve becomes broader and cardiac output measurements are artificially decreased. This is particularly likely to occur when pulmonary artery catheters with side-port extensions are placed in the internal jugular or subclavian veins but may also occur with peripherally placed lines. When possible, discontinue IV infusions at least 30 seconds before obtaining measurements or infuse fluids that are warmed to near body temperature. Warmed IV fluids also reduce or eliminate thermal stress to the patient.

8. *The rewarming phase following cardiopulmonary bypass.* As the patient vasodilates with warming, cooled peripheral blood returns to the central circulation. Consequently, blood returning to the heart may have differing temperatures, which cause rapid variations in pulmonary arterial blood and baseline drift. The overall effect is decreased cardiac output values. (See Box 11-1 for advantages and disadvantages of the thermodilution technique.)

Other Thermodilution Pulmonary Artery Catheters

Three new thermodilution pulmonary artery catheters have been introduced within the past two decades: a right ventricular ejection fraction catheter, a PA catheter that allows continuous thermodilution cardiac output measurements, and a PA catheter that continuously displays cardiac output, right ventricular end-diastolic volume, ejection fraction, stroke volume, and Svo_2 (see also Chapter 10).

7.5-French Right Ventricular Thermodilution Ejection Fraction Catheter

A rapid-response thermistor pulmonary artery catheter has been introduced from which cardiac output; right ventricular ejection fraction; and right atrial, right ventricular, pulmonary artery, and pulmonary artery wedge pressures may be obtained. Right ventricular end-systolic and end-diastolic volumes, as well as vascular resistances, also may be calculated. The catheter's rapid response thermistor permits measurement of beat-by-beat variations in pulmonary artery temperature following introduction of the cold injectate just proximal to the tricuspid valve. Arrhythmias, such as atrial fibrillations, pose a potential limitation owing to the extreme variability in diastolic filling time. However, because right ventricular ejection fraction is calculated every four to five beats, an "averaged" ejection fraction may be obtained. In patients with tricuspid regurgitation, an inaccurate right ventricular ejection fraction will be measured because the technique measures only forward flow. However, placement of the thermistor in the right atrium allows calculation of the regurgitant fraction.

8-French Filamented Pulmonary Artery Catheter for Continuous Cardiac Output Measurement

This pulmonary artery catheter provides continuous thermodilution cardiac output measurements that are calculated and displayed by its companion cardiac output computer. Every 30 seconds, the displayed cardiac output is updated and reflects the average pulmonary blood flow of the previous 3 to 6 minutes. Its graphic display illustrates cardiac output trends over time.

CCOmbo V Pulmonary Artery Catheter

The newest addition to the family of PA catheters, the CCOmbo V Pulmonary Artery Catheter (Edwards Lifesciences LLC, Irvine, California) continuously displays all of the parameters available with the right ventricular thermodilution ejection fraction catheter and the continuous cardiac output catheters, as well as displays right ventricular end-diastolic volume, stroke volume, and Svo_2. Also available are calculation and cross-calculation of hemodynamic and oxygenation parameters.

NONINVASIVE MEANS OF CALCULATING CARDIAC OUTPUT

Doppler Ultrasonography

Doppler velocimetry in combination with ultrasonic echocardiographic imaging may indirectly assess cardiac output. This technology measures stroke volume using the Doppler principle to assess blood flow velocity and echo imaging to assess aortic diameter. The results are then used to compute cardiac output.

A transducer projects an ultrasonic wave that is then reflected off moving red blood cells in the aorta. The wave is transmitted back to the transducer where an alteration in wave frequency can be sensed. Aortic diameter is accurately assessed as the ultrasonic waves are reflected off intrathoracic structures. Drawbacks render this technology impractical for clinical, bedside use. A single measurement is time consuming, taking 30 to 45 minutes. Serial trending therefore is impossible, and the effects of acute interventions, such as drug therapy, cannot be rapidly evaluated. This technology necessitates bulky equipment, and the study must be performed by an experienced operator.

Patient-related factors that interfere with accuracy of values, and therefore preclude the use of Doppler ultrasonography in the critical care setting, include anemia, tachycardia, thick chest walls, large sternal incisions, and tracheostomy or subcutaneous emphysema. The procedure is also rather cumbersome. As further refinements in this technique are developed, this technology may be more widely applied to bedside patient care.

Thoracic Electrical Bioimpedance and Impedance Cardiography

Thoracic electrical bioimpedance (TEB) is a noninvasive technology that uses computer algorithms to measure pulsatile changes (impedance) in the electrical conductivity

of the thorax. These pulsatile changes are then computer analyzed to determine stroke volume, cardiac output, indices of myocardial contractility, and afterload. The application of TEB technology for measuring cardiac hemodynamic function is termed *impedance cardiography.*

Principle

The amount of electrical energy that can flow through any substance relates to the size (in length and circumference) and the inherent conductivity of that substance. Certain substances are good conductors of electrical energy, whereas other substances impede (resist) the flow of energy. For example, air and bone are poor conductors (high impedance), whereas fluid (blood in the heart and great vessels of the thorax) is a good conductor (low impedance). To measure the electrical conductivity of an object, and the converse, its impedance, electrical energy of a known, constant voltage is introduced into that object. The amount of voltage is measured at a location (on the object) that is remote from the area where it was introduced. The difference in the amount of voltage between what was introduced and what was measured is an indicator of the impedance to the flow of energy through that object. If the object is the thorax, changes in impedance over time can be recorded in

Fiducial points determined from the ECG, dZ$_{CARDIAC}$, and dZ/dt tracings of a 28-year-old healthy female subject (supine position, HR = 61 bpm)

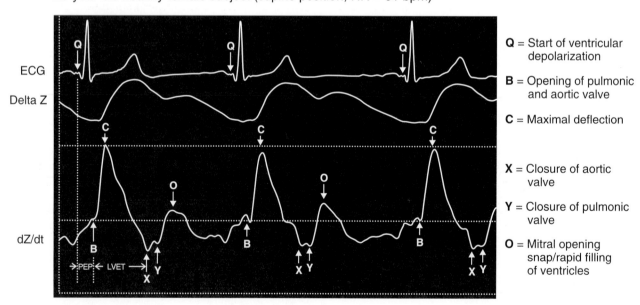

- Pre-ejection period (PEP) is measured from Q to B.
- Left-ventricular ejection time (LVET) is measured from B to X.

FIGURE 11-8 Simultaneous ECG and impedance waveform recordings with event markers. (Reprinted with permission: Cardiodynamics International Corp, San Diego, California).

numeric values and graphed as a waveform similar to an ECG waveform and correlated with the ECG (Figure 11-8).

In order to use this technology to measure the patient's hemodynamic status, baseline thoracic impedance is first established. Baseline impedance provides a measure of thoracic fluid content (the total of the intravascular, insterstitial, and intraalveolar fluids). Then, equations built into the bedside computer (Resaissance Technologies, Inc., Newtown, Pennsylvania; CardioDynamics International Corporation, San Diego, California) are used to calculate various hemodynamic indices from phasic changes in thoracic impedance as they relate to phases in the cardiac cycle. During systole, thoracic blood volume increases while electrical impedance decreases; in diastole, thoracic blood volume decreases while electrical impedance increases. The amount, direction, and timing of the pulsatile changes on the impedance waveform are then measured and computer analyzed to derive values for various cardiac hemodynamic functions.

Technique

Four (paired) specialized, self-adhering sensor-electrode pads (similar to ECG pads) are placed on the patient, one on either side of the base of the patient's neck and one on either side of the lower thorax (Figure 11-9). The sensor-electrode pads are then connected by cable to the computer module at the bedside. An alternating electrical current, which is not harmful and cannot be sensed by the patient, is introduced through the thorax through the voltage-delivering electrode pads and is measured through the corresponding sensor electrode pads. Blood pressure data are entered into the computer database and, along with impedance changes, are computer processed and displayed in graphic and numeric format on the computer screen in real time. The data can be downloaded or printed out for inclusion in the patient's electronic or hard-copy medical record.

Routinely displayed parameters include heart rate, blood pressure, mean arterial pressure, thoracic fluid content, cardiac output and index, acceleration index (how fast the change in ventricular blood volume and flow occurs), velocity index (maximum speed of blood flow), systolic time ratio, systemic vascular resistance and index, and left ventricular work index. The preejection period (ventricular filling time) and left ventricular ejection time are recorded, measured, and used to computer generate other parameters but are not routinely displayed.

Advantages and Disadvantages

The advantages of the system include obtaining continuous real-time hemodynamic data noninvasively (no risk to the patient) in a variety of health care settings, cost-effectiveness, immediately available hemodynamic data (minimal setup and no insertion time), and wide clinical application. For example, surgical patients may be hemodynamically evaluated preoperatively and monitored intraoperatively and postoperatively, including in the home setting after hospital discharge.

Like other techniques for hemodynamic evaluation, impedance cardiography has its limitations. The accuracy of impedance cardiography is variable in patients with sepsis and severe arrhythmias. Increased knowledge about the pathophysiology of these conditions, coupled with continued refinements in the technology, holds promise for overcoming these limitations.[17]

CONCLUSION

There is no "gold standard" method of determining cardiac output. Each cardiac output technique has inherent advantages and disadvantages and merely provides an *estimate* of cardiac output that is subject to margin(s) of error. See Box 11-1 for advantages and disadvantages of all methods of monitoring cardiac output. As in all monitoring techniques, serial trending with careful correlation with the patient's clinical and laboratory profile is essential to forming sound diagnostic and therapeutic judgments.

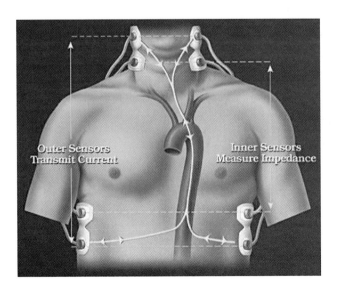

Outer Sensors
Transmit Current

Inner Sensors
Measure Impedance

FIGURE 11-9 A total of four specialized sensor electrode pads are placed. The outer distal portion of the pad contains the voltage-introducing electrodes, and the inner proximal portion of the pad senses the voltage changes. (Reprinted with permission: Cardiodynamics International Corp, San Diego, California).

REFERENCES

1. Fick A: Uber die Messung des Blutquantums in den Herzventrikeln, *Sitz der Physik-Med ges Wurzburg,* 1870.
2. Davies GG, Jebson PJR, Glascow BM, et al: Continuous

Fick cardiac output compared to thermodilution cardiac output, *Crit Care Med* 14:881, 1986.

3. Grossman W, Baim D: Blood flow measurements: the cardiac output. In *Cardiac catheterization and angiography,* ed 4, Philadelphia, 1991, Lea & Febiger.

4. Winniform MD, Lambert CR: Blood flow measurement. In Papine CJ, editor: *Diagnostic and therapeutic cardiac catheterization,* Baltimore, 1989, Williams & Wilkins.

5. Fegler G: Measurement of cardiac output in anesthetized animals by thermo-dilution method, *J Exp Physiol* 39:153, 1954.

6. Ganz W et al: A new technique for measurement of cardiac output by thermodilution in man, *Am J Cardiol* 27:392, 1971.

7. Yang SS, Bentivoglio LG, Maranchao V, et al: *Cardiac catheterization data to hemodynamic parameters,* Philadelphia, 1988, FA Davis.

8. Grose BL et al: Effect of backrest position on cardiac output measured by thermodilution method in acutely ill patients, *Heart Lung* 10:661, 1981.

9. Cline KJ et al: Effect of backrest position on pulmonary artery pressure and cardiac output measurements in critically ill patients, *Focus Crit Care* 18:383, 1991.

10. McCloy K et al: Effects of injectate volume on thermodilution measurements of cardiac output in patients with low ventricular ejection fractions, *Am J Crit Care* 8(2):86, 1999.

11. Medley RS et al: Comparability of the thermodilution cardiac output method: proximal injectate vs proximal infusion lumens, *Heart Lung* 21:12, 1992.

12. Levett JM, Replogle RL: Thermodilution cardiac output: a critical analysis and review of the literature, *J Surg Res* 27:392, 1979.

13. Snyder JV et al: Effects of mechanical ventilation on the measurement of cardiac output by thermodilution, *Crit Care Med* 10:677, 1982.

14. Harris J et al: The effect of the respiratory cycle on the reliability of thermodilution cardiac output measurements, *Heart Lung* 19:306, 1990 (abstract).

15. Stevens JH et al: Thermodilution cardiac output measurement: effects of the respiratory cycle on its reproducibility, *JAMA* 253:2240, 1985.

16. Grondelle AV et al: Thermodilution method overestimates low cardiac output in humans, *Am J Physiol* 245:H960, 1983.

17. DeMaria AN, Raisinghani A: Comparative overview of cardiac output measurement methods: has impedence cardiography come of age? *Congest Heart Failure* 6:7, 2000.

SUGGESTED READING

Banner TE: Invasive cardiac output measurement technology. In Civetta JM, Taylor RW, Kirby RR, editors: *Critical care,* ed 2, Philadelphia, 1992, JB Lippincott.

Bjoraker DG et al: Catheter thrombus artifactually decreases thermodilution cardiac output measurements, *Anesth Analg* 62:1031, 1983.

Boyson PG: Hemodynamic monitoring in the adult respiratory distress syndrome, *Clin Chest Med,* Jan 1982.

Gawlinski A: Cardiac output monitoring. In Chulay M, Gawlinski A, editors: *Hemodynamic monitoring series: protocols for practice,* 1997, AACN Critical Care.

Grossman W: Blood flow measurement: the cardiac output. In Grossman W, Baim DS, editors: *Cardiac catheterization: angiography and intervention,* Philadelphia, 1991, Lea & Febiger.

Hillis LD et al: Comparison of thermodilution and indocyanine green dye in low cardiac output or left-sided regurgitation, *Am J Cardiol* 57:1201, 1986.

Hines R, Griffin M: Pulmonary artery catheterization. In Lake C, Hines RL, Blitt CD, editors: *Clinical monitoring: practical applications for anesthesia and critical care,* Philadelphia, 2001, W.B. Saunders.

Kadota LT: Theory and application of thermodilution cardiac output measurement: a review, *Heart Lung* 14:605, 1985.

Lake C: Monitoring of ventricular function. In Lake C, editor: *Clinical monitoring,* Philadelphia, 1994, W.B. Saunders.

Marino PL: Thermodilution cardiac output. In *The ICU book,* Philadelphia, 1991, Lea & Febiger.

Shoemaker WC et al: Therapy of critically ill postoperative patients based on outcome predictions and prospective clinical trials, *Surg Clin North Am* 65(4):811, 1985.

Stetz CW et al: Reliability of the thermodilution method in the determination of cardiac output in clinical practice, *Am Rev Respir Dis* 126:1001, 1982.

Voyce SJ et al: Pulmonary artery catheters. In *Intensive care medicine,* ed 2, Boston, 1991, Little, Brown.

Wessel HU et al: Limitations of thermal dilution curves for cardiac output determination, *J Appl Physiol* 30:643, 1971.

Wetzel RC et al: Major errors in thermodilution cardiac output measurements during rapid volume infusion, *Anesthesiology* 68:308, 1988.

Wilson RF: Cardiovascular physiology. In *Critical care manual: applied physiology and principles of therapy,* Philadelphia, 1992, FA Davis.

Winniford MD, Lambert CR: Blood flow measurement. In Pepine CJ, editor: *Diagnostic and therapeutic cardiac catheterization,* Baltimore, 1989, Williams & Wilkins.

12

GLORIA OBLOUK DAROVIC

Monitoring Oxygenation

Hypoxia not only stops the machine, it wrecks the machinery.

JOHN SCOTT HALDANE, 1880

The average *resting* 70 kg adult consumes approximately 10^{18} (10 followed by 18 zeros) oxygen molecules per second to maintain oxidative metabolism for the support of life.[1] Far greater amounts of oxygen are needed to maintain the metabolic demands of strenuous activity. An effective system of oxygen delivery and cellular utilization is dependent on the normal and integrated function of the pulmonary and cardiovascular systems, as well as the ability of body cells to take up and consume oxygen in amounts proportionate to increases or decreases in metabolic activity.

Many conditions associated with critical illness or injury compromise cardiopulmonary function and cellular oxygen uptake and utilization, as well as alter systemic or regional tissue oxygen demands. One or a combination of various physiologic imbalances can cause regional or global tissue hypoxia, which is the final common pathway of all causes of death.

In the not so distant past, it was believed that hemodynamic stability and normal arterial blood gas levels indicate normal oxidative metabolism and physiologic integrity. However, conventional intensive care unit (ICU) bedside indices of cardiopulmonary function (blood pressure, respiratory depth and rate, cardiac output, pulmonary artery pressures, and arterial blood gases) are only pieces of the total complex physiologic picture of oxygen delivery and cellular respiration. Taken alone, ICU flow sheet "numbers" do not indicate whether cellular oxygen demand and consumption are systemically or regionally adequate for the continuance of normal cell and organ system function and viability of the patient.

Over the past three decades, various technologies have been developed that allow moment-to-moment bedside display of arterial and mixed venous oxygen saturations. Data derived from these technologies in conjunction with hemodynamic monitoring measurements now enable calculation of oxygen transport (supply) and consumption. This information has provided clinicians with a far more comprehensive means of assessing the balance of tissue oxygen supply and demand, as well as the adequacy of cellular oxygen metabolism. Should a problem in any of these variables develop, early identification, along with aggressive and effective treatment(s), guided by laboratory testing and monitoring data, may prevent hypoxic injury or damage.

This chapter describes physiologic effects of hypoxia, the normal and pathophysiologic variables that affect oxygen transport and metabolism, and the means by which the adequacy or inadequacy of oxidative metabolism can be clinically monitored and assessed. Factors that increase or decrease oxygen consumption of ICU patients will also be identified so that the threat of hypoxic insult can be minimized or prevented by modifying patient care activities to minimize the patient's systemic oxygen demands.

PHYSIOLOGIC EFFECTS OF HYPOXIA

Adequate energy is necessary to maintain normal cell and organ function, as well as support the varied activities of life. The amount of energy produced is determined by the metabolic rate, which, in turn, must be supported by the delivery of adequate amounts of glucose and oxygen to body cells. Depending on the amount of available oxygen, cells may metabolize by the energy-efficient aerobic pathway or the energy-inefficient anaerobic pathway.

Aerobic Metabolism

When cells metabolize in an oxygen-rich environment, the metabolism of glucose produces carbon dioxide (which is ultimately exhaled), water (which is added to the body's water pool), and adequate amounts of the high-energy compound adenosine triphosphate (ATP) (see Figure 16-2).

Anaerobic Metabolism

The term *hypoxia* applies when oxygen becomes unavailable or inadequate to meet tissue demands. Cells are then forced to metabolize anaerobically. The amount of ATP generated is reduced by approximately 97%, and lactic acid (rather than water and carbon dioxide) is released by cells. The energy crisis and accumulation of lactic acid are clinically evident as metabolic acidosis and organ dysfunction or failure.

Tissue hypoxia is an omnipresent threat to ICU patients because of the frequent incidence of severe cardiac, pulmonary, and metabolic problems that singly or in combination upset the balance of oxygen supply and demand, as well as cellular oxygen uptake and utilization.

Some of these conditions are discussed later in this chapter, as well as in the chapters relating to specific conditions such as multiple-system organ dysfunction.

OXYGEN SUPPLY, DEMAND, AND CONSUMPTION BALANCE

See Chapter 2 for further discussion and elaboration of the concepts and calculations of oxygen content, transport, and consumption, as well as the physiologic consequences of hypoxia.

Oxygen Supply

The flow rate of oxygen to tissue is variably termed *oxygen supply, oxygen delivery,* or *transport;* these terms are used in this text interchangeably. Normal or increased oxygen supply demanded by physiologic or emotional stress requires normal heart function, adequate amounts of hemoglobin, adequate arterial oxygen tension (PaO_2), adequate arterial oxygen saturation (SaO_2), and normal autonomic nervous system innervation (appropriately regionally dilating or constricting blood vessels).

Oxygen supply is calculated by taking into account cardiac output and the amount of oxygen in 100 ml of arterial blood (termed *oxygen content*). The oxygen content is calculated using the following formula.

$$Hgb \times SaO_2 \times 1.36 = \text{Oxygen content expressed in vol\%}$$

Normal values are 17 to 20 ml per 100 ml of whole blood (17 vol% to 20 vol%). Of the 17 to 20 ml of oxygen normally contained in arterial blood, 0.3 ml is dissolved in plasma and the remainder (16.7 to 19.7 ml) is bound to hemoglobin.

Oxygen transport is calculated using the following formula:

$$\text{Cardiac index} \times \text{Blood O}_2 \text{ content} \times 10 = \text{O}_2 \text{ transport in ml O}_2/\text{min/m}^2$$

The normal range for resting oxygen transport is 550 to 650 ml per minute per square meter of body surface area (unindexed oxygen transport in the average-sized adult is 900 to 1100 ml/min).

Oxygen transport is an overall assessment of oxygen availability to the entire body but does not ensure adequate regional oxygen supply to specific organ systems such as the gut, kidneys, or skeletal muscle.

Movement of Oxygen from Capillaries to Tissue

When the oxygen dissolved in plasma (PaO_2 equal to 90 to 100 mm Hg) and the oxygen bound to hemoglobin (SaO_2 equal to 97% to 99%) are transported to the capillary level, movement of oxygen to the cells depends first on the diffusion gradient between the capillary PO_2 and intracellular PO_2 (Figure 12-1).

The intracellular PO_2 averages 20 mm Hg. A normal PaO_2 of 100 mm Hg at the arterial end of the capillary bed establishes a diffusion gradient of 80 mm Hg, which drives diffusion of oxygen from the capillaries to the cells. The falling capillary PO_2 then stimulates hemoglobin to begin to desaturate, which facilitates continued movement of oxygen from plasma to cells. When blood reaches the venous end of the systemic capillary, the PvO_2 normally is 40 mm Hg, which stimulates hemoglobin to desaturate to an SvO_2 of approximately 65% to 75%. Generally, this normal

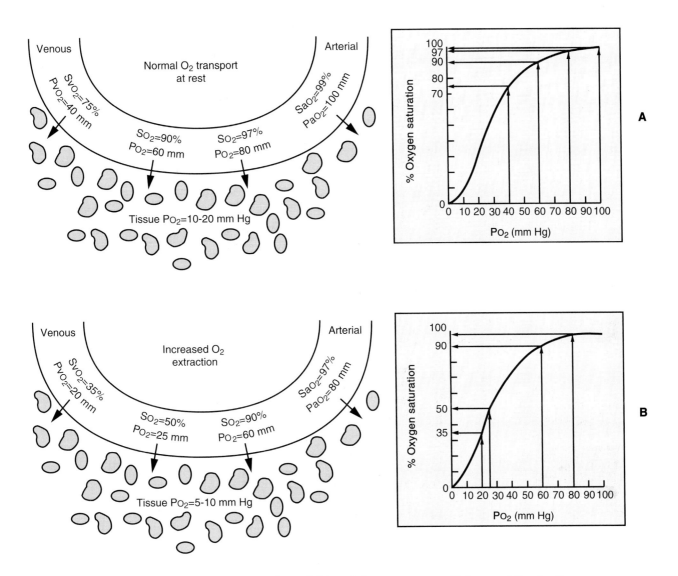

FIGURE 12-1 Oxygen transport to tissue. **A,** Normal O_2 transport at rest. **B,** Increased O_2 extraction.

range is typical of a patient with good balance between oxygen supply and demand. A monitored SvO_2 within the normal range implies that the patient has a normal partial pressure of oxygen in venous blood (40 mm Hg) and therefore has an effective diffusion gradient that supports continued movement of oxygen to cells at the venous end of the systemic capillaries. For example, mixed venous blood PO_2 of 40 mm Hg minus an intracellular PO_2 of 20 mm Hg equals a pressure gradient of 20 mm Hg that continues to drive oxygen from the venous end of systemic capillaries to cells.

If oxygen transport decreases or cellular oxygen demand increases, oxygen diffuses out of the capillaries more rapidly. In such a situation, the falling capillary PO_2 prompts hemoglobin to unload more oxygen, which decreases the SvO_2.

The oxyhemoglobin dissociation curve graphically illustrates what the hemoglobin saturation would be at a particular PO_2 (see Figure 12-1 and Figure 2-18). For example, a PO_2 of 25 mm Hg stimulates hemoglobin desaturation to approximately 50%, and a PO_2 of 20 mm Hg stimulates hemoglobin desaturation to approximately 35%.

A subnormal SvO_2 of 35%, as compared with a subnormal SvO_2 of 50%, not only suggests a much more severe oxygen supply/demand imbalance but also a venous PO_2 that results in a significantly decreased diffusion gradient for the movement of oxygen to body cells at the

TABLE 12-1
Factors That Affect Oxygen Consumption (Vo₂)

Conditions That Increase Vo₂	% Increase
Minor surgery	7
Fever (each 1° C)	10
Bone fracture	10
Agitation	16
Increased work off breathing	40
Severe infection	60
Chest trauma	60
Multiple organ failure	20–80
Shivering	50–100
Burns	100
Sepsis	50–100
Head injury, sedated	89
Head injury, not sedated	138

Medications That Increase Vo₂	% Increase
Norepinephrine (0.10–0.31 μg/kg/min)	10–21
Dopamine (5 μg/kg/min)	6
Dopamine (10 μg/kg/min)	15
Dobutamine	19
Epinephrine (0.10 μg/kg/min)	23–29

Procedures and Activities That Increase Vo₂	% Increase
Dressing change	10
Nursing assessment	12
Electrocardiogram	16
Physical examination	20
Visitors	22
Bath	23
Chest x-ray	25
Endotracheal suctioning	27
Turn	31
Chest physiotherapy	35
Weight on sling scale	36
Getting out of bed	39
Nasal intubation	25–40

Factors That Decrease Vo₂	% Decrease
Hypothermia (each 1° C)	10
Morphine sulfate IV push (0.5 mg/kg)	9–21
Morphine sulfate IV (0.2–0.5 mg/kg/hr)	21
Anesthesia	25
Anesthesia in burn patients	50
Assist/control ventilation	30
Propranolol in head injury	32
Neuromuscular blockade	Abolishes the increase in Vo₂ incurred by shivering

venous end of the systemic capillaries. *When the Pvo_2 is less than 20 mm Hg (oxygen saturation less than 32%), tissue oxygen extraction is no longer effective and anaerobic metabolism occurs followed by lactic acidosis. Patient deterioration and possibly death quickly follow unless appropriate clinical interventions are immediately instituted.*

Oxygen Demand and Consumption

Metabolic rate directly determines oxygen demand, and body tissue normally consumes the amount of oxygen demanded. Metabolic rate, in turn, is determined by neuro-hormonal factors, the presence or absence of disease, medications, and physical and emotional activity (Table 12-1).

The body of a resting, healthy adult of average size demands and consumes approximately 200 to 240 ml of oxygen per minute (115 to 160 ml/min/m² indexed values) to fuel the energy required for basal (normal, resting) metabolism. As metabolic rate and oxygen consumption increase or decrease, cardiac output and the amount of oxygen extracted from capillary blood likewise increase or decrease.

Tissue oxygen consumption cannot be directly measured. It can, however, be calculated taking into account cardiac output, hemoglobin level, and arterial and mixed venous oxygen saturation. The rationale is that if the amount of oxygen delivered to tissues is known, and the amount returning to the heart is known, the amount of oxygen consumed can be estimated. Oxygen consumption is calculated using the following formula:

$$\text{Cardiac index} \times 10 \times \text{Hgb} \times 1.36 \times (\text{Sao}_2 - \text{Svo}_2)$$
$$= \text{O}_2 \text{ consumption in ml O}_2/\text{min/m}^2$$

Mixed Venous Oxygen Content

Mixed venous blood samples are drawn from the proximal port of the pulmonary artery catheter. The oxygen saturation (Svo_2) may also be continuously sampled and displayed with the oximetric pulmonary artery catheter.

Mixed venous oxygen content and saturation are affected by cardiac output, metabolic rate, the environment of red blood cells (as it affects the oxyhemoglobin dissociation curve), and the hemoglobin level. The normal amount of oxygen consumed at rest is only approximately 25% of the amount delivered in arterialized blood. This leaves 75% of the oxygen remaining in the venous blood flowing into the pulmonary artery and is termed the *mixed venous reserve*. This "reserve" may be drawn on to maintain tissue oxygenation if either systemic oxygen demand increases (fever, strenuous exercise, shivering, seizure activity) or arterial oxygen content falls.

A normal balance between resting oxygen supply, demand, and consumption is illustrated in Figure 12-2. It should be noted again that the amount of oxygen delivered

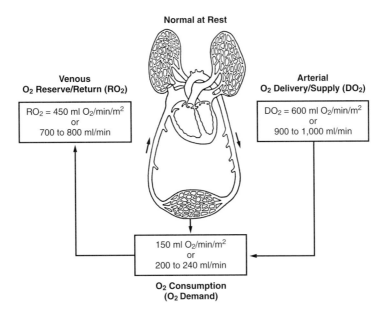

Normal at Rest

Venous
O₂ Reserve/Return (RO₂)

RO₂ = 450 ml O_2/min/m²
or
700 to 800 ml/min

Arterial
O₂ Delivery/Supply (DO₂)

DO₂ = 600 ml O_2/min/m²
or
900 to 1,000 ml/min

150 ml O_2/min/m²
or
200 to 240 ml/min

O₂ Consumption
(O₂ Demand)

FIGURE 12-2 Normal supply/demand balance at rest.

normally is four times the amount of oxygen consumed, and oxygen supply, demand, and consumption balance is therefore 4:1. Because tissues extract only 25% of delivered oxygen, the Svo_2 of 75% reflects the 4:1 balance and oxygen extraction of 25%.

Regional imbalances in oxygen supply and demand are not reflected in the Svo_2, the Sao_2, or any of the calculations used in assessing oxygenation status. This is because different organs consume oxygen at different rates at rest and during activity. Therefore the adequacy of regional oxygenation should be evaluated using physical assessment and laboratory studies specific to particular organ systems.

CONDITIONS THAT MAY COMPROMISE TISSUE OXYGENATION

A decrease in oxygen transport, a decrease in cellular oxygen uptake and utilization, or various metabolic abnormalities or toxicities may threaten tissue hypoxia. The more severe the condition and the more of the following conditions present in a given patient, the greater the threat of global or regional tissue hypoxia. Critically ill or injured patients commonly have several coexisting conditions.

Inadequate Rates of Blood Flow

Inadequate rates of blood flow result in regional or general deficiencies in the rate or volume of oxygenated blood perfusing body tissue and are termed *ischemic hypoxia*. Systemic causes include severe heart failure and all forms of shock. Regional causes include obstructive lesions of

blood vessels, such as coronary or cerebral thrombosis or spasm or patients with peripheral vascular disease.

Decreased Arterial Hemoglobin Oxygen Saturation

The underlying mechanism is inadequate transfer of oxygen from lungs to the hemoglobin molecule. The most common cause is hypoxemia (Pao_2 less than 60 mm Hg) and is termed *hypoxemic hypoxia*. Other causes include carbon monoxide poisoning and methemoglobinemia (see section on pulse oximetry).

Severe Anemia

The mechanism is a deficiency of hemoglobin molecules. Causes include hemorrhage, nutritional deficiencies, and hematopoietic problems (aplastic anemia, the leukemias) and are termed *anemic hypoxia*.

Excessive Tissue Oxygen Requirements

This hypoxic threat may occur when the efficiency of the normal oxygen transport mechanisms is outstripped by excessive oxygen demands. Causes include hypermetabolism due to extreme prolonged exercise; systemic inflammatory response syndrome or sepsis, delirium tremens, status seizure activity, thyroid storm, extreme fever, and malignant hyperthermia. However, patients who have minimal or no cardiac reserve (even though resting cardiac output may be acceptable) become vulnerable to hypoxia when even relatively minor increases in metabolic demand exceed the capacity of the impaired heart to transport oxygenated blood.

Inability of Body Cells to Take Up or Use Oxygen

This form of tissue hypoxia is termed *toxic hypoxia* and develops in patients who are septic or are suffering from cyanide or ethanol toxicity.

Impaired Oxygen Unloading at the Capillary Level

Causes include alkalemia, hypocarbia, administration of large amounts of banked blood, and systemic ateriovenous shunts (sepsis, cirrhosis).

COMPENSATORY MECHANISMS

When a systemic oxygenation deficit exists or is threatened, the following mechanisms are reflexively activated to maintain tissue oxygenation and normal organ function. The first two mechanisms can be activated acutely. The third (polycythemia) takes weeks to develop and is not available for the immediate needs of ICU patients. One or both of the acute compensatory mechanisms may be compromised in critically ill or injured patients. Therefore ICU patients are extremely vulnerable to the ravages of hypoxia.

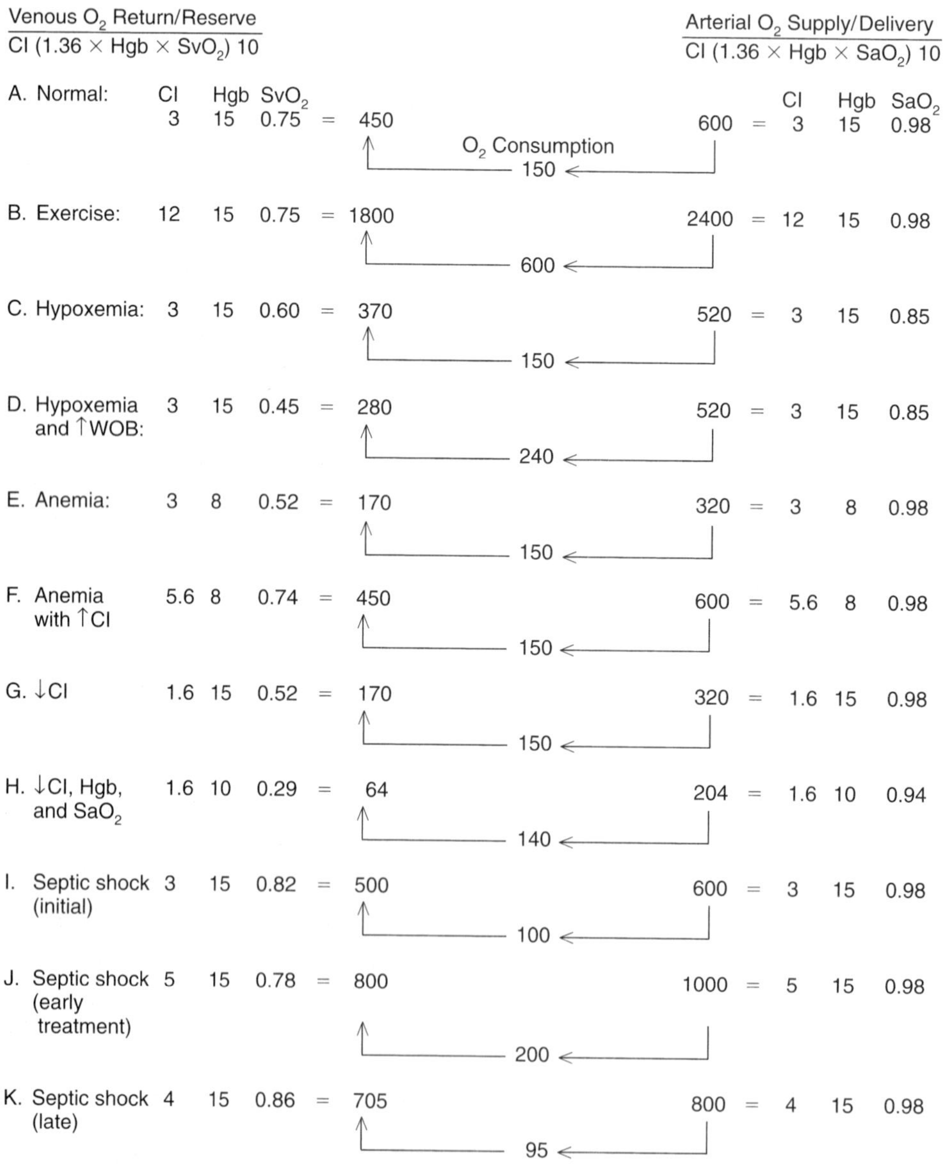

Venous O_2 Return/Reserve

$CI\ (1.36 \times Hgb \times SvO_2)\ 10$

Arterial O_2 Supply/Delivery

$CI\ (1.36 \times Hgb \times SaO_2)\ 10$

	CI	Hgb	SvO_2				CI	Hgb	SaO_2
A. Normal:	3	15	0.75	= 450	O_2 Consumption 150	600 =	3	15	0.98
B. Exercise:	12	15	0.75	= 1800	600	2400 =	12	15	0.98
C. Hypoxemia:	3	15	0.60	= 370	150	520 =	3	15	0.85
D. Hypoxemia and ↑WOB:	3	15	0.45	= 280	240	520 =	3	15	0.85
E. Anemia:	3	8	0.52	= 170	150	320 =	3	8	0.98
F. Anemia with ↑CI	5.6	8	0.74	= 450	150	600 =	5.6	8	0.98
G. ↓CI	1.6	15	0.52	= 170	150	320 =	1.6	15	0.98
H. ↓CI, Hgb, and SaO_2	1.6	10	0.29	= 64	140	204 =	1.6	10	0.94
I. Septic shock (initial)	3	15	0.82	= 500	100	600 =	3	15	0.98
J. Septic shock (early treatment)	5	15	0.78	= 800	200	1000 =	5	15	0.98
K. Septic shock (late)	4	15	0.86	= 705	95	800 =	4	15	0.98

FIGURE 12-3 Normal oxygen supply/demand balance and examples of supply/demand imbalance.

Increase Cardiac Output

The primary physiologic response to the increased oxygen demands imposed by stress is to increase oxygen delivery by proportionately increasing cardiac output. As Guyton[2] points out, "the tissues control the cardiac output in accordance with their need for oxygen." In Figure 12-3, a comparison may be made of *A,* normal supply/demand balance at rest, with *B,* wherein the oxygen demands of exercise quadruple tissue oxygen consumption.

A fourfold increase in cardiac output is required to maintain the physiologically acceptable oxygen supply/demand ratio of 4:1. As a result of compensatory increases in cardiac output, the SvO_2 is maintained in the normal range of 60% to 80%. This mechanism is used in anemic or hypoxemic patients and those with increased tissue oxygen demands. The healthy heart can increase output to as much as 15 to 25 L/min.

Extract More Oxygen from Hemoglobin within the Systemic Capillaries

There are two sets of circumstances during which more oxygen will be drawn from systemic capillaries. Consequently, the mixed venous oxygen content and saturation will fall below normal levels.

First and most commonly, if a person's metabolic rate increases (e.g., as a result of exercise, fever, shivering, seizure activity), a falling tissue PO_2 widens the diffusion gradient between tissue and capillary and prompts rapid movement of dissolved oxygen out of the systemic capillaries. The falling capillary PO_2, in turn, prompts hemoglobin to desaturate more rapidly.

Second, when tissue metabolism is normal but oxygen delivery is decreased due to inadequate blood flow, anemia, or hypoxemia, the metabolically active cells will continue to draw off oxygen from the capillaries at a normal rate. The falling capillary PO_2 will cause hemoglobin to desaturate more rapidly as it moves through the capillaries. In such patients, the oxygen saturation of mixed venous blood may be decreased from the normal values of 65% to 80% to levels as low as 32%. Below this level, anaerobic metabolism and metabolic acidosis ensue.

This mechanism is termed *drawing from the venous reserve* and is similar to drawing money from one's financial reserves during times of economic stress. The greater a person's financial cushion, the greater the margin of protection against bankruptcy. Similarly, the larger the patient's venous oxygen reserve, the greater the margin of safety to protect against hypoxic crisis.

Increase the Amount of Hemoglobin and Red Cell Mass

Polycythemia develops over weeks in persons with chronic hypoxemia, such as persons living at high altitude or those with chronic lung disease.

MONITORING TECHNIQUES FOR CONTINUOUSLY ASSESSING THE EFFECTIVENESS OF THE OXYGEN TRANSPORT AND UTILIZATION SYSTEMS

Measuring and monitoring arterial blood gases (ABGs) and, to a lesser extent, mixed venous blood gases (MVBGs) on an intermittent basis in patients with suspected or known acid-base, oxygenation, or ventilatory deficits have been common practices for several decades. Analysis is commonly performed at a hospital laboratory distant from the patient care unit. There is also a lag time of minutes to hours between the time of the blood draw and the time at which results become available to caregivers (institutionally variable). Thus there can be minimal or great disparity between the last measurement obtained and the patient's current physiologic condition. For example, intermittent ABG measurements are not likely to detect acute, severe hypoxemia that threatens cardiac arrest because arrest may occur in a matter of minutes of the onset of the severe hypoxemic episode.

Two technologies have been introduced within the past two decades to monitor the effectiveness of the oxygen transport and utilization systems. *Noninvasive pulse oximetry* provides a continuous, real-time, noninvasive, no-risk estimation of the oxygen saturation of hemoglobin within arteries proximal to the precapillary sphincters. Arterial oxygen saturation obtained by this method is abbreviated SpO_2. *Invasive mixed venous saturation (SvO_2) monitoring* provides a continuous, real-time means of estimating the amount of oxygen returning to the cardiopulmonary unit. The SvO_2 provides information that can be used in evaluating the efficiency of the cardiopulmonary unit, as well as cellular uptake and utilization of oxygen.

Continuous Monitoring of Arterial Oxygen Saturation (Pulse Oximetry)

Because it warns of arterial desaturation of many causes, the pulse oximeter has been a tremendous aid to monitoring patients in operating and recovery rooms, ICUs, stepdown units, outpatient surgical areas, and emergency departments. A normal SpO_2 indicates that oxygen is being delivered to the lungs, that the lungs are diffusing oxygen into the arterial blood, and that hemoglobin in binding with oxygen. Indications include detection and diagnosis of impending or actual hypoxemia in any patient in whom there is a known or suspected hypoxic risk and as a means of monitoring oxygen therapy, ventilatory support, or weaning from mechanical ventilation. *Normal pulse oximetry measurements do not guarantee that oxygen is being delivered to or used by body cells*.

Principle

A sensor, with a light-emitting diode and a light-receiving photodetector, is applied to the end of a finger, a toe, an earlobe, or the bridge of the nose. Two wavelengths of light, one red and one infrared, pass through the underlying, pulsating arterioles. Saturated hemoglobin absorbs more infrared light, whereas desaturated hemoglobin (also termed *reduced hemoglobin*) absorbs more red light. By sensing the differing intensities of red and infrared light passing through each jet of pulsating blood to the photodetector, the oximeter determines the percent of oxyhemoglobin against the percent of total hemoglobin. The percent of oxyhemoglobin is digitally displayed, and the strength of the pulsatile signal also appears on the oscilloscope of the companion computer module as waves that resemble the arterial waveform.

Normal and Abnormal Values

Normal arterial oxygen saturation values are 96% to 99%. Because oxygen saturation correlates with the adequacy of arterial oxygenation, all decreased values warn of hypoxic threat and require immediate investigation and intervention. However, patient tolerance to a decreased SpO_2 is variable. Healthy, young persons can tolerate saturation values in the high 60% to 70% range for long periods (as when acclimatized to high altitude). These values are never acceptable in hospitalized patients. Also, patients with severe chronic lung disease may maintain high values in the high 80% to low 90% range at rest, but cannot increase activity beyond minimal levels because of the chronic hypoxemia.

Because of decreased or absent compensatory mechanisms, vascular disease, or underlying organ dysfunction or failure, some critically ill patients may develop major problems with saturation values in the low 90% range. Generally, at SpO_2 values of 85% to 90% (PaO_2 less than 60 mm Hg), mild tissue hypoxia may be present regionally or globally. At 75% to 85% (PaO_2 less than 50 mm Hg), significant widespread tissue hypoxia is usually present. The clinician should promptly investigate possible causes, confirm displayed SpO_2 values less than 80 mm Hg with immediate blood gas analysis (laboratory CO-oximetry), and take immediate corrective actions. At 75%

or less (PaO_2 less than 40 mm Hg), severe hypoxemia threatens cardiac arrest within minutes and requires administration of 100% oxygen and other emergency interventions appropriate to the patient's clinical situation.

Sources of Error

Multiwavelength laboratory co-oximeters (CO-oximetry) have been long considered the "gold standard" of accuracy against which pulse oximeter studies are judged because they use more light wavelengths. Normally, the arterial oxygen saturation measurements from laboratory co-oximeters and pulse oximetry correlate reasonably well (see under Accuracy, later in this chapter).

Proper system setup and correct application of the sensor to the patient reduce the likelihood of flawed results (Box 12-1). Furthermore, clinicians must be aware of the sources of error inherent to the design principles and limitations of pulse oximetry in specific patient circumstances (Box 12-2).

Dyshemoglobins. Carboxyhemoglobin (CoHgb) and methemoglobin (MetHgb) do not transport oxygen. Laboratory co-oximeters distinguish the dysfunctional hemoglobins CoHgb and MetHgb from oxyhemoglobin and calculate only the percent of oxyhemoglobin. Pulse oximeters cannot distinguish dysfunctional hemoglobins from oxyhemoglobin and include them in the oxyhemoglobin measurement.

BOX 12-1
Procedural Tips for Pulse Oximetry

1. Inspect the sensor and cable for defects before application.
2. Choose a warm sampling site with good capillary refill. If the patient is intensely vasoconstricted or has peripheral vascular disease, use a nasal or earlobe sensor. Avoid application of the sensor to areas of edema or sites distal to an arterial line or automated blood pressure cuff.
3. Cleanse the intended monitoring site with alcohol.
4. Remove acrylic nails and black, blue, green, metallic, or thickly applied nail polish. Long fingernails prevent correct positioning of the finger under the diodes (inflexible probes).
5. Make sure that light-emitting and light-receiving sensors are oppositely aligned.
6. Following use, cleanse the sensor and cable with disinfectant (hospital protocol).

CoHgb levels are elevated in patients with carbon monoxide poisoning; however, the SpO_2 levels may appear acceptable while the patient is dying a hypoxic death. For example, in patients with CoHgb levels greater than 70%, the SpO_2 values may read greater than 90% while oxyhemoglobin levels are very low. MetHgb levels are increased in patients undergoing therapy with nitrates/nitrites, such as nitroglycerin; silver nitrate (burn therapy); phenacetin; sulfonamides; and anesthetics such as lidocaine, benzocaine, and prilocaine. MetHgb causes the SpO_2 to move toward 85%, although true arterial oxygen saturation may be considerably less and the patient may be showing dramatic clinical signs of hypoxia. Fetal hemoglobin does not affect the accuracy of pulse oximetry.

Differences between Manufacturers' Devices and Sensors. Calibration curves between manufacturers vary, and the output from the light-emitting diodes of sensors varies between types of sensors. The same oximeter and sensor should be used consistently for a patient unless a disposable sensor becomes defective.

BOX 12-2
Factors That Reduce the Accuracy of Oxygen Saturation Measurements (Spo$_2$) Using Pulse Oximetry

Poor Signal Detection

Poor probe positioning
Motion
Intense vasoconstriction or shock states that reduce
    pulsatile flow
Sensor applied to same limb as noninvasive blood pressure
    monitoring (weakness pulse during cuff inflation)
Sensor applied too tight

Falsely Lowered Spo$_2$

Some nail polishes
Very dark skin
Infrared heating lamps
Intravenously administered dyes (methylene blue, indigo
    carmine, indocyanine green)
Lipid infusions
Hemodilution, severe anemia (hematocrit $< 10\%$)
Venous pulsations present in the involved area

Falsely Raised Spo$_2$

Elevated COHgb, MetHgb levels
Intense surgical or fluorescent lights

Dislodgment or Poor Positioning of a Sensor. In this case, the light is shunted directly from the light-emitting diodes to the photodetector. This is termed the *penumbra effect.* The correct heart rate will be displayed, but the SpO_2 will be falsely low in normally oxygenated patients or falsely high in hypoxemic patients.

Use of Intravenous Dyes and Endogenous Pigments. Dyes, such as methylene blue, may produce sudden, significant decreases in SpO_2, although the SaO_2 is not really decreased and the patient is not at risk for hypoxic insult. Hyperbilirubinemia does not affect the accuracy of displayed values.

Weak Peripheral Pulses (Low Cardiac Output, Severe Vasoconstriction, or Severe Peripheral Vascular Disease). No pulse waveform or a damped waveform suggests poor signal quality; falsely low estimates will result. An ear or nose probe may be more reliable under these conditions.

Skin Pigmentation. Deeply pigmented skin may result in falsely lowered SpO_2 values. Consequently, SpO_2 measurements are more reliable in white patients than in black patients.

Nail Polish or Artificial (Acrylic) Nails. Nail polish has variable effects on SpO_2 measurements, usually producing false-low values. Opaque nail polish or acrylic nails can prevent the pulse oximeter from detecting any signal at all. The problem may be remedied by removing the nail polish; rotating the sensor 90 degrees so that the coated nail does not fall within the light path; or applying the sensor to the earlobe, the nose, or an unpolished toenail.

Patient Motion. Just as excessive patient movement can swamp an electrocardiogram tracing in a sea of artifact, so can movement due to restlessness, shivering, seizure activity, or tremors distort the signal and produce inaccurate readings.

High-Intensity Ambient Light. The light-receiving photodetector cannot distinguish one wavelength of light from another and therefore responds to intense room light (operating rooms, use of examining lights, etc.). Falsely elevated SpO_2 readings result. The problem can be eliminated by covering the sensor on the patient's finger or toe with a sheet.

Severe Anemia, Hemodilution (Hematocrit less than 10%). Although pulse oximetry is accurate over a wide range of hemoglobins, it becomes inaccurate with severe anemia.

Venous Pulses. The presence of venous pulsations, such as in patients with tricuspid regurgitation, may result in falsely lowered SpO_2 values.

Accuracy

Most pulse oximeter manufacturers claim an accuracy that is plus or minus 4% of true arterial saturations that are greater than 80%. This means that if the pulse oximeter displays an SpO_2 of 95%, the real value could be anywhere between 91% and 99%. Pulse oximetry measurements become less reliable between SaO_2 values of 50% and 70%. No accuracy is specified for SaO_2 values lower than 50%.[3-5]

Clinical Caveats

Normally, the pulse oximeter sensor produces no heat. If, however, the sensor of one manufacturer is connected to the oximeter of another manufacturer, heat or radiation may result in burns because the internal pin connections are different.

Also, tape-on sensors should be inspected frequently in patients at risk for regional swelling or generalized edema. As soft tissue becomes swollen, the inelastic adhesive wrapped around the finger can act as a tourniquet.

Limitations

Because of the shape of the oxyhemoglobin dissociation curve, pulse oximetry is a poor indicator of hyperox-

emia (PaO_2 greater than 100 mm Hg). It is also insensitive to hypoventilation if the patient is breathing supplemental oxygen. *When in doubt, verify the patient's oxygenation, ventilatory, and acid-base status with arterial blood gas measured by laboratory CO-oximetry.*

Continuous SvO_2 Monitoring

As stated earlier, SvO_2 reflects the ability of the cardiopulmonary unit to transport sufficient oxygen to meet body needs, as well as global cellular uptake and utilization of oxygen.

Principle

In 1981 Oximetrix (Abbott Critical Care Systems, Mountain View, California) introduced a fiberoptic pulmonary artery catheter. Edwards Critical-Care Division of Baxter Healthcare Corporation and Arrow International laboratories subsequently marketed a mixed venous oxygen saturation pulmonary artery catheter.

SvO_2 monitoring via the pulmonary artery catheter is measured by fiberoptic technology using reflectance spectrophotometry. A light source in the optical module transmits light to the tip of the pulmonary artery catheter where hemoglobin reflects the light relative to oxygen saturation. The reflected light is returned through the fiberoptics to the photodetector (light detector) contained in the optical module. The reflected light signals are then converted to electrical signals and transmitted to the SvO_2 computer (Figure 12-4). The computer interprets the signal, calculates the average of the SvO_2 levels of the previous 5 seconds, and displays an updated average every

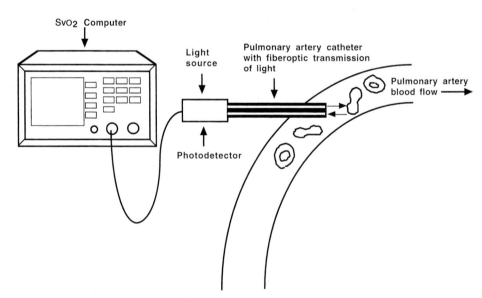

FIGURE 12-4 Reflection spectrophotometry. (Courtesy of Abbott Critical Care Systems, Mountain View, California.)

second. The computer screen also displays a trend recording, which can be set at 16-, 8-, 4-, 2-, or 1-hour intervals and can be accessed for the previous 72 hours of the patient's Svo_2 history.

Pulmonary Arterial Site for Measurement of Mixed Venous Oxygen Saturation

The oxygen saturation of venous flow from various organ systems varies because different organ systems have different metabolic needs. For example, the renal Svo_2 is approximately 90% (kidneys extract only 10% of the oxygen from capillary blood), myocardial Svo_2 is approximately 30% (70% oxygen extraction), and cutaneous Svo_2 is 90% (10% oxygen extraction). The venous oxygen saturation of blood within the pulmonary artery is an average of venous oxygen saturations from all parts of the body because venous blood mixes completely within the right ventricle.

General Insertion Guidelines and Avoidable Sources of Svo_2 Measurement Inaccuracy

Carefully read each manufacturer's recommendations for insertion and maintenance in the package insert. To ensure the accuracy of Svo_2 measurements, several steps must be taken. Before catheter insertion, a stability check of the computer and cable should be made. The body of the catheter should be left in its sterile package while the catheter connection is made to the optical cable. A simple "preinsertion" calibration of the catheter is then performed (manufacturer specific). Following this, the catheter is prepared as usual for insertion, the pressure lumina are irrigated and connected to transducers, the balloon and thermistor are checked for integrity, and the catheter is handled so that kinks that could damage or break the optics are avoided.

Once the catheter tip enters the circulation, the level of venous oxygen saturation, recorded from the anatomic location of the catheter tip, is displayed. Using the pressure waveforms as a guide, the pulmonary artery catheter tip is positioned in one of the main pulmonary artery branches. The light-intensity marker should be examined to ensure that the catheter is not too distally placed. If the catheter tip is close to the wedged position, the catheter is likely to illuminate the highly reflective vessel wall. This results in an increase in the intensity of light and a falsely high Svo_2 measurement. When necessary, the catheter should be repositioned until acceptable intensity markers are obtained.

If the catheter becomes kinked (not uncommonly at the point where the catheter is sutured to the skin, or where the catheter exits the introducer or protective sleeve), the emission of light can be interrupted. The intensity of light falls, indicating that the catheter must

be straightened. A sharp kink that breaks one or both of the optics results in a low-intensity light that cannot be corrected.

If the optic catheter is inserted without "preinsertion" calibration, or if the catheter becomes disconnected from the cable and is then reconnected, an in vivo recalibration must be performed. After checking for acceptable intensity markers, a mixed venous sample is *slowly* drawn. Box 12-3 outlines the technique for obtaining a mixed venous blood sample.

The Svo_2 of the mixed venous blood measured by laboratory CO-oximeter is then compared with the Svo_2 displayed on the computer. If values differ by more than 5%, the computer can be appropriately adjusted.

When patients must be transported, disconnection of the cable from the computer, rather than the catheter from the cable, avoids the need for in vivo calibration and mixed venous sampling later, when reconnection is made. A memory chip in the optical cable retains the previous calibration so that when the cable is reconnected to the computer, or connected to another Svo_2 computer, monitoring can resume without the need to recalibrate the catheter.

Accuracy

Older fiberoptic technology used a two-wavelength system. This was associated with an estimated error rate of 4% for accurately detecting oxyhemoglobin.[6] Improved optical processing through the introduction of a three-wavelength system showed improved measurements of oxyhemoglobin. Other improvements in Svo_2 technology include improvements in optical signal processing. Studies support the accuracy of Svo_2 monitoring compared with laboratory CO-oximetry measurements as long as there are no dysfunctional hemoglobins present.[7,8]

As mentioned earlier, laboratory CO-oximetry can distinguish CoHgb and MetHgb from oxyhemoglobin through the use of more light wavelengths.

Pulse oximeters are capable of detecting only the two functional hemoglobins. Similarly, fiberoptic technology used in pulmonary artery catheters detects only oxyhemoglobin and reduced hemoglobin. Consequently, Svo_2 measurements may be significantly flawed in patients suffering carbon monoxide poisoning or methemoglobinemia. Other factors that may reduce the accuracy of Svo_2 measurements are listed in Box 12-4.

It is important to remember that if proper setup procedures are followed and daily in vivo calibration is performed, the Svo_2 readings are generally accurate and reliable in patients with normal hemoglobins. The in vivo calibration procedure will vary between manufacturers. Check the manufacturer's manual for specific instructions.

BOX 12-3
Obtaining Mixed Venous Blood Gas Samples

Equipment
Anticoagulated blood gas syringe
Syringe cap
10 ml syringe for clearing line before sampling
10 ml syringe for clearing line after sampling
Cup of ice

Procedure
1. Wash hands.
2. Locate the sampling stopcock connected to the distal port of the pulmonary artery catheter.
3. Attach 10 ml syringe.
4. Turn stopcock OFF to the flush solution.
5. Using 10 ml syringe, aspirate 5 ml to clear the line of flush solution. Close stopcock to the halfway position. Remove and discard syringe.
6. Attach blood gas syringe.
7. Open stopcock again to the distal port and aspirate sample slowly. Aspirating too rapidly may "arterialize" the sample, withdrawing blood backward from the alveolar level, where blood is reoxygenated. Also, applying too much suction on the pulmonary artery may collapse the vessel, making it impossible to collect the sample.
8. Close stopcock and remove blood gas syringe. Hold syringe upright and expel any air in the syringe. Cap the syringe and roll it gently to mix the blood. Cap and submerge in ice immediately.
9. Attach sterile syringe to stopcock. Open stopcock to the flush solution, and irrigate into the syringe until stopcock is clear. Turn stopcock OFF to the sampling port. Remove and discard the syringe, and cap the port with sterile cap or plug.
10. Flush line until traces of blood are removed.
11. Check bedside oscilloscope to confirm presence of pulmonary artery waveform and patency of line.
12. Label the specimen/lab slip with the following:
    a. Patient name and identification number
    b. Type of sample: mixed venous blood gas
    c. Date and time sample was drawn
    d. Type and amount of oxygen therapy
    e. Patient's temperature
13. Expedite delivery of the sample to the laboratory.

BOX 12-4
Factors That May Reduce the Accuracy of Svo_2 Measurements

1. Neither a preinsertion nor an in vivo calibration performed
2. Light intensity calibration not performed at time of insertion
3. Optics bent or broken
4. Catheter tip close to or facing the wall of the pulmonary artery
5. Increased carboxyhemoglobin or methemoglobin

CLINICAL APPLICATIONS AND CONSIDERATIONS OF COMBINED ARTERIAL AND MIXED VENOUS OXYGEN SATURATION MONITORING

See the chapters related to patients with pulmonary or cardiovascular disease, multiple-system organ dysfunction, and shock. General and specific considerations of oxygen transport and consumption as evaluated by Sao_2 and Svo_2 monitoring are discussed here. The evaluation of the relationship of Sao_2 and Svo_2 pairs gives more information about the patient's circulatory and oxygenation status than use of one technique alone (Table 12-2).

Applications in Patients with Pulmonary Problems

Hypoxemia
Hypoxemia is a common finding in patients with acute and chronic pulmonary problems and may result in significant decreases in oxygen transport and cellular oxygen consumption (see Figure 12-3, C). Hypoxemic patient with adequate cardiac reserve increase cardiac output to maintain oxygen supply at physiologically acceptable levels. The following examples using the oxygen transport formula (assuming otherwise normal systems function and Svo_2) indicate the required cardiac index needed to sustain oxygen transport of 600 ml/min/m^2 at progressively decreasing arterial oxygen saturations levels.

Oxygen Delivery Do_2	=	Cardiac Index CI	× O_2 Content 1.36 × Hbg	× 10 Sao_2 × 10
600	=	3	15	0.98
600	=	3.06	15	0.94
600	=	3.19	15	0.90
600	=	3.95	15	0.80

TABLE 12-2
Examination of Arterial and Mixed Venous Oxygen Saturation Pairs*

Arterial Saturation	Mixed Venous Saturation	Causes
96%–99% (PaO$_2$ 90 to 100 mm Hg)	60%–80%	Normal physiology
<90% (PaO$_2$ < 60 mm Hg)	<60%	Hypoxemia due to very high altitude, alveolar hypoventilation, or pulmonary disease
Normal 96%–99%	<60%	Severe anemia (extreme exercise)
May be <96%–99%	<60%	Low-cardiac-output states, shock
Normal 96%–99%	>80%	Sepsis, carbon monoxide poisoning, methemoglobinemia, decreased levels of 2,3-diphosphoglycerate (banked blood), alkalosis, cyanide poisoning, ethanol poisoning

*Assuming FiO$_2$ of 21%, ambient air.

If compensatory increases in cardiac output are inadequate or work of breathing is increased, the SvO$_2$ will fall proportionate to the severity of the deficit in oxygen transport, as well as the increase in oxygen demand that parallels the work of breathing. In fact, to sustain the metabolic demands of work-stressed primary and accessory muscles of ventilation, oxygen consumption may be increased by 20% to 40%.[9-13] If, for example, greater oxygen demands raise oxygen consumption to 240 ml/min/m^2, but oxygen transport remains normal, the patient's SvO$_2$ would decrease to a level of approximately 45% (see Figure 12-3, *D*).

Effective treatment of hypoxemia and threats to cellular oxygen consumption requires removal of the cause of hypoxemia (if possible); oxygen therapy; and patient-supportive measures, such as mechanical ventilatory assistance and support of hemodynamic function (if compromised). The application of positive end-expiratory pressure (PEEP) may also be indicated but may be followed by a decrease in cardiac output. Improvement in both SaO$_2$ and SvO$_2$ following institution of PEEP implies that arterial oxygenation is increased without a corresponding decrease in cardiac output. If PEEP is associated with acceptable SaO$_2$ levels and a decrease in SvO$_2$, PEEP levels may have to be decreased or PEEP may have to be discontinued.

Potential Problems That May Develop with Management of Patients with Pulmonary Disease

Several intrinsic and care-related factors may produce decreases in both SaO$_2$ and SvO$_2$. The first factor is suctioning patients with or without an artificial airway. Airway suctioning not only decreases SaO$_2$ but also increases oxygen demands if the patient coughs, becomes agitated, or resists suctioning. One study found that the average increase in oxygen demand with endotracheal suctioning was 27%, with a range of 7% to 70%.[11] Another study of 189 critically ill patients found that despite preoxygenating with 100% oxygen and hyperinflating the patient's lungs three times with an anesthesia bag, the open method of suctioning resulted in a 5% decrease in SvO$_2$.[14] Using a closed method of suctioning, however, in which hyperoxygenation and hyperinflation on the ventilator were followed by suctioning with an in-line suction catheter, the continuously measured SvO$_2$ actually increased by 5%. These studies have supported the adoption of closed versus open suctioning technique in ICUs.

The second factor is accidental patient disconnection from the oxygen source or deliberate reductions in FiO$_2$. Abrupt, profound decreases in SaO$_2$ and SvO$_2$ may occur when the oxygen source is accidentally disconnected or the FiO$_2$ is decreased; when the ventilator malfunctions; or when endotracheal tubes become kinked, occluded, or dislodged. If equipment malfunction is a possibility, the patient should be manually bagged with 100% oxygen until the malfunction is corrected. The arterial (pulse oximeter) and mixed venous oxygen saturation may then be used to assess the effectiveness of bagging. If dislodgment of an endotracheal tube was the source of the problem, partial confirmation of proper placement of an endotracheal tube may be based on improvements in SaO$_2$ and SvO$_2$. The chest radiograph is necessary for absolute confirmation of proper endotracheal tube placement.

The third factor is an acute pulmonary event, such as pneumothorax. Pulmonary barotrauma is a common complication of mechanical ventilation, and patients with chronic obstructive pulmonary disease are also prone to spontaneous pneumothorax. If a chest tube is inserted for the treatment of pneumothorax, improvements in arterial and mixed venous saturations imply that the tube has been properly positioned and that the lung is being reinflated. Therapy for other acute pulmonary problems, such as pulmonary embolism, can likewise be evaluated with improvement in SpO_2 and SvO_2.

Assessment of Patient Status during Weaning from Ventilatory Support

Continuous arterial and mixed venous oxygen saturation monitoring assist in weaning patients from mechanical ventilation (in lieu of serial blood gas analysis). This simplifies the procedure, reduces diagnostic blood loss, and contains cost. A decrease in both arterial and mixed venous oxygen saturation by 10% or more is a reflection of the inability of the patient's lungs or ventilatory efforts to maintain arterial oxygenation.

Alternatively, a decrease in SvO_2 by greater than 10% with no change in arterial saturation implies either a significant decrease in cardiac output or a significant increase in the work of breathing. In either case, the weaning attempt should be abandoned while attempts are made to identify and correct the underlying defect.

Assessment of the Fraction of Intrapulmonary Shunt Using Arterial and Mixed Venous Saturation Measurements

See Chapter 2 for discussion of the intrapulmonary shunt and its effects on gas exchange. Assessment of the percentage of pulmonary shunt (percentage of cardiac output flowing past nonventilated alveoli) cannot be directly measured but can be estimated using the shunt equation discussed in Chapter 10. This can, however, be a time-consuming and laborious endeavor.

To simplify the procedure and the mathematics, the following technique using the SaO_2 and SvO_2 values may be used as a crude estimate of the intrapulmonary shunt fraction.

$$\text{Normal} = \frac{1 - SaO_2}{1 - SvO_2} = \frac{1 - 0.99}{1 - 0.75} = \frac{0.01}{0.25} = 4\%$$

For example:

$$\text{Mild shunt} = \frac{1 - 0.9}{1 - 0.6} = \frac{0.01}{1.0} = 25\%$$

$$\text{Moderate shunt} = \frac{1 - 0.85}{1 - 0.55} = \frac{0.15}{0.45} = 33\%$$

$$\text{Severe shunt} = \frac{1 - 0.8}{1 - 0.5} = \frac{0.2}{0.5} = 40\%$$

$$\text{Critical shunt} = \frac{1 - 0.8}{1 - 0.6} = \frac{0.2}{0.4} = 50\%$$

Examination of the formula reveals that the patients with severe degrees of intrapulmonary shunt (typically patients with acute respiratory distress syndrome [ARDS])

do not necessarily have SvO_2 levels that are correspondingly low. The reasons are discussed in the following section. However, the severely diseased lungs fail to resaturate the venous hemoglobin, thus producing low arterial oxygen saturations.

Application of Svo_2 Monitoring to Patients with Acute Respiratory Distress Syndrome

Refractory hypoxemia is the hallmark of ARDS. However, studies of patients with ARDS have shown that SvO_2 measurements may not correspond with the severity of hypoxemia.[15-17] This means that a "good SvO_2 measurement" does not necessarily mean that tissue oxygenation is "good." In the critical pulmonary shunt example shown earlier, the mixed venous oxygen saturation appears to be in a low-normal range at 60%. However, the patient's arterial saturation is only 80% and the fraction of intrapulmonary shunt is 50%. Why does the low SaO_2 not result in a proportionate decrease in SvO_2? Investigators have found that some patients with ARDS fail to take up or to use oxygen at the cellular level, thus leaving greater than anticipated amounts of oxygen in mixed venous blood.[15-17] They also have found that increasing oxygen transport (increasing cardiac output, oxygen content, or both) sometimes results in greater calculated tissue oxygen consumption. This phenomenon is termed *delivery-dependent oxygen consumption*. Two reasons have been proposed to explain why patients with severe ARDS fail to consume enough oxygen:

1. Severe hypoxemia may limit the ability of arterioles to successfully autoregulate regional blood flow to capillary beds. Some capillaries thereby receive too much oxygen, whereas others receive too little.
2. Systemic interstitial edema may limit diffusion of oxygen from systemic capillaries to cells.

It has been suggested that the therapeutic goal is to increase oxygen transport until oxygen consumption "plateaus" (additional increases in oxygen transport produce no further increases in oxygen consumption). Although initial reports suggested a favorable effect on morbidity and mortality, experience has failed to document benefit. Specific goals for hemodynamic support are unclear at this time and continue to be a topic of debate and controversy.

Assessment of Patients with Anemia and Hemorrhage

Despite a normal arterial PO_2, an adequate hemoglobin level is essential to maintaining adequate blood oxygen content and effective oxygen transport (see Table 2-7). Decreases in hemoglobin must be met with corresponding increases in cardiac output (which may to be several times normal) to maintain oxygen transport. This is commonly accomplished in critically ill patients by an increase in heart rate. In Figure 12-3, *E,* it should be noted that a patient with a *normal* cardiac index of 3 but a hemoglobin of 8 would deliver only 320 ml/min/m² of oxygen. If this patient has a resting oxygen demand of 150 ml/min/m², the oxygen supply would be only about two times the oxygen demand rather than four times. In this case, the supply/demand balance is 2:1, which is reflected by the decrease in Svo_2 to 52%.

In patients at risk for bleeding, an Svo_2 less than 50% and tachycardia are often the first clues to occult bleeding. Blood replacement or fluid therapy that increases oxygen transport so that Svo_2 rises above 50% implies that the oxygen supply/demand ratio is improved. Thus clinicians have time to investigate, identify, and begin definitive therapy of the source of bleeding.

Patients with anemia are able to maintain normal oxygen delivery, provided that they have adequate cardiac reserve. However, the cost in terms of heart work and oxygen consumption is high in light of the increased cardiac output necessary to sustain oxygen delivery. This is illustrated in the following calculations:

Oxygen Delivery Do_2	=	Cardiac Index CI	×	O_2 Content 1.36 × Hbg	×	10 Sao_2	×	10
600	=	3		15		0.98		
600	=	4.5		10		0.98		
600	=	5.6		8		0.98		
600	=	7.5		6		0.98		

Patients with compensated anemia develop tissue hypoxia secondary to any factor that reduces cardiac output or increases oxygen demand. For this reason, anemic patients with marginal cardiac reserve (such as the elderly) may require transfusion to correct the anemia before major operative procedures or following trauma.

Assessment of Patients with Heart Failure

Despite a normal Sao_2, if oxygen consumption remains constant, Svo_2 will fall with the development of heart failure proportionate to the severity of heart failure. The following formula for calculating oxygen transport indicates the effects of decreases in cardiac output on oxygen delivery:

Oxygen Delivery Do_2	=	Cardiac Index CI	×	O_2 Content 1.36 × Hbg	×	10 Sao_2	×	10
600	=	3		15		0.98		
500	=	2.5		15		0.98		
400	=	2.0		15		0.98		
300	=	1.5		15		0.98		
200	=	1.0		15		0.98		

If low cardiac output is compounded by anemia and hypoxemia, the patient is at triple clinical jeopardy (see Figure 12-3, *H*). The decrease in Svo_2 (29%) reflects the severity of the supply/demand imbalance. Consequent decreases in oxygen consumption are likely to be life threatening. Until one or all of the defects are corrected or modified, any avoidable activity known to increase oxygen demand, such as positioning or weighing, should be avoided. For example, in one study, turning a patient to a lateral position resulted in a 9% drop in Svo_2.[18] Another study, using patients with low ejection fractions, found that lateral positioning decreased Svo_2 by 8.5% for right lateral and 11.3% for left lateral position.[19] Both studies found that patients' Svo_2 returned to baseline within 5 minutes.

The effectiveness of therapies in patients with complicated or uncomplicated severe heart failure may be assessed by continuous Svo_2 monitoring. The efficacy of supportive therapies, such as the "best" pharmacologic therapy or optimal intraaortic balloon pumping timing, is indicated by the patient's improvement in continuously measured Svo_2 values, clinical status, and hemodynamic status.

Assessment of Patients at Risk for Increases in Oxygen Demand

Many factors are known to increase oxygen demand (see Table 12-1). Some are outside the caregiver's control and are part of the patient's underlying problem (trauma, sepsis), and some directly relate to patient care activities. In all cases, increases in oxygen demand increase hypoxic risk, particularly in unstable patients.

Continuously monitoring Svo_2 helps define high-risk patients whose oxygen demands are higher than normal and also those whose baseline oxygen transport is fixed and therefore cannot appropriately increase during times of stress.

Studies using continuous Svo_2 monitoring have documented that routine care increases metabolic activity and oxygen demands as evidenced by a fall in Svo_2.[20,21] Care activities can also reduce oxygen transport if, for example, a position change reduces venous return and cardiac output, or if suctioning reduces arterial oxygen content. Generally, an Svo_2 less than 50% helps identify patients who have a significant supply/demand imbalance and who are at risk for hypotensive crisis or serious arrhythmias.

Before beginning patient care activities that are known to increase oxygen demand, clinicians should consider measures that increase oxygen transport, such as temporarily increasing the Fio_2 for a few minutes before beginning the activity. Also, protective measures such as slowly turning the patient, staggering activities according to patient tolerance, coaching the patient to relax, and offering the patient encouragement may reduce oxygen demand. If the patient is in pain, an analgesic should be given before moving the patient and consideration should be given to sedating agitated patients. If the patient has a serious supply/demand imbalance (SvO_2 less than 40%), the activity should be postponed when possible until the condition is stabilized and tissue oxygenation is improved.

Overall, the magnitude of fall in SvO_2 that develops with activity in a given patient depends on the interrelationship of three factors: (1) the severity of a preexisting oxygenation deficit; (2) whether the patient has an adequate cardiac reserve to compensate for increases in oxygen demand; and (3) the level of increase in oxygen demand incurred with the specific activity. During the activity, the continuously monitored arterial saturation and SvO_2 measurements can be used to assess the patient's responses to specific care activities.

Many clinical conditions, similar to exercise, increase oxygen demand. Table 12-1 summarizes these conditions. This list may be used to estimate the metabolic rate of patients. For example, if a patient has a femur fracture, oxygen demand is increased by 10%. Two degrees of temperature elevation increases oxygen demand by 20%. If a patient has both problems, one would expect oxygen demand to be increased by 30%.

Resting O_2 demand	=	150 ml/min/m^2
Increased 30% with fracture and fever	=	+45
Current O_2 demand (estimate)	=	195 ml/min/m^2

By reviewing the multiple factors that increase oxygen demand, estimates in the magnitude of increases in oxygen demand can guide professionals caring for ICU patients by roughly estimating the metabolic burden imposed by their condition. Therapeutic and patient care activities that are tailored to decrease oxygen demand may make a significant contribution to reducing clinically evident and occult hypoxic episodes.

CONDITIONS ASSOCIATED WITH INCREASES IN SvO_2

"Normal" SvO_2 measurements may be misleadingly normal or elevated in severely ill ICU patients. In fact, elevations in the SvO_2 value may be the only indication that tissue hypoxia is ongoing despite all other numbers appearing reasonably "normal" or "acceptable" on the flow sheet. Sudden elevations may also indicate a sudden-onset life-threatening condition.

Oxygen that is returned to the heart is oxygen not used by the tissues. There are four reasons for SvO_2 measurements to be higher than normal:

1. The tissues were not exposed to blood flow as a result of a shunt, either a left-to-right intracardiac shunt or a systemic vascular shunt.
2. The hemoglobin failed to unload oxygen in response to falling oxygen saturation (increased affinity of hemoglobin for oxygen).
3. The diffusion distance from capillaries to cells is increased due to interstitial edema.
4. The cells are toxic and unable to take up and use oxygen.

For example, a patient with an anteroseptal myocardial infarction, whose SvO_2 suddenly increases, should be immediately suspected for development of ventricular septal defect (VSD). Usually, patients with a VSD shunt blood from the left ventricle to the right, thus increasing the SvO_2 of right ventricular and pulmonary arterial blood (see Chapter 21). The larger the defect, and the more profound and the greater the volume of left-to-right shunt, the more closely the SvO_2 will approximate the SaO_2. The efficacy of medical measures as a bridge to corrective surgery is demonstrated by a reduction in SvO_2, as the volume of the left-to-right shunt is reduced as well as observations in improvement in the patient's overall clinical and hemodynamic status.

Patients who have received large amounts of banked blood, who are hypothermic, or who are spontaneously or artificially hyperventilated increase the affinity of hemoglobin for oxygen (leftward shift in the oxyhemoglobin dissociation curve). Consequently, intracellular PO_2 falls and SvO_2 rises to 75% or slightly greater. If cellular activity and oxygen demand increase, it will be impossible for the cells to obtain access to the oxygen left tightly attached to the hemoglobin, which now returns "too saturated" to the heart. *Any condition that inhibits dissociation of oxygen from hemoglobin at the systemic capillary level must be avoided to maintain the integrity of the oxygen transport system.*

Increased SvO_2 measurements also are characteristic of patients with sepsis (see Figure 12-3, *I*). Possible causes include maldistribution of cardiac output, systemic arteriovenous shunting, decreased levels of 2,3-diphosphoglycerate, and defects in cellular oxygen uptake and utilization. Therapeutic goals for septic patients include at least a 50% increase in cardiac index (which, in turn, increases oxygen transport) and a tissue oxygen consumption greater than 170 ml/min/m^2 (see Figure 12-3, *J*). For patients in whom systemic oxygen consumption fails to respond to increases in oxygen transport (facilitated by volume loading and inotropic agents), the outcome is grim (see Figure 12-3, *K*).

Use of Continuous Spo$_2$ and Svo$_2$ Monitoring Combined with Cardiac Output Measurements

Pulse oximetry is a standard part of patient evaluation in ICUs. Coupled with cardiac output and Svo$_2$ measurements, the clinician is able to calculate oxygen transport and oxygen consumption, identify impending or actual global tissue hypoxia, determine the cause of hypoxic episodes, assess responses to treatment of hypoxia, and predict patient survival based on the underlying cause of tissue hypoxia and responses to therapy. For example, if a postoperative patient has a progressive increase in cardiac output from 5 L/min to 6.5 L/min from 8 AM to 9 AM, no Svo$_2$ monitoring, and the Spo$_2$ remained at 96% to 98%, the clinician would assume the patient is stable because all measurements are within the "normal" range. But if, by assessing the Svo$_2$ from 8 AM to 9 AM, the clinician notices a decrease from 77% to 60%, this decline suggests that oxygen demand increased during the past hour. By monitoring both Svo$_2$ and cardiac output, it becomes evident that even though the cardiac output increased, it was not enough to adequately supply needed oxygen to the patients. Attempts at treating the cause of increased tissue oxygen demands (possibly waking from general anesthesia and experiencing pain) can then be made with titrated anesthetic agents guided by Svo$_2$ measurements. If the Svo$_2$ fails to improve with anesthetic drugs, other causes of increased oxygen demand, such as shivering with rewarming, presence of visitors, and nursing activities, can be investigated and ruled out.

Evaluation of the combination of Svo$_2$ with continuous cardiac output monitoring, right ventricular end-diastolic volume, stroke volume, and ejection fraction is currently under evaluation to determine if patient outcome is improved over intermittent bolus technique (see Chapter 10). Advantages include elimination of the need for fluid boluses, thus reducing the risk of fluid overload and reducing nursing time with ritualistic bolus technique; ability to obtain real-time information of acute hemodynamic and physiologic change for time-appropriate clinical decision making; and ability to assess therapies with continuous feedback of the physiologic or hemodynamic effects of therapeutic interventions.

New Technologies for Monitoring Tissue Oxygenation

Other invasive and noninvasive techniques for monitoring tissue oxygenation have been and are currently being evaluated.

Continuous Indwelling Arterial Blood Gas Monitoring

This technology has been evolving since the 1950s. The intraarterial blood gas system uses a 20-gauge fiberoptic probe that senses pH, Pco$_2$, and Po$_2$. The attached blood gas monitor system provides either continuous in vivo ABG monitoring or on demand ex vivo ABG analysis. Studies of the accuracy of intraarterial blood gas monitoring have yielded conflicting results. Other limitations are their high cost and technical constraints. At the time of this writing, there are no commercially available units.

Point-of-Care Blood Gas Monitoring

This technology has been developing since the late 1970s and provides clinicians the capability of obtaining laboratory testing at the bedside. These ABG analyzers can also measure electrolytes, glucose, lactate, blood urea nitrogen, and hematocrit. They are small and portable, require a very small blood volume, and can repeat results every few minutes. They are self-calibrating and usually use a disposable cartridge. Limitations include high cost (disposable cartridges are expensive) and instrument maintenance. Quality control can also be labor intensive and confusing.

Transcutaneous Po$_2$ monitoring (Ptco$_2$)

The Ptco$_2$ is the oxygen tension of heated skin; the skin must be heated to a minimum of 43°C. This technology was originally used in the evaluation of Pao$_2$ of newborns. A heated electrode is placed on the surface of the skin, causing vasodilation of the dermal capillaries, which is thought to "arterialize" the underlying capillary blood. The Ptco$_2$ value follows trends in Pao$_2$ in patients with adequate tissue perfusion and decreases in tandem with Pao$_2$ in low-cardiac-output states. Therefore it is a good indicator of peripheral perfusion. Because of the risk of skin burns, calibration, warm-up time, and electrode maintenance, this technique is not commonly used clinically.

Transcutaneous Measurement of Local Tissue Oxygen Saturation (Sto$_2$)

This recently available technology, termed *near-infrared spectrometry (NIRS)*, uses specific, calibrated wavelengths of near-infrared light directed to varying tissue depths up to approximately 50 mm to noninvasively determine local tissue So$_2$ (Sto$_2$). The wavelengths of light, delivered via a fiber optic probe placed on the skin, scatter within the tissue and are absorbed relative to the amount of oxygen attached to the hemoglobin in arterioles, capillaries, and veins. The returned optical signal is analyzed and displayed the percent of oxyhemoglobin in the vascular bed. Whereas transcutaneous Po_2 measures only the Po_2 of skin, the spectrometer measures the oxygen saturation at differing tissue depths such as skin, subcutaneous tissue, and skeletal muscle. Because Sto_2 tracks local peripheral oxygenation, decreasing Sto_2 values correlate with decreasing oxygen availability. Sto_2 measurements of muscle (deltoid) and the stomach (at gastric surface) correlate with commonly used indices of shock such as lactate, oxygen delivery, and arterial base deficit. Clinical applications include assessment of oxygen delivery in patients with limb ischemia due to compartment syndrome or peripheral vascular disease and assessment of patients at risk for or being treated for shock (InSpectra Tissue Spectrometer, Hutchinson Technology, Hutchinson, Minnesota).

SUMMARY

Assessment of hemodynamic and pulmonary function using the pulmonary artery catheter, pulse oximetry, and arterial blood gas analysis has become routine in the care of the critically ill. The conventional cardiopulmonary profile, however, focuses on heart and lung performance, but not on how well the delivery of oxygen has met the demands of tissues. Continuous Svo_2 monitoring enhances patient evaluation potential and allows clinicians to detect and correct supply/demand imbalances before adverse consequences result.

REFERENCES

1. Tremper KK, Barker SJ: Monitoring of oxygenation. In Lake CL, Hines RL, Blitt CD, editors: *Clinical monitoring: practical applications for anesthesia and critical care,* Philadelphia, 2001, W.B. Saunders.
2. Guyton AC: *Textbook of medical physiology,* Philadelphia, 1991, W.B. Saunders.
3. Tobin MJ: Respiratory monitoring, *JAMA* 264:244, 1990.
4. Tremper KK, Barker SJ: Monitoring of oxygenation. In Lake CL, Hines RL, Blitt CD, editors: *Clinical monitoring: practical applications for anesthesia and critical care,* Philadelphia, 2001, W.B. Saunders.
5. Seguin P et al: Evidence for the need of bedside accuracy of pulse oximetry in intensive care units, *Crit Care Med* 28:3, 2000.
6. Ahrens T: Continuous mixed venous (Svo_2) monitoring: too expensive or indispensable? *Crit Care Nurs Clin North Am* 11:1, 1999.
7. Armaganidis A, Dhainant JF, Billard JL, et al: Accuracy assessment for three fiberoptic pulmonary artery catheters for Svo_2 monitoring, *Intensive Care Med* 20(7):484, 1994.
8. Bongard F, Lee TS, Leighton T, et al: Simultaneous in vivo comparison of two versus three wavelength mixed venous (Svo_2) oximetry catheters, *J Clin Monit* 11(5):329, 1995.
9. Fahey PJ, Harris K, Vanderwarf C: Clinical experience with continuous monitoring of mixed venous oxygen saturation in respiratory failure, *Chest* 86:748, 1984.
10. Kanak R, Fahey PJ, Vanderward C: Oxygen cost of breathing, *Chest* 87:126, 1985.
11. Harpin RP, Baker JP, Downer JP, et al: Correlation of the oxygen cost of breathing and length of weaning from mechanical ventilation, *Crit Care Med* 15:807, 1987.
12. Viale JP, Annat GJ, Bouffard YM, et al: Oxygen cost of breathing in postoperative patients, *Chest* 93:506, 1988.
13. Savino JA, Dawson JA, Agarwal N, et al: The metabolic cost of breathing in critical surgical patients, *J Trauma* 25:1126, 1985.
14. Clark AP et al: Effects of endoctracheal suctioning on mixed venous oxygen saturation and heart rate in critically ill adults, *Heart Lung* 19:552, 1990.
15. Lorente JA, Renes E, Gomez-Aguinaga MA, et al: Oxygen delivery-dependent oxygen consumption in acute respiratory failure, *Crit Care Med* 19:770, 1991.
16. Russell JA, Ronco JJ, Lockhat D, et al: Oxygen delivery and consumption and ventricular preload are greater in survivors than in nonsurvivors of the adult respiratory distress syndrome, *Am Rev Respir Dis* 141:659, 1990.
17. Weg JG: Oxygen transport in adult respiratory distress syndrome and other acute circulatory problems: relationship of oxygen delivery and oxygen consumption, *Crit Care Med* 19:650, 1991.
18. Winslow EH et al: Effects of a lateral turn on mixed venous oxygen saturation and heart rate in critically ill adults, *Heart Lung* 19:55, 1990.
19. Gawlinski A, Dracup K: Effect of positioning on Svo_2 in the critically ill patient with low ejection fraction, *Nurs Res* 47:5, 1998.
20. Swinamer DL, Phang PT, Jones RL, et al: Twenty-four hour energy expenditure in critically ill patients, *Crit Care Med* 15:637, 1987.
21. Weissman C, Kemper M, Damask MC, et al: Effect of routine intensive care interactions on metabolic rate, *Chest* 86:815, 1984.

SUGGESTED READINGS

Adrogue HJ, Madias NE: Arterial blood gas monitoring: acid-base assessment. In Tobin MJ, editor: *Principles and practice of intensive care monitoring,* New York, 1998, Mcgraw-Hill.

Appel PL, Kram HB: Tissue oxygen debt as a determinant of lethal and nonlethal postoperative organ failure, *Crit Care Med* 16:1117, 1988.

Astiz ME, Rackow EC, Falk JL, et al: Oxygen delivery and consumption in patients with hyperdynamic septic shock, *Crit Care Med* 15:26, 1987.

Barone JE, Snyder AB: Treatment strategies in shock: use of oxygen transport measurements, *Heart Lung* 20:81, 1991.

Bartlett RH: Oxygen kinetics and the art of physiological monitoring, *J Crit Care* 8:77, 1993.

Bartlett RH et al: Measurement of metabolism in multiple organ failure, *Surgery* 92:771, 1982.

Bartlett RH et al: Metabolic studies in chest trauma, *J Thorac Cardiovasc Surg* 87:503, 1984.

Bessey PQ: Editorial comment, *J Trauma* 33:67, 1992.

Bishop MH: Relationship between supranormal circulatory values, time delays, and outcome in severely traumatized patients, *Crit Care Med* 21:56, 1993.

Bishop MH, Wo CJ, Appel PS, et al: Effect of achieving optimal hemodynamic and oxygen transport values on the survival of severely traumatized patients, *Crit Care Med* 18:S68, 1991.

Burchell S, Yu M, Takiguchi S, et al: Evaluation of continuous cardiac output and mixed venous oxygen saturation catheter in critically ill surgical patients, *Crit Care Med* 25:3, 1997.

Cariou M et al: Continuous cardiac output and mixed venous oxygen saturation monitoring, *J Crit Care* 13:198, 1998.

Chiara O, Giomarelli PP, Biagioli B, et al: Hypermetabolic response after hyperthermic cardiopulmonary bypass, *Crit Care Med* 15:995, 1987.

Chiolero R et al: Effects of catecholamines on oxygen consumption and oxygen delivery in critically ill patients, *Chest* 100:1676, 1991.

Clifton GL, Robertson CS, Grossman RG, et al: The metabolic response to severe head injury, *J Neurosurg* 60:687, 1984.

Copel LC, Stolarik A: Impact of nursing care activities on SvO_2 levels of postoperative cardiac surgery patients, *Cardiovasc Nurs* 27:1, 1991.

Dorros G et al: Percutaneous transluminal valvuloplasty in calcific aortic stenosis: the double balloon technique, *Cathet Cardiovasc Diagn* 13:151, 1987.

Durbin CG, Kopel RF: Optimization of cardiac output in A-V sequential pacing using SvO_2 monitoring, *Anesthesiology* 71:A202, 1989.

Edwards JD: Oxygen transport in cardiogenic and septic shock, *Crit Care Med* 19:658, 1991.

Finch CA, Lenfant C: Oxygen transport in man, *N Engl J Med* 286:407, 1972.

Garr JL, Gentilello LM, Cole PA, et al: Monitoring for compartment syndrome using near-infrared spectroscopy: a noninvasive, continuous, transcutaneous monitoring technique, *J Trauma* 46:613, 1999.

Gettinger A, Detraglia MC, Glass DD: In vivo comparison of two mixed venous oxygen saturation catheters, *Anesthesiology* 70:373, 1987.

Gold WM: Pulmonary function testing. In Murray JF, Nadel JA, editors: *Textbook of respiratory medicine,* ed 3, Philadelphia, 2000, W.B. Saunders.

Greenburg AG: To transfuse or not to transfuse—that is the question! *Crit Care Med* 18:1045, 1990.

Hanning CD, Alexander-Williams JM: Pulse oximetry: a practical review, *BMJ* 311:311, 1995.

Headley JM: Invasive hemodynamic monitoring: applying advanced technologies, *Crit Care Nurs Q* 21:73, 1998.

Hess D: Respiratory monitoring. In Hurford WE, editor: *Critical care handbook of the Massachusetts General Hospital,* ed 30, Philadelphia, 2000, Lippincott Williams & Wilkins.

Horst HM et al: Factors influencing survival of elderly trauma patients, *Crit Care Med* 14:681, 1986.

Jubran A: Pulse oximetry. In Tobin MJ, editor: *Principles and practice of intensive care monitoring,* New York, 1998, McGraw-Hill.

Kupeli IA, Satwicz PR: Mixed venous oximetry, *Int Anesth Clin* 27:176, 1989.

Lee SE, Tremper KK, Barker SJ: Effects of anemia on pulse oximetry and mixed venous oxygen saturation in dogs, *Anesth Analg* 67:S130, 1988.

Liggett SB, St John RE, Lefrak SS: Determination of resting energy expenditure utilizing the thermodilution pulmonary artery catheter, *Chest* 91:562, 1987.

McGee WT, Veremakis C, Wilson GL: Clinical importance of tissue oxygenation and use of the mixed venous blood gas, *Res Medica* 4:15, 1988.

McKinley BA, Marvin RG, Cocanour CS: Tissue hemoglobin oxygen saturation during resuscitation of traumatic shock monitored using near infrared spectrometry, *J Trauma* 48:637, 2000.

McKinley BA, Parmley CL: Clinical trial of an ex vivo arterial blood gas monitor, *J Crit Care* 13:4, 1998.

Rackow EC, Astiz ME, Weil MH: Cellular oxygen metabolism during sepsis and shock, *JAMA* 259:1989, 1988.

Ralley FE, Wynands JE, Ramsay JG, et al: The effects of shivering on oxygen consumption and carbon dioxide production in patients rewarming from hypothermic cardiopulmonary bypass, *Can J Anaesth* 35:332, 1988.

Rasanen J, Downs JB, Malec RJ: Oxygen tensions and oxyhemoglobin saturations in the assessment of pulmonary gas exchange, *Crit Care Med* 15:1058, 1987.

Shibutani K, Olortegui G, Sanchala V, et al: The relationship between cardiac output and mixed venous oxygen saturation: an influence of timing and sampling, *Anesthesiology* 71:A378, 1989.

Shoemaker WC, Appel PL, Kram HB, et al: Prospective trial of supranormal values as therapeutic goals in high-risk surgical patients, *Chest* 94(6):1176, 1988.

Snyder JV: *Oxygen transport in the critically ill,* Chicago, 1987, Year Book.

Waite RM, Parsons D: Measurement of SvO_2, HR, and MAP in myocardial revascularization patients upon initial postoperative activity, *Crit Care Nurse* 11:87, 1990.

Walsh JM, Vanderwarf C, Hoschiet D, et al: Unsuspected hemodynamic alterations during endotracheal suctioning, *Chest* 95:162, 1989.

White KM et al: The physiologic basis for SvO_2 monitoring, *Heart Lung* 19:548, 1990.

Wolf YG, Cotev S, Perel A, et al: Dependence of oxygen consumption on cardiac output in sepsis, *Crit Care Med* 15:198, 1987.

CARE OF CRITICALLY ILL AND INJURED PATIENTS

13

ANAND KUMAR, ELIZABETH KRZYWDA, and GLORIA OBLOUK DAROVIC

Infusion-Related Sepsis

Technologic advances over the past three decades have resulted in increasingly complex medical and surgical therapies for the management of critically ill patients. Some of the most important advances have been in the area of vascular access for continuous hemodynamic monitoring, as well as infusion therapy for administration of fluids, drugs, total parenteral nutrition (TPN), and blood products. Hemodynamic monitoring and infusion therapy are dependent on stable vascular access through peripheral intravenous (IV), central venous, or intraarterial catheters.

Although continuous vascular access is one of the most essential modalities in modern-day medicine, it carries substantial and generally underappreciated potential for producing iatrogenic complications, the most important of which is blood-borne infection.

This chapter focuses on the pathogenesis, diagnosis, prevention, and management of infectious complications of intravascular cannulation and fluid infusion. In this text, the term *colonization* refers to the presence and growth of viable microorganisms on the mucosa, skin, or in situ catheter in the absence of infection. Colonization may or may not be a precursor of infection. *Infection* represents a microbial phenomenon characterized by an inflammatory response to the presence of microorganisms or the invasion of normally sterile host tissue by microorganisms. *Bacteremia* is the presence of viable bacteria in the blood (usually demonstrated by positive blood culture).[1] The term *catheter colonization* refers to the growth of significant numbers of organisms from the catheter surface in the absence of accompanying clinical symptoms. *Catheter infection* implies catheter colonization with accompanying

clinical manifestations suggestive of infection. *Nosocomial infection* is any infection acquired in the hospital. *Sepsis* represents the systemic response to infection (usually including various combinations of fever, tachycardia, tachypnea, and leukocytosis). This is typically associated with the presence of bacterial toxins or endogenous inflammatory mediators in the circulation. *Septicemia* is an older term, often used interchangeably with sepsis, frequently used to imply sepsis with presumed bacteremia. The general term *catheter-related sepsis* (CRS) refers to sepsis and septic complications specifically due to the presence of intravascular catheters. *Catheter-related bloodstream infection* (CR-BSI) is a related formal term that indicates the isolation of identical infectious organisms from a catheter segment and from blood in a patient with CRS. Another related formal term, *infusate-related bloodstream infection* (IR-BSI), is more specific, indicating isolation of the same organism from infusate and percutaneous blood cultures. In contrast, *infusion device–related sepsis* (IRS) is a highly inclusive general term that relates to all sepsis and septic complications secondary to invasive monitoring and therapeutic devices, including vascular catheters, fluid delivery systems, and infused solutions. Several of these terms are more precisely defined in the section on standardized microbiologic definitions of intravascular device–related infections.

Infusion-related sepsis is a relatively new concept. Until the 1960s, intravascular catheters or fluid systems were rarely considered by clinicians to be the infective source in septic patients.[2] In 1971, however, a nationwide epidemic of infusion-related *Enterobacter* bacteremia was traced to the contaminated parenteral products of one manufacturer.[3] Since that time, many additional infectious outbreaks have greatly enhanced awareness of the problem of infusion-related sepsis and have advanced our understanding of the epidemiology and pathogenesis of intravascular device–related infection.[3-5]

INCIDENCE

More than one half of the 40 million patients hospitalized in the United States each year receive some form of infusion therapy.[6] Since 150 million intravascular catheters, including 5 million pulmonary artery catheters, are sold annually in the United States, it is clear that many patients are intravascularly catheterized several times during the course of their illness. The true incidence of infusion-related sepsis is difficult to determine. Signs and symptoms of systemic sepsis are nonspecific, and local signs and symptoms are relatively uncommon. For this reason, clinicians often fail to consider the diagnosis of infusion-related sepsis. Over time, the infecting vascular catheter may be removed from a septicemic patient because it is no longer functional. The patient may then spontaneously recover. As a consequence, the primary infecting source is never identified. Alternatively, patients may die without the vascular septic source ever having been implicated or identified.

Available estimates suggest that almost 1 million vascular device–related infections occur annually.[7] The percent of intravascular catheters producing systemic bloodstream infection is estimated to be less than 1%. However, when this incidence rate is applied to the estimated 20 to 40 million patients who receive IV therapy, it is apparent that 300,000 to 400,000 recipients of such therapy acquire preventable bloodstream infections each year[8] (Figure 13-1). Half or more of these occur in the intensive care unit (ICU),[7] and more than one half of all epidemics of hospital-acquired (nosocomial) bacteremia and candidemia are shown to be infusion related.[4,9,10] Nosocomial infusion-related bacteremia or candidemia is associated with a twofold to threefold increase in attributable mortality rate.[9,11-13] Based on an attributable mortality rate of 3% to 25%, depending on the study,[14-16] between 500 and 4000 patients lose their lives to CRS each year in the United States.[17]

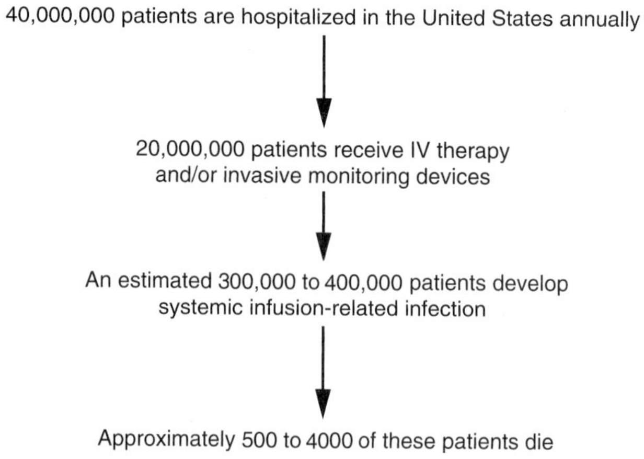

Hamory[5] reported that from 1975 to 1983, the specific microorganisms causing nosocomial bacteremias did not change. However, during that period, the proportion of primary bacteremias without an identifiable source caused by coagulase-negative staphylococci, usually *Staphylococcus epidermidis,* rose from 6.5% to 14.2%. The proportion of

40,000,000 patients are hospitalized in the United States annually

↓

20,000,000 patients receive IV therapy and/or invasive monitoring devices

↓

An estimated 300,000 to 400,000 patients develop systemic infusion-related infection

↓

Approximately 500 to 4000 of these patients die

FIGURE 13-1 The estimated incidence and mortality rate of infusion-related sepsis in hospitalized patients in the United States.

candidemias rose from less than 3.5% to 5.6% of primary bacteremias. Because these pathogens are among those most frequently implicated in IRS, Hamory[5] interpreted these findings as suggesting that most primary bacteremias and candidemias originate from intravascular devices. Other data from the Centers for Disease Control and Prevention (CDC) suggest that while the incidence of secondary bacteremia due to local infection (cellulitis, pneumonia, urinary tract infection, etc.) has remained constant, the incidence of primary nosocomial bloodstream infection (mostly central venous catheter related) has more than doubled over the last decade.[10,18] The cost of treating IRS in ICU patients rose from $8,000 per case in 1988 to $28,000 per case in 1994.[14,19,20]

In summary, catheter-related sepsis is often unsuspected by clinicians. Consequently, neither the catheter nor the infusate (fluid) given through the catheter is cultured.[2,4,21] Thus the true incidence of catheter-related sepsis is probably considerably higher than published estimates might suggest. The consequences of these infections are prolonged hospitalization, increased hospital cost, and, in up to 10% of the cases, a fatal outcome.[3-6]

STANDARDIZED MICROBIOLOGIC DEFINITIONS OF INTRAVASCULAR DEVICE–RELATED INFECTIONS

The CDC has published guidelines for prevention of intravascular device–related infections.[22] These guidelines also provide standardized microbiologic definitions for catheter-related infections. Definitions are not necessarily mutually exclusive. Infusion device–related infections are classified according to the following criteria and correlate with clinical syndromes.

Contamination

Contamination is the presence of microorganisms on the catheter taken to the laboratory for culture, inadvertently introduced while removing the catheter. Although a colony-forming unit (CFU) count of less than 15 colonies on semiquantitative culture suggests contamination, there is no definitive means of differentiating a contaminated specimen from a colonized or infected specimen. Diagnostic confusion is compounded by the fact that the most common contaminant, the most common colonizer, and the most common infecting organisms are coagulase-negative staphylococci. Therefore meticulous technique when collecting and preparing the specimen is essential to avoid diagnostic confusion.

Catheter Colonization

A positive semiquantitative (agar plate) culture showing bacterial growth greater than 15 CFU or quantitative (broth) culture greater than 1000 CFU of either the proximal or distal catheter segment in the absence of accompanying signs of inflammation at the catheter site is considered to be synonymous with colonization of the catheter.[20,22-29] Some authors have suggested that a quantitative culture of greater than 100 CFU is sufficient to define colonization rather than contamination.[28,29] Colonization may occur in the complete absence of notable clinical signs or symptoms. Positive semiquantitative cultures have a 15% to 40% concordance with concomitant bacteremia and are usually but not always associated with inflammation at the insertion site.

Catheter Infection

The term *catheter infection* indicates a positive semiquantitative or quantitative culture of the catheter in association with accompanying signs of local inflammation (e.g., erythema, warmth, swelling, or tenderness) at the device site.[22] In the absence of positive quantitative or semiquantitative cultures of a catheter segment, catheter infection can still be diagnosed when there is purulent drainage from the skin-catheter junction.

Exit Site Infection

Redness, tenderness, swelling, or purulence within 2 cm of the catheter exit site that may be associated with other signs of infection, including fever, indicates an exit site infection (infection at the catheter insertion site).[22] This is usually associated with catheter colonization and may be associated with CR-BSI.

Tunnel Infection

Redness, tenderness, and swelling in the tissues overlying the catheter tract and more than 2 cm from the catheter exit site indicate a tunnel infection. Associated signs of infection, including fever, may be present.[22]

Catheter-Related Bloodstream Infection

Catheter-related bloodstream infection is formally defined as isolation of the same organism (i.e., identical species, antibiogram) from a semiquantitative or quantitative catheter segment culture and from blood culture (preferably drawn from a peripheral vein) of a patient with clinical manifestations of bloodstream infection. Direct culture of the infusate should be negative. Clinical or autopsy microbiologic data should disclose no other apparent source of bacteremia. In the absence of laboratory confirmation, defervescence after catheter removal may serve as indirect evidence of CR-BSI.[22-26,30]

Infusate-Related Bloodstream Infection

Infusate-related bloodstream infection is formally defined as isolation of the same organism from infusate and from separate percutaneous blood cultures, with no other identifiable source of infection.[20,22,23,30] Typically, the patient has clinical and laboratory evidence of sepsis. Culture of the catheter is negative or isolates an unrelated organism. This term is much more specific than the term *infusion device–related sepsis* as used in this text.

CLINICAL SYNDROMES OF INFUSION-RELATED INFECTION

Four major clinical syndromes of IRS exist.

Asymptomatic Local Colonization of the Catheter, Colonization of the Catheter Hub, or Low-Level Colonization of the Infusate

In hospitalized patients, the skin and mucous membranes are often colonized with pathogenic, antibiotic-resistant bacteria. Colonization means that potentially pathogenic microorganisms are present, but evidence of both local tissue inflammation and systemic infection is absent. Consequently, the patient is asymptomatic. In the context of an intravascular catheter, colonization implies that there is no overt clinical consequence even though catheter or infusate cultures are positive. In hospitalized patients, between 5% and 25% of intravascular catheters cultured after routine removal demonstrate evidence of colonization. This condition is also occasionally referred to as *asymptomatic catheter infection*. Although this condition is intrinsically benign, it provides a biologic condition that favors development of bacteremia.

Symptomatic Local Infection

When the colonized microorganisms have invaded and infected the tissue, an inflammatory response may be evident as local redness, pain, swelling, heat, or purulence at the vascular access site. However, in severely debilitated or immune-compromised patients (patients with organ transplant, neutropenia, acquired immunodeficiency syndrome, etc.), these classic clinical findings may be minimal or absent. The infection may primarily involve the skin and surface soft tissue (exit site infection) or may involve the catheter tract (tunnel infection) with expressible purulence. Catheter cultures are positive although infusate cultures may be negative. Local infection may resolve or may become blood borne and progress to systemic infection.

Sepsis Arising from an Infected Catheter or from a Contaminated Infusate

Signs of local inflammation may or may not be present. Symptoms or signs of systemic infection are invariably present. Low-grade fever is a common symptom in patients with systemic infusion–related infection involving *S. epidermidis.* Other organisms may produce marked hyperthermia (pyrexia [fever]) or hypothermia, depending on the organism and on the patient's overall health, nutritional, and immune status. Other early septic symptoms and signs include changes in mental status, tachypnea, tachycardia, malaise, chills, myalgia, and fatigue. Elevations in blood glucose and changes in the white blood cell and platelet counts may be noted on laboratory examination. Blood cultures may be positive and, if so, should match the catheter or infusate culture. Septic shock is rare; however, contaminated infusate is more likely to be associated with shock than is catheter infection or CR-BSI.

Septic Thrombophlebitis, Septic Thrombosis of a Great Central Vein, or Septic Endarteritis of a Cannulated Artery

Each produces high-grade and unremitting bacteremia or fungemia with fulminant signs of overwhelming infection, which persist even after the catheter has been removed.[2,4,21] These are the most serious forms of catheter-related infection and usually originate from central venous catheters that have been used for prolonged periods in patients at high risk of nosocomial infection.[2,21] The cannulated segment of the vessel becomes filled by an infected thrombus. The clinical course is predictable—unremitting bloodstream infection that often proves fatal. Interestingly, patients with formation of pus at the infected, thrombosed site (suppurative

phlebitis) may develop signs and symptoms of systemic infection only after the catheter has been removed.[2] Culture of the catheter is positive. Organisms isolated from the blood, thrombus, or adjacent resected parts of the vessel should match those isolated from the catheter.

Local inflammation of a peripheral IV catheter, termed *peripheral phlebitis,* may be a harbinger of infection and warrants prompt removal of the catheter as a precaution.[2,21] However, most patients with infusion phlebitis do not develop catheter-related sepsis, and suppurative phlebitis of peripheral IV catheters is now extremely rare.[21] However, phlebitis can be an indicator of IR-BSI. For example, during a large nationwide epidemic of sepsis caused by contaminated fluids from one manufacturer, patients with IR-BSI had a higher incidence of phlebitis than patients who did not develop sepsis from the contaminated IV fluids.[3]

PATHOGENESIS OF INFUSION-RELATED SEPSIS

When a catheter is placed in a blood vessel, a fibrin sheath quickly develops around the catheter. The clot generally produces no circulatory problem but serves as a nidus for bacterial or fungal colonization (Figure 13-2).[2] Bacterial or fungal colonization of the intravascular device may occur via several mechanisms.

Migration of Cutaneous Flora down the Skin Tract to the Intravascular Catheter

Aerobic microorganisms of cutaneous origin, such as coagulase-negative staphylococcus (usually *S. epidermidis*), *Staphylococcus aureus,* enterococci, or *Candida,* gain intravascular access through the insertion wound. The insertion site is commonly colonized heavily by the patient's endogenous cutaneous flora or becomes colonized by microorganisms from the hands of the medical personnel inserting or manipulating the catheter.[2,20,21,23,31-33] Maki and co-workers,[20] in a prospective study of 234 central venous catheters, found that the majority of early infections of percutaneously inserted central venous catheters originated from the skin at the insertion site rather than contamination of the hub. Overall, in venous catheters, there is a strong correlation between skin microorganisms present on the catheter insertion site and microorganisms implicated in catheter-related sepsis based on molecular typing.[20,23,32,33] The most common organism found in catheter-related infection is *S. epidermidis,* the predominant aerobic species on the human skin. The risk of other, more pathogenic organisms rises with the pres-

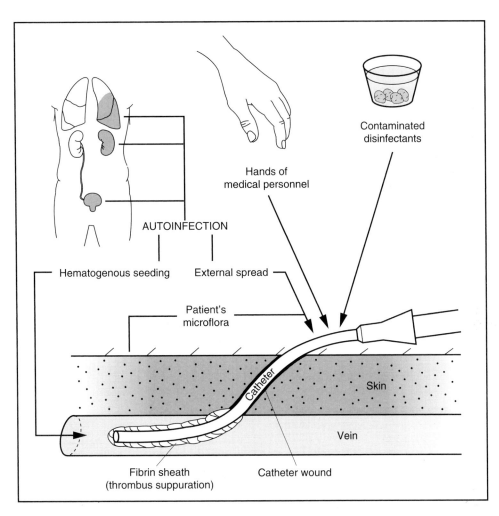

FIGURE 13-2 Potential sources of infusion-related sepsis. (Redrawn from *American Journal of Medicine*. Maki DG: Potential sources for infusion-related infection, *Am J Med* 70:719, 1981.)

ence and duration of severe illness. Traumatic or careless insertion technique increases the infectious risk.

Reliable disinfection of the insertion site with an effective skin antiseptic before insertion of an intravascular device would seem to be of great importance for prevention of infection. However, environmental contaminants or regrowth of the patient's suppressed endogenous flora can later invade the catheter wound and cause infection.[23]

Bloodstream Dissemination and Catheter Colonization with Microorganisms from a Distant Septic Focus

The vascular catheter may become colonized by hematogenous seeding from remote sites of infection. For example, if patients have *Escherichia coli* bacteremia from an intraabdominal source, vascular catheters may become seeded and

colonized with *E. coli*. The infected catheter may then, in turn, reseed the blood, thus propagating systemic infection even if the original septic focus has been eliminated. It has been suggested that CRS from certain organisms (yeast, enterococci, and enteric gram-negative organisms) may often result from hematogenous spread.[34,35]

Manipulation and Contamination of the Catheter Hub

The hub of the catheter also may be a potential source of catheter-related sepsis. Sitges-Serra and colleagues[36] have suggested that the hub of the central venous catheter, rather than the intracutaneous tract, is the most important source of microorganisms infecting the catheter and bloodstream. They reported little correlation between organisms found on the patient's skin and organisms found on the hub and on the catheter, but reported frequent contamination of catheter hubs and correlation with bacteremia. These investigators suggested that hubs became colonized during manipulation by clinicians. Maki and colleagues[20] confirmed the occurrence of hub contamination but were unable to demonstrate a major role in early catheter-related sepsis. Through the use of electron microscopy, Raad and colleagues[37] were able to demonstrate that hub contamination was the more likely mechanism of infection for long-term catheters (longer than 30 days). Skin contamination was more likely in catheters in place less than 10 days.

Although the role of hub contamination in CRS is unclear, *meticulous aseptic technique when manipulating the catheter hub, as well as limiting hub manipulation, is essential in reducing patients' septic risk.* The incidence and role of positive hub cultures in the pathogenesis of catheter-related infection with arterial catheters has not been investigated.

Contamination of the Delivery System

The catheter and hub are not the only elements of a vascular infusion that can produce infection. The delivery system, consisting of the fluid (infusate), stopcock, pressure transducer, and tubing, also can be a source of contamination, particularly epidemic nosocomial bacteremia (especially gram-negative bacteremia).[3-6]

Closed delivery systems are often deliberately disrupted for the addition of medications and electrolytes, as well as withdrawal of blood for laboratory studies by members of the ICU staff. Accidental disconnection or leaks in the closed system may also occur. Overall, any disruption of the closed system and manipulation of infusion fluids may introduce microorganisms into the system.

Arterial lines are particularly vulnerable to contamination because they are so heavily manipulated. In all monitoring systems, meticulous care of stopcocks, replacing the sterile protective caps after withdrawal of blood, and flushing the sampling port of remaining blood are essential to prevention of delivery system contamination.

Infusate contamination may also be a source of bacteremia or fungemia, but infusate-related infection can be identified only if the solution is cultured. This is rarely done in clinical practice because despite occasional epidemics, endemic bacteremia caused by extrinsically contaminated fluid during administration appears to be rare.[20,21,23] Based on anecdotal data, risk of infusate contamination may be higher with TPN and IV lipid emulsion–based medications such as propofol.[38-40]

DIAGNOSIS OF INFUSION-RELATED SEPSIS

Clinicians too often fail to consider the diagnosis of infusion-related sepsis because clinical signs and symptoms are generally indistinguishable from bloodstream infections arising from other sites, such as the urinary tract or lung. Sepsis from infected catheters and contaminated infusate also produce similar clinical features.[2] Generally, the diagnosis of catheter- or infusate-related infection should be considered whenever the patient has catheter insertion site or systemic signs or symptoms of infection, particularly if the patient has no other identifiable septic focus. Maki[9,21] has listed six clinical and three microbiologic findings that should alert the clinician to the possibility of infusion-related sepsis and prompt appropriate cultures and, in most cases, discontinuation of the infusion and removal of the catheter (Box 13-1).

BOX 13-1
Findings Suggestive of Infusion-Related Sepsis

Clinical
1. Intravascular device in place at time of onset of sepsis, bacteremia, or candidemia (especially central venous catheter)
2. Patient is an unlikely candidate for sepsis, being young or without underlying predisposing diseases
3. Inflammation or expressible purulence at the catheter insertion site
4. Primary bacteremia or candidemia without apparent source of local infection
5. Precipitous onset of overwhelming sepsis with shock (often indicative of massively contaminated infusate or intravascular suppuration)
6. Sepsis refractory to appropriate antimicrobial therapy or substantial improvement following removal of catheter or discontinuation of infusion

Microbiologic
1. Bacteremia caused by staphylococci (especially coagulase-negative staphylococci), *Bacillus* species, *Corynebacteria, Candida* species, and certain fungi or mycobacteria
2. Clusters of institutional outbreaks of sepsis due to *Enterobacter* species, *Serratia marcescens,* or *Pseudomonas* species other than *P. aeruginosa*
3. High-grade candidemia (greater than 25 CFU/ml peripheral blood)

Ideally, when CRS or IRS is suspected, several cultures should be obtained. These should include a blood culture drawn from the suspected catheter, one or more peripheral blood cultures (from separate venipuncture sites), and, if the clinical presentation warrants, culture of the infusate in broth. If the suspected catheter is removed, semiquantitative tip culture should be performed. Blood cultures should be drawn before antibiotic administration whenever possible. The technique for obtaining blood cultures is described in Box 13-2.

A firm diagnosis of IRS can be made only by demonstrating a colonized intravascular catheter or contamination of infusion solution, associated with culture-determined bacteremia or fungemia caused by the same microbial strain.[21] Negative catheter tip and infusion solution culture findings in the presence of bacteremia or fungemia strongly suggest that the IV device and solution are not the septic source.

When IRS is suspected, the catheter should be removed if possible (exceptions include limited situations involving surgically tunneled catheters or catheters that are unquestionably necessary and would be extremely high risk to replace; in such situations, treatment of the catheter in situ may be attempted). The intravascular segment of the catheter is severed aseptically and then cultured.[2,21] Catheter segments may be cultured semiquantitatively rather than using broth cultures (qualitative culture). The clinical interpretation of a positive catheter culture in liquid media is uncertain because a single contaminating organism acquired from the skin as the catheter is being removed can produce a positive culture.[24] Positive broth culture findings have not correlated well with signs of catheter site inflammation. The percent of catheters showing positive cultures in broth is often many times higher than the true rate of catheter-related sepsis.[24]

The semiquantitative culture technique described by Maki and colleagues[20] is now widely used to diagnose catheter-related infection.[5,25,26,32] (Technique for obtaining the catheter tip is described in Box 13-3.)

In the laboratory, the catheter is transferred to a blood agar plate labeled with the patient's name and catheter

---

BOX 13-2
Blood Culture Specimen Collection

Collect blood for culture by direct venipuncture and from different sites for subsequent blood cultures. A positive culture drawn from an intravascular catheter may be due to line colonization, not bacteremia.

Procedure

1. Remove the flip top from aerobic and anaerobic blood culture bottles. Scrub the rubber stoppers with an antiseptic prep pad (tincture of iodine is recommended over 10% providone-iodine).
2. Prepare the skin site for 1 minute with antiseptic starting at the center of the site and moving outward in a circular direction. Allow to dry. Repeat the iodine preparation a second time for another minute; allow to dry. Iodine may be removed following the preparation with an alcohol pad to improve visualization of the vein.
3. Wear sterile gloves while palpating the venipuncture site.
4. Perform venipuncture, withdrawing blood into a 20 or 30 ml syringe.
5. Do not change the needle before injecting blood into broth bottles because of the risk of inadvertent needle stick.
6. Inject 10 to 15 ml of blood into each aerobic and anaerobic bottle (the largest amount accommodated by the specific manufacturer's blood culture bottles because a large volume of blood for culture maximizes the sensitivity of the culture for diagnosis of bacteremia and candidemia).
7. Label and deliver the specimen to the laboratory immediately.
8. Broth with antibiotic binding resins may be preferred if antibiotic therapy was begun before collection of specimen.

BOX 13-3
Catheter Culture Specimen Collection

1. Wear goggles and nonsterile gloves.
2. Remove the dressings and cleanse the site with an antiseptic pledget.
3. Open a suture removal kit, remove nonsterile gloves, and put on sterile gloves.
4. Avoid skin contact while slowly removing the catheter.
5. Cut the catheter and transport the catheter segment(s), held by tweezers, to the sterile specimen container and drop inside. *Short catheters (arterial, peripheral venous):* Following catheter removal, aseptically cut the portion of the catheter that was within the vessel and transport it to the laboratory in a sterile container. *Long catheters (central venous or pulmonary artery):* Obtain two segments for culture: a proximal segment that began several millimeters inside the former skin-catheter interface and the tip of the catheter.
6. Label and send the specimen to the laboratory immediately.

type. Using flamed forceps, the catheter is rolled or smeared (if unable to be rolled) back and forth across the plate four times. A downward pressure is exerted on the catheter with the forceps to ensure that the entire catheter remains in contact with the agar plate. The plate is then incubated. Detecting 15 or more colonies growing on a semiquantitative plate is regarded as a positive culture. Positive semiquantitative cultures have a 15% to 40% concordance with concomitant bacteremia and are strongly associated with inflammation at the insertion site.[5,20,21,24-26,32]

The more arduous quantitative culture techniques using broth culture of catheter segments (greater than 100 to 1000 CFU defines true colonization) have proponents.[27-29] However, studies suggest that culture of the external surface of the catheter segment, which reflects the microbiologic status of the percutaneous wound and intravascular environment, distinguishes true catheter-related infection from contamination more reliably than the quantitative broth culture method.[24] Culturing catheters semiquantitatively also allows for more rapid identification of clinically significant isolates, because microbial growth usually occurs within 12 to 18 hours, whereas quantitative (broth) culture growth may take 24 to 48 hours. As a practical matter, most centers offer semiquantitative catheter culture rather than quantitative.

For those catheters that cannot be removed and safely replaced, comparison of quantitative peripheral and catheter-drawn blood cultures can make the diagnosis of catheter-associated bacteremia or fungemia (without catheter removal) with a sensitivity and specificity of approximately 90%.[9,19,41-43] Quantitative cultures of blood drawn from infected central venous catheters are usually 5 to 10 times higher than those from peripheral blood. Similarly, intraluminal brushes[44] and specialized staining of cytospin of lysed blood[45] drawn from infected central lines shows potential in diagnosis of CRS without removal of the catheter. However, these techniques make medical and economic sense only in assessment of long-term indwelling catheters where intraluminal colonization is likely and where the patient's condition makes removal and replacement of the intravascular catheter unacceptably risky.

A sudden onset of septic symptoms shortly after the start of infusion is suggestive of contamination of the intravenous fluid. *If infusate contamination is suspected, the infusion must be immediately terminated.* The entire infusate apparatus and infusate bag should be transported to the microbiology laboratory, where infusate is aseptically removed and cultured in broth.

Meticulous aseptic technique is likewise required for collecting and preparing both blood and catheter tip cultures. Contaminated blood or catheter tip cultures may result in a misdiagnosis of sepsis that lengthens the hospital stay and increases costs, as well as incurring the inappropriate use of antibiotics.

MICROORGANISMS ASSOCIATED WITH INFUSION-RELATED SEPSIS

CRS is associated with two major groups of organisms: those that are part of the normal skin flora (coagulase-negative staphylococci, *S. aureus, Bacillus* species, *Corynebacterium* species) and those organisms that are transferred from the hands of medical staff and equipment (*Pseudomonas aeruginosa, Acinetobacter* species, *Stenotrophomonas maltophila,* and *Candida* species). Certain microorganisms are so prevalent in catheter-related infection that their recovery from blood should substantially raise the suspicion that an intravascular catheter is the source. These include *S. aureus, S. epidermidis,* and *Candida*—the most common organisms in sepsis from infected catheters. For example, high-grade candidemia (greater than 25 CFU/ml of peripheral blood) indicates CRBSI in greater than 90% of cases.[46]

Contaminated infusate solution is strongly suggested by isolation of *Enterobacter cloacae, Enterobacter agglomerans,* or *Pseudomonas cepacia* because these are major pathogens in sepsis from contaminated fluid.[2-5,21] The latter gram-negative organisms are able to multiply rapidly in 5% dextrose in water solution.[2-4,21] For this reason, the use of dextrose-containing solutions as irrigants for intravascular monitoring catheters should be discouraged. Box 13-4 describes common pathogens associated with IRS.

Because *S. epidermidis* is a normal skin inhabitant, in the past, blood culture reports of *S. epidermidis* were

---

BOX 13-4
Common Microorganisms in Infusion-Related Sepsis

Infected Catheters
Coagulase-negative staphylococci (commonly *S. epidermidis*)
Candida
Staphylococcus aureus

Contaminated Fluids
Enterobacter cloacae
Enterobacter agglomerans
Pseudomonas cepacia

considered to be the result of skin contamination. Studies of central venous and peripheral venous catheter–related infections indicate that coagulase-negative staphylococci such as *S. epidermidis* are now the most common pathogens in IV catheter-related sepsis and one of the most important pathogens in infection of all types of percutaneous and implantable devices.* Coagulase-negative staphylococci are important nosocomial pathogens because of their increasing resistance to many commonly used antibiotic agents and their ability to adhere to and colonize vascular catheters. Many strains can withstand the application of topical antiseptics and can grow well on foreign bodies and disrupted epithelium.[2,4,21]

RISK FACTORS FOR INFUSION-RELATED SEPSIS

Understanding and consideration of the risk factors and sources of microorganisms predisposing patients to infusion-related infections may guide the development and implementation of control measures for prevention of these potentially lethal complications. The risk factors that predispose the patient to infusion-related sepsis include (1) patient factors, (2) therapy-related factors, and (3) catheter-specific factors (Box 13-5).

Patient Factors

Many patient and therapeutic factors predict an increased risk of nosocomial infection. Prospective studies have shown that patient age over 65; severe and numerous underlying diseases; sepsis; major trauma, surgery, or burns; invasive devices; underlying immune system dysfunction or immunosuppressive drugs; breakdown of anatomic barriers; and confinement in a critical care environment are associated with an increased risk of infection.[4,47-49] For the most part, these risk factors usually are not the cause of the infection but rather increase patient vulnerability to infection. Catheter-related infection is also more likely to occur if a catheter is inserted in a septicemic patient or if an inflammation (burn or traumatic injury) preexists or subsequently develops at the catheter insertion site.

Therapy-Related Factors

Overall, patients in ICUs have the highest risk profile for complicating infection. Most of these patients endure prolonged hospitalization and have serious underlying conditions associated with disease-related immune system impairment. Virtually all critically ill patients are exposed to multiple invasive procedures and monitoring equipment, and

*References 2, 4, 20, 21, 23, 31–33.

BOX 13-5
Risk Factors for Infusion-Related Sepsis

Patient-Related Factors
1. Extremes of age (neonates or age greater than 65 years)
2. Critical illness/sepsis
3. Remote active infection with coincident vascular catheter
4. Impaired host defenses
5. Major trauma
6. Major surgery
7. Major burn injury
8. Malnutrition
9. Immunosuppressive diseases (e.g., diabetes mellitus, uremia, chronic alcoholism, liver disease, neutropenia)
10. Interruption of anatomic barriers (e.g., severe psoriasis or eczema, major burns or wounds, mucositis)

Therapy-Related Factors
1. Catheter insertion or maintenance by other than a dedicated team
2. Multiple invasive devices
3. Hospitalization in intensive care unit
4. Use of immunosuppressive or antibiotic drugs
5. Use of total parenteral nutrition
6. Excessive time intervals (longer than 5 days) between replacement of components of the delivery system
7. Excessive time intervals between dressing changes (longer than 3 days) or failure to change dressings when soiled
8. Faulty decontamination of transducer between patients (reusable transducers)

Catheter-Specific Factors
1. Open surgical placement (cutdown rather than percutaneous)
2. Emergent rather than elective catheter insertion
3. Use of polyvinyl chloride or polyethylene catheters, polyurethane, or Teflon (for peripheral intravenous catheters)
4. Complex closed delivery system with multiple stopcocks and other ports
5. Interruption of closed fluid-filled system or need for catheter manipulation after initial insertion
6. Prolonged intravascular retention (longer than 5 days)
7. Suboptimal skin decontamination (2% chlorhexidine is superior to 10% providine-iodine or 70% alcohol)
8. Use of multilumen rather than single-lumen catheter (possible)
9. Failure to use antiseptic or antibiotic-bonded catheter
10. Failure to use catheter with silver-impregnated tissue cuff
11. Internal jugular rather than subclavian insertion site (femoral site risk intermediate)

many receive TPN or acute hemodialysis, both of which are associated with increased risk of IRS. Other therapeutic factors that may result in increased risk of catheter-related infection include prolonged supine positioning and suboptimal perianal hygiene, which allows for rapid dissemination of fecal organisms over the skin; care by multiple hospital personnel, which increases the risk of cross-contamination; and use of immunosuppressive drugs. Antibiotic therapy, common to nearly all ICU patients, increases the septic risk by destroying patients' normal bacterial flora. This allows colonization of skin and mucous membranes by the antibiotic-resistant pathogens indigenous to the ICU environment.

Catheter-Related Factors

Poor aseptic technique is unquestionably associated with risk of catheter or infusate infection. This is related not only to the technique of catheter insertion but also to the quality of aseptic technique during vascular line maintenance. Studies have shown that the use of a team specifically trained for catheter insertion and maintenance (termed *dedicated team*) can significantly reduce central venous catheter infection rates.[50-52] One study reported that the infection rate associated with central venous catheters for TPN before the establishment of a nutrition support team was 24.0%, whereas the infection rate during the 32 months the TPN team was used was only 3.5%.[50] Increased catheter longevity also appears to be a benefit of the dedicated IV team. Investigators in a study of the infection rate of peripheral venous catheters found a significantly lower rate of phlebitis (15%) and suppurative phlebitis (0.2%) with intravenous catheters inserted and maintained by a dedicated IV team compared with those inserted and maintained by the unit staff (30% and 1%, respectively).[52]

Traumatic vascular catheter insertion, frequently associated with emergency therapy, results in tissue damage that may serve as a nidus for infection. The compelling nature of a crisis situation often requires line insertion without strict adherence to sterile technique, which compounds the infectious risk. For these reasons, intravascular catheters placed during an emergency should be removed and replaced using aseptic technique as soon as the patient's condition is stabilized or within 24 hours.

The longer the vascular catheter is left in place, the greater the risk for local and systemic infection. An indwelling time longer than 5 days significantly increases the risk of catheter-related infection.[9,53]

A number of other factors are related to the infectious risk of specific types of intravascular catheters. These include catheter material, type of catheter placement (risk with cutdown greater than percutaneous), insertion sites for central venous placement (risk with internal jugular greater than subclavian), and type of catheter. The necessity of breaking the closed fluid-filled delivery system and the requirements for catheter manipulation compound any risk factors inherent to the specific type of catheter.

Catheter Material

There is increasing evidence that the material making up an intravascular catheter plays an important role in the pathogenesis of infusion-related infection. As mentioned earlier, a fibrin sheath, which favors bacterial growth, develops around vascular catheters following placement in the circulation. Fibrin formation increases if the catheter surface is not smooth and if the catheter is more reactive within the body (less inert). For this reason, polyvinyl chloride catheters, which are highly thrombogenic, are now available with heparin coating. The majority of catheters in the ICU are made from polyurethane, polyvinyl chloride, polyethylene, or silicone. Although they are thrombogenic, these materials are used by manufacturers because of favorable mechanical properties, including flexibility and tensile strength.

The major infectious risk factor is whether the catheter material provides an attractive surface for adherence by pathogenic microorganisms, such as *S. epidermidis*.[54,55] The majority of published research linking type of catheter material and infection risk has been done with peripheral intravenous catheters. In vitro studies have shown that Teflon, silicone, and polyurethane are more resistant to adherence by coagulase-negative staphylococci than polyvinyl chloride and polyethylene.[56,57] Although conflicting, current data do not support conclusions linking central venous catheter materials to risk of infection.[22]

The development of intravascular catheters and implantable devices that resist microbial adherence and fibrin formation, while retaining desired flexibility characteristics, must receive high priority. This goal remains a major challenge to manufacturers.

Technique for Catheter Placement

Catheter introduction using the Seldinger technique (catheter over a guide wire) for percutaneous catheter placement has almost completely replaced the cutdown technique for vascular access. Studies have clearly demonstrated that surgical cutdown insertion of vascular catheters substantially increases the risk of catheter-related infection.

Specific Central Venous Catheter Insertion Sites

Studies of pulmonary artery and central venous catheters have revealed that there is an increased risk of CRS with insertion in the jugular vein as compared with insertion in the subclavian vein.[58-60] This may be caused by heavier skin colonization with gram-negative rods and yeasts may be the result of the catheter being placed close to the openings of the respiratory tract (tracheostomy tube, nose, mouth). Placement in the femoral veins is generally not preferred because of the heavy growth of bacteria and yeast in the area, the likelihood of site contamination if the patient is involuntary of stool or incontinent of urine, the difficulty in keeping the groin dressing intact and sterile, and the difficulty in immobilizing the patient's leg as well as the risk of deep venous thrombosis incited by the presence of the catheter. Some data suggest an increased risk of infection with femoral venous catheterization compared with subclavian and internal jugular sites.[61] Peripheral placement in the antecubital fossa has generally required cutdown, which, as stated, increases the septic risk. Peripherally inserted central catheters (PICCs), in contrast, appear to be associated with a very low risk of infection.

SEPTIC RISK SPECIFIC TO TYPES OF VASCULAR CATHETERS

Central Venous Catheters

Catheter-related bacteremia or fungemia is the most frequent serious complication of these devices. In fact, 80% to 90% of intravascular device-related bacteremias and candidemias arise from central venous catheters,[10,60,62] and central venous catheterization is the single greatest risk factor for nosocomial candidemia.[11,63,64] The rate of catheter-related infection with central venous catheters is far higher than with peripheral venous catheters, which is in the range of 2% to 7%.*

Except for pulmonary artery catheters, central venous catheters generally have either single or triple lumina. Studies have reported inconsistent results regarding the risk of infection with single- versus triple-lumen catheters. For example, one study reported an incidence of catheter-associated bacteremia of 3.1% with triple-lumen catheters; all bacteremias were caused by *S. epidermidis*.[67] However, this study concluded that catheter-related infection occurred with similar frequency between single- and triple-lumen catheters. Another study, however, demonstrated that triple-lumen catheters were associated with an increased incidence of catheter-related sepsis (19%) compared with single-lumen catheters (3%).[68] An important factor to consider is that, in this latter study, the patients with triple-lumen catheters were more ill, and therefore at greater risk of catheter-related sepsis, than patients with single-lumen catheters.

Because of a lack of prospective, randomized comparative trials, there is still a great deal of controversy as to

the relative risks of infection associated with triple-lumen catheters as compared with single-lumen catheters. Intuitively, the more frequently the greater number of catheter ports are opened (adding medications, obtaining blood samples), the greater the opportunity for ambient microorganisms to enter the fluid system.

Among the variety of central venous catheters, hemodialysis catheters are associated with the highest risk of CRS (approximately 10%).[72-74] Peripherally inserted central venous catheters carry extremely low (less than 1%) risk of infection.[75] The lowest risk of infection is with cuffed, tunnelled, surgically implanted devices (e.g., Hickman, Brovian) with infection risks of 0.2% to 0.5%.[9] Other factors may affect the infection risk. If a central venous catheter is used for pressure measurement, pressure transducers may become colonized. On the other hand, a water manometer also imposes significant septic risk because the fluid may rise and spill over the top of the manometer during pressure measurements and may contaminate the internal system as the water column falls. For this and other reasons, use of water manometers is nearly obsolete.

Balloon Flotation Pulmonary Artery Catheters

Pulmonary artery catheters are widely used in diagnosis and management of critically ill and injured patients. Use of this highly invasive, long vascular catheter is associated with many potential complications (see Chapter 10). Septic complications of pulmonary artery catheters have been documented in many studies since their introduction into clinical medicine in the early 1970s. When evaluating published studies, however, it is difficult to distinguish contamination, colonization, and catheter-related infection from the available data. Consequently, the precise incidence of pulmonary artery catheter-related sepsis is difficult to determine. Some studies have reported a septic rate as high as 5.3%. In a study involving 297 Swan-Ganz catheters, Mermel and coworkers[58] estimated the rate of catheter-related sepsis to be 0.7%. These authors concluded that with "reasonable care" the risk of bacteremic infection is low, generally in the range of 1.0%. However, superficial consideration of this statistically low septic complication rate may minimize the scope of the problem. When the 1% infection rate is applied to the 1.5 million patients who receive pulmonary artery catheters in the United States annually, it suggests that 15,000 patients suffer pulmonary artery catheter-related sepsis. Also, the term *reasonable care* may be variably defined and practiced in different institutions, resulting in an equally variable pulmonary artery catheter infection rate.

Contamination of the pulmonary artery catheter may come from several sources, such as the pressure transducer or stopcocks, but, as with other intravascular

---

*References 20, 25, 26, 31–33, 35, 36, 65–71.

catheters, patients' skin is the single most important reservoir of microbes causing infection. In most cases, it is the catheter introducer that becomes primarily contaminated and not the body of the catheter.

The pulmonary artery catheter sepsis risk is related to the highly thrombogenic and bacterial adherence characteristics of the polyvinyl chloride catheter material. The intracardiac location of portions of the catheter also factors into the septic risk. For example, aseptic endocardial lesions were found at autopsy in 53% of cases with a pulmonary artery catheter in place; however, 7% had right-sided infective endocarditis.[76] The length of time the pulmonary artery catheter was left in place did not seem to be significantly related to the presence of endocardial lesions. The risk of infective endocarditis may be increased if there is an active septic focus or foci and bacteremia or fungemia during the period the pulmonary artery catheter is in place. Two cases of left ventricular abscess formation in patients with *S. aureus* bacteremia and pulmonary artery catheters also have been reported.[77]

The likelihood of introducing microorganisms into the sterile fluid-filled system is increased during cardiac output studies using the open technique (which has largely been replaced by the closed technique) and during blood withdrawal.

Catheter manipulation (advancement) also predisposes the patient to catheter-related sepsis. A sterile protective sleeve, which covers the external portion of the catheter, may offer some protection if catheter advancement is required. The question of how long and to what extent the sleeve ensures sterilization is uncertain. Gradual migration of organisms down the external surface of the catheter and through the distal end of the sheath clearly occurs and renders the "protected" area covered by the sheath nonsterile within hours to days.

Arterial Catheters

Arterial pressure monitoring is an essential component in the management of more than 80% of the 4 million to 5 million patients cared for in ICUs in U.S. hospitals each year. Like central venous catheters, catheter-related infection is generally the result of catheter contamination by the patient's skin flora or microorganisms from the hands of caregivers. Other significant sources of infection include the pressure transducer, which may become colonized, and the stagnant nature of the flush solution (3 ml/hr irrigation).

There is less information in the literature regarding the incidence and nature of infection with arterial catheters,

as contrasted with information available for peripheral and central venous catheters. Between 1969 and 1978 eight prospective studies identified only two bacteremias due to intraarterial monitoring systems. However, in most of these studies, arterial catheters were not regularly cultured; therefore these studies do not provide adequate information on the true risk of arterial catheter-related sepsis.

Later prospective studies, in which all of the intraarterial catheters studied were cultured using quantitative culture techniques, have better assessed the incidence of arterial catheter-related infection.[59,78-82] Rates of local infection ranged from 0.9% to 17.7%, and rates of catheter-associated bacteremia ranged from 0% to 4.6%. The relatively wide range of infection rates reflects, at least in part, differing patient populations studied and differing individual risk factors for nosocomial infection.

Maki and Ringer[23] conducted a prospective study of 489 percutaneously inserted arterial catheters in a large medical-surgical ICU, using microbiologic methods for identification of all potential sources of infusion-related infection. They found that the septic risk of local and bacteremic or fungemic catheter-related infection, as well as sepsis from contaminated catheter hubs and infusate, was very low, with local catheter-related infections at 3.1% and infusate- or hub-related infections at 0.8%. This is a rate of invasive infection threefold to sixfold lower than that encountered with central venous catheters used in similar ICU patients for a comparable period of in situ time.[13,20,83] These statistics are similar to the range reported for peripheral IV catheters.[23]

The aforementioned data should not lull the clinician into believing that intraarterial lines are at insignificant risk of septic complications. Sporadic epidemic outbreaks of nosocomial sepsis continue to plague unwary users of arterial pressure monitoring. Mermel and Maki[84] reviewed 23 epidemic outbreaks of nosocomial bloodstream infection traced to arterial pressure monitoring during the 1970s and 1980s. These institutional epidemics were extraordinarily insidious; epidemics investigated by the CDC since 1979 lasted 11 months on the average before being identified and controlled.[85] Very few practitioners, including critical care specialists, realize that the flush solution used for hemodynamic monitoring is vulnerable to contamination and is the most important cause of epidemic infusion-related gram-negative bacteremia in ICU patients.

Control measures to reduce the risk of line contamination for all hemodynamic monitoring fluid-filled systems are listed in Box 13-6.

BOX 13-6

Recommendations for Minimizing the Risk of Contamination of Fluid-Filled Catheter Systems

1. Minimize the manipulations of the system, especially for blood drawings. Do not break the closed system to position the patient or change patient gowns. Effective handwashing must be done before each manipulation; gloves provide additional protection.
2. Keep the number of stopcocks and connections in the fluid delivery system to a minimum.
3. Use disposable transducer assemblies when economically feasible, and resterilize reusable transducer components between patients.
4. Use saline rather than glucose-containing infusates for line irrigation.
5. Replace the entire monitoring system, including tubing, continuous flow device, bag of fluid, and transducer assembly, at prescribed intervals.
6. Avoid blood stagnation in all tubing and connections.
7. Protect sterility of all stopcock ports with the use of deadheads. If the sterility of a stopcock port or any component of a fluid system is in question, it should be replaced by a sterile component.

TREATMENT

Data suggest that many infected central venous catheters, particularly those infected with coagulase-negative staphylococci, can be effectively treated without catheter removal. However, there is a significant risk of recurrent bacteremia (approximately 20% after 3 weeks versus 3% if the catheter is removed).[86] Because the presence of an infected catheter puts the patient at risk for serious septic complications, including septic thrombosis and endocarditis, such an approach should be reserved only for those catheters that cannot be easily and safely replaced. As a general rule, any short-term intravascular catheter suspected of being the source of sepsis (unexplained fever, local inflammation, staphylococcal bacteremia or candidemia of uncertain origin) should be removed and replaced. Exceptions should be limited to those patients with severe coagulopathy or thrombocytopenia or exceptional problems with venous access where removal or replacement is not possible.

In contrast, CRS associated with surgically implanted catheters (e.g., Hickman, Broviac) can be assessed for in situ antibiotic treatment. If there is no evidence of a persistent exit site infection, tunnel infection, endocarditis, septic thrombosis, or septic shock; if the infecting organism is other than *Corynebacterium jeikeium, S. aureus, Bacillus* species, *Xanthomonas* species, yeast, fungus, or myocobacteria; and if bacteremia or candidemia has persisted for less than 3 days, an attempt at antibiotic treatment with retention of the catheter may be worthwhile.[9] Up to two thirds of CRS in surgically implanted catheters (apart from those conditions listed previously) may be cured with antibiotics administered through the device for 7 to 10 days.[64,87-92] Bacteremia, due to catheter-related sepsis, in such devices may be cured even more simply by locking a concentrated antibiotic-containing solution (usually vancomycin or an aminoglycoside) into the lumen of the catheter for 12 hours per day for 2 weeks.[93,94]

The role of local thrombolytics in in situ therapy of catheter-related infection is unclear. Some advocate such an approach as part of therapy of retained catheters because local thrombosis is known to be associated with catheter infections and should theoretically make it more difficult to clear an infection.[92,95] However, to date no randomized trial has been performed to definitively answer this question. For that reason, there are no uniformly accepted recommendations regarding this issue.

The question of how to handle asymptomatic colonization of intravascular catheters (semiquantitative count greater than 15 CFU) in the absence of positive blood cultures is problematic due to the lack of randomized trials. Catheter tip colony counts of greater than 15 CFU are clearly associated with increased risk of catheter-related bloodstream infections.[96] However, in the absence of clinical sepsis or documented bacteremia, most clinicians will not treat patients with antibiotics if catheter colonization or infection is found following catheter removal. On the other hand, such catheters are sometimes switched over a guide wire. If the original catheter tip grows greater than 15 CFU, any new catheter placed into the same site over a guide wire should be removed. Some authorities advise a brief course of antibiotic treatment in immunosuppressed patients and for certain organisms (*Candida* species, *S. aureus*).

Patients who have experienced high-grade catheter-related bacteremia or candidemia should always be assessed carefully for the development of late complications, including endocarditis or other metastatic infections.[9] This is particularly important for infections with *Candida* species and *S. aureus* and for those patients with intravascular prosthetic devices, including heart valves.

PREVENTION AND MANAGEMENT

Infection and infectious sequelae, such as sepsis and multiple-system organ failure, are the most common causes of death in surgical and trauma ICUs. It has been estimated that the ICU incidence of nosocomial sepsis is 24 times higher than that of general medical-surgical areas.[97] One major reason for this high incidence of nosocomial infection in the ICU is that invasive devices, which are a major risk factor for sepsis, are a standard part of ICU patient care; their use should therefore be kept to minimum. Once infected, nosocomial infection in the ICU may be more difficult to treat because antibiotic resistance is greater in bacteria colonizing humans and inanimate objects in ICUs than in general wards. *The importance of meticulously following sepsis prophylaxis in all aspects of patient care cannot be overstated.* Suggestions for infusion-related sepsis prophylaxis and management are discussed next.

Handwashing

Infusion-related infections may originate from microorganisms present on the hands of medical personnel inserting or manipulating the devices. The hands of the caregiver are a primary source of antibiotic-resistant bacterial contamination that causes nosocomial infection. Before and after manipulating any invasive device, vigorous rubbing together of all lathered hand surfaces for a minimum of 10 seconds (preferably for 30 seconds) is one of the oldest yet most important infection control measures. Unfortunately, handwashing continues to be done inconsistently or superficially by many health care professionals. A tendency to disregard this procedure because of the tedium of infection prophylaxis, particularly when one has an excessive or urgent workload, is common. Clinical practitioners must be disciplined in order to overcome this failure. Wearing gloves may provide an additional measure of patient safety when the closed fluid system requires disruption (changing connecting tubing or stopcocks, or aspiration of blood).

Handwashing soaps containing antiseptic are considerably more efficacious for "degerming" hands than are nonantiseptic soaps. It is yet to be determined whether antiseptic soaps also reduce the incidence of endemic nosocomial infection in patients.[98] Antiseptic handwashing soaps do not reduce the amount of time, friction, or water required for effective hand degerming. Consistent, careful handwashing technique and gloving also protects caregivers from acquiring transferable diseases such as hepatitis, acquired immunodeficiency diseases, and herpetic infections.

Dedicated Infusion Therapy Team

Many studies have conclusively demonstrated that the use of a dedicated infusion therapy team for intravascular catheter placement and care can substantially reduce the risk of IRS by up to eightfold.[50,99] If such a team is not possible, rigorous training of nurses and physicians involved in catheter insertion and care along with meticulous adherence to catheter care protocols can achieve similar results.[100,101]

Skin Disinfection of IV Catheter Sites

A strong relationship exists between microorganisms colonizing catheters and the skin at the catheter insertion site.[20,23,32,33] *Consequently, the importance of reliable suppression of the skin microflora with an antiseptic solution before catheter insertion and the follow-up care of the insertion site cannot be overemphasized.*

Before catheter insertion, the intended insertion site must be cleansed using an antiseptic soap, water, and friction. Friction is required to remove skin oil. However, too much friction may irritate or abrade the delicate, friable skin of debilitated or malnourished patients. Washing prepares the skin for the sterile skin preparation. If body hair at the intended insertion site is excessive, hair is removed (preferably by clipping because shaving may produce microabrasions that then become sites for bacterial growth).

The ideal agent for skin disinfection (nonirritating and effective in antimicrobial activity) has not yet been identified. In a study by Maki and colleagues,[102] insertion sites were disinfected with 70% alcohol, 10% povidone-iodine, or 2% aqueous chlorhexidine, by random allocation. Alcohol and povidone-iodine were equivalent in protection against infection but significantly less effective than chlorhexidine in preventing catheter-related infection.[102] Chlorhexidine deserves consideration as a first-line antiseptic for prevention of infection with percutaneously inserted intravascular devices of all types. Other studies demonstrate decreased risk of CRS with use of a topical polyantibiotic regimen (polymyxin B, neomycin, bacitracin) or mupirocin (an antistaphylococcal agent).[103,104] Future studies should examine other agents for cutaneous disinfection to improve the effectiveness and duration of flora suppression at the catheter insertion site. Even with adequate suppression of skin microflora at the time of insertion, the suppressed microorganisms can rapidly grow back and invade the wound.

Regardless of the type of solution chosen for skin preparation, the skin antiseptic is applied with sterile gloves in an expanding circular motion beginning at the proposed catheter insertion site to a diameter of approximately 9 to 10 inches. This is repeated in the same manner four times, changing forceps and gauze each time. The final application is allowed to dry to maximize antiseptic action and provide residual activity. Following the "prep," the operator puts on a new set of sterile gloves for insertion of the vascular catheter.

Surgical Aseptic Technique for Hemodynamic Monitoring Line Insertion

All intravascular lines for hemodynamic monitoring should be inserted under strict sterile technique. For central venous catheter insertion, the operator and assistant should wear gown, gloves, and mask, and the patient should be surgically draped. All those assisting in the room should wear a surgical mask and cap. When possible, the door to the room should be closed during the insertion procedure and the number of persons entering and leaving the room should be limited. The use of maximal barrier precautions has been shown to result in a highly significant fourfold to sixfold decrease in the risk of catheter-related infections.[39,58,105]

In patients who are spontaneously breathing, the face should be draped and turned away from the operative field during central line insertion. Likewise, the area should be protected from contamination from endotracheal or tracheal secretions or mist. Nearby tubing should be secured so that it does not fall into and contaminate the sterile field during the procedure. These site precautions also apply for dressing changes.

Intravascular Catheter Dressing Protocol

To prevent contamination of the insertion site, a sterile occlusive dressing should be applied. The dressing and not the tape should cover the wound. The date of catheter insertion should be recorded where it can be easily found, such as in the medical record and, if possible, directly on the dressing or tape.

As discussed earlier, there is a strong correlation between microorganisms present at the catheter insertion site and microorganisms implicated in catheter-related sepsis. In the past it was believed that frequent site dressing changes would reduce the incidence of catheter-related sepsis. However, studies regarding dressing material and frequency of dressing changes have produced conflicting results. At this point, the CDC has no recommendation on the frequency of dressing changes or the type of dressing material.[22] However, dressings should be changed whenever wet, soiled with drainage, or disrupted. Wet dressings particularly favor bacterial growth.

A semipermeable clear membrane dressing was introduced during the 1980s. Transparent dressings are less bulky and allow for visualization of the site while being vapor permeable and waterproof. Vasquez and Jarrad[106] studied one such dressing, Opsite, and found an overall catheter-related sepsis rate of 1% for the 100 patients studied. It was concluded that Opsite was a safe and cost-effective dressing for central venous catheters. Young and colleagues[107] compared a standard protocol of gauze changed three times per week with Opsite changed three times per week or every 7 to 10 days. Sepsis rates were low in all groups. It was concluded by these authors that Opsite could be safely left in place for up to 7 days. However, two studies have revealed a much higher incidence of catheter-related infection and sepsis when transparent dressings were used for central venous catheters.[108,109] Patients were found to have higher rates of colonization of the subcutaneous tract and subsequent bacteremia that coincided with microorganisms found at the catheter insertion site.[109] Bacterial colonization may actually be enhanced when moisture accumulates under the transparent dressing. Overall, further studies are required to determine safety and efficacy of transparent polyurethane dressings. Sterile gauze with an antimicrobial ointment is currently acceptable as an effective and economical dressing.

Regular maintenance and observation of the IV site are important for prevention or early detection of IV-related complications.[110] Intravenous sites should be inspected at least every 24 hours. If visual inspection is not possible, the insertion site should be gently palpated to detect pain, tenderness, or swelling. At each dressing change and at catheter removal, the insertion site should be observed for erythema, purulence, swelling, and tenderness.

Infusion System Protocols

Intraluminal antibiotic locks as part of routine catheter care may be effective in reducing intraluminal colonization and infection.[111,112] Antibiotics that can be locked into the infusion ports and reduce IRS include aminoglycosides and minocycline.[112] Vancomycin has been used but is not currently recommended due to the risk of the development of vancomycin-resistant organisms (especially enterococci).

Most infusion-related sepsis is, in fact, catheter-related sepsis. However, contamination of the infusate may occur, often in clusters. Historically, U.S. hospital practice has been to routinely replace the entire infusion delivery system on a 24- to 48-hour basis in order to reduce the risk from extrinsically contaminated fluid.[2] It was thought that frequent systems replacement minimizes the opportunity of any potential organisms in the infusate to grow to numbers large enough to cause adverse effects. However, studies suggest that infusate delivery systems do not require replacement more frequently than every 72 hours.[30,113,114] Exceptions may be made for infusion sets used for delivery of blood products, lipid emulsions, or arterial pressure monitoring where more frequent changes may be prudent.[9]

Catheter Design Improvements

Improvements in catheter design have been intrinsic to improvement in rates of CRS. Methods to prevent invasion of the transcutaneous tract by skin flora following catheter insertion have been studied. Surgically implanted, tunneled, Dacron-cuffed devices such as Hickman and Broviac catheters used for long-term vascular access are an example. Both tunneling and the cuff limit the migration of cutaneous microorganisms to the bloodstream. An attachable subcutaneous cuff constructed of a biodegradable collagen matrix impregnated with bactericidal silver was studied by Maki and colleagues.[20] They found that the silver-impregnated cuff can confer a threefold reduction of catheter-related infection with percutaneously inserted central venous catheters. Antiseptic hubs and in-line filters have also been studied.[9] Data suggest that the use of antiseptic (chlorhexidine and silver sulphadiazine) bonded and antibiotic (minocycline and rifampin) bonded catheters results in a threefold to fourfold reduction in the risk of CRS.[115-117] A single head-to-head comparison of the two types of catheter has favored the antibiotic-bonded device.[116,118]

Preferred Central Venous Catheter Insertion Site

Because studies of pulmonary artery and central venous catheters have shown that there is an increased risk of catheter-related sepsis with insertion in the jugular vein as compared with insertion in the subclavian vein,[58-60] the subclavian venous site is the preferred insertion site as it relates to the prevention of CRS. Recent data suggest an increased risk of CRS using the femoral insertion site.[17,61]

Duration of Intravascular Catheterization

Previous studies have indicated that the duration of vascular catheterization is related to the incidence of both catheter colonization and catheter-related sepsis.[79,119-122] Generally, an in situ duration of more than 72 hours significantly increases the risk of catheter-related infection. Consequently, it had been generally recommended that central venous catheters be changed routinely every 3 to 5 days (most clinicians use 5 days). Other studies support the theory that both arterial and pulmonary catheters can remain in place as long as needed, provided there are no signs or symptoms of catheter-related sepsis occurring more than 48 hours after catheter insertion, local signs of infection at the insertion site, or positive blood cultures.[58,61,84,123,124]

A special thank you to Charles E. Edmiston, PhD, CIC, Associate Professor of Surgery and Hospital Epidemiologist at the Medical College of Wisconsin and Froedtert Memorial Lutheran Hospital, Milwaukee, Wisconsin, for his review of this chapter upon the author's request.

If any of these signs or symptoms appear, or if a malfunctioning catheter is detected, a new catheter should be placed at a new site while the old one is removed. If placement of a catheter to a new site is problematic, guide wire exchanges can be done. Following a guide wire exchange, the original catheter must be cultured. If the culture is positive (more than 15 colonies), the newly inserted catheter should be removed. If the patient's condition still requires invasive hemodynamic monitoring, a new catheter must be inserted through a new insertion site. Neither approach (routine versus clinically indicated replacement) has won universal acceptance to date.

One disadvantage to using guide wire exchange in a febrile patient is the 24- to 48-hour time frame to obtain a negative culture. In addition, the new catheter may become contaminated in the exchange process. Guide wire exchanges should include a reprepping of the guide wire and site before placement of the new catheter.[125] Catheters also should be removed and reinserted in a new site when there is purulent drainage or cellulitis at the original skin puncture site.

As soon as patients' conditions no longer require invasive monitoring devices, catheters should be removed. Leaving intravascular catheters in place "in case something happens" increases the risk of infection, as well as all complications, and the likelihood that "something *will* happen."

REFERENCES

1. Bone RC, Balk R, Cerra FB, et al: ACCP/SCCM Consensus Conference: definitions of sepsis and organ failure and guidelines for use of innovative therapies in sepsis, *Chest* 101:1644, 1992.
2. Maki DG, Goldman DA, Rhame FS: Infection control in intravenous therapy, *Ann Intern Med* 79:867-887, 1973.
3. Maki DG, Rhame FS: Nationwide epidemic of septicemia caused by contaminated intravenous products, *Am J Med* 60:471, 1977.
4. Maki DG: Nosocomial bacteremia: an epidemiologic overview, *Am J Med* 70:719, 1981.
5. Hamory BH: Nosocomial bloodstream and intravascular device–related infections. In Wenzel R, editor: *Prevention and control of nosocomial infections,* Baltimore, 1987, Williams & Wilkins.
6. Maki DG: Infections due to infusion therapy. In Bennett JV, Brachman PS, editors: *Hospital infections,* Boston, 1986, Little, Brown.
7. Henderson DK: Intravascular device–associated infection: current concepts and controversies, *Infect Surg* 7:365, 1988.
8. Raad I, Darouiche RO: Catheter-related septicemia: risk reduction, *Infect Med* 13:807, 1996.
9. Maki DG: Infections caused by intravascular devices used for infusion therapy: pathogenesis, prevention, and management. In Bisno AL, Waldvogel FA, editors: *Infections*

associated with indwelling medical devices, Washington, DC, 1994, American Society for Microbiology.

10. Maki DG: The epidemiology and prevention of nosocomial bloodstream infections, *Prog Abstr Third Int Conf Nosocomial Infect* 1990 (abstract 3).

11. Komshian SV, Uwaydah AK, Sobel JD, et al: Fungemia caused by *Candida* species and *Torulopsis glabrata* in the hospitalized patient: frequency, characteristics, and evaluation of factors influencing outcome, *Rev Infect Dis* 3:379, 1989.

12. Maki DG: Nosocomial bactermia, *Am J Med* 70:183, 1981.

13. Maki DG, McCormack KN: Defatting catheter insertion sites in total parenteral nutrition is of no value as an infection control measure, *Am J Med* 83:833, 1987.

14. Heiselman D: Nosocomial bloodstream infections in the critically ill, *JAMA* 272:1819, 1994.

15. The Australian Study on Intravascular Catheter Associated Sepsis: Intravascular catheter associated sepsis: a common problem, *Med J Aust* 161:374, 1994.

16. Byers K, Adal K, Anglim A, et al: Case fatality rate for catheter-related bloodstream infections (CRBSI): a meta-analysis, *Infect Control Hosp Epidemiol* 16(2 suppl):23, 1995 (abstract).

17. Mermel LA: Prevention of intravascular catheter–related infections, *Ann Intern Med* 132:391, 2000.

18. Banerjee SN, Emori G, Culver RP, et al: Secular trends in nosocomial primary bloodstream infections in the United States, 1980-1989, *Am J Med* 91(suppl 3B):86S, 1991.

19. Raad I: Intravascular-catheter–related infections, *Lancet* 351:893, 1998.

20. Maki DG, Cobb L, Garman JK, et al: An attachable silver-impregnated cuff for prevention of infection with central venous catheters: a prospective randomized multicenter trial, *Am J Med* 85:307, 1988.

21. Maki DG: Infections associated with intravascular lines, *Current Topics in Infectious Diseases* 309, 1982.

22. Pearson ML, Hospital Infection Control Practice Advisory Committee: Guidelines for prevention of intravascular-device-related infections, *Infect Control Hosp Epidemiol* 17:438, 1996.

23. Maki DG, Ringer M: Evaluation of dressing regimens for prevention of infection with peripheral intravenous catheters, *JAMA* 258:2396, 1987.

24. Maki DG, Weise CE, Sarafin HW: A semiquantitative culture method for identifying intravenous catheter–related infection, *N Engl J Med* 296:1305, 1977.

25. Snydman DR, Murray SA, Kornfeld SJ: Total parental nutrition–related infections. Prospective epidemiologic study using semiquantitative methods, *Am J Med* 73:695, 1982.

26. Collignon PJ, Soni N, Pearson IY: Is semiquantitative culture of central vein catheter tips useful in the diagnosis of catheter–associated bacteremia? *J Clin Microbiol* 24:532, 1986.

27. Cleri DJ, Corrado ML, Seligman SJ: Quantitative culture of intravenous catheters and other intravascular inserts, *J Infect Dis* 141:781, 1980.

28. Sherertz RJ, Raad I, Belani A, et al: Three-year experience with sonicated vascular catheter cultures in a clinical microbiologic laboratory, *J Clin Microbiol* 28:76, 1990.

29. Raad I, Sabbagh MF, Rand KH, et al: Quantitative tip culture methods and the diagnosis of central venous catheter–related infections, *Diagn Microbiol Infect Dis* 15:13, 1992.

30. Band JD, Maki DG: Safety of changing intravenous delivery systems at longer than 24-hour intervals, *Ann Intern Med* 91:173, 1979.

31. McGeer A, Righter J: Improving our ability to diagnose infections associated with central venous catheters: value of Gram's staining and culture of entry site swabs, *Can Med Assoc J* 137:1009, 1987.

32. Snydman DR, Pober BR, Murray SA: Predictive values of surveillance skin cultures in total-parenteral-nutrition–related infection, *Lancet* 2:1385, 1982.

33. Bjornson HS, Colley R, Bower RH: Association between microorganism growth at the catheter insertion site and colonization of the catheter in patients receiving total parenteral nutrition, *Surgery* 92:720, 1982.

34. Kovacevich DS, Faubion WC, Bender JM, et al: Association of parenteral nutrition catheter sepsis with urinary tract infections, *J Parenter Enter Nutr* 10:639, 1986.

35. Pettigrew RA, Lang SDR, Haydock DA: Catheter-related sepsis in patients on intravenous nutrition: a prospective study of quantitative catheter cultures and guidewire changes for suspected sepsis, *Br J Surg* 72:52, 1985.

36. Sitges-Serra A, Linares J, Garau J: Catheter sepsis: the clue is the hub, *Surgery* 97:355, 1985.

37. Raad I, Costerton W, Sabharwal U: Ultrastructural analysis of indwelling vascular catheters: a quantitative relationship between luminal colonization and duration of placement, *J Infect Dis* 168:400, 1993.

38. Bennett SN, McNeil MM, Bland LA, et al: Postoperative infections traced to contamination of an intravenous anesthetic, propofol, *N Engl J Med* 333:147, 1995.

39. Goldman DG, Martin WT, Worthington JW: Growth of bacteria and fungi in total parenteral nutrition solutions, *Am J Surg* 126:314, 1973.

40. Freeman J, Goldmann DA, Smith NE, et al: Association of intravenous lipid emulsion and coagulase-negative staphylococcal bacteremia in neonatal intensive care units, *N Engl J Med* 323:301, 1990.

41. Ascher DP, Shoupe BA, Robb M, et al: Comparison of standard and quantitative blood cultures in the evaluation of children with suspected central venous line sepsis, *Diagn Microbiol Infect Dis* 15:499, 1992.

42. Benezra D, Kiehn T, Gold JWM, et al: Prospective study of infections in indwelling central venous catheters using quantitative blood cultures, *Am J Med* 85:495, 1988.

43. Vanhuynegem L, Parmentier P, Potvliege C: In situ bacteriologic diagnosis of total parenteral nutrition catheter infection, *Surgery* 103(2):114, 1988.

44. Markus S, Buday S: Culturing indwelling central venous catheters in situ, *Infect Surg* 13:157, 1989.

45. Rushforth JA, Hoy CM, Kite P, et al: Rapid diagnosis of central venous catheter sepsis, *Lancet* 342:402, 1993.

46. Telenti A, Steckelberg JM, Stockman L, et al: Quantitative blood cultures in candidemia, *Mayo Clinic Proc* 66:1120, 1991.

47. Craven DE, Kunches LM, Lictenberg DA: Nosocomial infections and fatality in medical and surgical intensive care unit patients, *Arch Intern Med* 148:1161, 1988.

48. Freeman J, McGowan JE: Risk factors for nosocomial infection, *J Infect Dis* 138:811, 1978.

49. Armstrong CW, Mayhall CG, Miller KB: Prospective study of catheter replacement and other risk factors for infection of hyperalimentation catheters, *J Infect Dis* 154:808, 1986.

50. Faubion WC, Wesley JR, Khalidi N, et al: Total parenteral nutrition catheter sepsis: impact of the team approach, *J Parenter Enter Nutr* 10:642, 1986.

51. Nelson DB, Kien CL, Mohr B: Dressing changes by specialized personnel reduced infection rates in patients receiving central venous parenteral nutrition, *J Parenter Enter Nutr* 10:220, 1986.

52. Tomford JW, Hershey CO, McLaren CE: Intravenous therapy team and peripheral venous catheter–associated complications: a prospective controlled study, *Arch Intern Med* 144:1191, 1984.

53. Mermel LA, Maki DG: Infectious complications of Swan-Ganz pulmonary artery catheters. Pathogenesis, epidemiology, prevention and management, *Am J Respir Crit Care Med* 149:1020, 1994.

54. Christensen GD, Simpson WA, Beachey EH: Adherence of slime-producing strains of *Staphylococcus epidermidis* to smooth surfaces, *Infect Immun* 37:318, 1982.

55. Peters G, Locci R, Pulverer G: Adherence and growth of coagulase-negative staphylococci on surfaces of intravenous catheters, *J Infect Dis* 146:479, 1982.

56. Sheth NK, Rose HD, Franson TR: In vitro quantitative adherence of bacteria to intravascular catheters, *J Surg Res* 34:213, 1983.

57. Sheth NK, Franson TR, Rose HD: Colonization of bacteria on polyvinyl chloride and Teflon intravenous catheters in hospitalized patients, *J Clin Microbiol* 18:1061, 1983.

58. Mermel LA, McCormick RD, Springman SR, et al: The pathogenesis and epidemiology of catheter-related infection with pulmonary artery Swan-Ganz catheters: a prospective study utilizing molecular subtyping, *Am J Med* 91:197S, 1991.

59. Pinilla JC, Ross DF, Martin T, et al: Study of the incidence of intravascular catheter infection and associated septicemia in critically ill patients, *Crit Care Med* 11:21, 1983.

60. Richet H, Hubert B, Netemberg G: Prospective multicenter study of vascular catheter–related complications and risk factors for positive central-catheter cultures in intensive care unit patients, *J Clin Microbiol* 28:2520, 1990.

61. Norwood S, Ruby A, Civetta J, et al: Catheter-related infections and associated septicemia, *Chest* 99:968, 1988.

62. Nystrom B, Olesen Larsen S, Daschner F, et al: Bacteremia in surgical patients with intravenous devices: a European multicentre incidence study, *J Hosp Infect* 4:338, 1983.

63. Bross J, Talbot GH, Maislin G, et al: Risk factors for nosocomial candidemia: a case-control study in adults without leukemia, *Am J Med* 87:614, 1989.

64. Wang EEL, Prober CG, Ford-Jones L, et al: The management of central intravenous catheter infections, *Pediatr Infect Dis* 3:110, 1984.

65. Capell S, Linares J, Sitges-Serra A: Catheter sepsis due to coagulase-negative staphylococci in patients on total parental nutrition, *Eur J Clin Microbiol* 5:40, 1985.

66. Linares J, Sitges-Serra A, Garau J: Pathogenesis of catheter sepsis: a prospective study with quantitative and semiquantitative cultures of catheter and hub segments, *J Clin Microbiol* 21:357, 1985.

67. Kelly CS, Ligas JR, Smith CA: Sepsis due to triple lumen central venous catheters, *Surg Gynecol Obstet* 163:14, 1986.

68. Pemberton LB, Lyman B, Lander V, et al: Sepsis from triple vs single-lumen catheters during total parenteral nutrition in surgical or critically ill patients, *Arch Surg* 121:591, 1986.

69. Padberg FT, Ruggiero J, Blackburn GL, et al: Central venous catheterization for parenteral nutrition, *Ann Surg* 193:264, 1981.

70. Bozzetti F, Terno G, Bonfanti G: Prevention and treatment of central venous catheter sepsis by exchange via a guidewire. A prospective controlled trial, *Ann Surg* 198:48, 1983.

71. Sitzmann JV, Townsend TR, Siler MC, et al: Septic and technical complications of central venous catheterization. A prospective study of 200 consecutive patients, *Ann Surg* 202:766, 1985.

72. Cheesbrough JS, Finch RG, Burden RP: A prospective study of the mechanisms of infection associated with hemodialysis catheters, *J Infect Dis* 154:579, 1986.

73. Pezzarossi HE, Ponce de Leon S, Calva JJ, et al: High incidence of subclavian dialysis catheter-related bacteremias, *Infect Control* 7:596, 1986.

74. Sherertz RJ, Falk RJ, Huffman KA, et al: Infections associated with subclavian Uldall catheters, *Arch Intern Med* 143:52, 1983.

75. Graham DR, Keldermans MM, Klemm LW, et al: Infectious complications among patients receiving home intravenous therapy with peripheral, central, or peripherally placed central venous catheters, *Am J Med* 91(suppl 3B):95S, 1991.

76. Rowley K, Clubb S, Smith W: Right-sided infective endocarditis as a consequence of flow-directed pulmonary artery catheterization, *N Engl J Med* 311:1152, 1984.

77. Becker RC, Martin RG, Underwood DA: Right sided endocardial lesions and flow directed pulmonary artery catheters, *Clev Clin J Med* 54:384, 1987.

78. Shinozaki T, Deane RS, Mazuzan JE: Bacterial contamination of arterial lines, *JAMA* 249:223, 1983.

79. Band JD, Maki DG: Infections caused by arterial catheters used for hemodynamic monitoring, *Am J Med* 67:735, 1979.

80. Singh S, Nelson N, Acosta I: Catheter colonization and bacteremia with pulmonary and arterial catheters, *Crit Care Med* 10:736, 1982.

81. Russell JA, Joel M, Hudson RJ: Prospective evaluation of radial and femoral artery catheterization sites in critically ill adults, *Crit Care Med* 11:936, 1983.

82. Damen J: The microbiological risk of invasive hemodynamic monitoring in adults undergoing cardiac valve replacement, *J Clin Monit* 2:87, 1986.

83. Maki DG, Will LR: Colonization and infection associated with transparent dressings for central venous, arterial, and Hickman catheters: a comparative trial. Proceedings and Abstracts of the 24th Intersci Conference on Antimicrobial Agents and Chemotherapy, 1984.

84. Mermel LA, Maki DG: Epidemic bloodstream infections from hemodynamic pressure monitoring: signs of the times, *Infect Control Hosp Epidemiol* 10:47, 1989.

85. Beck-Sague CM, Jarvis WR: Epidemic bloodstream infections associated with pressure transducers: a persistent problem, *Infect Control Hosp Epidemiol* 10:54, 1989.

86. Raad I, Davis S, Khan A, et al: Impact of central venous catheter removal on the recurrence of catheter-related coagulase-negative staphylococcal bacteremia, *Infect Control Hosp Epidemiol* 13:215, 1992.

87. Cappello M, De Pauw L, Bastin G, et al: Central venous access for haemodialysis using the Hickman catheter, *Nephrol Dial Transplant* 4:988, 1989.

88. Hartman GE, Shochat SJ: Management of septic complications associated with Silastic catheters in childhood malignancy, *Pediatr Infect Dis* 6:1042, 1987.

89. Johnson PR, Decker MD, Edwards KM, et al: Frequency of Broviac catheter infections in pediatric oncology patients, *J Infect Dis* 154:570, 1986.

90. Press OW, Ramsey PG, Larson EB, et al: Hickman catheter infections in patients with malignancies, *Medicine* 63:189, 1984.

91. Prince A, Heller B, Jevy J, et al: Management of fever in patients with central vein catheters, *Pediatr Infect Dis* 5:20, 1986.

92. Schuman ES, Winters V, Gross GF, et al: Management of Hickman catheter sepsis, *Am J Surg* 149:627, 1985.

93. Douard MC, Leverger G, Paulien R, et al: Quantitative blood cultures for diagnosis and management of catheter-related sepsis in pediatric hematology and oncology patients, *Intensive Care Med* 17:30, 1991.

94. Messing B, Peitra-Cohen S, Debure A, et al: Antibiotic-lock technique: a new approach to optimal therapy for catheter-related sepsis in home-parenteral nutrition patients, *J Parenter Enter Nutr* 12:185, 1988.

95. Jones GR, Konsler GK, Dunaway RP, et al: Prospective analysis of urokinase in the treatment of catheter sepsis in pediatric hematology-oncology patients, *J Pediatr Surg* 28:350, 1993.

96. O'Grady NP, Barie PS, Bartlett J, et al: Practice parameters for evaluating new fever in critically ill adult patients, *Crit Care Med* 26:392, 1998.

97. Wenzel RP, Osterman CA, Donowitz LG, et al: Identification of procedure-related nosocomial infections in high-risk patients, *Rev Infect Dis* 3:701, 1981.

98. Maki DG: Risk factors for nosocomial infection in intensive care, *Arch Intern Med* 149:301, 989.

99. Maki DG: Yes, Virginia, aseptic technique is very important: maximal barrier precautions during insertion reduce the risk of central venous catheter–related bacteremia, *Infect Control Hosp Edipemiol* 15:227, 1994.

100. Puntis JWL, Holden CE, Smallman S, et al: Staff training: a key factor in reducing intravascular catheter sepsis, *Arch Dis Child* 65:335, 1990.

101. Vanherweghem JL, Dhaene M, Goldman M, et al: Infections associated with subclavian dialysis catheters: the key role of nurse training, *Nephron* 42:116, 1986.

102. Maki DG, Alvarado CJ, Ringer M: A prospective, randomized trial of povidone-iodine, alcohol and chlorhexidine for prevention of infection with central venous and arterial catheters, *Lancet* 338:339, 1991.

103. Maki DG, Band JD: A comparative study of polyantitotic and iodophor ointments in prevention of vascular catheter–related infection, *Am J Med* 70:739, 1981.

104. Hill RL, Fisher AP, Ware RJ, et al: Mupirocin for the reduction of colonization of internal jugular cannulae—a randomised controlled trial, *J Hosp Infect* 15:311, 1990.

105. Raad I, Hohn DC, Gilbreath J: Prevention of central venous catheter–related infections using maximal barrier precautions during insertion, *Infect Control Hosp Epidemiol* 15:231, 1994.

106. Vasquez RM, Jarrad MM: Care of the central venous catheterization site: the use of a transparent polyurethane film, *J Parenter Enter Nutr* 8:181, 1984.

107. Young GP, Alexeyeff M, Russell DM, et al: Catheter sepsis during parenteral nutrition: the safety of long-term Opsite dressing, *J Parenter Enter Nutr* 12:365, 1988.

108. Conly JM, Grieves K, Peters B: A prospective randomized study comparing transparent and dry gauze dressings for central venous catheters, *J Infect Dis* 159:310, 1989.

109. Dickerson N, Horton P, Smith S, et al: Clinically significant central venous catheter infections in a community hospital: association with type of dressing, *J Infect Dis* 160:720, 1989.

110. Simmons BP: CDC guidelines for the prevention and control of nosocomial infections. Guidelines for prevention of intravascular infections, *Am J Infect Control* 11:183, 1983.

111. Schwartz C, Henrickson KJ, Roghmann K, et al: Prevention of bacteraemia attributed to luminal colonization of tunneled central venous catheters with vancomycin-susceptible organisms, *J Clin Oncol* 80:591, 1990.

112. Raad I, Buzaid A, Rhyne J, et al: Minocycline and ethylenediaminetetraacetate for the prevention of recurrent vascular catheter infections, *Clin Infect Dis* 25:149, 1997.

113. Buxton AE, Highsmith AK, Garner JS: Contamination of intravenous fluid: effects of changing administration sets, *Ann Intern Med* 90:764, 1979.

114. Gorbea HF, Snydman DR, Delaney A: Intravenous tubing with burettes can be safely changed at 48-hour intervals, *JAMA* 251:2112, 1984.

115. Maki DG, Stolz SM, Wheeler S, et al: Prevention of central venous catheter–related bloodstream infection by use of an antiseptic-impregnated catheter: a randomised, controlled trial, *Ann Intern Med* 127:257, 1997.

116. Raad I, Darouiche RO, Hachem R, et al: The broad spectrum activity and efficacy of catheters coated with minocycline and rifampicin, *J Infect Dis* 173:418, 1996.

117. Raad I, Darouiche RO, Dupuis J: Central venous catheters coated with minocycline and rifampin for the prevention of catheter-related colonization and bloodstream infection: a randomised, double-blind trial, *Ann Intern Med* 127:267, 1997.

118. Darouiche RO, Raad I, Heard SO, et al: A comparison of two antimicrobial-impregnated central venous catheters, *N Engl J Med* 340:1, 1999.

119. Gil RT, Krause JA, Thill-Baharozian MC: Triple vs single lumen central venous catheters, *Arch Intern Med* 149:1139, 1989.

120. Pinella JC, Ross DF, Martin T: Study of the incidence of intravascular catheter infection and associated septicemia in critically ill patients, *Crit Care Med* 11:21, 1983.

121. Roy O, Billiau V, Beuscart C: Nosocomial infections associated with long-term radial artery cannulation, *Intensive Care Med* 15:241, 1989.

122. Applefeld JJ, Caruthers TE, Reno DJ: Assessment of the sterility of long-term cardiac catheterization using thermodilution Swan-Ganz catheter, *Chest* 74:377, 1978.

123. Eyer S, Brummitt C, Crossley K: Catheter-related sepsis: prospective randomized study of three methods of long-term catheter maintenance, *Crit Care Med* 18:1073, 1990.

124. Snyder RH, Ardrer FJ, Endy T: Catheter infection: comparison of two catheter maintenance techniques, *Ann Surg* 208:651, 1988.

125. Krzywda EA, Andris DA, Edmiston CE: Catheter-related infection: diagnosis, etiology, treatment, and preventions, *Nutr Clin Pract* 14:178, 1999.

SUGGESTED READINGS

Conly JM, Grieves K, Peters B: A prospective randomized study comparing transparent and dry gauze dressings for central venous catheters, *J Infect Dis* 159:310, 1989.

Heiselman D: Nosocomial bloodstream infections in the critically ill, *JAMA* 272:1819, 1994.

Maki DG: Infections caused by intravascular devices used for infusion therapy: pathogenesis, prevention, and management. In Bisno AL, Waldvogel FA, editors: *Infections associated with indwelling medical devices,* Washington, DC, 1994, American Society for Microbiology.

Maki DG, Alvarado CJ, Ringer M: A prospective, randomized trial of povidone-iodine, alcohol and chlorhexidine for prevention of infection with central venous and arterial catheters, *Lancet* 338:339, 1991.

Maki DG, Weise CE, Sarafin HW: A semiquantitative culture method for identifying intravenous catheter–related infection, *N Engl J Med* 296:1305, 1977.

Mermel LA: Prevention of intravascular catheter–related infections, *Ann Intern Med* 132:391, 2000.

O'Grady NP, Barie PS, Bartlett J, et al: Practice parameters for evaluating new fever in critically ill adult patients, *Crit Care Med* 26:392, 1998.

Raad I: Intravascular-catheter–related infections, *Lancet* 351:893, 1998.

Raad I, Sabbagh MF, Rand KH, et al: Quantitative tip culture methods and the diagnosis of central venous catheter–related infections, *Diagn Microbiol Infect Dis* 15:13, 1992.

Wenzel RP, Osterman CA, Donowitz LG, et al: Identification of procedure-related nosocomial infections in high-risk patients, *Rev Infect Dis* 3:701, 1981.

14

GLORIA OBLOUK DAROVIC and ROBERT SIMONELLI

Pharmacologic Influences on Hemodynamic Parameters

Ideally, one therapeutic measure would correct all problems specific to a particular critical illness or injury. A single therapy would greatly simplify evaluation and predictability of treatment outcome. The reality, however, is that intensive care therapy uses a multifaceted approach that includes many drugs, as well as supportive devices such as mechanical ventilators. Drug therapy and intensive care support devices may directly or indirectly affect patients' hemodynamic status, as well as multiorgan function. The varied physiologic effects of the specific forms of intensive care polytherapy may be mutually synergistic or antagonistic. These factors often make evaluation of a single therapy measure, such as inotropic support of the heart, difficult. The difficulties in evaluating drug therapy are compounded by the fact that the effects of medication may be unpredictable because of differences in individual patients' constitutions, organ system reserves, and interplay of coexisting acute and chronic diseases. These factors affect drug metabolism and elimination and, as a consequence, the intensity and duration of action. The relationship of drug-patient-disease interactions is illustrated in Figure 14-1.

Medications commonly form the cornerstone of therapy in critically ill or injured patients. Considerations specific to intensive care unit (ICU) patient management include the following:

1. *The clinical and hemodynamic status of ICU patients often changes rapidly.* Because of the urgency of the patient's condition, effective drug concentrations must be achieved quickly. Consequently, a route of drug administration and a drug with rapid onset must be selected to allow prompt absorption and distribution, and rapid responsiveness at the tissue receptor sites.

2. *Most ICU patients have some degree of circulatory or metabolic dysfunction due to either their primary disease, their coexisting chronic diseases, or their stress response to critical illness.* These abnormalities may alter drug distribution or drug levels at target organs. Route of administration and drug dosage regimens must therefore be adjusted to accommodate these changes.

3. *Drug toxicities are poorly tolerated in critically ill or injured patients, who frequently have minimal or no physiologic reserve.* Avoidance of excessive drug dosing is extremely important.

4. *The polypharmacy of ICU therapy mandates that drug incompatibilities be investigated before drug administration.* Likewise, certain medications are incompatible with specific intravenous therapy solutions and may precipitate out of solution or may be rendered less active if administered through a "line" with an incompatible solution.

ROLE OF HEMODYNAMIC MONITORING IN INTENSIVE CARE UNIT DRUG THERAPY

Invasive hemodynamic monitoring has refined the evaluation and management of critically ill patients. The hemodynamic information obtained over the past several decades has led to further understanding of the complex

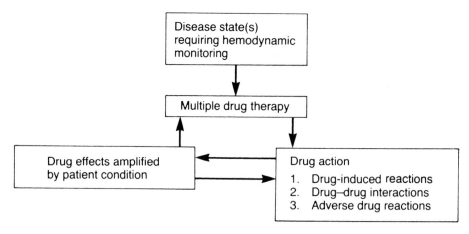

FIGURE 14-1 Interactions between the patient, the drug, and the disease.

interactions between critical illness and patient response to therapeutic interventions.

Invasive hemodynamic monitoring may assist evaluation of patient therapy by (1) helping to establish drug dose, efficacy, and the therapeutic end-point for medications that affect cardiopulmonary performance, and (2) helping to identify adverse drug-patient effects, drug-disease effects, and drug-drug effects.

This chapter is not intended to be a definitive treatise of critical care pharmacology. It does, however, discuss factors that affect drug absorption, distribution, metabolism, and excretion, as well as the mechanisms of actions of drugs commonly used in the ICU setting. Most of the drugs discussed are those that directly affect the circulatory system or those that may secondarily affect patient hemodynamics. The anticipated direction of changes in monitored hemodynamic parameters specific to each drug also are discussed, along with warnings or considerations specific to each medication.

FACTORS THAT DETERMINE DRUG ABSORPTION, DISTRIBUTION, METABOLISM, AND EXCRETION

The term *pharmacokinetics* refers to the association of route of administration with drug absorption, distribution, and availability at tissue receptor sites, as well as drug metabolic biotransformation and excretion. All aspects of pharmacokinetics affect the intensity of drug action in the body over a period of time. In the clinical setting, serum drug levels are used to evaluate drug pharmacokinetics. Drug dose and dosing in-

terval are then adjusted to the individual patient's needs.

Route of Administration

The patient's clinical status strongly determines the preferred route of administration. Oral, subcutaneous, or intramuscular routes are not indicated in patients with circulatory failure. In low-perfusion states, blood flow is diverted away from the gastrointestinal tract, as well as away from many skeletal muscle groups, subcutaneous tissue, and skin. If a drug is given orally or injected into peripheral tissue, absorption and onset of activity are unpredictably delayed. Because prompt drug intervention is important in critically ill patients, intravenous administration is preferred (Table 14-1).

Furthermore, after restoration of effective perfusion, drugs previously trapped in underperfused tissue may become mobilized, and the patient may become "dosed" at an inappropriate time. If multiple doses had been injected into peripheral tissue, wash-out of the drug at reperfusion may result in accidental overdose.

Rapid and total drug absorption is achieved only with the intravenous route. Generally, other parenteral routes are not used in critical care units.

Distribution

Normal circulatory function is required for effective drug distribution and concentration of the drug at appropriate tissue receptor sites. In patients with circulatory failure, the serum drug levels may be higher than expected for any given dose because of poor systemic tissue distribution. As a result, impaired drug uptake occurs at peripheral tissue receptor sites, along with decreased drug elimination.

TABLE 14-1
Routes of Drug Administration for Critical Care Patients

Route	Advantage	Disadvantage	Drugs	Use in ICU
Oral	Usually readily available	Slow, erratic, or no absorption	Many	None
Intramuscular, subcutaneous	Available	Slow, erratic absorption	Lidocaine	Arrhythmia management when IV route not available
			Epinephrine	Anaphylaxis
Peripheral, intravenous	Most drugs compatible with this route	Difficult to obtain access	Most	General
Central, intravenous	Can be placed in a severely hypotensive patient	Procedural risks	Many	General
Intratracheal	Available in intubated patients	Few data available	Epinephrine, lidocaine	During cardiac arrest when IV route not available
Intracardiac	Always available	Procedural risks	Epinephrine	When no other route is available

Elimination

All ingested or injected drugs must eventually be eliminated from the body. The liver and the kidneys are the primary organs of drug elimination, and their roles are briefly discussed.

Hepatic Clearance

Drugs cleared by the liver are metabolized (transformed) into inactive compounds that are ultimately excreted by the kidney, conjugated with another molecule to form an inactive water-soluble complex for urinary excretion, or excreted unchanged in the bile.

Hepatic drug clearance may be altered by several factors (Box 14-1). For example, splanchnic hypoperfusion, secondary to circulatory failure or the stress response to critical illness, reduces the effective rate of hepatic blood flow and drug clearance. Likewise, hepatic congestion and dysfunction, secondary to right heart failure, impairs drug clearance by the liver. In addition, a number of drugs, particularly those that affect the cytochrome P-450 system, can alter hepatic metabolism significantly.

Overall, hepatic hypoperfusion or hepatic dysfunction may result in altered and unpredictable drug elimination, serum drug levels, and drug effects. Because changes in hepatic drug clearance are among the most common causes of drug toxicities and intensified or reduced drug effects, serial drug levels should be obtained in high-risk patients. Drug doses or dosing intervals are then adjusted according to serum levels, which also are correlated with patients' clinical responses.

Renal Drug Excretion

Most drugs and toxins are ultimately excreted from the body by the kidneys. Drugs extracted by the kidneys are excreted unchanged in the urine or are first metabolized and conjugated by the liver to water-soluble forms for urinary excretion.

Drug excretion may be impaired because of prerenal failure (hypoperfusion of the kidneys); chronic or acute intrinsic renal disease, such as acute tubular necrosis (ATN); or postrenal failure (obstruction of the urinary tract) leading to hydronephrosis (Box 14-2). Renal dysfunction of any cause may result in decreased drug excretion and increased serum drug levels, intensified drug effects and prolongation of action, and a predisposition to drug toxicity. In patients with renal dysfunction, drug dosage regimens require careful adjustments based on the severity of the renal dysfunction, serial drug levels, and patients' clinical responses.

BOX 14-1
Factors That Influence Hepatic Clearance

Increase Hepatic Blood Flow/Increase Drug Clearance

Chronic respiratory disease
Glucagon
Drugs that increase cardiac output
Clinical situations that increase cardiac output

Hepatic Enzyme Inducers That Increase Clearance

Barbiturates
Phenytoin
Carbamazepine
Rifampin

Hepatotoxic Agents

Acetaminophen (high dose)
Anabolic steroids
Isoniazid
Nonsteroidal antiinflammatory agents
Phenothiazines
Tetracyclines
High-dose niacin

Decrease Hepatic Blood Flow/Decrease Drug Clearance

Hypotension
Volume depletion
Congestive heart failure
Advanced age
Circulatory collapse
Drugs that decrease cardiac output

Hepatic Enzyme Inhibitors That Decrease Clearance

Erythromycin
Isoniazid
Cimetidine
Ketoconazole

BOX 14-2
Factors That Influence Renal Excretion

Increase Renal Blood Flow (Increase Renal Excretion)

Expanded fluid volume
Low-dose dopamine
Agents that increase cardiac output
Loop diuretics

Renal Dysfunction (Decrease Renal Excretion)

Prerenal failure (hypoperfusion of the kidneys)
Renal failure (chronic or acute intrinsic disease)
Postrenal failure (obstruction of the urinary tract) leading to hydronephrosis

Nephrotoxic Agents (By Impairing Renal Function)

Aminoglycosides
Amphotericin
Cisplatin
Nonsteroidal antiinflammatory agents
Angiotensin-converting enzyme inhibitors
Vancomycin

Decrease Renal Blood Flow (Decrease Renal Excretion)

Reduced fluid volume
Vasopressors
Congestive heart failure
Nonsteroidal antiinflammatory agents
Shock

MECHANISMS OF ACTION OF CARDIOVASCULAR MEDICATIONS

Many medications used for ICU patients profoundly affect the performance of the cardiovascular system and hemodynamic measurements. These drugs induce direct or indirect changes within the myocardium, blood vessels, or both.

Pharmacologic modification of *cardiac function* involves one or more of the following factors: (1) changes in the force of myocardial contraction, referred to as positive (increased force) or negative (decreased force) inotropic effects; (2) changes in heart rate, referred to as increased or decreased chronotropic effects; (3) increasing or decreasing conduction velocity; and (4) altering the refractory period and automaticity of the myocardial cells through modification of the transmembrane action potential. Pharmacologic modification of the *blood vessels* includes decreases and increases in vascular smooth muscle tone (vasodilation and vasoconstriction, respectively).

Single drugs frequently produce several actions. Some actions are therapeutically desirable, whereas coexisting drug effects may be therapeutically counterproductive. For example, the potent inotropic action of norepinephrine (Levophed) is valuable in the management of patients with acute, severe heart failure. However, the desired inotropic effect is often offset by potent vasoconstrictor effects that increase left ventricular afterload and decreased systemic blood flow. Renal artery constriction and the associated threat of ischemic injury to the kidneys is particularly problematic in patients receiving norepinephrine. As a consequence of the multiplicity of drug actions, evaluation of the patient's risk-benefit response to the intended drug effect may be difficult.

Most of the cardiovascular support medications used in the ICU modify the physiology and biochemistry of the patient's cardiovascular system. Some of these drugs also have actions on bronchial smooth muscle and, as a consequence, effects on pulmonary function (discussed in the following section). In most cases, the drug effects are mediated by modifying autonomic nervous system influences on the heart and blood vessels or by treating arrhythmias by altering the transmembrane action potential. These mechanisms of action are briefly discussed later in this chapter.

PHARMACOLOGIC MODIFICATION OF AUTONOMIC NERVOUS SYSTEM INFLUENCES ON THE CARDIOVASCULAR SYSTEM

The sympathetic and parasympathetic branches of the autonomic nervous system profoundly affect cardiac output through their effects on the vascular tone, heart rate, myocardial contractility, and conduction velocity. Generally, progressive increases in drug dosing are associated with progressively intensified drug effects. Pharmacologic management of cardiovascular disease is mediated by augmenting (agonist) or blocking (antagonist) the actions of the sympathetic or parasympathetic nervous systems.

Drugs That Imitate the Cardiovascular Effects of the Sympathetic Nervous System (Agonists)

Nearly all sympathomimetic agents (drugs that mimic the actions of the sympathetic nervous system) are synthetic derivatives of natural substances released from the adrenal medulla (norepinephrine and epinephrine) and sympathetic nerve endings (norepinephrine).

Sympathomimetic agents act at special receptors, termed *adrenergic receptors,* located in effector cells in the heart, blood vessels, airways, and other tissues. Sympathomimetic drugs may directly or indirectly stimulate the sympathetic nervous system. Direct stimulation involves action of the agent at a sympathetic adrenergic receptor; indirect stimulation involves release of the endogenous sympathomimetic compounds that, in turn, exert action at a sympathetic adrenergic receptor. As stated, drugs used in patients with cardiovascular disease may therapeutically stimulate or blunt autonomic nervous system receptor responses.

Types of Sympathetic Nervous System Adrenergic Receptors

Sympathomimetic drugs act at special adrenergic receptor sites in effector cells; these are designated as alpha, beta, and dopaminergic receptors. These adrenergic receptors are further subdivided into alpha-1 and alpha-2 receptors, beta-1 and beta-2 receptors, and subclassifications of dopaminergic receptors.

Alpha Receptors. In general, alpha receptor stimulation results in potent constriction of vascular smooth muscle. The clinically observed effect is a generalized increase in systemic vascular resistance and blood pressure. There are no important alpha receptors in the heart.

Beta Receptors. Beta receptors are of two subtypes. Beta-1 receptors are located in and stimulate the myocardium, and beta-2 receptors are located in bronchial and vascular smooth muscle. Stimulation of beta-2 receptors results in bronchodilation and vasodilation. Overall, beta receptor stimulation is associated with positive inotropic and chronotropic effects, increased conduction velocity, increased automaticity in the conduction tissue and myocardial fibers, coronary and systemic vasodilation, and bronchodilation. This is noted clinically as an increase in heart rate and stroke volume, possibly ectopic arrhythmias, and decreased systemic vascular resistance. Airway resistance also decreases because of relaxation of bronchial smooth muscle.

Overall, alpha-adrenergic vasoconstrictor effects predominate over weaker beta vasodilator effects.

Dopaminergic Receptors. Dopaminergic receptors are activated by dopamine, which is a catecholamine formed in the body as an intermediate product in the synthesis of norepinephrine. Dopamine is an important central nervous system (CNS) neurotransmitter. Peripheral dopamine receptors exist within the myocardium, as well as in the renal, coronary, and intestinal blood vessels. When administered as a titrated drip, low-dose dopamine produces primarily dilation of the renal and mesenteric blood vessels. At intermediate doses, dopamine has a positive inotropic and chronotropic effect mediated by beta-1 stimulation, and in progressively higher doses, predominant alpha-adrenergic stimulation produces systemic vasoconstriction.

The location and primary effects of the adrenergic receptors are summarized in Table 14-2.

An easy way to remember the site of action of each beta receptor is

beta-1 = one heart; beta-2 = two lungs (airways)

TABLE 14-2

Classification, Location, and Primary Action of Adrenergic Receptors

Receptor	Location	Primary Action
Alpha-Adrenergic		
Alpha-1	Vascular smooth muscle	
	Arterioles and venules	Vasoconstriction
Alpha-2	Presynaptic nerve terminals	Feedback inhibition of catecholamine release, which results in peripheral vasodilation
Beta-Adrenergic		
Beta-1	Heart (myocardium)	Increased contractility
	SA node	Increased heart rate
	AV node	Increased conduction velocity
		Increased automaticity
Beta-2	Vascular smooth muscle	
	Arterioles and venules	Vasodilation
	Pulmonary, bronchial smooth muscle	Relaxation
Dopaminergic		
	Vascular smooth muscle (renal, coronary, mesenteric)	Vasodilation

Drugs That Block the Effects of the Sympathetic Nervous System (Antagonists)

Drug therapy may be used to block the alpha- or beta-adrenergic receptors of the cardiovascular system. The blunted sympathetic nervous system responses, in turn, result in an overall decrease in heart work and myocardial oxygen consumption.

Alpha-Adrenergic Blocking Agents

Drugs of this class, such as phentolamine, compete with endogenous alpha-adrenergic agonists for available alpha receptor sites. As a result, phentolamine produces vasodilation of both venous and arterial circulations. Thus systemic vascular resistance and blood pressure are lowered and venous return is decreased.

Beta-Adrenergic Blocking Agents

These drugs compete with beta-adrenergic agonists for available beta receptor sites. Some beta blocking agents, such as propranolol, block both beta-1 receptors (in the myocardium) and beta-2 receptors (in bronchial and vascular smooth muscle). The overall effect is a slowing of heart rate, decreased myocardial contractility, and inhibition of vasodilator and bronchodilator responses. This latter effect is highly undesirable in patients with hyperreactive airways and may worsen an asthmatic condition. For this reason, drugs that preferentially block beta-1 receptors, termed *cardioselective* drugs, have been developed and include metoprolol and atenolol.

Labetalol is a beta blocking agent with additional alpha blocking properties. As a result of the combined beta and alpha blocking effects, systemic vascular resistance and arterial pressure are reduced (alpha blocking effects) and the reflex tachycardia that commonly occurs with vasodilator therapy does not occur (beta blocking effects).

In general, stimulation or inhibition of each receptor type evokes a distinct change in cardiovascular function and hemodynamic measurements that may be predicted based on the known pharmacologic actions of that medication. However, the magnitude of specific drug responses is variable and is related to several factors.

Factors That Affect Individual Patient Responses to Drugs That Interact with the Autonomic Nervous System

In addition to the intrinsic receptor activity (agonist or antagonist) and drug dose, individual patient responses to the aforementioned medications depend on several other factors:

1. *The drug response is dependent on the relative proportion of receptor type and overall receptor density present in the various body tissues.* For example, the myocardium, which is rich with beta-1 receptors but has virtually no alpha receptors, would not be directly affected by a drug such as phenylephrine, which in therapeutic doses stimulates only alpha receptors. On the other hand, the peripheral vasculature, which has a

high concentration of alpha receptors, is very sensitive to the actions of phenylephrine.

2. *Sympathomimetic agonists and antagonists may stimulate reflex homeostatic mechanisms that, in turn, result in other cardiovascular changes.* For example, an alpha-induced increase in blood pressure usually results in a decrease in heart rate secondary to reflex vagal (parasympathetic) stimulation.

3. *Prolonged sympathomimetic drug therapy decreases the responsivity of patients' adrenergic receptors.* The decreased adrenergic response is the result of reduced tissue receptor sensitivity termed *down regulation.* In "down-regulated" patients, very high doses of a sympathomimetic agent may be necessary to overcome the acquired drug tolerance and maintain the desired therapeutic drug effect. Similarly, prolonged administration of antagonist drugs such as alpha or beta blocking agents may be associated with an increased receptor sensitivity, termed *up regulation.* Increased patient sensitivity to sympathetic nervous system stimulation may be noticed after the antagonist, such as a beta blocking agent, has been discontinued or a sympathomimetic agonist, such as epinephrine, is given. Meticulous drug dose titration is necessary in these sensitive patients.

Tables in this chapter include dosing charts for drugs given in the management of critical illness. Dosage ranges are applicable to most patients. However, in some down-regulated patients, drug doses much greater than those usually recommended are necessary. The need for increased drug dosing is based on *suboptimal* patient responses, as inferred by hemodynamic measurements and physical assessment findings. Alternatively, some patients require much lower doses than those recommended for their weight because of compromised hepatic and renal clearance or adrenergic receptor up regulation.

Drugs That Imitate the Cardiovascular Effects of the Parasympathetic Nervous System

Drugs in this category have profound depressant effects on cardiovascular function. They slow the rate of sinus nodal discharge and the rate of atrioventricular (AV) nodal conductivity to a level that may produce complete heart block or cardiac arrest. Parasympathomimetic drugs also produce marked vasodilation and decreases in systemic vascular resistance. The combined actions may be associated with profound hypotension. Overall, parasympathetic agonists have no clinical application. Atropine, which is commonly used in ICU patients, is a parasympathetic blocking agent that enhances the rate of discharge of the

sinus node and improves AV conduction. Consequently, the drug may be chosen for the treatment of symptomatic bradyarrhythmias or asystole.

ANTIARRHYTHMIC DRUG THERAPY

Arrhythmias that result in excessively rapid or slow heart rates, loss of the atrial contribution to ventricular filling, or distorted ventricular contractile dynamics are most likely to be associated with perfusion failure. The probability of arrhythmia-induced hemodynamic deterioration is further increased in patients with preexisting contractile failure (systolic dysfunction), valve disease, or coronary artery disease. Overall, the arrhythmic threat to the patient is related to (1) the likelihood of progression to a fatal arrhythmia, such as ventricular tachycardia spontaneously converting to ventricular fibrillation, and (2) how the arrhythmia is being clinically and hemodynamically tolerated. For example, a sinus tachycardia at a rate that results in anginal pain or signs of heart failure may be considered to be a greater threat to one patient than asymptomatic, hemodynamically stable ventricular tachycardia at the same ventricular rate in another patient.

Drug therapy is almost exclusively directed at the management of ectopic or reentry arrhythmias. Conduction disturbances are managed primarily by temporary or permanent pacemaker therapy. A discussion of the myocardial action potential and the normal sequence of cardiac excitation precedes the discussion of antiarrhythmic agents.

Transmembrane Action Potential

A brief description of the transmembrane action potential is included in this chapter. An understanding of how the myocardial cell is excited and how it returns to its resting state is necessary to understand and categorize the action of antiarrhythmic drugs.

Cardiac cells, like all body cells, have a difference between intracellular and extracellular ionic concentrations. Ion concentrations change dramatically within the cardiac cycle and are the mechanism underlying the cellular excitation/relaxation process. The difference in electrical potential between the inside and outside of the cell, created by the changing ionic gradient, is termed the *transmembrane action potential* (Figure 14-2). The transmembrane action potential may be graphically recorded in research laboratories using microelectrodes; one is impaled within the myocardial cell and the other impinges on the outer surface of the cell.

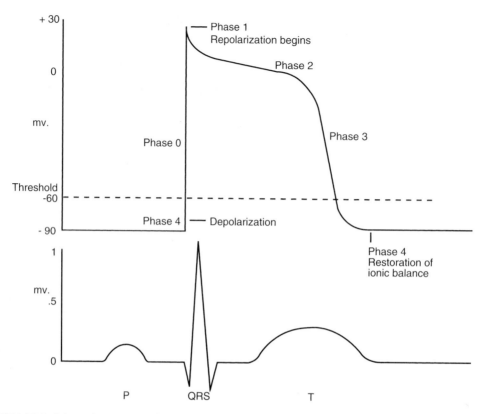

FIGURE 14-2 Schematic representation of ventricular myocardial cells' action potential. The recorded ECG is the sum of the action potentials of all myocardial cells. (Modified from Guntheroth WG: *Pediatric electrocardiography,* Philadelphia, 1965, W.B. Saunders.)

Phases of the Action Potential

The discussion begins with the resting myocardial cell. The cardiac cycle is then followed through excitation and back to the resting state (see Figure 14-2).

Phase 4—Immediately before Excitation. In the resting "polarized" state (phase 4), the sodium and calcium ion concentrations are much greater outside the myocardial cell than within, whereas potassium predominates within the cellular space. The inside of the cell is electronegative and the outside is electropositive, creating a transmembrane action potential of approximately −90 to −80 mV. Phase 4 correlates with the isoelectric line of the electrocardiogram (ECG).

Phase 0—Depolarization. With the onset of excitation "depolarization" of the myocardial cell, an abrupt change in the permeability of the cell membrane permits intracellular movement of positively charged sodium and calcium ions. The influx of positively charged ions then causes the inside of the cell to become relatively electropositive. The steep upstroke of the transmembrane action potential, to approximately +20 to +40 mV, brings the myocardial cell past its stimulation threshold, which is normally −60 mV. On passing the stimulation threshold, the myocardial cell becomes activated. Activation of a single myocardial cell also causes a longitudinal electrical potential difference that results in excitation of the adjacent cells of the myocardial fiber. In this manner, the wave of depolarization marches from cell to cell across the heart. Phase 0 corresponds to the QRS on the ECG.

Phase 1—Repolarization Begins. Following depolarization, the brief decrease in waveform positivity heralds the onset of cell relaxation repolarization.

Phase 2—Depolarization. The membrane potential is close to 0 mV and briefly remains so because of the continued slow influx of ionic calcium (see Figure 14-2). This plateau corresponds with the ST segment of the ECG.

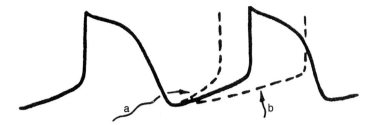

FIGURE 14-3 Action potential of pacemaking cell. Resting phase 4 spontaneously slopes toward the threshold. Increasing slope *(a)* produces acceleration; decreasing slope *(b)* produces slowing of pacemaker discharge rate. (From Marriott HJL: *Practical electrocardiography,* ed 8, Baltimore, 1988, Williams & Wilkins.)

Phase 3—Repolarization. The next phase is the phase of final recovery, during which the interior of the cell becomes electronegative as potassium moves out of the cell and the transmembrane action potential falls precipitously back to -80 to -90 mV. Phase 3 corresponds with the T wave on the ECG.

Phase 4—Restoration of Ionic Balance. This phase marks the return to the resting phase. The concentrations of sodium and potassium are readjusted by the action of the active transport mechanism of the cell wall (the sodium-potassium pump mechanism). The pump moves sodium out of and potassium into the cell, and the cell remains polarized, resting, and isoelectric until the arrival of the next wave of excitation.

Difference between Pacemaker and Contractile Cells

Many cardiac cells have *inherent automaticity,* which means the capability of spontaneous electrical discharge followed by contraction of myocardial fibers. These "automatic" cells are located in the sinus node, in certain cells of the atrium and AV node, and in the His-Purkinje system. The sinus node normally dominates as pacemaker because its spontaneous discharge rate is faster than those of other automatic cells.

The fundamental difference between myocardial "contractile" cells and automatic "pacemaking" cells is the automatic cell's ability to depolarize spontaneously during phase 4 and undergo spontaneous, cyclic excitation. The resting phase 4 slopes spontaneously toward threshold, usually -60 mV, and a new excitation wave is sent to the heart. An increased slope produces acceleration of the pacemaker discharge rate, whereas a decreased slope is associated with the slowing of the pacemaker discharge rate (Figure 14-3). However, any myocardial fiber is capable of generating a conducted impulse. The sinus node remains the pacemaker of the heart so long as (1) the sinus node and the conduction system function normally and (2) the sinus node generates impulses faster than any other portion of the myocardium.

Sequence of Cardiac Excitation

As mentioned earlier, the excitatory impulse that depolarizes and then animates the heart is initiated and discharged by the sinus node. At rest, the sinus node discharges at a rate of 60 to 100 beats per minute. The depolarizing impulse then spreads rapidly downward through the atria and enters the AV node, which is the only normal conduction pathway between the atria and the ventricles. Impulse propagation then proceeds through the His-Purkinje system and spreads to all parts of the ventricles (Figure 14-4).

A normal excitation sequence and an associated synchronous cardiac contractile pattern are generally associated with a hemodynamically effective stroke volume and cardiac output. The depolarization currents associated with some arrhythmias deviate from the normal conduction pathway and may be associated with distorted myocardial contractile dynamics and reduced stroke volume. Arrhythmias result from disturbances in impulse formation (originating in areas of abnormal myocardium) competing for primary pacemaker activity, disturbances in impulse conduction, or both.

Pharmacologic Management of Ectopic and Reentrant Arrhythmias

The objectives of antiarrhythmic therapy are restoring normal heart action by reducing ectopic cardiac pacemaker activity, normalizing the heart rate in patients with conduction defects, and altering the refractory period of reentrant conduction tissue pathways. Drug therapy is the cornerstone in management of most cardiac arrhythmias. As mentioned, conduction disturbances are managed by temporary or permanent pacemaker therapy.

The antiarrhythmic agents are classified according to their electrophysiologic properties and effect on the cardiac action potential (Table 14-3).

Class I

Drugs in this class are sometimes called "membrane stabilizing" agents because they inhibit the fast sodium channels of the cell membrane. In this way, class I agents decrease phase 0 of the rapid depolarization of the action potential. Class I agents are often subdivided according to the specific characteristics of fast sodium channel inhibition.

Class I-A. This class of drugs includes quinidine, procainamide, and disopyramide. Repolarization is delayed and there is a prolongation of the action potential.

Class I-B. This class of drugs includes lidocaine, mexiletine, and phenytoin. Repolarization is accelerated and the action potential is abbreviated.

Class I-C. This class includes flecainide and propafenone. There is a marked inhibition of conduction through the His-Purkinje tissue and, as a result, QRS prolongation.

Class II

This group of drugs includes the beta blockers such as propranolol. They exert their effects by blocking sympathetic nervous system effects on the cardiovascular system and have no specific effects on ion transport and action potential.

Class III

This class of drugs includes amiodarone, bretylium, sotalol, ibutilide, and the newest antiarrhythmic available, dofetilide. These agents inhibit repolarization, causing a prolongation of the action potential duration.

Class IV

This class of antiarrhythmic agents includes the calcium-channel blockers such as verapamil and diltiazem. These drugs exert their antiarrhythmic effect by inhibiting movement of ionized calcium across the slow calcium channel, particularly at the AV node. This results in a depression of phase 4 depolarization.

In summary, through selective mechanisms, antiarrhythmic drugs restore normal cardiac rhythm by either decreasing excitability and automaticity of cardiac cells or altering the refractory period of abnormal conduction pathways (that enable the propagation of reentrant tachyarrhythmias) while only minimally affecting the electrical activity in the normal portions of the myocardium. The associated hemodynamic drug effects vary with the specific drug and each patient's underlying cardiovascular function.

TABLE 14-3

Classification and Action of Antiarrhythmic Agents

Class	Electrophysiologic Effect	Agents
I	Depresses phase 0; depresses either phase 4 or prolongs effective refractory periods	Lidocaine, quinidine, procainamide, phenytoin
II	Blocks beta receptors	Propranolol, labetalol, esmolol atenolol, metoprolol
III	Prolongs effective refractory period, action potential duration	Bretylium, amiodarone, sotalol, ibutalide, dofetilide
IV	Blocks calcium channels	Verapamil, diltiazem

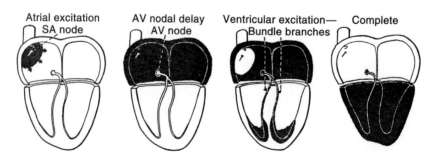

FIGURE 14-4 Excitation of the heart is normally initiated by an impulse that is generated by the SA node and that spreads rapidly in all directions through the atrial musculature. After a slight delay at the AV node, impulses are conducted by the Purkinje system into the ventricles, where the wave of excitation spreads from the endocardial surfaces through the ventricular musculature.

INTRAVENOUS MEDICATIONS COMMONLY USED FOR HEMODYNAMIC SUPPORT OF CRITICALLY ILL OR INJURED PATIENTS

The following medications are commonly used in management of critically ill or injured patients. Drug activity, indications, available intravenous (IV) preparations, dosage recommendations, drug elimination, specific parameters to monitor, as well as specific precautions or important drug-disease interactions are described for each medication.

The recommended dose ranges may not be appropriate for all patients. Doses much higher or, in some cases, lower than the usual range may be required and are gauged by each patient's clinical and hemodynamic responses. Vigilant monitoring of up-regulated or down-regulated patients is of particular importance, especially when the patient is receiving very high drug dosages. A summary of the expected change in hemodynamic parameters with some of these medications appears in Table 14-4. Many of the cardiovascular drugs have multiple actions; for example,

TABLE 14-4
Effect on Hemodynamic Parameters of Selected Common Intravenous Medications for Monitored Patients

	HR	MAP	PAP	PWP	CVP	SVR	SV	CO
Vasodilating Agents								
Nitroglycerin	0/↑	↓	↓	↓	0/↓	↓	↑	↑
Nitroprusside	↑	↓	↓	0/↓	0/↓	↓	↑	↑
Hydralazine	↑	↓	↓	0/↓	0/↓	↓	↑	↑
Trimethaphan	↑	↓	↓	0/↓	0/↓	↓	↑	↑
Vasopressor Agents								
Phenylephrine	0/↓	↑	↑	↑	↑	↑	↓	↑/↓
Mixed-Activity Agents								
Epinephrine	↑	↑	↑	↑	↑	↑/↓	↑/↓	↑
Norepinephrine	0/↑	↑	↑	↑	↑	↑	↑/↓	↑/↓
Dopamine	0/↑	0/↑	0/↑	0/↑	0/↑	0/↑	↑/↓	↑
Inotropic Agents								
Dobutamine	0/↑	0/↑	0	0/↓	0/↑	0/↓	↑	↑
Isoproterenol	↑	0/↑	0/↑	0/↓	0/↓	0/↓	↑	↑
Amrinone	0/↑	↓	↓	↓	0/↓	↓	↑	↑
Milrinone	0/↑	↓	↓	↓	0/↓	↓	↑	↑
Digoxin	↓	0	0/↓	0/↓	0/↓	↑	↑	↑
Antiarrhythmic Agents								
Lidocaine	0	0/↓	0/↓	0	0	0/↓	0	0/↑
Procainamide	0	↓	0/↓	0/↓	0/↓	0	0	0/↓
Propranolol*	↓	↓	0/↓	0/↑	0/↓	0/↑	↑	↓
Atenolol*	↓	↓	0/↓	0/↑	0/↓	0	↑	↓
Metoprolol*	↓	↓	0/↓	0/↑	0/↓	0	↑	↓
Labetalol*	↓	↓	↓	↓	↓	↓	↑	↓
Esmolol*	↓	↓	↓	0/↑	0/↓	0	↑	↓
Bretylium	↑/↓	0	0	0	0	0	0	0
Verapamil	↓	0/↓	0/↓	0/↑	0/↓	↓	0	↑/↓
Diltiazem	0/↓	0/↓	0/↓	0/↑	0/↓	↓	0	↑/↓

KEY: 0, Little or no change; ↑, increase; ↓, decrease.

CO, cardiac output; *CVP,* central venous pressure; *HR,* heart rate; *MAP,* mean arterial pressure; *PAP,* pulmonary artery pressure; *PWP,* pulmonary artery wedge pressure; *SV,* stroke volume; *SVR,* systemic vascular resistance.

*The effect of beta blocking agents on CO is variable and depends to a great extent on preexisting left ventricular function. Beta blocker use in patients with diastolic dysfunction and an increased heart rate results in an increase in CO secondary to increased filling time. In contrast, beta blocker use in patients with decompensated systolic dysfunction may result in a decrease in CO and worsening of heart failure.

digoxin is both a positive inotropic and an antiarrhythmic drug. The various drug actions for each medication are discussed, although the specific drug appears in one general drug category in this chapter.

The authors recommend that the drugs described, particularly the vasoactive agents, be infused via a central venous line. This precautionary measure prevents the tissue injury that may occur secondary to accidental extravasation through a peripheral IV catheter and also ensures predictable bioavailability. Any drug solution that is discolored should not be used. Also, therapy with all titratable agents should not be discontinued abruptly but should be tapered gradually, guided by careful monitoring.

The authors also recommend that when potent vasoactive agents are being infused, the patient should be in a critical care unit and that the arterial pressure should be continuously monitored via intraarterial line. If invasive blood pressure monitoring is not possible, frequent blood pressure measurements (every 3 to 5 minutes) via automated devices are required. The accuracy of machine-acquired measurements should also be periodically cross-checked using the manual technique. These precautionary measures reduce the risk of sudden increases or decreases in blood pressure that may be poorly tolerated, particularly by patients with cerebral or coronary vascular or cardiac diseases. The adjunctive invasive or noninvasive measurement of cardiac output is indicated for many of the medications listed in this chapter when used in patients with potential or actual hemodynamic instability.

Vasodilator Agents

Nitroglycerin

Nitrates relax venous and, to a lesser degree, arterial smooth muscle. Venodilation, in turn, is associated with a marked reduction in *preload*. The slight arterial dilator effect produces a *slight* decrease in systemic vascular resistance (*afterload* reduction) that, in turn, is associated with an increase in stroke volume. Reflex tachycardia may occur in response to vasodilation. Nitroglycerin also dilates the epicardial and collateral coronary arteries while preserving coronary autoregulation so that coronary blood flow is not shunted away from ischemic myocardium (coronary steal).

Uses. Nitroglycerin is most often used to control chest pain, mild-to-moderate hypertension, and congestive heart failure due to ischemic heart disease (angina pectoris and myocardial infarction).

Preparations. Tridil, Nitrostat IV, Nitro-Bid, nitroglycerin injection, 0.5 mg/ml, 0.8 mg/ml, 5 mg/ml, 10 mg/ml in dilution for titration administration.

Dosing. Continuous infusion beginning at 5 to 10 μg/min. This dose is increased every 5 minutes until blood pressure, wedge pressure response, or relief of pain is obtained. Dosage increments may be increased by 10 μg/min if necessary. There is no maximal dose of nitroglycerin, but most clinicians believe that if 200 μg/min does not provide relief of hypertension or ischemic pain, doses higher than that are unlikely to be of any benefit. In these cases, it may be prudent to carefully add or change to a more potent titratable drug such as sodium nitroprusside.

Pharmacokinetics. The onset of nitroglycerin's hypotensive effect is approximately 1 to 5 minutes; the duration of effect is 5 to 10 minutes. The therapeutic effect for relieving chest pain may be up to 30 minutes. Nitroglycerin undergoes hepatic metabolism.

Monitoring. Monitor blood pressure (BP), heart rate (HR), and ECG for worsening or resolution of ischemic changes. Pulmonary artery pressure (PAP) and pulmonary artery wedge pressure (PWP) should be monitored in hemodynamically unstable patients.

Cautions. Latent or overt hypovolemia may be associated with a marked reduction in blood pressure. Hypotension may, in turn, worsen myocardial ischemia. Restoration of circulatory volume by fluid loading generally stabilizes the patient's response to nitroglycerin. Occasionally, bradycardia and severe hypotension occur during IV infusion (Bezold-Jarisch reflex). If this occurs, the drug should be stopped and the patient's legs elevated. If bradycardia and hypotension persist, IV atropine and fluid challenges are required to stabilize the patient's condition. Other undesirable effects of nitroglycerin include headache because of direct cerebral vasodilation and development of tolerance with long-term use. Hypoxemia results from ventilation-perfusion mismatch (perfusion in excess of ventilation), induced by pulmonary vasodilation in areas of nonventilated or poorly ventilated alveoli.

Sodium Nitroprusside

Nitroprusside is an extremely potent direct-acting dilator of both veins and arteries of the systemic, coronary, pulmonary, and renal circulations. Decreased *preload,* mediated by venodilation, is associated with reduced right and left ventricular filling volume and pressure (right atrial and PWP, respectively), reduced size and wall stress of both ventricles, and reduced pulmonary vascular congestion and therefore pulmonary artery pressures. Decreased *afterload* (mediated by arteriolar dilation) results in a reduction in systemic and pulmonary vascular resistance and an increase in stroke volume. Both preload and afterload reduction decrease myocardial oxygen consumption. Reflex tachycardia may result from the decreased blood pressure.

Uses. Nitroprusside is given for the immediate reduction of blood pressure in emergencies such as hypertensive encephalopathy, catecholamine crisis, and pulmonary edema secondary to systemic hypertension. Nitroprusside is used also as a balanced (preload and afterload) unloading agent in patients with refractory congestive heart failure with or without myocardial infarction. Nitroprusside is more likely to cause coronary steal than nitroglycerin and is therefore *not* the drug of choice in controlling blood pressure or managing heart failure in patients with ischemic heart disease.

Preparations. Nipride, Nitropress, and others, powder for injection 50 mg per vial to be diluted for titration administration.

Dosing. Continuous infusion, beginning at 0.3 μg/kg/min and titrated for BP or hemodynamic effect. A dose of 10 μg/kg/min is considered the usual maximal dose and should be given only for several minutes before being decreased. The usual maximum maintenance dose is 2 μg/kg/min. The drug is photosensitive and degrades rapidly in light. Consequently, the IV bag should always be covered with metal foil or another opaque material. It is not necessary to cover the drip chamber and the tubing.

Pharmacokinetics. The onset of activity of nitroprusside occurs within 30 to 60 seconds. Blood pressure begins to rise almost immediately after discontinuation of therapy and reaches pretreatment levels within 1 to 10 minutes. Nitroprusside is rapidly metabolized in the presence of red blood cells. The ferrous ion in the nitroprusside molecule reacts rapidly with the sulfhydryl compounds in the red blood cells, resulting in the release of cyanide. Cyanide is further metabolized in the liver to thiocyanate. The thiocyanate is excreted in the urine with a half-life of 2.7 to 7 days in patients with normal renal function.

Monitoring. The HR, PAP, PWP, BP (preferably using an intraarterial line), and acid-base balance are monitored.

Cautions. Nitroprusside is contraindicated in patients with compensatory hypertension due to arteriovenous shunt or hypertension due to coarctation of the aorta. Vigilant bedside hemodynamic monitoring is indicated, especially in patients who have decreased hepatic or renal

function and in patients who are severely debilitated. Nitroprusside may result in or may worsen hypoxemia by dilating the pulmonary arterioles and increasing ventilation/perfusion mismatch.

Patients receiving nitroprusside also should be observed for signs of thiocyanate and cyanide toxicity. Signs of thiocyanate toxicity include weakness, rashes, tinnitus, lactic acidosis, blurred vision, seizures, psychotic behavior, and mental confusion. Metabolic acidosis is one of the earliest signs of plasma accumulation of the cyanide radical. Ideally, nitroprusside therapy should not exceed 48 hours, but the drug may be continued for longer periods if necessary. Daily thiocyanate levels are recommended for patients receiving nitroprusside for more than 48 hours.

Hypovolemia should be suspected in patients in whom a labile blood pressure requires frequent, small dose adjustments for control. In these patients, diuretic therapy or an additional vasodilator stimulus such as warming may result in precipitous, severe hypotension. Restoration of normal intravascular volume is usually associated with stabilization of blood pressure at a relatively constant nitroprusside drip rate.

Nitroprusside should *not* be used alone for blood pressure control in patients with dissecting aortic aneurysm or traumatic aortic dissection. The increased force of the left ventricular pressure pulse increases shearing forces on the injured aortic wall and, as a result, perpetuates aortic injury. If nitroprusside is being considered for blood pressure control in these clinical situations, the patient *must* have effective beta-1 blockade treatment before beginning the nitroprusside drip.

Trimethaphan*

Trimethaphan is a ganglionic blocking agent that blocks transmission of impulses at the sympathetic and parasympathetic ganglia by competing with acetylcholine for cholinergic receptors. This action results in vasodilation, decreased systemic vascular resistance, and decreased blood pressure. Trimethaphan has been unavailable from the manufacturer for some time now, but there has been some consideration for making the drug available again in the future.

Uses. Trimethaphan is given for the immediate reduction of blood pressure in patients with hypertensive emergencies. Trimethaphan also is given for controlling blood pressure and the rate of left ventricular pressure rise in patients with acute dissection of the aorta or traumatic rupture of the aorta.

---

*Trimethaphan has been removed from the market since the writing of this chapter.

Preparations. Arfonad 50 mg/ml to be diluted for titration administration (must be refrigerated).

Dosing. Initial doses of 0.5 to 1.0 mg/min are recommended for treating hypertensive emergencies. Gradual increases can be made every 1 to 2 minutes until the desired blood pressure is achieved. Doses greater than 6.0 mg/min are not routinely used. In patients with dissecting aortic aneurysms, dosage adjustments are made to maintain systolic blood pressure at approximately 100 to 120 mm Hg.

Pharmacokinetics. The onset of the hypotensive effect occurs within 30 to 60 seconds, and the duration of effect is 10 to 15 minutes. Trimethaphan undergoes pseudocholinesterase (enzymatic) metabolism and is excreted by the kidney.

Monitoring. The BP, HR, PAP, PWP, respiration rate, and urine output are monitored.

Cautions. Trimethaphan is associated with many side effects because of its nonselective blocking effects on the autonomic nervous system. The adverse effects tend to be dose related. Trimethaphan causes urinary retention, orthostatic hypotension (the patient should never be raised suddenly to a sitting position; likewise, placing patients in a recumbent position may require an increase in the drip rate), tachycardia, angina, anorexia, nausea, vomiting, dry mouth, and weakness. Large doses have been associated with apnea and respiratory arrest.

Warnings. Sodium nitroprusside and trimethaphan are both extremely potent, rapid-acting hypotensive agents that may produce a precipitous drop in blood pressure. If patients are not vigilantly monitored, severe hypotension may lead to major ischemic injuries or death. Accidental hypotension resolves within 1 to 10 minutes of discontinuation of the drugs. During this period, placing the patient in a leg-elevated position may increase blood pressure by augmenting venous return. If, at any time, hypotension persists after discontinuation of either agent, the drug is not the cause. The true cause, such as hypovolemia, must be immediately investigated.

Hydralazine

Hydralazine is a direct-acting dilator of smooth muscle. The primary effect is arterial dilation, with minor venodilator effects. Pulmonary and renal vascular resistance also decrease. Systemic vasodilation results in decreased systemic vascular resistance, decreased arterial pressure, increased stroke volume, and increased rate of left ventricular pressure rise. Reflex tachycardia may occur secondary to vasodilation.

Uses. Hydralazine is given in the management of moderate to severe hypertension and severe congestive heart failure.

Preparations. Apresoline, 20 mg/ml.

Dosing. Bolus administration of 5 to 10 mg until the desired effect is attained or a maximal single dose of 20 mg. The drug should be given cautiously in patients whose circulatory volume and status are uncertain. In these patients, injection of a maximal single dose of 20 mg may be associated with severe hypotension in the ensuing 5- to 20-minute period. Therefore dosing in small increments and waiting 15 to 20 minutes for the maximal response is recommended.

Pharmacokinetics. The onset of action for hydralazine is 5 to 20 minutes, and the duration of effect is approximately 2 to 6 hours. Hydralazine is metabolized by the liver.

Monitoring. BP and HR should be monitored.

Cautions. Blood pressure must be checked frequently and immediately after administration because it may begin to fall within a few minutes of injection. The maximal blood pressure decrease may occur within 10 minutes. The drug dose must be decreased in patients with liver dysfunction, low cardiac output, and severe renal dysfunction. The "hyperdynamic" circulatory changes (increased rate of left ventricular pressure rise and stroke volume) produced by hydralazine may be dangerous in patients with certain cardiovascular disorders.

Hydralazine should be used with caution in patients with *coronary artery disease* because the reflex tachycardia produced by the drug may produce anginal attacks or acute myocardial infarction. Hydralazine also is contraindicated in patients with *rheumatic mitral valve disease* because the drug may increase pulmonary artery pressures. Hydralazine is *not* recommended for blood pressure control in patients with *dissecting aortic aneurysm* because the increased rate of left ventricular pressure rise stresses the dissecting aortic segment and worsens aortic injury and propagates dissection. Finally, because postural hypotension may occur with hydralazine, the drug should be given with caution in patients with *cerebrovascular disease.*

Enalaprilat

Enalaprilat (Vasotec IV) is the activated form of enalapril and is currently the only angiotensin-converting enzyme (ACE) inhibitor available for parenteral administration. Enalaprilat dilates both veins and arteries and therefore reduces both preload and afterload.

Uses. Enalaprilat is given to rapidly reduce blood pressure, to "unload" patients with low cardiac output, or in the treatment of heart failure when oral therapy is not feasible.

Preparations. Enalaprilat IV, 1.25 mg/ml, 2.5 mg/ml.

Dosing. The usual dosage range is 0.625 to 2.5 mg every 6 to 8 hours via IV push. The maximum recommended dose is 5 mg every 6 hours.

Pharmacokinetics. The onset of the antihypertensive effect is 0.5 to 4 hours, but may be earlier, especially after multiple doses. The duration of effect is approximately 6 hours. Enalaprilat is renally eliminated.

Monitoring. The BP and serum creatinine are monitored.

Cautions. Enalaprilat is contraindicated in patients with bilateral renal artery stenosis and should be used with caution in those with unstable renal function because ACE inhibitors may cause a worsening of renal function. Patients may develop hyperkalemia while receiving enalaprilat, especially if their renal function is compromised. Rarely, enalaprilat causes angioedema.

Nicardipine

Nicardipine is a calcium channel blocker in the dihydropyridine class. Its hemodynamic and electrophysiologic effects resemble those of nifedipine.

Uses. Parenteral nicardipine is most often used for short-term treatment of hypertension. It may be an effective alternative to other agents, including sodium nitroprusside, in patients who do not respond to or tolerate other agents.

Preparations. Cardene IV, 2.5 mg/ml. Nicardipine must be diluted before being administered, and a final concentration of 0.1 mg/ml is recommended in the product information. There are some data available regarding more concentrated solutions for use in fluid-restricted patients, but these are not recommended by the manufac-

turer. Nicardipine is compatible with 0.9% saline and 5% dextrose, but it should not be diluted in lactated Ringer's solution and is not compatible with sodium bicarbonate (5%) solution.

Dosing. Initial therapy is 5 mg/hr, with adjustments of 2.5 mg/hr made every 5 or 15 minutes, depending on how rapidly blood pressure control needs to be achieved. The maximum recommended dose is 15 mg/hr. Once blood pressure is controlled, the lowest effective maintenance dose should be given. Most patients are maintained with doses of 3 to 5 mg/hr.

Pharmacokinetics. Intravenous nicardipine decreases blood pressure within 1 minute of administration, and the effect may persist for several hours or more once the infusion has been discontinued. Nicardipine undergoes extensive liver metabolism.

Monitoring. The HR and BP are monitored.

Cautions. Nicardipine IV is generally well tolerated, and most side effects are expected consequences of vasodilation.

Epoprostinol

Epoprostinol is a naturally occurring prostaglandin possessing potent vasodilating properties.

Uses. The major use of epoprostinol is primary pulmonary hypertension. Several studies have shown it to be effective when other vasodilators have failed. Epoprostinol has also been used for short-term management of secondary pulmonary hypertension in the hospitalized patient.

Preparations. Flolan, 0.5 mg/vial, 1.5 mg/vial lyophilized powder for injection. Epoprostinol is supplied as a freeze-dried powder that must be diluted with a *special diluent* before administration. The diluent can be obtained through the distributor of the epoprostinol. The resultant solution should be protected from light and discarded after 8 hours at room temperature. Infusions can be used for up to 24 hours if two frozen 6-ounce gel packs (changed every 12 hours) in a cold pouch are used. The product information contains instructions on how to prepare specific amounts of epoprostinol.

Dosing. The initial recommended dose of epoprostinol is 2 ng/kg/min. The dose is titrated by 2 ng/kg/min every 15 minutes until dose-limiting hemodyamic or adverse effects occur. These include hypotension, nausea, vomiting, and headache. The mean maximum dose that was well tolerated in clinical studies was approximately 8 ng/kg/min.

Pharmacokinetics. Epoprostinol has a rapid onset of effect and short duration of action. Cardiovascular effects subside within 5 minutes following discontinuance of an infusion. The drug is hydrolyzed in the plasma.

Monitoring. Monitor HR, BP, and PAP as needed in patients in the acute care setting.

Cautions. Patients receiving epoprostinol experience dose-related decreases in systemic blood pressure and increases in heart rate. Other side effects include facial flushing, hyperglycemia, nausea, vomiting, and abdominal discomfort. Epoprostinol is contraindicated in patients with congestive heart failure secondary to severe left ventricular dysfunction.

Vasopressor Agents

Vasopressors are given to patients with hypotension and shock because of systemic vasodilator reactions or in patients in whom all other therapeutic measures, such as volume replacement or inotropic support, fail to increase mean arterial pressure. The drugs most commonly given possess some degree of alpha receptor agonist properties. Patients receiving vasopressor medications have intense systemic vasoconstriction and therefore may appear pale and cool to touch. Because of the tremendous risk of ischemic tissue injury in the event of drug extravasation, these drugs, ideally, should be infused through a central venous catheter. If demands of an emergency situation do not allow time for placement of a central line but the drug is urgently needed, check integrity of the IV site frequently until a central line can be placed. A thin layer of nitroglycerin paste has been effective in countering the local effects of extravasated pressor agents.

Phenylephrine

Phenylephrine is a sympathomimetic amine that acts by direct stimulation of alpha-adrenergic receptors in the systemic vasculature. Vasoconstriction, in turn, increases both systolic and diastolic blood pressure. Phenylephrine also produces an indirect effect by release of norepinephrine from cell storage sites.

Uses. Phenylephrine is used in the treatment of hypotension because of systemic vasodilator reaction (neurogenic shock, septic shock, or anaphylactic shock)

that persists after adequate fluid replacement. The drug also may be helpful in maintaining adequate cerebral perfusion in patients after vascular surgery such as carotid endarterectomy.

Preparations. Neo-Synephrine, 10 mg/ml to be diluted for titration administration.

Dosing. The drug may be initially infused at 50 to 100 μg/min. The drug is titrated to the desired hemodynamic effect. The usual infusion rate is 40 to 60 μg/min.

Pharmacokinetics. The onset of action occurs within seconds in most patients. The duration of effect is 5 to 20 minutes. Phenylephrine is eliminated by tissue uptake and hepatic metabolism.

Monitoring. The HR, BP, cardiac output (CO), PWP, renal function, and acid-base balance should be monitored.

Cautions. Decreased stroke volume and increased cardiac work (secondary to increased afterload) and reflex bradycardia may induce or exacerbate circulatory failure or myocardial ischemia. Prolonged administration of this potent vasoconstrictor drug may result in peripheral ischemia and tissue necrosis in the fingers, ears, and toes, particularly in patients with peripheral vascular disease.

Mixed-Activity Agents (Vasopressor and Inotropic)

Epinephrine

This drug is a direct-acting catecholamine with alpha- and beta-adrenergic stimulating effects. Beta effects predominate at low doses and alpha vasoconstrictor effects predominate at higher doses. The low-dose beta effects cause vasodilation, cardiac stimulation, and bronchial smooth muscle relaxation.

Uses. Epinephrine is chosen most often in the management of cardiac arrest because of its alpha-adrenergic receptor stimulating effects. Intense systemic vasoconstriction increases central aortic and therefore coronary and cerebral perfusion pressures. Epinephrine also is used in the management of patients with either severe bronchospasm bradycardia or heart block. The drug should be avoided in patients with cardiogenic shock due to myocardial ischemia because of the dramatic drug-induced increases in cardiac work and myocardial oxygen consumption.

Preparations. Adrenalin and others, 1 mg/ml (1:1000) and 0.1 mg/ml (1:10,000).

Dosing. When given by constant IV infusion, an initial starting dose of 1 to 2 μg/min is recommended. The usual maximal dose is 8 μg/min. The dose is adjusted for desired patient effects and is not specifically altered for any particular disease or condition. In the management of *cardiac arrest,* epinephrine is usually administered intravenously, but it also may be given directly into the tracheobronchial tree via an endotracheal tube. The recommended initial IV dose is 1 mg, which may be repeated every 3 to 5 minutes as needed. Higher doses of epinephrine (5 mg or approximately 0.1 mg/kg) may be considered only if the 1 mg dose has failed. For endotracheal delivery, drug administration 2 to 2.5 times the recommended IV dose may be required (2 to 2.5 mg in 10 ml of normal saline). Some clinicians recommend much higher doses (10 mg) than those that now appear in the literature, but studies have not demonstrated a definite survival benefit with these doses; therefore they should not be routinely used.

Pharmacokinetics. The physiologic effects of epinephrine are seen within seconds of administration. The duration of effect is approximately 1 to 2 minutes. Epinephrine is eliminated by cellular reuptake and general peripheral tissue metabolism.

Monitoring. The HR, BP, CO, PWP, and urine output should be monitored.

Cautions. Epinephrine should be administered via a central venous line because local tissue necrosis may result if extravasation occurs. Cardiac arrhythmias and tachycardia may be seen with epinephrine because of the intrinsic arrhythmogenic and chronotropic effects of the drug. Epinephrine in conjunction with digoxin or certain anesthetics (halothane and cyclopropane) increases the likelihood of arrhythmias.

Vasopressin

Vasopressin is included in this section of the chapter because it has been added to the most recent advanced cardiac life support (ACLS) guidelines as an alternative agent to epinephrine in the setting of ventricular fibrillation/pulseless ventricular tachycardia.

Uses. In addition to its use in the code setting, vasopressin is used in the treatment of diabetes insipidus and as adjuvant treatment in the management of acute massive hemorrhage associated with ruptured esophageal varices, peptic ulcer disease, esophagogastritis, and other gastrointestinal (GI) abnormalities.

Preparations. Pitressin, 20 units/ml; generic vasopressin preparations are also available.

Dosing. A one-time dose of 40 units given by IV push is recommended in the ACLS guidelines. The longer half-life of vasopressin allows for less frequent dosing compared with epinephrine. The usual dose in the treatment of diabetes insipidus is 5 to 10 units given intramuscularly or subcutaneously 2 to 4 times a day as needed. Dosages may range from 5 to 60 units daily. When vasopressin is being given by the IV route in the management of GI bleeding, a low dose should be started to minimize side effects and titrated up as necessary. Initial doses of 0.2 to 0.4 units/min are often used and titrated to 0.9 units/min. Intraarterial infusions of 0.1 to 0.5 units/min have been used.

Pharmacokinetics. Vasopressin has a plasma half-life of 10 to 20 minutes. It is rapidly destroyed in the liver and kidneys. Vasopressin is degraded by trypsin in the GI tract and therefore cannot be given orally.

Monitoring. Monitor ECG for arrhythmias; HR, BP; electrolytes and fluid intake and output, especially when vasopressin is being given for indications other than in a code.

Cautions. Vasopressin may cause circumoral pallor, sweating, tremor, abdominal cramps, nausea, vomiting, and belching. Large doses may produce increased blood pressure, bradycardia, minor arrhythmias, heart block, decreased cardiac output, and other cardiovascular effects. Vasopressin should be used cautiously in patients with seizure disorders, migraine, asthma, heart failure, vascular disease, renal disease, or other conditions in which rapid additions to the extracellular fluids may be deleterious.

Norepinephrine

Norepinephrine is a catecholamine with predominant alpha-1 and some beta-1 adrenergic stimulation. Norepinephrine causes constriction of all systemic arterioles except those of the coronary and cerebral circulations and produces direct inotropic and chronotropic cardiac stimulation.

Uses. Norepinephrine may be given in the treatment of cardiogenic shock. Although the drug increases myocardial contractility, this effect is often offset by the systemic vasoconstrictor effects (afterload increase) that limit any rise in stroke volume. Increases in afterload may increase myocardial oxygen requirements, which may be a significant problem in ischemic heart disease. Norepinephrine also may be used to treat hypotension that persists after adequate fluid replacement or refractory hypotension not due to hypovolemia, such as that in septic shock. In these patients, the beneficial effect of the drug is to increase aortic diastolic pressure and thereby improve coronary and cerebral perfusion. Renal, abdominal visceral, and skeletal muscle blood flow are sacrificed, however, and hypoperfusion of these tissue beds predisposes large masses of body tissue to ischemia.

Preparations. Levophed, 1 mg/ml to be diluted for titration administration.

Dosing. Initial infusion of 8 to 12 μg/min; titrated to desired effect. The maintenance dose is generally reduced to 2 to 4 μg/min. Because of the ischemic risk to the renal and splanchnic bed, the smallest effective dose should be administered for the shortest possible amount of time.

Pharmacokinetics. The onset of activity of norepinephrine occurs within 1 to 2 minutes, and the duration of effect is approximately 1 to 2 minutes. The drug is eliminated by cellular reuptake and general peripheral tissue metabolism.

Monitoring. The ECG is monitored for signs of arrhythmias. HR, BP, and CO are also monitored. Urine output also should be closely monitored because of the drug's renal artery constrictive effects.

Cautions. Administration should be via a central vein. Phentolamine is not commercially available.

Dopamine

Dopamine is a catecholamine with alpha, beta, and dopaminergic stimulation. At doses less than 3 μg/kg/min, dopaminergic stimulation results in dilation of the mesenteric and renal vasculature. Although renal and mesenteric blood flow and cardiac output increase at low-dose infusions, heart rate and blood pressure are not significantly affected. At doses of 3 to 10 μg/kg/min, cardiac stimulation results in greater myocardial contractility and heart rate without predictably increasing the blood pressure. Doses higher than 10 μg/kg/min result predominantly in alpha stimulation and generalized vasoconstriction, including the renal and mesenteric vessels. At this point, blood pressure increases and there is generally no elevation in stroke volume. Overall, at high dose levels, the actions of dopamine become more like those

of norepinephrine. Note also that these dose ranges and anticipated effects are generalizations. Individual patients' responses may be highly variable and depend on up or down regulation of the specific adrenergic receptors.

Uses. Dose-adjusted dopamine is used in the management of congestive heart failure (increased inotropic effect), hypotension (increased inotropic and vasoconstrictor effects), and prerenal insufficiency (increased renal blood flow). Dopamine is the vasopressor favored for hypotension *not* due to hypovolemia because of its dopaminergic (renal dilator) effects. Dopamine is generally not recommended for patients with pulmonary congestion or edema because the *venoconstrictor* effects of the drug may increase venous return, pulmonary blood flow, and left ventricular end-diastolic pressure. As a result, pulmonary edema may be produced or worsened.

Preparations. Inotropin and others, 40, 80, and 160 mg/ml to be diluted for titration administration.

Dosing. Initial infusions of 1 to 4 μg/kg/min, titrated for desired effects. The desired maintenance range is less than 20 μg/kg/min. In hypotensive emergencies, the starting dose is 5 μg/kg/min.

Pharmacokinetics. The onset of action occurs within 1 to 5 minutes after dopamine administration, and the duration of effect is approximately 10 minutes. Dopamine is metabolized in the plasma and tissues.

Monitoring. The HR, BP, ECG (for arrhythmias), PWP, CO, and urine output should be monitored. Tachycardia and ventricular arrhythmias have been reported with high doses of dopamine.

Cautions. Dopamine should be administered via a central venous line. If that is not possible, care should be taken to avoid extravasation because local tissue injury and necrosis may result. Monoamine oxidase inhibitors (psychotropic antidepressant agents) potentiate the effects of dopamine. Patients known to have been on these drugs within the past 2 to 3 weeks should receive initial dopamine doses not greater than 10% of the usual dose. These patients require fastidious drug titration.

Warning. All of the aforementioned drugs described are potent, rapid-acting agents. Vigilant monitoring is required for administration because sudden, uncontrolled blood pressure increases may result in cerebrovascular accident and myocardial ischemia. Uncontrolled hypertension also increases capillary oozing in surgical or trauma patients and increases stress on vascular suture lines or aneurysms.

Vasopressor agents, through their peripheral vasoconstrictor properties, may significantly decrease blood flow to areas of the circulation. As a consequence of stasis of blood in the constricted vessels, vascular thrombosis and decreased blood flow to the organs of drug elimination may affect the elimination of concomitantly administered drugs. If these vasoconstrictor drugs are given over extended periods, variable degrees of ischemic injury may occur throughout the body. Tissue ischemia is of particular concern in patients with underlying peripheral vascular disease or in patients with diabetes mellitus. Therapy with all agents should not be discontinued abruptly but, rather, should be gradually tapered while carefully assessing the patient's clinical and hemodynamic responses.

Inotropic Drugs

Inotropic drugs are indicated in the management of low-cardiac-output syndromes, particularly when heart failure is the result of impaired ventricular contractility (systolic dysfunction). As a direct consequence of increased myocardial contractility and improved ventricular emptying, stroke volume and forward blood flow increase. This effect, in turn, results in a decrease in ventricular size and end-systolic and end-diastolic blood volumes. Systemic venous and pulmonary vascular congestion also are alleviated.

Ionized calcium is an integral component of muscle contraction. The available inotropic agents improve myocardial contractility by increasing intracellular ionized calcium levels. Different classes of inotropic drugs increase intracellular calcium by different mechanisms. For example, *digitalis* preparations work by inhibiting the sodium-potassium ATPase pump, which results in an increased influx of calcium across the slow (calcium) channel. Amrinone and milrinone are phosphodiesterase inhibitors. They inhibit the metabolism of cyclic adenosine monophosphate (cAMP), which, in turn, results in an increase in ionized intracellular calcium. Beta-adrenergic agonists such as dopamine increase cAMP production, resulting in increased intracellular calcium.

Dobutamine

Dobutamine is a synthetic catecholamine and a potent inotropic agent that has primarily beta-adrenergic effects.

The increase in stroke volume is mediated by a primary increase in myocardial contractility (beta-1 effect), as well as secondary effects such as a decrease in systemic vascular resistance (beta-2 effect) and reflex vasodilation due to the increase in stroke volume. Increases in blood pressure observed with dobutamine are due solely to the inotropic properties (increases in stroke volume). Because dobutamine does not significantly increase blood pressure, the beneficial hemodynamic effects are difficult to evaluate without a pulmonary artery catheter and cardiac output studies.

Uses. Dobutamine is given to increase cardiac output in the short-term management of severe congestive heart failure. Dobutamine is most commonly indicated for patients with severe systolic dysfunction who maintain a near-normal or normal blood pressure. For patients with heart failure complicated by hypotension, a medication with a vasoconstrictor effect, such as dopamine, is preferable to dobutamine.

Preparations. Dobutrex, 12.5 mg/ml to be diluted for titration administration.

Dosing. Initial infusion of 2.5 μg/kg/min; titrated for effect to a maximal infusion rate of 20 μg/kg/min. Maintenance infusion rates are 2.5 to 10 μg/kg/min, and higher doses are rarely required.

Pharmacokinetics. The usual onset of activity is 1 to 2 minutes, with a peak effect in 10 minutes. The drug effects cease shortly after the drug is discontinued. Dobutamine is metabolized in the liver and other tissues, and the conjugated metabolites are then excreted by the kidney.

Monitoring. The ECG is monitored for tachycardia and arrhythmias. The BP, CO, and PWP are also monitored to guide therapy.

Cautions. Increased heart rate and ectopic beats are dose-related problems (increasing with increasing doses) but are seen less frequently than with epinephrine, norepinephrine, or dopamine.

Pharmacologic Properties of Dopamine versus Dobutamine. The actions of and indications for dopamine and dobutamine are frequently confused. The differences between the two inotropic drugs are as follows:

- Dobutamine does not exert a constrictor effect on the systemic arteries and veins, whereas dopamine does. In fact, with dobutamine, systemic vascular resistance may fall as a reflex response to increased stroke volume and direct vasodilating properties. Consequently, dobutamine does not significantly increase blood pressure or venous return, whereas dopamine does.

- Dobutamine has no direct dilator effect on the renal or mesenteric blood vessels.
- Dobutamine is less arrhythmogenic than dopamine, and significant increases in heart rate rarely occur with dobutamine.

Isoproterenol

Isoproterenol is a synthetic catecholamine with potent pure beta-1 and beta-2 adrenergic effects. The beta-1 effects increase myocardial contractility (positive inotropic effects) and increase heart rate (positive chronotropic effects). As a result, stroke volume, cardiac output, and myocardial work and oxygen consumption are significantly increased. The tremendous increase in myocardial oxygen consumption is a major drawback, particularly when the drug is administered to patients with ischemic heart disease. The beta-2 effects result in systemic and pulmonary vasodilation and, as a result, a reduction in vascular resistances of the two circulations. Unfortunately, systemic vasodilation seems to be somewhat selective and tends to redistribute blood flow to nonvital organs, such as skin and skeletal muscle, and therefore tends to shunt blood from the coronary, cerebral, and renal circulations. Isoproterenol also causes bronchodilation through its relaxing action on bronchial smooth muscle.

Uses. The clinical use of isoproterenol is quite limited. Treatment with this drug is discouraged in patients with ischemic heart disease. The current indications are for *temporary* treatment of hemodynamically significant bradyarrhythmias, until pacemaker therapy can be initiated, and for refractory torsades de pointes (polymorphous ventricular tachycardia). Today, however, other drugs (such as atropine for the bradyarrhythmias and magnesium for torsades de pointes) or other interventions (such as external or temporary transvenous pacemakers) are given as first-choice agents for these conditions. In selected cases, isoproterenol also may be chosen for treatment of refractory bronchospasm, particularly during anesthesia. It has also been used in cardiac transplant patients to increase heart rate.

Preparations. Isuprel and others, 0.05 or 0.2 mg/ml to be diluted for titration administration.

Dosing. Initial infusions of 0.5 μg/min are most commonly used; dose is titrated to desired effect, with most patients responding to doses of 2 to 20 μg/min. Boluses of 0.2 to 0.6 μg/kg may be given in extreme cases, such as profound bradyarrhythmias, but adverse effects are more likely to occur at higher doses.

Pharmacokinetics. The onset of action is seen within 30 to 60 seconds, and the duration of effect is variable, lasting from 8 to 50 minutes. Isoproterenol is eliminated primarily by tissue uptake and peripheral metabolism and by direct conjugation.

Monitoring. The HR, BP, PWP, CO, and ECG for arrhythmias, which could include any ectopic rhythms, should be monitored.

Cautions. Cardiac rhythm disturbances often occur with IV use. Isoproterenol is particularly *contraindicated* in patients with severe coronary disease because of the tremendous increase in myocardial oxygen consumption associated with it. Other undesirable effects include the possibility of hypotension (beta-2 dilating effects), nervousness, headache, and sweating.

Amrinone

Amrinone is a bipyridine phosphodiesterase inhibitor that has positive inotropic and both arterial and venodilating effects. Stroke volume is increased as a result of both the inotropic and afterload-reducing effects of the drug. The potent balanced vascular dilating properties of amrinone may produce a severe hypotensive episode, particularly if the patient has had a recent myocardial infarction or hypotension at the onset of amrinone therapy.

Uses. Amrinone is used in the short-term management of congestive heart failure and other low-cardiac-output syndromes (such as those following open heart surgery) that are refractory to conventional therapy.

Preparations. Inocor, 5 mg/ml, in a 20 ml ampule. Amrinone should not be added to dextrose-containing solutions because this may result in a reduction of the drug's potency.

Dosing. A bolus loading dose of 0.5 to 1.5 mg/kg over 2 to 3 minutes is followed by an infusion of 5 to 10 μg/kg/min. The total dose should not exceed 10 mg/kg/day, although some continued response may be observed with increasing doses.

Pharmacokinetics. Increases in cardiac output are seen within 2 to 5 minutes after the bolus dose, with a peak effect at 10 minutes. The duration of effect is approximately 30 minutes to 2 hours. Amrinone is metabolized and conjugated in the liver and excreted in the urine.

Monitoring. The ECG is monitored for arrhythmias, the platelet count for thrombocytopenia, and urine output for assessment of renal perfusion. The HR, BP, CO, and PWP are also monitored to guide therapy.

Cautions. Careful monitoring and dose adjustments are required to prevent excessive tachycardia and hypotension. Careful consideration in dosing is required in hepatic or renal dysfunction. Reversible thrombocytopenia has been associated with high-dose therapy or therapy continued for more than several days. The drug is contraindicated in patients who are hypersensitive to bisulfites because administration may cause allergic responses, including anaphylactic reactions or mild to severe asthmatic episodes. Sulfite sensitivity is more common in asthmatic patients.

Milrinone
Milrinone is a bisulfite phosphodiesterase inhibitor similar to amrinone in its positive inotropic and vasodilating properties. Milrinone is approximately *15 to 20 times* more potent than amrinone, and clinical studies have reported significantly less thrombocytopenia with milrinone as compared with amrinone.

Uses. Milrinone is given for the short-term management of patients with myocardial dysfunction and high systemic vascular resistance that is refractory to conventional therapy (postoperative cardiac surgical patients, shock).

Preparations. Primacor, 1 mg/ml in dilution.

Dosing. An initial loading dose of 50 μg/kg given over 10 minutes by IV infusion is recommended. This is followed by a maintenance infusion of 0.375 to 0.750 μg/kg/min.

Pharmacokinetics. An increase in cardiac output often is seen within 5 to 15 minutes after a dose of milrinone. Milrinone is primarily excreted unchanged by the kidney; however, a small percentage of the drug is metabolized by the liver.

Monitoring. The HR, BP, CO, PWP, and ECG for arrhythmias, urine output, and platelet count for thrombocytopenia are monitored.

Cautions. Dosing adjustments may be necessary in patients with serious renal dysfunction. Hypotensive episodes may develop because of the balanced vasodilating properties; therefore the drug should be carefully titrated and the patient should be vigilantly observed and monitored during drug administration. Administration of the bolus dose more slowly than recommended by the product literature (e.g., over 20 minutes) may be necessary in patients with low baseline blood pressure. As with amrinone, the drug is contraindicated in patients with bisulfite hypersensitivity.

Digoxin
The digitalis preparations are the oldest and most widely administered inotropic medications. However, of the available inotropic drugs, digitalis preparations are the least potent, are the most diversely toxic, and are of limited value when given alone in treating patients with sudden exacerbations of chronic heart failure or in patients with acute, severe heart failure. The toxic-to-therapeutic ratio of digitalis is narrow, and the risk of toxicities is even greater in patients with hypokalemia, hypomagnesemia, acid-base abnormalities, hypoxemia, or acute cardiac injury and in elderly patients.

Digoxin is a relatively weak positive inotropic drug that is commonly administered in the treatment of chronic heart failure. Digoxin also prolongs the refractory period of the AV node, enhances vagal tone, and slows the ventricular response in atrial flutter or fibrillation. ICU patients receiving catecholamine infusions or patients with sympathetic nervous system stimulation may be somewhat refractory to the antiarrhythmic effects of digoxin. The cardiac-slowing effects of digitalis preparations are caused, in part, by increased vagal (parasympathetic) effects that may be overridden in patients with increased sympathetic nervous system activity. In these patients, beta blockade (sympathetic nervous system inhibition) or direct AV nodal slowing by calcium-channel blocking agents, such as verapamil or diltiazem, is more likely to control the ventricular rate of atrial flutter or fibrillation.

Uses. Digoxin is given predominately in the management of chronic congestive heart failure. Digoxin also is used to control the ventricular rate in patients with atrial fibrillation or atrial flutter and sinus tachycardia due to heart failure.

Preparations. Lanoxin, 0.25 mg/ml; the 2 ml vial contains 0.5 mg.

Dosing. For patients not previously digitalized, a loading dose of 0.25 to 0.50 mg (7 to 14 μg/kg) is given as a slow IV bolus. This is followed by 0.125 to 0.25 mg doses every 4 to 8 hours until a total of 0.75 to 1.50 mg has been given over 24 hours. Maintenance doses of 0.125 to 0.375 mg are given daily and adjusted to serum digoxin levels and patients' clinical response. Overall, this dosage regimen should be adjusted to the individual patient's drug response, underlying condition, and digoxin levels. Normal serum levels for digoxin are 1 to 2 ng/ml, but therapeutic or even subtherapeutic levels (less than 0.8 ng/ml) do not exclude toxicity. There is no established digoxin level that documents toxicity. Values must be interpreted relative to the presence of coexisting factors that augment or blunt digitalis effect (serum electrolyte levels, acid-base imbalances, hypoxemia, myocardial injury) and the patient's clinical presentation.

Pharmacokinetics. The onset of action is 5 to 30 minutes, a significant response may be noted within 30 to 60 minutes, and the peak response generally occurs in approximately 4 to 6 hours. The duration of effect is variable and may persist for days after the drug has been discontinued. Digoxin is mainly excreted in the urine as unchanged drug; there is a variable amount of hepatic metabolism. The half-life is 36 hours in patients with normal renal function, and the half-life may be up to 18 days in anephric patients.

Monitoring. The HR, ECG for arrhythmias, digoxin levels, and renal function should be monitored. In therapeutic doses, digoxin may cause slight prolongation of the PR interval, shortening of the QT interval, and ST segment depression. These electrocardiographic effects are not a quantitative measure of the degree of digitalization.

Cautions. The patient's heart rate should be assessed before the administration of digoxin; if the heart rate is below 60 beats per minute, the drug should be withheld until the decision to give or omit the dose is made by the provider in charge. Digoxin possesses a narrow therapeutic-to-toxic index, especially when the patient has physiologic abnormalities such as electrolyte imbalances (see earlier). Dosage adjustment is necessary for patients with renal insufficiency. Keen observation for the early detection of digitalis toxicity is extremely important because the cardiovascular effects of digitalis toxicity may rapidly become life threatening. Digoxin toxicity (as it affects the heart) is associated with various arrhythmias, such as AV conduction disturbances; bradyarrhythmias; atrial tachycardia with block; accelerated junctional rhythm; multiformed premature ventricular contractions (PVCs) or frequent PVCs, particularly

ventricular bigeminy with first-degree AV block; and ventricular tachycardia. In fact, *any single type or combination of arrhythmias in a digitalized patient should alert the clinician to the possibility of cardiac manifestations of digitalis toxicity.*

Extracardiac signs of digoxin toxicity include GI effects such as anorexia, nausea, and vomiting; CNS effects such as headache, fatigue, malaise, inappropriate behavior, drowsiness, and generalized weakness; visual abnormalities such as disturbances in color perception (yellow- or green-tinted vision), seeing halos around bright lights, blurred vision, and photophobia; and variable effects on serum potassium. Drugs such as quinidine, calcium-channel blockers, and amiodarone decrease the volume of distribution of digoxin, which results in increased serum concentrations. As a result, concomitant use of any of these drugs with digoxin may result in digoxin toxicity if serum digoxin concentration monitoring or dosage adjustments are not performed. *Patients who are hypokalemic or hypomagnesemic are at increased risk for digoxin toxicity because a deficiency in these electrolytes sensitizes the myocardium to digitalis toxicity. Hypercalcemia increases the risk of digitalis toxicity.*

Treatment of digitalis toxicity includes (1) immediately discontinuing administration of digoxin; (2) correcting physiologic abnormalities such as electrolyte disturbances, hypoxemia, and acid-base abnormalities; and (3) antiarrhythmic therapy such as lidocaine (Xylocaine) and consideration of digitalis antibody fragments (Digibind) if digitalis-induced arrhythmias are life threatening. A dose of 60 mg of Digibind will bind approximately 1 mg of digoxin.

Antiarrhythmic Drugs

See the section earlier in this chapter on antiarrhythmic therapy.

Lidocaine (Class I-b)

Lidocaine has, for decades, been the antiarrhythmic drug of choice for treatment of acute ventricular arrhythmias but is currently a second-tier choice for some ventricular arrhythmias. Lidocaine works by suppressing both Purkinje system automaticity and spontaneous depolarization of the ventricles. At therapeutic concentrations, little drug activity occurs at the sinoatrial (SA) or AV nodes. There is a variable effect on the refractory period and the action potential duration. Lidocaine may slightly decrease myocardial contractility, cardiac output, and blood pressure, but this cardiodepressant effect is usually not clinically significant.

Uses. Lidocaine now appears in the ACLS algorithm for stable ventricular tachycardia (as a choice second to amiodarone), which is associated with acute myocardial ischemia or injury. This drug no longer appears in the algorithm for ventricular fibrillation or unstable ventricular tachycardia, but its use would be acceptable in the resuscitation attempt. Lidocaine may also be used in the management of some ventricular arrhythmias not associated with a myocardial infarction, such as those due to digitalis toxicity. *Prophylactic administration of lidocaine is not recommended in patients with uncomplicated myocardial ischemia or infarction without ventricular ectopy.*

Preparations. Xylocaine and others are available in 2, 4, and 8 mg/ml for infusion and 10, 40, 100, and 200 mg/ml for injection.

Dosing. A loading bolus of 1 mg/kg is given to rapidly attain a therapeutic drug level. Additional boluses of 0.5 to 1.5 mg/kg are then given, as necessary, every 5 to 10 minutes to a total of 3 mg/kg (210 mg for the average 70 kg person). Following the initial bolus administration, an IV infusion of 0.5 to 4 mg/min, mixed in 5% dextrose in water, is initiated. No greater than 300 mg should be administered over any 1-hour period. Dosing adjustments are made based on serum drug levels, the patient's clinical response, and evidence of CNS toxicity.

Pharmacokinetics. Antiarrhythmic activity is seen within 45 to 90 seconds after drug administration; the duration of effect is 12 to 15 minutes after a single bolus injection. Lidocaine is metabolized by the liver, and the metabolites are excreted in the urine.

Monitoring. The ECG and serum drug levels (to evaluate for signs of drug toxicity) should be monitored. Patients with toxicity often have CNS symptoms (in order of severity related to drug levels) of perioral paresthesias, feelings of dissociation, dizziness, numbness, slurred speech, drowsiness, agitation or lethargy, hearing difficulty, confusion, muscle twitching, seizures, hypotension, and respiratory arrest. Prolongation of the PR interval and QRS complex and the appearance or aggravation of arrhythmias also are indications to stop therapy.

Cautions. Drug toxicity is more likely to occur in patients with decreased cardiac output (heart failure or shock), hepatic dysfunction, or renal dysfunction; in elderly patients; in patients with low body weights; or in patients also receiving beta blockers (e.g., propranolol) or cimetidine.

Administration of smaller loading doses (50% to 75% of the usual loading dose) and lower infusion rates (0.5 to 1 mg/min), as well as monitoring lidocaine levels, should be strongly considered in patients prone to lidocaine toxicity. Lidocaine also should be administered with caution in patients with any form of heart block. The drug is contraindicated in patients who do not have an artificial pacemaker who have severe degrees of SA, AV, or intraventricular heart block.

Procainamide (Class I-a)

Procainamide is used in the management of atrial reentry and ectopic arrhythmias, including ventricular ectopic arrhythmias; wide QRS tachyarrhythmias of uncertain cause; paroxysmal supraventricular tachycardia (PSVT) unresponsive to vagal maneuvers and administration of adenosine; and rapid atrial fibrillation with Wolff-Parkinson-White syndrome. Procainamide decreases conduction velocity and automaticity in atrial and ventricular conduction tissue. It may also be considered when repeated defibrillation attempts, epinephrine and vasopressin, and amiodarone have failed to convert ventricular fibrillation or unstable ventricular tachycardia or for patients with recurrent ventricular tachycardia.

Uses. In the ICU setting, procainamide is given primarily for stable wide QRS tachycardia of unknown origin in patients with normal cardiac function.

Preparations. Pronestyl, 100 and 500 mg/ml.

Dosing. A bolus of procainamide is given at 20 to 50 mg/min until (1) the arrhythmia is suppressed, (2) the QRS widens to greater than 50% of its previous duration, (3) hypotension develops, or (4) a total of 17 mg/kg (not to exceed 1 g total) has been given. The loading dose is then followed by an infusion of 1 to 6 mg/min. An alternative method of infusing a loading dose of procainamide involves giving 0.5 to 1.0 g by IV drip infusion at a rate not faster than 20 mg/min. Drug dosing levels may require adjustment downward in patients with impaired hepatic or renal function. *Sudden hypotension may develop if procainamide is injected too rapidly.*

Pharmacokinetics. Approximately 60% of the dose is hepatically metabolized to an active form, *N*-acetyl procainamide (NAPA). Some degradation by plasma cholinesterase occurs; the remainder is excreted unchanged in the urine. NAPA is eliminated by renal excretion.

Monitoring. The BP must be closely monitored during bolus or IV drip administration because of the drug's potential hypotensive effect. Closely monitor CO, HR, and ECG for arrhythmias and widening of QRS complex, AV block, and ventricular ectopy. Prolongation of the PR and QT intervals also may occur as a result of procainamide toxicity.

Serum procainamide and NAPA (the primary metabolite) levels should be monitored in patients with renal and hepatic failure and in patients receiving greater than 3 mg/min for longer than 24 hours. Complete blood counts should be evaluated routinely because of the possibility of procainamide-related leukopenia or agranulocytosis, which may become fatal.

Cautions. Procainamide is contraindicated in patients with preexisting QT prolongation or torsades de pointes. Administration of procainamide to these patients may result in refractory ventricular tachyarrhythmias. The drug should be given with extreme caution in patients with preexisting borderline hypotension or significantly widened QRS complexes.

Beta Blocking Agents (Negative Inotropic, Negative Chronotropic, Antihypertensive, Antiarrhythmic Agents)

Propranolol (Class II)

Propranolol is a nonselective beta-adrenergic antagonist that prevents catecholamine-induced cardiac stimulation. This effect results in decreased automaticity, reduced rate of sinus nodal discharge, prolonged AV nodal conduction time, and decreased myocardial contractility.

Uses. Propranolol has been administered in the acute management of refractory supraventricular and ventricular arrhythmias, especially those associated with catecholamine excess or digitalis toxicity, angina, and hypertension. The drug also is recommended for management of arrhythmias and hypertensive crisis due to cocaine overdose. However, caution should be used in patients with cocaine overdose with known or suspected coronary artery disease because the unopposed alpha-adrenergic stimulation may result in coronary artery spasm.

Propranolol is not indicated as a first-line antiarrhythmic drug for ventricular arrhythmias. Nor is propranolol a first-line agent for supraventricular tachyarrhythmias. However, propranolol may be given to patients with arrhythmias who have not responded to IV lidocaine, procainamide, amiodarone, verapamil, adenosine, or digoxin.

Propranolol also may be helpful for patients with recurrent arrhythmia-induced arrests when other antiarrhythmic drugs have failed or when sinus tachycardia precedes each

arrest. In patients who fail to remain in a hemodynamically stable heart rhythm, the stress of the cardiac arrest or exogenous administration of epinephrine may contribute to a hyperadrenergic state that predisposes them to recurrent fatal ventricular arrhythmias.

Propranolol is also given in treating symptoms of acute and chronic ischemic heart disease and dilated and hypertrophic cardiomyopathy.

Preparations. Inderal, 1 mg/ml.

Dosing. A bolus of 0.5 to 3.0 mg at a rate not faster than 1 mg/min may be given initially. This dose may be repeated after 2 minutes if the desired effect has not been achieved. Additional doses should be given at intervals of at least 4 hours to avoid toxicity. Alternatively, an IV drip may be started at an initial infusion rate of 1 mg/hr and titrated to therapeutic effect. The maximal infusion rate is 3 mg/hr.

Pharmacokinetics. The onset of activity after IV administration is 1 to 5 minutes; the duration of effect is 10 to 20 minutes. Propranolol elimination is by hepatic metabolism.

Monitoring. The HR, BP, CO, and ECG for arrhythmias, such as bradycardia or heart block, should be monitored. Serum levels are not usually of value in assessing the drug's therapeutic effect because patients may require individualized drug concentrations owing to different levels of circulating catecholamines and beta-adrenergic receptor activity.

Cautions. Propranolol should not be given if patients have heart block, bradycardia, hypotension, or asthma. The drug's beta-2 blocking effects may predispose susceptible patients to status asthmaticus attacks. Propranolol (IV) should be used with extreme caution if verapamil (IV) has been given within the preceding 30 minutes. These agents are synergetic and may produce severe bradycardias or asystole. Propranolol metabolism is extremely sensitive to changes in hepatic blood flow and enzyme activity. Propranolol also decreases blood flow to the liver and may slow the metabolism of other drugs that are metabolized by the liver. Consequently, hepatic hypoperfusion secondary to propranolol may result in elevated serum concentrations of other prescribed drugs and predispose the patient to drug toxicity. Because of the drug's negative inotropic effect, propranolol may precipitate congestive heart failure in those with underlying ventricular dysfunction.

Atenolol (Class II)

Atenolol is a beta-1 selective (cardioselective) adrenergic blocking agent with pharmacologic properties similar to the beta-1 blocking effects of propranolol and other beta blockers.

Uses. Like propranolol, atenolol has been administered in the acute management of hypertension and ischemic heart disease. It also is used to reduce the risk of cardiovascular death in the patient experiencing a myocardial infarction.

Preparations. Tenormin, 0.5 mg/ml.

Dosing. In patients with acute myocardial infarction, an initial loading dose of 5 mg is given over 5 minutes. If well tolerated, a second bolus of 5 mg is given in 10 minutes at the same rate. Patients then should then be given oral therapy by administration of a 50 mg tablet 10 to 30 minutes after the second bolus. Dosing recommendations for other indications have not been established for IV atenolol.

Pharmacokinetics. The effect on heart rate is seen within 1 minute; it peaks within 5 minutes and is negligible by 12 hours. The duration of effect may be significantly shorter in some patients. Atenolol is excreted unchanged by the kidney. Little or no hepatic drug metabolism occurs.

Monitoring. The HR, BP, CO, and ECG (for arrhythmias such as bradycardia or heart block) should be monitored.

Cautions. Atenolol should not be given in patients with heart block, bradycardia, hypotension, or pulmonary edema secondary to heart failure. Because atenolol is a beta-1 selective agent, it may be better tolerated when given in low doses to a patient with a history of asthma or peripheral vascular disease. Atenolol decreases hepatic blood flow and therefore may alter the metabolism of drugs cleared by the liver.

Metoprolol (Class II)

Metoprolol is a beta-1 selective adrenergic blocking agent with similar pharmacologic activity to other beta blockers, including atenolol.

Uses. See atenolol.

Preparations. Lopressor, 1 mg/ml.

Dosing. An initial IV regimen recommended for patients with acute myocardial infarction, to decrease my-

ocardial oxygen consumption and infarct size, consists of three 5 mg doses administered *slowly* at 2-minute intervals. If the loading regimen is well tolerated, an oral regimen of 50 mg every 6 hours for 48 hours should be initiated 15 to 30 minutes after the last IV dose. Following this, the usual oral dose is 50 to 100 mg given twice daily. Dosing recommendations for other indications are not well established for IV metoprolol.

Pharmacokinetics. The onset of effect is seen within 10 minutes after an IV dose. This effect usually persists for 5 to 8 hours, depending on the dose administered. Metoprolol is primarily metabolized in the liver to inactive metabolites.

Monitoring. The HR, BP, CO, and ECG should be monitored for dysrhythmias, such as bradycardia and heart block.

Cautions. See atenolol.

Esmolol (Class II)

Esmolol is a short-acting beta-1 selective adrenergic blocking agent with a rapid onset of action following IV administration. Because of a very short drug half-life, both beneficial and untoward drug effects are short lived. This is advantageous in some situations, such as in patients with acute myocardial infarction, when beta blockade may be indicated, but questions exist that drug effects may be poorly tolerated owing to preexisting heart failure or asthma. The brief drug effect therefore serves as a minitherapeutic drug trial.

Uses. Esmolol is administered in the short-term management of supraventricular tachyarrhythmias, ventricular arrhythmias due to excessive sympathetic nervous system stimulation, and hypertensive crisis with or without acute myocardial infarction.

Preparations. Brevibloc, 10 mg/ml; concentrate 250 mg/ml in dilution.

Dosing. Esmolol is given by IV infusion. Therapy is usually initiated by giving a loading dose of 500 μg/kg/min for 1 minute, followed by an infusion of 50 μg/kg/min over a 4-minute period. If the desired therapeutic effect is not achieved, a repeat bolus of 500 μg/kg/min for 1 minute can be given, followed by an infusion of 100 μg/kg/min for 4 minutes. Repeat boluses and increased infusions up to 200 μg/kg/min may be administered until the desired therapeutic effect is achieved.

Pharmacokinetics. The effects of esmolol are seen within 5 minutes, and the duration of action is usually 20 to 30 minutes. Esmolol is rapidly metabolized by red blood cell esterases. Terminal half-life is approximately 9 minutes.

Monitoring. The ECG should be monitored for HR and various degrees of heart block. The BP should be closely monitored because hypotension is relatively common with the drug.

Cautions. Esmolol should be used with caution, if at all, in patients with hypotension, bradycardia, heart block, uncontrolled congestive heart failure, or a history of asthma.

Labetalol (Class II)

Labetalol is a beta-adrenergic blocking agent—similar in this respect to propranolol but with additional alpha-1 adrenergic blocking properties. As a result of these two effects, there is a reduction in catecholamine-induced cardiac stimulation and direct vasodilation. Therefore systemic vascular resistance and arterial pressure are reduced, and the reflex tachycardia usually expected with vasodilators does not occur. The beta blocking effects also blunt the rate of left ventricular pressure rise usually associated with vasodilator drugs. This effect, in turn, reduces stress on the aortic wall and makes labetalol valuable in managing hypertensive crisis as a result of dissecting aortic aneurysm or traumatic dissection of the aorta.

Uses. Labetalol is used in the management of hypertensive crisis, hypertension associated with dissecting aortic aneurysm, traumatic aortic dissection, and severe angina. Labetalol also may be used in cocaine-induced hypertensive crisis and arrhythmias.

Preparations. Trandate, Normodyne, 5 mg/ml.

Dosing. A bolus of 20 mg IV is followed by incremental dosing of 20 mg every 10 minutes until the desired therapeutic effect is noted or a total dose of 2 mg/kg is given. A full therapeutic response is usually observed within 5 to 10 minutes of the IV dose. An infusion of 2 mg/min may then be started to sustain the drug effect.

Labetalol is not a titratable drug, and the effect of increases in the IV drip rate may not be noted for approximately 10 minutes. Likewise, diminution of the drug effect may not be noted for several hours following reduction in dose or discontinuation of the drug.

Pharmacokinetics. The hypotensive effect is usually seen within 2 to 5 minutes, peaks at 10 minutes, and persists for 2 to 6 hours after IV administration in most patients. Labetalol is metabolized in the liver; drug metabolites are excreted in the urine and bile. A small amount of labetalol is excreted unchanged in the urine, and dosage reduction is necessary in patients with creatinine clearances less than 10 ml/min. Half-life is 5 to 8 hours.

Monitoring. The HR, BP, CO, and ECG (for arrhythmias such as bradycardia or heart block) should be monitored.

Cautions. Dosage reduction may be required in patients with hepatic dysfunction or hepatic hypoperfusion. Adverse reactions, such as orthostatic hypotension and light-headedness, are related to alpha blockade. Potential beta blockade reactions include bronchospasm, decreased myocardial contractility and stroke volume, and bradycardia. These adverse reactions are dose related. The patient should not quickly be raised to a sitting position during labetalol therapy and for at least 1 to 2 hours after the last dose.

Amiodarone (Class III)

Amiodarone is an extremely potent and effective antiarrhythmic agent for treatment of supraventricular and ventricular arrhythmias, as well as supraventricular tachyarrhythmias and tachyarrhythmias associated with accessory conduction pathways, such as Wolff-Parkinson-White syndrome.

Amiodarone is a class III antiarrhythmic agent that prolongs the duration of the myocardial transmembrane action potential, increases the refractory period, and does not affect the resting membrane potential. Amiodarone also inhibits beta- and alpha-adrenergic cardiovascular stimulating effects, which may contribute to the antiarrhythmic activity.

Uses. Amiodarone currently is indicated for the treatment of recurrent, life-threatening ventricular arrhythmias (ventricular fibrillation and recurrent hemodynamically unstable ventricular tachycardia) that are refractory to defibrillation, epinephrine, and vasopressin. Recent literature shows that amiodarone may be more effective than other agents when used first line. The newest guidelines for ACLS recommend that IV amiodarone be considered the antiarrhythmic of first choice in the management of ventricular fibrillation or pulseless ventricular tachycardia. In these cases the recommended dose is 300 mg given as an IV push, with additional 150 mg boluses given as necessary. This regimen can be followed by a loading infusion for a total dose not to exceed 2.2 g in 24 hours. Amiodarone also has been used in the management of refractory atrial arrhythmias such as atrial fibrillation.

Preparations. Cardarone and generic brands, 200 mg tablets; injection, Cardarone IV 150 mg/ampule.

Dosing. Bolus doses of 150 mg administered over 10 minutes are given in the management of stable ventricular arrhythmias. The bolus is followed by an infusion of 1 mg/min for 6 hours and then an infusion of 0.5 mg/min for 18 hours. If the patient is unable to tolerate oral therapy, the infusion should be continued at a rate of 0.5 mg/min until oral therapy is feasible or it is determined that further amiodarone therapy is unnecessary. Oral dosing of 200 to 600 mg/day maintains suppression of malignant arrhythmias. Chronic dosing with 300 mg/day or less is associated with significantly fewer side effects.

Pharmacokinetics. Definitive information related to the onset of action and duration of activity of IV amiodarone is not available at this time. Amiodarone is extensively metabolized in the liver. Dosing adjustments should be considered in patients with hepatic dysfunction, but recommended guidelines are not available.

Monitoring. Hypotension is the primary complication of IV therapy. In addition to frequent BP monitoring, HR, CO, ECG, and hepatic enzymes should be monitored. This drug increases the serum levels of other antiarrhythmics and digoxin. If present, these drugs must be carefully monitored with both clinical assessment and serum drug levels. Because of the long half-life (9 to 50 days), monitoring is prolonged. Slight increases in the PR and QT intervals may occur after chronic therapy. QT prolongation induced by the drug is associated with an increased risk of ventricular arrhythmias such as torsades de pointes. The QRS duration may be unchanged or increased.

Cautions. Amiodarone should be given with caution in patients receiving calcium and beta blocking agents because sinus arrest or AV nodal block may result. Amiodarone should be administered through a central line if the concentration of the solution is greater than 2 mg/ml. Adverse effects include serious pulmonary fibrosis, ocular keratopathy, heart failure, peripheral neuropathy, mental status changes, thyroid abnormalities, and elevation of hepatic enzymes. A nonserious but bizarre side effect is a blue-gray skin discoloration. The noncardiac side effects

are most often associated with long-term therapy and are of little concern when used acutely.

Calcium-Channel Blocking Agents (Antiarrhythmic, Negative Inotropic, Negative Chronotropic, Vasodilator)

Verapamil (Class IV)

Verapamil is a calcium-channel blocking agent that inhibits the transmembrane influx of calcium ions into myocardial cells and vascular smooth muscle. Decreased intracellular calcium, in turn, inhibits the myocardial contractile process (negative inotropic effect), relaxes vascular smooth muscle (decreases systemic vascular resistance), increases refractoriness, and slows conduction at the AV node.

Uses. Parenteral verapamil is a second-line agent, in patients with an adequate blood pressure and normal left ventricular function, after adenosine in the management of reentrant tachyarrhythmias (narrow QRS) that require AV nodal conduction for perpetuating tachyarrhythmias. Verapamil also may be given to control the ventricular response in patients with supraventricular arrhythmias, including multifocal atrial tachycardia and atrial flutter and fibrillation.

Preparations. Calan, Isoptin, 2.5 mg/ml.

Dosing. A bolus of 0.075 to 0.15 mg/kg (usually 2.5 to 10 mg) is given over 2 minutes (or 3 to 4 minutes in elderly or debilitated patients). If the arrhythmia persists and there is no adverse drug effect, doses of 2.5 to 10 mg may be repeated every 15 to 30 minutes until a desired effect is achieved or a maximum of 20 mg is given. Because of the vasodilatory effects, hypotension may occur if the drug is injected too rapidly or if administered even at recommended rates in elderly or debilitated patients. *Consequently, slow injection while vigilantly monitoring blood pressure and ECG are mandatory during drug administration.*

Pharmacokinetics. The hemodynamic effects of verapamil peak within 5 minutes and persist for 10 to 20 minutes. The effect on the AV node is seen within 1 to 2 minutes, peaks at 10 to 15 minutes, and often lasts for 30 to 60 minutes. Delayed AV nodal conduction may persist much longer in some patients. Verapamil is metabolized by the liver and is highly dependent on hepatic function and blood flow.

Monitoring. The HR, BP, ECG for arrhythmias, and hepatic function should be monitored. Bradycardia and various degrees of heart block are associated with verapamil. The length of the PR interval correlates with serum verapamil concentrations. Serum drug level monitoring is rarely required.

Cautions. Verapamil should not be administered if the patient is bradycardic or hypotensive. P waves may be unidentifiable in rapid sinus tachycardia. This normal compensatory tachycardia may *appear* to be an ectopic supraventricular rhythm. In a clinical setting in which sinus tachycardia is appropriate (fever, hypovolemia) or even necessary to sustain cardiac output (severe heart failure), verapamil should *never* be used to slow the heart rate. Rather, management of sinus tachycardia is directed at the underlying cause, such as restoration of circulatory volume or treatment of heart failure. The drug also should be given with caution in patients with sick sinus syndrome and those receiving beta blocking agents or digoxin. Verapamil may increase the serum concentrations of digoxin when the two are provided concomitantly. The dose of verapamil should be reduced in patients with decreased hepatic blood flow or hepatic dysfunction.

Diltiazem (Class IV)

Diltiazem is a calcium-channel blocker that is used to terminate reentrant tachyarrhythmias. Like most drugs of this class, diltiazem increases refractoriness at the AV node and slows AV nodal conduction. The drug also has vasodilating and myocardial depressant properties. Compared with verapamil, diltiazem is less likely to precipitate heart failure and hypotension, and the degree of drug interaction with digoxin is less than that with verapamil.

Uses. Diltiazem is indicated for the control of ventricular rate in patients with atrial fibrillation or atrial flutter or after a trial of adenosine for rapid conversion of PSVT to normal sinus rhythm.

Preparations. Cardizem injectable, 5 mg/ml; 25 and 50 mg vials (must be refrigerated).

Dosing. An initial slow bolus of 0.25 mg/kg body weight (usually not more than 20 mg) is recommended. If the desired response is not achieved within 15 minutes, a second bolus of 0.35 mg/kg of actual body weight (usually not more than 25 mg) should be slowly injected. An infusion of 5 to 15 mg/hr then may be started to maintain control of the ventricular rate. The infusion is not recommended to be administered for more than 24 hours.

Pharmacokinetics. The peak hemodynamic effects of IV diltiazem are seen within 5 to 7 minutes. The duration of effect after single doses is 10 to 20 minutes. Diltiazem undergoes extensive hepatic metabolism.

Monitoring. Monitor BP for signs of heart failure and ECG for bradyarrhythmias.

Cautions. Second- or third-degree heart block may occur secondary to diltiazem's effect on the AV node. Patients with serious left ventricular dysfunction or clinical heart failure should be monitored closely because diltiazem may be associated with significant depression in myocardial contractility. Decreases in BP, particularly during bolus administration, have occasionally resulted in significant hypotension.

Adenosine

Adenosine is a naturally occurring substance (nucleoside) found in body cells in the form of adenosine triphosphate (ATP). The drug depresses sinus automaticity, alters repolarization of atrial tissue, and slows conduction through the AV node.

Uses. Because most forms of paroxysmal supraventricular tachyarrhythmias are perpetuated by a reentry pathway involving the AV node, adenosine is effective in terminating these arrhythmias. In fact, it is the drug of choice in treating symptomatic PSVT. However, adenosine does not organize the chaotic atrial activity characteristic of atrial flutter or fibrillation. Therefore, if the arrhythmia is *not* due to reentry pathways involving the AV or sinus node, adenosine does not terminate the arrhythmia but merely temporarily reduces the ventricular responses, which may help clarify the ECG diagnosis.

Preparations. Adenocard, 3 mg/ml.

Dosing. An initial dose of 6.0 mg is given as a rapid push (1 to 3 seconds). This should be followed immediately by a 20 ml saline flush to prevent trapping of the drug in the IV tubing or connections, where it rapidly breaks down. If the response is not adequate after 1 to 2 minutes, a second bolus of 12 mg is recommended. If the desired response is still not achieved, another 12 mg bolus is recommended. If after a total dose of 30 mg (6 mg + 12 mg + 12 mg = 30 mg) the arrhythmia persists, alternative therapy should be considered.

Pharmacokinetics. The onset of adenosine's effects is within 20 to 30 seconds, and the duration of effect is less than 10 seconds.

Several drug or physiologic interactions may affect individual patient susceptibility to the drug. Patients with increased sympathetic nervous system tone are likely to require higher than recommended doses of adenosine. Higher doses also may be needed for patients receiving theophylline (aminophylline) because this drug blocks the receptor responsible for adenosine's effects. Patients receiving dipyridamole (Persantine) probably should have alternative antiarrhythmic therapy selected because dipyridamole may prolong or potentiate the degree of AV block produced by adenosine.

Because of adenosine's extremely short duration of action, a longer-acting drug may be necessary to maintain normal sinus rhythm once conversion to normal sinus rhythm has been achieved.

Adenosine is rapidly metabolized in red blood cells and vascular epithelium by a deamination process. Adenosine also undergoes phosphorylation in red blood cells.

Monitoring. Monitor HR, BP, and ECG (for signs of arrhythmias). Sinus bradycardia, sinus pauses lasting several seconds, and ventricular ectopy are common after termination of the supraventricular tachycardia with adenosine. Because of adenosine's brief action, usually few or no adverse hemodynamic effects occur.

Cautions. This drug must be given via a peripheral IV line because injection into a central venous site may result in asystole. Adverse reactions and side effects generally resolve spontaneously within 1 to 2 minutes and are usually of no clinical consequence. Adenosine is a mild bronchoconstrictor and cutaneous vasodilator. Consequently, transient flushing, hypotension, coughing, chest discomfort, and dyspnea may occur. Peripherally administered adenosine has resulted in brief periods of asystole. Adenosine should be avoided in patients with sick sinus syndrome, AV block, or asthma.

Other Medications Commonly Used in Intensive Care Units

Theophylline

Theophylline is a xanthine derivative that is a nonselective phosphodiesterase inhibitor that causes bronchial and vascular smooth muscle relaxation. The drug also stimulates the central respiratory drive, stimulates diuresis, and increases diaphragmatic strength, thus rendering the diaphragm less susceptible to fatigue in patients with acute or chronic dyspnea.

Cardiovascular effects include positive inotropic and chronotropic actions. The cardiac stimulant effects in conjunction with pulmonary and systemic vasodilation may significantly increase right and left ventricular output. Theophylline also may increase mucociliary clearance. Theophylline has a narrow therapeutic-to-toxic window; therefore it is not a first-choice drug in the treatment of acute bronchospasm.

Uses. Patients with severe asthma, chronic bronchitis, and chronic obstructive pulmonary disease (COPD) who fail to respond to selective beta agonist therapies such as albuterol are candidates for this therapy.

Preparations. Many preparations of theophylline (its salt form is aminophylline) are available for oral, rectal, inhalant, or IV use. For IV use, ampules or vials containing 250 mg in 10 ml or 500 mg in 20 ml are available.

Dosing. A loading dose of 6 mg/kg is given *slowly* over 15 to 30 minutes in patients with no recent theophylline therapy. The bolus injection is followed by a continuous infusion of 0.2 to 0.9 mg/kg/hr. When patients are known to take long-term theophylline preparations but have no clinical evidence of toxicity or when patients have physiologic risk factors that tend to increase serum theophylline levels (erythromycin, propranolol, caffeine, cimetidine, congestive heart failure, cor pulmonale, advanced age), one half of the loading dose should be cautiously administered.

Pharmacokinetics. The onset of theophylline's activity is 15 to 30 minutes after IV administration. Theophylline is metabolized by the liver. The rate of hepatic drug metabolism is highly variable and may be increased (yielding a suboptimal therapeutic response) or decreased (predisposing to toxicity) by many factors (Box 14-3).

Because hepatic metabolism of this drug is so patient variable, careful monitoring for clinical evidence of theophylline toxicity coupled with serum theophylline levels is extremely important for safe and effective patient management. The therapeutic range of serum theophylline is 10 to 20 μg/ml; however, theophylline levels tend to correlate poorly with toxicity. Some patients may have normal serum theophylline levels but have strong clinical signs of theophylline toxicity, whereas other patients may have elevated serum theophylline levels with no clinical evidence of drug toxicity. In these latter patients, normal serum drug levels may be associated with suboptimal clinical response.

Monitoring. The HR, BP, CO, ECG, serum theophylline levels, and hepatic function should be monitored.

BOX 14-3
Factors That Influence Theophylline Levels

Factors That Decrease Theophylline Levels
Phenobarbital
Cigarette smoking
Hypermetabolism, such as hyperthyroidism

Factors That Increase Theophylline Levels
Liver disease
Heart failure, cor pulmonale
Viral infections
Advanced age
Caffeine
Erythromycin
H_2 blockers
Phenytoin
Propranolol
Oral contraceptives
Ciprofloxacin

Cautions. Theophylline toxicity, which manifests as nausea, vomiting, diarrhea, excitability, tremors, restlessness, and sinus tachycardia, is relatively common. Advanced toxicity may be clinically evident as sinus tachycardia greater than 120 to 130 beats per minute, ventricular ectopy, and agitation. Severe theophylline intoxication manifests as grand mal seizures and ventricular tachycardia or fibrillation. As mentioned, signs of toxicity may be present with normal serum drug levels, particularly in elderly patients.

There is no antidote to theophylline; however, serial administration of activated charcoal, given either as a retention enema or orally, facilitates drug clearance (GI dialysis). This factor is related to the apparent ability of the intestinal mucosa to act as a dialysis membrane when charcoal is in the lumen of the gut.

Cimetidine

Cimetidine is a histamine receptor blocking agent that reduces gastric acid secretion by inhibiting the action of histamine on the parietal cells. Cimetidine also inhibits hepatic microsomal enzyme function and reduces blood flow through the liver. These hepatic factors result in increased levels of many medications with hepatic elimination (e.g., warfarin).

Uses. Cimetidine is given in treatment and prevention of duodenal and gastric ulcer disease and in prevention of stress-induced gastritis or ulceration.

Preparation. Tagamet, 150 mg/ml.

Dosing. Cimetidine must be diluted before IV administration. The usual IV dosage of cimetidine is 300 mg every 6 to 8 hours, although daily doses up to 2.4 g have been administered. When given as an intermittent IV injection, cimetidine should be administered over a period of not less than 5 minutes.

Pharmacokinetics. Inhibition of gastric acid secretion occurs within 15 to 60 minutes of an IV dose of cimetidine. This effect lasts approximately 4 to 6 hours. There are approximately equal amounts of hepatic metabolism and renal excretion of unchanged drug. The dosage interval should be increased in patients with renal or hepatic dysfunction so that patients with creatinine clearances below 30 ml/min should have a recommended dosing interval of at least 12 hours.

Monitoring. Careful monitoring is needed for drug effects and drug levels of other medications patients may be receiving that require hepatic elimination. Hypotension may result from rapid IV bolus administration.

Cautions. Hallucinations and delirium may occur, particularly in elderly patients. Cardiac arrhythmias, bradycardia, and cardiac arrest have been reported following IV injection.

Ranitidine

Ranitidine is a histamine receptor blocker similar in activity to cimetidine. That is, it is an inhibitor of the action of histamine at the histamine H_2 receptors. Ranitidine's effect on hepatic metabolism of other drugs appears to be significantly less than that of cimetidine.

Uses. Ranitidine is given in the treatment and prevention of duodenal and gastric ulcer disease and prevention of stress-induced gastritis and ulcerations.

Preparations. Zantac, 25 mg/ml.

Dosing. Ranitidine is given by intermittent IV infusion in doses of 50 mg every 6 to 8 hours. Ranitidine is usually diluted in at least 20 ml of solution before administration. A total daily dose of greater than 400 mg is not recommended. Continuous IV infusions of 6.25 mg/hr (150 mg/day) also may be used for dosing. For the treatment of hypersecretory states such as Zollinger-Ellison syndrome, 1 to 2.5 mg/kg/hr infusions have been administered.

Pharmacokinetics. The inhibition of gastric acid secretion occurs within 1 hour of IV ranitidine administration. The duration of effect is approximately 6 to 8 hours. Ranitidine is primarily metabolized by the liver, with some drug being excreted unchanged via glomerular filtration and tubular secretion. The dosage interval should be increased in patients with renal dysfunction.

Monitoring. Careful monitoring of other drugs that undergo hepatic metabolism is recommended, but as stated earlier, the possibility of such effects is less with ranitidine than with cimetidine.

Cautions. Mental confusion, agitation, and hallucinations have been reported, particularly in severely ill, elderly patients. As with cimetidine, arrhythmias and asystole may rarely occur following IV injection.

Famotidine

Famotidine is a histamine receptor blocker with pharmacologic activity similar to that of cimetidine and ranitidine.

Uses. Famotidine is used in the treatment and prevention of duodenal and gastric ulcers, the prevention of stress-induced gastritis and ulcerations, and the treatment of hypersecretory states such as Zollinger-Ellison syndrome.

Preparation. Pepcid IV, 10 mg/ml, 2 ml vial (must be refrigerated).

Dosing. Famotidine is given as a slow IV injection or IV infusion in doses of 20 mg every 12 hours. It is recommended that the drug be diluted (usually in 5 to 10 ml for IV injection and 100 ml for infusion in solution) before being administered. Dosing adjustment is recommended in patients with renal insufficiency.

Pharmacokinetics. Famotidine inhibits gastric acid secretion within 1 hour following administration; peak effects are seen within 0.5 to 3 hours, and the inhibition lasts approximately 10 to 12 hours. The drug undergoes some hepatic metabolism after IV administration, but most IV famotidine is excreted unchanged by the kidney.

Monitoring. Famotidine appears to have less effect on the hepatic metabolism of other drugs than cimetidine and ranitidine. However, patients receiving drugs that undergo hepatic metabolism should be monitored more closely than usual for signs of toxicity while receiving famotidine.

Cautions. Famotidine is generally well tolerated, with an overall incidence of adverse effects similar to that of ranitidine. CNS effects such as confusion, depression, and hallucinations have been reported in less than 1% of patients. Other adverse effects include pruritus, urticaria, abnormal liver function studies, cardiac arrhythmias, palpitations, and AV block.

Furosemide

Furosemide is a high-potency diuretic that inhibits reabsorption of sodium, water, and chloride from the ascending limb of the loop of Henle. It also decreases reabsorption of sodium and water and increases potassium excretion in the distal renal tubule. Because of the renal vasodilatory effects of the drug and subsequent increased renal blood flow, patients receiving drugs eliminated by renal excretion may have decreased serum level and suboptimal therapeutic drug effects.

An additional therapeutic effect of furosemide is the nearly immediate increase in venous capacitance. In patients with cardiogenic pulmonary edema, preload reduction is the mechanism by which clinical improvement occurs within minutes following furosemide administration before diuresis begins.

Uses. Furosemide is given in the management of cardiogenic pulmonary edema, congestive heart failure, hypertensive emergencies, acute or chronic renal failure, and other conditions characterized by fluid retention.

Preparations. Lasix, 10 mg/ml, in vials of 20, 40, and 100 mg.

Dosing. For acute pulmonary edema or hypertensive emergencies, the typical initial dose is 20 to 80 mg by slow (over 2 to 3 minutes) IV push. If no response occurs in 30 to 60 minutes, the dose may be increased in increments of 20 to 40 mg. Patients resistant to high doses of furosemide may benefit by the addition of 5 mg of metolazone (Zaroxolyn) or 500 mg of chlorothiazide (Diuril) given 30 to 60 minutes before the furosemide because these agents may produce a synergistic effect with furosemide. Patients not responding to intermittent boluses of furosemide may benefit from a continuous infusion of the drug.

In a nonemergency situation, an IV injection or intermittent infusion of 0.5 to 2 mg/kg may be provided one to four times daily, with dose increases of 0.25 to 0.5 mg/kg as the patient's condition requires. Continuous infusion doses of 5 to 20 mg/hr are used most often. Dosages up to 6.0 g/day have been reported in the literature.

Pharmacokinetics. The onset of diuresis by IV route is 5 to 15 minutes, peaks within 20 to 60 minutes, and lasts for approximately 2 hours. Furosemide is eliminated by hepatic metabolism and renal excretion.

Monitoring. The BP and HR; urine output; serum potassium, sodium, chloride, and magnesium levels; and acid-base status should be monitored. Furosemide may alter serum levels of other drugs that are excreted renally; therefore drug levels and clinical effects of such drugs also should be monitored.

Cautions. Furosemide is a potent diuretic, and, although commonly given in the management of conditions of ICU patients, it is not a benign medication. Numerous cautions specific to its use include the following:

1. Administration of furosemide may lead to profound diuresis and electrolyte loss, which may result in clinically significant fluid depletion and electrolyte imbalances. A low urine output in an ICU patient should be considered the result of hypovolemia until proved otherwise. Administration of furosemide to "force diuresis" in the context of patients with marginal fluid depletion may lead to hypovolemic shock and the possibility of vascular thrombosis, particularly in elderly patients.
2. Loop diuretics may cause urine potassium losses greater than 100 mEq/L, as well as significant losses of magnesium, sodium, and chloride. Serum potassium levels should be evaluated following furosemide-induced diuresis, and serum electrolyte panels should be performed periodically on patients receiving loop diuretic therapy.
3. Tinnitus, reversible or permanent hearing impairment, and reversible deafness have been associated with overly rapid IV administration of higher than usual doses of furosemide or administration in patients with renal impairment.
4. Patients with sulfonamide sensitivity may show allergic reactions to furosemide.
5. Furosemide IV solution should not be administered if it is discolored.

Bumetanide

Bumetanide is a sulfonamide-type loop diuretic that is structurally similar to furosemide and shares many of the same uses and properties. Bumetanide is a more potent diuretic (approximately 40 times the potency of furosemide) and may be effective in patients refractory to furosemide. The manufacturer claims that patients who exhibit hypersensitivity reactions to furosemide may tolerate bumetanide, but others believe that cross-sensitivity is likely because of the structural similarities of the drugs. Bumetanide is considered to be less ototoxic than furosemide.

Uses. Bumetanide is given in the management of pulmonary edema, congestive heart failure, hypertensive emergencies, acute or chronic renal failure, and conditions characterized by fluid retention.

Preparations. Bumex, 0.25 mg/ml, in 2 and 4 ml vials.

Dosing. Initial IV doses are 0.5 to 1.0 mg. Doses can be repeated every 2 to 3 hours as needed. The recommended maximal daily dose is 10 mg, but higher doses have been given in the intensive care setting.

Pharmacokinetics. The onset of activity of bumetanide occurs within minutes, peaks within 1 to 2 hours, and persists for 2 to 3 hours. Bumetanide is partially metabolized in the liver, with these metabolites and unchanged drug excreted primarily by the kidney.

Monitoring. The BP, fluid status, electrolytes (particularly potassium, sodium, magnesium, and chloride), and acid-base status should be monitored.

Cautions. Bumetanide, like furosemide, may cause electrolyte depletion, dehydration, metabolic alkalosis, hypotension, hyperuricemia, and transient rises in blood urea nitrogen and serum creatinine. The drug should be used cautiously in patients with known sensitivity to sulfonamides.

Midazolam

Midazolam is a short-acting, water-soluble CNS depressant benzodiazepine that produces antianxiety, sedative, hypnotic, skeletal muscle relaxant, and anticonvulsant effects.

Uses. Midazolam may be administered for anesthesia induction or preanesthetic sedation and as a hypnotic. In ICU patients, the drug is most commonly used to achieve conscious sedation to facilitate placement of central circulatory catheters, intubation, and mechanical ventilatory support. Midazolam is commonly given also for sedative effects in restless, combative, or agitated patients after hypoxemia, hypercarbia, perfusion failure, and an intracranial process following brain injury have been ruled out as the underlying cause. In many clinical situations, midazolam may be preferable to diazepam owing to its rapid, nonpainful induction, lack of venous irritation, and relatively short duration of action.

Preparations. Versed injection, 1 and 5 mg/ml, available in 2, 5, and 10 ml vials.

Dosing. Before IV dosing, the availability of resuscitative equipment and trained personnel for the maintenance of airway and ventilatory support, as well as cardiovascular support, is encouraged. Doses of 1 to 2.5 mg, by slow IV injection, may be given immediately before the intended procedure or for induction of a sedated state. The dose may be titrated in small increments every 2 to 5 minutes until the desired sedative effect is achieved. To maintain the desired sedative effect over a long period, a bolus of midazolam may be followed by a continuous infusion. The usual bolus dose in such situations is 1 to 5 mg, followed by an infusion of 1 to 10 mg/hr. IV doses of midazolam must be decreased for elderly or debilitated patients.

Pharmacokinetics. The onset of action of midazolam is 1 to 3 minutes, and the duration of effect is 30 to 80 minutes after a single dose. The drug undergoes extensive liver metabolism.

Monitoring. The BP, HR, ECG for arrhythmias, respiratory rate, and tidal volume, as well as level of consciousness, should be monitored.

Cautions. Vital sign changes that are frequently observed following IV administration include decreased respiratory rate and tidal volume, as well as variations in blood pressure. Profound hypotension and apnea may develop in elderly or debilitated patients. Midazolam has also been associated with a slight decrease in mean arterial pressure and cardiac output in the general patient population. Alterations in heart rhythm such as ventricular ectopy or nodal rhythm may occasionally develop. Patients with pulmonary disease, hepatic and renal dysfunction, severe fluid and electrolyte imbalance, or shock and trauma should receive midazolam in very small doses, if at all, and it should be injected very slowly. Rarely, paradoxic reactions may occur following IV administration of the drug. The incidence of headache, oversedation, drowsiness, confusion, and respiratory depression is similar to that associated with other benzodiazepines.

Flumazenil

Flumazenil is a benzodiazepine antagonist approved for the reversal of the sedative effects of benzodiazepines. It competes for and blocks the γ-aminobutyric acid (GABA) receptors, which are the CNS receptor sites of action for all benzodiazepines. Flumazenil does not antagonize the effects of opioids, barbiturates, ethanol, or other CNS depressants.

Uses. Flumazenil is given to reverse the sedative effects of benzodiazepines, thus speeding the patient's recovery from CNS sedation and shortening the monitoring period. Flumazenil may be administered after various procedures. It is used to reverse the sedation associated with suspected or known benzodiazepine overdose. However, flumazenil has not yet been approved by the Food and Drug Administration (FDA) to reverse the respiratory depression associated with benzodiazepines.

Preparation. Romazicon, 5 and 10 ml multiple-use vials, each containing 0.1 mg/ml of flumazenil.

Dosing. For reversal of sedation, an initial IV dose of 0.2 mg over 15 seconds is recommended. If the desired effect is not noted within 45 seconds, additional doses of 0.2 mg can be given every 60 seconds to a total dose of 1.0 mg. Most patients respond to doses of 0.6 to 1.0 mg. If resedation occurs, additional doses of no more than 1.0 mg (given as 0.2 mg/min) can be administered every 20 minutes as necessary. No more than 3 mg should be provided in 1 hour. For the initial management of suspected or known benzodiazepine overdose, the recommended dose is 0.2 mg IV over 30 seconds. If the desired effect is not seen within 30 seconds, an additional dose of 0.3 mg can be given over 30 seconds. Further additional doses of 0.5 mg administered over 30 seconds at 1-minute intervals up to a cumulative dose of 3 mg may be given. Most patients respond to doses of 1 to 3 mg. In patients not responding to 3 mg of flumazenil, the major cause of sedation is probably not a benzodiazepine.

Pharmacokinetics. The onset of reversal usually is seen within 1 to 2 minutes after the injection is given. Peak effects occur within 6 to 10 minutes. The duration and degree of reversal are related to the plasma concentration of the benzodiazepine and the dose of flumazenil. Flumazenil undergoes hepatic metabolism, and the metabolites are excreted in the urine.

Monitoring. The CNS status, respiratory rate, and cardiovascular status are monitored. Patients who have received flumazenil for reversal of sedation should be monitored for resedation, respiratory depression, or other residual effects of benzodiazepines for up to 2 hours after flumazenil administration.

Cautions. The most common serious adverse effect reported is seizures. Seizure occurs most often in patients receiving benzodiazepines for seizure control, those physically dependent on benzodiazepines, or those who have ingested large amounts of other drugs. Flumazenil also should be administered with caution in patients with head injury because of the risk of seizures and because of altered cerebral blood flow in those who have received benzodiazepines. Other commonly observed adverse effects include dizziness, pain at the injection site, increased sweating, headache, abnormal or blurred vision, nausea and vomiting, agitation, and emotional lability. Flumazenil is not recommended in patients with serious cyclic antidepressant overdoses as manifested by motor abnormalities, arrhythmias, anticholinergic signs, and cardiovascular collapse at presentation. The availability of flumazenil does not diminish the need for prompt respiratory support in the event of hypoventilation associated with benzodiazepines. Flumazenil also should not be given until the effects of neuromuscular blocking agents have been reversed.

Propofol

Propofol is an intravenously administered sedative-hypnotic agent for induction and maintenance of anesthesia or sedation. It is chemically unrelated to any opioid, barbiturate, or benzodiazepine used for anesthesia or sedation. Propofol is only slightly water soluble and therefore is formulated in a white oil in water emulsion.

Uses. Propofol is administered for rapid induction and maintenance of anesthesia or sedation. This agent can be used as part of a balanced anesthesia technique for inpatient and outpatient procedures. It also has been approved in critically ill or injured patients for sedation and control of mechanical ventilatory support.

Preparations. Diprivan, 20, 50, and 100 ml ready-to-use vials, each containing 10 mg/ml of propofol.

Dosing. For intubated, mechanically ventilated adult patients, ICU sedation should be initiated slowly with a continuous infusion to titrate to desired clinical effect and to minimize hypotension. When indicated, initiation of sedation should begin at 5 μg/kg/min, with increments of 5 to 10 μg/kg/min (maximum dose of 50 μg/kg/min) until the desired level of sedation is achieved. A minimum of 5 minutes between adjustments is important to allow peak effects to occur. Bolus doses of 10 or 20 mg may be given to rapidly increase the depth of sedation, but they should not be given to patients in whom hypotension is likely.

For induction of anesthesia, most patients require 2.0 to 2.5 mg/kg every 10 seconds until the onset of anesthesia. Maintenance of anesthesia is accomplished with a continuous infusion of 100 to 200 μg/kg/min for most patients. Clinicians should note that elderly, debilitated, or severely ill patients may require lower doses to achieve the desired effect.

Pharmacokinetics. Propofol has an extremely short duration of action and produces hypnosis within 40 seconds of the start of an injection. The recovery from the effect is seen within 10 minutes of stopping the drug. Propofol should be tapered, at approximately 5 μg/min decrements, rather than abruptly discontinuing in patients receiving long-term or high-dose therapy. Abrupt cessation can result in abrupt awakening, anxiety, and restlessness. Duration of effect is dose related, with larger doses providing longer periods of sedation or anesthesia. Propofol undergoes liver metabolism, and inactive metabolites are then excreted by the kidney.

Monitoring. The HR, BP, ECG, and signs of hypersensitivity should be monitored.

Cautions. Hypotension and bradycardia are the most common cardiovascular side effects associated with propofol. In some cases, these effects are related to overly rapid administration of the drug. Decreases in cardiac output also may occur. Other cardiovascular effects such as AV block and atrial fibrillation have been reported, but a causal relationship between the drug and the arrhythmias has not been proven. Other effects include burning and stinging at the injection site, myalgia, flushing and pruritus, hypertonia, dystonia, and hyperlipemia. *Resuscitative and suction equipment, an endotracheal intubation tray, and oxygen must be available in the immediate area. Vital signs should be assessed immediately before beginning administration, and the patient should be assessed frequently for signs of decreased cardiac output, hypotension, and bradycardia.*

Propofol should not be used in patients with increased intracranial pressure or impaired cerebral circulation because it may cause substantial decreases in mean arterial pressure and consequently substantial decreases in cerebral perfusion pressure.

Morphine Sulfate

Morphine sulfate is the most widely administered narcotic analgesic and has various physiologic effects. It is an extremely potent analgesic that also allays anxiety and creates a sense of well-being. These actions reduce the levels of circulating catecholamines and the tendency toward arrhythmias in acute myocardial infarction.

Morphine also exerts a direct depressant effect on the respiratory system; respiratory rate is affected more than tidal volume. A dose of 0.15 mg/kg of morphine (approximately equal to 10 mg for the average-sized person) increases P_{CO_2} by approximately 3 mm Hg in normal persons.

Morphine, via a venodilatory effect, produces an increase in venous capacitance. This, in turn, decreases pulmonary artery blood flow and pressure and left ventricular end-diastolic volume and pressure (preload). The drug induces mild systemic arteriolar dilation, which, by reducing afterload, improves stroke volume and decreases heart work. Morphine has a negative chronotropic effect. The cardiopulmonary effects of morphine are useful in patients with acute myocardial ischemia or pulmonary edema. Morphine reduces heart work and oxygen consumption while decreasing pulmonary vascular congestion and pressures.

Uses. Uses include those for acute ischemic myocardial pain secondary to unstable angina pectoris or acute myocardial infarction; acute cardiogenic pulmonary edema; severe pain associated with trauma; burn injury; visceral pain; and as an adjunct to benzodiazepines for sedation and control in patients receiving mechanical ventilatory assistance, particularly patients who resist ventilatory assistance ("buck the vent"). Morphine is *strongly* recommended for its consciousness-blunting effect when neuromuscular blocking agents are needed to facilitate controlled mechanical ventilation.

Preparations. 5, 10, or 15 mg per ampule.

Dosing. For the relief of pain, the drug is given in 2 to 3 mg increments every 5 to 30 minutes according to the patient's symptoms or observed clinical responses. Morphine also may be given as an IV drip at 1 to 5 mg/hr in conjunction with benzodiazepines or neuromuscular blocking agents for patients receiving mechanical ventilation.

Pharmacokinetics. An IV injection is associated with immediate effects. Plasma levels decrease rapidly within the first hour and subsequently remain low and decline over the next 8 hours. Elderly patients are more sensitive to the nervous system effects of morphine; therefore, in these patients, a standard dose may be 1.5 times lower than that for younger persons.

Monitoring. The BP, HR, respiratory rate, and level of consciousness should be monitored.

Cautions. Important caveats relative to morphine "use and misuse" include the following:

1. Some practitioners believe that morphine "masks" myocardial ischemic pain and consequently interferes with evaluation of relief in treatment with nitroglycerin or thrombolytic therapy. However, pain severely stresses the patient psychologically and physiologically, which further increases serum catecholamine levels. These cardioexcitatory hormones, in turn, increase heart work and myocardial oxygen consumption and predispose to propagation of myocardial ischemia and arrhythmias. *Morphine sulfate should be given to patients with acute myocardial ischemia if the pain fails to resolve with other therapeutic measures.*

2. Because of its respiratory depressant effects, morphine should be given cautiously in nonventilated patients with acute or chronic severe pulmonary disease such as asthma, COPD, or pneumonia.

3. Morphine should not be given to hypovolemic or hypotensive patients. Patients with suspected or known blood loss or illness, such as sepsis, associated with reduced intravascular volume may develop severe hypotension following injection of morphine. In these patients, IV fluid administration and normalization of circulating plasma volume are recommended before morphine administration.

All patients at risk for respiratory depression or hypotension who are to receive morphine should have naloxone or resuscitative equipment available.

Fentanyl

Fentanyl is a short-acting, potent, synthetic opiate agonist. It shares the actions of other opiate agonists. When given in equipotent doses it has the same potential to cause respiratory depression as meperidine and morphine, but it does not appear to be as potent a vasodilator as morphine. It possesses little hypnotic activity, and histamine release is rare.

Uses. As an analgesic preoperatively, during surgery, and in the immediate postoperative period; as an anxiolytic and sedative before short procedures; and as an analgesic/sedative in the ICU patient.

Preparations. Fentanyl injection, 50 μg/ml; also available as lozenge and transdermal (patch) preparations.

Dosing. The usual dose for analgesia or sedation is 25 to 100 μg IV push; continuous infusions of 25 to 100 μg/hr are used in some patients. Patches are available that deliver 25, 50, 75, and 100 μg/hr, although these are most often used to manage chronic pain.

Pharmacokinetics. The onset of analgesia or sedation is almost immediate after an IV dose, is delayed 7 to 8 minutes after an intramuscular injection (rarely used), and is delayed 12 to 24 hours after patch administration. The duration of effect after a single IV dose is 30 to 60 minutes. Fentanyl is extensively metabolized by the liver.

Monitoring. As with other opiates, BP, HR, respiratory rate, and level of consciousness should be monitored.

Cautions. Fentanyl is an extremely potent opiate with a significant potential for respiratory depression and oversedation. Patients should receive the lowest effective dose to accomplish the goals of therapy. It should be given very cautiously to those patients not on a ventilator. Naloxone and resuscitative equipment should be available.

Neuromuscular Blocking Agents

Neuromuscular blocking agents are commonly used in the hospital setting to produce skeletal muscle relaxation during procedures of short duration, such as endotracheal intubation and endoscopic examination. These medications also are useful in the longer term for patients who physically resist mechanical ventilatory assistance ("buck the vent"). These agents are particularly helpful when controlled mechanical ventilation is indicated to decrease a patient's oxygen consumption. Neuromuscular blocking may also be used to decrease energy demands and oxygen expenditure in patients who have status epilepticus and tetanus, as well as to prevent shivering in febrile patients who require cooling devices. Pharmacologically paralyzed patients appear to be in coma or asleep, but unless neurologically impaired, consciousness and cognition are intact. Consequently, *provision of sedation and analgesia is absolutely necessary and humane.* Tachycardia, hypertension, diaphoresis, SpO_2 and SvO_2 decrease, and tearing, particularly with noxious stimuli such as endotracheal suctioning, are signs of inadequate sedation or analgesia. However, the absence of these autonomic signs does not rule out inadequate sedation. Consequently, brief, periodic reversal of neuromuscular blockade should be considered as a means of assessing adequacy of sedation and analgesia.

Monitoring the Level of Neuromuscular Blockade

The patient receiving this highly sophisticated and complex pharmacologic therapy must be carefully monitored for drug underdosing or overdosing. Several techniques are available. Inadequate neuromuscular blockade (NMB) is easily evaluated by observing the patient for efforts to resist the mechanical ventilator, a decreased SvO_2 and possibly decreased SpO_2, abnormal airway pressure curves and compliance tests, and sporadically elevated peak inspiratory pressures. However, this technique does not evaluate for drug overdosing and myopathy.

Patient responses to *peripheral nerve stimulation* are useful because they enable identification of the need for additional NMB, as well as identify inadvertent drug overdosing and myopathy. Peripheral nerve stimulation should be done at baseline with the patient sedated to determine the level of stimulation required during therapeutic paralysis. The level of NMB is determined by individual patient needs and preference of the level of paralysis desired by the prescribing physician (such as high-dose drug therapy needed to produce diaphragmatic paralysis). Peripheral nerve stimulation techniques include the following:

1. *Electrical stimulation of the ulnar nerve at the wrist.* Upon delivery of graded electrical current by a generator, response of the adductor pollicis muscle is evidenced by thumb adduction. Tension and twitch height decrease with increasing depth of NMB.
2. *The response to train-of-four twitches* (supramaximal electrical stimuli at a frequency of 2 Hz repeated at intervals of no less than 10 seconds apart via a generator). Elimination of the fourth, third, second, and first responses correlate to 75%, 80%, 90%, and 100% depression of the first twitch and increased level of NMB, respectively.

Acetylcholine is a neurotransmittor that acts at the myoneural junction. Muscle relaxants exert their action by one of two possible mechanisms: (1) by binding with acetylcholine receptors at the neuromuscular junction termed *depolarizing relaxants* or (2) by preventing the acetylcholine from binding to the receptors termed *nondepolarizing relaxants.* These actions, in turn, prevent depolarization and subsequent contraction of muscle fibers.

Succinylcholine

Succinylcholine is a depolarizing neuromuscular blocking agent.

Uses. Succinylcholine is given when paralysis of short duration is desired. It is administered principally during endotracheal intubation, endoscopic examination, and certain orthopedic manipulations. Because of its short duration, many practitioners consider succinylcholine the agent of choice for procedures lasting 3 minutes or less. It is preferred also when rapid onset of action is important, such as during emergency intubation.

Preparations. Anectine and others, 20, 50, and 100 mg/ml.

Dosing. The usual adult dose for short procedures is 0.5 to 1 mg/kg given over 10 to 30 seconds. Additional doses may be administered as needed. For prolonged procedures, an IV infusion delivering 0.5 to 10 mg/min may be administered.

Pharmacokinetics. The time to onset of activity for succinylcholine is 30 to 60 seconds; the duration of clinical effect is 6 to 20 minutes. Succinylcholine is rapidly metabolized, primarily by plasma pseudocholinesterases, to pharmacologically less active compounds. A small fraction of succinylcholine is excreted unchanged in the urine.

Monitoring. The BP, HR, electrolytes, and level of paralysis should be monitored.

Cautions. Patients receiving succinylcholine for prolonged periods may experience profound paralysis. Bradyarrhythmias and other arrhythmias have been reported, especially in children. Hyperkalemia may result from potassium release from muscle cells during the initial depolarization; a small rise in serum potassium (0.5 to 1 mEq/L) is commonly noted with routine use of the drug. Clinically significant hyperkalemia predisposing the patient to cardiac arrest may occur with major trauma or burn injuries, intraabdominal infections, and closed head injuries. Some patients may complain of myalgias following succinylcholine therapy. Succinylcholine may increase intracranial pressure and intraocular pressures and may also trigger malignant hyperthermia in genetically predisposed patients.

Pancuronium

Pancuronium is a synthetic nondepolarizing neuromuscular blocking agent. This agent, like vecuronium and atracurium, produces skeletal muscle paralysis by blocking the action of acetylcholine on the end plate of the myoneural junction.

Uses. Pancuronium is administered most often to produce muscle relaxation *after* induction of anesthesia, but it also is administered in the ICU setting to facilitate controlled ventilation, as well as the conditions described earlier.

Preparations. Pavulon and others, 1 and 2 mg/ml.

Dosing. For endotracheal intubation, 0.06 to 0.1 mg/kg doses are given IV. Additional doses of 0.01 mg/kg may be administered every 25 to 60 minutes if a prolonged effect is desired. For muscle relaxation for controlled mechanical ventilation, doses of 0.015 mg/kg may be administered. An alternative to intermittent dosing is infusion at a rate of 0.35 μg/kg/min.

Pharmacokinetics. The onset of action occurs within 2 to 3 minutes for pancuronium; the clinical effects begin to subside 35 to 45 minutes after the drug is discontinued. Pancuronium is mainly excreted unchanged by the kidneys, although hepatic metabolism is involved to some extent. The duration of effect may be prolonged in patients with impaired renal or hepatic function.

Monitoring. Monitor BP, HR, renal function, and level of paralysis.

Cautions. Because pancuronium has a slight sympathomimetic effect, the drug may cause a slight increase in heart rate and blood pressure. Most patients tolerate these effects well, but those with hemodynamic instability may not. Pancuronium may cause an increase in cardiac output.

Vecuronium

Vecuronium is a synthetic nondepolarizing neuromuscular blocking agent that shares the muscle relaxant properties of other nondepolarizing neuromuscular blockers such as pancuronium.

Uses. Vecuronium is generally administered in the same clinical situations as pancuronium (see previous discussion). Vecuronium offers the advantage of minimal cardiovascular effects (little or no effect on heart rate and blood pressure), shorter duration of action, and minimal cumulative effects.

Preparations. Norcuron, 10 mg vial; powder for reconstitution.

Dosing. Vecuronium is given by IV injection or continuous infusion. Initial doses for intubation are 0.08 to 0.1 mg/kg given 2 to 5 minutes before the procedure.

Continuous infusions are usually administered at a rate of 0.5 to 1.5 μg/kg/min.

Pharmacokinetics. The onset of activity for vecuronium is 2 to 4 minutes; the duration of clinical effect is 30 to 60 minutes. Vecuronium undergoes liver metabolism, and at least one of the metabolites possesses neuromuscular blocking properties. The kidney is responsible for excreting the metabolites and a small fraction of unchanged drug.

Monitoring. Monitor BP, HR, and level of paralysis.

Cautions. Vecuronium is usually well tolerated, with most side effects being mild and transient. Patients with severe renal dysfunction may experience a prolonged effect. Vecuronium should be administered with caution in patients with hepatic dysfunction.

Atracurium

Atracurium is a nondepolarizing neuromuscular blocking agent with effects on skeletal muscle similar to those of pancuronium and vecuronium.

Uses. Atracurium is useful in the same clinical situations as pancuronium and vecuronium. The duration of neuromuscular blockade is similar to that of vecuronium.

Preparations. Tracrium, 10 mg/ml (must be refrigerated).

Dosing. Initial doses of 0.4 to 0.6 mg/kg may be given IV, 2 to 5 minutes before the procedure. Continuous infusions of 5 to 9 μg/kg/min have been used to provide continuous neuromuscular blockade.

Pharmacokinetics. The onset of effect for atracurium occurs within 2 to 5 minutes; the duration of effect is 35 to 60 minutes. Atracurium undergoes rapid metabolism by nonhepatic and nonrenal mechanisms that may be impaired by acidosis or hypothermia. Hepatic metabolism and renal excretion appear to play minimal roles in the elimination of atracurium.

Monitoring. The BP, HR, and level of paralysis should be monitored. Because of drug-related histamine release, atracurium may result in hypotension when large boluses are given rapidly.

Cautions. Atracurium may decrease blood flow slightly, possibly secondary to histamine release. The by-products of metabolic breakdown may accumulate in patients with renal insufficiency, possibly causing CNS excitation. Patients with asthma may experience an exacerbation of the disease because of the histamine release associated with atracurium administration.

Cisatracurium

Cisatracurium is a newer nondepolarinzing neuromuscular blocking agent of intermediate onset and duration of action. It is similar to atracurium in its clinical application and pharmacokinetics, but it is not associated with significant histamine release and therefore does not cause flushing, peripheral vasodilation, decreases in mean arterial pressure, or wheezing.

Preparations. Nimbex, 2 and 10 mg/ml. Nimbex must be refrigerated and protected from light before use.

Dosing. For skeletal muscle blockade in the ICU setting, the usual dosage range is 0.5 to 10 μg/kg/min. Bolus doses of 0.1 mg/kg may be necessary to quickly achieve the desired effect.

NOTE: Cisatracurium is similar to atracurium in that elimination is not dependent on hepatic or renal function.

Monitoring. Monitor HR, BP, and level of paralysis.

General Caveats for Use of Neuromuscular Blocking Agents

1. *Many accidental or induced factors may potentiate neuromuscular blockade.* Electrolyte imbalances such as low serum sodium, potassium, calcium, and magnesium potentiate neuromuscular blockade. Respiratory acidosis and metabolic alkalosis also increase the effects of these drugs. Drugs commonly given in critical care that increase neuromuscular blocking effects include antiarrhythmic agents and antibiotics, such as aminoglycosides, tetracycline, and clindamycin.
2. *Coughing and clearance of respiratory secretions, and the corneal reflex, are eliminated.* Fastidious attention to tracheobronchial hygiene and protection of the eyes are essential to prevent more complications.
3. *The patient is pharmacologically rendered apneic.* Accidental disconnection from the mechanical ventilator leads to "disconnect" death within minutes. Monitor alarms must be carefully set and kept constantly on. However, mechanical alarm systems may fail or be accidentally turned off. Therefore a caregiver must remain in immediate proximity of the patient paralyzed with NMB.

4. *Muscle paralysis profoundly decreases heat production.* Paralyzed patients commonly have a rapid drop in body temperature, particularly when cooled. Additional blanketing may be necessary prevent heat loss and maintain a normal body temperature.

Glycoprotein IIb IIIa Receptor Inhibitors

Glycoprotein IIb IIIa receptor inhibitors are antiplatelet agents that bind to the receptor involved in the final common pathway of platelet aggregation. These agents include abciximab (Reopro), tirofiban (Aggrastat), and eptifibatide (Integrilin).

Uses. Glycoprotein IIb IIIa inhibitors are used to decrease acute thrombotic closure of coronary arteries after percutaneous coronary interventions. Tirofiban and eptifibatide are also used in the treatment of acute coronary syndromes without percutaneous coronary interventions.

Preparations. Abciximab: Most references recommend administering the bolus dose from a separate syringe. The bolus dose should be filtered using a sterile, nonpyrogenic, low-protein-binding 0.2 or 0.22 μm filter. The infusion is prepared with 5% dextrose or 0.9% saline. This should also be filtered as described previously or at the time of administration with a similar in-line device. Abciximab should be administered through a separate intravenous line whenever possible.

Tirofiban: Tirofiban is available as a solution that must be further diluted before it can be administered. The solution is prepared by adding 50 or 100 ml of concentrated tirofiban to 250 or 500 ml of 5% dextrose or 0.9% saline to achieve a final concentration of 50 μg/ml. The bolus and maintenance doses can be administered from the infusion bag. Tirofiban is also available in premixed bags of 50 μg/ml.

Eptifibatide: Eptifibatide is available as a premixed solution in 100 ml vials with a final concentration of 0.75 mg/ml.

Dosing. Abciximab: A bolus of 0.25 mg/kg should be administered 10 to 60 minutes before the start of percutaneous coronary intervention, followed by a continuous infusion of 0.125 μg/kg/min (maximum of 10 μg/min) for 12 hours. Infusions have been given for up to 24 hours in patients with unstable angina who are scheduled to undergo percutaneous coronary angioplasty within 24 hours.

Tirofiban: A bolus infusion of 0.4 μg/kg/min for 30 minutes is followed by an infusion of 0.1 μg/kg/min for 24 to 96 hours. Patients with severe renal impairment (creatinine clearance of 30 ml/min or less), including those requiring hemodialysis, should receive half the usual rate of tirofiban.

Eptifibatide: A bolus of 180 μg/kg given over 1 to 2 minutes followed by an infusion of 2 μg/kg/min for 24 to 96 hours is the most commonly used regimen for acute interventions. In patients with creatinine concentrations between 2 and 4 mg/dl, the recommended dose is a bolus of 135 μg/kg given over 2 minutes followed by an infusion of 0.5 μg/kg/min. Eptifibatide is not recommended for patients with more severe renal impairment, including those requiring hemodialysis. The lower dose regimen may be used in elective angioplasty.

Pharmacokinetics. Abciximab: A rapid, dose-dependent inhibition of platelet aggregation is seen after bolus administration. The half-life of abciximab is less than 10 minutes, but platelet function recovers slowly over 48 hours or longer.

Tirofiban: Platelet aggregation is inhibited within 5 minutes after initiation of an infusion. Platelet function returns to pretreatment levels within 4 to 8 hours after discontinuance of a tirofiban infusion. Tirofiban is excreted primarily unchanged by the kidney.

Eptifibatide: Significant inhibition of platelet aggregation is seen soon after administration of the bolus dose. Platelet function returns to pretreatment levels within 4 hours after discontinuance of an infusion. Eptifibatide is excreted by the kidneys.

Monitoring. Patients must be monitored closely for signs of bleeding while on glycoprotein IIb IIIa inhibitors; this is particularly important because most are also receiving aspirin and many are receiving heparin concomitantly. Pretreatment platelet counts are necessary because *a platelet count less than 100,000 is a contraindication to the use of glycoprotein IIb IIIa inhibitors.* Patients receiving abciximab should have platelet counts performed 2 to 4 hours after the bolus dose and at 24 hours or at the time of discharge, whichever is earlier. Patients receiving tirofiban should have platelet counts performed 6 hours after the bolus dose and daily thereafter while on the drug. Patients receiving eptifibatide should have platelet counts performed daily while on the drug.

Cautions. The most common side effect associated with glycoprotein IIb IIIa inhibitor therapy is bleeding. The likelihood is greater in patients receiving concomitant heparin therapy or those having received thrombolytics. As stated earlier, platelet counts less than 100,000 are a contraindication to glycoprotein IIb IIIa therapy. Other contraindications include active internal bleeding; recent (within 6 weeks) GI or genitourinary bleeding of clinical significance; history of cerebrovascular accident (CVA) within 2 years or CVA with significant neurologic deficit; bleeding diathesis; administration of oral anticoagulants within 7 days, unless the prothrombin time is less than 1.2 times control; recent (within 6 weeks) major surgery or trauma; intracranial neoplasm; arteriovenous malformation or aneurysm; severe uncontrolled hypertension; presumed or documented history of vasculitis; and use of IV dextran before percutaneous coronary intervention or intent to use it during intervention. The usual precautions for avoiding bleeding complications in patients receiving drugs affecting coagulation should be employed in patients receiving glycoprotein IIb IIIa receptor inhibitors.

DISCUSSION

In many ICU situations, a rapid change in clinical status does not permit measurements of drug concentrations in the blood, even when means of measurement are available. Decisions on drug dosing must be made on the basis of patients' clinical and hemodynamic status. Table 14-4 lists the expected hemodynamic changes induced by individual

TABLE 14-5
Vasoactive Agent Dosages and Uses

Drug	Indication	Dose	Monitoring
Epinephrine	Cardiac arrest	IV: 0.5–1.0 mg over 1 min IT: 1 mg Tracheal route: 2–2.5 mg in 10 ml normal saline	Heart rate and blood pressure; local tissue necrosis if drug extravasation occurs, ECG, urine output *PWP, CO
	Hypotension that is refractory to fluid administration	1–8 μg/min IV, titrate for effect	
Norepinephrine	Hypotension	4–8 μg/min IV, titrate for effect	Heart rate and blood pressure, ECG, urine output,*CO, local tissue necrosis if extravasation occurs
Phenylephrine	Shock	100–200 μg/min initially, 40–60 μg/min maintenance	Heart rate, blood pressure, acid-base, local tissue necrosis if extravasation occurs *CO, PWP
Dopamine	Circulatory failure	1–2 μg/kg/min IV, titrate for effect up to a maximum of 50 μg/kg/min	Heart rate, and blood pressure; cardiac output; renal function, local tissue necrosis if extravasation occurs
Dobutamine	Circulatory failure	2–2.5 μg/kg/min IV, titrate for effect to a maximum of 20 μg/kg/min	Heart rate and blood pressure; ECG, *CO, PWP
Isoproterenol	Bradycardia, AV heart block	0.5–5.0 μg/min IV, titrate for effect	Heart rate and blood pressure, ECG, *PWP, CO
Nitroglycerin	Angina, heart failure, hypertension	5–10 μg/min, titrate for effect	Heart rate and blood pressure, *PAP, PWP
Nitroprusside	Hypertension, heart failure	0.5–2 μg/kg/min; titrate for effect	Heart rate, blood pressure, signs of cyanide and thiocyanate toxicity, *PAP, PWP
Trimethaphan	Hypertension, heart failure	0.5–1 μg/min; titrate for effect	Heart rate and blood pressure, respiratory rate, urine output, *PAP, PWP
Hydralazine	Hypertension, heart failure	5–10 mg; repeat as needed	Heart rate and blood pressure, liver function

CO, cardiac output; *ECG*, electrocardiogram; *PWP*, pulmonary capillary wedge pressure; *PAP*, pulmonary artery pressure.

*These are recommended for measurement if the patient has a pulmonary artery catheter in place.

drugs. This information may be helpful in predicting dosage requirements or dosage adjustments for medications currently in use, as well as for subsequent therapeutic agents provided in combination. Table 14-5 lists common vasoactive agents and their general indications and dosages.

This chapter describes some pharmacologic agents commonly used in critical care patient management. Many more drugs may be selected for ICU patients; however, it is beyond the scope of this text to include all the drugs that may be used in the critical care setting.

All drugs are toxins, and this fact must be acknowledged and respected when selecting drugs and monitoring effects. One of the most fundamental responsibilities of health care professionals is to inflict no injury on the patient while attempting to palliate or heal. However, the nature of some diseases, and drugs in treatment of disease, requires that some variable degree of untoward effects be tolerated for the greater good—cure or significant relief of suffering. Knowledge of the nature of therapeutic agents and vigilant monitoring may keep the number and level of untoward drug effects to an absolute minimum.

SUGGESTED READINGS

Adult advanced cardiac life support, *Circulation* 102(suppl 1): 2000.

Benet LZ, Massoud N, Gambertoglio JG: *Pharmacokinetic basis for drug treatment,* New York, 1984, Raven Press.

Braunwald E: *Heart disease: a textbook of cardiovascular medicine,* ed 5, Philadelphia, 1997, W.B. Saunders.

Chernow B: *The pharmacological approach to the critically ill patient,* ed 3, Baltimore, 1994, Williams & Wilkins.

DiPiro JT, Talbert RL, Yee RC, et al: *Pharmacotherapy: a pathophysiologic approach,* ed 4, Stamford, 1999, Appleton & Lange.

Drug information 2000, 2000, American Society of Hospital Pharmacists.

Harrison TR: *Principles of internal medicine,* ed 14, New York, 1998, McGraw-Hill.

Kress JP, Pohlman AS, O'Connor MF, et al: Daily interruption of sedative infusions in critically ill patients undergoing mechanical ventilation, *N Engl J Med* 342:1471, 2000.

Luer JM: Sedation and neuromuscular blockade in patients with acute respiratory failure, *Crit Care Nurse* 20:84, 2000.

Parrillo JE et al: Septic shock in humans. Advances in the understanding of pathogenesis, cardiovascular dysfunction and therapy, *Ann Intern Med* 113:227, 1990.

Rackow EC, Astiz ME: Pathophysiology and treatment of septic shock, *JAMA* 266:548, 1991.

Shoemaker WC, Ayers S, Grenvick A, et al, editors: *Textbook of critical care,* ed 3, Philadelphia, 2000, W.B. Saunders.

Tobin MJ: *Principles and practices of intensive care monitoring,* New York, 1998, McGraw-Hill.

Winter ME: *Basic clinical pharmacokinetics,* ed 2, Spokane, 1988, Applied Therapeutics.

15

GLORIA OBLOUK DAROVIC

Intraaortic Balloon Counterpulsation

Shock developing as a complication of acute myocardial infarction is typically due to infarct extension. Mortality rates have been dismally high (in the range of 70% to 85%),[1] because standard medical management does not stop progression of the ischemic process.

The concept of and instrumentation for mechanically assisting severely compromised hearts was spearheaded by the Kantowitz brothers[2] and further developed by others through the 1950s and 1960s.[3,4] During this time period it was also realized that a significant percent of patients undergoing open-heart surgery could not be weaned from cardiopulmonary bypass due to severe dysfunction of the surgically stunned heart. Reports of intraaortic balloon pump stabilization of patients with cardiogenic shock, as well as successful weaning from cardiopulmonary bypass, began appearing in the late 1960s.[5,6] In the 1970s, the intraaortic balloon pump began to gain clinical acceptance. In the subsequent decades it was found that, despite intraaortic balloon pump stabilization, the short- and long-term survival of acute myocardial infarction shock patients is determined by the severity of underlying coronary artery disease, the level of left ventricular dysfunction, and the speed with which definitive revascularization procedures (when possible) are instituted. Patients with immediate revascularization achieve early survival rates as high as 93%.[7]

DEFINITION

The *intraaortic balloon pump* (IABP) is a mechanical cardiac assist device that benefits patients with actual or potential life-threatening circulatory problems. Intraaortic balloon counterpulsation (IABC) reduces the resistance to left ventricular ejection and increases coronary and systemic blood flow. Patient management of this sophisticated, invasive device is complex and cannot be adequately covered in a single chapter.

In fact, comprehensive coverage of all the ramifications of care fills an entire textbook. For this reason, the reader is referred to the manufacturers' instruction materials for use, as well as textbooks that are devoted entirely to comprehensive clinical application and patient management of intraaortic balloon pumping.[8,9]

This chapter discusses, in overview, the following topics: the principles underlying balloon counterpulsation, the effect of balloon counterpulsation on the arterial waveform, indications and contraindications, triggers and timing of balloon inflation/deflation cycles, balloon pressure waveforms, physical assessment considerations, and risks and complications. Focus is on principles and assessment of balloon inflation/deflation timing using the arterial pressure waveform. This is because proper timing of inflation/deflation cycles is one of the most important prerequisites for attaining hemodynamic benefit and salvaging ischemic mycocardium.

PRINCIPLES UNDERLYING BALLOON COUNTERPULSATIONS

A catheter is advanced into the aorta, most commonly via a femoral artery insertion site, until the catheter tip lies just distal to the left subclavian artery. A 30, 40, or 50 ml sausage-shaped balloon is located at the distal end of the catheter so that, when in place, the inflated balloon fills the descending thoracic aorta. All manufacturers have sizing recommendations for their products based on the patient's height and body surface area; the usual inflation volume is 40 ml. The bottom of the balloon lies just above the renal arteries. The proximal end of the balloon catheter is attached to a computerized console, which, in turn, is connected to the electrocardiogram (ECG) and arterial pressure monitor or cable. The balloon is inflated and deflated with helium synchronous with phases of the cardiac cycle by a computerized pump housed within the IABP console.

Hemodynamic Benefits

Circulatory benefits occur during both systole and diastole. The dual benefit is difficult or impossible to achieve with standard pharmacologic management of patients with cardiogenic shock that cannot be easily remedied medically (e.g., tachyarrhythmias or bradyarrhythmias, acidemia, drug effects).

Diastole

Balloon *inflation* at the onset of diastole increases aortic diastolic pressure to a level higher than systolic pressure and also displaces a volume of blood equal to its inflation volume. A portion of the displaced blood perfuses the cerebral and coronary circulations. Because 75% to 80% of coronary perfusion occurs during diastole, the diastolic pulse of blood improves perfusion to normal as well as jeopardized areas of myocardium. There are also potential increases in the size of the coronary collateral circulation.

Forward displacement of blood also improves renal, mesenteric, and generalized systemic flow. When correlated with the simultaneously obtained ECG, the period of balloon inflation usually relates to the period from the crest of the T wave to the next R wave (Figure 15-1). Because electromechanical delays may be highly variable in humans, particularly those having received controlled hypothermia (open heart surgery), ECG (electrical) markers are not precise indicators of the onset of mechanical diastole and systole. Consequently, balloon inflation/deflation cycles should be timed using the arterial waveform landmarks and pressure responses.

Systole

Deflation of the balloon occurs at the end of isovolumetric contraction (just before opening of the aortic valve) and is maintained until the onset of diastole. This period coincides with the R wave to the crest of the T wave on the ECG. The rapid diastolic inflation of the balloon and displacement of blood leaves a void (proportional to the size of the balloon) when the balloon

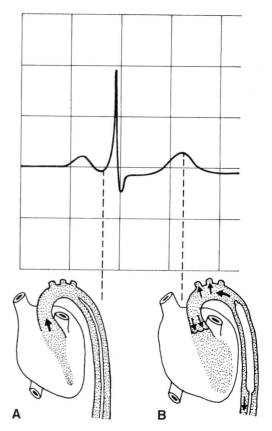

FIGURE 15-1 Schematic representation of the ECG and mechanical sequence of balloon counterpulsation. **A,** Systole. Deflation of the balloon coincides with the R wave. The resulting decrease in aortic pressure reduces impedance to left ventricular ejection. **B,** Diastole. The balloon inflates with closure of the aortic valve, which corresponds to the crest of the T wave on the ECG. Balloon inflation increases pressure in the aorta, thus increasing coronary and systemic perfusion.

deflates. Therefore a potential intraaortic vacuum is created that decreases aortic end-diastolic pressure below the patient's baseline value. Benefits include (1) decreased resistance to opening the aortic valve and left ventricular ejection (decreased afterload), (2) decreased myocardial work and oxygen consumption, (3) increased stroke volume and cardiac output, and (4) decreased left ventricular preload (measured as pulmonary artery wedge pressure [PWP]).

The rate of IABP assist ranges from one balloon inflation/deflation cycle for each cardiac cycle (1:1 ratio) to as few as one cycle for every eight cardiac cycles (1:8 ratio; manufacturer variable). Generally, IABP support is begun using a 1:1 ratio. The ratio of cardiac assist cycles is then gradually reduced, according to the patient's

BOX 15-1
Indications and Contraindications for Intraaortic Balloon Pump Therapy

Indications

As a bridge to reperfusion therapies in patients with cardiogenic shock

Unstable angina

As a bridge to emergent surgery in patients with acute cardiac defects, such as ventricular septal defect and acute mitral regurgitation

As a bridge to cardiac transplant

Perioperative support of high-risk cardiac and general surgical patients

Weaning from cardiopulmonary bypass

High-risk (multiple-vessel disease, poor left ventricular function) patients undergoing elective percutaneous coronary angiography or angioplasty

Pharmocologically refractory ventricular arrhythmias complicating acute myocardial infarction

Recurrent postinfarction angina

Contraindications (Absolute)

Aortic regurgitation

Thoracic or abdominal aneurysm

End-stage diseases

Brain death

Severe coagulopathy

Dissecting aortic aneurysm

Contraindications (Relative)

Severe aortic or femoral atherosclerosis

Symptomatic peripheral vascular disease

---

clinical and hemodynamic tolerance, until the device is discontinued.

Indications and Contraindications

Appropriate indications and contraindications for IABP circulatory support are listed in Box 15-1.

TECHNIQUE OF CATHETER PLACEMENT

When originally introduced in 1969, the catheter could only be placed by surgical cutdown technique. The percutaneous approach, which became available during the early 1980s, allows placement in approximately 5 minutes by experienced operators. The procedure may be performed at the patient's bedside or in the cardiac catheterization laboratory. *Thorough familiarity with manufacturer's*

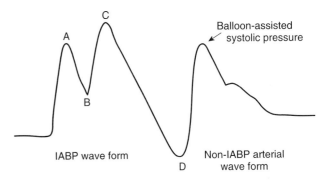

FIGURE 15-2 Balloon waveform showing the first hump *(A)*, first dip *(B)*, second hump *(C)*, and second dip *(D)*.

instructions is essential because as new catheters are being introduced, each has specific variations in insertion technique and precautions. Refer to appropriate texts for a general overview of catheter placement.[10-12]

EFFECTS OF THE INTRAAORTIC BALLOON PUMP ON THE ARTERIAL WAVEFORM

The effects of balloon pumping on the arterial waveform are dramatic changes from the normal single pressure rise (systole) followed by a single fall (diastole) (see Chapter 7, Figure 7-1).

During balloon counterpulsation, a double-hump and double-dip pattern is inscribed on the arterial waveform (Figure 15-2):

- *The first hump (A)* is the normal peak systolic pressure.
- *The first dip (B)* correlates with aortic valve closure and should be V shaped.
- *The second hump (C), termed diastolic augmentation or peak diastolic pressure (PDP),* is produced by balloon inflation and ideally raises diastolic pressure to a level higher than the systolic pressure. The mechanically induced increase in diastolic pressure optimizes coronary and systemic blood flow.

There are several circumstances in which diastolic augmentation (the second hump) may be equal to or less than systolic pressure (the first hump) and may result in suboptimal therapeutic effects. This may occur when the patient's stroke volume is high or very low; the balloon is positioned too low in the aorta; the patient is hypovolemic or has low systemic vascular resistance; the balloon inflation volume is inadequate relative to the size of the patient's aorta; late balloon inflation occurs; or the patient is hypertensive. The underlying cause of decreased peak diastolic pressure should be corrected (when possible) with appropriate measures, such as fluid repletion or repositioning of the balloon. Placement of a balloon that is too small for the patient may warrant replacement with a new catheter with a larger balloon. If the balloon inflation volume is too low (e.g., a 35 ml inflation volume for a 40 ml balloon), inflation volume should be carefully added while assessing the IABP waveform for appropriate pressure responses.

The *second dip (D)* relates to balloon deflation just before the next systole and should also be V shaped. Deflation of the balloon reduces end-diastolic pressure by approximately 15 mm Hg and the ensuing systolic pressure (assisted systolic pressure) by 5 to 10 mm Hg. In patients with cardiogenic shock, the assisted systolic pressure may be decreased by 20 mm Hg.

TRIGGERS FOR BALLOON INFLATION AND DEFLATION

The computer within the IABP console requires a physiologic signal, termed a *trigger,* from the patient that is used to indicate the beginning of cardiac cycles and also assesses the length of R-R intervals. The pneumatic system within the console then appropriately deflates and inflates the balloon in synchrony with the patient's cardiac cycles. The two principle modes of triggering use either the ECG or the arterial pressure waveform. Both signals can be directly obtained from the patient or indirectly obtained by "slaving" from the bedside monitor via cables. The signals are then cable-fed into the IABP console for analysis.

It is preferable to obtain signals directly from the patient because of the variability in software analysis of ECG or arterial line signals by different console models, as well as the risk of disrupting counterpulsation due to cable problems (accidental disconnect, defective cables).

Electrocardiogram-Derived R Wave

The ECG lead is connected to and analyzed by the IABP computer. The ECG lead selected should display an R wave that is larger than the P or T waves. The balloon automatically deflates in synchrony with the R wave. However, precise timing is usually set by the operator. From the trigger signal and length of R-R intervals, the IABP computer automatically determines the point of onset of balloon inflation, which typically coincides with the crest of the T wave (Table 15-1) (see Figure 15-1).

In other words, the period of balloon deflation is related to the period from the R wave through approximately the crest of the T wave, and the period of balloon inflation relates to the period from the crest of the T wave through the next QRS complex. It is important to select the ECG

lead with the most pronounced R wave. Triggering problems are commonly due to low-amplitude R waves, electrical interference (artifact), or disconnected electrodes.

Several other ECG triggering modes allow selection of the most reliable trigger signal for specific patient conditions such as demand or 100% paced rhythms, grossly irregular rhythms (atrial fibrillation), or patients with wide QRS complexes. The number of trigger modes varies among manufacturers and also varies relative to vintage of models from the same manufacturer. *It is essential that details and indications for trigger modes for specific IABP models be obtained from the manufacturer.*

Upstroke of the Arterial Pressure Waveform

This trigger mode may be used when the ECG signal is distorted by artifact (during transport, restless patients). It is also used in the operating room because electrocautery can interfere with the signal. A fairly sharp upstroke with a pulse pressure of at least 40 mm Hg is usually necessary for reliable arterial triggering but is dependent on the console used. Some manufacturers' newer models can use a lower pulse pressure for triggering.

TIMING OF INFLATION/DEFLATION CYCLES

There are two means of precisely timing inflation/deflation cycles to optimize hemodynamics and coronary blood flow. In both, a trigger (as listed previously) is used by the IABP console to identify cardiac cycles.

TABLE 15-1
Phases of the Cardiac Cycle

Phase	Benefit	ECG Correlate
Inflation (diastole)	Increased coronary, systemic, and brain blood flow Increased collateral myocardial blood flow	Crest of T wave through onset of next QRS complex
Deflation (systole)	Decreased afterload Decreased preload (PWP) Decreased myocardial work and oxygen consumption Increased stroke volume and cardiac output	From R wave through crest of T wave

Conventional Timing

This form of timing is based on the duration of balloon *inflation* throughout diastole. Because diastolic time intervals vary with the length of cardiac cycles, this form of timing requires a regular rhythm and relatively consistent heart rate (regular diastolic intervals) for effective timing. Conventional timing is discussed at length because it initially was the only form of timing available and remains the most common timing mode used clinically.

Real Timing

Real timing is based on rapid, automatic balloon *deflation* at the onset of systole with deflation maintained throughout systole. Because systolic intervals remain constant regardless of rate and rhythm, effective pumping is maintained despite irregular heart rhythms and significant changes in heart rate. See references 13 and 14 for elaboration on this form of timing.

When using conventional timing, the precise moment of onset of balloon inflation/deflation is fine-tuned using the arterial pressure waveform. Poor timing not only results in suboptimal circulatory benefits, but may also be harmful. It is essential to have a clearly defined, artifact-free arterial waveform for selecting timing landmarks and evaluating arterial pressure responses.

When the intended ratio will be 1:1, pumping is first set at a 1:2 ratio in order to assess arterial waveform timing landmarks and pressure responses by comparing IABP arterial pressure waveforms and non-IABP waveforms. Switches or dials on the console permit adjustments to inflation/deflation timing. The arterial waveforms are then carefully evaluated during several cardiac cycles. When the operator is satisfied with both triggering and timing, the console is set to a 1:1 pumping ratio to assist each cardiac cycle.

Timing should be rechecked using a hard copy of the IABP pressure tracing, every 1 to 2 hours, whenever there is a greater than 20% change in heart rate, a change in cardiac output or triggering mode, or the development or worsening of arrhythmias.

For each timing check, the console should be returned to the 1:2 pumping ratio (Figure 15-3). The hard copy of the timing check is then attached to the chart.

Inflation Timing

Because the dicrotic notch heralds the onset of diastole, it is used as a landmark for balloon inflation. The onset of balloon inflation is evidenced as the upstroke of diastolic augmentation. When using a radial artery catheter or IABP central lumen to obtain the arterial waveform, the upstroke should be adjusted to occur 40 ms (one little square on graph paper) before the dicrotic notch. The upstroke should occur 120 ms (three little squares) before the dicrotic notch if a femoral arterial line is used; however, use of this distal site is discouraged for IABP pressure monitoring. When balloon inflation is properly timed, the dicrotic notch is not visible and the point of onset of the upstroke of diastolic augmentation inscribes a V shape (Figure 15-4).

Deflation Timing

Deflation timing is assessed by arterial pressure responses, not waveform landmarks. There are two pressure responses to assess for effective deflation timing:

1. *The aortic end-diastolic pressure, following the balloon inflation/deflation cycle, should be lower than the preceding unassisted aortic end-diastolic pressure. This event, which should be V shaped, should also be*

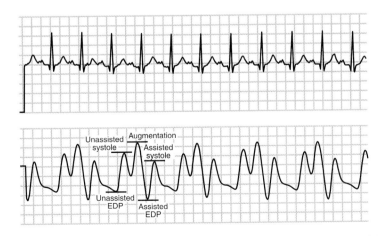

FIGURE 15-3 Sample documentation of ECG and IABP waveforms (1:2 ratio).

the lowest point on the IABP-assisted and unassisted blood pressure curves.

2. *The systolic peak that occurs after the balloon inflation/deflation cycle should be lower than the previous unassisted systolic peak* (Figure 15-5).

If all of these landmark/pressure response criteria are not fulfilled, adjustments are made on the console control panel to bring the points of inflation and deflation to those recommended to maximize hemodynamic benefits.

Errors in Timing

The points of balloon inflation and deflation may be either too early or too late. Only one error per balloon inflation/deflation cycle may be present, such as early balloon inflation. Double errors, such as both early or late inflation *and* early or late deflation, may be present. The hemodynamic and clinical consequences to the patient depend on the number and types of errors.

Early Balloon Inflation

With early balloon inflation, the upstroke of peak diastolic pressure greater than one little square before the dicrotic notch is visible for radial line placement. This error results in premature closure of the aortic valve. The consequences include an increase in aortic pressure, which increases afterload and myocardial oxygen consumption; impaired ventricular emptying, which results in reduced stroke volume and increased PWP; and a potential for aortic regurgitation. *This is a potentially dangerous timing error and may result in perfusion failure, myocardial ischemia, or pulmonary edema* (Figure 15-6).

Late Balloon Inflation

The dicrotic notch is visible with late balloon inflation. This results in a less than optimal diastolic augmented pressure and reduces the time period for

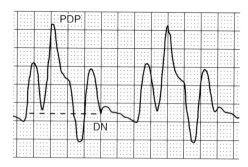

FIGURE 15-4 Optimal inflation timing landmark; 1:2 inflation-to-deflation ratio. *PDP,* peak diastolic pressure; *DN,* dicrotic notch.

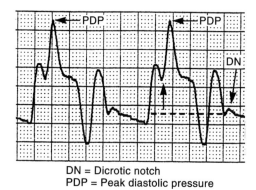

DN = Dicrotic notch
PDP = Peak diastolic pressure

FIGURE 15-6 Early balloon inflation. Note that the upstroke *(arrow)* of peak diastolic pressure occurs approximately nine little squares before the onset.

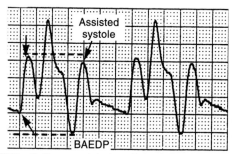

BAEDP = Balloon-assisted aortic end-diastolic pressure

FIGURE 15-5 Proper deflation timing responses on arterial waveform; 1:2 inflation-to-deflation ratio.

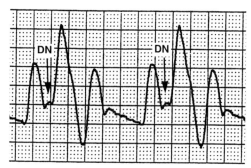

DN = Dicrotic notch

FIGURE 15-7 Late balloon inflation. Notice that a significant portion of the dicrotic notch *(arrows)* is visible.

augmented diastolic perfusion of the cerebral, coronary, and systemic circulations. The point of onset of the up-stroke of diastolic augmentation is U rather than V shaped. This error in timing is not dangerous, but the patient does not receive maximum benefit from IABC (Figure 15-7).

Early Balloon Deflation

This error results in a premature termination of diastolic augmentation. This is then followed by aortic pressure equilibration back to baseline before the next systole. A U rather than the desired V shape is inscribed before the next systolic upstroke. A brief shelf just before the next systolic upstroke may be noted in patients with heart rates less than 90 beats per minute (Figure 15-8). The ensuing systolic pressure may be equal to the previous unassisted systolic pressure. Early deflation results in suboptimal hemodynamic benefits because left ventricular afterload is not decreased and the time period for augmented diastolic perfusion is shortened. Retrograde flow from the higher-pressure coronary, renal, and carotid ar-teries into the lower-pressure aorta may be clinically evi-dent as transient angina or light-headedness.

Late Balloon Deflation

The balloon remains partially or completely inflated at the beginning of the next systole. Identifying features include a balloon-assisted aortic end-diastolic pressure that is greater than the unassisted aortic end-diastolic pressure and a depressed slope of the systolic upstroke of the next beat (assisted systole). Obstruction of the aorta by the inflated balloon as the aortic valve is opening in-creases afterload. Consequently, the velocity of ventricu-lar ejection, ejection time, and stroke volume are de-creased, which results in the depressed slope of the next systolic upstroke. *Late deflation is an extremely danger-ous timing error because the left ventricle must eject against the resistance imposed by the inflated balloon.* Myocardial work and oxygen consumption increase while stroke volume decreases. The combined effects may re-sult in hemodynamic deterioration and myocardial is-chemia (Figure 15-9).

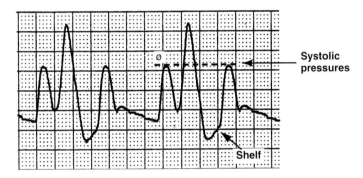

FIGURE 15-8 Early balloon deflation. Notice the U shape rather than V shape of the waveform and inscription of a brief shelf *(arrow)* before the next systole.

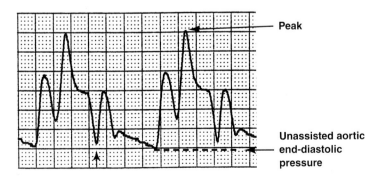

FIGURE 15-9 Late balloon deflation. Note that the balloon-assisted aortic end-diastolic pressure *(arrow)* is greater than the unassisted balloon aortic end diastolic pressure.

PHYSICAL ASSESSMENT CONSIDERATIONS FOR PATIENTS BEING MAINTAINED ON THE INTRAAORTIC BALLOON PUMP

Intraaortic balloon counterpulsation creates significant hemodynamic and physical assessment changes that appear to conflict with traditional thinking and experience. These changes must be considered when interpreting physical assessment findings.

Blood Pressure Changes

Normally, there are two reference points in blood pressure measurement: the systolic and diastolic pressures. There are five reference points of blood pressure measurement when the patient is on a 1:2 ratio of balloon pumping (Figure 15-10). There are three reference points when the patient is on a 1:1 ratio (Figure 15-11).

When the blood pressure is measured via *intraarterial line,* bedside monitors average the systolic and peak augmented diastolic pressure readings and display them as the systolic pressure. The balloon-assisted end-diastolic pressure is displayed as the diastolic pressure. Consequently, the displayed systolic and diastolic readings do not correlate with what the patient's blood pressure would be off the balloon pump. If hemodynamics are optimized with proper IABP timing, the systolic value displayed is higher and the diastolic value lower than the patient's true blood systolic and diastolic values.

When the blood pressure is measured using the *auscultatory (cuff) technique,* the first audible Korotkoff sound is produced by diastolic augmented pressure, which is the highest pressure driving blood throughout the cardiac cycle. The disappearance of Korotkoff sounds relates to the balloon-assisted aortic end-diastolic pressure. In other words, both the appearance and disappearance of Korotkoff sounds are IABP-related diastolic events. This concept may seem bizarre to clinicians learning care of IABP patients.

When patients are receiving titratable vasoactive drugs, mean arterial pressure (MAP) is commonly used for adjusting drug dosing. As with all hemodynamic measurements, the MAP must be evaluated in conjunction with other hemodynamic, physical assessment, and laboratory data. The following caveats must also be considered when evaluating the MAP in patients being maintained on the IABP.

Pressure measurements of the same intraarterial blood pressure monitoring source (either the bedside monitor console or the IABP console) must be used when titrating vasoactive drugs. When serially obtaining and evaluating any monitoring information, consistency of technique is essential to effective trend analysis and appropriate therapies.

Bedside monitors tend to underestimate the true MAP because they cannot distinguish peak diastolic augmented pressure as an independent pressure, nor do they include assisted systolic pressure in the calculation.

Calculation of the Pulse Pressure

Normally the pulse pressure is calculated by subtracting the diastolic arterial pressure from the systolic pressure. In IABP patients, pulse pressure is calculated by subtracting the balloon-assisted end-diastolic pressure from diastolic augmented pressure.

Arterial Pulse Rate

Both the patient's systolic pressure and diastolic augmented pressure produce palpable peripheral pulses. Consequently, the pulse rate at arterial sites (radial, brachial) will be twice that counted by auscultating the heart or that digitally displayed on the ECG monitor. For example, if the patient with a heart rate of 80 beats per minute is receiving IABC at a 1:1 ratio, the pulse rate counted while auscultating the heart and digitally displayed on the bedside ECG monitor will be 80 beats per minute. However, because of the two pulsatile flow component of each cardiac cycle induced by counterpulsation, the palpated peripheral pulse rate will be 160 beats per minute.

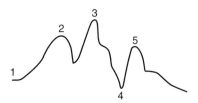

FIGURE 15-10 1:2 ratio. *1,* Patient aortic end-diastolic pressure. *2,* Patient systolic pressure. *3,* Augmented diastolic pressure. *4,* Balloon-assisted aortic end-diastolic pressure. *5,* Assisted systolic pressure.

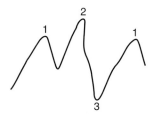

FIGURE 15-11 1:1 ratio. *1,* Assisted systolic pressure. *2,* Peak diastolic pressure. *3,* Assisted aortic end-diastolic pressure.

Effects of the Intraaortic Balloon Pump on Cardiac Auscultation

The sounds made by rhythmic balloon inflation/deflation may swamp heart sounds, making evaluation of heart sounds difficult. Identification of low-frequency sounds, such as S_3 and S_4 sounds, may be impossible.

Briefly suspending balloon counterpulsation when auscultating the heart, lungs, and gastrointestinal tract is generally well tolerated. However, the pump should immediately be resumed if chest pain develops or the patient's blood pressure begins to fall.

BALLOON PRESSURE WAVEFORM

Helium is the gas used for aortic balloon inflation. Because it is a light gas, transfer time from balloon to pump is less than it would be with other gases, such as CO_2.

A characteristic gas pressure waveform, recorded from an in-line transducer located between the helium drive system and the balloon, is inscribed as helium moves into and out of the intraaortic balloon. The waveform is then displayed on the pump console screen. Changes from the normal balloon pressure waveform morphology indicate problems within the console, balloon, or catheter or specific patient problems.

Five components normally make up the balloon pressure waveform (Figure 15-12).

1. Baseline

This is the pressure measured at the end of balloon deflation; the expected value is usually 2.5 mm Hg but may be up to 10 mm Hg depending on the type of pneumatics the specific manufacturer's pump employs. All of the helium must return from the balloon to the pump system in order for the baseline to return to the 2.5 to 10 mm Hg level.

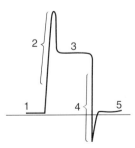

FIGURE 15-12 Balloon pressure waveform. *1,* Baseline. *2,* Rapid balloon inflation and overshoot artifact. *3,* Balloon pressure plateau. *4,* Rapid deflation and undershoot artifact. *5,* Return to the balloon pressure baseline.

Gas leakage causes the baseline to drop below normal, whereas a restriction to gas flow, causing a balloon overfill, may elevate the baseline above acceptable limits. When the pump is in the "off" mode, the baseline is at zero.

2. Rapid Balloon Inflation and Overshoot Artifact

Gas rapidly moving into the balloon normally produces a steep vertical upstroke and sharp overshoot artifact. Overshoot artifact is not a true pressure change within the vascular system but, rather, reflects pressure generated within the balloon lumen.

3. Balloon Pressure Plateau

The plateau pressure represents the internal pressure generated to keep the balloon inflated throughout diastole and is achieved when the balloon is fully inflated and pressure equilibrium is reached inside and outside the balloon. Therefore the plateau pressure correlates with diastolic augmented pressure within a variance of ±25 mm Hg for adult patients and ±10 mm Hg for pediatric patients.

Patient-related causes of variations in the height and width of the pressure plateau include changes in heart rate and blood pressure.

Changes in Heart Rate

The width of the plateau correlates with the length of diastole (narrow plateau with tachyarrhythmias and wide plateau with bradyarrhythmias) (Figure 15-13). If the cardiac rhythm is irregular, such as in atrial fibrillation or frequent atrial or ventricular ectopy, the balloon pressure plateau will have varying widths. *If the width of the pressure plateau does not correlate with the patient's heart rate, there may be a significant error in timing.* Immediately set timing to a 1:2 ratio and evaluate timing landmarks and pressure responses on the arterial waveform. Use real timing if available.

Change in Blood Pressure

The height of the pressure plateau increases in hypertensive patients and decreases in hypotensive patients (Figure 15-14).

4. Rapid Deflation and Undershoot Artifact

Gas rapidly moving from the balloon to the closed system produces a steep, verticle downstroke and undershoot artifact. As with the overshoot artifact, this is not a true intravascular pressure but a reflection of helium movement from the intraaortic balloon into the pump.

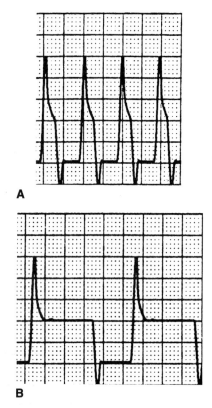

FIGURE 15-13 A, Tachycardia. **B,** Bradycardia. (Courtesy of Arrow International, Reading, PA 19605).

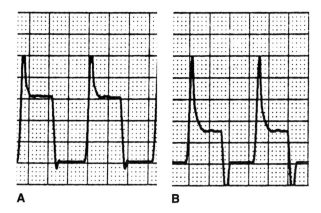

FIGURE 15-14 Changes in blood pressure. **A,** Hypertensive. **B,** Hypotensive. (Courtesy of Arrow International, Reading, PA 19605).

5. Return to the Balloon Pressure Baseline

This portion of the balloon pressure waveform indicates full deflation of the balloon.

CAUSES OF ABNORMAL BALLOON PRESSURE WAVEFORM MORPHOLOGY

There are two causes of abnormalities in the balloon pressure waveform. Both will initiate a console alarm and require troubleshooting. The baseline may be either above or below the normal baseline.

Restriction to Gas Flow within the Closed System

In this circumstance, the baseline is above or below acceptable limits and the pressure plateau is heightened. Widening of the peak inflation and deflation artifacts are valuable indicators of gas transmission problems. When the intraluminal cross-sectional area of the catheter is decreased, gas transmission is delayed and is reflected by widened overshoot and undershoot artifacts.

Sources of restriction to gas flow include a kink in the plastic connection tubing or catheter, such as that caused by a steep angle of balloon catheter insertion; tight sutures around the catheter insertion site; condensation of moisture within the catheter and balloon; malposition of the balloon within the aortic lumen; inadvertent balloon placement within the medial layer of the aortic wall, as may happen with aortic dissection; the tail of the balloon has not exited the catheter insertion sheath; presence of blood or dried blood particles within the balloon and catheter; the balloon has not fully unfurled with initiation of pumping; and patient episodes of extreme restlessness with straining, Valsalva maneuver, or strenuous coughing.

Helium Leak

The gas leak, which causes the pressure baseline to fall, may be within the balloon, the connecting tubing, or the IABP console. This is a potentially dangerous problem because of the risk of systemic or cerebral helium embolization.

Balloon pump consoles in current use in the United States display continuous, real-time ECG, balloon pressure, and arterial waveforms. However, the pneumatic, alarm, and display systems differ among manufacturers. It is the responsibility of practitioners to become familiar with specifics of IABP models in use at their institution.

TYPES AND CAUSES OF ABNORMAL BALLOON PRESSURE WAVEFORMS

Low Balloon Pressure Plateau

A low balloon pressure plateau could be caused by hypotension; hypovolemia; low systemic vascular resistance; a balloon sized too small for the patient, or low balloon

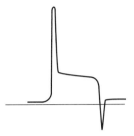

FIGURE 15-15 Low balloon pressure plateau.

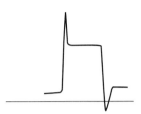

FIGURE 15-17 Balloon pressure baseline elevation.

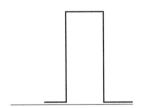

FIGURE 15-16 High balloon pressure plateau.

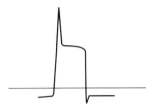

FIGURE 15-18 Balloon pressure baseline depression.

inflation volume; or a balloon positioned too low in the aorta (Figure 15-15).

High Balloon Pressure Plateau

In a high balloon pressure plateau, the top of the plateau may be squared or rounded and may be associated with loss of peak inflation and deflation artifacts. Causes include hypertension, a balloon too large for the aorta, or a restriction to gas flow within the system (Figure 15-16).

Balloon Pressure Baseline Elevation

A balloon pressure baseline elevation may be caused by a restriction of gas flow or gas system overpressurization (Figure 15-17).

Balloon Pressure Baseline Depression

A balloon pressure baseline depression usually indicates a helium leak. Other possible causes not related to a helium leak include inappropriate timing settings (early inflation or late deflation) that do not permit enough time for gas to return to the console or a mechanical defect that causes failure to autofill.

In addition to activation of the alarm system, the console will automatically stop balloon pumping to avoid the risk of systemic or cerebral helium embolization (Figure 15-18).

COMPLICATIONS AND RISK FACTORS

Complications may develop during catheter placement, while the catheter is in situ, and during or after catheter re-moval (Box 15-2). Risk factors include the presence of peripheral vascular disease, insulin-dependent diabetes, female gender (probably due to smaller-caliber vessels), hypertension, presence of atherosclerotic plaque within the aorta, history of cigarette smoking, coronary artery disease, obesity, low cardiac index, and postoperative insertion. The complication rate ranges from 6% to 46%.[15,16] The incidence of complications can be minimized by limiting IABP use to patients with well-accepted indications, using meticulous catheter insertion and IABP management technique, and vigilant patient monitoring and assessment.

CONCLUSION

The intraaortic balloon pump is a palliative device, not a cure. The major values of the IABP are to enhance patient stabilization before, during, or after operative or cardiac catheterization procedures, as well as a temporizing measure that "buys time" in patients with cardiogenic shock. Cardiac catheterization can then be performed in preparation for revascularization or corrective procedures.

Achieving the best possible outcome for the IABP patient while minimizing patient risk requires user familiarity with the specifics of manufacturer IABP console models and catheters, catheter insertion technique, and trigger and timing principles, as well as meticulous, comprehensive patient evaluation and care. However, even in the most capable hands, there is the potential for unavoidable complications in patients with severe peripheral vascular disease or severe, irreversible cardiac disease.

BOX 15-2
Complications of Intraaortic Balloon Pumping

During Insertion

Aortic dissection

Dislodgement of plaque or obstruction of the femoral artery
by the catheter

Arterial perforation

During Pumping

Limb ischemia (most frequent complication)

Systemic or cerebral embolization of gas, plaque, or
catheter thrombi

Thrombocytopenia

Local or systemic infection

Aortic rupture

Helium emboli from the intraaortic balloon or central
lumen of the catheter

Air emboli from inadvertent entry of air during flushings
of the central lumen when used for blood draws
(practice discouraged)

Intensive care unit psychosis

Bleeding at the insertion site

Hemodynamic compromise due to poor balloon
inflation/deflation timing

Obstruction of major vessels (renal, left subclavian) by a
malpositioned intraaortic balloon

Compartment syndrome

During or after Catheter Removal

Dislodgement and embolization of plaque or catheter
thrombus

Site bleeding

Intraaortic balloon entrapment

Infection

REFERENCES

1. Goldberg RJ et al: Temporal trends in cardiogenic shock complicating acute myocardial infarction, *N Engl J Med* 340:1162, 1999.
2. Krantrowitz A, Krantrowitz A: Experimental augmentation of coronary blood flow by retardation of the arterial pressure pulse, *Surgery* 34:678, 1953.
3. Clauss RH, Birtwell WC, Albertal G, et al: Assisted circulation: I. The arterial Counterpulsator, *J Thorac Cardiovasc Surg* 41:447, 1961.
4. Moulopoulos SD, Topaz S, Kolff WJ: Diastolic balloon pumping (with carbon dioxide) in the aorta—a mechanical assistance to the failing circulation, *Am Heart J* 63:669, 1962.
5. Kantowitz A, Tjonneland S, Freed PS, et al: Initial clinical experience with intraaortic balloon pumping in cardiogenic shock, *JAMA* 203:135, 1968.
6. Buckley MJ, Lenbach RC, Kastor JA, et al: Hemodynamic evaluation of intraaortic balloon pumping in man, *Circulation* 46(suppl II):130, 1970.
7. Allen BS, Rosenkranz E, Buckberg GD, et al: Studies in prolonged regional ischemia: VI. Myocardial infarction with left ventricular power failure: a medical/surgical emergency requiring urgent revascularization with maximal protection of remote muscle, *J Thorac Cardiovasc Surg* 98:691, 1989.
8. Quall SJ: *Comprehensive intraaortic balloon counterpulsation,* ed 2, St Louis, 1993, Mosby.
9. Current nursing issues in intraaortic balloon pumping, *Crit Care Nurs Clin North Am* 8: 1996.
10. Cutler BS: The intraaortic balloon and counterpulsation: technique of insertion. In Irwin RS et al, editors: *Procedures and techniques in intensive care medicine,* ed 2, Philadelphia, 1999, Lippincott Williams & Wilkins.
11. Quall SJ: Balloon insertion techniques. In *Comprehensive intraaortic balloon counterpulsation,* ed 2, St Louis, 1993, Mosby.
12. Poore BJ: Intraaortic balloon counterpulsation. In Hurford WE, editor: *Critical care handbook of the Massachusetts General Hospital,* ed 3, Philadelphia, 2000, Lippincott Williams & Wilkins.
13. Cadwell CA, Hobson KS, Tettis S, et al: Clinical observations with real timing, *Crit Care Nurs Clin North Am* 8(4):357, 1996.
14. Cadwell C, Tyson G: Real timing. In Quall S, editor: *Comprehensive intraaortic balloon counterpulsation,* ed 2, St Louis, 1993, Mosby.
15. Richenbacher WE, Peirce WS: Management of complications of intraaortic balloon counterpulsation. In Waldhausen JA, Orringer MB, editors: *Complications in cardiothoracic surgery,* St Louis, 1991, Mosby.
16. Stavarski DH: Complications of intra-aortic balloon pumping: preventable or not preventable? *Crit Care Clin North Am* 8(4):409, 1996.

SUGGESTED READINGS

Bates ER, Stomel RJ, Hochman JS, et al: The use of intraaortic balloon counterpulsation as an adjunct to reperfusion therapy in cardiogenic shock, *Int J Cardiol* 65(suppl 1):171, 1998.

Hochman JS, Boland J, Sleeper LA, et al: Current spectrum of cardiogenic shock and effect of early revascularization on mortality: results of an international registry: SHOCK Registry Investigators, *Circulation* 91:873, 1995.

Hochman JS et al: Early revascularization in acute myocardial infarction complicated by cardiogenic shock, *N Engl J Med* 341:625, 1999.

Klein LW: Intraaortic balloon pumping. In Parrillo JE, Bone RC, editors: *Critical care medicine: principles of diagnosis and management,* St Louis, 1995, Mosby.

Pae W, Miller CA, Matthews Y, et al: Ventricular assist devices for postcardiotomy cardiogenic shock, *J Thorac Cardiovasc Surg* 104:541, 1992.

Pae WE, Pierce WS: Intraaortic balloon counterpulsation, ventricular assist pumping and the artificial heart. In Baue AE et al, editors: *Glenn's thoracic and cardiovascular surgery,* East Norwalk, CT, 1991, Appleton & Lange.

Richenbacher WE, Pierce WS: Assisted circulation and the mechanical heart. In Braunwald E, editor: *Heart disease: a textbook of cardiovascular medicine,* ed 5, Philadelphia, 1997, W.B. Saunders.

Urban P et al: A randomized evaluation of early revascularization to treat shock complicating acute myocardial infarction: the (Swiss) Multicenter trial of Angioplasty for Shock— (S)MASH, *Eur Heart J* 20:1030, 1999.

16

CORY M. FRANKLIN and GLORIA OBLOUK DAROVIC

Monitoring the Patient in Shock

More than 100 years ago, the eminent physiologist John Scott Haldane described shock as "a rude unhinging of the machinery of life." As we enter the twenty-first century, the poignant accuracy of that description remains unchallenged. Although the shock syndromes are the most dramatic and critical situations encountered in clinical practice, shock is a notoriously difficult condition to define and often goes unrecognized in its early stages. This is because the early clinical manifestations may be subtle and often manifest differently, relative to the precipitating event (hemorrhage, anaphylaxis, spinal cord injury, systemic infection).

Shock, a problem of circulatory insufficiency and altered metabolism, is never a primary diagnosis. Rather, it is a physiologic adaptation to a potentially life-threatening physical insult. Shock reflects the body's attempt to preserve its most vital functions. The most consistent features in all forms of shock are capillary hypoperfusion (microcirculatory failure) and widespread abnormalities in cell metabolism that ultimately result in a diminution of the life-generating forces within the cells. Therefore, for the purpose of this discussion, *shock* is defined as circulatory insufficiency, which typically coexists with disordered metabolism, resulting in diffuse disturbances in cellular function. Diffuse cellular dysfunction, in turn, is clinically expressed as sudden-onset multiple-organ dysfunction. Depending on the magnitude of the primary illness or injury, as greater numbers of cells become impaired and damaged, major organ dysfunction or failure may constitute a threat to the patient's life.

The pathophysiology, signs, symptoms, hemodynamic profiles, and specific treatments for shock depend on the underlying cause. Five general etiologic categories of shock—hypovolemic, cardiogenic, septic, neurogenic, and anaphylactic—are described later in this chapter. A final classification of "other" is briefly discussed whereby shock may be precipitated by various physiologic abnormalities such as severe endocrine dysfunction. Although useful in describing precipitating mechanisms and specific pathophysiology, rigid categorization by "cause" oversimplifies the clinical concept of shock because several precipitating factors often coexist in each patient. For example, septic shock may be complicated by severe hypovolemia (hypovolemic shock), as well as profound myocardial depression (cardiogenic shock). These coexisting causes of shock collectively complicate the patient's clinical, hemodynamic, and treatment profile.

This chapter first discusses the pathophysiology of shock at the cellular and microcirculatory level. This is followed by a description of organ system responses to shock. The stages of shock are then presented, followed by a discussion of general diagnostic and therapeutic principles. The last and major portion of the chapter focuses on the elaboration of the distinctive clinical, pathophysiologic, hemodynamic, and treatment features specific to each of the five etiologic categories of shock.

PATHOPHYSIOLOGY

The capillary-cellular junction is the "site of action" where oxygen and nutrients are delivered to body tissues and metabolic waste is removed (Figure 16-1).

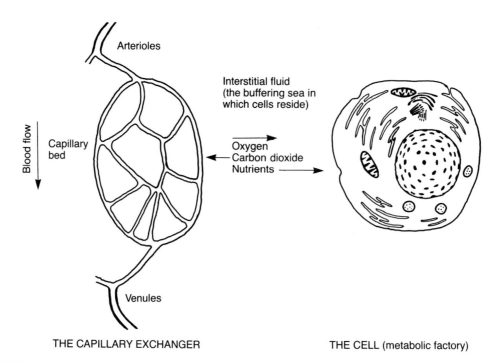

FIGURE 16-1 The site of dysfunction in shock is the capillary–interstitial fluid–cell interface. Organs are highly complex aggregates of billions of specialized cells. Abnormalities at this critical junction are associated with the signs and symptoms of organ dysfunction observed in patients in shock.

Each type of shock results in reduced capillary blood flow, thus creating the potential for diffuse ischemic hypoxia. The hypoxic risk is compounded by biochemical and neurohumoral factors that interfere with cellular uptake and utilization of oxygen. The effect of hypoxia on the basic structural unit of life, the cell, is discussed first. This is then expanded to the pathophysiology of hypoxia on the vascular endothelium and major organ systems.

The Cell in Shock

Normal cell, organ system, and total body function all depend on the cell's ability to continuously generate energy (adenosine triphosphate [ATP]) (Figure 16-2).

Considerable amounts of the energy produced by the cell drive a membrane pump that maintains an ionic gradient across the cell wall. Intracellular sodium and potassium levels are kept constant at approximately 10 and 140 mEq/L, respectively, whereas extracellular sodium and potassium levels are maintained at 140 and 4 mEq/L, respectively. The maintenance of this transcellular ionic gradient is critical to determining cell size, shape, and function (Figure 16-3).

Hypoxic Energy Crisis

When confronted with an oxygen-poor environment as a result of hypoxemia or perfusion failure, the cell is forced to dead-end in the initial (anaerobic) portion of the Kreb's cycle (step 1). Anaerobic metabolism is associated with a nearly twentyfold decrease in cellular energy production (2 moles of ATP generated through the anaerobic pathway versus 36 moles of ATP generated via the completed aerobic pathway). Energy-inefficient anaerobic metabolism causes a cellular energy crisis. Initially, the sodium-potassium pump mechanism fails, and various cells (renal, cerebral cortical neurons, hepatic) begin to lose their specialized functions. In patients in early shock, this manifests as subtle signs and symptoms of organ dysfunction that may not appear obvious to the casual observer.

Effect on the Sodium-Potassium Pump. The energy-deprived sodium-potassium pump permits extracellular potassium to leak to the intracellular space. Reciprocally, sodium followed by water enters the cells; cells then swell and become irregular in shape (Figure 16-4).

Failure of the membrane ionic pump also results in abnormal distribution of other ions, particularly calcium, across the cell membrane. This results in further cellular and mitochondrial dysfunction. The cascade of cell dysfunction is exacerbated by an accumulation of lactic acid and a decrease in intracellular pH. As large areas of

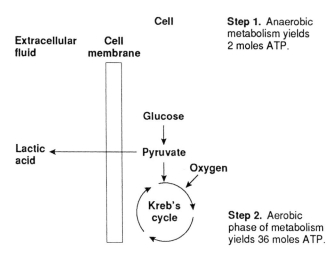

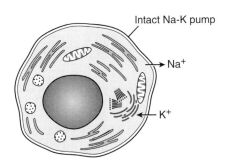

FIGURE 16-3 Normal cell.

FIGURE 16-2 The two-step process of intracellular glucose metabolism. Step 1—anaerobic metabolism. One mole of glucose is metabolized to pyruvate, which, in the absence of oxygen, is converted to lactic acid and two moles of adenosine triphosphate (ATP). This high-energy compound enables cells to transport substances across their membrane, maintain normal cell shape, synthesize materials, and maintain their specialized functions, such as contraction of myocardial cells. Thus ATP is the energy currency that drives life forces. Step 2—aerobic metabolism. In this oxygen-dependent process, pyruvate is converted to acetyl-CoA, which enters the Kreb's cycle to produce carbon dioxide (which is ultimately exhaled), water (which is added to the body's water pool), and 36 moles of ATP. Therefore oxidative metabolism results in a twentyfold increase in energy production to fuel normal organ function and the life of the organism. (From Darovic GO, Rokowsky JS: Shock. In Patrick ML et al, editors: *Medical-surgical nursing: pathophysiological concepts,* ed 2, Philadelphia, 1991, JB Lippincott.)

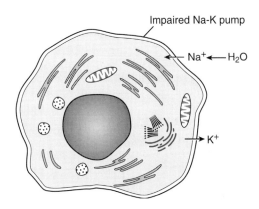

FIGURE 16-4 Cell in shock.

body tissue metabolize anaerobically, blood lactate levels progressively rise, while bicarbonate and body base are consumed to neutralize excess lactic acid. Thus the patient develops metabolic acidosis.

Effect on Capillary Function. The hypoxic chain of events feeds on itself as capillary endothelial cells begin to swell. Endothelial swelling has three harmful effects:
1. The swollen cells encroach on and narrow the capillary lumina, which further reduces blood flow.
2. Sludging of blood (clumping of red blood cells, white blood cells, and platelets) compounds tissue ischemia by plugging the capillary lumina.
3. The normally tight capillary intracellular junctions widen and become intracellular clefts. As capillary wall integrity is lost, intravascular fluid begins to leak from the blood vessels to the tissue spaces (third-

space losses). The increase in interstitial fluid blocks diffusion of whatever oxygen might otherwise be available to cells.

Ultimately a point of no return is reached when lysosomes (i.e., intracellular vacuoles that contain highly caustic enzymes) rupture owing to the unstable cellular environment. The cell then autolyses. The release of vasoactive metabolites and lysozymes from the dying cell, in turn, stimulates an inflammatory reaction accompanied by an accumulation of activated phagocytes. Phagocytosis further perpetuates cell injury and the lytic cycle. Depending on the number and distribution of cells lost, clinically significant organ damage may follow (Figure 16-5).

Organ Systems in Shock

Body organs are highly complex aggregates of billions of specialized cells. The organ dysfunction that is clinically apparent in patients in shock represents the collective dysfunction of billions of individual cells. The consequences of shock on major organ systems are briefly described in Box 16-1.

Between the extremes of intact and functioning organs (minor illness or injury) and life-threatening organ damage and dysfunction in profound shock are many possible clinical gradations. The individual person's response to an event inciting shock is also variable. Each person's response depends on the presence or absence of preexisting chronic disease, drug use, biologic age, individual physiologic characteristics, magnitude of underlying illness or injury, and time period over which the shock process develops.

Reperfusion Injury

Severe, sustained hypoperfusion results in irreversible ischemic organ damage, particularly in those organs whose metabolic rates and oxygen consumption are greatest, such as the brain, heart, liver, and kidneys. Damage to viable cells is made worse during tissue reperfusion and is termed *reperfusion injury.*

Nitric oxide (NO) is a physiologic vasoactive agent that normally plays an important role in regulating blood flow. During reperfusion following an ischemic event, endothelial and inflammatory cells release increased amounts of NO. A cascade of biochemical events results in abnormal oxygen metabolism, which, in turn, increases production of cytotoxic substances and toxic oxygen radicals such as superoxide anion, hydrogen peroxide, and the hydroxyl radical. These substances cause loss of cell membrane integrity and destruction of membrane-associated transport functions. Thus the cycle of cell injury and death is replayed. The lungs are particularly vulnerable to injury because they receive the total systemic venous return. Consequently, they are exposed to all circulating inflammatory mediators, oxygen radicals, and other cytotoxins. This explains why the first organ that typically shows clinical signs of dysfunction following resuscitation is the lungs.

Neurohumoral, Biochemical, and Metabolic Responses to Shock

Any severe physical or psychologic stress induces an altered physiology that is biologically designed to support the host (stress response). The magnitude of this fight-or-flight response is generally proportional to the severity of the stress. Numerous neurohumoral agents are interrelated to produce the normal stress response (Table 16-1).

Neurohumoral responses include stimulation of the sympathetic nervous system; anterior pituitary stimulation of the adrenocorticotropic hormone (ACTH)–

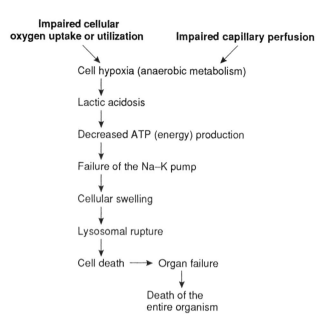

Impaired cellular oxygen uptake or utilization   **Impaired capillary perfusion**

Cell hypoxia (anaerobic metabolism)

Lactic acidosis

Decreased ATP (energy) production

Failure of the Na–K pump

Cellular swelling

Lysosomal rupture

Cell death ⟶ Organ failure

Death of the entire organism

FIGURE 16-5 The hypoxic sequence of cellular events in shock.

endorphin system and stimulation of release of other hormones, such as thyroid-stimulating hormone (TSH) and growth hormone (GH); posterior pituitary release of antidiuretic hormone (ADH); and activation of the renin-angiotensin system. It is beyond the scope of this chapter to detail the complex actions and interactions of these systems; however, the overall effects are the following:

- Supporting cardiac output by increasing heart rate and contractility
- Producing systemic vasoconstriction to distribute the supported cardiac output to core organs necessary for immediate survival
- Retaining salt and water to maintain circulating plasma volume
- Mobilizing metabolic fuels such as glucose and lipids for energy production

Researchers have identified the importance of other vasoactive and immune mediators that are systemically activated or released in people with major illness or injury. These biochemical agents, which mediate the inflammatory response to tissue injury, include complement, cytokines such as cachectin (tumor necrosis factor), interleukins, interferon, prostaglandins, leukotrienes, and thromboxane. Mediator substances are intended to facilitate resolution of injury and promote wound healing. However, systemic activation of these systems can be tolerated only briefly. If

BOX 16-1
Organ Systems in Shock

Nonvital Organs
Gastrointestinal Tract

Altered permeability due to ischemic damage; translocation of enteric bacteria and toxins into the systemic circulation

Decreased motility leading to paralytic ileus

Ulceration of the gastric and intestinal lining

Impaired absorption of nutrients such as carbohydrates and protein

Release of a myocardial depressant factor from ischemic pancreas

Skeletal Muscle

Production of large amounts of lactic acid from ischemic muscle contributes to metabolic acidosis

Catabolism of muscle as source of energy

Respiratory muscle fatigue and possible subsequent respiratory failure

Immune System

Impaired immune system function

Increased susceptibility to infection

Skin

Increased risk of pressure ulcer formation

Impaired wound healing

Liver

Initially, glycogen breakdown and the formation of glucose from noncarbohydrate sources (gluconeogenesis) is accelerated. This results in an increased blood glucose.

If shock is sustained, carbohydrate stores are depleted and gluconeogenesis is impaired.

Hypoglycemia follows.

Protein and fat metabolism are altered.

Hepatic conversion of lactic acid may be impaired and contributes to metabolic acidosis.

Bile formation from bilirubin and bile excretion is reduced. Serum bilirubin is increased and mild jaundice results.

Impaired ability to neutralize bacterial toxins and other metabolites such as ammonia.

Inability of Kupffer cells to clear circulating bacteria and cellular breakdown products.

Kidneys

Initially, the glomerular filtration rate falls. Aldosterone and antidiuretic hormone cause the kidney to conserve salt and water. Altogether, the kidneys produce a small amount of concentrated urine with a low urine sodium.

A prolonged reduction in renal blood flow may lead to acute tubular necrosis (ATN). A profound reduction in renal blood flow may result in renal cortical necrosis and permanent renal failure.

Hematologic

Platelets and clotting factor levels may be subnormal due to the following:

1. Clotting factor consumption due to systemic activation of the coagulation cascade (disseminated intravascular coagulation)
2. Hemodilution secondary to volume replacement
3. Platelet dysfunction (without thrombocytopenia), which may develop with hypothermia or sepsis

Lungs

The number of ventilated alveoli that are not perfused (West zone 1) increases. Because nonperfused alveoli cannot participate in gas exchange, oxygenation of blood may become impaired.

Weak or ineffective ventilatory movements impair alveolar ventilation. Carbon dioxide retention and hypoxemia may result.

Prolonged hypoperfusion, pulmonary capillary microthrombi formation, and release of mediator substances may lead to the acute respiratory distress syndrome (ARDS).

Vital Organs
Heart

Initially, sympathetic nervous stimulation increases the rate and force of ventricular contraction

Later, poor coronary blood flow and release of myocardial depressant factor result in contractile failure

Predisposition to arrhythmias

Possibility of subendocardial or transmural infarction

Brain

Initial excitation of the CNS from stress-mediated adrenalin and norepinephrine release

Progressive decreases in cerebral function with inadequate cerebral perfusion

Occasionally, due to hypoperfusion of the brainstem, vasomotor and ventilatory control may fail

Ultimately, brain cell ischemia results in a local buildup of lactic acid, movement of sodium and water into the brain causing cerebral edema, cell membrane destruction, neurotransmitter failure, and finally irreversible brain damage

Inadequate blood flow to any organ produces functional impairment. Decreases in blood flow and dysfunction occur first in those tissues not essential for immediate survival. Cardiac and cerebral hypoperfusion develop only when physiologic compensatory mechanisms are depleted.

TABLE 16-1
Major Neurohumoral Agents Released in Shock

Agent	Source	Actions
Norepinephrine	Peripheral nerve endings; adrenal medulla	Vasoconstriction Increases force of cardiac contraction Stimulates liver and pancreas to increase blood glucose Stimulates free fatty acid release
Epinephrine	Adrenal medulla	Increases skeletal muscle and splanchnic blood flow (physiologic doses) Increases force of myocardial contraction Increases heart rate Stimulates peripheral tissues to increase blood glucose Stimulates free fatty acid release
Angiotensin II	Lungs convert to active form	Vasoconstriction Stimulates release of aldosterone
Antidiuretic hormone (ADH/Vasopressin)	Synthesis by hypothalamus; release by posterior pituitary	Stimulates water reabsorption by the kidneys
Aldosterone	Adrenal cortex	Stimulates sodium and water reabsorption by the kidneys
Cortisol	Adrenal cortex	Permissive for catecholamine actions Suppresses immune and inflammatory responses Promotes protein catabolism Increases blood sugar by stimulating gluconeogenesis

activation is sustained or exaggerated, it ultimately destroys the body these systems were intended to protect (see Chapter 17, sections on the systemic inflammatory response syndrome and multiple-system organ failure).

The various neurohumoral mechanisms elicited in shock, however, are a physiologic double-edged sword. Whereas hemodynamics and metabolism are altered to protect immediate patient survival and promote resolution of injury, the sustained activation of these survival-oriented mechanisms cannot be physiologically tolerated. Ultimately, activation of these mechanisms becomes incompatible with long-term (days to weeks) survival (Figure 16-6).

An example occurs when the underlying problem causing shock, such as massive trauma or systemic infection, cannot be immediately corrected or therapy is suboptimal. Subclinical circulatory insufficiency and mediator release and activation may persist although the patient's condition appears to be stable. As a consequence of the ongoing physiologic stress, the sustained, clinically subtle neurohumoral and metabolic responses eventually result in progressive destruction of multiple organ systems and eventually lead to "death in slow motion"—the syndrome of multiple-system organ dysfunction or failure within the

ensuing weeks. *The importance of early recognition of shock, coupled with aggressive and effective stabilization of the patient and treatment of the underlying cause, cannot be overstated.*

STAGES OF SHOCK

Blood pressure measurements are determined by the degree of tone in the systemic arterial circulation (systemic vascular resistance [SVR]) and cardiac output. Normally, decreases in either of these factors are reflexively offset by compensatory increases in the other factor, and blood pressure is maintained within a hemodynamically acceptable range (Figure 16-7).

However, factors that significantly decrease cardiac output (heart failure, hypovolemia, extreme tachyarrhythmias or bradyarrhythmias) or factors that produce a significant systemic vasodilator reaction (barbiturate overdose, systemic infection, anaphylactic reactions, spinal cord injury) can lead to hypotension.

Any severe injury or illness that threatens to cause a significant drop in blood pressure also threatens homeostasis and perfusion to vital organs. To maintain immedi-

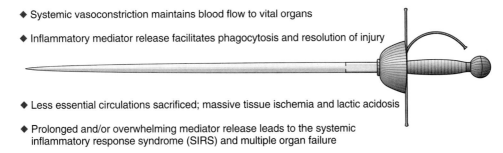

◆ Systemic vasoconstriction maintains blood flow to vital organs

◆ Inflammatory mediator release facilitates phagocytosis and resolution of injury

◆ Less essential circulations sacrificed; massive tissue ischemia and lactic acidosis

◆ Prolonged and/or overwhelming mediator release leads to the systemic inflammatory response syndrome (SIRS) and multiple organ failure

FIGURE 16-6 The "double-edged sword" of compensatory changes in shock.

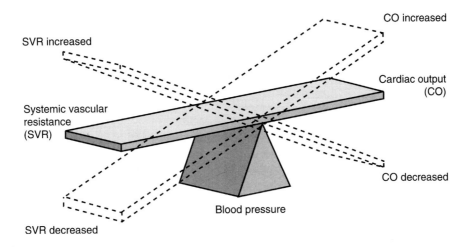

FIGURE 16-7 The effects of cardiac output and systemic vascular resistance on blood pressure.

ate survival, the body reflexively alters cardiovascular function. If, however, the underlying illness or injury is not corrected and the patient's circulation is not properly supported, the survival responses become maladaptive and cardiovascular function deteriorates. The progressive changes in cardiovascular function are discussed next. The changes discussed are typical of hypovolemic shock, which is the most common cause of shock. The compensatory vasoconstrictive responses are absent or attenuated in patients with hypotension due to vasodilator reactions. This is because the hemodynamic problem *causing* hypotension is inappropriate vasodilation.

Phase I—Compensated Shock

Because hypotension threatens blood flow to *all* organ systems, when blood pressure falls, the cardiovascular system undergoes compensatory changes that initially support or increase ventricular performance and favor shunting of the supported cardiac output to the heart and brain. Adaptive compensation includes the following responses:

1. *Heart rate and myocardial contractility increase to optimize cardiac output and mean arterial pressure.*

The positive inotropic and chronotropic effects are mediated by catecholamines released as part of the stress response.

2. *Systemic venous constriction displaces blood from the veins, thereby augmenting venous return and ventricular filling.* Enhanced ventricular filling, in turn, supports stroke volume and cardiac output. Venoconstriction is perhaps the most significant compensatory mechanism in patients with shock associated with low cardiac output. Constriction of the systemic veins accounts for the decreased visibility and progressive disappearance of veins on the dorsum of the hands, feet, and extremities of patients in this stage of shock.

3. *Constriction of the systemic arteries shunts blood away from nonvital organs, such as skin, skeletal muscle, and abdominal viscera, and directs the oxygenated blood flow toward the "vital" heart and brain.* Peripheral hypoperfusion accounts for the cool, pale skin; muscle weakness; decreased urine output; and gastrointestinal dysfunction noted in "shocky" patients. Vasoconstriction helps maintain blood pressure (arterial pressure equals cardiac output times systemic vascular resistance).

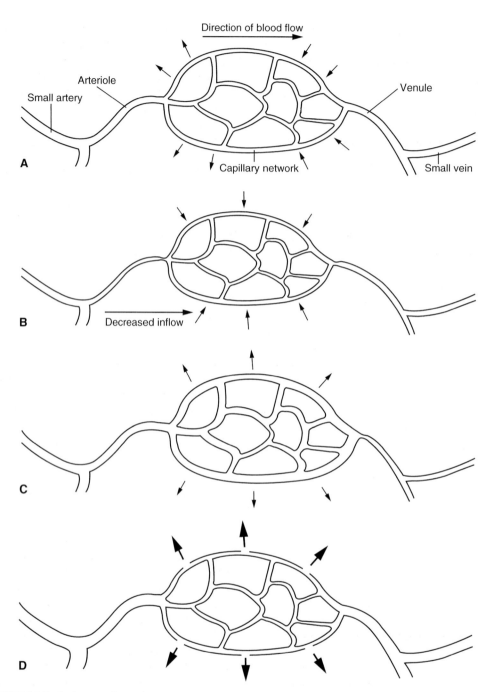

FIGURE 16-8 A, A normally perfused capillary in which net outflow of fluid into the tissue space equals net inflow *(arrows).* **B,** Compensated shock. Arteriolar constriction is greater than constriction of the venules and small veins. This reduces net capillary blood flow and filling. As a result, capillary hydrostatic pressure falls, which, in turn, favors movement of fluid from the tissue space to the vascular space *(arrows).* This is termed *transcapillary refill.* **C,** Decompensated shock. Precapillary sphincters relax secondary to acidosis and hypoxia, but postcapillary sphincters remain constricted. The increased capillary inflow relative to impaired outflow coupled with weakening of the capillary walls results in extravasation of plasma water and a decrease in plasma volume. **D,** Irreversible shock. Passive dilation of the arterioles and venules favors pooling of resuscitative fluids in the vascular space. The severely damaged capillary walls also allow a massive leak of fluid into the extravascular space *(large arrows.)*

Constriction of the arterioles, however, produces a "dam" in front of the systemic capillaries. Consequently, blood flow and hydrostatic pressure within the capillary lumina fall (Figure 16-8, *B*).

The decrease in capillary hydrostatic pressure that results promotes the movement of fluid from body tissue into the vascular space. For example, rapid blood loss (approximately 1500 ml within 1 hour) is associated with an approximately 400 to 600 ml transcapillary fluid shift from the interstitium to the vascular space. This fluid shift thus partially offsets the plasma volume deficit. Intravascular volume augmentation, in turn, increases venous return and cardiac output. However, if bleeding continues, the extravascular (tissue) fluid reservoir ultimately becomes depleted. This is noted clinically in the characteristic sunken, haggard face and dry mucous membranes of the patient in shock. Because the nonvital tissue mass is approximately 75% of total body mass, the anaerobic metabolism occurring in this large area of tissue results in metabolic (lactic) acidosis.

At this stage of shock, the patient's blood pressure may be maintained within numerically acceptable levels. On casual observation, the patient's appearance may be unremarkable. However, careful physical examination may disclose the subtle signs of early shock—increased heart rate, cool hands and feet, disappearing peripheral veins, and pallor. Serial measurements of urine output usually indicate oliguria (urine output less than 0.5 to 1.0 ml/kg/hr). The patient also may appear restless and anxious because of excitation of the central nervous system by the stress-mediated hormones epinephrine and norepinephrine.

During this period, correction of the primary problem (such as control of hemorrhage) and supportive therapy (such as volume repletion) are usually met with a favorable patient outcome and no permanent sequelae.

Phase II—Decompensated Shock

When the shock stimulus is of sufficient magnitude to overwhelm the aforementioned compensatory mechanisms, the patient becomes hypotensive. Blood flow to the vital organs is critically reduced. Cerebral and myocardial ischemia is clinically apparent as marked deterioration in mental status, cardiac rhythm disturbances, ischemic ST-T wave changes, and critical reductions in cardiac output evidenced as a diminution or absence of peripheral pulses.

The now intense sympathetic nervous system–mediated vasoconstriction is clinically evident as waxen, cold, clammy skin; pale mucous membranes and nail beds; and progressively diminishing urine output. Lactic acid continues to pour from greater masses of more intensely underperfused, ischemic tissue, and metabolic acidosis worsens.

Because local tissue hypoxia and acidosis are better tolerated by the muscle lining of veins than by the musculature of arteriolar sphincters, precapillary constriction is relaxed. As a result of arteriolar relaxation and venular constriction, the amount of blood flowing *into* the capillary bed exceeds the amount of blood flowing *out of* the capillaries (Figure 16-8, *C*.) This results in an increase in capillary hydrostatic pressure and, in turn, forces fluid out of the now weakened, damaged capillary walls into the interstitial space. Fluid extravasation worsens existing deficits in circulating plasma volume. The capillary-cell interface, which is normally the "site of action" that sustains oxidative metabolism and life, now becomes the primary "site of dysfunction." If the primary illness or injury is not rapidly treated, the chances for patient survival rapidly decline.

Phase III—Irreversible Shock

Intense or prolonged systemic tissue hypoxia may impair the vascular responses that maintain arterial pressure. As a consequence, hypotension worsens and a vicious cycle ensues. Severe systemic hypoperfusion eventually leads to physical and functional changes in the cardiovascular system that ultimately become incompatible with life. Patients in advanced shock resemble a "bag of water" with leaky, porous capillaries that are unable to hold resuscitative fluids. Arterioles and venules tend to passively dilate, and resuscitative fluid pools in the peripheral circulation. Venous return and cardiac output remain unacceptably low despite massive, aggressive fluid challenges as a consequence of the capillary leak and peripheral vascular pooling (Figure 16-8, *D*).

Profound organ damage supervenes. Shock-damaged pulmonary capillaries allow plasma to enter the lungs, which stiffen and become poor diffusers of respiratory gases. Renal tubules become necrotic, and oliguria becomes refractory to fluid and diuretic therapy. The ischemic lining of the gastrointestinal tract becomes ulcerated and necrotic and therefore releases intestinal bacteria and toxins to the blood, termed *translocation*. Consequently, the patient may appear "septic," and the poorly perfused myocardium loses contractile power.

No laboratory tests or clinical markers can unequivocally identify this stage of shock. However, arterial lactate levels reflect the degree of total body anaerobic metabolism and therefore perfusion failure. When lactate levels rise from the normal 1 to 2 mM/L to greater than 8 mM/L, the chances for patient survival decrease dramatically. Successful resuscitation becomes unlikely at this stage. Some patients, however, may be effectively resuscitated and may survive in the short term, only to die later from multiple-system organ failure.

Although the aforementioned cardiovascular responses follow a continuum, the rate of progression is determined by patient-related factors, whether or not the underlying problem has been corrected, and the rate and appropriateness of resuscitative measures.

In summary, it is a mistake to regard shock as simply hypotension or poor capillary perfusion. Rather, it is an extremely complex altered physiologic condition involving many compensatory adaptations. Depending on the primary problem, varying combinations of microcellular, biochemical, hormonal, metabolic, and hemodynamic factors produce the clinical and pathologic entity we know as shock.

DIAGNOSIS OF SHOCK

The early diagnosis of shock is usually not difficult if the clinician keeps two principles in mind: (1) *no sign or symptom is absolutely specific for shock,* and (2) *not all patients with shock have identical signs and symptoms.* For example, some patients are remarkably alert and lucid despite advanced shock. Furthermore, the diagnosis should never be ruled out because a single finding, such as hypotension or tachycardia, is not present. In fact, in compensated shock

the patient's blood pressure may be higher than normal because of compensatory systemic vasoconstriction. Tachycardia also is not invariably present (Box 16-2).

Vital sign abnormalities and laboratory findings depend on the underlying cause of shock. The constellation of signs and symptoms is highly variable, depending on when in the course of the illness the patient is being examined. In the earliest and most reversible stages of shock, clinical findings may be subtle or absent. The classic description of a shocky patient—one with hypotension; tachycardia; tachypnea; cool, clammy, pale, or dusky skin; mental obtundation; markedly decreased urine output; and diminished or absent peripheral pulses—is classic only for the late (decompensated) stage that is common to all causes of shock. This classic clinical picture warns of impending death. At this stage, even aggressive, state-of-the-art therapy may be ineffective.

Clinical Caveats to Diagnosis and Patient Exceptions to the Clinical Picture of Shock

- Young, healthy patients have highly effective compensatory vasoconstrictor responses and may maintain normal blood pressure despite severe reductions in cardiac

---

BOX 16-2
Areas of Assessment for Patients at Risk of Shock

Level of Consciousness and Mentation
Assess for changing level of consciousness or changes in mentation such as irritability, anxiety, inappropriate behavior, impaired mental functioning.

Arterial Pressure
Assess changes in systolic and diastolic values, pulse pressure, and quality of Korotkoff sounds, and track mean values when possible.

Pulses
Assess rate, volume, rhythm, and differences at various sites. For example, with the development of hypotension, the pulses are lost first at the distal sites. If the radial pulse can be palpated, the systolic pressure is at least 80 mm Hg. If the femoral pulse can be palpated, the systolic pressure is at least 70 mm Hg; and if the carotid pulse can be palpated, the systolic pressure is at least 60 mm Hg.

Respirations
Assess rate, depth, and rhythm, whether labored or effortless.

Cutaneous
Assess for temperature, color, turgor, and presence or absence of sweat. Evaluate color and moistness of mucous

membranes, and evaluate capillary refill. The temperature of the big toe, the farthest peripheral site in the body from the heart, can be helpful for evaluating the patient's perfusion status. Because a decreasing cardiac output (hypovolemic and cardiogenic shock) will constrict vessels to this area in the preshock or compensated stages of shock, a patient who has a warm big toe is unlikely to have a low cardiac output. The reverse is not necessarily true. A shock patient with a cold big toe may have either a high cardiac output (septic shock, neurogenic shock) or a low cardiac output (hypovolemic shock, cardiogenic shock, late-stage anaphylactic shock). Cold toes are also a normal finding in people in a cold environment, those with severe peripheral vascular disease, and fatigued or anxious people.

Veins
Assess for visibility of peripheral and neck veins.

Urine
Assess color, volume output, and specific gravity. Severe shock with fluid resuscitation may require urine flow checks every 15 minutes.

output and tissue perfusion. In fact, some physically fit patients may maintain normal blood pressure until cardiopulmonary arrest. The clinician should not be lulled into a false sense of security because the patient is young and was previously in a good state of health. Young patients should be monitored as vigilantly and managed as aggressively as those with decreased reserve, because when they suddenly "crash," the ischemic damage and disability incurred must be borne through many decades. In addition, major organ system reserve lost as a result of the shock incident may ultimately become clinically significant, with further loss of functional reserve with aging.

- Systemic vasoconstriction may maintain blood pressure without significant compensatory increases in heart rate. Tachycardia may not be classically present because (1) preexisting conduction system disease or long-term pharmacologic therapy, such as beta blockade, severely limits appropriate increases in heart rate; (2) preexisting slow resting heart rates in athletically inclined people may increase from 40 to 50 beats per minute and still be within normal range (60 to 100 beats per minute); and (3) heart rates may not rise in response to hemorrhage if the patient is recumbent and at rest. Bradycardia accompanied by syncope has been reported in previously healthy people with a 1500 to 2000 ml blood loss (40% blood loss).[1] The bradycardia may be the result of conduction system ischemia secondary to reduced coronary blood flow, or it may be vagally mediated.

- Most patients in shock have pallor, cool and clammy skin, restlessness, or irritability as the first indicators of shock. This should put the clinician on alert that the patient is in shock until proved otherwise. Exceptions include the following:

  1. Patients who are ethanol intoxicated or those with cirrhosis have lost the capacity to constrict the blood vessels. Consequently, they maintain skin perfusion despite falling cardiac output, and their blood pressure tends to fall early in shock. These patients are exquisitely sensitive to vasodilating agents and may "crash" at relatively low-level volume loss or low doses of analgesics, nitroglycerin, and other vasodilating agents.

  2. Patients in septic shock may not develop vasoconstriction even though they are in severe perfusion failure.

  3. Hypotension in patients with neurogenic and anaphylactic shock is produced by a massive, inappropriate vasodilator reaction. Consequently, these patients may have warm, pink skin despite an inadequate systemic perfusion. The patient with neurogenic shock also is likely to be bradycardic.

Any patient who appears to have a sense of well-being not justified by reality should be immediately investigated. Naturally released opiates (endorphins and enkephalins), released in response to intense stress, reduce pain and produce a euphoric state. Consequently, severely ill or injured patients may deny distress or may appear not to be distressed. Hypoxemia also may be associated with an inappropriate sense of well-being.

- Patients with coronary artery disease who develop shock may exhibit signs and symptoms of myocardial ischemia before vital sign changes. These patients are especially at risk for myocardial infarction and hypotension due to decreased cardiac reserve.

- Hemodynamic "numbers" should be assessed not only for normal versus abnormal values, but also for appropriate versus inappropriate responses. For example, it is appropriate to be tachypneic, tachycardic, and hyperglycemic in response to major blood loss, but it is highly inappropriate to maintain normal measurements. Failure of the patient to develop the anticipated compensatory mechanisms to a shock stimulus predicts early clinical deterioration or collapse.

Box 16-2 shows major areas of patient assessment and the most common diagnostic findings of patients in shock. An important principle to remember is that *assessment and hemodynamic measurement trends are more important than isolated pieces of patient information.* Vigilance and thorough, serial examination of the patient are essential to early identification and intervention of the underlying and secondary problems. Both are major factors in determining patient outcome.

Type-Specific Diagnostic Problems

Regardless of the cause of shock, the situation cannot be corrected unless the underlying problem is identified and addressed. In the three most commonly encountered causes of shock—hemorrhagic, septic, and cardiogenic—diagnostic "minefields" exist to confound even the most seasoned clinician. In hemorrhagic (hypovolemic) shock, it is critical that the site of bleeding be identified with certainty so that appropriate surgical intervention, whether simple suture repair of a disrupted vessel or corrective abdominal or thoracic surgery, can be quickly undertaken. Blunt trauma to the abdomen or chest poses a diagnostic dilemma. Experienced clinicians are aware of the potential for massive blood loss from trauma to the spleen or an unsuspected fractured pelvis or femur.

Cardiogenic shock, although most commonly caused by a massive myocardial infarction, also can result from massive pulmonary embolism, pericardial disease, pericardial tamponade, or cardiomyopathy. A sudden deterioration in the condition of a patient with myocardial infarction also may be the result of papillary muscle rupture or acute ventricular septal defect that, while difficult to diagnose on clinical examination, is amenable to lifesaving surgical intervention. Septic shock poses the greatest problem in immunocompromised patients, who may not have the classic signs and symptoms of infection.

To minimize the aforementioned problems, remember the basics. Have a high index of suspicion in patients with a possible risk factor for shock; take a thorough history; perform meticulous serial physical examinations, with close attention to changes in hemodynamic trends; and conduct frequent reassessments and appropriate diagnostic investigations, including radiographs, laboratory tests, ultrasound examinations, and computed tomography.

GENERAL PRINCIPLES OF THERAPY

Type-specific shock therapies are presented with each cause of shock (see the following section). However, some management principles are common to all patients in shock. Overall, the goals of therapy are to correct the primary problem, support the cardiovascular system, and maintain adequate oxygen delivery while reducing the patient's oxygen demands. Frequent or continuous hemodynamic monitoring assists diagnosis and assessment of the patient's responses to therapy. General monitoring and therapeutic measures include correcting the primary problem; ensuring an adequate airway, ventilation, and arterial oxygenation; providing fluid resuscitation; correcting acid-base abnormalities; maintaining recumbency with 30-degree elevation of the legs; providing inotropic support when evidence of heart failure is present; and attempting to keep the patient's temperature within a normal range.

Correct the Primary Problem

If the underlying problem causing shock, such as hemorrhage or septic focus, is left uncorrected, the best that can be achieved with supportive measures is "buying time." Affected patients still have a very high, albeit delayed, rate of mortality.

Ensure an Adequate Airway and Adequate Ventilation and Arterial Oxygenation

Inadequate alveolar ventilation combined with circulatory failure warns of physiologic disaster. Maintenance of an adequate tidal volume and ventilatory rate may mean instituting ventilatory assistance. The presence of an artificial airway, such as an endotracheal tube, also enables airway suctioning as needed. The need for mechanical ventilation is often heralded by a poorly compensated metabolic acidosis demonstrated on arterial blood gases. If the ventila-

tory response to the metabolic acidosis of shock appears to be insufficient, it may mean mechanical ventilation is necessary. Failure to recognize this trend may result in respiratory arrest, followed by cardiovascular collapse.

Mechanical ventilation facilitates improved alveolar ventilation and decreases or eliminates the patient's work of breathing, particularly when the breathing has been labored. The increase in respiratory muscle oxygen consumption due to the increased work of breathing can be met only by augmented blood flow. In patients with reduced cardiac output, anemia, or hypoxemia, the oxygen consumption and blood flow requirements of overworked respiratory muscles may further deprive other vital organs of their needed oxygen supply. A sudden or gradual decrease in respiratory muscle oxygen supply may lead to ventilatory failure and respiratory arrest.

Even patients in shock who appear to be breathing adequately require oxygen therapy for several reasons. Tissue oxygen demands may be twice normal as a result of the increases in oxygen consumption mediated by the stress response. In addition, shock-related pulmonary dysfunction occurs very quickly and may significantly impair arterial oxygenation. Also, shock that results from hemorrhage further reduces blood oxygen content by decreasing hemoglobin levels. If cardiac output also falls, oxygen delivery may become dangerously inadequate.

Administration of oxygen to maintain a PaO_2 of at least 80 to 100 mm Hg (saturation of 95% to 99%) is essential to providing patient support and to minimizing the ischemic sequelae that result from anaerobic metabolism. *In patients with known or probable hypovolemia, caution must be exercised when initiating positive pressure ventilation, particularly with positive end-expiratory pressure (PEEP). The ventilator-induced increases in intrathoracic pressure may impede venous return and reduce cardiac output.*

Hemodynamic Monitoring

Monitoring techniques commonly used in evaluating patients in shock are the following.

Arterial Pressure Monitoring

Blood pressure measurements obtained by ausculation and palpation are notoriously inaccurate in patients with low pulsatile flow or intense vasoconstriction. In these patients, vascular vibrations under the cuff may be too weak to be heard or palpated (see Chapter 7). Cohn[2] demonstrated an average 33.1 mm Hg difference between cuff and intraarterial pressures in patients with low stroke volumes and high SVR. The cuff pressure reading commonly *underestimates* the true intraarterial pressure. In most patients, an unobtainable cuff pressure indicates a systolic pressure less than 50 to 60 mm Hg. In a small group of patients with unobtainable cuff pressures, however, the blood pressure may actually be normal or high. In these patients, inappropriate therapies, such as treatment with vasopressors, may be instituted and may result in stroke or myocardial infarction. If an arterial line has not yet been placed, the Doppler technique detects vascular vibrations that approximate the systolic pressure.

Because significant discrepancies between cuff and intraarterial pressures occur in patients with low stroke volume and severe vasoconstriction, *intraarterial pressure monitoring is indicated in all patients with shock not rapidly responsive to therapy.* Another important advantage of the intraarterial line is that it provides arterial access for blood gas analysis and other laboratory studies. Arterial catheters may be placed in the radial, brachial, axillary, femoral, or dorsalis pedis arteries. In most patients, the catheter can be placed percutaneously. This insertion technique, compared with cutdown, reduces the risk of catheter-related infection. When it is technically feasible, a smaller artery, usually the radial artery, is the preferred site for placement because of the advantage of less bleeding. However, radial arterial systolic pressure can exceed central aortic systolic pressure by approximately 10 to 20 mm Hg, and radial diastolic pressure similarly underestimates central aortic diastolic pressure. *Mean arterial pressure is relatively constant, regardless of arterial sampling site. Therefore trends in mean arterial pressure (rather than systolic and diastolic measurements) should be used for hemodynamic evaluation.*

Central Venous Pressure Monitoring

The central venous pressure (CVP) measures pressure in the superior vena cava, which in turn correlates with mean right atrial pressure and right ventricular end-diastolic pressure. This invasive monitoring technique assesses circulating blood volume and the heart's ability to accept therapeutic fluid challenges. Normal CVP measurements are 3 to 11 cm H_2O (0 to 8 mm Hg).

Evaluation of isolated CVP measurements is not as meaningful as observation of patient responses to fluid challenge. Generally, fluid resuscitation should continue until the blood pressure has been stabilized and clinical evidence exists of adequate tissue perfusion (warm extremities, color improvement, brisk capillary refill, full peripheral pulses, clear sensorium, normal urine flow rates, and resolution of metabolic acidosis). Rapid rises in CVP measurements that do not decrease toward normal within several minutes are strongly suggestive of fluid overload. If, however, the CVP fails to increase or increases and then falls within 5 minutes, this is suggestive of continuing hypovolemia and possible ongoing fluid losses (see Chapter 9, section on assessment and management of intravascular volume status).

Measurements of CVP do not always correlate with fluid requirements in critically ill or injured patients because increases in pulmonary vascular resistance (due to hypoxemia, acidemia, massive pneumothorax) may be associated with normal or high CVP readings despite hypovolemia. In these cases, the high CVP measurements reflect right ventricular failure due to abnormally high right ventricular outflow resistance (afterload).

In patients receiving vasopressors, the CVP also may be misleadingly high relative to the true circulating blood volume. Intense venoconstriction of the small veins and venules displaces venous blood to the central circulation and tends to produce central circulatory pressure measurements that are disproportionately high relative to the actual circulating blood volume. Although CVP measurements usually change in the same direction as pulmonary artery wedge pressure (PWP) measurements, CVP is the last central circulatory pressure to change in primary left ventricular dysfunction (see Chapter 9, Figure 9-2). Therefore CVP is not always a direct or a precise means of assessing left heart function. Use of this technique to monitor fluid replacement and cardiac function is therefore generally reserved for young patients with good cardiopulmonary function who have incurred uncomplicated trauma or illness.

Pulmonary Artery Catheter

The pulmonary artery catheter is indicated for use in elderly or chronically ill patients with shock and poorly compliant hearts, in patients with shock of uncertain cause, and in patients with hypotension and circulatory failure unresponsive to conventional therapy. The pulmonary artery catheter is the most invasive tool for assessing hemodynamics and also carries the highest attendant risks; therefore its use must be weighed against anticipated benefits after the patient's needs have been carefully evaluated. The pulmonary artery catheter provides a means of assessing systemic and pulmonary vascular resistance, intravascular fluid volume, and right and left ventricular function. This catheter also provides a means of sampling blood from the pulmonary artery for measurement of mixed venous oxygen saturation (SvO_2), as well as calculation of oxygen transport (delivery), oxygen consumption, and intrapulmonary shunt fraction.

Provide Fluid Resuscitation

Hypovolemic shock is the most common type of shock. Most other forms of shock also have some hypovolemic components. Consequently, the most fundamentally effective treatment measures for most types of shock are restoration of circulating plasma volume and control of fluid loss. Considerations for fluid resuscitation include venous access, choice of fluid, and hematocrit level.

Venous Access

Adequate venous access is essential. Each patient in shock should have at least two large-bore intravenous catheters in place for delivery of fluids and medications. More than one catheter is necessary because (1) signifi- cant fluid volume resuscitation may be necessary; (2) some medications given for the treatment of shock may be incompatible when infused together; and (3) one catheter may become dislodged or clotted.

Recommendations on the size and location of in- travascular catheters vary. Catheters placed in hemor- rhagic shock must be of a much larger caliber than those placed in cardiogenic shock because the rate and volume of fluid infused are much greater (Table 16-2).

There is no universally preferred catheter placement site. In trauma, it is desirable to avoid insertion near the site of injury. In patients with decompensated hemor- rhagic shock, saphenous vein cutdown allows use of a large-bore catheter and is distant from important struc- tures that may be inadvertently damaged during emer- gency catheter insertion. A saphenous vein catheter, like any invasive device placed under emergency conditions, should be removed and replaced with a new catheter (us- ing appropriate sterile technique) as soon as the patient's condition is stable.

Choice of Fluid for Volume Resuscitation

The type of fluid lost generally determines the type of fluid used for replacement. When hemorrhage is the cause of shock, blood component therapy supplemented with isotonic crystalloid infusion is the mainstay of therapy (Table 16-3).

If hemorrhage is not the cause of hypovolemia, iso- tonic crystalloid electrolyte solutions, such as Ringer's lactate or normal saline solutions, or colloid solutions are the fluids of choice.

TABLE 16-2
Relative Flow Rates for Variously Sized Catheters*

Catheter Size	Flow (ml/min)
8.5 French × 12 cm†	108
8.0 French × 13 cm†	96
14 gauge × 5.7 cm	94
14 gauge × 13.3 cm	83
16 gauge × 5.7 cm	83
16 gauge × 13.3 cm	57
16 gauge × 20 cm	25
18 gauge × 4.3 cm	55

From Sacchetti A: Large-bore infusion catheters (Seldinger technique of vascular access). In Roberts JR, Hedges JR, editors: *Clinical proceedings in emergency medicine*, Philadelphia, 1985, W.B. Saunders.

*These flow rates are only comparative and represent the rate of emptying of 1 L bottles of normal saline solution over a gradient of 3 m. The ab- solute rate of flow of these catheters in variable and is determined by the clinical situation.

†Cook Corp. High-Flo Desilets-Hoffman sheaths.

TABLE 16-3
Estimated Fluid and Blood Requirements* (Based on Patient's Initial Presentation)

	Class I	Class II	Class III	Class IV
Blood loss (ml)	Up to 750	750–1500	1500–2000	≥2000
Blood loss (% blood volume)	Up to 15%	15%–30%	30%–40%	≥40%
Pulse rate	<100	>100	>120	≥140
Blood pressure	Normal	Normal	Decreased	Decreased
Pulse pressure (mm Hg)	Normal or increased	Decreased	Decreased	Decreased
Capillary refill test	Normal	Positive	Positive	Positive
Respiratory rate	14–20	20–30	30–40	>35
Urine output (ml/hr)	≥30	20–30	5–15	Negligible
CNS—mental status	Slightly anxious	Mildly anxious	Anxious and confused	Confused, lethargic
Fluid replacement (3:1 rule)	Crystalloid	Crystalloid	Crystalloid + blood	Crystalloid + blood

*For a 70 kg male patient.

Modified with permission from American College of Surgeons Committee on Trauma: *Advanced trauma life support student manual,* ed 6, Chicago, 1997, American College of Surgeons.

Optimal Hematocrit

Some degree of hemodilution may be well tolerated and actually may enhance capillary perfusion owing to decreased blood viscosity. The optimal hematocrit is patient dependent and has been the subject of controversy. Generally, patients with adequate cardiopulmonary function in whom there is minimal risk of further bleeding may be maintained with hematocrit values in the mid-20% range. Patients with cardiac or pulmonary disease and patients who are at risk of further bleeding should probably be given transfusions to reach a hematocrit of 30%.

Head-injured patients should undergo transfusion to reach a hematocrit in the range of 30% to 33%. This value optimizes blood viscosity while maintaining a fairly high oxygen-carrying capacity to minimize the likelihood of secondary hypoxic injury to the traumatized brain tissue.

Administration of blood and blood products should be limited because of the risk of blood-borne disease.

TABLE 16-4

Approximate Distribution of 1 Liter of Various Intravenous Fluids in Body Compartments after 1 to 2 Hours of Infusion

Isotonic Saline Solutions (Ringer's Lactate, Normal Saline)	Distribution
Intracellular volume	−100 ml
Total extracellular volume	1100 ml
Interstitial volume	825 ml
Plasma volume	275 ml

5% Dextrose in Water	Distribution
Intracellular volume	660 ml
Total extracellular volume	340 ml
Interstitial volume	255 ml
Plasma volume	85 ml

Colloid Solutions (5% Albumin)	Distribution
Intracellular volume	0 ml
Total extracellular volume	1,000 ml
Interstitial volume	500 ml
Plasma volume	500 ml

Whole Blood	Distribution
Intracellular volume	0 ml
Total extracellular volume	1,000 ml
Interstitial volume	0 ml
Plasma volume	1,000 ml

Adapted from Carlson RW, Rattan S, Haupt MT: Fluid resuscitation in conditions of increased permeability, *Anesth Rev* 17(suppl 3), 1990.

Of the crystalloid solutions, Ringer's lactate has the electrolyte composition closest to that of plasma. Generally, lactate in this solution accepts hydrogen ions and is then converted, by the Krebs cycle, to carbon dioxide and water. However, patients with poor hepatic blood flow or inadequate ventilation probably should not receive Ringer's lactate for volume repletion, because lactate will be poorly metabolized or retained carbon dioxide may contribute to acidemia.

Blood component or colloid solutions, such as 5% albumin or hydroxyethl starch (Hetastarch 6%, Pentastarch 5%), expand circulating volume two to three times more than isotonic crystalloid. However, isotonic crystalloids (Ringer's lactate, normal saline) are far less expensive, are readily available, carry no risk of disease transmission or allergic reactions, and replace fluids and electrolytes lost from the tissue space.

Morbidity and mortality rates do not seem to differ significantly between colloid- and crystalloid-treated patients, although controversy exists. Approximately 70% to 80% of crystalloid solution volume is lost from the intravascular to the extravascular compartments within 20 minutes of administration; therefore the total volume of crystalloid required for filling the intravascular space is three to four times greater than the estimated volume loss. See Table 16-4 for estimates of distribution of various intravenous fluids in body compartments following infusion.[3] It has been theorized that the large volume of extravasated fluid may contribute to pulmonary and systemic edema and may compromise patient outcome. The final judgment in the crystalloid versus colloid debate in the management of patients in shock has not yet been made.

Successful resuscitation from shock probably is related more closely to early identification and correction of the underlying patient problem and the rapidity of fluid volume replacement than to the specific type of fluid used.

Correct Acid-Base Abnormalities

Metabolic acidosis as a result of shock generally tends to correct with restoration of adequate tissue perfusion and oxygenation. If, however, the pH remains less than 7.20 despite optimal cardiopulmonary support, administration of sodium bicarbonate should be considered. If the patient is being mechanically ventilated, mild acidemia can be corrected by mild hyperventilation rather than by administration of sodium bicarbonate. In either case, "overshoot alkalosis" must be carefully avoided. Alkalemia impairs oxygen unloading at the tissue level, reduces ionized calcium and magnesium levels, and predisposes the patient to central and peripheral nervous system irritability.

Maintain Patient Recumbency with a 30-Degree Elevation of the Legs

This position is recommended particularly for patients in shock when hypovolemia is a suspected cause or associated factor (Figure 16-9). In trauma patients in whom there is possible spinal injury, the legs should not be elevated until it is determined that the lumbar spine is free of injury.

Elevation of the lower extremities returns the relatively large volume of blood, normally sequestered in the leg veins, to the central circulation. When the most physiologically beneficial position is in question (such as when pulmonary edema complicates cardiogenic shock), most patients intuitively and spontaneously assume or request the position of comfort that is most physiologically advantageous for them. Never force patients into a position that they resist.

Provide Inotropic Support When Evidence of Heart Failure Is Present

The inotrope of choice is related to the underlying problem and hemodynamic profile. For example, because of its vasodilator properties, dobutamine (Dobutrex) is the inotrope of choice in patients with a low cardiac output but normal or increased blood pressure, whereas dopamine (Intropin) is the preferred inotrope in patients with hypotension and low cardiac output because it has both venous and arterial constriction properties. (A detailed discussion of the various inotropes and their properties can be found in Chapter 14.)

Attempt to Keep the Patient's Temperature within a Normal Range

Body temperature is normally maintained by balancing heat production against heat loss. This balance fails in patients in shock because of (1) the generalized decrease in heat (energy) production and (2) the potential for increased heat loss as a result of rapid administration of room-temperature intravenous solutions or refrigerated banked blood. Many patients also are exposed for assessment or observation. A room temperature that is comfortable for a fully clothed

person is often too cold for a naked patient who must generate extra body heat to maintain body temperature. The problem of heat loss is compounded if the patient is in wet (blood-, urine-, or solution-soaked) linen.

Chilled people normally shiver as a means of generating body heat. The muscle activity that accompanies shivering increases carbon dioxide production and requires an increase in cardiac output three to four times normal to meet the greater muscle oxygen demand. Accidental cooling imposes the additional physiologic demand of cold stress on a massively stressed patient whose physiologic resources may be nearly depleted. Hypothermia, most frequent in patients with hypovolemic shock, also predisposes to coagulopathies and immunosuppression.

Core temperature is usually decreased relative to the duration and severity of shock (in patients without sepsis) and how well the patient is protected from accidental cooling. Generalized cellular function usually becomes depressed when body temperature falls below 95.6° F (35° C). Hypothermia may be clinically apparent as slowing of heart rate and breathing, development of cardiac arrhythmias, and presence of hypotension. Refractoriness to therapy for shock and failure to clot appropriately may be due to the fact that the patient is hypothermic. Maintaining normal body temperature in shock patients by conserving body heat is extremely important. Avoidance of unnecessary exposure to cool air and wet linen, prevention of the patient from remaining naked for "ongoing assessment," and infusion of heated intravenous solutions are essential body temperature conservation measures.

CLASSIFICATION OF SHOCK BY CAUSE

Shock is classified by five etiologic categories—hypovolemic, septic, anaphylactic, neurogenic, and cardiogenic. This chapter also contains a brief discussion of other possible causes. The discussion of specific types of shock that follows focuses on the anticipated direction of pathophysiologic, hemodynamic, clinical, and laboratory changes rather than absolute values. *In the individual patient, coexisting disease and complicating factors may alter or even reverse the anticipated direction of change.*

Hypovolemic Shock

Hypovolemic shock is the result of a critical reduction in circulating intravascular volume. Inadequate tissue perfusion and diffuse ischemic hypoxia result. An associated interstitial fluid volume deficit also may be present. Hypovolemia is the most common cause of shock, and it frequently complicates other forms of shock.

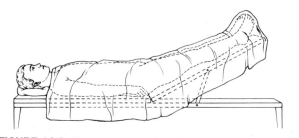

FIGURE 16-9 The recommended position for patients in shock.

Causes

Intravascular volume depletion may result from blood loss, third-space fluid shifts, or dehydration (Table 16-5).

Pathophysiology

Intravascular volume loss reduces venous return to the heart, which in turn reduces ventricular filling and stroke volume. The cardiovascular effects of hypovolemia are illustrated in Figure 16-10.

The patient's pathophysiologic response, hemodynamic profile, and clinical presentation are related to the type and amount of fluid lost, the rapidity of volume loss, the length of time the fluid loss continues, and the adequacy of fluid repletion.

The person initially may maintain a normal mean arterial pressure and remain "compensated." However, with continued or massive fluid loss, decompensation and hypotension ensue. The stages of shock described earlier in this chapter classically apply to hypovolemic shock.

Compensated Shock

In compensated shock, vasoconstriction and hypoperfusion are localized to the peripheral, nonvital tissue. Although this stage may initially be well tolerated, if not corrected, prolonged perfusion deficits to bowel, kidney, and skeletal muscle eventually lead to organ dysfunction and lactic acidosis. Mediator substance activation or release may sustain or worsen the shock syndrome.

TABLE 16-5
Causes of Hypovolemic Shock

Cause	Description
Hemorrhage	
Wound hemorrhage	Laceration of a vein or artery, open wounds
	Hemorrhage at fracture sites
	Fractured pelvis may be associated with 1500 ml blood loss *before* increase in abdominal girth can be measured; fractured femur may be associated with 500–1000 ml blood loss *before* increase in thigh girth can be measured
Gastrointestinal (GI)	Upper GI and proximal colon bleeding may produce burgundy-colored stool; distal colon (rectal) bleeding may produce red stool; hematemesis (vomiting of blood) may be bright red, dark red and clotted, or coffee ground (altered by gastric secretions); melena (black, tarry stools) may not appear for some time after the onset of upper GI bleeding
Hemothorax	Laceration of major vessel may result in accumulation of 1–2 L of blood within the thorax
Intraabdominal bleeding	Laceration, erosion, or rupture of intraabdominal vessels may result in sudden, massive intravascular blood loss
Saline or Combined Saline and Water Loss	
Gastrointestinal losses	Protracted vomiting or diarrhea leads to hypotonic fluid loss
High fever	Hyperventilation and evaporative losses of hypotonic fluid from skin may exceed 500–1500 ml/day beyond normal
Excessive sweating	Seen clinically during alcohol withdrawal (especially delerium tremens), seizures, hot environment; moist skin without beads of sweat can cause loss of 1–3 L of hypotonic fluid within 24 hr; drenched sweats can cause hypotonic fluid loss exceeding 4 L/day
Diuretics	Sudden, massive response to a potent diuretic such as furosemide can precipitate hypovolemic shock; chronic losses may lead to water deficit
Polyurea	Secondary to osmotic loads (hyperglycemia, mannitol) or diabetes insipidus
Third-Space Fluid Shifts	
Soft tissue trauma (swelling)	Losses are relative to the size and severity of the area of trauma
Sepsis	Capillary leak is most pronounced in the infected area; however, generalized systemic losses also occur
Peritonitis/intestinal obstruction	8–10 L of fluid can translocate into loops of injured or inflamed bowel
Ascites	Progressive accumulation of ascites fluid can exceed 2–3 L
Large-area burn injuries	Increased capillary permeability occurs throughout the body but is greatest in the burn area

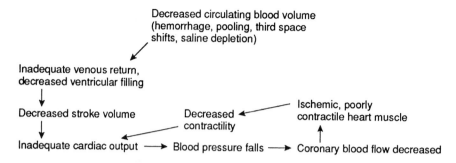

FIGURE 16-10 Effects of hypovolemia on ventricular filling and cardiac function. (From Darovic GO, Rokowsky JS: Shock. In Patrick ML et al, editors: *Medical-surgical nursing: pathophysiological concepts,* ed 2, Philadelphia, 1991, JB Lippincott.)

Hemodynamic Profile

Arterial Pressure Measurement and Waveform. Systemic vasoconstriction maintains or elevates diastolic pressure. Systolic pressure may be maintained at greater than normal, normal, or near-normal levels. The pulse pressure narrows and reflects the decrease in stroke volume. Isolated numbers, as a guide to the patient's hemodynamic status and tissue perfusion, may be misleading. An example is using a systolic pressure of 90 to 100 mm Hg as a cutoff point for the diagnosis of shock. Although the systolic pressure driving blood to core organs may be 90 to 100 mm Hg or higher, large areas of tissue may be receiving minimal blood flow because of regional vasoconstriction. The interrelationship of all hemodynamic measurements, the relationship to the patient's clinical presentation, and the changes in response to treatment provide more meaningful assessment tools than isolated numbers.

The arterial waveform may appear damped. Cyclic variations in waveform amplitude also may exist. These relate to changes in intraventricular volume and stroke volume within the respiratory cycle (pulsus paradoxus) (see Chapter 5, Figure 5-4). Ordinarily, the inspiratory fall and expiratory rise in left ventricular filling volume do not produce significant changes in stroke volume and arterial pressure. In hypovolemic patients, the relatively small expiratory increase in left ventricular filling volume (steep portion of the ventricular function curve) may be associated with a significant increase in stroke volume, which, in turn, is reflected in the momentarily widening pulse pressure and increase in systolic pressure.

Systemic Vascular Resistance. This calculated measurement is often elevated owing to generalized systemic arteriolar constriction.

Pulmonary Vascular Resistance. This value is usually within the normal range.

Central Venous Pressure and Right Atrial Pressure. These measurements are usually decreased because venous return is decreased. However, compensatory venoconstriction may produce values that are misleadingly high relative to the actual amount of plasma volume lost.

Pulmonary Artery Pressure and Pulmonary Artery Wedge Pressure. These measurements are usually below normal and reflect the reduction in pulmonary intravascular volume and left ventricular filling volume. The morphology of the pulmonary artery waveform is usually unchanged, but it may be slightly damped. Pulsus paradoxus also is usually observed in the pulmonary artery waveform.

Cardiac Output. This measurement may be slightly decreased owing to reduced ventricular filling, or cardiac output may be maintained in the normal range by sympathetic nervous system stimulation. At this stage, decreases in stroke volume are generally offset by compensatory increases in heart rate.

Mixed Venous Oxygen Saturation. The SvO_2 measurement may be decreased owing to hypoperfusion of large areas of tissue or anemia if hemorrhage is the cause of hypovolemia.

Clinical Presentation

Mentation. Patients are typically alert and lucid. Mild anxiety, irritability, and restlessness also may be present as a result of the excitatory effects of catecholamines on the central nervous system. Frequently the patient complains of thirst.

Cutaneous Manifestations. The patient's complexion is usually pale and the extremities may be cool and clammy, although the trunk is typically warm and dry.

Capillary Blanch (Refill) Test. This assessment technique is performed by depressing the patient's fingernail, thereby squeezing blood from the underlying capillary bed. Normally, after release of pressure, the color returns in less than 2 seconds. Because of poor peripheral capillary perfusion in patients in compensated shock, the return to color takes longer than 2 seconds (positive test).

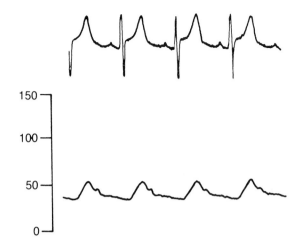

FIGURE 16-11 Arterial pressure tracing from a 50-year-old man in hemorrhagic shock. Note the damped-appearing waveform, slurred upstroke (inotropic component of the waveform), and narrow pulse pressure.

Heart Rate and Peripheral Pulses. The heart rate usually increases above 100 beats per minute to maintain cardiac output. The volume of the pulses may be weak due to the diminishing stroke volume ejected into the systemic circulation.

Neck Veins. The external jugular veins are typically collapsed and invisible when the patient is in the supine position (the external jugular veins are normally slightly distended in the supine position). The peripheral veins on the dorsum of the hands and feet gradually become non-palpable and difficult to see.

Respiratory Rate and Character of Breathing. The patient is typically tachypneic (20 to 30 breaths per minute). Ventilatory movements are commonly visible.

Urine Output. Urine output may be decreased to 20 to 30 ml/hr. Urine sodium is low, and the specific gravity is greater than 1.025 because sodium and water are being reabsorbed by the kidney. Recent use of diuretics invalidates urine output as an assessment tool.

Acid-Base Levels. Significant base deficit (minus 5 mEq of HCO_3 per liter or more) reflects poor tissue perfusion, anaerobic metabolism, and lactic acid production. An increase in serum lactate is a grim indicator of the hypoxic insult being borne by many cells despite apparent hemodynamic stability. Nevertheless, the arterial pH may be maintained at normal levels by the compensatory respiratory alkalosis or even may be in the alkalemic range (greater than 7.45). Trauma, pain, and stress are potent stimuli to ventilation, and respiratory alkalosis may override the metabolic effects of shock.

Decompensated Shock

Decompensated shock usually occurs with an acute intravascular volume loss greater than 30%. In a 70 kg person whose normal blood volume is 5000 ml, this represents a loss greater than 1500 ml. Smaller people require smaller fluid losses to produce this level of shock, whereas larger people may remain compensated with larger volume deficits.

When compensatory mechanisms are maximized and fluid losses continue, systolic pressure falls. Therefore a falling systolic pressure does not represent the onset of shock but rather a level of shock in which compensatory mechanisms are exhausted. At this stage, blood flow to the body as a whole, including heart and brain, may be severely compromised.

Hemodynamic Profile

Arterial Pressure. The measurements are now in a conventionally unacceptable range—that is, a significant drop in arterial pressure occurs in a patient known to be previously hypertensive, or a systolic pressure less than 90 to 100 mm Hg occurs in a previously normotensive patient. The pulse pressure also is narrowed.

Pulsus paradoxus is usually visible on the arterial waveform. The slurred upstroke and decreased rate of rise of the arterial waveform (inotropic component) reflect the diminished force of left ventricular ejection. The waveform also appears damped (Figure 16-11).

Clinical Presentation

Mentation. Patients with decompensated shock are typically anxious and confused and may have changes in affect. With worsening of shock, mental changes may progress to obtundation, stupor, and eventually coma.

Cutaneous Manifestations. The skin is pale with waxen mucous membranes and nail beds. The face of the patient in decompensated shock is typically ashen, gray, and haggard. The skin is cool to touch and clammy over most of the body.

Capillary Blanch (Refill) Test. The test is positive at the nail bed. Following compression and then rapid release of skin over the chest, capillary refill of the underlying skin may also be delayed.

Heart Rate and Peripheral Pulses. The heart rate is typically greater than 120 beats per minute and the pulses are weak and thready. Pulses may not be palpable at distal arteries (radial, brachial, pedal).

Neck Veins. The neck veins, as well as peripheral veins, are collapsed.

Respiratory Rate and Character of Breathing. Tachypnea, in the range of 30 to 40 breaths per minute, is common. The absence of compensatory hyperventilation indicates that disease, drugs, or trauma has altered or blunted the normal ventilatory response to stress or hypoperfusion. Such patients are at high risk for ventilatory failure. The source of the problem must be rapidly identified and corrected. If correction is not possible, mechanical ventilatory assistance is indicated.

Urine Output. Urine flow rates may fall to less than 15 ml/hr.

Acid-Base Disorders. The accumulation of lactic acid overrides respiratory alkalosis. Metabolic acidosis (pH less than 7.35) typically predominates in the later stages of shock.

Systemic Vascular Resistance. This measurement continues to be increased (in proportion to the amount of compensatory arteriolar constriction present) until very late in the course of shock. When compensatory mechanisms fail, vascular tone is lost and blood vessels passively dilate; SVR then falls.

Pulmonary Vascular Resistance. Hypoxemia and acidemia, which accompany decompensated shock, have potent pulmonary vasoconstrictor effects. The degree of increase in pulmonary vascular resistance therefore relates to the severity of shock. A marked increase in pulmonary vascular resistance is an ominous sign.

Central Venous Pressure and Right Atrial Pressure. Progressive intravascular volume losses produce greater decrements in right atrial pressure and CVP. Patients with acute, profound hemorrhage may have measurements as low as -8 to -10 mm Hg.

Pulmonary Artery Pressure and Pulmonary Artery Wedge Pressure. These measurements remain low. The rate of rise of the upstroke of the pulmonary artery waveform may be delayed and slurred, and the narrowed pulse pressure correlates with decreased right ventricular stroke volume. The pulmonary artery waveform usually appears damped. If increased pulmonary vascular resistance accompanies hypovolemic shock, the pulmonary artery diastolic (PAd) pressure is more than 4 mm Hg greater than the pulmonary artery wedge pressure (widening of the PAd-PWP gradient).

Cardiac Output. This measurement is decreased primarily as a result of the decreased stroke volume that occurs secondary to reduced ventricular filling. Myocardial depression caused by toxic metabolites or poor coronary blood flow further impairs ventricular function, which, in turn, results in greater falls in cardiac output. At this level of shock, tachycardia is inadequate to maintain cardiac output at acceptable levels.

Mixed Venous Oxygen Saturation. Measurements are decreased as a result of hypoperfusion, lower arterial oxygen content, or both. Arterial oxygen content may be decreased as a result of the hypoxemia and anemia that frequently accompany hemorrhagic shock.

Treatment

The goals of treatment are correction of the primary problem and supportive patient care. Steps are taken to (1) ensure adequate ventilation and oxygenation, (2) identify and stop the source of fluid loss, and (3) restore intravascular volume. (See general guidelines for management of shock.)

Pain medications generally should be withheld from trauma patients until vascular access is secured, fluid therapy has begun, and hypovolemia is resolved. Opiates inhibit arteriolar constriction and have venodilator properties. Therefore an analgesic-induced increase in venous capacitance may result in a severe, sudden drop in blood pressure in a previously normotensive patient with maximal or near-maximal compensatory venoconstriction. If opiate analgesics are absolutely necessary, it is recommended that they be administered in small, frequent doses while the patient is carefully and vigilantly monitored.

Septic Shock

Septic shock (systemic infection associated with hypotension) is caused by a wide variety of infectious agents. Bloodstream invasion by these microorganisms can precipitate sepsis and septic shock, especially when microbial invasion is abetted by defects in the patient's immune mechanisms.

Causes

Many infectious agents can cause the clinical picture of sepsis and septic shock. The infecting agents may be viruses, spirochetes, parasites, *Rickettsia,* common fungi such as the *Candida* species, and gram-negative or gram-positive bacteria. However, gram-negative bacilli, such as *Escherichia coli, Pseudomonas aeruginosa, Proteus mirabilis, Enterobacter cloacae,* and *Haemophilus parainfluenzae,* as well as *Cirtobacter* and *Klebsiella* species, are the most common causes of hospital infection and septic shock. Nonetheless, other microorganisms play a significant role in the incidence of infectious disease. Because *Staphylococcus epidermidis* is frequently the cause of vascular line sepsis, and the exotoxin of *Staphylococcus aureus* and group A streptococci produces toxic shock syndromes, clinicians are reminded that the importance of septic shock is not specific to gram-negative bacteria.

Also, fungi, such as those of the *Candida* species, are the most common cause of opportunistic infections in medical and surgical intensive care units (ICUs). It is frightening to consider that the incidence of these infections has increased dramatically within the past 10 years. The *Candida* species are now the fourth most common microorganisms isolated from blood cultures.

Predisposing Factors

Many factors predispose patients to systemic infection, and these can be grouped according to (1) patient factors that affect immune response, (2) primary infections that can be especially virulent, and (3) iatrogenic (hospital-acquired) causes (Table 16-6).

The patient's underlying disease or physical condition is of paramount importance in determining the outcome of sepsis and septic shock. Malignancies, extremes of age, diabetes mellitus, uremia, cirrhosis, and asplenia can impair immune competence. Patients with immune incompetence have a much greater risk of death from septic shock because they are more susceptible to and less likely to contain infection; they are less likely to manifest the classic clinical signs of infection (thus making early diagnosis and treatment difficult); and their impaired defense mechanisms make recovery less likely.

Pathophysiology

High circulating levels of bacterial antigens and bacterial toxins, which are the result of the presence and growth of microorganisms in the blood, activate a number of metabolic pathways. These activated pathways, in turn, result in the systemic release of various biochemical *inflammatory mediators* that interact to produce the pathophysiologic cascade that characterizes the septic process. Fundamentally, the pathophysiology represents various aspects of the normal immune response, such as activation of complement, kinin, coagulation, and fibrinolytic systems, as well as release of various other mediator substances, such as cytokines (see Chapter 17, Box 17-3) and vasodilator substances such as bradykinin, nitric oxide (NO), prostaglandin E_2, and prostacyclin.

In sepsis, systemic uncontrolled and exaggerated immune system activation occurs and results in profound changes in metabolic, cardiovascular, pulmonary, and hemostatic function. Immune system anarchy leads to a state wherein the body cannot control its own inflammatory, metabolic, and hemodynamic responses. Physiologic chaos and organ destruction follow. Prominent pathophysiologic features are hypovolemia; coagulopathies; abnormalities in cellular oxygen demand, uptake, and utilization; maldistribution of cardiac output; abnormalities in ventricular performance; and pulmonary vascular changes.

Hypovolemic Components to Sepsis. Hypovolemia plays a critical role in septic shock and has two components:
1. *Biochemical mediator–induced systemic vasodilation.* This results in relative hypovolemia (the intravascular

---

TABLE 16-6
Factors Predisposing to Septicemia

Inadequate Immune Response	Primary Infections	Iatrogenic Sources
Granulocytopenia	Pneumonia	Indwelling vascular or urinary catheters
Diabetes mellitus	Urinary tract infection, especially	Instrumentation of the urinary tract
Liver disease	following instrumentation	Extensive major abdominal or pelvic
Neoplasms	Female genital tract	surgery
Neonates	Cholecystitis	Implantation of prosthetic heart valves or
The elderly (over 60 years of age)	Peritonitis	other implantable devices
Alcoholics	Burn or other large wound infections	
Renal failure	Abscess	
Pregnancy		
Protein-calorie malnutrition		
Massive trauma/shock states		
Use of immunosuppressive drugs (patients with organ transplant and autoimmune diseases)		
Congenital or acquired immune system deficiencies		

volume is inadequate relative to the expanded size of the vascular compartment).
2. *Biochemical mediator–induced capillary permeability.* Plasma-rich fluid leaks from the vascular to tissue spaces through porous capillaries. Intravascular losses can exceed 200 ml/hr.

Although total body water may be normal or even increased if the patient receives intravenous replacement fluids, the fluids are often being shifted into areas of body where they are nonfunctional, resulting in systemic or pulmonary edema.

Coagulation Abnormalities. Systemic, accelerated, and simultaneous activation of the clotting and fibrinolytic systems develops. This is essentially the pathophysiologic description of disseminated intravascular coagulation (DIC). Affected patients are disposed to two seemingly paradoxic phenomena:
1. *Diffuse intravascular coagulation.* Clots inappropriately form at an accelerated rate; most are within capillary lumina. The inappropriate formation of countless capillary microthrombi further compromises nutrient blood flow, which in turn predisposes the patient to diffuse ischemic tissue injury.
2. *Systemic hemorrhage.* Formation of the countless capillary thrombi depletes plasma coagulation factors such as platelets and fibrinogen. Essentially, plasma (which is coagulable) is being transformed into serum (which is noncoagulable). At the same time, the fibrinolytic system is systemically activated for eventual dissolution of the clots. Fibrin split products (which are end products of fibrinolysis and are potent inhibitors to clotting) are then released into the bloodstream. The patient becomes systemically autoanticoagulated and is therefore predisposed to systemic bleeding. When diffuse hemorrhage complicates DIC, the hypovolemic component of septic shock is compounded.

Abnormalities in Oxygen Requirements, Oxygen Uptake, and Utilization. The oxygen needs of septic patients are typically greater than normal due to hypermetabolism of diffusely inflamed tissue. This, in turn, demands the hyperdynamic circulation that is characteristic of septic patients who are not hypotensive.

Under normal conditions, as well as in other forms of circulatory abnormalities, cellular oxygen consumption is appropriate to cellular metabolic need. Furthermore, oxygen consumption remains normal despite decreases in oxygen delivery until oxygen delivery falls to approximately one half the normal value. However, at or below this critical level, cellular oxygen consumption is forced to fall because delivery becomes grossly inadequate.

However, patients with sepsis have defects in taking up or metabolizing available oxygen despite normal oxygen delivery. This, in turn, predisposes them to cellular hypoxia. Proposed mechanisms include (1) abnormalities in red blood cell function that favor retention of oxygen by hemoglobin, (2) mitochondrial injury, and (3) arteriovenous shunts. Abnormal cellular uptake or utilization of oxygen is manifested by elevated mixed venous oxygen saturations, clinical evidence of ischemic organ dysfunction, and possibly lactic acidosis.

Maldistribution of Cardiac Output. Increases in cardiac output serve as a compensatory mechanism to maintain arterial pressure and maximize oxygen delivery to hypermetabolic tissue. However, the increased cardiac output may not be appropriately distributed, and thus blood flow may not be suitable to meet local tissue needs. On the one hand, blood flow through mediator-induced vasodilated areas (such as skin and skeletal muscle) may exceed the metabolic requirements of these relatively inactive tissues. On the other hand, blood flow to highly active organs (such as abdominal viscera) may be inadequate to support oxidative metabolism.

Microscopic vascular channels that open from arterioles to venules, termed *anatomic shunts,* also may be present in septic patients and divert the augmented cardiac output around the capillary bed.

Abnormalities in Ventricular Performance. Cardiac output is generally normal or even greater than normal during the initial stages of sepsis. However, myocardial systolic and diastolic dysfunction is present, despite the supernormal cardiac output.

The *systolic (contractile) dysfunction* is characterized by a decrease in ejection fraction. A normal stroke volume is usually maintained by compensatory ventricular dilation, which in turn allows increases in both end-diastolic and end-systolic volumes (Figure 16-12). The augmented cardiac output is thought to be the result of increases in heart rate. If the patient fails to recover, cardiac output may not fall to subnormal levels until very late in the septic course.

The contractile defect, which is reversible at 7 to 10 days following resolution of sepsis, is thought to result from a blood-borne myocardial depressant factor, which is released from ischemic splanchnic tissue.

ACUTE PHASE OF SEPTIC SHOCK

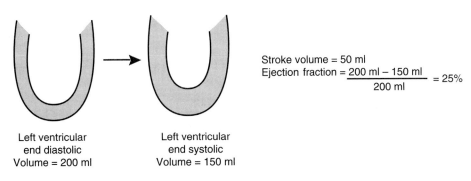

Stroke volume = 50 ml

$$\text{Ejection fraction} = \frac{200 \text{ ml} - 150 \text{ ml}}{200 \text{ ml}} = 25\%$$

Left ventricular
end diastolic
Volume = 200 ml

Left ventricular
end systolic
Volume = 150 ml

RECOVERY PHASE OF SEPTIC SHOCK

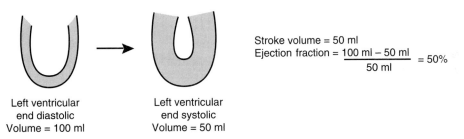

Stroke volume = 50 ml

$$\text{Ejection fraction} = \frac{100 \text{ ml} - 50 \text{ ml}}{50 \text{ ml}} = 50\%$$

Left ventricular
end diastolic
Volume = 100 ml

Left ventricular
end systolic
Volume = 50 ml

FIGURE 16-12 Schematic representation of ventricular performance changes during the acute and recovery periods of septic shock in humans. (With permission from Parrillo JE et al: Septic shock in humans: advances in the understanding of pathogenesis, cardiovascular dysfunction and therapy, *Ann Intern Med* 113:228, 1990.)

Diastolic dysfunction is characterized by decreased ventricular compliance. This abnormality makes judgments of left ventricular end-diastolic volume by evaluation of PWP difficult for the following reason. Ventricular end-diastolic pressures may be disproportionately high relative to end-diastolic volumes, because the stiff, unyielding ventricular walls cannot accommodate any end-diastolic volume without a greater than usual end-diastolic pressure. Consequently, normal PWP measurements may be inadequate to support cardiac output. In fact, patients with sepsis generally require increased PWP measurements (in the range of 12 to 15 mm Hg) to maintain an adequate cardiac output.

Pulmonary Vascular Changes. Increased pulmonary vascular resistance, evidenced by pulmonary hypertension and widening of the pulmonary artery diastolic to pulmonary artery wedge pressure (PAd-PWP) gradient, occurs in some septic patients. The mechanisms that dispose a patient to pulmonary hypertension are not well understood. Theories include pulmonary vascular plugging by microthrombi, pulmonary vasoconstriction mediated by

activated components and products of the immune system, and hypoxemia. When severe, pulmonary hypertension can limit or reduce right ventricular stroke volume by increasing afterload.

Generally, the clinical presentation of septic patients is similar, regardless of the offending microorganism. Sepsis due to some gram-positive bacteria may have distinctive clinical features (see the section on gram-positive shock syndromes).

Clinical and Hemodynamic Profiles in Septic Patients

Sepsis is generally classified into hyperdynamic and hypodynamic cardiovascular phases (Figure 16-13). These phases are *not* distinct and fixed but rather are dynamic and depend on moment-to-moment changes in intravascular fluid volume and cardiac function. A patient's condition may fluctuate between the hyperdynamic and hypodynamic phases in the course of the disease. This depends on the time-related magnitude of bloodstream microbial seeding from the infected locus, the adequacy of treatment, and the individual patient's responses to the disease and treatment.

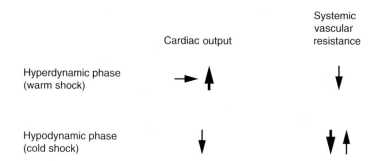

FIGURE 16-13 Hemodynamic phases in sepsis. The *heavy arrows* indicate the more commonly encountered response.

Hemodynamic assessment is complicated further because of the multiplicity of possible coexisting complications, such as hypovolemia, ventricular failure, and pulmonary hypertension.

Hyperdynamic Phase (Warm Shock). The term *systemic inflammatory response syndrome* (SIRS) describes the clinical manifestations of sepsis, as well as the conditions other than sepsis that are associated with a massive systemic inflammatory response that occurs secondary to a variety of insults or sepsis. Physiologic insults include diseases such as pancreatitis, as well as the initial period following major trauma, major burn injury, and major surgery. Systemic inflammatory response syndrome is manifested by two or more of the following conditions:

- Temperature greater than 38° C or less than 36° C
- Heart rate greater than 90 beats per minute
- Respiratory rate greater than 20 breaths per minute or $Paco_2$ less than 32 mm Hg
- White blood cell count greater than 12,000 cells/ml^3, or less than 4000 cells/ml^3, or greater than 10% immature cell (band) forms

Sepsis is always associated with SIRS, but SIRS may be present in the absence of an infectious process. Box 16-3 lists the nomenclature specific to the septic syndromes, as well as the features that should alert the clinician to evidence of systemic infection and altered organ function.

Clinical Presentation. Clinical signs other than those listed in the following may indicate the septic source. For example, headache and nucal ridgidity indicate central nervous system infection; abdominal pain and tenderness indicate peritonitis; urinary frequency, dysurea, or flank pain indicates urinary tract infection; and cough and purulent sputum indicate respiratory tract infection. Clinical signs may also aid early detection of the type of microorganism causing sepsis. The appearance of a generalized rash, sore throat, bloodshot eyes, muscle aches, mental status changes, a "strawberry tongue," fever, a wound that looks unremarkable, and recent use of a tampon indicate toxic shock syndrome due to *S. aureus*. Blood cultures may be negative.

Likewise, the presence of shock, fever, confusion, soft tissue infection with or without necrotizing fasciitis or myositis, multiple-organ dysfunction, and a generalized "sunburnlike" rash (10% of cases) strongly indicates infection with group A streptococci.

Mentation. Patients frequently complain of malaise and "not feeling well," aching, and tiredness. Confusion, restlessness, intellectual impairment, irritability, hostility, flattened affect, or delirium also may be present. These changes may be consistently maintained or may alternate with periods of apparently normal mental function.

Cutaneous Manifestations. Because vasodilation is a prominent feature of hyperdynamic sepsis, the skin is warm and may be flushed. However, the complexion of most septic patients appears sallow rather than pink despite vasodilation.

Heart Rate and Character of Pulse. Tachycardia is typical, and the pulses are bounding.

Respiratory Rate and Character of Breathing. The respiratory rate is greater than 20 breaths per minute, and breathing is noticeable. *Hyperventilation inappropriate to apparent stimulus is an important clinical indication that a patient may be septic, and the condition should be immediately investigated.*

Urine Output. If intravascular volume is not replaced at a rate equal to losses, urine output decreases.

Acid-Base Values. Respiratory alkalosis, due to hyperventilation, is a classic finding in early sepsis.

Body Temperature. Fever may be accompanied by shaking chills. Elderly or severely debilitated patients may

BOX 16-3
Definitions and Clinical Characteristics of Systemic Inflammatory Response Syndrome and Septic Syndromes

Infection—an inflammatory response to the presence of microorganisms or the invasion of normally sterile host tissue by those organisms

Bacteremia—the presence of viable bacteria in the blood

Sepsis/septicemia—the systemic inflammatory response to invasion by microorganisms

Severe sepsis—sepsis associated with hypotension or hypoperfusion or dysfunction of at least one organ, such as acute respiratory failure, oligurea, mental status changes, or lactic acidosis

Septic shock—sepsis with hypotension, despite adequate fluid resuscitation, in conjunction with the presence of perfusion abnormalities, which may include, but are not limited to, lactic acidosis, oliguria, or an acute alteration in mental status. Patients who are on inotropic or vasopressor agents may not be hypotensive at the time that perfusion abnormalities are measured

Hypotension—A systolic blood pressure less than 90 mm Hg or a reduction of greater than 40 mm Hg from baseline in the absence of other causes for hypotension

Refractory septic shock—hypotension that persists longer than 1 hour despite adequate fluid resuscitation

fail to increase body temperature in response to infection and, instead, may even become hypothermic. Hypothermia portends a poor prognosis.

The hyperdynamic phase may last from hours to weeks, depending on the amount of inoculum and virulence of infecting microorganisms contaminating the blood and on the host's age, resistance, constitution, and cardiovascular reserve. A critical determinant of the patient's ability to maintain the hyperdynamic circulation is the ability of the heart to maintain cardiac output commensurate with the expanding size of the vascular bed, fluid losses, and increased metabolic needs.

Hemodynamic Profile. The hyperdynamic phase is characterized by a normal-to-high cardiac output and decreased systemic vascular resistance (systemic vasodilator reaction).

Arterial Pressure. Blood pressure may be in the near-normal range or slightly decreased. There may be an orthostatic fall in blood pressure (fall in systolic pressure greater than 10 mm Hg on rising). The inotropic compo-

nent of the arterial waveform may have a rapid, steep upstroke.

Systemic Vascular Resistance. Measurements of SVR are below normal due to generalized vasodilation. The specific agents responsible for decreased systemic vascular tone are unknown, but they are thought to be the result of locally or systemically released inflammatory mediators.

Pulmonary Vascular Resistance. This calculated value may be in the normal range or increased depending on various cardiopulmonary factors, such as cardiogenic pulmonary edema or the adult respiratory distress syndrome (ARDS).

Central Venous Pressure and Right Atrial Pressure. Measurements may be decreased owing to the intravascular volume loss or the expanded size of the vascular bed. Decreases in right ventricular compliance may result in pressure measurements that are disproportionately high relative to actual circulating blood volume.

Pulmonary Artery Pressure and Wedge Pressure. Decreased measurements are the result of third-space fluid losses and systemic vasodilation. An increase in pulmonary artery systolic and diastolic pressure with a widening of the PAd-PWP gradient indicates an increase in pulmonary vascular resistance. The PWP may not correlate well with left ventricular filling volume in a patient with diastolic dysfunction (stiff ventricle).

Cardiac Output. Cardiac output is typically elevated because of the hyperdynamic circulation demanded by the increased tissue oxygen requirements and the decreased systemic vascular resistance (afterload). The cardioadaptive response to sepsis increases cardiac output and heart work to a level similar to that which occurs with strenuous exercise. In contrast to strenuous exercise, this level of heart work is maintained for days or weeks as the debilitating effects of sepsis continue to weaken the patient. Patient outcome depends, in part, on the capability of the heart to maintain the prolonged high output and therefore maximize oxygen delivery to hypermetabolic tissue.

Mixed Venous Oxygen Saturation. This measurement is usually greater than normal (greater than 75%) and reflects impaired cellular oxygen uptake or utilization (or both).

Hypodynamic Phase (Cold Shock). This phase is characterized by a falling cardiac output and increased systemic vascular resistance. In some patients, systemic vascular resistance may remain decreased.

When the heart no longer maintains cardiac output at a level sufficient to compensate for the systemic vasodilation or intravascular volume losses, hypotension follows. Cardiac decompensation may occur because

(1) preload falls below a critical level (hypovolemia); (2) due to cardiac disease, cardiac output is unable to increase beyond a particular level despite increased physiologic demands; and (3) sepsis-induced myocardial depression develops.

Occasionally, intravascular volume loading may restore preload and ventricular performance to a level necessary to normalize blood pressure. In such patients, a hyperdynamic circulation may be reestablished. However, if sepsis continues, volume loading eventually produces no significant increase in ventricular performance because of severe myocardial depression (Figure 16-14).

Systemic vascular resistance may remain low during the hypodynamic phase. In some patients, compensatory vasoconstriction may increase systemic vascular resistance and may produce the clinical picture of cold shock.

Overall, the hypodynamic phase is associated with profound changes in systemic perfusion that result in ischemic dysfunction and rapid damage to multiple organ systems.

Clinical Presentation

Mentation. The patient's level of consciousness falls and may end in stupor or coma. The rate of cerebral deterioration correlates with the rate of cardiovascular deterioration.

Cutaneous Manifestations. The patient's skin is typically cold, clammy, and pale, with peripheral mottling and cyanosis. Gangrenous skin lesions may be present if the patient develops florid DIC.

Heart Rate and Character of Pulse. Tachycardia continues, but the pulses become weak and thready and may become imperceptible at peripheral arteries.

Neck Veins. The normally visible extremity veins are usually collapsed.

Respiratory Rate and Character of Breathing. Although the patient may be tachypneic, ventilatory movements usually become shallow. Altered breathing patterns, such as Cheyne-Stokes respirations, also may be present.

Urine Output. Urine flow rates may be reduced to the point of anuria.

Acid-Base Values. The rapid accumulation of lactic acid overrides the effects of hyperventilation, and metabolic

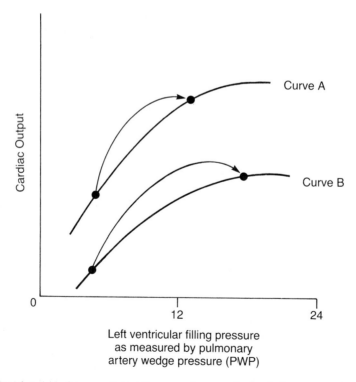

FIGURE 16-14 Deterioration of myocardial performance from septic shock. In *curve A,* the patient is in septic shock without myocardial depression. The decrease in cardiac output is the result of low ventricular filling volume/pressure. Volume loading restores heart function to normal. In *curve B,* the patient is volume depleted but also has myocardial depression. Volume loading fails to restore cardiac performance to an acceptable level.

acidosis prevails. Weak, ineffective ventilatory movements may produce a combined respiratory and metabolic acidosis. *Combined respiratory and metabolic acidosis is an absolute indication for endotracheal intubation and mechanical ventilation because this condition predicts cardiopulmonary collapse.*

Hemodynamic Profile

Arterial Pressure. Hypotension may occur suddenly or over a period of hours. The damped arterial waveform may show a sloped and slowed inotropic component.

Systemic Vascular Resistance. Vascular resistance may remain low, or the patient may be vasoconstricted in response to hypotension. Terminally, SVR may fall to extremely low levels and become unresponsive to vasoconstrictor drugs.

Pulmonary Vascular Resistance. This measurement is likely to be increased to very high levels, particularly in patients with ARDS.

Central Venous Pressure and Right Atrial Pressure. On the one hand, right ventricular failure due to increases in pulmonary vascular resistance or left ventricular failure may elevate these measurements. On the other hand, hypovolemia or decreased right ventricular compliance decreases these values.

Pulmonary Artery Pressure and Wedge Pressure. The direction of change in these measurements can be highly variable as a result of the many abnormalities that frequently coexist in septic patients. Varying combinations of factors make interpretation of these measurements difficult. For example, pulmonary artery pressure and PWP tend to be low if hypovolemia is a dominant problem. By comparison, severe left ventricular dysfunction and failure tend to elevate these measurements. In addition, simultaneous elevations in pulmonary artery systolic and diastolic pressures with a widening of the PAd-PWP gradient are related to elevations in pulmonary vascular resistance.

Cardiac Output. Measurements of cardiac output typically fall over time with the progression of the disease.

Mixed Venous Oxygen Saturation. This measurement is variably affected late in sepsis. The mixed venous oxygen saturation may remain increased because of decreased cellular uptake and utilization of oxygen. Coexisting perfusion failure may override this effect and decrease mixed venous oxygen saturation. Therefore it is possible for the mixed venous oxygen saturation to be increased, decreased (depending on which defect predominates), or normal. In patients with septic shock, however, normal values do not reflect a normal physiologic status but are more likely the result of two physiologic abnormalities oppositely influencing the absolute value.

Treatment. The goals of treatment are identification and elimination of the septic focus, appropriate antibiotic therapy, and measures directed at patient support. Treatment measures are not listed in order of importance. All are important and must be aggressively addressed to maximize patient outcome.

- Maintenance of adequate ventilation and oxygenation. Endotracheal intubation and mechanical ventilation may be necessary.
- Culture and sensitivity of blood, urine, wound drainage, indwelling catheters, and all other possible sites of infection.
- Fluid replacement directed at restoring intravascular volume and ventricular filling pressures to levels that maximize cardiac output.
- Correction of acid-base abnormalities.
- Vasopressor or inotropic drug therapy is indicated in patients in whom blood pressure or cardiac output cannot be maintained by fluid administration alone. Drug therapy is then titrated to optimize the patient's hemodynamic status. Dopamine (Intropin) is commonly used because of its dopaminergic effects, which can increase urine output; dobutamine (Dobutrex) is usually not indicated because of its vasodilator effects; and norepinephrine's (Levophed's) inotropic and vasoconstrictor effects may be useful.
- Intravenous administration of broad-spectrum antibiotics ensures more rapid onset of action and more predictable blood levels than oral or intramuscular dosing. Selection of antibiotics is based on the pathogens known to be prevalent in the observed site of infection, Gram stain smears, and antibiotic sensitivity patterns of flora endogenous to the hospital. Typically, two drugs with activity against gram-negative organisms and *S. aureus* are selected, especially in patients with granulocytopenia. In a patient with suspected sepsis in whom an obvious source is not evident, it is critically important to institute broad-spectrum antibiotic therapy as soon as all cultures are done.
- Removal of the septic focus may require incision and drainage of an abscess, debridement of necrotic or grossly infected tissue, or simply removal of an infected vascular catheter. *The importance of this measure cannot be overemphasized because sepsis continues to ravage the patient until the septic source is eliminated.*
- Treatment for temperatures greater than 102° F (38.5°C) should first begin with antipyretics. If these drugs are inadequate or ineffective, cooling blankets may be necessary.

Investigational Therapies. Despite the extensive research and attention to the problem of hospital-related sepsis and the rapidly expanding number of clinically available antibiotics, the overall incidence of sepsis is increasing and the mortality rate is not decreasing. It seems likely that hope for the future lies in the development of therapies directed at prevention or modification of the complex pathophysiology that characterizes the septic syndromes.

Although high-dose glucocorticoids (methylprednisolone, 30 mg/kg) were routinely recommended and provided throughout the 1970s and 1980s in the treatment of sepsis and septic shock, these antiinflammatory agents have fallen from therapeutic grace. Two multicenter, prospective, double-blind studies have shown that, at best, steroids offer no therapeutic advantage.[4,5] At worst, steroid-treated patients with preexisting renal disease had significantly increased morbidity and mortality rates compared with placebo-treated patients. Currently, *steroids are not recommended in the management of sepsis or septic shock,* although research continues to evaluate the possible therapeutic efficacy of these drugs.

Other experimental therapy agents include antiserum to endotoxin and inflammatory mediator substances, such as tumor necrosis factor and interleukin-1, opiate antagonists, and nonsteroidal antiinflammatory agents. Newer therapies currently being evaluated include bactericidal/permeability increasing protein, lipid A antagonists, and a high-density lipoprotein lipid emulsion that appears to neutralize endotoxin.[6]

Anaphylactic Shock

Anaphylactic shock is the result of an exaggerated systemic allergic reaction to an antigenic substance. Anaphylactic reactions are particularly common in hospitalized patients because of the frequent use of diagnostic and therapeutic antigenic substances.

Causes

A large and varied number of substances are capable of producing anaphylactic reactions. These include anesthetic and analgesic agents, foods, drugs, blood products, diagnostic agents, and venoms (Box 16-4).

Anaphylactic reactions occur more commonly in people with a history of multiple allergies. These people may have a genetically acquired inability to control the immune reaction to certain stimuli. However, anaphylactic reactions also may occur in those with no allergic history.

Pathophysiology

A serious anaphylactic reaction is the culmination of a series of immunologic events. Exposure to an anti-

genic agent (reagin) results in the production of immunoglobulin E (IgE) antibodies. Specific sites on the IgE antibodies bind to the antigen. Next, the IgE molecule attaches to the cell-surface membrane of circulating basophil and tissue mast cells that are found in the respiratory tract, the gastrointestinal tract, and the skin. These cells then become "sensitized" to the antigen. When exposure to the antigen is repeated, the antigen combines with IgE antibodies and activates surface receptors on basophil and mast cells. This process initiates a sequence of biochemical events that leads to the release of mediator substances into the extracellular fluid. These mediator substances include histamine, prostaglandins, kinins, slow-reacting substances of anaphylaxis, platelet activating factor, complement fragments, components of the coagulation cascade, products of the lipoxygenase pathway, and products of arachidonic acid metabolism.

Some substances, such as iodinized radiocontrast material, may directly activate the surface receptors on mast cells and basophils. This means that no prior exposure is required for an anaphylactic reaction to occur. These nonimmunologic reactions are termed *anaphylactoid reactions.* Anaphylactic and anaphylactoid reactions are clinically and hemodynamically indistinguishable.

Systemic release of vasoactive mediator substances produces systemic or pulmonary capillary permeability defects that result in profound third-space fluid losses clinically manifested as severe, generalized swelling and, occasionally, acute pulmonary edema. Mediator-induced coronary vasoconstriction may result in myocardial ischemia or infarction. Patients may develop tachyarrhythmias or conduction disturbances. A generalized arteriolar dilator reaction results in precipitous hypotension. Strong smooth muscle constriction predisposes the patient to bronchospasm and intense abdominal cramping, nausea, vomiting, or diarrhea. Initially, cardiac output increases secondary to the decreases in systemic vascular resistance. However, with progression of the syndrome, cardiac function deteriorates. Systemic activation of the coagulation cascade may result in a mild coagulopathy or, in some patients, fulminant DIC.

Hypovolemia plays a critical role in the hypotension and cardiovascular collapse and has two components: dilation of the vascular bed, which results in a relative hypovolemia, and increased capillary permeability, which results in a functional loss of intravascular volume into the tissue spaces.

Although the hemodynamic and clinical responses may vary from individual to individual, those reactions of a particular individual to a specific antigenic substance

---

BOX 16-4
Agents Commonly Causing Anaphylaxis

Antibiotics
Penicillin and penicillin analogs
Aminoglycosides
Cephalosporins
Tetracyclines
Amphotericin B

Nonsteroidal Antiinflammatory Agents
Salicylates
Colchicine
Ibuprofen

Venoms
Bees
Wasps
Hornets
Yellowjackets
Fire ants
Snakes
Spiders

Local Anesthetics
Lidocaine (Xylocaine)
Procaine

Diagnostic Agents
Iodinized radiocontrast material

Hormones
Insulin
Adrenocorticotropic hormone
Vasopressin

Pollens
Ragweed
Grass

Foods
Eggs
Dairy products
Nuts
Legumes
Shellfish
Citrus fruit
Chocolate
Grains

Dextrans
Rheomacrodex

Narcotic Analgesics/Anesthetics
Thiopental
Morphine
Codeine
Meprobamate

Extracts Used in Desensitization
Blood and Blood Products
Gamma globulin
Plasma
Whole blood

Miscellaneous Drugs
Protamine
Iodides
Thiazide diuretics
Parenteral iron
Heparin

---

tend to recur. The severity and rate of progression of the reaction depend on the amount of the antigen introduced, the route of ingestion, and the allergic potential of the antigen to the individual.

Differential Diagnosis

The time relationship of the onset of symptoms and antigenic exposure is an important diagnostic clue. Bronchospasm and hematuria are nearly pathognomonic of anaphylactic shock. Evaluation of serum histamine, tryptase, and IgE levels helps confirm an acute, antibody-mediated reaction.

Clinical Presentation

Initial symptoms may occur within seconds after exposure to the antigenic substance, but they may be delayed by as much as 1 hour.

Mentation. The patient may complain of pounding in the head, dizziness, or a feeling of impending doom. Restlessness, disorientation, or obtundation may rapidly proceed to coma or seizure activity.

Cutaneous Manifestations. The complexion is variably affected. Hives and itching are common. Because anaphylaxis represents a vasodilator reaction, the patient's skin may be flushed, diaphoretic, and warm. In patients with profound circulatory collapse, the skin is typically ashen. There may be considerable swelling of subcutaneous and mucous tissue.

Heart Rate and Character of Pulse. The heart rate is rapid and may be irregular as a result of rhythm disturbances. The pulses may initially be bounding but then diminish in amplitude.

Airway Response. Cough, runny nose, nasal congestion, hoarseness, and dysphonia are common. Two patterns of airway response are commonly encountered:

1. *Upper airway obstruction due to edema of the larynx, epiglottis, or vocal cords.* Sensations of tightness or a lump in the throat that cannot be cleared with coughing are signs of lesser degrees of airway obstruction or edema. With obstruction of 70% or more of the upper airway, an inspiratory crowing noise (stridor) and dyspnea may precede death by suffocation. *Stridor is an absolute medical emergency and demands emergency intubation.*

2. *Lower airway obstruction due to diffuse bronchoconstriction.* This is characterized by wheezing and profound expiratory effort. Suprasternal, substernal, intercostal, and supraclavicular retractions may be noted as the patient forces rapid inspiration to provide more time for the difficult exhalation. The intercostal spaces may bulge on exhalation.

None of the aforementioned airway responses or one or both of these two responses (upper and lower airway obstruction) can be seen in any patient.

Pulmonary Response. Patients may show clinical evidence of pulmonary edema. Edema fluid, with albumin concentrations identical to those of plasma, may be suctioned from the patient's airways. A pulmonary capillary permeability defect is the likely cause because pulmonary edema occurs in the presence of a low PWP (see Chapter 18). An associated increase in pulmonary vascular resistance, reflected as an increase in PAd-PWP gradient, may be present.

Gastrointestinal Response. The patient may experience nausea, vomiting, intense abdominal cramping, or diarrhea.

Hemodynamic Profile

Arterial Pressure. Systolic and diastolic pressures fall because of vasodilation and intravascular fluid loss. Hypotension can be sudden and dramatic.

Systemic Vascular Resistance. Systemic vasodilation results in a profound generalized decrease in vascular resistance.

Pulmonary Vascular Resistance. Measurements may be normal or elevated as a result of hypoxemia or mediator-induced effects on the pulmonary vasculature.

Central Venous Pressure and Pulmonary Artery and Wedge Pressures. Loss of intravascular volume (third-space shifts) and expansion of the size of the vascular bed proportionately reduce these measurements.

Cardiac Output. Cardiac output may be increased initially as a result of decreased afterload, but then it rapidly falls as a result of reductions in ventricular filling volume, as well as myocardial ischemia due to coronary hypoperfusion. If present, rhythm disturbances further impair cardiac performance.

Mixed Venous Oxygen Saturation. Levels fall below normal when circulatory collapse or severe hypoxemia is present.

Treatment

Treatment of anaphylactic shock involves removal or discontinuation of the offending antigen when applicable and provision of an adequate airway, ventilation, and oxygenation. Upper airway obstruction may require intubation or emergency tracheotomy. Epinephrine is the primary mainstay of pharmacologic therapy. For mild anaphylactic reactions, aqueous epinephrine 1:1000 is given 0.3 to 0.5 ml, intramuscularly or subcutaneously. The dose may be repeated at 5- to 10-minute intervals. For severe reactions, 1 to 5 ml of the 1:10,000 aqueous solution is administered intravenously. This may need to be followed by a continuous infusion of 1 to 4 μg/min. For potentially *life-threatening reactions,* a tourniquet may be placed above the site of introduction of the antigen when applicable (venomous stings and bites). Injection of epinephrine, 0.1 to 0.2 ml of a 1:1000 solution, into the site of antigen introduction may reduce the systemic absorption of venom.

Antihistamines and corticosteroids are useful additions to, but not replacements for, epinephrine. Benadryl is given at an intravenous dose of 25 to 50 mg. Hydrocortisone, 100 to 200 mg intravenously, inhibits the runaway immune response. However, the maximal effect may not be apparent for 4 to 6 hours. Bronchospasm may be treated with intravenous theophylline (Aminophyllin), 5 to 6 mg/kg injected slowly over a 15- to 30-minute period. Rapid administration of this drug may worsen the tachycardia and cardiac ectopic activity, produce seizures, and induce vomiting.

Hypovolemia is corrected with crystalloids or colloids, titrated to maintain an adequate blood pressure. This may require massive amounts of fluids, occasionally as much as 2 to 3 L over a 15-minute period. If hypotensive, the patient is placed in a supine position with a 30-degree elevation of the legs. Persistent hypotension may require vasopressors with alpha-adrenergic activity such as norepinephrine or phenylephrine.

Neurogenic Shock

Neurogenic shock is shock that results from damage to or dysfunction of the sympathetic nervous system.

Causes

Neurogenic shock may be produced by spinal cord damage or pharmacologic blockade of the sympathetic nervous system at the level of T6 or higher. Hypotension due to brain damage or head injury does not occur unless death is imminent or damage is to the brainstem, in which case the patient is apneic.

Typically, arterial systolic pressure rises with increases in intracranial pressure associated with head injury (Cushing response). If a patient with head injury develops hypotension, another cause of hypotension (such as hemothorax, hemoperitoneum) must be aggressively sought, identified, and treated.

Pathophysiology

The neurons of the sympathetic nervous system located in the thoracolumbar portion of the spinal cord depend on stimulation from the brain for maintenance of vasoconstrictive and cardioaccelerator reflexes. The brainstem stimulatory impulses must first traverse the cervical and high thoracic segments of the spinal cord before exiting the central nervous system.

High spinal cord damage or pharmacologic blockade (spinal anesthesia) interrupts the brainstem-mediated vasoconstrictor and cardioaccelerator impulses. The consequent loss of sympathetic nervous system control of arterioles results in a massive vasodilator reaction and pooling of blood in the peripheral circulation. These reactions create relative hypovolemia, a decrease in venous return to the heart, and a consequent decrease in cardiac output. Bradycardia may accentuate hypotension because interruption of the positive chronotropic effects of the sympathetic nervous system leaves the negative chronotropic influences of the parasympathetic (vagal) system unopposed. The higher the level of damage to the cord, the greater the anticipated decrease in arterial pressure and heart rate.

Clinical Presentation

Mentation. Changes in mentation (confusion, lethargy, stupor) may accompany falls in arterial pressure.

Cutaneous Manifestations. The patient's skin is typically warm, pink, and dry and reflects the vasodilated state.

Heart Rate and Character of Pulse. Because of the loss of cardioaccelerator influences in the heart, bradycardia is common in patients with neurogenic shock. The pulse may be normal or of low volume.

Respiratory Response. Paralysis of the intercostal and abdominal muscles often occurs in patients with cervical spinal cord lesions. Paralysis makes ventilation entirely dependent on the diaphragm. Affected patients may exhibit paradoxic respirations. With inspiration the abdomen rises and the thorax collapses as the diaphragm descends. With expiration the abdomen descends and the thorax expands as the diaphragm rises. With high cervical spine lesions or brainstem injury, the patient is likely to be apneic.

Temperature Regulation. Loss of the ability to sweat and passive dilation of the cutaneous vascular bed impair these aspects of the normal thermoregulatory mechanism. Therefore the body temperature of patients with cervical spinal cord lesions tends to equilibrate with that of the environment. This is termed *poikilothermia*. Affected patients must be protected from chilling or overheating.

Patients in neurogenic shock have two significant differences in presentation that are contrary to the "classic" findings of patients in shock: (1) the skin is usually warm and pallor is absent, and (2) the bradycardia persists despite hypotension. In victims of trauma, these findings should immediately suggest injury to the cervical or high thoracic spinal cord. In affected patients, *strict cervical immobilization (such as that employed during endotracheal intubation) is critical to preventing further injury to the spinal cord.*

Hemodynamic Profile

Arterial Pressure. If the patient is maintained in a supine position, the systolic pressure may not fall below 100 mm Hg. Patients with high spinal cord dysfunction are very sensitive to position changes, and profound decrements in stroke volume and blood pressure may occur if the upper portion of the patient's body is elevated.

Systemic Vascular Resistance. Massive vasodilation occurs because of the loss of sympathetic nervous system control of resistance vessels (arterioles). Consequently, SVR falls.

Central Venous Pressure and Pulmonary Artery and Wedge Pressures. These measurements are decreased as a result of the relative hypovolemia.

Cardiac Output. Decreases in cardiac output may occur because of decreases in ventricular filling volume or bradycardia.

Mixed Venous Oxygen Saturation. As cardiac output decreases, this measurement likewise decreases owing to systemic hypoperfusion.

Treatment

The first treatment principle of neurogenic shock is that adequate arterial oxygenation be maintained. This may require insertion of an artificial airway while maintaining strict stabilizing support of the cervical spine, ventilatory support, or both. Crystalloid (electrolyte) solution should be infused at a rate sufficient to maintain a systolic pressure above 100 mm Hg. If injury to the lumbar spine has been ruled out, elevation of the legs may restore an acceptable arterial pressure. Sinus bradycardia secondary to cervical spinal cord injury usually does not require therapy. However, if the heart rate falls below 40 beats per minute or if nodal or ventricular escape rhythms predominate, intravenous atropine, 1.0 mg, may be given in anticipation of mechanical pacemaker placement.

Cardiogenic Shock

Cardiogenic shock (pump failure) occurs when the heart is unable to maintain a cardiac output sufficient to meet the metabolic needs of major organ systems. The organ dysfunction that results begets more deleterious physiologic changes, and a rapid, progressive, downward clinical course follows. Cardiogenic shock is the most severe form of heart failure and is associated with mortality rates in the range of 50% to 100%. Rather than diagnostic reliance on specific hemodynamic measurements alone, clinical and laboratory indications of systemic underperfusion also should be used in evaluating patients for cardiogenic shock.

Although cardiogenic shock is most commonly the result of severely decreased cardiac output, it also may develop in patients with a normal or elevated cardiac output. This may occur when problems, such as anemia, sepsis, hyperthyroidism, or multiple arteriovenous fistulas, require an increased cardiac output, but the patient's heart is unable to mount or maintain an output commensurate with these increased physiologic needs. For example, an anemic patient who normally requires a cardiac output of 10 L/min to maintain adequate resting tissue oxygenation may exhibit signs of shock if cardiovascular disease acutely limits cardiac output to 6 L/min.

Causes

The most common cause of cardiogenic shock is acute myocardial infarction. Discussion of the hemodynamic profile and clinical findings will be specific to cardiogenic shock in acute myocardial infarction. Cardiogenic shock also may be seen in the end stage of many forms of heart disease and a variety of other causes. Predisposing factors include the following:

1. *Acute myocardial infarction* (AMI). Shock is estimated to occur in 10% to 15% of patients who enter the hospital with myocardial infarction. Autopsy studies of cases of AMI cardiogenic shock have demonstrated destruction of 40% to 50% of the total left ventricular muscle mass. Severe triple-vessel disease (70% to 80% obstruction of the three main coronary arteries) is common. If a patient has had preexisting myocardial ischemic damage or another heart disease that has compromised cardiac function, the amount of acute ischemic damage necessary to produce shock may be considerably less than 40%. Cardiogenic shock may also be the result of severe right ventricular damage and dysfunction.

2. *Cardiomyopathy and pericardial disease.* Many types of cardiomyopathy and restrictive pericardial disease, such as pericardial tamponade, may result in an acute or a progressive reduction in cardiac performance that results in shock.

3. *Tachyarrhythmias.* Healthy hearts generally tolerate rapid heart rates well. However, tachycardia may result in shock in patients with preexisting deficiencies in cardiac performance. Rapid heart rates reduce coronary perfusion and ventricular filling time and increase myocardial work and oxygen consumption proportionate to increases in heart rate.

4. *Loss of the atrial contribution to ventricular filling.* In patients with abnormal ventricular function, arrhythmias that result in asynchrony between atria and ventricles (ventricular tachycardia, complete atrioventricular block) or the absence of atrial contraction (atrial fibrillation) may significantly reduce cardiac output.

5. *Bradyarrhythmias.* Shock may result when the heart rate falls in patients whose stroke volume cannot increase proportionately to maintain cardiac output. This may occur in hypovolemic patients or in patients with fibrotic or ischemic heart disease. Bradycardia with signs of shock is particularly common in elderly patients with conduction system disease.

6. *Substances or factors that depress myocardial function.* Acidemia; severe hypoxemia; hypocalcemia; hyperkalemia; hypomagnesemia; and drugs such as beta blockers and calcium-channel blocking agents, quini-

dine, and procainamide have negative inotropic effects. Therefore these factors may result in severe hypoperfusion and shock, particularly in patients with preexisting systolic dysfunction.

7. *Structural heart defects or obstruction to a major pulmonary or systemic blood vessel.* Rupture of the intraventricular septum, grossly abnormal valve function, large intracardiac ball-valve thrombus, rupture of the free wall of the left ventricle, vena caval compression by tumor or hematoma, or massive pulmonary embolism may produce shock because all of these conditions may severely reduce systemic blood flow.

8. *Sequela to major surgery (particularly cardiac surgery) or trauma.* The hemodynamic and metabolic changes that occur as a result of major surgery may predispose the patient to severe cardiac dysfunction.

Pathophysiology

Cardiogenic shock as a result of AMI represents progressive hemodynamic and metabolic deterioration. Myocardial infarction is a dynamic process that involves progressive myocardial necrosis that extends outward from the subendocardium into the surrounding injured and ischemic ventricular myocardium.

In patients with coronary artery disease, coronary blood flow is critically dependent on coronary perfusion pressure (aortic diastolic pressure minus central venous pressure). Therefore a decrease in aortic diastolic pressure may result in an abrupt and often severe fall in coronary blood flow. The "critical" hemodynamic values at which this occurs are patient variable. In some chronically hypertensive people with severe coronary artery disease, symptoms of myocardial ischemia may develop with aortic diastolic pressures within ranges considered "normal." Reductions in coronary blood flow predispose patients to more ischemic myocardial damage and dysfunction, establishing the vicious cycle illustrated in Figure 16-15.

Inadequate coronary and systemic blood flow, in turn, forces anaerobic metabolism that results in metabolic (lactic) acidosis. Other metabolic effects include increases in plasma levels of glucose and free fatty acids mediated by the sympathetic nervous system (stress) response.

Clinical Presentation

Overall, the patient appears gravely ill. This appearance is commonly accompanied by the patient's perception of impending doom.

Mentation. Depending on the severity of circulatory failure, the patient may be restless, apprehensive, confused, irritable, obtunded, or stuporous.

Cutaneous Manifestations. The patient's skin is typically pale, cool, and clammy, with peripheral cyanosis. The complexion may appear ruddy in patients who fail to vasoconstrict to a level appropriate to decreases in cardiac output.

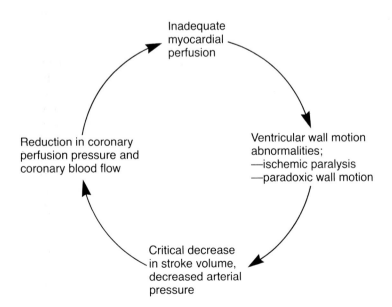

FIGURE 16-15 The self-perpetuating vicious cycle of progressive myocardial damage and dysfunction in AMI shock.

Heart Rate and Character of Pulse. The heart rate is usually greater than 90 beats per minute and may, in part, compensate for the decreased stroke volume. Bradyarrhythmia complicating AMI (sinus bradycardia, junctional rhythm, heart block) frequently causes further deterioration in the hemodynamics. Other disturbances in rhythm (premature atrial beats, atrial fibrillation, premature ventricular beats, ventricular tachycardia) frequently complicate cardiogenic shock. The peripheral pulses are typically weak and thready.

Heart Sounds. The heart sounds are weak and muffled because of the decreased ventricular contractile dynamics (which diminishes the audibility of S_1) and possible decreased diastolic pressure in the aorta (which diminishes S_2). Atrial and ventricular gallops are invariably present, but may be barely audible or inaudible.

Palpation of the Precordium. It may be difficult to perceive precordial activity in the patient because of the weakened ventricular contractions. If heart failure has developed suddenly in a patient with a previously healthy heart, the apex beat is likely to occupy the normal location or may be only slightly displaced leftward. In patients with more long-standing heart failure (several days), the apex beat of the dilated heart is displaced downward and to the left. Wall motion abnormalities and atrial and ventricular gallops, if present, may not be palpable in hypotensive patients.

Neck Veins. The external jugular veins are visibly distended from primary or secondary right ventricular failure.

Respiratory Rate and Character of Breathing. Irregularities in the breathing pattern may coexist with tachypnea. If pulmonary edema is present, the patient also complains of dyspnea. The overall increased work of breathing, which is caused by the development of pulmonary edema, diverts a greater percent of cardiac output to the respiratory muscles. This further reduces blood flow to other major organ systems.

Lung Sounds. In patients with pulmonary edema with alveolar flooding, bilateral adventitious lung sounds are diffusely audible. Otherwise, the lungs are clear.

Urine Output. The patient produces a small volume of concentrated urine—usually less than 30 ml/hr. Recent diuretic therapy invalidates urine output and specific gravity as assessment parameters.

Acid-Base Changes. Metabolic acidosis, hypoxemia, and hypocapnia are typical laboratory findings. The severity of these abnormalities is related to the severity of shock.

Hemodynamic Effects

Two forms of myocardial dysfunction occur during an acute ischemic attack: contractile failure (systolic dysfunction) and a decrease in myocardial compliance (diastolic dysfunction). Both have significant hemodynamic implications.

Systolic Dysfunction May Result in a Significant Decrease in Stroke Volume and Significant Reflex Increases in Systemic Vascular Resistance. Regional contractile defects (hypokinesis, akinesis, dyskinesis) compromise ventricular function proportionate to the size and extent of ventricular ischemic involvement. The resulting decrease in stroke volume is associated with a compensatory increase in SVR. Vasoconstriction serves two purposes: (1) to shunt the decreased stroke volume to vital organs and (2) to support mean arterial pressure.

Systemic vasoconstriction reduces blood flow to large areas of tissue. As it becomes more difficult for blood to flow beyond the constricted arterioles into the capillary bed, it becomes more difficult for the left ventricle to eject blood into the arterial circulation. This is particularly true for a compromised left ventricle. Therefore stroke volume and cardiac output are further decreased, whereas myocardial oxygen requirements are increased.

Some patients with AMI develop abnormal vascular reflexes, and thus systemic vascular resistance may increase only slightly or may actually decrease. In affected patients, significant hypotension may be present, although cardiac output may not be significantly reduced. This abnormal vascular response has been attributed to the activation of left ventricular stretch receptors that are more numerous within the inferior wall of the left ventricle. Stimulation of stretch receptors, in turn, causes stimulation of vagal receptors that produce slowing of heart rate and vasodilation. Hypotension and bradycardia follow as a result. This is the so-called Bezold-Jarisch reflex and is seen more commonly in patients with inferior wall infarctions.

Diastolic Dysfunction (Decreased Ventricular Compliance) Impairs Ventricular Filling and Alters the Ventricular Volume/Pressure Relationship. Because of stiff, unyielding left ventricular walls, for any given ventricular filling volume the filling pressure (as reflected by PWP) is higher than it would be normally. Because intraventricular end-diastolic volume, not pressure, determines ventricular output, a significant reduction in the patient's cardiac output may occur with little or no change in the measured PWP.

Hemodynamic Profile

Arterial Pressure. A systolic pressure of less than 80 to 90 mm Hg is characteristic of, but not a necessary prerequisite for, cardiogenic shock. A patient known to be previously hypertensive may have a significant fall in arterial pressure, but the absolute systolic pressure may exceed 90 mm Hg. The arterial waveform appears damped and has a diminished inotropic component. The slurred upstroke and delayed rate of rise reflect the reduced force of ventricular contraction and decreased acceleration of blood flow into the aorta.

Systemic Vascular Resistance. Sympathetic nervous system stimulation may increase SVR to greater than 2000 dynes/sec/cm^{-5}. As mentioned, the SVR of some patients may increase only slightly or may even be in the low-normal range. In end-stage cardiogenic shock, SVR falls and cannot be restored.

Pulmonary Vascular Resistance. If hypoxemia or acidemia is present, this measurement is increased. If the patient's condition is complicated by pulmonary edema, pulmonary vascular resistance may increase to levels sufficient to produce right ventricular failure.

Central Venous Pressure and Right Atrial Pressure. These measurements are elevated in patients with ischemic involvement of the right ventricle. In patients with pure left ventricular involvement, these measurements are elevated only if pulmonary artery pressures are sufficiently high to produce right ventricular failure.

Pulmonary Artery Pressure and Wedge Pressure. Because ischemic disease more commonly involves the left ventricle, the PWP is usually elevated in patients with cardiogenic shock. Pulmonary artery pressure, and then right ventricular pressures, may ultimately increase as blood is dammed in the vascular and cardiac structures proximal to the failing left ventricle. However, some patients have relatively low PWP measurements because of fluid losses from diuretic therapy, nausea and vomiting, or diaphoresis. In these patients, carefully monitored fluid challenges (preload augmentation) may significantly improve myocardial performance and cardiac output.

When right ventricular ischemic failure is the predominant problem, pulmonary blood flow and left ventricular filling are inadequate. As a result, pulmonary artery pressures and PWP decrease, and left ventricular stroke volume likewise decreases. Right ventricular failure also results in anatomic distortion of the heart. In health, the left ventricular end-diastolic pressure is slightly higher than the right—4 to 12 mm Hg and 0 to 8 mm Hg, respectively. In patients with right ventricular failure, the right ventricular end-diastolic pressure becomes greater than that of the left ventricle and shifts the intraventricular septum toward the left ventricle. Septal shift, in turn, may narrow the left ventricular outflow tract and may diminish the systolic and diastolic volume capacity of the left ventricle. This, in turn, distorts the left ventricular volume/pressure relationship (see Chapter 18, Figure 18-1). Consequently, measured PWP may be misleadingly high, relative to ventricular end-diastolic volume.

Cardiac Output. Ischemic ventricular dysfunction is associated with a decrease in the force of the isovolumetric and ejection phases of systole, which results in a decrease in stroke volume and cardiac output.

Mixed Venous Oxygen Saturation. Measurements fall relative to the severity of perfusion failure as the venous oxygen reserve is drawn on to maintain tissue oxygen needs. This measurement may be further reduced if arterial oxygen content is reduced by hypoxemia.

Treatment

Goals in the management of AMI shock are to (1) improve myocardial oxygen supply by increasing aortic diastolic pressure and coronary blood flow, as well as ensuring adequate arterial oxygenation; (2) decrease myocardial oxygen requirements by decreasing heart work; and (3) optimize cardiac output and systemic perfusion.

The following measures are instituted to fulfill these goals.

Maintain Adequate Ventilation and Arterial P_{O_2} Greater Than 80 mm Hg (O_2 Saturation Greater Than 95%). If there is any question about the adequacy of ventilation, the patient should be intubated and assisted with mechanical ventilation.

Restore Coronary Perfusion. Immediate reperfusion of damaged myocardium may not only salvage jeopardized muscle but also restore cardiac function and reverse shock. In this respect, clot-dissolving agents, such as streptokinase and tissue plasminogen activator, are routinely used to dissolve thrombi that may have acutely occluded coronary vessels. However, it is becoming more common for patients with myocardial infarction who are in cardiogenic shock to be taken to the catheterization laboratory for angiography of the coronary vessels, as a means of defining the extent of the precipitating lesion, and restoring flow via angioplasty or stenting. Coronary artery bypass has also been used as treatment for cardiogenic shock in patients with multiple-vessel disease. Stabilization with the intraaortic balloon pump is recommended before, during, and after both interventions.

Relieve Pain and Provide Rest for the Patient. Morphine titrated in small doses at frequent intervals is generally regarded as the drug of choice for treating AMI pain. Morphine analgesia reduces sympathetic nervous system stimulation, thereby decreasing the potential for arrhythmias, as well as myocardial and systemic oxygen requirements. Other effects of morphine include diminishing diaphoresis and fluid losses; reducing preload, which decreases myocardial oxygen demands and relieves pulmonary vascular congestion; and inducing a sense of well-being to facilitate patient rest.

Control Rhythm Disturbances. Conduction disturbances may be managed with pacing or atropine. Antiarrhythmic agents for the treatment of ectopic arrhythmias are to be used cautiously because of their potential myocardial depressive effect.

Optimize Ventricular Filling Volume and Pressure. Hypovolemia secondary to nausea, vomiting, diuretic therapy, third-space losses, or diaphoresis may complicate AMI shock. Because preload is an important determinant of ventricular performance, ventricular filling may have to be increased by fluid challenges to right atrial pressure or PWP levels that optimize right or left ventricular performance.

In patients with heart disease, the filling pressures required to optimize cardiac output are typically greater than those considered as the upper normal limit for the involved ventricle. In patients with AMI, a left ventricular filling pressure of approximately 15 to 18 mm Hg may be required to increase cardiac output and restore arterial pressure to acceptable levels. With right ventricular impairment, a filling pressure as high as 15 mm Hg may be required to optimize right ventricle output and left ventricular filling.

If, however, the left ventricular filling pressure exceeds 20 to 22 mm Hg or if pulmonary edema is present, diuretics or venodilator agents may be required to lower preload to a level more beneficial for the individual patient.

Make Pharmacologic Adjustments in Systemic Vascular Resistance. Low cardiac output is commonly accompanied by compensatory increases in SVR, which,

unfortunately, elevates the left ventricular afterload. Drugs that dilate the systemic arteries ease left ventricular emptying. Consequently, stroke volume is increased and systemic perfusion is improved, whereas myocardial work and oxygen consumption are decreased. When these drugs are given to patients in severe left ventricular failure, the increase in stroke volume may offset the vasodilator effects on the arterial pressure, and mean arterial pressure may remain unchanged or actually may rise. Vasodilator therapy should not be attempted in patients with systolic pressures of less than 90 mm Hg, however, because of the risk of a further drop in blood pressure that could seriously compromise coronary or cerebral blood flow.

As a counterpoint, patients with severe hypotension may require treatment with drugs that increase systemic vascular resistance; most of these drugs are also positive inotropic agents. Although medications that increase systemic vascular resistance may further decrease stroke volume and systemic perfusion (by increasing ventricular outflow resistance), the maintenance of a central aortic pressure compatible with adequate coronary and cerebral perfusion is of paramount importance for the immediate support of the patient's life. A measurement commonly used clinically is a minimum mean arterial pressure of 55 mm Hg. However, *the fact that this is a minimum mean arterial pressure for normal people is emphasized because chronically hypertensive patients or those with severe coronary or cerebral vascular disease may experience significant reductions in myocardial or cerebral blood flow at mean arterial pressure measurements that are normal or slightly below normal.*

Provide Inotropic Support for the Heart. Drugs that improve cardiac output by increasing myocardial contractility may have the undesirable effect of increasing automaticity, myocardial oxygen requirements, or SVR. The concomitant administration of a vasodilator agent, such as nitroprusside (Nipride), may offset the vasoconstrictive effect of the commonly used inotropes, thereby further increasing cardiac output and peripheral blood flow. Box 16-5 lists vasoactive medications that also have inotropic effects. (See Chapter 14 for a discussion of the properties of inotropic agents used in the ICU setting.)

Digitalis, a relatively weak inotrope, is generally not a first-line agent in the treatment of shock. Metabolic and oxygenation abnormalities associated with shock predispose patients to potentially lethal digitalis-induced arrhythmias.

Implicit in the discussion of pharmacologic management of cardiogenic shock is an understanding that any anticipated benefit also may carry a risk. For example, if

---

BOX 16-5
Vasoactive Agents with Inotropic Effects

Inotropic Agents That Have a Vasoconstrictor Effect on the Peripheral Vasculature

Epinephrine (Adrenalin)
Norepinephrine (Levophed)
Dopamine (Intropin)—at doses usually greater than
  20 μg/kg/min
Digitalis—mild

Inotropic Agents That Have a Vasodilator Effect on the Peripheral Vasculature

Isoproterenol (Isuprel)
Dobutamine (Dobutrex)
Dopamine (Intropin)—at low to moderate doses
Amrinone (Inocor)
Milrinone (Primacor)
Dopexamine (experience in the United States is limited,
  not yet approved by the Food and Drug Administration)

---

vasodilators are given for ventricular unloading, coronary perfusion pressure may drop below a critical level, thereby increasing myocardial ischemia. If, however, arterial pressure is raised with vasoconstrictors to improve coronary perfusion pressure, systemic blood flow may be sacrificed. The higher afterload may also increase myocardial oxygen requirements enough to exacerbate ischemia. *The individual patient's hemodynamic profile dictates the pharmacologic approach, and the patient's clinical response (level of ischemic pain, mental status, skin color, urine output) determines whether the overall pharmacologic effect is beneficial or harmful.*

Institute Therapy with the Intraaortic Balloon Pump (Balloon Counterpulsation). The intraaortic balloon pump is a mechanical counterpulsation device that benefits patients in cardiogenic shock by reducing afterload and increasing coronary and systemic blood flow (see Chapter 15). With improvement in systemic perfusion, major organ function improves. Clinical evidence is an increase in urine output, mentation improvement, intestinal motility return, and resolution of lactic acidosis. In many patients, initiation of intraaortic balloon pumping is quickly followed by startling clinical improvement and reversal of shock. Occasionally, however, as balloon pumping is discontinued, some patients whose condition appeared to be stable during balloon counterpulsation suddenly experience clinical and hemodynamic deterioration.

Some patients expire suddenly during or following balloon counterpulsation. The clinical deterioration observed in these patients may be a result of massive cardiac damage that occurred before institution of balloon pumping. For this reason, *it is recommended that the intraaortic balloon counterpulsation be instituted as early in the acute ischemic episode as possible before severe ventricular damage occurs.* Indeed, the intraaortic balloon pump in the management of cardiogenic shock is most successful when it is applied early in acute unstable myocardial infarction, preferably before hemodynamic deterioration occurs. Surgical correction of any anatomic defects, such as ventricular septal rupture or coronary revascularization in conjunction with balloon pumping, offers the greatest long-term benefits.

Ventricular Assist Devices. The term *ventricular assist device* (VAD) is used to describe a variety of mechanical pumps (roller, centrifugal, pulsatile) that may be used to replace the function of either the right or left ventricle.

Whereas the intraaortic balloon pump improves the ratio between myocardial oxygen supply and demand, reduces the workload of a failing ventricle (typically the left), and modestly supports the circulation, the VAD entirely replaces the function of either the right or left ventricle. For the right ventricle, blood is withdrawn from the right atrium and mechanically driven into the pulmonary circulation. For the left ventricle, blood is withdrawn from either the left ventricular apex or left atrium and returned to the ascending aorta via the VAD.

The VAD was initially used for patients with postcardiotomy cardiogenic shock; VAD support can also be used as a bridge to transplantation. Some patients with AMI shock have also had VADs placed for stabilization of the circulation to allow cardiac catheterization and surgical corrective procedures. Use of these devices is currently limited to teaching and research facilities.

OTHER CATEGORIES OF SHOCK

Shock also may occur in association with a wide variety of physiologic abnormalities. On occasion, hypoglycemia, severe endocrine dysfunction, and drug overdose can be associated with shock syndromes. It is beyond the scope of this text to present a discussion of the numerous other causes of shock. In each, the precipitating event has to be identified, the hemodynamic pattern determined, and the specific underlying cause appropriately treated.

In summary, although shock may be considered to be the final common pathway in most forms of death, the focus of treatment should be directed at the fact that many

TABLE 16-7

Guidelines to Anticipated Hemodynamic Changes in Several Types of Shock

Disorder	Arterial Pressure	Pulse Pressure	Systemic Vascular Resistance	Pulmonary Vascular Resistance	Central Venous Pressure	Pulmonary Artery Pressure	Pulmonary Wedge Pressure	Cardiac Output	SvO₂
Hypovolemic									
Compensated	~	↓	↑	~	↓	↓	↓	~↓	↓
Decompensated	↓	↓	↑	↑	↓	↑~↓	↓	↓	↓
Septic*									
Hyperdynamic	~↓	↓~↑	↓	~↑	↓~	↑~↓	~↓	↑	~↑
Hypodynamic	↓	↓	↑~↓	↑	↓~↑	↑~↓	↑~↓	↓	↓~↑
Anaphylactic	↓	↓	↓	~↑	↓	↓	↓	↓	↓
Neurogenic	↓	↓	↓	~	↓	↓		~↓	↓
Cardiogenic	↓	↓	↑~↓	↑	~↑	↑	↑	↓	↓

*The hemodynamic profiles of hyperdynamic and particularly hypodynamic septic shock are quite variable. The magnitude and direction of change of hemodynamic measurements may be affected by coexisting problems or complications. KEY: ↑, increase; ↓, decrease; ~, no change.

shock states can be reversed. Indeed, the "rude unhinging of the machinery of life" often can be repaired and functional survival restored with appropriate diagnosis and therapy. Table 16-7 summarizes the hemodynamic profiles of the various types of shock described in this chapter.

REFERENCES

1. Shenkin HA, Cheney RH, Covons SR, et al: On the diagnosis of hemorrhage in man. A study of volunteers bled large amounts, *Am J Med Sci* 208:421, 1944.
2. Cohn JN: Blood pressure measurements in shock, *JAMA* 199:972, 1967.
3. Carlson RW, Rattan S, Haupt MT: Fluid resuscitation in conditions of increased permeability, *Anesth Rev* 17(suppl 3): 1990.
4. Bone RC, Fisher CJ, Clemmer TP, et al: A controlled clinical trial of high-dose methylprednisolone in the treatment of severe sepsis and septic shock, *N Engl J Med* 317:653, 1987.
5. Veterans Administration Systemic Sepsis Cooperative Study Group: Effect of high dose glucocorticoid therapy on mortality in patients with clinical signs of systemic sepsis, *N Engl J Med* 317:659, 1987.
6. Goldfarb RD, Parker TS, Levine DM, et al: Dose-dependent improvements in survival and cardiovascular status in porcine septic shock by infusion of phospholipid rich emulsion, 2000 (abstract).

SUGGESTED READINGS

Abou-Khalil, Scaelea TM, Trooskin SZ, et al: Hemodynamic responses to shock in young trauma patients: need for invasive monitoring, *Crit Care Med* 22:633, 1994.
Astiz ME, Rackow EC, Weil EC: Circulatory shock. In Carlson RW, Geheb MA, editors: *Principles and practice of medical intensive care,* Philadelphia, 1995, W.B. Saunders.
Chow JL, Baker K, Bigatello LM: Hypotension and shock. In Hurford WE, senior editor: *Critical care handbook of the Massachusetts General Hospital,* ed 3, Philadelphia, 2000, Lippincott Williams & Wilkins.
Darovic G, Rokowsky JS: Shock. In *Medical-surgical nursing: pathophysiologic concepts,* Philadelphia, 1991, JB Lippincott.
Dunham CM, Frankenfield D, Belzberg H, et al: Inflammatory markers: superior predictors of adverse outcome in blunt trauma patients? *Crit Care Med* 22:667, 1994.
Falk JL, O'Brien JF, Kerr R: Fluid resuscitation in traumatic hemorrhage shock, *Crit Care Clin* 8:323, 1992.
Ferguson DW, Abboud FM: The pathophysiology, recognition, and management of shock. In Hurst JW et al, editors: *The heart,* ed 7, New York, 1990, McGraw-Hill.
Ganong WF: Cardiovascular hemostasis in health and disease. In *Review of medical physiology,* ed 19, Stamford, 1999, Appleton & Lange.
Guyton A: Circulatory shock and physiology of treatment. In *Textbook of medical physiology,* ed 8, Philadelphia, 1996, W.B. Saunders.
Holcroft JW, Robinson MK: Shock. In *American College of Surgeons care of the surgical patient,* vol I, *Critical care,* New York, 1993, Scientific American Medicine.
Jiminez EJ: Shock. In Civetta JM, Taylor RW, Kirby RR, editors: *Critical care,* ed 3, Philadelphia, 1997, Lippincott-Raven.
Kruse JA: Lactic acidosis. In Carlson RS, Geheb MA, editors: *Principles and practice of medical intensive care,* Philadelphia, 1993, W.B. Saunders.
Kumar A, Parillo JE, Bone RC, editors: *Critical care medicine: principles of diagnosis and management,* St Louis, 1995, Mosby.
Reilly PM, Schiller HJ, Bulkley GB: Reactive metabolites in shock. In *American College of Surgeons care of the surgical patient,* vol I, *Critical care,* New York, 1993, Scientific American Medicine.

Rubertson S: Resuscitation. In Grenvik A et al, editors: *Textbook of critical care,* Philadelphia, 1996, W.B. Saunders.

Shoemaker WC: Shock states: pathophysiology, monitoring, outcome prediction, and therapy. In Shoemaker W et al, editors: *Textbook of critical care medicine,* Philadelphia, 1989, W.B. Saunders.

Weil MH, von Planta M, Rackow EC: Acute circulatory failure (shock). In Braunwald E, editor: *Heart diseases: a textbook of cardiovascular medicine,* Philadelphia, 1988, W.B. Saunders.

Wilson RW: Shock. In *Critical care manual,* ed 2, Philadelphia, 1992, FA Davis.

Hypovolemic Shock

Shamji FM, Todd TRJ: Hypovolemic shock, *Crit Care Clin* 1:609, 1985.

Shenkin HA, Cheney RH, Covons SR, et al: On the diagnosis of hemorrhage in man: a study of volunteers bled large amounts, *Am J Med Sci* 208:421, 1944.

Septic Shock

Abraham E, Matthay MA, Dinarello CA, et al: Consensus conference definitions for sepsis, septic shock, acute lung injury, and acute respiratory distress syndrome: time for a reevaluation, *Crit Care Med* 28:232, 2000.

Alia I, Esteban A, Gordo F, et al: A randomized and controlled trial of the effect of treatment aimed at maximizing oxygen delivery in patients with severe sepsis or septic shock [see comments], *Chest* 115:453, 1999.

Astiz ME, Rackow EC: Septic shock, *Lancet* 351:1501, 1998.

Balk RA: Severe sepsis and septic shock. Definitions, epidemiology, and clinical manifestations, *Crit Care Clin* 16:179, 2000.

Balk RA: Pathogenesis and management of multiple organ dysfunction or failure in severe sepsis and septic shock, *Crit Care Clin* 16:337, 2000.

Barriere SL, Guglielmo BJ: Gram-negative sepsis, the sepsis syndrome, and the role of antiendotoxin monoclonal antibodies, *Clin Pharmacokinet* 11:223, 1992.

Briegel J, Forst H, Haller M, et al: Stress doses of hydrocortisone reverse hyperdynamic septic shock: a prospective, randomized, double-blind, single-center study [see comments], *Crit Care Med* 27:723, 1999.

Casey LC: Immunologic response to infection and its role in septic shock, *Crit Care Clin* 16:193, 2000.

Fein AM, Calalang-Colucci MG: Acute lung injury and acute respiratory distress syndrome in sepsis and septic shock, *Crit Care Clin* 16:289, 2000.

Frank ED: Septic shock. 1964 [classic article], *Int Anesthesiol Clin* 37:129, 1999.

Hardaway RM: The etiology and treatment of traumatic and septic shock, *Compr Ther* 25:330, 1999.

Hardaway RM: A review of septic shock, *Am Surg* 66:22, 2000.

Hatherill M, Tibby SM, Hilliard T, et al: Adrenal insufficiency in septic shock, *Arch Dis Child* 80:51, 1999.

Jindal N, Hollenberg SM, Dellinger RP: Pharmacologic issues in the management of septic shock, *Crit Care Clin* 16:233, 2000.

Klosterhalfen B, Bhardwaj RS: Septic shock, *Gen Pharmacol* 31:25, 1998.

Kumar A, Haery C, Parrillo JE: Myocardial dysfunction in septic shock, *Crit Care Clin* 16:251, 2000.

Lowry SF: Sepsis and its complications: clinical definitions and therapeutic prospects, *Crit Care Med* 22:S1, 1994.

Lundberg JS, Perl TM, Wiblin T, et al: Septic shock: an analysis of outcomes for patients with onset on hospital wards versus intensive care units [see comments], *Crit Care Med* 26:1020, 1998.

Meduri GU: New rationale for glucocorticoid treatment in septic shock, *J Chemother* 11:541, 1999.

Mizock BA: Metabolic derangements in sepsis and septic shock, *Crit Care Clin* 16:319, 2000.

Murphy K et al: Molecular biology of septic shock, *New Horiz* 6:181, 1998.

Reyes WJ, Brimioulle S, Vincent JL: Septic shock without documented infection: an uncommon entity with a high mortality, *Intensive Care Med* 25:1267, 1999.

Schelling G, Stoll C, Kapfhammer HP, et al: The effect of stress doses of hydrocortisone during septic shock on posttraumatic stress disorder and health-related quality of life in survivors, *Crit Care Med* 27:2678, 1999.

Shands KN, Schmid GP, Dan BB, et al: Toxic shock syndrome in menstruating women—association with tampon use and *Staphylococcus aureus* and clinical features in 52 cases, *N Engl J Med* 303:1436, 1980.

Smith AL: Treatment of septic shock with immunotherapy, *Pharmacotherapy* 18:565, 1998.

Stevens RA: The occurrence of *Staphylococcus aureus* infection with a scarlatiniform rash, *JAMA* 88:1957, 1927.

Suffedini AF: Current prospects for the treatment of clinical sepsis, *Crit Care Med* 22:S12, 1994.

Taylor RW: Sepsis, septic syndrome and septic shock. In Civetta JM, Taylor RW, Kirby RR, editors: *Critical care,* ed 2, Philadelphia, 1992, JB Lippincott.

Ziegler EJ et al: Treatment of gram-negative bacteremia and septic shock with HA-IA human monoclonal antibody against endotoxin, *N Engl J Med* 324:429, 1991.

Anaphylactic Shock

Haupt MT, Carlson RW: Anaphylactic and anaphylactoid reactions. In Shoemaker W et al, editors: *Textbook of critical care,* Philadelphia, 1989, W.B. Saunders.

Hollingsworth HM, Giansiracusa DF, Upchurch KS: Anaphylaxis. In Rippe JM et al, editors: *Intensive care medicine,* ed 2, Boston, 1991, Little, Brown.

Levy JH: *Anaphylactic reactions in anesthesia and intensive care,* ed 2, Boston, 1992, Butterworth Heinemann.

Neurogenic Shock

Gennarelli T, Trunkey DD, Blaisdell FW: Trauma to the central nervous system. In *American College of Surgeons care of the surgical patient,* vol I, *Critical care,* New York, 1993, Scientific American Medicine.

Cardiogenic Shock

Akyurekli MD et al: Effectiveness of intra-aortic balloon counterpulsation on systolic unloading, *Can J Surg* 23:122, 1984.

Alpert JS, Becker RC: Cardiogenic shock: elements of etiology, diagnosis, and therapy, *Clin Cardiol* 16:182, 1993.

Alpert JS, Becker RC: Mechanisms and management of cardiogenic shock, *Crit Care Clin* 9:205, 1993.

Andrews WR, Arnold JM, Sibbald WJ: Threatened reinfarction. Effective therapy using streptokinase with reversal of cardiogenic shock, *Chest* 98:495, 1990.

Barry WL, Sarembock IJ: Cardiogenic shock: therapy and prevention, *Clin Cardiol* 21:72, 1998.

Bartel AG: Resuscitation from cardiogenic shock by direct angioplasty and 23-hour balloon inflation using a coronary perfusion balloon, *J Invasive Cardiol* 6:241, 1994.

Bates ER: Coronary angioplasty in cardiogenic shock, *Rev Port Cardiol* 18(suppl 1):I71, 1999.

Bates ER, Stomel RJ, Hochman JS, et al: The use of intraaortic balloon counterpulsation as an adjunct to reperfusion therapy in cardiogenic shock, *Int J Cardiol* 65(suppl 1):S37, 1998.

Bates ER, Topol EJ: Limitations of thrombolytic therapy for acute myocardial infarction complicated by congestive heart failure and cardiogenic shock, *J Am Coll Cardiol* 18:1077, 1991.

Bengtson JR, Kaplan AJ, Pieper KS, et al: Prognosis in cardiogenic shock after acute myocardial infarction in the interventional era, *J Am Coll Cardiol* 20:1482, 1992.

Berger PB, Holmes DR Jr, Stebbins AL, et al: Impact of an aggressive invasive catheterization and revascularization strategy on mortality in patients with cardiogenic shock in the Global Utilization of Streptokinase and Tissue plasminogen activator for Occluded coronary arteries (GUSTO-I) trial. An observational study, *Circulation* 96:122, 1997.

Berger PB, Tuttle RH, Holmes DR Jr, et al: One-year survival among patients with acute myocardial infarction complicated by cardiogenic shock, and its relation to early revascularization: results from the GUSTO-I trial, *Circulation* 99:873, 1999.

Beyersdorf F, Buckberg GD: Myocardial protection in patients with acute myocardial infarction and cardiogenic shock, *Semin Thorac Cardiovasc Surg* 5:151, 1993.

Califf RM, Bengtson JR: Cardiogenic shock, *N Engl J Med* 330:1724, 1994.

Chaterjee S, Rosenweig J: Evaluation of intra-aortic balloon counterpulsation, *J Thorac Cardiovasc Surg* 61:405, 1971.

Chilian WM, Marcus ML: Phasic coronary blood flow velocity in intramural and epicardial coronary arteries, *Circ Res* 50:775, 1982.

Chou TM et al: Cardiogenic shock: thrombolysis or angioplasty? *J Intensive Care Med* 11:37, 1996.

Craver JM, Hatcher CR: The percutaneous intraaortic balloon pump. In Hurst JW, editor: *The heart,* New York, 1990, McGraw-Hill.

Daily EK: Use of hemodynamics to differentiate pathophysiologic causes of cardiogenic shock, *Crit Care Nurs Clin North Am* 1:589, 1989.

Dzavik V, Burton JR, Kee C, et al: Changing practice patterns in the management of acute myocardial infarction complicated by cardiogenic shock: elderly compared with younger patients, *Can J Cardiol* 14:923, 1998.

Feld H: New treatment strategies for cardiogenic shock in acute MI. Management options depend on the availability of a cath lab, *J Crit Illn* 7:1277, 1992.

Gacioch GM, Ellis SG, Lee L, et al: Cardiogenic shock complicating acute myocardial infarction: the use of coronary angioplasty and the integration of the new support devices into patient management [see comments], *J Am Coll Cardiol* 19:647, 1992.

Gawlinski A: Saving the cardiogenic shock patient, *Nursing* 19:34, 1989.

Goldberg RJ, Samad NA, Yarzebski J, et al: Temporal trends in cardiogenic shock complicating acute myocardial infarction, *N Engl J Med* 340:1162, 1999.

Goldenberg IF: Nonpharmacologic management of cardiac arrest and cardiogenic shock, *Chest* 102(5 suppl 2):596S, 1992.

Hasdai D, Holmes DR Jr, Califf RM, et al: Cardiogenic shock complicating acute myocardial infarction: predictors of death. GUSTO Investigators. Global Utilization of Streptokinase and Tissue-plasminogen activator for Occluded coronary arteries, *Am Heart J* 138(1 pt 1):21, 1999.

Hochman JS, Boland J, Sleeper LA, et al: Current spectrum of cardiogenic shock and effect of early revascularization on mortality. Results of an International Registry. SHOCK Registry Investigators [see comments], *Circulation* 91:873, 1995.

Hochman JS, Sleeper LA, Godfrey E, et al: Should we emergently revascularize occluded coronaries for cardiogenic shock: an international randomized trial of emergency PTCA/CABG-trial design. The SHOCK Trial Study Group, *Am Heart J* 137:313, 1999.

Hochman JS, Sleeper LA, Webb JG, et al: Early revascularization in acute myocardial infarction complicated by cardiogenic shock. SHOCK Investigators. Should we emergently revascularize occluded coronaries for cardiogenic shock [see comments], *N Engl J Med* 341:625, 1999.

Hollenberg SM, Kavinsky CJ, Parrillo JE: Cardiogenic shock, *Ann Intern Med* 131:47, 1999.

Kovack PJ, Rasak MA, Bates ER, et al: Thrombolysis plus aortic counterpulsation: improved survival in patients who present to community hospitals with cardiogenic shock, *J Am Coll Cardiol* 29:1454, 1997.

Leor J, Goldbourt U, Reicher-Reiss H, et al: Cardiogenic shock complicating acute myocardial infarction in patients without heart failure on admission: incidence, risk factors, and outcome. SPRINT Study Group, *Am J Med* 94:265, 1993.

Levine GN, Hochman JS: Thrombolysis in acute myocardial infarction complicated by cardiogenic shock, *J Thromb Thrombolysis* 2:11, 1995.

McGhie AI, Golstein RA: Pathogenesis and management of acute heart failure and cardiogenic shock: role of inotropic therapy, *Chest* 102(5 suppl 2):626S, 1992.

Menon V, Hochman JS: Reference guide to cardiogenic shock complicating acute myocardial infarction, *J Thromb Thrombolysis* 9:95, 2000.

Moosvi AR, Khaja F, Villanueva L, et al: Early revascularization improves survival in cardiogenic shock complicating acute myocardial infarction [see comments], *J Am Coll Cardiol* 19:907, 1992.

Moscucci M, Bates ER: Cardiogenic shock, *Cardiol Clin* 13:391, 1995.

Moulopoulos SD, Stamateolopoulos SF, Nanas JN, et al: Effect of protracted dobutamine infusion on survival of patients in cardiogenic shock treated with intraaortic balloon pumping, *Chest* 103:248, 1993.

Mueller HS: Management of acute myocardial infarction. In Shoemaker W et al, editors: *Textbook of critical care,* Philadelphia, 1989, W.B. Saunders.

Mueller HS: Role of intra-aortic counterpulsation in cardiogenic shock and acute myocardial infarction, *Cardiology* 84:168, 1994.

O'Neal PV: How to spot early signs of cardiogenic shock, *Am J Nurs* 94:36, 1994.

Perez-Castellano N, Garcia E, Serrano JA, et al: Efficacy of invasive strategy for the management of acute myocardial infarction complicated by cardiogenic shock, *Am J Cardiol* 83:989, 1999.

Reedy JE, Swartz MT, Raithel SC, et al: Mechanical cardiopulmonary support for refractory cardiogenic shock, *Heart Lung* 19(5 pt 1):514, 1990.

Robinson N: Cardiology update. Cardiogenic shock, *Nurs Stand* 8:48, 1993.

Seydoux C, Goy JJ, Beuret P, et al: Effectiveness of percutaneous transluminal coronary angioplasty in cardiogenic shock during acute myocardial infarction, *Am J Cardiol* 69:968, 1992.

Shawl FA et al: Emergency percutaneous cardiopulmonary bypass support in cardiogenic shock from acute myocardial infarction, *Am J Cardiol* 64:967, 1989.

Stomel RJ, Rasak M, Bates ER: Treatment strategies for acute myocardial infarction complicated by cardiogenic shock in a community hospital, *Chest* 105:997, 1994.

Teba L, Banks DE, Balaan MR: Understanding circulatory shock. Is it hypovolemic, cardiogenic, or vasogenic? *Postgrad Med* 91:121, 1992.

Wojner AW: Assessing five points of the intra-aortic balloon pump waveform, *Crit Care Nurse* 14:48, 1994.

17

BARRY A. MIZOCK and GLORIA OBLOUK DAROVIC

Monitoring the Patient with Multiple-System Organ Dysfunction

HISTORICAL PERSPECTIVE

The syndrome of multiple-system organ failure (MSOF) has its historical basis in the management of patients having suffered severe trauma. Awareness of MSOF arose paradoxically as the result of advances in supportive therapy. This can be illustrated by reviewing the epidemiology of combat-related death during modern times. Before World War II, the major cause of death was hemorrhagic shock. During World War II and the Korean War, advances in transfusion therapy reduced the rate of death due to blood loss and enabled the initial stabilization of soldiers who would otherwise have died. Renal failure then emerged as a major cause of death. The hemodialyzer was invented in 1938 by Kolff; however, it was not introduced into the United States until the late 1940s and was not effectively used by the military until the time of the Vietnam War. It was during this time that a syndrome of posttraumatic pulmonary edema with oxygenation failure, termed *Da Nang lung* and now known as acute respiratory distress syndrome (ARDS), became recognized as a major cause of death. During the 1970s, the management of patients with ARDS was greatly facilitated by the application of positive end-expiratory pressure (PEEP) during mechanical ventilation. Although PEEP was noted to improve oxygenation, a significant decrease in mortality rate did not occur. Thus it appeared that technologic advances in organ support did not appreciably alter mortality rates in severe traumatic injury.

The initial report of MSOF is attributed to Skillman and co-workers,[1] who in the late 1960s described concurrent respiratory failure, sepsis, and jaundice in intensive care unit (ICU) patients with erosive gastritis. Tilney and colleagues[2] subsequently recognized sequential system failure following surgical treatment of ruptured abdominal aortic aneurysm. By the mid-1970s, posttraumatic MSOF was well described. In 1992 a consensus conference of the American College of Chest Physicians and the Society of Critical Care Medicine proposed that the term *multiple-organ dysfunction syndrome* (MODS) replace MSOF.[3] This recommendation acknowledged the fact that the term *multiple-organ dysfunction syndrome* better represents the continuum of organ dysfunction that exists clinically.

Multiple-organ dysfunction syndrome is the major cause of death in surgical and trauma ICUs and also in noncardiac medical ICUs. The incidence of MODS is difficult to determine because of the variability in definitions and scoring systems in clinical practice. In 1985 Knaus and colleagues[4] revealed that 49% of critically ill patients experience failure of one organ system before ICU discharge and 15% experience failure of more than one organ system. The average ICU stay of patients with MODS is 21 days. Survivors may require rehabilitation lasting 10 to 12 months with costs of $500,000 or more. The toll in human suffering, permanent disability, and lost lives is incalculable.

Our present inability to make a significant impact on the outcome of patients with severe illness or injury underscores the futility of treating isolated organ dysfunction without controlling the systemic pathophysiology that underlies multiple organ dysfunction or failure. This is the therapeutic goal for the future.

BOX 17-1
Definitions of Organ System Failure

Cardiovascular Failure (Presence of One or More of the Following)

Heart rate $\leq$ 54 beats per minute

Mean arterial blood pressure $\leq$ 49 mm Hg (systolic blood pressure < 60 mm Hg)

Occurrence of ventricular tachycardia or ventricular fibrillation or both

Serum pH $\leq$ 7.24 with $PaCO_2$ $\leq$ 49 mm Hg

Respiratory Failure (Presence of One or More of the Following)

Respiratory rate $\leq$ 5 breaths per minute or $\geq$ 49 breaths per minute

$PaCO_2$ $\geq$ 50 mm Hg

Arterial-alveolar oxygen tension difference $\geq$ 350 mm Hg

Dependent on ventilator or continuous positive airway pressure on the second day of organ system failure

Renal Failure (Excludes Patients on Chronic Dialysis) (One or More of the Following)

Urine output $\leq$ 479 ml/24 hr or $\leq$ 159 ml/8 hr

Serum blood urea nitrogen $\geq$ 100 mg/100 ml

Serum creatinine $\geq$ 3.5 mg/100 ml

Hematologic Failure (Presence of One or More of the Following)

White blood cell count $\leq$ 1000/mm³

Platelets $\leq$ 20,000/mm³

Hematocrit $\leq$ 20%

Hepatic Failure (Presence of Both of the Following)

Bilirubin > 6 mg%

Prothrombin time > 4 seconds over control in absence of systemic anticoagulation

Neurologic Failure

Glasgow Coma Score $\leq$ 6 (in absence of sedation)

From Knaus WA, Wagner DP: Multiple systems organ failure: epidemiology and prognosis, *Crit Care Clin* 5:223, 1989.

DEFINITION

Multiple-organ dysfunction is a syndrome of sequential organ system dysfunction that follows resuscitation from severe traumatic, medical, or surgical insult. If the underlying cause is not corrected or the patient is not properly supported, organ failure may follow. The organs involved are frequently distant from the primary area of injury or infec-

tion. MODS is characterized by the presence of deteriorating organ function in an acutely ill patient such that homeostasis cannot be maintained without medical intervention.

EPIDEMIOLOGY

As mentioned, approximately 15% of patients admitted to the ICU will meet criteria for failure of more than one organ. The single strongest predictor for the development of MODS is the severity of disease or injury at the time of ICU admission. The next most important risk factor is the diagnosis of sepsis or respiratory infection. Advanced age also predisposes a patient to the development of MODS.

DIAGNOSTIC CRITERIA FOR ORGAN SYSTEM DYSFUNCTION AND FAILURE

The laboratory and clinical parameters that constitute the diagnostic criteria for MODS have not been standardized. A number of scoring systems currently exist that enable assessment of organ dysfunction (e.g., Multiple Organ Dysfunction Score, Sequential Organ Failure Assessment, Logistic Organ Dysfunction System).[5] The severity of MODS is typically assessed based on clinical or laboratory evidence of dysfunction in six organ systems: respiratory, coagulation, hepatic, cardiovascular, central nervous, and renal. The system created by Knaus and Wagner[6] is shown in Box 17-1 (organ failure is diagnosed if the patient has one or more of the findings listed in Box 17-1 during a 24-hour period regardless of other values). Table 17-1 outlines the stages of organ dysfunction that precede overt failure.

The finding that critical illness, particularly of a septic nature, is the major risk factor for MODS is compatible with the hypothesis that the syndrome has an identifiable inciting event, termed *activator*, that persists and serves as the stimulus for metabolic responses that predispose a patient to organ dysfunction. The term *systemic inflammatory response syndrome* (SIRS) was proposed to incorporate the concept that either infectious or noninfectious processes could serve as activators for systemic inflammation, which may then progress to MODS[3] (Box 17-2).

PATHOPHYSIOLOGY

The pathophysiologic features of MODS are related to a systemic inflammatory response that can be triggered by a variety of events. Tissue inflammatory reactions to localized injury and systemic responses to major surgery, major trauma, severe burn, injury, or sepsis are similar. Inflamed

TABLE 17-1
The Multiple Organ Dysfunction Score

Organ System	Score				
	0	1	2	3	4
Respiratory[a] (PO_2/FiO_2 ratio)	>300	226-300	151-225	76-150	≤75
Renal[b] (serum creatinine)	≤100	101-200	201-350	351-500	>500
Hepatic[c] (serum bilirubin)	≤20	21-60	61-120	121-240	>240
Cardiovascular[d] (PAR)	≤10.0	10.1-15.0	15.1-20.0	20.1-30.0	>30.0
Hematologic[e] (platelet count)	>120	81-120	51-80	21-50	≤20
Neurologic[f] (Glasgow Coma Score)	15	13-14	10-12	7-9	≤6

[a]The PO_2/FiO_2 ratio is calculated without reference to the use or mode of mechanical ventilation, and without reference to the use or level of positive end-expiratory pressure.

[b]The serum creatinine concentration is measured in μmol/L, without reference to the use of dialysis.

[c]The serum bilirubin concentration is measured in μmol/L.

[d]The pressure-adjusted heart rate (PAR) is calculated as the product of the heart rate (HR) multiplied by the ratio of the right atrial (central venous) pressure (RAP) to the mean arterial pressure (MAP): PAR = HR × RAP/MAP.

[e]The platelet count is measured in platelets m 10^{-3}.

[f]The Glasgow Coma score is preferably calculated by the patient's nurse and is scored conservatively (for the patient receiving sedation or muscle relaxants, normal function is assumed, unless there is evidence of intrinsically altered mentation).

tissue, in conditions such as peritonitis, pancreatitis, or acute lung injury, may be considered a wound because resolution and healing depend on the same biochemical processes as does healing in any wound.

The evolutionary benefit of the inflammatory response is to contain and control local infection, clear cellular debris and foreign material, and support wound healing. This is accomplished in part by the production of *mediators,* substances derived from either bacterial products (e.g., endotoxin) or manufactured by the host (e.g., complement) that cause tissue inflammation. When infection or injury is severe, this local inflammatory response becomes manifest *systemically* due to the entry of regionally produced mediators into the circulation and their consequent effects on distant organs.

The list of mediators produced during critical illness is constantly growing (Box 17-3). Although mediator production is beneficial in resolving tissue injury or infection, prolonged mediator production eventually becomes maladaptive. MODS may therefore be best viewed as a state of physiologic dysregulation (i.e., the failure of normal feedback mechanisms to regulate a physiologic process) leading to organ dysfunction that results from prolongation of the systemic inflammatory response.

Normally, inflammation is regulated so that it is appropriate to the degree of tissue injury and "turns off" as

---

BOX 17-2
Predisposing Factors to Systemic Inflammatory Response and Multiple-System Organ Failure

Imposed Risk Factors
Severe, multiple trauma, especially with peritoneal spillage or prolonged intestinal ischemia
Active infection, especially intraabdominal*
Large-area, deep-tissue burns
Complex emergency or elective surgical procedures
Pancreatitis
Presence of devitalized tissue
Unstable major lower extremity fractures
Shock or persistent subclinical hypoperfusion
Aspiration of gastric contents
Multiple blood transfusions

Patient-Related Risks
Advanced age (65 years or older)
Preexisting major system disease
Presence of underlying immunosuppression (acute or chronic renal or hepatic disease, alcoholism, acquired immune disease)
Poor nutrition status

*Sepsis is the most frequent cause of ARDS and MODS.

injured tissue resolves and heals. This is due in large part to a counterbalancing process that has been termed the *compensatory antiinflammatory response syndrome* (CARS); it results from production of antiinflammatory mediators such as interleukin-4, interleukin-10, and transforming growth factor–beta.[7] CARS may be viewed as a mechanism that prevents excessive inflammation. The physiologic state in which SIRS and CARS are balanced has been termed the *mixed antagonistic response syndrome* (MARS); it is conceptually similar to the normal interaction between the coagulation and fibrinolytic systems.[7] Prolonged critical illness may result in an imbalance between inflammatory and antiinflammatory processes. Patients in whom inflammation is dominant manifest organ dysfunction, whereas excessive production of antiinflammatory mediators results in an immunosuppressed state with increased susceptibility to infection. The details of the local and systemic responses to injury or infection and the pathophysiologic progression to MODS are discussed in the following sections.

Local Tissue Injury and Inflammation

Tissue injury or infection results in the local production and release of vasoactive and immune mediators that originate from products of leukocytes, platelet aggregation, vascular endothelial injury, and tissue factors. Mediator production is triggered by the presence of antigenic substances such as microorganisms, tissue trauma products, bacterial toxins, and aggregated immunoglobulins. Mediator release produces a local inflammatory response evidenced as heat, redness, swelling, and pain. The magnitude of this reaction is influenced by the severity of injury, the amount of necrotic tissue, and the presence or absence of infection. Identification and understanding of the actions of varied endogenous inflammatory mediator substances are continuously expanding. Box 17-3 lists some of the mediators involved in the inflammatory response.

Systemic Inflammatory Response Syndrome

If tissue injury is severe or massive, inflammatory mediators (see Box 17-3) are released into the bloodstream by the primary focus of injury or infection. Neurohormonal mediators, such as glucagon, epinephrine, insulin, and cortisol, are also considered to play a significant role in the metabolism of SIRS and MODS. Products of the arachidonic acid pathway (e.g., prostaglandins, thromboxanes, leukotrienes), cytokines, and toxic oxygen radicals are important mediators of the inflammatory response. Arachidonic acid metabolites are derived from phospholipids contained in cellular membranes. They are vasoconstrictive and chemotactic, they aggregate platelets, and they promote adhesion of leukocytes to endothelial surfaces. Cytokines are hormonelike molecules produced by a variety of cells (e.g., leukocytes, endothelial cells) that enable cell-to-cell communication and determine the magnitude and duration of the systemic response to injury or infection. Certain cytokines (e.g., interleukin-1, interleukin-6, tumor necrosis factor [TNF]) play a major role in determining the metabolic response to critical illness. Toxic oxygen radicals (e.g., superoxides, peroxides) are released by neutrophils during inflammation. They are important in bacterial killing but also may cause damage to vascular endothelium, cell membranes, and mitochondria. The clinical diagnosis of SIRS is discussed in the section on clinical presentation and course.

The physiologic consequence of systemic inflammation is that metabolism and energy expenditure are globally accelerated, caloric requirements are increased, and body temperature is usually elevated proportionate to the severity of injury. For example, patients with major burn injury typically have markedly increased caloric needs and body temperatures as high as 102° F (39° C) even in the absence of infection. Organ function becomes accelerated, the systemic vessels are generally dilated, and resting cardiac output is greater than normal. The hyperdynamic circulation enhances oxygen delivery to injured tissue for the support of wound healing.

Overall, physiology is altered and adapted to promote resolution of injury and host survival. The systemic metabolic response to massive injury or illness ideally turns off as the inciting event is eliminated and tissue injury is resolved.

Progression to Multiple Organ Dysfunction

Unresolved critical illness or injury, particularly when complicated by sepsis, prolongs the hypermetabolic response. The inflammatory response (SIRS) then becomes amplified and refractory to antiinflammatory mediators. The crossover point when the repair-oriented homeostatic process becomes malignant (highly injurious and uncontrolled) is impossible to identify. A constellation of physiologic abnormalities, which coexist and interrelate, develops.

There are two major mechanistic theories for organ dysfunction during prolonged SIRS. The first theory *(malignant intravascular inflammation)* states that SIRS promotes the production of mediators that result in endothelial injury and microvascular thrombosis. This in turn compromises tissue perfusion, resulting in organ dysfunction. The second theory *(cytopathic hypoxia)* attributes organ dysfunction to cellular hypoxia resulting from mitochondrial injury.

Uncontrolled Intravascular Inflammatory Response

Release of certain mediators results in microvascular injury and formation of microthrombi in organs remote from the initial site of injury or infection (see Box 17-3). Such mediators include toxic oxygen radicals (e.g., superoxides, peroxides), metabolites of arachidonic acid (e.g., leukotrienes, thromboxanes), platelet activating factor, products of platelet lysis, activated Hageman factor, and plasminogen proactivator, as well as products of kinin and complement system activation. Injury and thrombosis in the microvascular bed results in capillary leak, interstitial edema, tissue hypoperfusion, and organ dysfunction. This process may represent a subclinical form of disseminated intravascular coagulation that has been termed *malignant intravascular inflammation.*[8]

Impaired Oxygen Utilization

One of the more important metabolic abnormalities seen in patients with MODS is a progressive fall in systemic oxygen consumption due to a defect in cellular oxygen utilization. Although this process has been attributed to arteriovenous shunting, it is more likely that it results from mediator-induced cellular injury that interferes with mitochondrial oxygen uptake and utilization. This phenomenon is termed *cytopathic hypoxia.*[9]

This process is prominent in the liver, where deteriorating mitochondrial function is reflected by impairment in hepatic energy (adenosine triphosphate [ATP]) production. Ketone bodies (acetoacetate, beta-hydroxybutyrate) are synthesized in hepatic mitochondria, and measurement of these ketones in the plasma can be used to provide an index of the functional status of this organelle. Patients with worsening MODS characteristically demonstrate a progressive decrease in the normal ratio (greater than 0.7) of acetoacetate to beta-hydroxybutyrate in the plasma; values less than 0.25 are universally fatal.

Abnormalities in Carbohydrate, Fat, and Protein Metabolism

The systemic inflammatory response is accompanied by an increase in metabolic rate and caloric expenditure; a hyperdynamic cardiovascular response; and major alterations in the metabolism of carbohydrates, fat, and protein. All appear to be designed to support tissue repair. Cytokines (e.g., interleukin-1, TNF) and hormones (e.g., glucagon, epinephrine) are important determinants of these metabolic alterations.

Various metabolic pathways show evidence of defective feedback inhibition, termed *metabolic dysregulation,* due to the ongoing mediator formation.

Carbohydrate Metabolism. During critical illness, certain cytokines promote increased cellular uptake of glucose in wound and in tissues concerned with immune function, such as lung, spleen, gut, and skin. Increased cellular glucose uptake serves to stimulate anaerobic conversion of glucose to pyruvate (glycolysis) by a mechanism that can be likened to "pouring gasoline on a fire;" this in turn results in increased formation of pyruvate (see Chapter 16, Figure 16-2). Pyruvate is formed at a rate exceeding that which can be metabolized in the Krebs cycle; this results in increased lactate formation and hyperlactatemia. Although tissue hypoxia is the major mechanism for increased glycolysis during shock, patients with SIRS or MODS have increased glycolysis in the absence of tissue hypoxia. This process, termed *aerobic glycolysis,* serves to meet the increased energy demands of cells (e.g., neutrophils, macrophages) that satisfy their ATP requirements via glycolysis. Therefore, in SIRS and MODS, increases in the blood lactate concentration reflect the severity of hypermetabolism rather than tissue hypoperfusion. It is important to appreciate this concept when lactate is used as a tool to assess the hemodynamic status of patients with SIRS or MODS.

Hyperglycemia is common during SIRS and MODS and results from insulin resistance that is both *central* (i.e., increased hepatic glucose production that is not suppressed by physiologic concentrations of insulin) and *peripheral* (i.e., decreased insulin-stimulated glucose uptake in tissues such as skeletal muscle).

Patients with terminal sepsis and MODS may occasionally experience hypoglycemia due to cytokine-mediated suppression of hepatic glucose production.

Alterations in Lipid Metabolism. The stress associated with critical illness or injury induces an increase in the breakdown of fat, which results in the release of free fatty acids (FFAs). Uptake of FFAs from the bloodstream is also decreased; this promotes hyperlipidemia. Critical illness or injury is also associated with hepatic fat deposition and fatty liver. As mentioned, ketogenesis may also be decreased during MODS.

Protein Metabolism. Severe sepsis, burn, or trauma promotes catabolism of skeletal muscle and visceral protein. The catabolic response is often associated with urine urea nitrogen losses in excess of 20 g daily. Glucocorticoids and cytokines are probably the most important mediators of protein catabolism during stress. Prolonged protein catabolism ultimately results in a significant loss of lean body mass that has been termed *autocannibalism.*

In summary, the altered metabolism associated with critical illness is directed toward promoting resolution of injury. The increased energy demand in wound and in tissues involved in the immune response is satisfied glycolytically even in the absence of tissue hypoxia. The hypermetabolic state is also characterized by prominent protein catabolism that parallels the severity of illness or injury and is commonly associated with significant urinary protein wasting and loss of lean body mass.

Patients who are recovering from MODS exhibit a progressive decrease in the severity of hypermetabolism and proteolysis. Conversely, patients with deteriorating organ function show evidence of progressive metabolic deregulation that results from continuing mediator formation and defective feedback inhibition.

Stimuli That Drive Mediator Formation, Hypermetabolism, and Inflammatory Responses

The precise nature of the stimulus or stimuli that result in the prolonged hypermetabolism and inflammatory responses associated with SIRS and MODS have not been clearly established. It is likely that the etiology is multifactorial. Potential mechanisms include ongoing stimulation by untreated activators (e.g., persistent infectious or inflammatory foci); complicating secondary activator events (massive blood transfusions, recurrent episodes of hypotension); or persistant regional (e.g., splanchnic) hypoperfusion. These factors, in turn, result in sustained mediator formation and release. Ultimately, organ damage develops (Figure 17-1).

Hypoperfusion of the Abdominal Viscera and Bacterial Overgrowth of the Gut

Hypoperfusion of the splanchnic vascular bed and overgrowth of pathogenic flora within the gastrointestinal tract have been referred to as the potential "motors" that drive the systemic inflammatory response and MODS.[10]

The gut is highly vulnerable to ischemia due to its high oxygen demand relative to oxygen delivery. Patients with critical illness may develop locally acquired cellular defects in oxygen extraction or local vascular sensitivity to circulating vasoconstrictors; this may result in ischemic injury of the abdominal viscera despite hemodynamic and metabolic profiles that indicate adequate oxygen delivery. The process whereby bacteria or endotoxins move across the intestinal wall is termed *translocation* (Figure 17-2). A limited amount of translocation occurs in normal individuals. The presence of splanchnic ischemia markedly increases gut permeability and translocation. Critically ill patients often have overgrowth of the gut with antibiotic-resistant intestinal bacterial flora secondary to administration of broad-spectrum antibiotics; this increased intestinal bacterial load also increases the rate of translocation. Translocated bacteria and endotoxin subsequently enter the portal vein and lymphatics and are taken up by hepatic macrophages (Kupffer cells). Persistent simulation of Kupffer cells promotes production of mediators that suppress hepatic protein synthesis. Increased translocation also accounts for the increased frequency of bacteremia in patients with MODS without a septic source.

The interaction between gut hypoperfusion, translocation, and organ dysfunction has been incorporated in the "two-hit" theory of MSOF.[11] This theory postulates that patients who typically develop MODS often have a period of tissue hypoperfusion that is followed by a second, often minor complication. Based on this theory, the first "hit" is inadequate systemic oxygen delivery that is associated

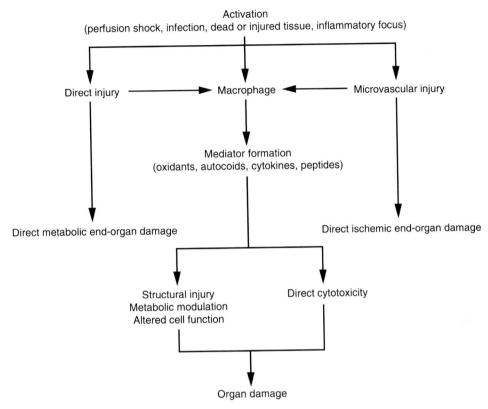

FIGURE 17-1 The cascade of the systemic inflammatory response and mechanisms of cell injury and metabolic regulation. (Adapted from Bihari DJ, Cerra FB: *Multiple organ failure,* Fullerton, CA, 1989, Society of Critical Care Medicine.)

with splanchnic hypoperfusion. Ischemic gut serves as the site where neutrophils are "activated" (e.g., more likely to produce toxic oxygen radicals). They are then released into the bloodstream and ultimately localize in other organs (e.g., lung). Subsequently, a second "hit" (e.g., bacteremia) promotes local neutrophil release of oxygen radicals that damage adjacent capillary endothelium and result in organ damage. It has been suggested that the pulmonary capillary leak and ARDS, which commonly herald the onset of MODS, may be the consequence of this process.

Immune System Incompetence

As mentioned previously, critical illness is associated with an inflammatory response that is counterbalanced by production of antiinflammatory mediators. When the antiinflammatory response becomes excessive, immunosuppression and increased risk of infection result. In addition, certain drugs (e.g., corticosteroids, antineoplastics), preexisting diseases (e.g., malnutrition, chronic renal failure, cirrhosis), and invasive devices

(e.g., intravenous catheters) also increase the susceptibility to infection.

In summary, the pathophysiology of MODS relates to a systemic inflammatory response that is prolonged, perhaps secondary to splanchnic ischemia and intestinal bacterial overgrowth. This in turn promotes organ dysfunction as the result of leukocyte-mediated endothelial injury and mitochondrial dysfunction. A variety of alterations in carbohydrate, fat, and protein metabolism accompany SIRS and MODS.

The development of MODS may be represented as a cascade of events consisting of *activation of the inflammatory response, release of inflammatory mediators,* and *organ dysfunction or failure* (see Figure 17-1).

HEMODYNAMIC PROFILE

The hemodynamic profile of patients with the hypermetabolic response to critical illness and MODS can be variable in intensity and depends on the nature and duration of illness at presentation, as well as patient-related factors such

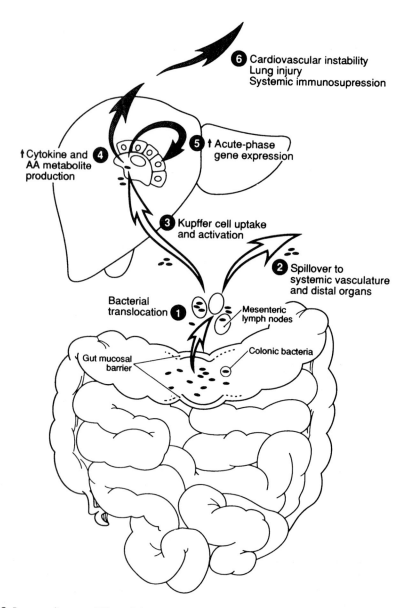

6 Cardiovascular instability
Lung injury
Systemic immunosupression

5 ↑ Acute-phase
gene expression

↑ Cytokine and **4**
AA metabolite
production

3 Kupffer cell uptake
and activation

2 Spillover to
systemic vasculature
and distal organs

Bacterial
translocation **1**

Mesenteric
lymph nodes

Colonic bacteria

Gut mucosal
barrier

FIGURE 17-2 Increased permeability of the gut resulting in translocation of bacteria and toxins is thought to play a major role in the perpetuation of the multiple organ failure syndrome. (Redrawn with permission from Matuschak GM: Multiple system organ failure. In Hall JB, Schmidt GA, Wood LDH, editors: *Principles of critical care,* New York, 1992, McGraw-Hill.)

as underlying heart disease and age. The hemodynamic profile follows a physiologic time course that is accompanied by the aforementioned metabolic abnormalities that evolve and deteriorate with time.[12,13] Most patients with SIRS and early MODS have a hyperdynamic circulation that can be described as a *balanced stress response state* (stage 1). Patients with uncontrolled risk factors, such as unremitting, severe sepsis, typically move into a *state of unbalanced vascular tone* characterized by profound vasodilation

(stage 2). Ultimately, they enter a *state of severe cardiopulmonary failure* that is unresponsive to therapeutic support (stage 3).

Certain patients may follow an atypical course; for example, patients with preexisting heart disease may initially have signs and symptoms of heart failure *(cardiogenic state).* The details of these stages are discussed next. The anticipated directions of change of measured variables are summarized in Table 17-2.

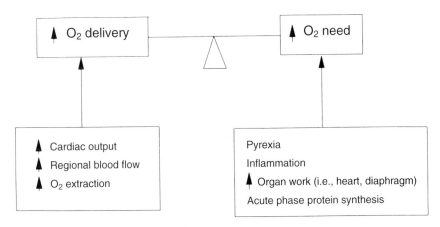

FIGURE 17-3 The hypermetabolic state elicits a hyperdynamic circulatory response which increases oxygen delivery as a means to satisfy increased oxygen need. (Adapted from Bern A, Sibbald WJ: Circulatory dynamics of multiple organ failure, *Crit Care Clin* 5:234, 1989.)

TABLE 17-2
Anticipated Direction of Change of Hemodynamic Measurements

	Blood Pressure	Systemic Vascular Resistance	Pulmonary Vascular Resistance	Pulmonary Artery Pressure	Pulmonary Artery Wedge Pressure	Cardiac Output	Svo₂
Stage 1	—	↓	− ↑	− ↑	—	↑	—
Stage 2	↓	↓ ↓	↑	↑	− ↑	↑ ↑	↑
Stage 3	↓ ↓	↓ ↓	↑ ↑	↑ ↑	− ↑	↓	↑

The magnitude of direction of change is indicated by the number of arrows. These serve only as general guidelines. Coexisting factors such as hypovolemia may accentuate or oppose the anticipated direction of change.

Stage 1

Most patients with severe illness or injury, who have been successfully resuscitated, initially manifest a hyperdynamic state characterized by systemic vasodilation and increased cardiac output. This cardiovascular state serves to deliver additional blood flow to injured tissue for the support of wound healing (Figure 17-3). Vasodilation is considered the primary event; nitric oxide appears to play a major role in this process. The increase in cardiac output is *proportional* to the degree of vasodilation. Blood pressure is maintained despite systemic vascular resistance (SVR) in the range of 800 dynes/sec/cm^{-5}. Consequently, hypotension is unusual. Increased stroke volume and cardiac output also occur from positive inotropic effects of catecholamines. Oxygen delivery and consumption (Vo₂) are typically increased. Adequate tissue perfusion is reflected in normal or high-normal arteriovenous oxygen content difference (AVDo₂) and a normal Svo₂. Metabolic acidosis is not present, although blood lactate concentration may be increased (see laboratory section later in this chapter).

As stated previously, cardiac output fails to increase in some patients. This may be due to underlying heart disease or secondary to negative inotropic effects of circulating myocardial depressant factors. Failure to increase cardiac output in response to vasodilation often results in hypotension and lactic acidosis. This is usually rapidly followed by death.

Stage 2

Stage 2 is characteristic of patients with deteriorating organ function. The SVR is markedly reduced, often to values of 400 dynes/sec/cm^{-5} or less. Hypotension is common despite cardiac output three to four times normal; pharmacologic support may be required to maintain the arterial pressure within an acceptable range. Some patients die suddenly without experiencing the transition to a low-cardiac-output state.

This stage is also marked by clinical and laboratory evidence of reduced oxygen consumption that is the result of impaired cellular oxygen extraction. Patients with sepsis or severe liver disease most commonly display this abnormality. Clinically, patients in stage 2 show further evidence of multiple organ dysfunction, progressive narrowing of the arteriovenous oxygen difference (secondary to decreased oxygen extraction), and hyperlactatemia. The Svo_2 is typically normal or even elevated because of defective oxygen extraction (see laboratory section later in this chapter).

Pulmonary hypertension and increased pulmonary vascular resistance (PVR) may be seen with concomitant respiratory failure. The elevated PVR is thought to be due to pulmonary vasoconstriction or pulmonary microthrombus formation. However, left ventricular failure also can cause elevated pulmonary artery pressures with or without increases in pulmonary vascular resistance. Pulmonary hypertension accompanied by an increased pulmonary artery diastolic to wedge pressure gradient (greater than 5 to 7 mm Hg) suggests "active" pulmonary vasoconstriction or microvascular disease. On the other hand, maintenance of a normal diastolic to wedge pressure gradient is consistent with "passive" pulmonary hypertension due to left ventricular failure. Generally, persistent and progressive pulmonary hypertension is a poor prognostic sign. Metabolic abnormalities, such as hyperglycemia, insulin resistance, negative nitrogen balance, and decreased hepatic protein synthesis, become pronounced during stage 2.

Stage 3

Stage 3 is the hemodynamic stage characteristic of patients in frank multiple organ failure who are no longer responsive to pharmacologic or mechanical support measures. Cardiac output is reduced, SVR is very low, mean arterial pressure is less than 50 mm Hg, and lactic acidosis is evidenced on blood gas analysis. Death usually follows.

CLINICAL PRESENTATION AND COURSE

MODS is usually preceded by an acute inciting (activator) event that is associated with a variable period of hypotension. Following resuscitation, a latent period of hours to days occurs during which the patient appears to be stable and doing well by the usual clinical criteria. Systemic inflammation is heralded by the appearance of fever, leukocytosis, tachycardia, and tachypnea.

The clinical diagnosis of SIRS requires the presence of two or more of the following conditions: (1) temperature greater than 38° C or less than 36° C; (2) heart rate greater than 90 beats per minute; (3) respiratory rate greater than 20 breaths per minute or $Paco_2$ less than 32 mm Hg; or (4) white blood cell count greater than 12,000/mm^3, less than 4000/mm^3, or greater than 10% immature (band) forms.[3] Although these findings suggest the presence of infection, nonseptic activators of the inflammatory response can produce an identical picture. Indeed, approximately one third of patients who develop MODS never have bacteremia or obvious septic focus during the disease course.

Generally, clinical findings of MODS are variable and depend on the patient's underlying disease, the number of organ systems involved, and the severity of organ dysfunction. Although the clinical findings of MODS are patient dependent, the syndrome usually develops in one of three clinical patterns:

1. *Acute respiratory failure as a secondary event.* This pattern is most commonly seen in surgical ICUs, trauma patients, or burn patients. Lung injury manifested by noncardiogenic pulmonary edema and ARDS occurs 12 to 24 hours following an initial insult such as severe trauma or major surgery. Other organ failures then progressively and sequentially emerge over a period of 7 to 14 days. During this time, continually worsening hemodynamics, with increasing requirements for pharmacologic support, and renal failure become prominent. At this advanced stage, the prognosis is extremely poor (mortality rate greater than 80%).

2. *Acute respiratory failure as a primary event.* This pattern is more commonly seen in the medical ICU. Acute lung injury (ARDS) occurs as the *primary* event owing to gastric aspiration, viral pneumonia, or bacterial pneumonia. Progressive and sequential organ failure then occurs within 2 to 4 days of the primary insult.

3. *Major organ failure without pulmonary involvement.* This is the least common pattern. Progressive liver and renal failure develop in the absence of obvious pulmonary dysfunction or injury.

The following assessment findings are generally observed in patients with MODS.

Mentation

Patients may be irritable, agitated, lethargic, apathetic, or confused early in the course of the syndrome. Later, they may progress to obtundation and coma due to an encephalopathy that is metabolic in origin. The diagnosis of MODS-related encephalopathy is often missed due to concomitant use of mechanical ventilation and use of sedatives and paralytic agents.

Cutaneous Manifestations

The skin is typically warm. However, vasoconstricted patients have cool, pale, or dusky extremities. The complexion is usually sallow; jaundice suggests the presence of hepatic dysfunction. Generalized edema, secondary to large-volume crystalloid fluid resuscitation, a diffuse capillary leak, and hypoalbuminemia, is common. Impaired wound healing, persistent wound infection, decubitus ulcers, impaired formation of granulation tissue, and wound dehiscence are other cutaneous manifestations of MODS. Gangrene of digits or patchy infarcts of the skin (purpura fulminans) may occur in the setting of disseminated intravascular coagulation (DIC).

Body Temperature

Elevations in body temperature are common and appear to be cytokine mediated. The fever may be due to the presence of multiple sites of phagocytic stimulation, such as surgical or traumatic wounds, hematomas, or crush injuries, or from stress-induced metabolic alterations (e.g., increased fatty acid–triglyceride cycling). A normal or subnormal temperature is atypical and may indicate sepsis, severe immune system dysfunction, hypothyroidism, or malnutrition. Fever that is disproportionately high relative to the level of injury indicates sepsis.

Heart Rate and Character of Pulse

Patients are typically tachycardic with strong bounding pulses that reflect the hyperdynamic response to infection or injury. With the advent of cardiovascular failure, peripheral pulses become weak. Bradycardia or the appearance of supraventricular or ventricular tachyarrhythmias may compromise the patient's circulatory function.

Respiratory Status

Noncardiogenic pulmonary edema with oxygenation failure (ARDS) is commonly the first manifestation of MODS. Tachypnea with diffuse crackles and wheezes is generally found on examination (see Chapter 18).

Urine Output

Involvement of the kidneys may be associated with high- or low-output renal failure. Oliguria is the more common clinical finding.

Acid-Base Abnormalities

Respiratory alkalosis is the most common acid-base abnormality in stage 1 and 2 MODS. Increased lactate with or without concomitant metabolic acidosis commonly occurs at stages 2 and 3. Stage 3 also may be associated with respiratory acidosis as pulmonary failure progresses.

LABORATORY EXAMINATION

There is no specific laboratory test for MODS; the following abnormalities are commonly seen.

Complete Blood Count, Prothrombin Time, Partial Thromboplastin Time

Critical illness and MODS are often associated with alterations in the complete blood count and coagulation profile. Anemia, which is usually multifactorial, is common. Fragmented red blood cells, termed *schistocytes,* may be noted on microscopic examination. The white blood cell count is generally elevated but may be inappropriately low. Thrombocytopenia generally results from increased consumption of platelets secondary to immune mechanisms or DIC. Hepatic dysfunction or DIC may cause elevation of the prothrombin and partial thromboplastin times and predisposes the patient to bleeding.

Serum Bilirubin

As MODS progresses, liver involvement is marked by progressive direct hyperbilirubinemia. Serum transaminases, alkaline phosphatase, and ammonia may likewise be elevated. Correctable causes of hyperbilirubinemia such as calculus or acalculus cholecystitis or a hemolytic reaction should also be considered.

Serum Albumin

Serum albumin is often reduced during SIRS and MODS. In contrast to malnutrition, the hypoalbuminemia accompanying critical illness relates to factors other than deficient protein intake. Cytokine-induced suppression of albumin synthesis, albumin catabolism, dilution hypoalbuminemia, and third-space losses are major causes of hypoalbuminemia during critical illness or injury. Overall, the lower the serum albumin and total protein levels, the greater the level of generalized edema and the greater the risk of complications and death. Large supplemental doses may become necessary to maintain an albumin level within the normal range. However, the benefit of albumin supplementation during critical illness is controversial. If supplemental albumin is administered, the serum albumin level is prognostically unreliable.

Serum Triglycerides

Serum triglycerides may be elevated during SIRS and MODS due to both increased synthesis and decreased clearance. Hypertriglyceridemia may become clinically manifest as lipemic serum, particularly in patients who are receiving intravenous lipids. If serum triglyceride levels exceed 400 mg/dl, fat infusion should be reduced or discontinued.

Glucose

Hyperglycemia in the range of 250 to 325 mg/dl and glucose intolerance are common and can be attributed to increased hepatic glucose production, as well as insulin resistance in skeletal muscle. The degree of glucose intolerance commonly parallels the severity of hypermetabolism. A minority of patients with sepsis or severe underlying liver disease may become hypoglycemic because of depressed glucose production.

Although mild to moderate hyperglycemia (160 to 225 mg/dl) may be beneficial in promoting glucose uptake, hyperosmolarity is undesirable because it promotes hypovolemia and electrolyte imbalance, as well as increases the risk of infection. Significant hyperglycemia (greater than 250 mg/dl) may necessitate administration of regular insulin to keep blood glucose below 225 mg/dl.

Serum Cortisol

Occult hypoadrenalism has been described in critically ill patients who become vasopressor dependent. This process may be cytokine mediated. Serum cortisol analysis typically reveals a submaximal adrenal response evidenced at baseline or stimulated serum cortisol (less than 20 μg/dl). Administration of exogenous corticosteroids to these patients often enables vasopressor weaning.

Electrocardiogram

The prolonged hyperdynamic state characteristic of SIRS and MODS places a severe stress on the heart and predisposes the patient to arrhythmias, repolarization abnormalities, conduction disturbances, and transient ischemic changes. They appear to be more common when underlying sepsis is the cause of the hypermetabolic state. The term *myocardial distress syndrome* has been proposed to describe this association. Mild elevations in cardiac troponin may occur in septic patients as the result of mediator-induced myocardial injury.

Chest Radiograph

Some patients have a fairly normal film, whereas others manifest dense, homogeneous bilateral pulmonary infiltrates consistent with ARDS. Radiologic manifestations of pulmonary barotrauma (pneumothorax, subcutaneous and pulmonary interstitial emphysema) may be seen in patients receiving high levels of PEEP. Infiltrates due to pneumonia may be difficult to identify in the presence of the radiographic "whiteout" of full-blown ARDS.

Blood Lactate

Although an increased blood lactate level (normal is less than 2 mM/L) is often attributed to tissue hypoperfusion, hyperlactatemia during SIRS and MODS is more often the result of hypermetabolism. This condition has been termed *stress hyperlactatemia* and is largely due to increased lactate production secondary to accelerated aerobic glycolysis (see alterations in carbohydrate metabolism) in wounds and macrophage-rich tissues such as lung. This is in contrast to the lacticacidemia, secondary to tissue hypoxia, typical of patients with circulatory shock. Impaired hepatic clearance of lactate may also play a role in hyperlactatemia during critical illness. For example, stressed patients with underlying cirrhosis may have a higher blood lactate than noncirrhotic patients despite a similar rate of lactate production.

The lack of specificity of blood lactate as an index of tissue hypoperfusion limits its diagnostic utility. Concomitant measurement of pyruvate with calculation of the lactate/pyruvate (L/P) ratio has been proposed as a means to increase the specificity of lactate as an index of tissue hypoxia. Hyperlactatemia secondary to inadequate oxygen delivery is typically associated with an increased L/P ratio (greater than 10:1 to 15:1); the ratio is normal in the setting of augmented aerobic glycolysis secondary to SIRS and MODS. Although this approach is theoretically attractive, its diagnostic value appears to be limited. The blood lactate concentration provides useful prognostic information in circulatory shock; the mortality rate is increased in those patients who fail to demonstrate a progressive decrease in lactate during hemodynamic resuscitation.

Mixed Venous Oxygen Saturation (Svo$_2$)

The mixed venous oxygen saturation (Svo$_2$) is the oxygen saturation in mixed venous blood. It is generally obtained by aspirating blood from the distal port of a pulmonary artery catheter. The Svo$_2$ provides an index of the relationship between oxygen delivery and oxygen demand; decreased oxygen delivery is manifested by a decrease in the Svo$_2$ (less than 70%). However, it is difficult to determine the critical value of Svo$_2$ that defines inadequate oxygen delivery. In addition, patients with SIRS/MODS often have abnormalities in oxygen extraction that blunt the expected fall in Svo$_2$ consequent to decreased cardiac output. In some hypoperfused patients with MODS, the Svo$_2$ may therefore be normal.

Oxygen Flux Test

The oxygen flux test has been proposed as a means to assess the adequacy of tissue perfusion. The test is performed by increasing oxygen delivery using volume loading, blood transfusion, inotropes, or vasodilators and noting the response of oxygen consumption. A positive test (e.g., an increase in oxygen consumption concomitant with an increase in oxygen delivery) supports the presence of tissue hypoxia. Unfortunately, the oxygen flux test has a number of drawbacks that limit its utility in the clinical setting. (See Table 17-1 for laboratory assessment parameters of the severity of MSOF.)

MANAGEMENT

Our understanding of the origin and pathophysiology of MODS remains incomplete. This is reflected in unacceptably high morbidity and mortality rates. Currently, prevention and treatment of MODS are oriented toward intervening at three levels: activator (source) control, limitation of mediator formation, and organ support.

Activator Control

This approach is directed at elimination or modification of initiating conditions. Common activators of the systemic inflammatory response are circulatory shock and inflammatory foci such as necrotic or infected tissue.

1. *Aggressive resuscitation from circulatory shock.* One of the most common events preceding MSOF is circulatory shock; the risk for MODS is related to the severity and duration of global or regional tissue hypoxia. Measures essential in preventing MODS include early identification of the shock stimulus, correction of the underlying cause (this may require immediate surgical intervention), aggressive hemodynamic resuscitation, and maintenance of adequate ventilation and oxygenation. Unfortunately, there are no gold standards for use in assessing tissue hypoxia. It is therefore difficult to guarantee that clinically undetectable areas of regional hypoperfusion (e.g., the splanchnic circulation) do not persist despite apparently adequate hemodynamic resuscitation. This is particularly true when insensitive resuscitative endpoints are used, such as urine output and blood pressure. The limitations of lactate, Svo_2, and the oxygen flux test as markers of tissue hypoperfusion have been previously discussed. Alternative approaches such as tonometry are reviewed later in this chapter.

2. *Elimination of the inflammatory or septic focus* (see also Chapter 16). Wounds with necrotic tissue, grossly contaminated material, or foreign debris do not heal and are invitations to local or systemic infection. Prompt surgical debridement of necrotic or infected tissue and drainage of purulent matter are critical in preventing the prolonged activator stimulus that leads to MODS. If the patient has active infection, antibiotic therapy guided by appropriate sensitivity testing should be directed toward the most likely microorganisms.

Multiple antibiotics are frequently necessary. However, it is not uncommon for patients with MODS to be culture negative despite signs of infection. In such patients, clinical signs of systemic infection may result from a noninfective etiology such as products of tissue injury. In contrast, positive blood cultures, particularly during the late stages of MODS, are often secondary to transient bacteremia resulting from bacterial translocation rather than from a serious infectious focus.

3. *Prevention of infectious complications.* Secondary infections resulting from the use of devices, such as endotracheal and nasogastric tubes and intravenous and urinary catheters, may prolong the hypermetabolic response and lead to MODS. It is beyond the scope of this text to discuss strategies to prevent infection. However, meticulous adherence to standard techniques of infection control is essential. Frequent wound cleansing and dressing changes and meticulous care of intravenous catheter insertion sites are important in preventing infectious complications. The presence of unexplained fever should be considered as catheter sepsis until proven otherwise and should prompt collection of appropriate cultures, catheter replacement, and empiric antibiotic therapy. Nasogastric tubes and urinary catheters should be removed as soon as feasible. The ability of prophylactic antibiotic decontamination of the gut to decrease the incidence of nosocomial infections and the complications associated with their development has been investigated. A reduction in the incidence of nosocomial pneumonia was noted, but there was no clear effect on mortality rate.[14]

Limitation of Mediator Formation

The systemic manifestations of the septic syndrome are caused by a wide variety of inflammatory mediators. A number of therapeutic strategies have been explored as a means to decrease mediator synthesis or neutralize or block their effect, thereby improving patient survival.

During the 1970s and 1980s, high-dose glucocorticoids (methylprednisolone, dexamethasone) were used in sepsis or endotoxemia to limit mediator formation and inflammatory response. Results in animals were promising; however, human studies have not demonstrated efficacy. Steroid therapy in sepsis is currently not recommended.

Administration of antibodies to the lipid A core of the endotoxin molecule or of analogues to compete with endotoxin for binding to macrophage receptors has been investigated as prophylaxis for gram-negative shock, as well as the treatment of established infection. Animal studies investigating the use of antibodies to cytokines that mitigate their deleterious effects on organs, such as antibodies to TNF, also have shown promise. Unfortunately, human studies have been disappointing. At present, there is no Food and Drug Administration–approved mediator antagonist available for clinical use.

Recent studies have indicated that mediator formation may be modulated using various immunonutrients. This approach is discussed in the following section.

Patient and Organ Support Measures

Most of the support measures discussed in this section do not directly affect the inflammatory response. However, following elimination or control of the initiating activator, they may prevent further insult and provide the time needed to allow the patient to heal spontaneously. It is important to appreciate that organ support is not without hazard (e.g., hypotension or barotrauma may result from mechanical ventilation with high levels of PEEP). Therefore the use of these supportive modalities mandates careful monitoring.

Metabolic Support

Nutritional pharmacology is a relatively new field that incorporates the concept that certain nutrients possess pharmacologic effects that may be therapeutic. The term *immunonutrients* has been proposed to describe these substances. A variety of immunonutrients have been investigated, such as branched-chain amino acids, arginine, glutamine, and nucleotides. Encouraging results were recently reported with administration of an enteral feeding solution supplemented with fish oil–derived fatty acids (omega-3 fatty acids) to patients with SIRS and ARDS.[15] This supplemented formula was compared with a standard vegetable oil–based formula. Patients receiving the fish oil–based product demonstrated improved oxygenation, decreased ventilator time, and decreased incidence of new organ failures relative to the standard formula. Various vitamins, such as vitamins C and E, and other substances, such as selenium and *N*-acetyl-L-cysteine, have also been used in patients with sepsis and ARDS in an effort to decrease oxidative injury secondary to production of toxic oxygen radicals. However, to date, no antioxidant has been conclusively proven to control toxic oxygen radical–mediated injury in a clinical trial.

Hemodynamic Support

As stated previously, persistent regional tissue hypoperfusion is one of the major stimuli that perpetuates the hypermetabolic state and contributes to the progression of MODS. Patients at risk for organ failure may benefit from invasive monitoring to optimize tissue perfusion and oxygen delivery (Box 17-4). Unfortunately, the hemodynamic end-points for successful resuscitation from circulatory

---

BOX 17-4
Monitoring for Hemodynamic Support

Pulmonary artery catheterization for measurement of central circulatory pressures (right atrial, pulmonary artery, and pulmonary arterial wedge pressures), cardiac output by thermodilution, calculated systemic and pulmonary vascular resistances, and measurement of mixed venous oxygen saturation
Arterial catheterization for continuous measurement of arterial pressure, as well as measurement of arterial blood gases
Calculated blood oxygen content, transport, and consumption
Serum lactate levels
Gastric tonometry

---

shock have not been agreed on. Although achieving standard clinical end-points of resuscitation (e.g., restoration of urine output and normalization of vital signs) may suggest that systemic perfusion is restored, occult regional hypoperfusion may nevertheless persist. The use of resuscitation directed toward achieving "supranormal" hemodynamic end-points has been explored as a means to improve regional perfusion during hemodynamic resuscitation. Although initial reports suggested a favorable effect on outcome,[16] other studies have failed to document benefit and in some cases have indicated increased mortality rates.[17] The optimal goals for hemodynamic resuscitation are therefore unclear at this time.

Gastrointestinal Tonometry to Evaluate Perfusion Status. The gastrointestinal tract is particularly vulnerable to ischemia during critical illness. Gastrointestinal tonometry can be used to provide information regarding the adequacy of splanchnic blood flow. A gastric tonometer is a nasogastric tube with a balloon tip that is used to measure the partial pressure of carbon dioxide in the gastric lumen. The lumenal gastric CO_2 correlates with the intramucosal gastric CO_2 ($PgCO_2$), which can be used to calculate the intramucosal pH (pHi) (Figure 17-4). Inadequate splanchnic blood flow results in mucosal hypoperfusion, local accumulation of carbon dioxide, and a fall in pHi. It has been suggested that an increase in the gap between the $PgCO_2$ and the PCO_2 of an arterial blood sample is a better indicator of gut hypoperfusion than a low pHi.[18]

Gastrointestinal tonometry has been used in patients with circulatory shock as a means to direct the adequacy of hemodynamic resuscitation. However, studies have failed to consistently demonstrate beneficial effects in

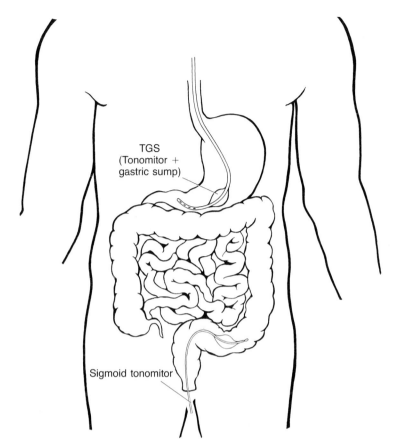

FIGURE 17-4 The tonometric intramucosal pH monitoring device, located in either the stomach or the sigmoid colon, assesses the viability and integrity of the gut mucosal tissue. (Courtesy of Tonometrics, Inc., Hopkinton, MA.)

reducing ICU stay, the development of MODS, or mortality rates.[19] Nevertheless, this technique may be useful in determining prognosis. A study in trauma demonstrated that patients with a low pHi 24 hours after admission had an increased likelihood of developing MODS.[20]

Ventilatory Support

Patients with MODS commonly are hypoxemic as the result of ARDS or pneumonia. In addition to improving gas exchange, mechanical ventilation also decreases the work of breathing and energy demand of the respiratory muscles. This may improve oxygenation in other organs. Appropriate sedation may also reduce oxygen demand.

Excessive airway pressures should be avoided because overdistention may harm previously undamaged alveoli and stimulate local cytokine production. Tracheostomy should be performed when mechanical ventilatory support is prolonged to promote patient comfort and decrease work of breathing.

Conservation of Patient Energy

Patients with hypermetabolism commonly are febrile. Significant energy can be lost as radiated heat if the patient is uncovered; this is particularly important in patients with burn injury. If fever exceeds physiologically acceptable levels (generally more than 102° F), antipyretics should be given to reduce body temperature. Surface cooling with cooling blankets may produce shivering, particularly with very low blanket temperatures, and is generally no more effective than antipyretics.[21,22] Shivering is undesirable because of associated increases in metabolic rate and oxygen demand. The use of cooling blankets should be reserved for patients with significant fever (greater than 104° F) who do not respond to antipyretics.

Provision of Time for Rest and Sleep

Patients in the ICU are frequently sleep deprived because of stimulation by physicians, nurses, and other hospital personnel and by the constant light and noise. Sleep deprivation in combination with the stress of critical illness may result in mental disturbances such as confusion, irritability, and occasionally psychosis. Sleep deprivation also may contribute to physiologic deterioration. Provision of "sheltered" time for sleep and rest (particularly at night) is an important consideration in patient care. Complete bed baths and linen changes when the patient and linen are not soiled are not important to a favorable patient outcome, and time spent in these routine, cyclic activities may be better devoted to allowing the patient time to sleep.

Patient Orientation to Time and Routine

The absence of normal time cues and round-the-clock ICU routine may add to the patient's confusion. Patients should be regularly oriented to time, date, and location, and they should be given simple explanations relative to care activities. Wall clocks are also helpful.

PROGNOSIS

Because current therapeutic options are supportive rather than corrective, the prognosis of MODS is poor. The individual patient's prognosis depends on several factors:

1. The severity of the underlying diseases and the time-related responses to therapy (a surgically correctable lesion versus viral pneumonia).
2. The specific organs involved. The organ system that carries the worst prognosis is the central nervous system; it has a death risk of approximately 40% when involved alone. All other organ systems are approximately equal in their impact on outcome.
3. The greater the number of organ failures and the longer their durations, the worse the prognosis. In 1989 Knaus and Wagner[6] analyzed more than 5000 critically ill patients in the United States and France and found that a single organ system failure persisting for more than 3 days was associated with a hospital mortality risk of 40%. A persistent two-organ failure for more than 3 days was associated with a 60% risk of hospital death. Three or more system failures lasting for more than 3 days resulted in a mortality rate approaching 100%.
4. Individual patient factors that increase the risk of MODS and portend a poor outcome include advanced age (65 years or older); alcoholism; and preexisting disease, such as renal or hepatic disease or malnutrition.

REFERENCES

1. Skillman JJ, Bushnell LS, Goldman H, et al: Respiratory failure, hypotension, sepsis and jaundice, *Am J Surg* 117:523, 1969.
2. Tilney NL, Bailey GL, Morgan AP: Sequential system failure after rupture of abdominal aortic aneurysms: an unsolved problem in postoperative care, *Ann Surg* 178:117, 1973.
3. American College of Chest Physicians/Society of Critical Care Medicine Consensus Conference: Definitions for sepsis and organ failure and guidelines for the use of innovative therapies in sepsis, *Crit Care Med* 20:864, 1992.
4. Knaus A, Draper EA, Wagner DP, et al: Prognosis in acute organ system failure, *Ann Surg* 202:685, 1985.
5. Vincent JL, Ferreira F, Moreno R: Scoring systems for assessing organ dysfunction and survival, *Crit Care Clin* 16:353, 2000.
6. Knaus A, Wagner DP: Multiple systems organ failure: epidemiology and prognosis, *Crit Care Clin* 5:221, 1989.
7. Bone RC: Sir Isaac Newton, sepsis, SIRS, and CARD, *Crit Care Med* 24:1125, 1996.
8. Pinsky MR, Matuschak GM: Multiple systems organ failure, *Crit Care Clin* 5:195, 1989.
9. Fink M: Cytopathic hypoxia in sepsis, *Acta Anaesthesiol Scand Suppl* 110:87, 1997.
10. Meakins JL, Marshall JC: The gastrointestinal tract: the "motor" of multiple organ failure, *Arch Surg* 121:197, 1986.
11. Faist E, Baue AE, Dittmer H, et al: Multiple organ failure in polytrauma patients, *J Trauma* 23:775, 1983.
12. Siegel JH, Cerra FB, Coleman B, et al: Physiological and metabolic correlation in human sepsis, *Surgery* 86:163, 1979.
13. Cerra FB, Border JR, McMenamy RH, et al: Multiple systems organ failure. In Cowley RA, Trump BF, editors: *Pathophysiology of shock, anoxia, and ischemia,* Baltimore, 1982, Williams & Wilkins.
14. Heyland D, Cook DJ, Jaeschke R, et al: Selective decontamination of the digestive tract: an overview, *Chest* 105:1221, 1994.
15. Gadek JE, DeMichele SJ, Karlstad MD, et al: Effect of enteral feeding with eicosapentaenoic acid, γ-linolenic acid, and antioxidants in patients with acute respiratory distress syndrome, *Crit Care Med* 27:1409, 1999.
16. Shoemaker W, Appel PL, Kram HB, et al: Prospective trial of supranormal values in survivors as therapeutic goals in high-risk surgical patients, *Chest* 94:1176, 1988.
17. Hayes MA, Timmins AC, Yau EHS, et al: Elevation of systemic oxygen delivery in the treatment of critically ill patients, *N Engl J Med* 330:1717, 1994.
18. Schlichtig R, Mehta N, Gayowski TJ: Tissue-arterial P_{CO_2} difference is a better marker of ischaemia than intramural pH (pHi) or arterial pH-pHi difference, *J Crit Care* 11:51, 1996.
19. Gomersall CD, Joynt GM, Freebairn RC, et al: Resuscitation of critically ill patients based on the results of gastric tonometry: a prospective, randomized, controlled trial, *Crit Care Med* 28:607, 2000.
20. Kirton OC, Windsor J, Wedderburn R, et al: Failure of splanchnic resuscitation in the acutely injured trauma patient correlates with multiple organ system failure and length of stay in the ICU, *Chest* 113:1064, 1998.

21. O'Donnell J, Axelrod P, Fisher C, et al: Use and effectiveness of hypothermia blankets for febrile patients in the intensive care unit, *Clin Infect Dis* 24:1208, 1997.

22. Caruso CC, Hadley BJ, Shukla R, et al: Cooling effects and comfort of four cooling blanket temperatures in humans with fever, *Nurs Res* 41:68, 1992.

SUGGESTED READINGS

Abraham E, Matthay MA, Dinarello CA, et al: Consensus conference definitions for sepsis, septic shock, acute lung injury and acute respiratory distress syndrome: time for a reevaluation, *Crit Care Med* 28:232, 2000.

Balk RA: Pathogenesis and management of multiple organ dysfunction or failure in severe sepsis and septic shock, *Crit Care Clin* 16:33, 2000.

Barton R, Cerra FB: The hypermetabolism multiple organ failure syndrome, *Chest* 96:1153, 1989.

Baue AE, Durham R, Faist E: Systemic inflammatory response syndrome (SIRS), multiple organ dysfunction syndrome (MODS), multiple organ failure (MOF): are we winning the battle? *Shock* 10:79, 1998.

Beal AL, Cerra FB: Multiple organ failure syndrome in the 1990s. Systemic inflammatory response and organ dysfunction, *JAMA* 271:226, 1994.

Bessey PQ: Metabolic response to critical illness. In Holcroft JW, Wilmore DW, Meakins L, et al, editors: *Care of the surgical patient,* vol 1, New York, 1989, Scientific American Medicine.

Bihari DJ: Acute liver failure–the ultimate cause of multiple organ systems failure? *Intens Crit Care Dig* 5:39, 1986.

Bihari DJ: Prevention of multiple organ failure in the critically-ill. In Vincent JL, editor: *Update in intensive care and emergency medicine,* Berlin, 1987, Springer-Verlag.

Demling R, LaLonde C, Saldinger P, et al: Multiple-organ dysfunction in the surgical patient: pathophysiology, prevention, and treatment, *Curr Probl Surg* 30:345, 1993.

Doig CJ, Sutherland LR, Sandham JD, et al: Increased intestinal permeability is associated with the development of multiple organ dysfunction syndrome, *Am J Respir Crit Care Med* 158:444, 1998.

Evans TW, Smithies M: ABC of intensive care: organ dysfunction, *BMJ* 318:1606, 1999.

Feltis BA, Wells CL: Does microbial translocation play a role in critical illness? *Curr Opin Crit Care* 6:117, 2000.

Fernandes CJ Jr, Akamine N, Knobel E: Cardiac troponin: a new serum marker of myocardial injury in sepsis, *Intensive Care Med* 25:1165, 1999.

Fiddian-Green RG: Associations between intramucosal acidosis in the gut and organ failure, *Crit Care Med* 21:S103, 1993.

Groeneveld ABJ, Nauta JJP, Thijs LG: Peripheral vascular resistance in septic shock: its relation to outcome, *Intensive Care Med* 14:141, 1988.

Gutierrez G, Palizas F, Doglio G, et al: Gastric intramucosal pH as a therapeutic index of tissue oxygenation in critically ill patients, *Lancet* 339:195, 1992.

Hanique G, Dugernier T, Laterre PF, et al: Significance of pathologic oxygen supply dependency in critically ill patients: comparison between measured and calculated methods, *Intensive Care Med* 20:12, 1994.

Heys SD, Walker LG, Smith I, et al: Enteral nutritional supplementation with key nutrients in patients with critical illness and cancer: a meta-analysis of randomized controlled clinical trials, *Ann Surg* 229:467, 1999.

Hurley R, Chapman MV, Mythen MG: Current status of gastrointestinal tonometry, *Curr Opin Crit Care* 6:130, 2000.

Keller GA, West MA, Cerra FB, et al: Macrophage-mediated modulation of hepatocyte protein synthesis, *Arch Surg* 121:1199, 1986.

Kreimeier U, Peter K: Strategies of volume therapy in sepsis and systemic inflammatory response syndrome, *Kidney Int* 53:S75, 1998.

Kumar A, Haery C, Parrillo JE: Myocardial dysfunction in septic shock, *Crit Care Clin* 16:251, 2000.

Landow L, Andersen LW: Splanchnic ischaemia and its role in multiple organ failure, *Acta Anaesthesiol Scand* 38:626, 1994.

Le Gall JR, Klar J, Lemeshow S, et al: The logistic organ dysfunction system, *JAMA* 276:802, 1996.

Livingston DH: Management of the surgical patient with multiple system organ failure, *Am J Surg* 165:8S, 1993.

Livingston DH, Mosenthal AC, Deitch EA: Sepsis and multiple organ dysfunction syndrome: a clinical-mechanistic overview, *New Horizons* 3:257, 1995.

Marshall JC, Cook DJ, Christou NV, et al: Multiple organ dysfunction score: a reliable descriptor of a complex clinical outcome, *Crit Care Med* 23:1638, 1995.

Marston A, Bulkley GB, Fiddian-Green RG, et al: *Splanchnic ischemia and multiple organ failure,* St Louis, 1989, Mosby.

Matuschak GM, Rinaldo JE, Pinsky MR, et al: Effect of end-stage liver failure on the incidence and resolution of the adult respiratory distress syndrome, *J Crit Care* 2:162, 1987.

Mizock BA: Metabolic derangements in sepsis and septic shock, *Crit Care Clin* 16:319, 2000.

Moore EE, Moore FA, Franciose RJ, et al: The postischemic gut serves as a priming bed for circulating neutrophils that provoke multiple organ failure, *J Trauma* 37:881, 1994.

Norton LW: Does drainage of intraabdominal pus reverse multiple organ failure? *Am J Surg* 149:347, 1985.

Ozawa K, Aoyama H, Yasuda K, et al: Metabolic abnormalities with postoperative organ failure, *Arch Surg* 118:1245, 1983.

Ranieri VM, Suter PM, Tortorella C, et al: Effect of mechanical ventilation on inflammatory mediators in patients with acute respiratory distress syndrome, *JAMA* 282:54, 1999.

Soni A, Pepper G, Wyrwinski PM, et al: Adrenal insufficiency occurring during septic shock: incidence, outcome, and relationship to peripheral cytokine levels, *Am J Med* 98:266, 1995.

Third European Consensus Conference in Intensive Care Medicine: Tissue hypoxia: how to detect, how to correct, how to prevent, *Am J Respir Crit Care Med* 154:1573, 1996.

Uusaro A, Russell JA: Could anti-inflammatory actions of cate-cholamines explain the possible beneficial effects of supra-normal oxygen delivery in critically ill surgical patients? *Intensive Care Med* 26:99, 2000.

Van Leeuwen PD, Boermeester MA, Houdijk AP, et al: Clinical significance of translocation, *Gut* 35:S28, 1994.

Vincent JL, Moreno R, Takala J, et al: The SOFA (Sepsis-related Organ Failure Assessment) score to describe organ dysfunc-tion/failure, *Intensive Care Med* 22:707, 1996.

West MA, Keller GA, Hyland BJ, et al: Hepatocyte function in sepsis: Kupffer cells mediate a biphasic protein synthesis response in hepatocytes after exposure to endotoxin or killed *Escherichia coli, Surgery* 98:388, 1985.

Wheeler AP, Bernard GR: Treating patients with severe sepsis, *N Engl J Med* 340:207, 1999.

Zhang H, Slutsky AS, Vincent JL: Oxygen free radicals in ARDS, septic shock and organ dysfunction, *Intensive Care Med* 26:474, 2000.

18

GLORIA OBLOUK DAROVIC

Monitoring Patients with Acute Pulmonary Disease

The primary functions of the respiratory system are to transfer oxygen from the atmosphere to blood and then to cells and to transfer carbon dioxide from the cells to blood and then to the atmosphere. The system fails when these functions are not performed adequately to meet the metabolic needs of the body. Respiratory failure as a result of pulmonary dysfunction or dysfunction of the anatomic structures that support ventilation may occur as an acute or a chronic condition that ultimately deteriorates and becomes life threatening. Acute and chronic forms of respiratory failure may be divided into three categories determined from blood gas measurements: hypoxemic, hypercapnic, and mixed (hypoxemic and hypercapnic). Each category has many causes, and multiple causes may coexist in a given patient.

1. The *hypoxemic* type is defined as a PaO_2 of less than 60 mm Hg while the person is at rest and breathing room air at sea level. The $PaCO_2$ may be normal or decreased. Hypoxemic failure is generally due to one or both of two possible pathophysiologic mechanisms. The first is ventilation/perfusion mismatch, such as intrapulmonary shunts (pneumonia, atelectasis, cardiogenic or permeability pulmonary edema) or increased alveolar dead space (pulmonary embolism, shock states). The second is a severe reduction in the diffusion capacity due to advanced pulmonary fibrosis (end-stage acute respiratory distress syndrome [ARDS], chronic obstructive pulmonary disease [COPD]).

2. The *hypercapnic* type is defined by a $PaCO_2$ of greater than 50 mm Hg (when the patient is not inhaling sup-

plemental oxygen). This type may be the result of alveolar hypoventilation (obstructive airway diseases, chest wall abnormalities, paralytic diseases, respiratory depression). Hypoxemia always occurs in association with significant hypercapnia.

3. The *mixed* type usually results from advanced hypoxemic respiratory failure or when the patient becomes profoundly fatigued from the work of breathing and is near collapse.

Both abnormalities in blood gases have deleterious effects on cell function. Compensatory adaptations of *acute hypoxemia* include an increase in cardiac output, hyperventilation, decreases in the mixed venous oxygen reserve, and systemic and arterial hypertension. *Chronic hypoxemia* is compensated by polycythemia and an increase in 2,3-diphosphoglycerate (2,3-DPG), decreases in the mixed venous oxygen reserve, and varying degrees of systemic and pulmonary hypertension.

Acute hypercapnea produces respiratory acidosis. When hypercapnia lasts for a few days, the serum bicarbonate level increases to offset the respiratory acidosis and bring the patient's pH within an acceptable range (compensated respiratory acidosis).

This chapter first defines *acute respiratory failure.* Acute and chronic pulmonary hypertension and respiratory muscle fatigue commonly coexist with and complicate acute respiratory failure. For these reasons, the causes and effects of acute and chronic pulmonary hypertension on cardiac structure and function (cor pulmonale), as well as the potent role of the work of breathing on patient outcome, are presented. The remainder of the chapter is devoted to discussion of the causes, pathophysiology, hemodynamic effects, patient evaluation, and management of acute pulmonary embolism; exacerbation of COPD; and high-pressure (cardiogenic) and permeability (ARDS) pulmonary edema.

ACUTE RESPIRATORY FAILURE

Acute respiratory failure (ARF) is a potentially life-threatening, rapidly developing failure of the pulmonary system to maintain oxygenation or carbon dioxide homeostasis (Table 18-1).

ARF is the result of a variety of diseases or injuries that may be pulmonary, cardiac, anatomic, neuromuscular, or systemic in origin. Most patients with acute respiratory failure have had normal pulmonary function before hospitalization. However, some patients have a history of chronic lung disease and significant baseline blood gas abnormalities. In these patients, *acute respiratory failure* is defined as an abrupt deterioration in their previous condition.

Acute respiratory failure is one of the most common life-threatening problems in hospitals. It is present in the majority of intensive care unit (ICU) patients and is usually associated with pulmonary hypertension. However, pulmonary hypertension can occur as an isolated disorder (primary pulmonary hypertension).

TABLE 18-1
Diagnostic Criteria for Acute Respiratory Failure (ARF)

Parameter	Normal	ARF
Respiratory rate	8 to 16 beats/min	>28 beats/min
Pao_2 mm Hg (room air)	90 to 100 mm Hg	<60 mm Hg
$Paco_2$ mm Hg	35 to 45 mm Hg	>55 mm Hg
Ratio of dead space to tidal volume (V_D/V_T)	0.3	>0.5
Intrapulmonary shunt fraction (Q_S/Q_T)	5 to 8%	>20%
Compliance (ml/cm H_2O)	100	<20
Alveolar-arterial oxygen difference (A-aDo_2) on Fio_2 100%	25 to 65	>450

Pulmonary Hypertension as a Condition Associated with Some Cardiac and Pulmonary Disorders

Acute and chronic pulmonary diseases, as well as some cardiac diseases, are commonly associated with elevated pulmonary artery systolic and diastolic pressures (pulmonary hypertension). Pulmonary hypertension is considered to be present when the patient's mean pulmonary artery pressure exceeds 20 mm Hg (normal values are 8 to 15 mm Hg). Pulmonary hypertension is considered severe when mean pressures exceed 40 mm Hg. Unlike systemic arterial pressures, pressures within the pulmonary arteries are not accessible for noninvasive study. Consequently, measurement of pulmonary arterial pressures is possible only with invasive technologies such as the flow-directed pulmonary artery catheter.

Causes of Pulmonary Hypertension
The normal pulmonary circulation is a capacious and highly distensible vascular bed that offers little resistance to blood flow. Therefore pulmonary artery systolic and diastolic pressures are normally low. The normally low-resistance pulmonary circulation may gradually or acutely become a high-resistance circulation as a result of distortion of lung tissue and vascular structures because of chronic, progressive cardiopulmonary disease; pulmonary vasoconstriction due to hypoxemia and acidemia; or acute or chronic pulmonary vascular obstructive disease. Pulmonary artery systolic and diastolic pressures increase in proportion to the increase in pulmonary vascular resistance in order to maintain blood flow through the lungs and maintain adequate left heart filling.

Classifications
Pulmonary hypertension is classified by the anatomic site of flow disturbance. *Precapillary and capillary pulmonary hypertension* result directly from disease or dysfunction of the lungs. *Postcapillary pulmonary hypertension* usually results from left heart disease or, rarely, pulmonary venous obstruction.

Precapillary and Capillary Pulmonary Hypertension. This condition, also termed *active pulmonary hypertension,* results from increases in pulmonary vascular resistance, which is the result of one or a combination of three factors. The first is increased pulmonary vascular tone resulting from hypoxemic or acidemic vasoconstriction. The second is vascular obstruction, which results in a loss in the cross-sectional area of the pulmonary vascular bed as in patients with pulmonary embolism. In the third, structural changes in the pulmonary arterioles, which include hypertrophy, hyperplasia, tortuosity, and stricture up to and including the pulmonary capillary bed, increase pulmonary vascular resistance and pulmonary artery pressures (Figure 18-1).

In patients with precapillary and capillary hypertension, the force of right ventricular ejection, and therefore pulmonary artery systolic pressure, increases to drive blood across the pulmonary circulation. Pulmonary artery diastolic pressure is elevated because of the resistance to diastolic blood flow. However, left ventricular end-diastolic, left atrial, and pulmonary venous pressures (as measured by pulmonary artery wedge pressure) are normal if left heart function is normal. In these patients, the pulmonary artery diastolic to wedge pressure (PAd-PWP) gradient is greater than 4 mm Hg and increases in tandem with increases in vascular resistance. Assuming no associated problems (e.g., hypoxemia, acidemia), if the patient's left heart pressures rise, pulmonary artery systolic and diastolic pressures likewise rise, but the preexisting PAd-PWP gradient is unaffected. For example, if a patient with COPD with a pulmonary artery diastolic pressure of 35 mm Hg and a pulmonary artery wedge pressure (PWP) of 10 mm Hg (gradient of 25 mm Hg) develops left ventricular failure, the PWP may rise to 22 mm Hg and the pulmonary artery diastolic pressure may passively rise to approximately 47 mm Hg (gradient of 25 mm Hg).

Conditions that result in tremendous increases in pulmonary blood flow, such as left-to-right intracardiac shunts, also result in elevations in pulmonary artery pressures. If chronic, these conditions eventually result in adaptive hypertrophic changes in the pulmonary blood vessels, which in turn cause greater elevations in pulmonary artery pressures. If the intracardiac shunt, such as a congenital ventricular septal defect, is corrected, the secondary hypertrophic changes and pulmonary hypertension may persist for months to years or may never resolve.

Postcapillary Pulmonary Hypertension. This condition, also termed *passive pulmonary hypertension,* typically results from disease or failure of the left side of the heart. Left atrial and pulmonary venous pressures increase and, as a result, pulmonary artery systolic and diastolic pressures passively increase. In these patients, the PAd-PWP gradient is typically less than 4 mm Hg.

If the postcapillary type becomes chronic (such as that which occurs with mitral stenosis), structural pulmonary arteriolar changes (hyperplasia and hypertrophy) eventually develop and add a precapillary component that further elevates pulmonary artery systolic and diastolic pressures. In such patients, pulmonary artery pressures may eventually approximate systemic blood pressure levels (Figure 18-2).

Other rare postcapillary causes of pulmonary hypertension include occlusive disease of the pulmonary veins such as by thrombotic problems, constricting mediastinitis, and tumors. All cause a variable degree of obstruction to pulmonary venous blood flow and a passive increase in pulmonary artery pressures.

Both precapillary and postcapillary pulmonary hypertension increase right ventricular workload and may eventually lead to right ventricular failure.

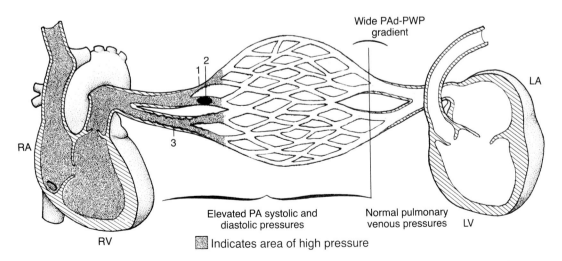

FIGURE 18-1 Precapillary pulmonary hypertension. *1,* Pulmonary arteriolar constriction (increased pulmonary vascular tone). *2,* Obstruction of pulmonary artery (i.e, embolism). *3,* Structural changes in pulmonary arterioles. The illustration indicates right ventricular failure secondary to the pulmonary hypertension.

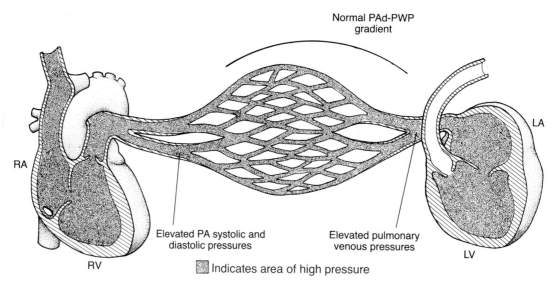

FIGURE 18-2 Postcapillary pulmonary hypertension. *Shaded areas* represent areas of high pressure. The illustration indicates right ventricular failure secondary to the high pulmonary artery pressure.

Extrapulmonary Factors That Influence Patient Outcome in Acute Respiratory Failure

Two important extrapulmonary factors require clinical consideration because they may singly or jointly affect patient outcome. These factors include the effects of pulmonary disease on cardiac function (cor pulmonale) and respiratory muscle fatigue.

Heart-Lung Interaction

Clinical and academic appreciation for the importance of the right ventricle has long been overshadowed by the role of the muscular, powerful left ventricle. Over the past 20 years, however, there has been a growing appreciation that right ventricular dysfunction plays a major role in the course of common cardiopulmonary diseases such as pulmonary embolism, COPD, and mitral stenosis.

The normally poorly muscled right ventricle is designed to eject into the low-resistance, low-pressure pulmonary circulation. However, if mean pulmonary artery pressure suddenly exceeds 35 to 45 mm Hg—as may occur in patients with massive pulmonary embolism; acute, severe hypoxemia; and acidemia—the right ventricle is unable to generate a systolic pressure high enough to provide adequate blood flow through the lungs. Right ventricular dilation and failure follow. Right ventricular dilation, in turn, results in widening of the tricuspid valve annulus. As a consequence, the valve leaflets may not close completely during systole. Acute tricuspid regurgitation then worsens the patient's hemodynamic and clinical picture.

If the patient also becomes hypotensive or hypoxemic, right ventricular dysfunction is compounded by myocardial ischemia, particularly in patients with right coronary artery disease. The hemodynamic consequences of acute and chronic right ventricular pressure overload are discussed later.

Cardiac Dysfunction Induced by Lung Disease (Cor Pulmonale). The term *cor pulmonale* means right ventricular hypertrophy, dilation, or failure due to pulmonary hypertension caused by disease of the lungs. By definition, this excludes dysfunction or distortion of the right ventricle that results from left heart disease or failure.

Chronic Cor Pulmonale. In those patients with chronic lung disease, a progressive rise in pulmonary vascular resistance imposes a gradually increasing systolic pressure load on the right ventricle. However, there is a corresponding progressive increase in right ventricular size. The adaptively hypertrophied and dilated right ventricle gradually becomes capable of generating systolic pressures as high as 70 to 90 mm Hg in order to eject a normal stroke volume into the high-resistance pulmonary circulation. When the underlying lung disease reaches a critical level or when a complication such as pulmonary embolism or pneumonia imposes an additional systolic pressure burden, the previously compensated right ventricle fails.

Four categories of pulmonary disease eventually result in chronic cor pulmonale:

1. *Chronic obstructive pulmonary disease* accounts for greater than 80% of patients with chronic cor pulmonale.

2. *Pulmonary fibrosis* occurs in patients with emphysema or chronic pulmonary inflammatory conditions such as tuberculosis and bronchiectasis.
3. *Thoracic musculoskeletal disorders* such as severe kyphoscoliosis, massive obesity, and muscular dystrophy that comprise ventilatory movements and lung function.
4. *Idiopathic primary pulmonary hypertension* is characterized by disease and distortion of the pulmonary vessels without an apparent cause.

Acute Cor Pulmonale. *Acute cor pulmonale* is defined as right heart strain and failure that results from acute pulmonary hypertension. Acute cor pulmonale is most commonly the result of massive pulmonary embolism.

Effects of Right Ventricular Failure on Left Ventricular Function. Although the right and left ventricles perfuse different circulations, the function of one ventricle is strongly affected by the function of the other ventricle because both are bonded by a common pliable intraventricular septum, the nondistensible pericardium, and muscle fibers that cross both ventricles. As a consequence of anatomic bonding, right ventricular failure profoundly affects left ventricular function via several mechanisms. First, a decreasing right ventricular stroke volume is immediately met by a proportionate decrease in left ventricular stroke volume. In other words, as the right ventricle fails, the outputs of both ventricles are brought into balance within a few heartbeats.

As the right ventricle continues to fail to empty adequately, the progressive increase in right ventricular end-systolic and end-diastolic blood volume shifts the intraventricular septum into the left ventricular cavity. Septal shift, in turn, alters the internal shape of the left ventricle and reduces its end-systolic and end-diastolic volume capacity (Figure 18-3).

The change in left ventricular cavity shape and size compromises systolic and diastolic function and alters the normal left ventricular filling volume/pressure relationship. This means that the measured left ventricular end-diastolic pressure (PWP) is greater than that which would be expected for any given end-diastolic volume. The clinical implication is that a patient's PWP measurement may be in the normal or greater than normal range (suggesting an acceptable ventricular filling volume), but the end-diastolic volume may be inadequate to support an acceptable stroke volume. Because of the misleadingly normal or greater than normal PWP, the unwary clinician may not realize that the decreased stroke volume is due to decreased left ventricular filling (hypovolemia).

In summary, acute and chronic changes in the pulmonary vasculature induced by hypoxemia, acidemia, or obstruction may cause profoundly adverse effects on cardiac function and hemodynamic status.

In addition, there are cardiac-related factors that may cause hemodynamic measurements to be misleading in patients with cor pulmonale. For example, a chronically strained, hypertrophied right ventricle is relatively stiff. As a result, the measured right atrial or central venous pressure may be greater than normal (even though intracardiac volumes are normal) and may lead the unwary clinician to think that the patient is in heart failure when, in fact, stroke volume is normal. In other words, the patient is not in heart failure despite elevated right atrial or central venous pressures.

On the other hand, right ventricular failure that occurs suddenly in an otherwise normal, highly compliant right ventricle may not be immediately associated with elevated end-diastolic pressures because the thin-walled ventricle can dilate to accommodate the increased volume without immediate elevations in end-diastolic pressure. Heart failure may then be present despite normal intracardiac pressures. The recognition of right heart failure in patients with acute and chronic lung disease requires an awareness of a probable cause for heart failure (i.e., identify the high-risk patient), as well as astute observation for changes in the patient's clinical status and careful evaluation of other hemodynamic and laboratory data.

Work of Breathing and Respiratory Muscle Fatigue

Acute respiratory failure, not caused by paralytic problems, is invariably associated with increased work of breathing. To maintain adequate alveolar ventilation and sustain the work of normal or labored breathing, the inspiratory and expiratory muscles must have strength and endurance, as well as adequate nutrient blood flow.

Except for the heart, the intercostal muscles and diaphragm are the only muscles on which life depends. Therefore respiratory muscle fatigue leading to failure threatens the patient's life. There are two causes of respiratory muscle fatigue:

1. *A workload beyond the capacity of normal ventilatory muscles.* This may occur in patients with very high airway resistance, such as that in status asthmaticus, and in patients with very low chest wall or lung compliance, such as those with circumferential thoracic burns or pulmonary edema.
2. *A limitation or reduction of the muscle's intrinsic work capacity or energy supply.* One or both of two possible factors may be the cause. First, the work capacity

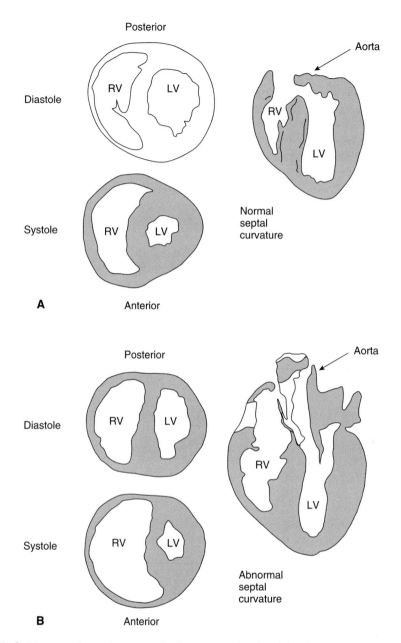

FIGURE 18-3 A, The normal septal curvature in the cross-sectional and longitudinal views in systole and diastole. The intraventricular septum is normally curved toward the right ventricle. **B,** With distention of the failing right ventricle, the septum is deviated toward the left ventricle and may additionally encroach on the left ventricular outflow tract. *RV,* right ventricle; *LV,* left ventricle. (Adapted from Weber KT, Janicki JS, Shroff SG, et al: The cardiopulmonary unit. The body's gas transport system, *Clin Chest Med* 4:101, 1983.)

of the diaphragm and intercostal muscles may fall below normal because of physiologic imbalances such as hypokalemia, hypocalcemia, hypomagnesemia, paralytic disease, and muscle deconditioning due to prolonged periods of mechanical ventilatory support.

Second, effective ventilatory muscle contraction depends on the constant aerobic generation of the energy currency, adenosine triphosphate (ATP), from oxygen and foodstuffs. When oxygen availability is reduced because of hypoxemia or circulatory failure or when the patient is profoundly malnourished, the capacity of the muscles of ventilation to generate energy may fall short of work requirements. Patients may not be able even to sustain the work of normal, quiet breathing.

Another important clinical consideration is that when the respiratory muscle's need for oxygen is high but circulatory function is impaired (as may occur in patients with acute pulmonary edema, massive pulmonary embolism, sepsis, and shock syndromes), significant amounts of blood may be diverted to the work-stressed ventilatory muscles. As a result, other vital organs become further deprived of nutrient flow, and the risk of ischemic multiple-organ dysfunction or damage is increased.

Clinical Signs and Symptoms of Respiratory Muscle Fatigue. Normally, the chest and abdomen rise and fall synchronously with breathing. With the onset of respiratory muscle fatigue, the patient's chest and abdomen move in opposite directions during both inspiration and expiration. This produces a rocking movement to the patient's respiratory efforts; respiratory movements also become rapid and spastic in appearance (see Chapter 3, section on chest/abdominal synchrony and respiratory muscle fatigue). The patient, if able to talk, typically complains of dyspnea; hypoxemia and hypercarbia will be noted on blood gas analysis.

Mechanical ventilation relieves the problem by improving alveolar ventilation and oxygen supply while taking over the patient's work of breathing. This reduces the blood flow requirements of the respiratory muscles and increases the proportion of cardiac output available to other organs. Intubation with ventilatory assistance also eliminates the risk of respiratory arrest, which usually occurs when the patient succumbs to exhaustion.

CAUSES OF ACUTE RESPIRATORY FAILURE

The causes of acute respiratory failure that commonly occur in critically ill or injured patients are discussed in this chapter. Although the inciting events may differ, the aforementioned principles as related to pulmonary hypertension, cor pulmonale, and respiratory muscle failure apply to all.

Pulmonary Embolism

A pulmonary embolism is a plug that has impacted and partially or totally occluded all or a portion of the pulmonary circulation. The plug may be air, tumor, amniotic fluid, septic or fat embolism, injected particulate matter (intravenous drug abusers), or foreign body, such as a broken portion of a vascular catheter. More than 90% of pulmonary emboli are blood clots. These clots most commonly form in the deep veins of the lower extremities such as the iliac or femoral veins or in the inferior vena cava. Clots also may originate in the pelvic veins in patients with pelvic inflammatory disease or abdominal malignancy. Alternatively, they may develop in the right heart of the patient with atrial fibrillation or dilated right heart. Clots that develop in the deep veins below the knee are usually of little consequence.

Superficial thrombophlebitis noted as a tender, red "venous cord" poses little embolic risk unless the associated clot extends into the major, deep veins. Such extension is suggested by swelling of the involved leg.

Upper extremity venous thrombosis may develop in ventilated patients with coexisting regional trauma, neoplasm, and implanted pacemakers. Central venous catheters pose additional risk for superior vena caval, axillary, or subclavian venous thrombosis, as well as the superior vena caval syndrome. These clots may dislodge and become pulmonary emboli.

Classification of Pulmonary Emboli

A *massive pulmonary embolism* involves the main pulmonary trunk, the right or left main pulmonary artery, or two or more lobar branches (Figure 18-4).

The term *submassive pulmonary embolism* is related to embolic material that produces lesser degrees of vascular obstruction.

Incidence

Pulmonary embolism is a common pulmonary complication in hospitalized patients. The exact incidence of pulmonary embolism in ICU patients is difficult to ascertain. However, it is the most commonly misdiagnosed, serious acute illness because the signs and symptoms of pulmonary embolism are very similar to those of other major cardiopulmonary disorders. Pulmonary embolism is estimated to be the third most common cause of death in the United States; in many cases the finding of pulmonary embolism is made at autopsy. Although accurate figures are impossible to come by, it was estimated in 1975 (most recently published estimate) that the annual incidence of pulmonary embolism in the United States was approximately 630,000.[1] Of these patients, approximately 11% die within the first hour. Of the initial survivors, an estimated 71% are not correctly diagnosed; of these, 30% die. Of the 29% of initial survivors who are correctly diagnosed, only 8% die. These statistics underscore the importance of an early correct diagnosis and appropriate therapy.

Although no current estimates are available, evidence suggests that the incidence of pulmonary embolism is

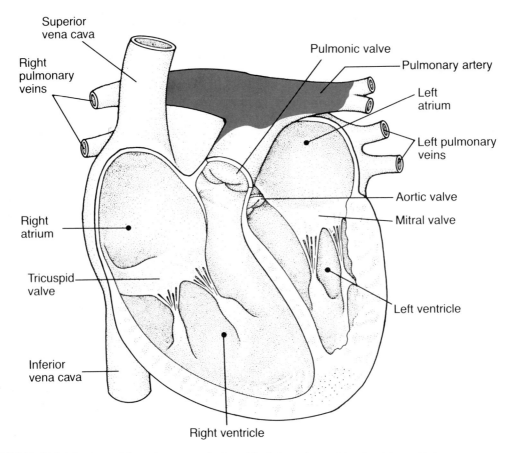

Superior
vena cava

Pulmonic valve

Pulmonary artery

Right
pulmonary
veins

Left
atrium

Left pulmonary
veins

Aortic valve

Right
atrium

Mitral valve

Tricuspid
valve

Left ventricle

Inferior
vena cava

Right ventricle

FIGURE 18-4 Massive saddle pulmonary embolism *(shaded area)* overrides the right and left main pulmonary arteries; note right ventricular dilation. The hemodynamic effect is complete blockade of the central circulation and cardiovascular collapse. The clinical corollary is sudden death.

increasing. The proposed reasons for the apparent increase are (1) the generally larger and sicker patient population, (2) the prolongation of life in metastatic disease, (3) the increased use of oral contraceptives, (4) the larger elderly population, and (5) the increased recognition of pulmonary embolism.

Predisposing Factors

More than 100 years ago, Rudolf Virchow, a pathologist, proposed a triad of factors that favors venous clot formation: damage to the vascular lining (endothelial injury), venous stasis, and hypercoagulability.[2]

1. *Direct activation of the clotting mechanism by alterations or damage to the vascular lining.* Venous clot formation may occur following venipuncture; distention of or trauma to a vein; or as a result of inflammatory vascular disease, atherosclerosis, or varicose veins.

2. *Venous stasis.* Poor blood flow, in turn, delays the wash-out of activated clotting factors from damaged

or altered veins. Venous stasis commonly occurs in people who are on prolonged bed rest, those who sit for long periods of time, or traumatic spinal cord–injured patients with leg paralysis (the first 2 weeks after injury is the period of greatest risk). Other patients at risk include the morbidly obese; patients in congestive heart failure or shock; and patients with dehydration, hypovolemia, and abdominal tumors because of vascular compression adjacent to the tumor mass. The atrial chambers also are susceptible to clot formation within a few days of the onset of atrial fibrillation.

3. *Hypercoagulability.* A hypercoagulable state has been linked with pregnancy; carcinoma; fever; oral estrogen therapy; polycythemia vera; hyperhomocysteinemia; systemic lupus; deficiencies in antithrombin III, protein C or protein S, and plasminogen; the antiphospholipid antibody syndrome; mutations in factor V (Leiden mutation) or mutations of the prothrombin gene; and

---

BOX 18-1

Risk Factors for Deep Venous Thrombosis and Pulmonary Embolism

- Previous episode of thromboembolism
- Prolonged immobility or paralysis
- Malignant disease, particularly carcinoma of the breast, pancreas, lung, ovary-uterus, stomach, and bowel
- Morbid obesity
- Pregnancy and the postpartum period
- Oral estrogen use
- Congestive heart failure
- Varicose veins, atherosclerosis, phlebitis
- Advanced age (over 60 years of age)
- Hematologic deficiencies (antithrombin III, protein C and protein S, plasminogen)
- The presence of antiphospholipid antibody, hyperhomo-cysteinemia, or factor V (Leiden) or prothrombin mutations
- Trauma or surgery, particularly to the hips, lower limbs, and spine*
- Indwelling central venous catheters; embolization is especially likely to occur on catheter withdrawal
- Dehydration
- Hypovolemia
- Fever
- Atrial fibrillation
- Open prostatectomy
- Cerebrovascular accident
- Systemic lupus
- Polycythemia vera

*Reconstructive surgeries to the hip and knee carry the highest overall single risk of deep venous thrombosis and pulmonary embolism.

immediate postoperative, posttrauma, and postpartum periods.

The more risk factors (listed in Box 18-1) that coexist in an individual patient, the greater the risk for deep venous thrombus and subsequent pulmonary embolism. Because critically ill or injured patients have a multiplicity of risk factors, many ICU patients develop pulmonary embolisms that adversely affect their clinical course and contribute to death.

Once formed, the venous clot may be lysed by the proteolytic activity of the fibrinolytic system. Scar tissue may also infiltrate the clot, which then becomes a part of the vessel wall (organized thrombus). Alternatively, the clot may fragment or become dislodged by sudden changes in venous pressure associated with standing, walking, straining at stool, coughing, or sneezing.

Once dislodged, the flow of blood directs the clot up the vena cava and through the right heart, and the clot reaches the pulmonary circulation within seconds.

Pathophysiology

Obstruction of the pulmonary arterial circulation results in disturbances in lung function, as well as hemodynamic abnormalities. The degree of cardiopulmonary abnormalities depends on the size and location of the embolized vessel, the completeness of occlusion, and the presence and severity of acute or chronic underlying disease. If the patient is critically ill or injured, a pulmonary embolism usually produces a more dramatic clinical picture and more life-threatening consequences than an embolism of the same size in an otherwise healthy person.

Pulmonary Abnormalities

Several abnormalities collectively contribute to blood gas abnormalities. If significant in magnitude, hypoxemia results.

Ventilation in Excess of Perfusion (Increased Dead Space Volume). Ventilation of the involved lung segment is wasted because nonperfused lung tissue cannot participate in gas exchange. If the patient's minute ventilation were to remain constant, the $Paco_2$ would rise. However, tachypnea and hyperventilation, which typically occur as reflex responses to local lung changes, more than compensate for the wasted ventilation. Consequently, the patient's $Paco_2$ usually falls. Diffuse bronchoconstriction, which is mediated mostly by platelet-derived serotonin, also develops and reduces ventilation to the well-perfused areas of the lung. Impaired alveolar ventilation, in turn, predisposes patients to diffuse microatelectasis, as well as perfusion in excess of ventilation. If significant in magnitude, both defects result in hypoxemia.

The bronchi distal to the pulmonary embolus further constrict owing to the local release of biochemical agents (serotonin, histamine) from the lung itself.

Perfusion in Excess of Ventilation (Shunt Units). There are two reasons for the development of shunt units. First, diffuse bronchoconstriction, mediated by the local release of serotonin and histamine, develops and reduces ventilation to the well-perfused areas of the lung. Impaired alveolar ventilation, in turn, predisposes patients to diffuse microatelectasis. Second, a significant local surfactant deficiency and regional atelectasis occur within 24 hours of the embolic event. Both increase overall lung shrinkage and worsen hypoxemia.

No Ventilation or Perfusion (Silent Units). Fewer than 10% of pulmonary emboli result in *pulmonary infarction* because of the double (bronchial and pulmonary arterial) vascular supply to the lung. Pulmonary infarction is more likely to develop in patients with compromise to both pulmonary and bronchial circulations, such as occurs in patients with pneumonia, pulmonary hypertension, systemic hypotension, intrathoracic malignancies, heart failure, and COPD. Lung tissue in the infarcted area of lung is essentially dead and is neither ventilated nor perfused. Pulmonary infarction is characterized by ischemic necrosis of alveolar walls and localized inflammatory response. On chest radiograph this appears as a localized infiltrate.

Low Mixed Venous Oxygen Content. This cause of hypoxemia develops only in patients with massive pulmonary embolism and low cardiac output. Because venous blood is presented to the pulmonary circulation with less than normal venous oxygen content, it leaves the lungs and returns to the systemic circulation with less than normal arterial oxygen content.

Opening of a Patent Foramen Ovale. In a small but significant percent of the population, the foramen ovale is closed but may be opened if right atrial pressure exceeds left atrial pressures, as happens in massive pulmonary embolism. The consequent right-to-left atrial shunt results in hypoxemia that is unresponsive to oxygen therapy.

Hemodynamic Abnormalities

Occlusion of pulmonary arteries results in a decrease in the cross-sectional area of the pulmonary circulation, and, if significant, an increase in the resistance to blood flow through the lungs results. Because of the immense size of the pulmonary circulation and the high level of distensibility of the pulmonary vessels, small pulmonary emboli usually have no hemodynamic consequences. In such patients, right ventricular output is redirected to the unoccluded pulmonary vessels, which passively dilate to accommodate blood flow. As a result, vascular resistance and pulmonary artery pressures remain normal.

A greater than 40% to 50% reduction in the size of vascular bed (which occurs in patients with massive pulmonary embolism) requires an increase in pulmonary artery pressure to maintain blood flow through the significantly diminished cross-sectional area of the pulmonary circulation. Pulmonary artery pressures may increase acutely or chronically. For example, if acute massive pulmonary embolism occurs, the patient develops acute pulmonary hypertension. On the other hand, pulmonary vascular obstruction may develop gradually, if the pulmonary

circulation is sporadically and progressively "showered" by small clots over the course of the patient's primary illness or the patient's lifetime. In such a patient, pulmonary hypertension usually develops gradually.

In patients with major pulmonary vascular obstruction, the pulmonary artery systolic and diastolic pressures are elevated but the pulmonary capillary hydrostatic pressure and left heart pressure (as estimated by PWP) are normal if the patient is without heart disease. *Widening of the PAd-PWP gradient is characteristic of the precapillary pulmonary hypertension associated with massive pulmonary embolism.*

The increase in pulmonary vascular resistance, in turn, increases the systolic workload and oxygen consumption of the right ventricle. If mean pulmonary artery pressures increase beyond 35 to 45 mm Hg, the right ventricle fails because the normally thin-walled right ventricular is not anatomically or physiologically designed to acutely accept heavy pressure loads. With the advent of right ventricular failure, pulmonary blood flow and left ventricular filling are reduced, cardiac output falls, and right atrial and right ventricular end-diastolic pressures increase. Hypoxemia originally due to the pulmonary embolism is exacerbated by the presence of circulatory failure. The acutely failing right ventricle dilates, and, if dilation is significant, the development of acute tricuspid regurgitation compounds the hemodynamic deterioration.

In patients with preexisting heart or lung disease, hemodynamic deterioration occurs with less than 40% to 50% pulmonary vascular obstruction (submassive pulmonary embolism).

Clinical Presentation

The information in Table 18-2 supports the statement that no single sign or symptom is diagnostic of pulmonary embolism. In fact, the signs and symptoms and laboratory values are highly inconsistent among affected patients and often mimic other cardiopulmonary diseases. A high index of suspicion for a patient with risk factors for deep venous thrombosis and pulmonary embolism is essential for early recognition and appropriate therapy.

Dyspnea and tachypnea are the most common presenting signs and symptoms, and their sudden appearance should alert the clinician to the possibility of acute pulmonary embolism. However, if a paralyzed patient is being maintained on mechanical ventilation, it is impossible to evaluate for these important pulmonary embolic clues. In addition, tachypnea and dyspnea are common to patients with other conditions, such as cardiogenic and ARDS pulmonary edema, pneumonia, COPD, and nonspecific reactions to physiologic or mental stress. These factors

TABLE 18-2
Frequency of Signs and Symptoms in 327 Patients with Documented Pulmonary Embolism

Signs	Percent
Respiratory rate greater than 16/min	92
Rales (crackles)	58
Increased pulmonic component of the second heart sound (S₂)	53
Pulse greater than 100/min	44
Temperature greater than 37.8° C	43
Phlebitis	32
Gallop rhythm	34
Diaphoresis	36
Edema	24
Heart murmur	23
Cyanosis	19

Symptoms	Percent
Chest pain	88
Pleuritic (typically, sharp and stabbing)	74
Nonpleuritic (substernal, may mimic myocardial infarction	14
Dyspnea	84
Apprehension	59
Cough	53
Hemoptysis	30
Sweats	27
Syncope	13

From Bell WR, Simon TL, Demetes DL: The clinical features of submassive and massive pulmonary emboli, *Am J Med* 62:358, 1977.

contribute to the assessment problems that delay the timely and accurate diagnosis of pulmonary embolism.

Palpation of the Precordium. Right ventricular activity may be palpable over the right or left sternal borders in patients with massive pulmonary embolisms. The right ventricular thrust correlates with the forceful right ventricular contractions that result from pulmonary hypertension.

Hemodynamic Profile

The sudden, unexplained development of pulmonary hypertension with a widened PAd-PWP gradient or sudden elevation in central venous pressure (CVP) in any invasively monitored patient should alert the clinician to the possibility of a massive pulmonary embolism. Patients with submassive pulmonary emboli may have no significant hemodynamic changes.

Arterial Pressure. In most cases, there is no change from the patient's normal values; a systolic pressure less than 100 mm Hg develops in less than 3% of patients. When a significant drop in blood pressure does occur, it usually signifies a massive pulmonary embolism causing acute cor pulmonale. When hypotension is present, it appears that the decrease in blood pressure is greater than that expected for the level of fall in cardiac output. This exaggerated fall in arterial pressure is thought to be the result of impaired baroreceptor reflexes. The cause of the altered reflex response is not known.

Systemic Vascular Resistance. Systemic vascular resistance is increased in patients with circulatory failure due to massive pulmonary embolism.

Pulmonary Vascular Resistance. The increase in pulmonary vascular resistance is proportional to the degree of cross-sectional obstruction of the pulmonary arterial bed and is also related to the presence or severity of hypoxemia and acidemia.

Central Venous Pressure or Right Atrial Pressure. Elevation of the right atrial (RA) pressure and CVP occurs in patients with massive pulmonary embolism and reflects right ventricular failure. An increased-amplitude *a* wave may be observed in the right atrial waveform; it reflects increased resistance to filling the failing right ventricle during atrial systole (Figure 18-5).

Pulmonary Artery and Wedge Pressures. An increase in pulmonary artery systolic and diastolic pressure occurs in patients with massive pulmonary embolism. The PWP may be in the normal range or may be decreased because of impaired left ventricular filling. The increased PAd-PWP gradient correlates with elevations in pulmonary vascular resistance (Figure 18-6). The hemodynamic diagnosis may be difficult, however, in patients with preexisting cardiopulmonary disease. For example, patients with underlying COPD or ARDS have preexisting pulmonary hypertension and widened PAd-PWP gradients, and patients with coexisting left heart dysfunction have elevations in both pulmonary artery and wedged pressures.

The contour of the pulmonary artery waveforms is unchanged, although in patients with severe right ventricular dysfunction, a pulmonary artery pulsus alternans may be observed.

Cardiac Output. A decrease in cardiac output occurs in patients with massive pulmonary embolism. In a previously

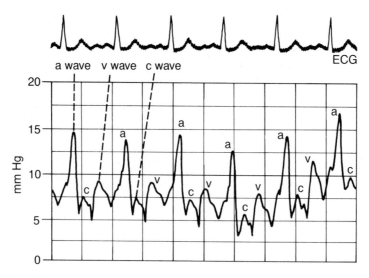

FIGURE 18-5 Right atrial pressure tracing taken from a patient with a massive pulmonary embolism. Note the increased-amplitude a waves.

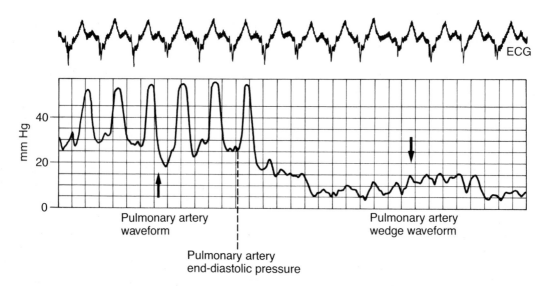

FIGURE 18-6 Pulmonary hypertension secondary to a massive pulmonary embolism. Note the increased pulmonary artery diastolic to wedge pressure (PAd-PWP) gradient. Note also the respiratory-induced variation in the waveform baseline due to the patient's dyspnea.

healthy person, if the pulmonary circulation is obstructed by more than 75%, the cardiac index falls below 2.5 L/min/m² and the patient may become hypotensive. In a critically ill or injured patient, far lesser degrees of pulmonary vascular obstruction may be associated with life-threatening circulatory failure.

If the patient becomes hypotensive, ischemic myocardial dysfunction (due to coronary hypoperfusion) is likely to produce an even greater decrease in cardiac output.

Mixed Venous Oxygen Saturation. Mixed venous oxygen saturation (Svo_2) is decreased if circulatory failure or hypoxemia complicates pulmonary embolism.

Laboratory Studies and Other Diagnostic Tests
Tests Specific for Diagnosis of Deep Venous Thrombosis. Pulmonary embolism is a complication of deep venous thrombosis (DVT) and is not a primary illness. Therefore an important component of the diagnostic

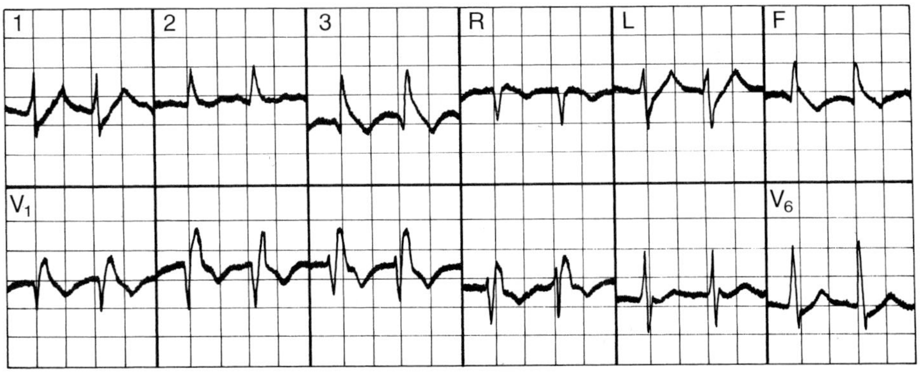

FIGURE 18-7 Acute cor pulmonale from a patient with massive pulmonary embolism. Note the T-wave inversion in the inferior (III, aVF) and anteroseptal (V1-4) leads, the S wave in lead I, the Q wave in lead III, and right bundle branch block. (From Marriott HJL: *Practical electrocardiography,* ed 7, Baltimore, 1983, Williams & Wilkins.)

workup for patients suspected of pulmonary embolism is to document the underlying disease—thrombi in the major deep veins. There is also concern that additional deep venous thrombi may also become emboli. However, approximately 30% of patients with pulmonary embolism show no evidence of DVT on laboratory examination. Thus negative study findings may be false and do not necessarily rule out the possibility of DVT and acute pulmonary embolism. The laboratory search for DVT includes iodine-125 fibrinogen uptake, impedance plethysmography, contrast venography, duplex ultrasonography, and magnetic resonance imaging.

The "classic" clinical findings such as Homan's sign (calf pain with flexion of the knee and dorsiflexion of the ankle), Moses' sign (pain with compression of the calf against the tibia), and swelling of the involved leg are infrequent and nonspecific.

There is no diagnostic test specific for pulmonary embolism, but the following tests may be helpful. Most tests are nonspecific, and coexisting abnormalities may produce positive results unrelated to pulmonary embolism. Conversely, all diagnostic test results may be negative in patients with pulmonary embolism.

Tests for Diagnosis of Pulmonary Embolism

Electrocardiogram. The electrocardiogram (ECG) may be completely normal, or there may be only nonspecific ST-T wave abnormalities and sinus tachycardia. The effects of the excessive pressure load on the right heart imposed by a *massive* pulmonary embolism are manifested as a sudden development of an S wave in standard lead I, a Q wave in standard lead III, and an inverted T wave in standard lead III (S1, Q3, T3) (Figure 18-7).

Sudden-onset, complete or incomplete bundle branch block or supraventricular or ventricular arrhythmias should raise the index of suspicion of pulmonary embolism in high-risk patients. Generally, the ECG is more useful to rule out cardiac conditions that clinically mimic pulmonary embolism, such as acute myocardial infarction, than in diagnosis of embolism. Thus diagnostic use of the ECG in pulmonary embolism is one of exclusion of other conditions with a similar clinical presentation.

Chest Radiograph. Radiographic abnormalities may vary considerably, and a preembolic film is helpful for making comparisons. The chest radiograph in patients with pulmonary embolism may be completely normal. Important changes to look for include (1) elevation of the affected side hemidiaphragm (due to loss of lung air volume secondary to bronchoconstriction, microatelectasis, and lung shrinkage); (2) unexplained densities (pulmonary infarction), more common in the peripheral and dependent lung fields; (3) pleural effusion; (4) dilated central pulmonary artery; (5) abrupt cutoff of a pulmonary artery with distention of the proximal portion of the vessel; and (6) locally decreased vascular markings.

Lung Perfusion Scan. A completely normal perfusion scan rules out pulmonary embolism with the same degree of certainty as a pulmonary angiogram.[3] False-positive scans may be obtained in patients with other causes of perfusion defects, such as localized hypoxic vasoconstriction due to mucous plugging or pneumonia, blebs, tumors, or redistribution of pulmonary blood flow due to congestive heart failure.

Ventilation Scan. Addition of the ventilation scan increases specificity to the perfusion scan. For example, patients with a recent pulmonary embolism usually have normal ventilation in the areas of perfusion defects, whereas patients with mucous plugs, pneumonia, or tumors have ventilation and perfusion defects within the same area of lung. However, total occlusion of a pulmonary vessel, over days, may result in atelectasis of the involved alveoli, as well as pulmonary infarction. In these patients, ventilation and perfusion defects may be present.

The most frequently referenced study evaluating the diagnostic value of ventilation/perfusion scans, the Prospective Investigation of Pulmonary Embolism Diagnosis indicated that normal lung scans make the probability of pulmonary embolism very unlikely.[3] Also, 87% of patients with multiple, segmental-sized areas of perfusion defects without corresponding ventilation abnormalities (high probability) had pulmonary emboli and increased to 96% with high clinical probability. However, from 15% to 30% of patients with low probability do have pulmonary embolism. Conclusions from this study are that pulmonary embolism is very unlikely in patients with normal lung scans and that a low-probability scan does not exclude pulmonary embolism. Overall, the presence of pulmonary embolism cannot be ruled out with perfusion scanning alone.

Echocardiography. The detection of a dilated right arium; a dilated akinetic right ventricle or right ventricle with regional wall motion abnormalities and normal motion of the apical wall; or flattening or deviation of the intraventricular septum toward the left ventricle suggests the possibility of pulmonary embolism. When properly performed, transesophageal echocardiography has shown sensitivity and specificity rates greater than 90% in detecting main pulmonary trunk and right and left main pulmonary emboli.[4] Echocardiography is also helpful in ruling out other conditions with similar clinical findings such as right ventricular infarction, endocarditis, pericardial tamponade, and aortic dissection.

Blood Gases. Approximately 13% of patients with documented pulmonary embolism have a PaO_2 above 80 mm Hg, and 6% have a PaO_2 greater than 90 mm Hg while breathing room air. The PaO_2 is less than 60 mm Hg in approximately 35% of patients with documented pulmonary embolism. A PaO_2 less than 50 mm Hg in a patient with previously normal blood gas values indicates that greater than 50% of the pulmonary arterial tree is obstructed and that pulmonary hypertension is present.[5] The problem is that the evaluative capability of this laboratory measurement is blurred because acute or chronic hypoxemia preexists in most ICU patients with cardiopulmonary dysfunction. Therefore this test is not particularly useful.

However, hypocapnia and respiratory alkalosis are typically present because of the hyperventilation that accompanies pulmonary embolism. Even in chronically hypercarbic patients (COPD), an acute reduction in $PaCO_2$ from baseline values often develops at the onset of an acute pulmonary embolism.

Dead Space to Tidal Volume Ratio. The dead space to tidal volume ratio (VD/VT) measures the volume of "wasted ventilation." In healthy people, this is related only to inhaled air that fills the tracheobronchial tree and constitutes approximately one third of tidal volume (VD/VT of 0.3). In people with pulmonary embolism, the ratio is increased relative to the size of ventilated but nonperfused lung. This test is diagnostically specific and sensitive for pulmonary embolism when arterial blood gases are withdrawn simultaneously with *carefully* measured and analyzed expired air. The end-tidal carbon dioxide is also typically decreased.

Contrast-Enhanced Spiral or Electron-Beam Computed Tomography and Magnetic Resonance Imaging. Both tests have the advantages of being minimally invasive and enabling diagnosis of chest diseases that have clinical presentations similar to those of pulmonary embolism. Both tests can identify large emboli in the larger pulmonary arteries. Negative tests do not, however, exclude the presence of subsegmental emboli. Disadvantages to both are the requirement for patient transport; requirement of a 24-second breath hold, which is difficult for tachypneic and dyspneic patients; and exposure to contrast material in patients with renal insufficiency. In these patients, clinicians should consider directly proceeding to pulmonary angiography in order to minimize exposure to contrast material if computed tomography is followed by angiography.

Pulmonary Angiography. Because critically ill or hemodynamically unstable patients tolerate diagnostic studies and transportation poorly, consideration should be given to bedside angiography as the initial study. Pulmonary angiography is the definitive and most reliable study, but it too has pitfalls and associated risks. Angiography should be performed within 1 week of the embolic event; otherwise, resolution of the clot may occur and may yield a false-negative study. Also, false-negative results may be obtained from patients with very small emboli.

Positive angiographic findings include intraluminal filling defects from incomplete vascular obstruction by the clot and pulmonary arterial cutoffs from complete vascular obstruction. Other angiographic findings that may be present (but are not considered diagnostic) include local flow abnormalities, asymmetric vascular filling or localized tortuosity, and tapering of blood vessels.

Angiography is the most invasive diagnostic study. Serious complications include life-threatening arrhythmias, vascular injury, cardiopulmonary arrest, and allergic reactions to contrast material. The complication risks are higher in patients with renal insufficiency, pulmonary hypertension, or critical illness or injury.

Other Diagnostic Clues. Because diagnostic and clinical criteria are so nonspecific for pulmonary embolism, the following clinical markers may be helpful in arriving at a timely diagnosis:

1. Sudden, severe hypoxemia with normal pulmonary compliance suggests a pulmonary vascular problem.
2. A sudden increase in pulmonary vascular resistance and pulmonary artery pressures with widening of the pulmonary artery diastolic to wedge pressure gradient points to an acute pulmonary vascular problem.

Prevention

DVT is the primary problem, and pulmonary embolism is a complication of this problem. Prophylaxis for the underlying problem includes anticoagulation and prevention of venous stasis.

Low-Dose Anticoagulation. Low-dose unfractionated heparin, 5000 U every 8 to 12 hours, is started 2 hours before surgery or at the institution of bed rest (onset of illness) and continues until the patient is ambulatory. The rationale for this approach is that low-dose heparin therapy inhibits thrombin formation but produces minimal risk of bleeding. Although prophylactic anticoagulation with low-dose heparin is currently regarded as state-of-the-art management of patients at high risk of thromboembolic disease, one multicenter study found that prophylaxis for venous thromboembolism is still underused, particularly in nonteaching hospitals.[6] Alternatively, the recently Food and Drug Administration (FDA)–approved fractionated heparin, dalteparin (Fragmin), may be given at a 5000 U subcutaneous dose once daily. Advantages include more predictable dose-response characteristics and no need for anticoagulation monitoring.

Prevention of Venous Stasis. Impaired blood flow in the lower extremities is prevented by frequent changes in the patient's position. Positioning is adjusted so that there is no extreme knee or hip flexion.

Intermittent inflation of pneumatic leggings (sequential compression devices) simulates the pumping action of active leg muscles and enhances venous return. There are no risks associated with these devices, although some patients find them annoying. This method is popular in ICUs, but it does not prevent thigh and pelvic vein thrombosis, particularly following hip surgery.

The application of compression stockings is thought to prevent DVT by decreasing the cross-sectional area of veins by external compression. This, in turn, increases the velocity of blood flow. The important clinical point is that these *must* be kept smooth, otherwise a tourniquet effect may produce venous stasis. Although commonly done, the simultaneous use of graduated compression stockings and intermittent pneumatic compression leggings does not produce a synergetic augmentation of deep venous blood flow.

Treatment

The goals in treating patients with acute pulmonary embolism are the support of the vital functions, relief of the symptoms, reduction of the extent of pulmonary vascular obstruction, and prevention of the recurrent deep venous embolization. Treatment guidelines include the following measures:

1. *Correction of hypoxemia.* Oxygen therapy should be provided if hypoxemia is present.
2. *Anticoagulation.* Prompt anticoagulation with unfractionated heparin is the treatment of choice for most patients with thromboembolic disease. Heparin does not directly lyse the clot or clots, but it does interfere with clot formation at several steps in the coagulation cascade. These actions prevent the formation of more clots or distal extension of the existing clots. In patients with normal coagulation profiles, heparin is usually given as an initial 80 U/kg intravenous bolus followed by a continuous infusion of 18 U/kg/hr for a minimum of 4 to 5 days. Heparin requirements may be considerably higher than normal for patients in the first few days following pulmonary embolism, however, because antithrombin III (heparin cofactor) levels tend to fall in patients with an acute thromboembolic process. The partial thromboplastin time of 1.5 to 2 times control values (46 to 70 seconds) should be achieved within 24 hours and maintained for 5 to 7 days with 5 days of overlap with warfarin (Coumadin) therapy.

    At the time of publication of this text, enoxaparin sodium (Lovenox) has been FDA-approved for treatment of DVT or DVT with pulmonary embolism. Dalteparin (Fragmin) has not. Check with the hospital pharmacy for availability and dosing of specific anticoagulants.

3. *Fluid therapy.* Fluid therapy and volume expansion targeted to maintain RA pressures of 15 to 20 mm Hg may be indicated in hypotensive patients to restore left ventricular filling pressure to a level sufficient to maintain left ventricular filling, stroke volume, and systemic perfusion. Care must be taken to avoid overdistention of the right ventricle (RA pressure greater than 20 mm Hg). Right ventricular diastolic pressure/volume overload

predisposes to right ventricular ischemia and shift of the intraventricular septum into the left ventricle.

4. *Pharmacologic stabilization of the cardiovascular system*. Inotropic agents, such as dobutamine or dopamine, may improve right (or possibly left) ventricular performance. Vasopressor therapy may be required in patients with hypotension that persists despite volume expansion.

5. *Positioning the patient with the involved lung in either a dependent or nondependent position*. Hypoxemia may depend on the patient's position if the pulmonary embolism involves only one lung because gravity influences the ventilation/perfusion relationship of both lungs. There seems to be no predictability as to whether positioning the patient with the involved lung side up or down is more beneficial. Therefore experimenting with different patient positions while observing pulse oximetric or blood gas changes may be helpful in determining which position (or positions) most relieves the hypoxemia. Routine position changes are still necessary, with avoidance of the position that results in the worst SpO_2.

6. *Thrombolytic therapy*. Fibrinolytic agents accelerate lysis of clots, whereas traditional heparin therapy only prevents extension of preexisting clots or formation of more thrombi. Generally, it takes the intrinsic fibrinolytic system approximately 2 to 4 days to lyse the clot. Acceleration of clot lysis using thrombolytic agents reduces lysis time to a few hours. Indications include proximal DVT, massive pulmonary emboli, or emboli causing hemodynamic instability. Some also recommend lytic therapy for patients with echocardiographic evidence of right ventricular dysfunction and severe hypoxemia despite maximun oxygen supplementation. Thrombolysis quickly alleviates the pulmonary hypertension and right heart failure associated with involvement of more than 50% of the pulmonary circulation. The risk of bleeding associated with the use of these drugs outweighs the anticipated benefit in patients with submassive pulmonary embolism and no hemodynamic compromise.

    Absolute contraindications include actual or strong probability of intracranial bleeding or other bleeding. Relative contraindications are surgery or trauma within the past 10 days.

    Currently available thrombolytic agents and recommendations for dosing change rapidly. Therefore the hospital pharmacy department should be consulted for current treatment guidelines.

7. *Pulmonary embolectomy*. Surgical removal of the pulmonary embolism requires cardiopulmonary bypass and is reserved for patients with massive pulmonary embolism who remain hemodynamically unstable despite thrombolytic therapy or who have contraindications to thrombolytic therapy. This emergency procedure has an operative mortality rate of up to 60% because patients are taken to the operating suite while their condition is unstable. Patients usually also have coincident severe medical or surgical problems.

8. *Interruption of blood flow through the inferior vena cava (IVC)*. There are several types of vena caval filters, including the three types of Greenfield filters, the Bird's-nest filter, the Simon nitinol filter, and the Vena Tech filter. These devices prevent further pulmonary embolization of leg or pelvic vein thrombi. Indications include patients who bleed with anticoagulation, patients with contraindications to anticoagulation, patients following pulmonary embolectomy, and patients in whom emboli recur despite adequate anticoagulation. Complications include vascular injury at the time of device insertion, venous thrombosis at the insertion site, filter dislodgement and embolization into the heart, thrombosis of the filter that causes IVC obstruction, and erosion of the filter through the vena caval wall.

9. *Minimize psychologic stress*. This measure is important because stress is associated with increased platelet adhesiveness, which may produce or exacerbate a hypercoagulable state. Stress is also known to predispose patients to other physiologic abnormalities (arrhythmias, hypertension), all of which complicate and worsen the patients' clinical and hemodynamic conditions.

Chronic Obstructive Pulmonary Disease

Chronic obstructive pulmonary disease is a catchall term used to describe significant airflow limitations in patients with a varying combination of chronic bronchitis and emphysema. An asthmatic component frequently complicates COPD. All three conditions are variably interrelated and also may potentiate each other. One disease can predominate over the others and may be identified by the patient's history and clinical characteristics. Figure 18-8 and Table 18-3 outline distinguishing characteristics of chronic bronchitis and emphysema.

Chronic Bronchitis
Chronic bronchitis is a diagnosis based on a history of productive cough on most days of each week for at least 3

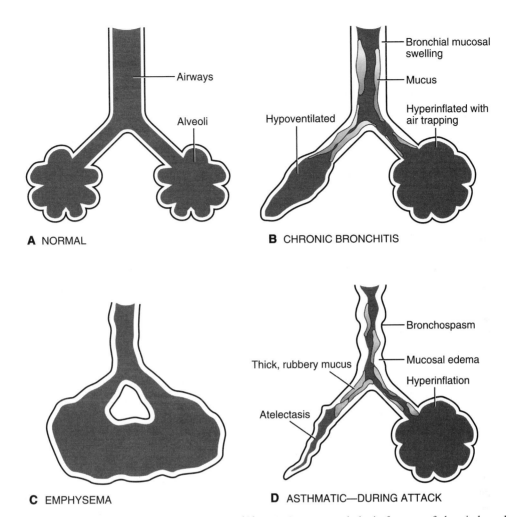

FIGURE 18-8 Comparison of a normal lung unit **(A)** with the gross pathologic features of chronic bronchitis **(B),** emphysema **(C),** and asthma during an attack **(D).**

TABLE 18-3
Clinical Features of Chronic Bronchitis and Emphysema

Clinical Characteristics	Chronic Bronchitis	Emphysema
Body/build complexion	Cyanotic, dependent edema, "blue bloater"	Thin, normal complexion, "pink puffer"
Breathing	Modest dyspnea	Severe dyspnea, pursed-lip on exhalation
Sputum production	Copious	Minimal
Lung compliance	Normal	High compliance, "floppy lungs"
Airway resistance	Increased	Increased at end-expiration
Cor pulmonale	Common	End-stage disease
Intrapulmonary shunt	Ycs	No
Ventilation/perfusion mismatch	Yes	Yes
Age at onset of symptoms	40 to 50	50 to 70
Clinical course	Progressive with remissions and exacerbations	Progressive

Emphysema and chronic bronchitis may occur in pure form. However, chronic bronchitis and emphysema commonly coexist in varying degrees. An asthmatic component frequently complicates COPD.

months of the year for 2 or more consecutive years (Figure 18-8, *B*). The disease is characterized by exacerbating and remitting inflammatory swelling of the bronchial mucosa and increased mucus production that exacerbates and remits. If the inciting inflammatory stimulus, such as cigarette smoke, is removed early in the course of the disease, airway mucosal changes are reversible. However, continued bronchial irritation and inflammation eventually lead to irreversible terminal airway obstruction and alveolar damage. Pulmonary fibrotic changes also develop over time. Chronic hypercarbia and hypoxemia result from severely impaired alveolar ventilation. Wheezing is variable in people with chronic bronchitis, coarse crackles generally relocate or clear with coughing, and the intensity of breath sounds is usually loud. Central cyanosis is often present and may be dramatic in patients with severe disease. A history of cigarette smoking is invariably present.

Emphysema and chronic bronchitis may exist in pure form. However, chronic bronchitis, emphysema, and asthma commonly coexist in varying degrees.

Emphysema

Emphysema is a condition characterized by partial airflow obstruction within the small bronchioles during expiration (Figure 18-8, *C*). Air trapping results in progressive enlargement of the distal air spaces and destruction of the alveolar walls. These events lead to a reduced number and an enlarged size of air spaces distal to the terminal bronchioles. In other words, several small normal alveoli merge to become one large alveolus. Overall, these changes result in a reduction in the surface area of the alveolar-capillary membrane; in hyperinflated lungs; and in the loss of the natural elastic recoil property of the lungs that allows outward expansion of the patient's chest wall (barrel chest). Damage is irreversible, and symptoms do not occur until more than one third of the terminal airways and alveoli have been destroyed.

Emphysema can be presumed to be present in barrel-chested patients who complain of relentless dyspnea. A history of cigarette smoking is usually present. On physical examination dramatically decreased breath sounds are noted, wheezing is high pitched and heard at end-expiration, and cyanosis is usually absent because the arterial Po_2 is usually sufficient to sustain near-normal hemoglobin saturation.

Both chronic bronchitis and emphysema are closely linked to cigarette smoking, inhaled pollutants, or both. Individual susceptibility to these risk factors is variable. In some people, a genetically acquired deficiency of serum antiproteolytic activity (α_1-antitrypsin deficiency) is associated with an increased incidence of COPD, even in the absence of identifiable risk factors.

Asthma

Asthma is defined as episodic hyperreactivity of the airways in response to exposure to numerous stimuli (Figure 18-8, *D*). During the asthma attack, airway hyperreactivity is manifest as bronchial mucosal swelling, increased mucus production, and intense bronchial smooth muscle contraction (bronchospasm). Between attacks, the airways and lungs are usually normal. Over time, severe, frequently occurring attacks result in lung tissue changes similar to those of emphysema. Wheezing and cough are the hallmarks of asthma attacks; however, cough may be chronically present. Lung sounds are usually loud.

One type of asthma is triggered by exposure to an antigenic substance (allergic asthma) such as pollens, foods, and animal danders and is common in children and young adults. In another type the attack is triggered by nonspecific stimuli such as a gust of cold air, exercise, and respiratory infections. This type commonly manifests for the first time in middle age (intrinsic asthma, adult-onset asthma). Patients with COPD commonly have characteristics of both allergic and intrinsic asthma.

Pathophysiology

Poorly ventilated alveoli either fail to be efficient gas-exchanging units (ventilation/perfusion mismatch) or shrink and collapse and do not participate in gas exchange at all (shunt units). Patients with COPD, particularly with dominance of the bronchitic component, have varying degrees of ventilation/perfusion mismatch and intrapulmonary shunting. Chronic hypoxemia, hypercarbia, and respiratory acidosis with compensatory metabolic alkalosis are characteristic of the patient's baseline condition. Any factor that increases ventilation/perfusion mismatch or shunt fraction worsens the patient's clinical status and blood gas measurements.

For COPD patients, acute respiratory failure is determined by blood gas analysis as a sudden significant drop in Pao_2 or rise in $Paco_2$ (or both), particularly if hypoxemia or hypercarbia disposes patients to complications, such as myocardial ischemia, or even death.

Consequences of Airflow Obstruction. The expiratory flow limitations characteristic of COPD patients result in two problems. The first problem, which is a chronically increased work of breathing, is the result of two factors: (1) expiration becomes an effort because emphysematous lungs are nonelastic and bronchitic airways are narrowed by swelling or mucus, and (2) intrapulmonary air trapping decreases the expiratory reserve volume and increases the residual volume, functional residual capacity, and total lung volume. Because the patient begins each breath on overinflated lungs, the inspiratory muscles are at a mechanical disadvantage and must generate more inspiratory force. One can experience this extraordinary work by first inhaling, holding his or her breath, and then continuing to breathe on top of the original breath. However, only inspiratory work is perceived in this experiment. The patient with COPD experiences unrelenting inspiratory *and* expiratory work.

Because of the chronically increased work of breathing, patients are more prone to respiratory muscle fatigue when stressed by exercise, illness, or injury.

The second problem is the development of positive end-expiratory pressure (PEEP). Expiratory flow obstruction is sufficient to favor alveolar air trapping that, in turn, makes end-expiratory pressure positive throughout the patient's thorax. This phenomenon has been termed *intrinsic end-expiratory pressure (intrinsic PEEP), occult PEEP,* or *auto-PEEP.* The presence of intrinsic PEEP may decrease cardiac output by a tamponade-like effect on both ventricles, which interferes with ventricular filling, as well as by external compression of the thoracic portions of the vena cava, which decreases venous return. Increased intrathoracic pressure as a result of air trapping can also increase pulmonary vascular resistance by compressing pulmonary vessels. Air trapping and intrinsic PEEP are usually made worse in patients receiving mechanical ventilation who have copious secretions of mucus. The mucous plug acts as a ball valve and allows delivery of air to the terminal airways and alveoli under positive pressure ventilation, but alveolar air cannot escape past the plug during passive expiration.

Pulmonary Hypertension in Patients with Chronic Obstructive Pulmonary Disease. Secondary to pulmonary vasoconstriction induced by hypoxemia, pulmonary artery systolic and diastolic pressures rise and the PAd-PWP gradient widens in proportion to the increased pulmonary vascular resistance. Pulmonary hypertension also develops because of the reduction in the size of the pulmonary capillary bed as a result of destructive vascular changes. A fibrotic process also develops around the arterioles that distorts the structure and elastic characteristics of these vessels.

As pulmonary vascular resistance increases with progression of the disease, the right ventricle may initially maintain a compensated cardiovascular status through hypertrophic adaptation to the greater systolic pressure load, but, with progression in the disease, it may eventually fail. Acute respiratory failure of any cause may suddenly present the compensated or failing right ventricle with an intolerable pressure load. Right ventricular failure then either develops or is made worse.

Clinical Indications of Deterioration in Patients with Chronic Obstructive Pulmonary Disease

Acute, significant patient deterioration may be signaled by increasing dyspnea, wheezing, and sputum production; alterations in mental status; headache due to cerebrovascular dilation (if hypercarbia is severe enough); and/or the effects of hypoxia or acidosis on the cardiovascular system (acute right ventricular failure, tachycardia, arrhythmias, or myocardial ischemia or infarction).

Common Causes of Acute Respiratory Failure in Patients with Chronic Obstructive Pulmonary Disease

The natural progression of COPD may reach an endpoint with a clinical presentation identical to that of acute respiratory failure. Almost any systemic, cardiovascular, or pulmonary illness or injury also can tip the clinical picture of chronically compromised COPD patients toward life-threatening acute respiratory failure.

Pulmonary Infection. Infection accounts for approximately one half of COPD patients admitted to the hospital with acute respiratory failure. Patients typically complain of increasing dyspnea and cough with purulent sputum production. Respiratory infection may or may not be accompanied by the usual systemic signs of infection (fever or increased white blood cell count). The most commonly isolated pathogens include *Haemophilus influenzae, Streptococcus pneumoniae,* and *M. catarrhalis.* Pneumonia also may be viral in origin or may be the result of gram-negative bacteria, particularly in immunologically compromised, long-term hospitalized, or recently hospitalized patients.

Left Ventricular Failure. Left ventricular failure worsens pulmonary dysfunction by increasing pulmonary vascular blood volume. The subsequent rise in pulmonary capillary hydrostatic pressure (measured by PWP) favors the development of pulmonary edema that, in turn, worsens pulmonary gas exchange and increases the work of breathing. Patients in the COPD age group commonly have systemic hypertensive, valvular, or ischemic heart disease, all of which predispose them to acute pulmonary edema. In these patients, the clinical diagnosis of pulmonary edema is made difficult because the usual signs and symptoms (tachypnea, dyspnea, crackles, wheezes) are always present in COPD. The sound of a gallop rhythm may be completely swamped by crackles and wheezes.

Generally, the aforementioned chronic signs and symptoms worsen with the advent of pulmonary edema.

Acute Pulmonary Embolism. This is a common complication in patients with COPD due to the chronic presence of risk factors such as a sedentary lifestyle, increased blood viscosity, and coexisting heart failure. Patients with COPD who show sudden worsening of symptoms or hypoxemia with a slight fall rather than rise in $PaCO_2$ should be suspected of having acute pulmonary embolism.

With the passage of time, sporadic pulmonary embolic episodes take their toll as more of the pulmonary circulation is progressively obstructed and functionally lost because of organized thrombi. This effect intensifies pulmonary hypertension, which worsens chronic cor pulmonale.

Injudicious Use of Narcotic or Sedative Agents. Opiate analgesics and sedatives blunt the ventilatory drive. Because COPD patients at peak function may barely be able to maintain marginal arterial oxygenation and carbon dioxide elimination, the administration of drugs that blunt the ventilatory drive risks placing patients in a severely decompensated state.

Chest or Abdominal Surgery or Trauma. Surgical or traumatic pain limits ventilatory movements (splinting) and may result in significant deterioration in arterial blood gas concentrations.

Injudicious Use of Oxygen in a Spontaneously Breathing Patient. Although oxygen supplementation is important in treating patients with acute respiratory distress, the clinical challenge is giving the most effective dose safely. In patients with a chronically elevated $PaCO_2$, oxygen administration may worsen hypercarbia. This has been attributed to the fact that a chronically elevated $PaCO_2$ causes the chemoreceptors to become insensitive to carbon dioxide. The patient's primary drive to breathe then becomes hypoxemia. Correction of hypoxemia with supplemental oxygen eliminates the only consistent stimulus to breathe. As a result of hypoventilation, arterial carbon dioxide levels acutely rise and produce central nervous system depression that may end in stupor or coma (termed *CO_2 narcosis*). However, speculation now exists that acute hypercarbia in these circumstances is the result of altered ventilation/perfusion relationships and not decreased ventilatory drive. Whatever the actual mechanism, administration of excessive oxygen to COPD patients is known to worsen hypercarbia. Generally, an FiO_2 sufficient to maintain an oxygen saturation of approximately 90% is the therapeutic goal in managing spontaneously breathing, chronically hypercarbic patients.

Pulmonary Barotrauma. Barotrauma is the result of the escape of air from airways or alveoli that have ruptured because of increased intraalveolar pressures—likened to bursting of a hyperinflated balloon. Clinical problems develop when air escapes the ruptured alveolus, dissects through lung tissue, and then eventually enters the pleural space (pneumothorax), pericardial space (pneumopericardium), or mediastinum (pneumomediastinum).

The hyperinflated, highly compliant lungs of patients with COPD are particularly susceptible to barotrauma and pneumothorax. If a significant pneumothorax (greater than 20% lung involvement) develops, clinical deterioration is typically sudden and severe. Critically ill or injured patients are at particular risk for barotrauma because of the frequent insertion and presence of central venous lines; use of mechanical ventilation with high mean airway pressures; and bouts of strenuous coughing, gagging, or retching. A significant pneumothorax usually causes immediate chest pain, but it may be painless, particularly in critically ill or injured patients who are heavily narcotized. Other signs and symptoms include shortness of breath, possible arrhythmias, and circulatory or respiratory deterioration. The "shunted" venous blood that flows through the collapsed lung segment does not exchange with air and compounds the patient's baseline hypoxemia.

Very small pneumothoraxes, which do not progress over time and produce no hemodynamic compromise, usually do not require chest tube insertion. If the patient is being mechanically ventilated, however, chest tube evacuation of air is required to prevent enlargement of the pneumothorax.

A simple pneumothorax may progress to *tension pneumothorax,* particularly in mechanically ventilated patients. Progression to tension pneumothorax results in sudden circulatory and respiratory collapse. Rapidly developing massive subcutaneous emphysema may also develop. *Tension pneumothorax is an absolute medical emergency because patients typically die within minutes.* Emergency therapy is chest tube or needle evacuation of the air that is under high pressure and is lifesaving (see Chapter 9, section on complications; pneumothorax).

Sepsis and the Systemic Inflammatory Response Syndrome. The hypermetabolic state imposed by systemic infection and the systemic inflammatory response syndrome (SIRS) increases tissue oxygen demands and carbon dioxide production. Both place additional burdens on the chronically compromised pulmonary system. Respiratory failure usually follows.

Decreased Respiratory Muscle Strength and Endurance. Decreased respiratory muscle strength and endurance may occur as a result of acquired neuromuscular disease, neuromuscular blockade due to drugs, muscular weakness due to decreased oxygen delivery (anemia, circulatory failure, worsening of preexisting blood gas abnormalities), electrolyte abnormalities (hypomagnesemia, hypophosphatemia, hypocalcemia, hypokalemia), and malnutrition.

Clinical Presentation

Clinical findings in people with COPD are highly variable and depend on the stage of the disease; the amount of bronchotic, emphysematous, and asthmatic involvement; the presence or absence of heart failure; and complicating factors, such as infection.

Mentation. In patients with uncomplicated COPD, the level of mentation is normal. However, patients may exhibit personality characteristics, such as irritability and manipulative, dependent behaviors, that are common in patients with chronic, debilitating illness.

Acute changes in cerebral function, such as lethargy, slurred speech, confusion, and emotional instability, accompany sudden deterioration in blood gases. If hypercarbia is severe enough, there may be sufficient cerebral vasodilation to increase intracranial pressure. The patient may then complain of headache, and swelling of the optic nerve head may be noted on funduscopic examination of the patient's eyegrounds.

Cutaneous Manifestations. Central cyanosis and a ruddy complexion are common in patients with predominantly bronchitic involvement. Because patients with COPD tend to be vasodilated, the trunk and extremities are warm and the patient's palms may be erythematous.

Heart Rate and Character of Pulse. Greater than normal resting heart rates are frequently present due to hypoxemia, hypercapnia, and increased work of breathing. The peripheral pulses are usually strong.

Heart Sounds. An early sign of pulmonary hypertension is an accentuation of the pulmonic component of the second heart sound. A high-pitched systolic ejection click (from accentuated right ventricular ejection vibrations) also may be heard over the pulmonic area. A right-sided S_3, which is best heard near the lower left sternal border or in the epigastrium, signifies right ventricular failure. It may be difficult to hear the heart sounds over the left side of the chest because of the damping effect of air in the patient's hyperinflated lungs. Although heart sounds may be audible over the epigastrium, they also may be overshadowed by the presence of loud crackles and wheezes.

Palpation of the Precordium. The apex beat is difficult to palpate because of the increased anteroposterior dimensions of the patient's thorax (barrel chest). Right ventricular thrusts may be felt over the right or left lower sternal border and signify forceful right ventricular activity as a response to pulmonary hypertension.

Neck Veins. If the patient develops right ventricular failure, venous distention and dependent edema also develop. If heart failure is severe, an enlarged, pulsatile liver can be palpated. However, the neck veins may be distended in some COPD patients without right ventricular failure because of the prolonged, forced expiratory effort.

Respiratory Rate and Character of Breathing. The respiratory rate is typically greater than normal. Labored breathing, commonly through pursed lips, may be present only with exertion but is present even at rest in people with advanced disease. The patient prefers a sitting position, bent forward, and commonly uses the accessory muscles of breathing.

Lung Sounds. Crackles and wheezes are commonly heard diffusely over both lung fields. In people with severe disease, adventitious sounds may be audible even without a stethoscope. On the other hand, a quiet chest may be heard in some people with severe COPD due to severe airflow limitation.

Acid-Base Values. Patients with pure emphysema tend to hyperventilate and maintain near-normal arterial oxygen tensions—hence the name "pink puffers." Late in the course of the disease, the $PaCO_2$ drops below 60 mm Hg.

Patients with pure bronchitis are hypoxemic and have an increased $PaCO_2$; generalized edema develops with the onset of right ventricular failure—hence the name "blue bloaters." Most patients have a varying combination of both conditions and are therefore "blue puffers." The severity of pulmonary hypertension and cor pulmonale in COPD is closely related to the severity of the hypoxemia and usually becomes apparent when the resting PaO_2 falls below 45 mm Hg.

Hemodynamic Profile

The hemodynamic profile of uncomplicated COPD is described. Changes in these measurements, with the imposition of complications, are specific to the complicating event such as sepsis, pneumothorax, pulmonary embolism, or acute pulmonary edema.

Arterial Pressure. Systemic arterial pressure is not significantly affected by COPD. However, in patients with severe bronchospasm, there may be an increase in the magnitude of the cyclic systolic blood pressure change that normally occurs with breathing (see Chapter 5; pulsus paradoxus).

The reason for exaggerated systolic pressure changes is the severe airflow limitation, in which expiration becomes more prolonged and forceful. Because of the sustained and increased intrathoracic pressure, venous return becomes significantly reduced. During labored inspiration, the abrupt drop in intrathoracic pressure is associated with a sudden increase in venous return. The marked intrathoracic pressure swings of COPD result in abrupt changes in left ventricular stroke volume and therefore systolic pressure during each respiratory cycle. A systolic pressure difference greater than 15 mm Hg during each breath is typical of the pulsus paradoxus noted in patients with severe airflow limitation of any cause.

Systemic Vascular Resistance. This calculated measurement is decreased in proportion to the degree of hypoxemic and hypercapnic vasodilation present.

Pulmonary Vascular Resistance. This measurement is typically increased to a level proportionate to the degree of hypoxemia, acidemia, and anatomic distortion of the pulmonary circulation secondary to pulmonary fibrosis or pulmonary emboli.

Central Venous Pressure and Right Atrial Pressure. These measurements usually remain within the normal range or are only slightly elevated if the hypertrophied right ventricle remains compensated. With the development of significant right ventricular failure, CVP and right atrial pressures rise. A prominent a wave may be observed in the right atrial wave form because of the resistance to filling the hypertrophic, failing right ventricle during atrial systole. The *x* descent also becomes more brisk and more conspicuous.

Pulmonary Artery and Wedge Pressure. Pulmonary artery systolic and diastolic pressures increase in proportion to elevations in pulmonary vascular resistance. Mean pulmonary artery pressures of 80 mm Hg are not uncommon in patients with advanced COPD (normal is 8 to 15 mm Hg). The approximately eightfold increase over normal mean values is proportionately far greater than in-

creases ever encountered in the systemic circulation with either chronic or emergency hypertension. A proportionate increase in systemic arterial pressure would result in a mean arterial pressure of approximately 700 to 800 mm Hg. Any factor that increases cardiac output (fever, catecholamines, sepsis, shivering, seizure activity, exercise) results in further elevations in pulmonary artery pressure. This is because the constricted or damaged pulmonary blood vessels cannot distend and accommodate the increased right ventricular output.

The pulmonary artery diastolic pressure no longer reflects the left atrial or left ventricular end-diastolic pressure. The higher PAd-PWP gradient is the result of blood gas or anatomic changes in the pulmonary vessels that increase resistance to diastolic runoff of blood through the pulmonary circulation. In the wedged position, there is no runoff of blood distal to the inflated balloon, and the catheter tip measures only left atrial pressure. The left heart pressures, as estimated by the PWP, are normal unless the patient also has left heart disease.

Obtaining an accurate PWP reading, however, may be difficult because of the positive intrathoracic pressures induced by the combination of pursed-lip breathing, intrinsic PEEP, and forced expiration that is typical of patients with COPD. PWP measurements may be misleadingly elevated secondary to the positive intrathoracic pressure effects. This phenomenon can lead the unwary clinician to believe that the patient is developing heart failure when this is not what is happening or that the patient is normovolemic when the patient may actually be hypovolemic. In COPD patients, certainty of the accuracy of the PWP may be impossible. Therefore analysis of PWP trends coupled with observed changes in the patient's clinical condition is necessary.

Cardiac Output. This resting measurement is usually normal but is fixed. The distorted pulmonary vessels cannot accommodate stress-induced increases in blood flow, and, as a result, they cannot provide stress-demanded increases in left heart filling.

Mixed Venous Oxygen Saturation. The Svo_2 measurement is typically decreased in proportion to the level of arterial hypoxemia, heart failure, or both.

Laboratory Studies and Other Diagnostic Tests
Electrocardiograph. Low QRS voltage and poor precordial R wave progression are common findings. In patients with cor pulmonale, there is usually evidence of right axis deviation, right ventricular hypertrophy (prominent R waves in the anterior precordial leads and deep S waves in the left precordial leads). A right bundle branch

block may also be present. Atrial arrhythmias are common, and ventricular arrhythmias also may develop in severely hypoxic patients.

Chest Radiograph. Changes develop late in the course of COPD. Overinflation of the lungs (noted as very black lung fields), with flattening of the hemidiaphragms and widening of the intercostal spaces, is typical of patients with advanced emphysema. Enlargement of the pulmonary artery trunk and right and left main pulmonary artery branches and attenuation of the peripheral branches are evidence of pulmonary hypertension. Radiographic evidence of the right ventricular enlargement becomes evident only after considerable dilation has occurred. Blebs (intrapleural collections of air) and bullae (lung air spaces) are characteristic findings of COPD.

Hematology. Chronic hypoxemia results in a compensatory increase in the red blood cell count and hemoglobin concentration.

Pulmonary Function Tests. These tests may be used as a guide to assessment and management of expiratory airflow limitations. Pulmonary function tests include forced expiratory spirometry (forced expiratory volume in 1 second [FEV_1]); lung volumes (total lung capacity, functional residual capacity, residual volume); volume-pressure relationships; diffusion capacity; and arterial blood gases.

Treatment

Therapy of COPD is directed at treatment or prevention of infection, improvement in airflow, control of correctable components of the disease (hypoxemia, hypercapnia, cardiovascular problems), and avoidance of factors that may worsen the condition, such as cigarette smoking, environmental pollutants, and sedatives. The following directives are specific for care in the acute care setting.

Improvement in Arterial Oxygenation. Oxygen therapy serves three important purposes:
1. *Improving systemic oxygen availability.*
2. *Improving alveolar oxygenation and reducing pulmonary hypertension.* In fact, the pulmonary artery pressures may decrease significantly with improvement in alveolar oxygenation and the blood oxygen content. With long-term, low-flow oxygen therapy, right ventricular hypertrophy may be stabilized or even reversed.
3. *Improving arterial oxygenation and decreasing hypoxemia-related bronchoconstriction.* These, in

turn, improve alveolar ventilation and ventilation/perfusion relationships.

Generally, patients do best if the arterial PaO_2 is 55 to 60 mm Hg with a hemoglobin saturation of approximately 90%. Because an improvement in arterial PaO_2 may blunt the patient's hypoxemic ventilatory drive, a rise in $PaCO_2$ may occur with oxygen administration. This is not grounds for alarm as long as the patient remains lucid, is easily arousable, has satisfactory cardiovascular function, and has an arterial pH not less than 7.25. In spontaneously breathing patients, oxygen is given by nasal cannula starting at 1 to 2 L/min or by an air entrainment mask (Venturi mask) starting at an FiO_2 of 30%. At the onset of oxygen administration, the patient's clinical status and blood gas measurements should be evaluated frequently to determine if increases or decreases in FiO_2 are required. Pulse oximetry, though useful in assessing oxygenation, does not provide information about carbon dioxide retention. Between blood gas measurements, the patient should be vigilantly watched for signs of CO_2 narcosis, such as lethargy, confusion, flushing, sweating, headache, slurred speech, twitching, or stupor.

Improvement in Airflow. Measures that promote meticulous bronchial hygiene, such as percussion, effective coughing, and suctioning, are essential and are discussed in the following section. Further improvement in airflow may necessitate corticosteroid therapy to reduce airway inflammation and edema. Corticosteroids are thought to increase intracellular cyclic adenosine monophosphate (cAMP), which produces bronchodilation and inhibits synthesis of cyclic guanidine monophosphate (cGMP), which produces bronchoconstriction.

Inhaled sympathomimetic bronchodilators, such as metaproterenol (Alupent, Metaprel), terbutaline (Brethaire), albuterol (Proventil, Ventolin), and isoetharine mesylate (Bronkosol), are commonly used and have selective bronhcodilating action on the bronchial tree with minimal cardiovascular effects (beta-2 activity). This is a distinct advantage over the older, nonselective bronchodilators, such as epinephrine (Adrenalin) and isoproterenol (Isuprel), which also have cardiovascular stimulant effects (beta-1 activity). Beta-1 receptor stimulation may be particularly harmful when given to patients with ischemic heart disease, which commonly coexists in elderly patients. Inhaled anticholinergic drugs such as glycopyrrolate (Robinul) and ipratropium bromide (Atrovent) are direct bronchodilators via their parasympatholytic effect.

Intravenous theophylline (aminophylline) is a drug also used in managing COPD patients. In addition to its bronchodilating effect, it increases mucociliary clearance and improves ventilatory drive, although these effects are weak.

It is speculated that the drug also improves right ventricular performance and renders the diaphragm less susceptible to fatigue. However, *careful evaluation of serum levels is important, because toxicity may develop despite administration within the recommended dose range.* Typically, the COPD or critically ill patient has several characteristics that are known to decrease theophylline metabolism and increase blood levels, such as advanced age, coexisting heart failure, hepatic dysfunction, severe acute illness, viral infections, certain drugs (macrolides, fluoroquinolones, cimetidine, propranolol) and cor pulmonale.

Because theophylline is a central nervous system and cardiovascular stimulant, signs of toxicity include sinus tachycardia, ectopic atrial and ventricular activity, restlessness, and seizures. Nausea and vomiting also may occur. The therapeutic range of serum theophylline is 10 to 20 μg/ml. Seizures and cardiac arrhythmias are likely to occur at serum levels greater than 25 μg/ml.

Some patients have intolerable side effects to the aforementioned medications. Patients with structural changes to the airway walls may not respond adequately to standard medications. Medications such as magnesium, cyclosporine, and methotrexate are occasionally used in such patients. Helium-oxygen (heliox) may be used to facilitate oxygenation in patients with upper airway obstruction due to postextubation edema.

Clearance of Tracheobronchial Secretions. A strong cough is the most effective method of clearing secretions. For this the patient must sit upright because coughing in the supine or partially upright position is difficult and may result in ineffective clearance of secretions. Provision of adequate hydration; sputum liquefying agents, such as potassium iodide; or mucolytic agents, such as acetylcysteine (Mucomyst), and inhalation of a heated aerosol make the sputum less viscous and easier to cough up. Nasotracheal suction, bronchoscopy, chest percussion, and postural drainage may be required when the cough is ineffective or mucus is thick and impacted in the airways.

Antibiotics. Because pneumonia is the most common cause of deterioration in COPD patients, broad-spectrum antibiotics directed toward *S. pneumoniae, H. influenzae,* and *M. catarrhalis* (the most common infecting agents in COPD) are started before the results of sputum cultures are available. Because of evolving antibiotic-resistant bacterial strains and antibiotic resistance specific to institutions, the hospital pharmacologist may need to be consulted for the most effective antibiotic coverage. The choice of drugs may also have to be tailored to a specific patient's requirements, such as immune system suppression.

Pulmonary Vasodilators. The sudden development of congestive heart failure in previously compensated COPD patients implies that either ventilation/perfusion mismatch has worsened hypoxemic and acidemic vasoconstriction or pulmonary embolism has obstructed the pulmonary vascular bed to produce a level of pulmonary hypertension sufficient to cause right ventricular failure. Oxygen and bronchodilators may sufficiently reduce pulmonary hypertension by relief of hypoxemic vasoconstriction. Other direct pulmonary vasodilating agents include beta-adrenergic agonists, such as isoproterenol (Isuprel); alpha-adrenergic antagonists, such as nitroprusside (Nipride) or hydralazine (Apresoline); angiotensin-converting enzyme inhibitors, such as captopril; calcium-channel blockers, such as nifedipine or diltiazem; and prostaglandin I_2 (Flolan). Patients should be carefully assessed during therapy because many of these vasodilating drugs may produce systemic hypotension and tachycardia, and they worsen hypoxemia by dilating the pulmonary arterioles in areas of alveolar consolidation, collapse, or edema. Perfusion to these nonventilated areas increases the shunt fraction.

Mechanical Ventilation. There are two options for mechanical ventilatory support:

1. *Noninvasive positive pressure ventilation (NPPV).* This technique may be used if the patient does not require an artificial airway or secretion clearance. Noninvasive ventilatory assistance using the cuirass chest piece or the poncho wrap may be provided. Oronasal masks are preferable to nasal cannulas to prevent oxygen leak from the mouth.

2. *Mechanical ventilatory support requiring an endotracheal intubation.* This therapeutic option is avoided whenever possible because of the difficulties encountered in weaning patients, as well as the problems related to barotrauma. The decision to provide ventilatory support is based on the patient's mental and physical status rather than on blood gas measurements alone.

An additional and a potentially lethal problem associated with mechanical ventilatory assistance is the creation of a profound metabolic alkalosis. This complication occurs when a chronically hypercarbic patient is mechanically ventilated and the tidal volume and respiratory rate are adjusted to bring the $Paco_2$ into the "normal" range of 35 to 45 mm Hg. However, patients with chronic carbon dioxide retention develop an increase in serum bicarbonate, as a renal compensatory mechanism to maintain serum pH within a physiologically acceptable range (compensatory metabolic alkalosis). Overly vigorous mechanical ventilatory assistance and sudden reduction in the $Paco_2$ toward "normal" values risks severe metabolic alkalosis because it takes days for kidneys to readjust the bicarbonate levels downward toward normal. Severe alkalemia leads to tetany and convulsions. Low-grade alkalemia also causes hypoventilation and is a possible reason for the inability to wean COPD patients off the ventilator using intermittent mandatory ventilation or a T-piece.

The assist-control mode is preferred when ventilatory muscle rest is desired. Levels of auto-PEEP should be monitored closely because excessive auto-PEEP can decrease cardiac output. Resetting the ventilator with a reduced rate, higher inspiratory flows, and increased expiratory time helps reduce development of this problem. Ventilatory management and weaning of COPD patients is complex and is beyond the scope of this text to detail. See references 7 and 8 for more detailed discussion of this topic.

Pulmonary Edema

Pulmonary edema literally means "swollen lungs." By a more conventional academic definition, pulmonary edema is an abnormal accumulation of fluid outside of the vascular space of the lung. The excessive fluid may be in the interstitial space (which is made up of the connective tissue that surrounds airways), blood vessels, lymphatics, and alveoli.

Pulmonary Fluid Dynamics and Lymphatic Pumping

All body tissue has continuous two-way movement of fluid between the intravascular and interstitial space across the capillary membranes. This is the means by which nutrients are delivered to the cells and nongaseous metabolic wastes are removed. The factors that determine the intravascular versus extravascular fluid volume are the oppositely directed forces of osmotic and hydrostatic pressures in both spaces and the permeability (porosity) characteristic of the capillary membrane (see Chapter 4, section on capillaries). Normally, a greater overall force directs fluid *out* of the systemic and pulmonary capillaries. In the lungs, this results in the movement of approximately 10 to 20 ml of fluid per hour *into* the lung tissue. If allowed to accumulate, this fluid would ultimately result in suffocation. To offset fluid accumulation within the lungs, the pulmonary lymphatic network acts as a skimming pump and returns this watery extract of plasma to the venous circulation. If greater than normal amounts of fluid enter the lungs, the lymphatic pumping capacity can increase approximately 10 times to maintain the lungs in their normal, relatively dry state. However, when the amount of fluid entering the lungs outstrips the lymphatic capacity to remove it, pulmonary edema develops.

Pulmonary fibrosis distorts and chokes off lymphatic channels, and, in affected patients, clearance of lung water is impaired. Disorders that lead to obliteration of the lymphatics, such as lymphangitic carcinomatosis, also severely impair clearance of lung water. Generally, in patients with impaired pulmonary lymphatic pumping, the threshold for developing pulmonary edema of any cause is lowered. Severely affected patients may develop acute pulmonary edema with minimal provocation.

Sequence of Formation of Pulmonary Edema

The sequence of formation of pulmonary edema is the same regardless of the cause. Three progressive pathophysiologic, radiologic, and clinical phases are discussed.

Phase 1—The Compensated Phase. There is an increase in the amount of fluid moving from the pulmonary capillaries into the lung tissue due to one or a combination of physiologic disturbances (see discussions of the causes of pulmonary edema). Because of the compensatory increase in lung lymph flow, there is no measurable increase in lung fluid volume because incoming and outgoing fluid is kept in balance (Figure 18-9). Other than a mild increase in respiratory rate (which is thought to augment lymphatic drainage by a massaging effect on lymphatic vessels), there are no other clinical findings. The patient's chest radiograph is normal. At this stage, pulmonary edema is not clinically detectable, and it goes unrecognized. In an absolute sense, this is not pulmonary edema because there is no increase in lung water. However,

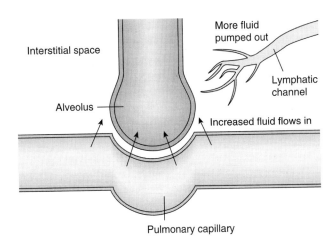

FIGURE 18-9 Compensated pulmonary edema. Increased movement of fluid influx into the lungs is met with a proportionate increase in pulmonary lymphatic fluid clearance, and lung fluid balance is normal.

this stage does represent an abnormality in pulmonary fluid dynamics. The cause may spontaneously resolve, and the normal state is then reestablished. If there is no resolution to the underlying problem and the patient's underlying disease does not worsen, the patient plateaus at this level, which becomes the new, resting steady state. On the other hand, if the underlying condition worsens, pulmonary edema may progress to phase 2.

Phase 2—Interstitial Pulmonary Edema. When the pumping capabilities of the lymphatics are overwhelmed by the additional influx by fluid, fluid first accumulates in pools in the loose connective tissue surrounding blood vessels and airways (Figure 18-10). At this point, the alveoli remain dry and gas exchange remains acceptable, albeit with a mild drop in arterial Po_2. The accumulating interstitial edema compresses the terminal airways and terminal pulmonary vessels. As a result of the decreased intraluminal diameter, airway and vascular resistances are increased in the involved lung areas. Because of increased vascular resistance, blood flow is directed away from areas of edema, causing poor matching of alveolar ventilation with capillary perfusion. Normally, an increase in pulmonary venous pressure (PWP) to 18 to 20 mm Hg produces interstitial edema, although this threshold is considerably less in hypoproteinemic patients and those with ARDS (see the section on hemodynamic effects and the section on exceptions to pulmonary edema PWP thresholds).

Clinical signs are minimal; the lungs are usually clear to auscultation, an occasional hacking cough may be present, and dyspnea is not perceived while at rest. However, the rate of breathing increases (20 to 24 breaths per minute) because sensory nerve endings in the alveolar walls, termed *J receptors,* become excited by the increase in lung fluid and trigger reflex tachypnea.

Because of the absent or minimal clinical findings, the diagnosis can be made for certain only by chest radiograph. The initial radiographic finding is pulmonary vascular congestion with visualization of the blood vessels in the upper third of the upright chest film (termed *cephalization of blood flow*). Then movement of edema fluid into the tissue surrounding blood vessels produces a clouding and poor definition of the vascular markings. The lung fields have a hazy appearance. The interlobar septa (which separate the secondary lobules of the lung) become edematous and produce linear densities, which were originally described by Kerley.[9] Peripherally located Kerley B lines are short, horizontal, white lines that extend out a few centimeters from the pleural edges and are seen most commonly at the lung bases. Kerley A lines are centrally located, are longer than B lines, and may course in any direction.

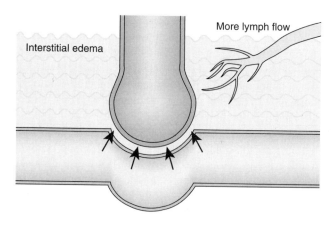

FIGURE 18-10 Interstitial pulmonary edema. Increased movement of fluid into the lungs *(arrows)* cannot be compensated for by increased lymphatic pumping. Fluid accumulates in the connective tissue.

With worsening of the patient's underlying condition, pulmonary edema may progress to phase 3.

Phase 3—Alveolar Flooding. Normally, an increase in pulmonary venous pressure to greater than 25 mm Hg is associated with marked increases in fluid movement from the blood vessels into the lungs. The continuous fluid inflow, which is not matched by removal, eventually saturates the interstitial space. The excess lung water then breaks through the terminal airways and alveolar walls and accumulates in the alveoli. In normal adults, the interstitial space can maximally accommodate 200 to 300 ml of fluid, and thus substantial fluid collects in the lungs before alveolar flooding occurs. Therefore the first clinically recognizable signs and symptoms of pulmonary edema do not reflect early pulmonary edema but rather its most advanced stage—alveolar flooding (Figure 18-11).

Fluid first accumulates at the corners of some alveoli. This small amount of fluid increases surface tension, and, as the alveolus rapidly shrinks, gas is replaced by pulmonary edema fluid. The characteristic of alveolar flooding is such that alveoli are either completely air filled or completely fluid filled. This creates a tissue mosaic of functional (aerated) and nonfunctional (fluid-filled) alveoli. Hypoxemia is multifactoral and is the result of (1) "shunting" of venous blood past flooded alveoli, (2) mismatching of alveolar ventilation to capillary perfusion, and (3) impaired diffusion of oxygen across the edematous alveolar-capillary membrane. However, diffusion block contributes least to hypoxemia.

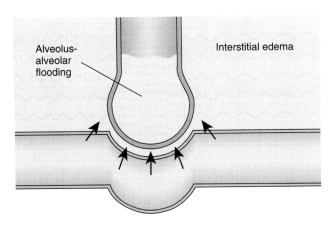

FIGURE 18-11 Alveolar edema. The air spaces flood with fluid *(arrows)*.

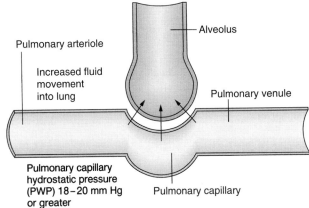

FIGURE 18-12 Schematic illustration of the alveolar-capillary unit. A greater than normal capillary hydrostatic pressure (estimated clinically by PWP) results in increased movement of plasma water into the extravascular space *(arrows)*.

The point at which dyspnea is perceived depends on the patient's sensitivity to body sensations, activity level, and tolerance to discomfort. With the advent of alveolar flooding, the rate and depth of breathing increase and crackles become apparent. Initially, they are fine (with a sound similar to Velcro opening) and are heard near the peak of inspiration. Fine crackles are thought to be produced when the walls of small airways and alveoli that were stuck together by fluid at end-expiration "pop" open during inhalation. As fluid moves into the larger airways, the auscultated sound takes on a coarse and then a gurgling quality. With progression of airway flooding, gurgling becomes expiratory, as well as inspiratory. If the edema fluid reaches the level of the trachea, gurgling is audible without a stethoscope, and edema foam can easily be coughed up.

As the number of fluid-filled alveoli increases, the lungs become stiffer, the work of breathing increases, and the vital capacity and other lung volumes decrease. The patient's arterial PaO_2 measurement continues to decrease. Airway mucosal edema and reflex bronchospasm increase resistance to airflow, and wheezing becomes apparent. Initially, $PaCO_2$ is decreased secondary to hyperventilation. However, if the patient becomes overcome with exhaustion, ventilatory movements become inadequate and the $PaCO_2$ climbs to normal and then increased levels.

Radiographically, whiteouts (infiltrates, opacities) in the lungs appear as alveolar air is replaced by fluid. The distribution of infiltrates varies with the type of pulmonary edema.

Types of Pulmonary Edema

Pulmonary edema is classified according to the mechanisms that produce increased fluid movement across the pulmonary capillary membrane. This may be the result of an imbalance in the hydrostatic and protein osmotic pressures or increased permeability of the pulmonary capillary membrane. These are discussed as isolated events. In the ICU patient with multisystem dysfunction, however, pulmonary edema is commonly caused by several overlapping mechanisms.

High-Pressure (Cardiogenic, Hydrostatic) Pulmonary Edema. The most common form of pulmonary edema is the result of volume and pressure overload of the pulmonary circulation. This is usually due to left heart dysfunction or failure—hence the term *high-pressure or cardiogenic pulmonary edema.* An abnormally elevated pulmonary capillary hydrostatic pressure (as clinically estimated by PWP or left atrial pressure) increases fluid movement out of the capillaries and into the lung tissue (Figure 18-12).

When the amount of fluid entering the lung is greater than the lymphatics' capacity to remove it, x-ray or physical signs of pulmonary edema develop. This typically occurs when the PWP exceeds 18 to 20 mm Hg. Generally, the higher the measured PWP, the greater the fluid flux into the lung and the more dramatic the patient's clinical presentation.

Causes. In most patients, high-pressure pulmonary edema is caused by a passive increase in pulmonary intravascular volume and pressure due to elevated left heart pressures (passive pulmonary hypertension). Elevated left heart pressure is most commonly the result of ischemic disease of the left ventricle; however, some patients have no cardiac disease or dysfunction. Causes include the following:

1. *Intravascular volume overload.* In this circumstance, there is fluid overload of the entire cardiovascular system, which results in a generalized increase in pressures throughout the cardiac and vascular structures. Intravascular fluid overload may be the result of rapid overtransfusion, fluid retention as in appropriate antidiuretic hormone secretion, or oliguric renal failure (Figure 18-13).

2. *Increased pulmonary venous pressure.* Obstructive diseases involving the pulmonary veins are rare but may cause generalized or localized pulmonary edema. The elevated pulmonary venous pressure is passively transmitted back to the pulmonary capillaries. Pulmonary venous hypertension may be the result of mediastinitis with scarring, mediastinal tumor, or pulmonary venous thrombosis (Figure 18-14).

3. *Increased left atrial pressure.* In this circumstance, mean left atrial pressure is elevated because of flow obstruction at the mitral valve (stenosis) or regurgitant flow through an incompetent mitral valve during systole. The elevated left atrial pressures, in turn, are reflected back throughout the pulmonary circulation. Less common causes include prosthetic mitral valve dysfunction, left atrial myxoma, and large left atrial thrombus. In affected patients, left ventricular function may or may not be normal (Figure 18-15).

4. *Increased left ventricular end-diastolic pressure.* In patients with left ventricular dysfunction, the elevated left ventricular end-diastolic pressure (LVEDP) is passively reflected back to the left atrium, pulmonary veins, and pulmonary capillaries. Fluid under high pressure then transudates from the capillaries into the lungs (Figure 18-16).

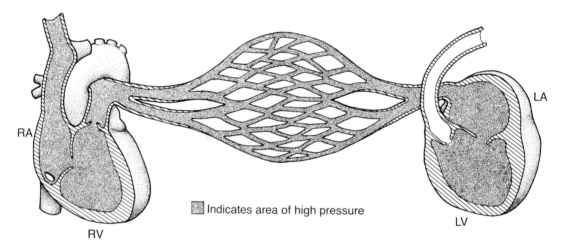

Indicates area of high pressure

FIGURE 18-13 Pulmonary edema due to generalized intravascular volume overload.

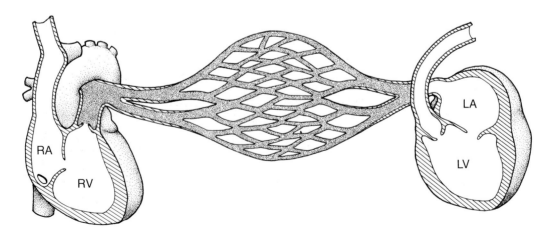

FIGURE 18-14 Pulmonary edema due to increased pulmonary venous pressure.

Increased LVEDP may be the result of ischemic heart disease, including angina; acute myocardial infarction; cardiomyopathy; pericardial diseases, including constrictive pericarditis and cardiac tamponade; aortic valvular disease, including aortic stenosis, aortic regurgitation, and dysfunctional prosthetic aortic valve; mitral regurgitation; hypertensive emergencies, including pheochromocytoma crisis, dissecting aortic aneurysm, and malignant hypertension; arrhythmias producing heart failure; and decompensating high-cardiac-output states, including severe anemia, thyrotoxicosis, atrioventricular fistula, sepsis, SIRS, and extreme fever.

Because high pressure pulmonary edema is most commonly the result of heart disease, particularly ischemic disease, the remaining discussion focuses on cardiogenic pulmonary edema.

Factors That Precipitate Acute Cardiogenic Pulmonary Edema

The most common causes of cardiogenic pulmonary edema are a sudden left ventricular ischemic event (which may be painless), an exacerbation of preexisting heart failure, or a cardiac catastrophe such as a massive myocardial infarction or an acute ventricular septal defect. Factors known to predispose patients with chronic heart disease to acute pulmonary edema include excessive or rapid intravenous fluid transfusion; sodium excess; physical exertion; intolerable elevations in blood pressure; noncompliance with prior drug therapy;

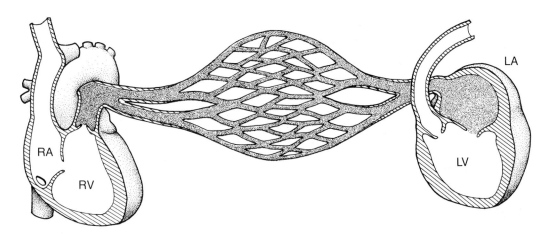

FIGURE 18-15 Pulmonary edema due to increased left atrial pressure.

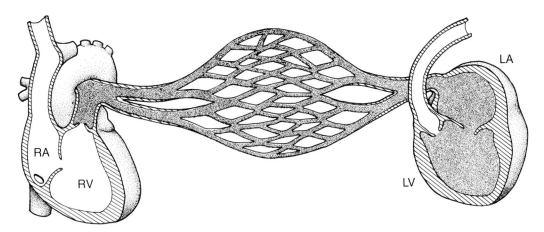

FIGURE 18-16 Pulmonary edema due to increased left ventricular end-diastolic pressure.

or emotional stress, such as anger, fear, or intense anxiety.

Pathophysiology

A number of pathophysiologic features are interrelated to culminate in a life-threatening imbalance between systemic and myocardial oxygen supply and demand. On the *oxygen supply* side of the imbalance, fluid accumulation in the lung results in shunt units (fluid-filled alveoli) and poor matching of alveolar ventilation with capillary perfusion. Both disturbances lower the arterial Po_2 in proportion to the amount of interstitial and alveolar edema. If cardiac output also is subnormal (myocardial ischemia, severe valvular disease), oxygen transport is further decreased. In other words, hypoxemia *and* perfusion failure combine to reduce systemic and myocardial oxygen supply.

Many factors also contribute to the *oxygen demand* side of the imbalance. Stiff, edematous lungs require a greater inspiratory force to maintain a physiologically acceptable tidal volume. At the same time, airway narrowing increases the effort associated with exhalation. The progressively increasing respiratory rate characteristic of worsening pulmonary edema further adds to the work of breathing and respiratory muscle oxygen demand.

The feeling of breathlessness and accumulation of secretions creates a sensation of suffocation. The intense fear and anxiety that naturally result, as well as systemic underperfusion, heighten sympathetic nervous system activity. The stress response that results, in turn, causes potent systemic vasoconstriction and increased heart rate and contractility and produces a generalized increase in metabolism and oxygen demand. In other words, the patient requires progressively more oxygen but paradoxically is getting progressively less. At the same time, the failing heart is required to work harder. If this cycle is not interrupted, the patient ultimately succumbs to exhaustion and dies of suffocation (Figure 18-17).

Hemodynamic Effects

Dysfunction of the left heart leading to pulmonary edema is usually associated with two hemodynamic problems: (1) systemic underperfusion and (2) blood volume/pressure overload of the pulmonary circulation.

Systemic Underperfusion. If there is a loss of ventricular contractile power (acute myocardial ischemia), blood flow obstruction (mitral or aortic stenosis), or regurgitant flow (mitral or aortic regurgitation), the heart may not be able to maintain a sufficient output to meet the metabolic demands of the body. Compensatory sympathetic nervous system–induced vasoconstriction helps maintain mean arterial pressure and blood flow to core organs de-

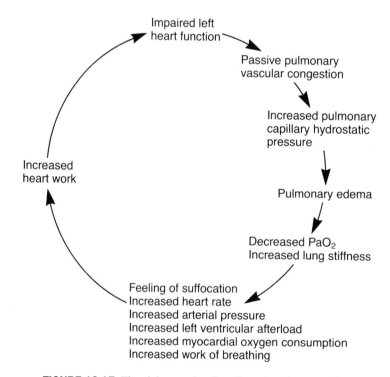

FIGURE 18-17 The vicious cycle of cardiogenic pulmonary edema.

spite the reduction in cardiac output. However, increased systemic vascular resistance elevates left ventricular afterload, and, as a result, stroke volume drops while myocardial oxygen consumption rises. The combined effects potentiate preexisting myocardial ischemia and heart failure.

Volume and Pressure Overload of the Pulmonary Circulation. Elevations in pulmonary intravascular volume and pressure may result from one or both cardiac factors:

1. The left heart is unable to pump out all the blood brought to it. Consequently, blood passively accumulates in the pulmonary circulation. This is commonly described as the congestive component of left heart failure that may result from any form of left heart disease.
2. An acute reduction in left ventricular compliance, typically due to an acute ischemic attack, suddenly elevates ventricular end-diastolic pressure. The elevated pressure is reflected back to the pulmonary capillaries.

Regardless of the initiating mechanisms, an increase in left ventricular end-diastolic pressure (PWP) greater than 18 to 20 mm Hg is met with an increase in movement of fluid into the lungs. As PWP increases, progressively greater extravascular fluid shifts occur. Generally, an acute elevation of PWP to 35 mm Hg is associated with massive transudation of fluid into the lungs and is incompatible with life beyond a few hours.

Exceptions to the Pulmonary Edema Threshold. There are three exceptions to the hydrostatic pressure threshold for the development of pulmonary edema.

Patients with Slow-Onset, Long-Standing Elevations in Left Atrial Pressure. Patients with mitral stenosis or chronic mitral regurgitation may tolerate a very high PWP rather well. This is because several compensatory mechanisms gradually develop and protect the patient from pulmonary edema even when left atrial pressure is as high as 35 mm Hg. These pulmonary edema "safety factors" include supernormal pulmonary lymph flow; diminished permeability of the pulmonary capillary membrane; and reactive constriction of the pulmonary arterioles, which reduces the volume of blood flowing into the pulmonary capillaries, veins, and left atrium (see Chapter 22). In these patients, a "normal" PWP of 4 to 12 mm Hg indicates profound, possibly life-threatening hypovolemia. This point reemphasizes that "normal" hemodynamic measurements may not be "acceptable" for all patients based on their underlying pathology.

Patients with Low Plasma Protein Concentrations. Hypoproteinemic or hypoalbuminemic patients may develop pulmonary edema (termed *hypo-oncotic pulmonary edema*) at relatively low pulmonary capillary hydrostatic pressures. Low plasma protein levels decrease the threshold pulmonary capillary hydrostatic pressure at which fluid begins to accumulate in the lung (Figure 18-18).

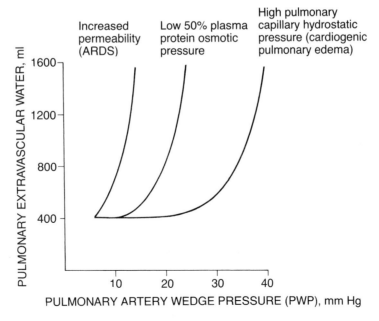

FIGURE 18-18 Threshold pulmonary capillary hydrostatic pressure levels at which fluid accumulates in the lung with various physiologic or hemodynamic abnormalities.

In a classic study, Guyton and Lindsey[10] demonstrated that when the plasma protein concentration was reduced to approximately 50% of normal by plasmapheresis, pulmonary edema developed at a PWP of 11 mm Hg. Consequently, the pressure threshold (PWP) known to produce pulmonary edema may be less than 18 to 20 mm Hg in many critically ill or injured patients, many of whom are known to be severely hypoproteinemic. Patients with chronic hepatic or renal disease (hypoalbuminemia) and protein-wasting enteric disorders also may develop fulminant pulmonary edema with relatively mild heart failure or fluid overload.

Patients with a Porous Pulmonary Capillary Membrane. Patients suffering from ARDS develop pulmonary edema with "normal" PWP measurements because of the extreme permeability of the pulmonary microcirculation. This syndrome is described later in this chapter.

Clinical Presentation

The clinical presentation of patients with pulmonary edema varies and depends on the stage of pulmonary edema and the severity of the underlying problem. In the earlier stage (interstitial pulmonary edema), the patient may be entirely asymptomatic or may experience only exertional dyspnea, occasional cough, mild tachypnea, and possibly orthopnea, whereas in the severe, late stage, the patient may be moribund. The clinical presentation discussed next is typical of patients with advanced pulmonary edema (alveolar flooding).

Mentation. Patients who can talk typically describe a sensation of suffocation sometimes associated with prostration. When able, patients intuitively sit upright and may indicate that the supine position is intolerable. The patient is usually very anxious and also may be irritable, belligerent, or even combative. Obtundation is an ominous sign because it usually is a consequence of severe hypoxemia or acidemia (or both).

Cutaneous Manifestations. If pulmonary edema is the result of low cardiac output, the skin is typically cool and clammy. The patient's complexion is typically pale, and central cyanosis may be mild or the skin may appear dusky. In patients with pulmonary edema due to high-cardiac-output states (volume overload, arteriovenous fistulas, extreme fever), the skin is usually warm, moist, and pink.

Heart Rate and Character of Pulse. Weak peripheral pulses and tachycardia accompany pulmonary edema due to heart failure. Ectopic arrhythmias such as premature ventricular contractions or bursts of ventricular tachycardia may occur as a direct consequence of the underlying heart disease, high circulating catecholamine levels, or hypoxemia and disturbances in arterial pH. However, the rapid pulse may be bounding in patients with high-cardiac-output conditions.

Auscultation of the Chest. Crackles begin in the dependent portions of the lungs and progressively extend upward to varying heights, such as the level of the midscapulae. Wheezing (cardiac asthma) is commonly the result of edema around the bronchi, bronchial mucosal swelling in upright patients, and reflex bronchospasm. The adventitious sounds may obscure the S_3 and S_4 gallops that are characteristic of a failing, noncompliant ventricle. In patients with very severe pulmonary edema, gurgling may be heard across the room; this is appropriately termed the ominous *death rattle*.

Palpation of the Precordium. If pulmonary edema is the result of chronic heart failure, the apex beat is displaced downward and to the left, covers a large area, and is sustained. The apex beat may occupy the normal midclavicular space if the patient developed sudden left ventricular failure (massive myocardial infarction, mitral valvular disruption) or if the patient developed pulmonary edema as the result of stiffness, not contractile failure, of an acutely ischemic left ventricle.

Neck Veins. Right heart failure, if present, usually develops secondary to left heart failure. In these patients, the external jugular veins are visibly distended and reflect the elevated systemic venous blood volume and pressure. In patients with chronic right heart failure, the liver and spleen are usually tender and enlarged because of passive congestion. If right heart failure develops suddenly, there also may be severe right upper quadrant pain caused by sudden hepatic distention that stretches the fibrous capsule of the liver.

Respiratory Rate and Character of Breathing. The first and often only clinical indication of interstitial pulmonary edema is an increase in the patient's respiratory rate. With the development of alveolar flooding, respirations become labored and rapid (26 to 46 breaths per minute). The nares are usually flared. Intercostal, suprasternal, supraclavicular, and substernal retractions reflect the generalized increased negative intrathoracic pressure required for inspiration. There may also be audible grunts with each expiratory effort. The patient may not be able to speak in complete sentences; a gasp between each syllable indicates severe, potentially life-threatening respiratory distress. The expectorated or suctioned sputum is typically frothy because of the mixture of pulmonary edema fluid and air. The froth may be clear and colorless, but it is more likely to be peach colored or red streaked. This coloration occurs with the addition of blood to the edema fluid that results from pulmonary capillary rupture.

Acid-Base Values. Patients with circulatory failure have metabolic acidosis. However, the pH may be in the alkalemic or normal range because tachypnea produces overriding respiratory alkalosis. When the patient cannot maintain the work of breathing, respiratory acidosis prevails and the patient develops a combined metabolic/respiratory acidosis (a very ominous sign). Hypoxemia is always present in patients with alveolar flooding.

Hemodynamic Profile

Patients with severe heart failure should have an arterial line, a pulmonary artery catheter, and possibly a Foley catheter (if the patient is uncooperative, unconscious, or incontinent) placed so that hemodynamic measurements and urine output can be accurately evaluated. However, if a patient without these devices develops acute pulmonary edema, insertion should be delayed until acute respiratory distress is relieved with aggressive therapy. Insertion of a pulmonary artery and Foley catheter usually requires that the patient be supine. Unfortunately, this position can be lethal for patients with alveolar flooding.

Arterial Pressure. The blood pressure is typically elevated unless the patient is in cardiogenic shock. In fact, an extremely elevated blood pressure may have *caused* pulmonary edema. The waveform may appear damped if there are significant reductions in stroke volume and therefore pulse pressure. A falling blood pressure is often due to an acute cardiac insult.

Systemic Vascular Resistance. This measurement is typically elevated due to systemic vasoconstriction (stress response).

Pulmonary Vascular Resistance. Early increases in left atrial pressure result in the opening of pulmonary vascular channels in the uppermost portions of the patient's lungs (West zones 1 and 2). Vascular recruitment reduces pulmonary vascular resistance by enlarging the cross-sectional area of the pulmonary circulation. However, the initial decrease in pulmonary vascular resistance is almost immediately overridden by the decrease in the intraluminal size of pulmonary blood vessels, caused by the pools of perivascular fluid. Later, with the development of alveolar flooding, hypoxemic pulmonary vasoconstriction further increases pulmonary vascular resistance.

Central Venous Pressure or Right Atrial Pressure. These measurements may be normal if the right ventricle is able to increase contractile performance commensurate with increased afterload. However, when the mean pulmonary artery pressure exceeds 35 to 45 mm Hg, the previously normal right ventricle usually fails. CVP values greater than 15 mm Hg (20 cm H_2O) are not uncommon in patients with cardiogenic pulmonary edema. If right ventricular failure develops, a dominant a wave may be observed in the right atrial waveform. It reflects the increased resistance to right ventricular filling during atrial systole.

Pulmonary Artery and Wedge Pressure. The PWP is greater than 18 mm Hg in a person with a previously normal left atrial pressure, or the PWP is higher than baseline values in the person with chronically elevated left atrial pressures, such as those associated with mitral stenosis. The pulmonary artery systolic and diastolic pressures passively rise in tandem with increases in PWP. Hypoxemia or acidemia induces pulmonary vasoconstriction and widens the PAd-PWP gradient.

The contour of both the pulmonary artery pressure and PWP waveforms is unchanged unless the primary disturbance produces an altered waveform, such as giant v waves in patients with mitral regurgitation.

Cardiac Output. A decrease in cardiac output is typical of pulmonary edema due to left heart dysfunction. However, cardiac output may be normal or even increased if pulmonary edema is the result of intravascular volume overload or a high-cardiac-output condition such as arteriovenous fistula or thyroid storm.

Mixed Venous Oxygen Saturation. This measurement (SvO_2) is decreased because of systemic hypoperfusion, hypoxemia, or both.

Laboratory Studies and Other Diagnostic Tests

If the patient is in extremis, immediate therapy takes precedence over obtaining laboratory tests. Otherwise, the following laboratory studies are immediately evaluated.

Electrocardiograph. Changes are noted specific to the cause of the pulmonary edema, such as ischemia or infarct patterns. Hypertrophy or "strain" patterns commonly are related to hypertensive or valvular heart disease.

Chest Radiograph. Roentgen rays that strike the x-ray film cause it to be blackened when developed. Normal lung tissue is well aerated, and the lung fields therefore appear relatively black. Water within the lungs and pulmonary vessels impedes passage of roentgen rays to the x-ray films and therefore appears white.

One of the earliest radiographic findings of heart failure and elevated PWP is the redistribution of blood flow from gravity-dependent areas of lung (the bases) to the least gravity-dependent zones of the lung (the apices). This is detected as white, vascular markings that extend up to the apices. However, this can be detected only on a film taken with the patient upright. In films commonly taken on supine patients in the ICU, blood flow is uniform from apex to base.

Interstitial edema is evident by white cuffs of fluid around blood vessels and airways, Kerley A and B lines, and a hazy appearance in the areas immediately adjacent to the mediastinum (perihilar haze). The findings just described are subtle but important indicators of a possible impending pulmonary crisis.

With the progression to alveolar flooding, cloudlike pulmonary infiltrates (whiteouts) begin to form and are more prominent in the central areas, whereas the peripheral regions of the lung are relatively clear. This distribution of edema resembles the outstretched wings of a butterfly and is therefore commonly referred to as a "butterfly-wing" pattern (Figure 18-19).

Pleural effusion also may occur and blunts the costophrenic angles. Heart size is enlarged if the primary defect is chronic ventricular failure. In a patient with an acute event, cardiomegaly may not be evident for several days because the stiff pericardium cannot dilate acutely to accommodate a rapidly failing and enlarging heart. For information concerning interpretation of chest radiographs, see Box 18-2.

There are other limitations of the chest radiograph in diagnosing pulmonary edema due to left heart dysfunction. A known diagnostic lag period exists in which pulmonary artery pressures may be elevated but edema may not be apparent on the chest radiograph. Alternatively, it may take 12 to 48 hours for radiographic evidence of pulmonary edema to clear after therapy has stabilized cardiac function and normalized hemodynamic measurements.

Chemistries. Arterial blood gases, complete blood count, serum electrolyte values, renal function studies (blood urea nitrogen, serum creatinine), serum albumin, and total protein should be immediately assessed in patients experiencing acute pulmonary edema. In patients already hospitalized who have prior chemistry panels

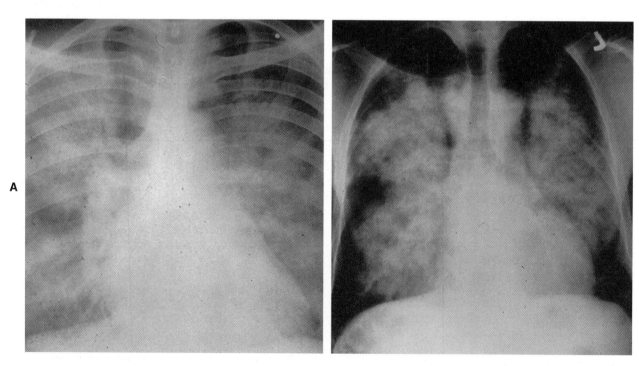

A   **B**

FIGURE 18-19 Chest radiographs of two patients with cardiogenic pulmonary edema with bilateral air space edema (alveolar flooding). Note the butterfly-wing distribution to the edema most conspicuous in **B** as well as an increase in heart size in both **A** and **B**. (Courtesy of the late Dr. Leo Schamroth and Dr. H.J.L. Marriott.)

available, only arterial blood gas analysis is usually required for patient evaluation.

Echocardiography. Patients admitted to the hospital with acute pulmonary edema should have the condition investigated with echocardiography and Doppler assessment to determine left ventricular size, thickness, and performance characteristics. Determinations of ventricular function, as well as the presence or absence of acute valvular regurgitation or ventricular septal defect, are cornerstones to developing effective therapeutic strategies.

Management

In young or otherwise healthy people with pulmonary edema due to inadvertent, intravenous fluid overload, supplemental oxygen, fluid restriction, or diuretic therapy usually resolves the process quickly.

Acute pulmonary edema, sometimes termed *flash pulmonary edema,* is the most dramatic and terrifying consequence of left heart failure. The prognosis is good if pulmonary edema is not the result of end-stage or overwhelming heart disease and is aggressively and effectively treated. If not promptly diagnosed and effectively treated, it may rapidly lead to death. Therapeutic strategies de-

---

BOX 18-2
Difficulties in Interpretation of Intensive Care Unit Chest Radiographs

Chest films taken in the ICU are notoriously difficult to evaluate because of the following factors:
1. In portable anteroposterior or supine films taken in the ICU, heart size is magnified.
2. The patient is usually unable to "hold" the deep breath and maintain an optimal body position for film taking. Frequently, patients slide down or to one side or the thorax becomes rotated.
3. Mechanical ventilation with high lung volumes, particularly with PEEP, may cause underestimation of the severity of pulmonary edema by hyperinflating the flooded alveoli. Hyperinflated, air-filled alveoli allow penetration of roentgen rays, whereas fluid-filled alveoli do not.
4. Coexisting pulmonary diseases such as pneumonia or ARDS (which also white out the lung fields) may render detection or evaluation of subtle findings or even gross fluid infiltrates impossible.
5. Variations in technique relative to different x-ray technicians. All efforts should be made to standardize techniques as much as possible.

---

pend, in part, on the underlying cause. The following general measures are indicated in patients with acute or chronic heart disease.

Maintain Adequate Arterial Oxygenation. Supplemental oxygen is given to maintain a PaO_2 of at least 65 mm Hg. Continuous positive airway pressure applied with a tight-fitting face mask (1) alleviates the work of breathing by reducing the required inspiratory force generated by the patient, (2) reduces the shunt fraction by distending and recruiting alveoli, and (3) corrects ventilation/perfusion mismatch.

Patients who are unconscious, uncooperative, or exhausted require intubation and positive pressure ventilation with the application of PEEP. PEEP improves arterial oxygenation by hyperinflating the lungs. Lung expansion provides a greater functional alveolar-capillary surface area for the diffusion of respiratory gases (Figure 18-20, *B, C, D*).

Place the Patient in a Sitting Position with Feet Down. Patients spontaneously assume the sitting position if able. Seating the patient front-to-back in a simple, armless chair provides support for the upper body and allows serial auscultation of the patient's back (Figure 18-21).

The upright position is critical to patient management because three fourths of the blood displaced to the dependent parts of the body comes from the pulmonary circulation. This results in an approximately 25% reduction in pulmonary blood volume. As a result, pulmonary capillary hydrostatic pressure and fluid movement into the lung decrease. Alternatively, placing the upright patient supine to obtain the ECG or hemodynamic measurements may produce intolerable overload of the central circulation and risks suffocation by lung fluid or risks cardiopulmonary arrest.

It is common to find patients in acute pulmonary edema in the emergency department and critical care units being managed in a semi-Fowler's or high Fowler's position while on a cart or bed. This position has two disadvantages:
1. With the legs held horizontally, the force of gravity is not maximized to unload the cardiopulmonary unit.
2. Patients typically slip down and do not remain in the high Fowler's position longer than about 5 minutes. If patients are unable to sit upright at the side of the bed or in a chair, they should be placed in an upright position while in bed. The patient probably has to be "pulled up" frequently; however, *the therapeutic importance of the upright position cannot be overstated.* A pillow placed vertically between the scapulae also brings the shoulders back and facilitates effective ventilatory movements in bedridden patients.

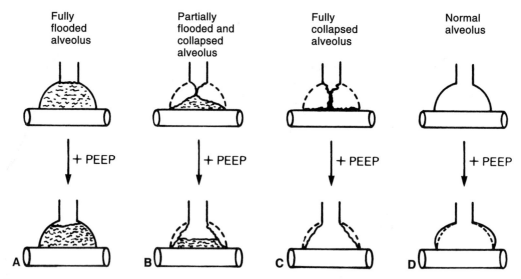

FIGURE 18-20 The lungs in stages 3 and 4 of ARDS consist of normal regions with air-filled alveoli, regions in which alveoli are collapsed or partially fluid filled (recruitable), and regions where alveoli are completely fluid filled (nonrecruitable). The following schematic representation shows the effects of PEEP on all regions of lung in ARDS. **A,** PEEP has no effect on completely fluid-filled alveoli. **B,** PEEP redistributes fluid and expands alveoli that are partially filled with fluid and collapsed. **C,** PEEP expands fully atelectatic alveoli. **D,** PEEP distends normal alveoli. The *broken lines* represent normal alveolar size and shape. (From Lankin PN: Clinical management, overview of therapy and prognosis of ARDS. In Carlson RW, Geheb MA, editors: *Principles and practice of medical intensive care,* Philadelphia, 1993, W.B. Saunders.)

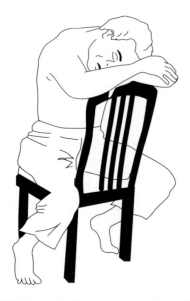

FIGURE 18-21 Posture instinctively assumed by patients in acute cardiogenic pulmonary edema. (From Marriott HJL: *Bedside cardiac diagnosis,* Philadelphia, 1993, JB Lippincott.)

Morphine Sulfate. When carefully administered intravenously in 3 to 5 mg increments to a possible total of 15 mg, morphine sulfate has several beneficial effects. The opiate promotes a sense of well-being. Thus the sympathetically induced arteriolar and venous constriction is diminished; preload, afterload, and heart work are reduced; and stroke volume is increased.

Caveats to Morphine Therapy. The patient should be carefully observed for respiratory depression because of the drug's central nervous system-depressant effects. Morphine should be avoided in the patient with decreased consciousness, hypotension, or COPD.

Preload Reduction. Although morphine sulfate has venodilator effects, additional preload reduction may require a diuretic such as furosemide (Lasix), which also acts as an immediate venodilator. Venodilation also may be accomplished with nitroglycerin given sublingually, topically, or intravenously.

Caveats to Diuretic and Venodilator Therapy. Therapeutic diuresis and venodilation should be performed with caution because both decrease left ventricular filling pressure and stroke volume. Consequently, if blood pressure falls significantly, hypotension worsens the imbalance of systemic and myocardial oxygen supply and demand.

Afterload Reduction. The arterial dilator action of nitroprusside (Nipride) reduces systemic vascular resistance, which helps increase stroke volume while decreasing myocardial work and oxygen consumption. In fact,

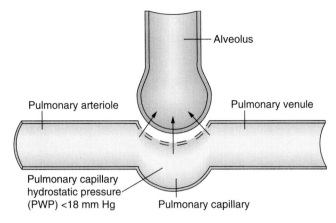

FIGURE 18-22 Schematic of the alveolar-capillary unit in ALI/ARDS. The pulmonary capillary membrane is damaged and freely allows a leak of plasma and the formed elements of blood into the extravascular space.

cardiac output may double with nitroprusside use, whereas PWP may be reduced by as much as 30%. Nitroprusside also has venodilator properties and is generally helpful in the management of patients in pulmonary edema, particularly when the patient is hypertensive.

Positive Inotropic Agents. By increasing cardiac output, these drugs improve perfusion of the systemic circulation and may reduce preload by increasing stroke volume. Dobutamine (Dobutrex) is preferred in patients with normal or elevated blood pressure and high systemic vascular resistance. Dopamine (Intropin) is indicated in patients who are hypotensive (systolic pressure less than 90 mm Hg). Phosphodiesterase inhibitors (e.g., milrinone [Primacor]), which have both vasodilator and inotropic effects, should also be considered.

Supportive, Reassuring Environment for the Patient. The most immediate and compelling need in life is to breathe. A feeling of suffocation provokes intense fear, which, in turn, stimulates or augments the stress response. Ironically, intense fear and the stress response are known to precipitate or exacerbate pulmonary edema. Thus a virulent cycle is established. Although caring for patients with acute pulmonary edema is also stressful for clinicians, all efforts must be made to provide a supportive and comfortable milieu. For example, reassuring patients that they will not be left alone and holding their hand when they are frightened establishes a meaningful, nurturing contact with the caregiver and may significantly reduce their anxiety.

Permeability Pulmonary Edema

Permeability pulmonary edema is a severe form of acute respiratory failure that occurs in people of all ages with or without preexisting lung disease. The patient has signs and symptoms of pulmonary edema despite a low to normal pulmonary capillary hydrostatic pressure (PWP).

In 1992 the American-European Consensus Conference defined diagnostic criteria for two stages of the same process.[11] *Acute lung injury* (ALI) is clinically characterized by an intense inflammatory response and fibrosis of lung tissue to infectious or noninfectious insults. Pathophysiologic and clinical characteristics are diffuse alveolar damage, increased permeability of the pulmonary capillary membrane that allows a leak of protein-rich fluid into the interstitial and alveolar spaces (Figure 18-22), hypoxemia that is poorly responsive to oxygen supplementation, increasing dyspnea and tachypnea, and a progressive decrease in lung compliance. The *acute respiratory distress syndrome* (ARDS) describes the end stage of ALI based on hypoxemic criteria.

As with multiple-system organ dysfunction (MSOD), there are no specific diagnostic tests for either ALI or ARDS. The diagnosis is strongly considered if the following criteria are fulfilled in a patient with signs and symptoms of pulmonary edema:

1. Acute onset of respiratory distress with no other reason for hypoxemia and radiographic findings such as cardiogenic pulmonary edema
2. Diffuse, bilateral infiltrates on frontal chest radiograph
3. Severe refractory hypoxemia: PaO_2/FiO_2 ratio equal to or less than 300 regardless of PEEP level (ALI) and PaO_2/FiO_2 less than 200 mm Hg regardless of PEEP level (ARDS)
4. Pulmonary artery wedge pressure equal to or less than 18 mm Hg or, if there is no pulmonary artery catheter, no clinical evidence of elevated left atrial pressures

---

BOX 18-3

Alternative Names for Permeability Pulmonary Edema (Acute Respiratory Distress Syndrome)

Descriptive of Pathophysiologic Features

Acute respiratory distress syndrome (ARDS)
Adult hyaline membrane disease
Congestive atelectasis
Noncardiogenic pulmonary edema
Progressive respiratory distress
Respiratory insufficiency syndrome
Stiff lung
Wet lung
White lung
Liver lung

Descriptive of Clinical Setting

Shock lung
Transplant lung
Posttransfusion lung
Da Nang lung
Septic lung

Throughout this chapter, for simplicity's sake, the acronym ARDS is uniformly used for permeability pulmonary edema.

The use of the aforementioned diagnostic criteria may be complicated because multisystem disease and coexisting pulmonary problems are frequently present in ICU patients.

Although ARDS can occur in critically ill infants and children, ARDS was given the alternative name "adult hyaline membrane disease" because the histologic changes are similar to those noted in the lungs of premature neonates with the infant respiratory distress syndrome. However, ARDS has been known by many other names, and the incidence of the syndrome was increasingly recognized in severely ill or injured patients from the late 1960s through the 1980s. Some names are descriptive of the conditions that predispose patients to ARDS, and some names describe the pathophysiologic process. Alternative names for permeability pulmonary edema are listed in Box 18-3.

Predisposing Factors

The lung damage characteristic of ARDS is the result of a systemic inflammatory response induced by massive tissue damage, inflammation, or infection. The various predisposing factors are listed in Box 18-4. In fact, ARDS is the pulmonary expression of SIRS and MSOD (see Chapter 17).

The likelihood of developing ARDS is compounded by the addition of other predisposing factors; the incidence of ARDS with one risk factor is approximately 25%, with two risk factors is 45%, and with three risk factors is 85%.[12]

Incidence and Mortality Rate

The incidence of ARDS is not clear because diagnostic criteria have not been standardized and because of nonuniformity of study populations reported. The annual incidence is estimated to be about 100,000 to 250,000 cases per year in the United States[11,13] and 2% to 3% of all ICU admissions.[14,15]

The mortality rate is estimated to be in the range of 20% to 60%, but if ARDS occurs secondary to unremitting sepsis or viral pneumonia, the mortality rate is closer to 90% to 95%.

Although more than 50 causes of ARDS have been identified, *sepsis is the most important cause in hospitalized patients.*

Pathophysiology

The common denominator in all patients with ARDS is a serious insult to the body that directly or indirectly targets the lungs. When not the result of direct lung injury, such as aspiration of gastric contents or smoke inhalation, the mechanisms that provoke lung damage appear to be systemic biochemical and immunologic abnormalities. These abnormalities, in turn, secondarily affect the lungs and other major organ systems through blood-borne inflammatory and vasoactive mediators (see Chapter 17).

Therefore ARDS is not an isolated, single disease. The inflammatory cascade involving systemic mediator activation and release affects multiple organ systems, not just the lung. Because clinical indications of lung injury and edema typically precede evidence of other major organ dysfunction, the first and most dramatic clinical signs and symptoms of MSOD result from lung dysfunction.

A major mechanism implicated in the permeability and inflammatory edema characteristic of the lungs of ARDS patients is systemic complement activation. The theory is that complement-activated leukocytes, such as polymorphonuclear neutrophils, are attracted to the pulmonary microcirculation where they release proteolytic enzymes and toxic oxygen radicals that directly injure the capillary-alveolar membrane, as well as lung tissue. Other variably activated or inactivated homeostatic systems that produce lung injury include the coagulation cascade; the cyclooxygenase, leukotriene, and cGMP pathways; cytokines and chemokines; and nitric oxide.

The formation of platelet microthrombi results in capillary endothelial cell damage and occlusion.

Biochemically induced damage and disruption of the pulmonary capillary membrane produce progressively enlarging spaces between the pulmonary capillary endothelial cells. These vascular "pores" allow a fluid leak from the capillary to the interstitial spaces despite low-to-normal pulmonary intravascular pressures, hence the terms *permeability pulmonary edema* and *noncardiogenic pulmonary edema*. The amount of extravascular lung water may be increased three to eight times normal. The vascular pores become large enough to allow formed elements of blood (such as red blood cells) and plasma proteins (such as albumin and fibrinogen) to escape into the extravascular space. Therefore the protein content of the pulmonary edema fluid and interstitial protein osmotic pressure are nearly identical to those of plasma.

Because of the extreme porosity of the pulmonary capillary membrane, the pulmonary capillary hydrostatic pressure, as estimated by PWP, becomes a critical factor in determining fluid movement into the lungs. Pulmonary edema develops at normal PWP pressures and can be catastrophic with even relatively mild fluid overload or heart failure (Figure 18-23; also see Figure 18-18).

The hypoxemia of ARDS is not only the result of alveolar flooding. Abnormalities in airway reactivity, thrombotic occlusion of the pulmonary capillaries, small airway closure, and mediator attack on the lung's surfactant system result in diffuse microatelectasis. These abnormalities cumulatively result in a lung tissue montage of variably disturbed matching of alveolar ventilation to capillary blood flow. Some lung units are overventilated relative to perfusion (increased dead space), whereas other units are underventilated relative to perfusion. Because of mediator-induced blunting of the pulmonary vasoconstrictive response to hypoxemia, mixed venous blood is freely "shunted" through areas of atelectasis or alveolar flooding.

Pathologic changes in lung tissue occur in a predictable pattern and are divided into an early exudative phase that is followed by a proliferative phase characterized by progressive lung fibrosis.

Early Exudative Phase (First 24 to 48 Hours of the Original Insult). This phase is characterized by damage to the pulmonary capillary membrane. This damage, in turn, results in progressively increasing interstitial and then alveolar edema. Inflammatory cells, red blood cells, and plasma proteins also eventually spill into the lung tissue and alveoli. Type I alveolar cells, which normally line most of the alveolus, are sensitive to this process and are destroyed, leaving a denuded alveolar membrane. Finally,

---

BOX 18-4

Causes of Permeability Pulmonary Edema (Acute Respiratory Distress Syndrome)

Shock
All types

Trauma
Direct lung injury
Nonthoracic trauma
Fracture of the long bones

Inhalation of Noxious Substances
Aspiration of gastric contents
Near-drowning (fresh or salt water)
Irritant gases
Smoke inhalation
Sustained high FiO_2 (50% to 60% or greater)

Infectious Causes
Viral or bacterial pneumonia
Septicemia

Drug Overdose
Heroin
Methadone
Acetylsalicylic acid (aspirin)
Barbiturates
Colchicine
Propoxyphene (Darvon)
Chlordiazepoxide (Librium)

Hematologic Disorders
Massive blood transfusion
Disseminated intravascular coagulation
Prolonged cardiopulmonary bypass
Thrombotic thrombocytopenic purpura
Leukemia

Metabolic Disorders
Diabetic ketoacidosis
Uremia
Pancreatitis

Miscellaneous
Eclampsia
Air or amniotic fluid emboli
Radiation
Heatstroke

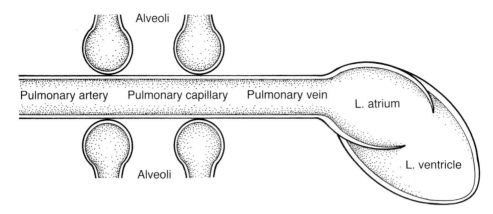

FIGURE 18-23 In diastole, there is a continuous open passage from the left ventricle to the right pulmonary arteries. Therefore pulmonary artery diastolic and wedge pressures approximate pulmonary capillary hydrostatic pressure, pulmonary venous pressure, left atrial pressure, and left ventricular end-diastolic pressure. Because pulmonary capillary hydrostatic pressure is an important determinant of fluid movement into the lung, reducing PWP reduces fluid flux into the lung in ARDS.

aggregates of plasma proteins, fibrin, and cellular debris precipitate and begin to adhere to the denuded alveolar surface, forming a hyaline-like membrane. The edematous, congested lungs provide an ideal environment for bacterial growth, predisposing the patient to bacterial pneumonia.

Proliferative and Fibrotic Phase (Ensuing 3 to 10 Days of Insult). This stage is characterized by alveolar cell replacement and formation of fibrous connective tissue. Type II alveolar cells begin to proliferate and ultimately cover the alveolar walls. Hyaline membranes organize and line the alveoli, alveolar ducts, and terminal bronchioles. The alveolar septa become progressively thickened. Fibrotic changes usually begin by the end of the first week. If the systemic inflammatory stimulus leading to lung injury is unrelenting, the microscopic appearance and gross appearance of the edematous, hemorrhagic, fibrotic lungs ultimately become unrecognizable as lung tissue. At autopsy, the lungs frequently look like and have the consistency of liver, hence the origin of the name *liver lung.*

Not all patients progress through the full pathologic spectrum. Some patients recover within the course of the disease if the inciting insult is self-limiting or therapeutically corrected and the systemic inflammatory response resolves. In these patients, lung regeneration and resolution require weeks to months. If, however, the ARDS trigger is ongoing (such as in uncontrolled sepsis), lung pathology progresses to end-stage fibrosing alveolitis. However, the majority of ARDS patients do not die directly from irreversible respiratory failure but rather from multisystem organ failure (MSOF). Table 18-4 lists

features that distinguish high-pressure (cardiogenic) from permeability (ARDS) pulmonary edema.

Hemodynamic and Clinical Course of Acute Respiratory Distress Syndrome

Regardless of the inciting insult that triggers ARDS, the evolution of unremitting ARDS predictably follows four distinct but overlapping hemodynamic and clinical phases that relate to progressive lung pathology.

Injury (the Initiating Insult). This first stage is usually associated with biochemical, immunologic, and perfusion abnormalities as the body attempts to "adapt and survive" in response to the insult. These abnormalities initiate a systemic inflammatory response that leads to vascular damage and the beginning of the pulmonary capillary leak.

Clinical Presentation. Unless associated thoracic or upper airway trauma is present, there is no evidence of respiratory distress and the lungs are clear to auscultation. There may be slight tachypnea or tachycardia. These variably accompany severe injury or illness, which makes evaluation of these signs difficult.

Hemodynamic Profile. This is specific to the type of injury (massive trauma, burn injury, systemic infection, pancreatitis, drug overdose, and so on). If the patient is being invasively monitored, a widening of the pulmonary artery diastolic to wedge pressure gradient may be noted and reflects increased pulmonary vascular resistance.

Laboratory and Other Diagnostic Tests

Chest Radiograph. The chest film is typically normal in the absence of other complicating problems such as hemothorax and pneumothorax.

TABLE 18-4

Features Distinguishing Hydrostatic (High-Pressure), Hypo-Oncotic, and Permeability Pulmonary Edema

Type of Pulmonary Edema	Response to Oxygen Administration	PWP, LA Pressure	Associated Trauma Serious Illness	Edema Fluid to COP or Plasma Protein Ratio	Hospital Mortality Response to Treatment
Hydrostatic (high pressure)	Good	High	Only incidental	Less than or equal to 60%	Good, unless overwhelming cardiac disease is present
Hypo-oncotic	Good	Normal	Underlying disease producing hypoproteinemia	Less than or equal to 60%	Good
Permeability (ARDS)	Poor (refractory hypoxemia is typical)	Low or normal; high if heart failure is also present or if there is fluid overloading	Always	Greater than or equal to 60%	Poor

LA, left atrial; *PWP*, pulmonary artery wedge pressure; *COP*, colloid osmotic pressure.

Arterial Blood Gases. The Po_2 is slightly below the patient's normal values. In the case of previously normal arterial oxygenation, a Pao_2 of 75 to 90 mm Hg may be anticipated while the patient is breathing room air (Fio_2 of 0.21). The calculated intrapulmonary shunt fraction is usually in the normal range of 5% to 8%. The $Paco_2$ is decreased relative to the degree of hyperventilation accompanying the physiologic and psychologic stress.

Mixed Venous Oxygen Saturation. The Svo_2 may be in the normal range or may fall if hypoxemia or a perfusion deficit accompanies the insult.

Latent Period (Following Patient Stabilization for Injury or Critical Illness). This second stage of apparent clinical stability may last from 12 to 24 hours. During this early exudative phase, a protein-rich fluid leaks into the interstitium of the lung through the pulmonary capillary "pores." The interstitial edema decreases lung compliance, compresses peripheral airways, and, as a result, increases airway resistance. However, the increased work of breathing typically is not perceived by the patient at this time. In many patients, ARDS resolves during this phase if the initiating insult is eliminated or controlled. In such patients, the presence of ARDS may never have even been suspected.

Clinical Presentation. The patient's chest is clear to auscultation, although some fine, high-pitched crackles may be audible. There is no declared or apparent respira-tory distress. Respiratory rates of 20 to 24 breaths per minute are an early, subtle clinical indication of an evolving virulent pulmonary problem.

Hemodynamic Profile

Pulmonary Artery and Wedge Pressure. Further widening of the PAd-PWP gradient develops and reflects increases in pulmonary vascular resistance. It is believed that pulmonary vasoconstriction is induced by mediators such as thromboxane A_2, leukotrienes, and serotonin, which are produced by white blood cells and platelets. Inhibition of nitric oxide (a vasodilator) production has also been implicated.

Laboratory and Other Diagnostic Tests

Chest Radiograph. Lung volumes may be slightly decreased. The appearance of the lung fields may be consistent with interstitial pulmonary edema. Subtle, diffuse "ground-glass" infiltrates may be noted on close inspection of the film.

Arterial Blood Gases. The Po_2 decreases, and it may approximate 65 to 80 mm Hg while the patient is breathing room air. Although this value is considered physiologically acceptable, it is not "normal" for a previously healthy person. The calculated intrapulmonary shunt fraction is approximately 10% to 15%. The Pco_2 decreases to approximately 30 to 40 mm Hg due to tachypnea.

Mixed Venous Oxygen Saturation. The Svo_2 typically remains within acceptable "normal" measurements if the patient is not experiencing perfusion failure or sepsis.

Acute Respiratory Failure. Approximately 24 to 48 hours after the trigger insult, it becomes clinically evident in the third stage that the patient is in respiratory distress. Proteinaceous edema fluid and formed elements of blood enter both the interstitial space and the alveoli. Increased thickness of the alveolar-capillary membrane begins to impair diffusion of oxygen, and the increasingly edematous and atelectatic lungs become more difficult to expand with inhalation. The increased work of breathing is perceived by the patient, who now complains of shortness of breath. Diffuse microatelectasis and alveolar edema raise the shunt fraction to approximately 20% to 30%.

Clinical Presentation. If not on a mechanical ventilator, the patient complains of dyspnea and may be anxious and restless. The respiratory rate may be approximately 26 to 32 breaths per minute. High-pitched end-expiratory crackles are heard throughout the lungs. The presence of bronchial breath sounds over the lung tissue indicates the consolidation and fibrosis characteristic of this process.

Hemodynamic Profile. The PWP may remain essentially within normal limits unless cardiovascular disease coexists or heart failure compounds the problem. Marked mediator-induced pulmonary hypertension is present, and the PAd-PWP gradient is significantly increased. The magnitude of the gradient directly correlates with risk of death. A mean pulmonary artery pressure greater than 35 to 45 mm Hg also predisposes the patient to acute right ventricular failure (cor pulmonale). In this case, circulatory failure exacerbates the pathologic progression of ARDS. Hypoxemia also augments the severity of pulmonary hypertension.

The patient usually has the hyperdynamic circulation (decreased systemic vascular resistance and increased cardiac output) characteristic of the systemic inflammatory response syndrome and MSOF. The supernormal cardiac output also may accentuate pulmonary hypertension. The calculated shunt fraction also increases because as cardiac output rises, greater amounts of blood perfuse the "shunt units" of the lungs.

Laboratory and Other Diagnostic Tests

Chest Radiograph. Airless lung tissue on x-ray films appears white. Patchy, scattered whiteouts appear and begin to coalesce diffusely throughout the lungs. In fact, the lungs may become nearly completely "whited out" (this inspired one of the alternative names, "white lung"). The diffuse infiltrates are due to the accumulation of lung fluid, diffuse microatelectasis, and beginning fibrotic changes. There is generally an absence of cardiomegaly, as well as an absence of the typical "butterfly" distribution of edema noted in patients with cardiogenic pulmonary edema.

Rather, the infiltrates are usually evenly distributed from the central to peripheral lung areas (Figure 18-24).

Asymmetry of infiltrates between lung fields may be observed if the initiating cause of ARDS was asymmetric (aspiration or trauma) or in patients with preexisting lung disease (bullae).

Arterial Blood Gases. The Po_2 continues to fall and approximates 50 to 60 mm Hg on room air. The shunt fraction is increased to 20% to 30%. Unfortunately, it is common to take first serious notice of the blood gas analysis when the numbers are outside the physiologically acceptable limits. Earlier careful evaluation of blood gas findings and subtle clinical signs would have revealed the developing problem *before* severe respiratory failure. The Pco_2 decreases to approximately 20 to 35 mm Hg owing to increasing tachypnea.

Mixed Venous Oxygen Saturation. The Svo_2 continues to fall relative to worsening hypoxemia.

Severe Respiratory Failure (End-Stage Disease). Gross distortion of the lung tissue is present in the fourth or end stage. The number of functional, perfusing pulmonary capillaries is markedly reduced as a result of microthrombotic obstruction. Aggregates of plasma proteins, cellular debris, and fibrin form thick hyaline membranes. In advanced disease, dense, irregular fibrous tissue bands replace alveolar-capillary membranes and alveolar duct

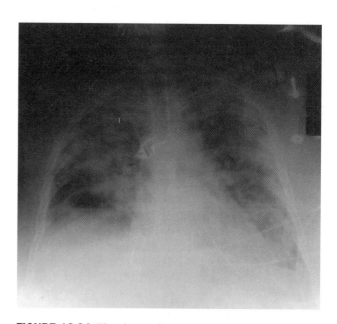

FIGURE 18-24 The chest radiograph in a patient with ARDS 3 days after drug overdose. Note the homogeneous distribution to the infiltrates giving a "whited-out" appearance throughout both lung fields.

surfaces. Lung compliance is usually profoundly decreased secondary to pulmonary edema; fibrosis; and massive, diffuse microatelectasis.

Clinical Presentation. If the patient is not on a mechanical ventilator, the dramatically increased work of breathing can be appreciated at a glance. The patient is typically using accessory muscles to generate wider swings in intrathoracic pressure to move air into increasingly stiff lungs and out through diffusely diseased airways. The exaggerated swings in intrathoracic pressure reflect on the vasculature of the thorax and produce a swinging baseline to the pulmonary artery and wedge waveforms. Intercostal, suprasternal, substernal, and supraclavicular retractions are evident. Diaphoresis, central cyanosis, mental obtundation, and nasal flaring are apparent. Diffuse high-pitched wheezes and crackles continue. Breath sounds diminish and reflect decreased movement of air through the narrowed airways and atelectatic lungs. The patient's respiratory rate may be in the range of 32 to 44 breaths per minute; expiratory grunting is common. The tremendously increased work of breathing, coupled with extreme hypoxemia, is incompatible with life. For this reason, patients are typically supported with mechanical ventilation. The peak inspiratory pressures that are required to deliver tidal volumes of 10 to 15 ml/kg progressively increase from values of 20 to 30 cm H_2O (early in the course of ARDS) to levels as high as 80 to 110 cm H_2O in patients with severe, late disease. Increased tracheobronchial secretions or pleural fluid may contribute to greatly increased peak inspiratory pressures and should be ruled out.

High mean and peak airway pressures and tidal volumes may lead to volutrauma and barotrauma that are clinically evident as subcutaneous emphysema, pneumomediastinum, or pneumothorax. New approaches, termed *lung-protective* and *pressure-limited* strategies, have been proposed to protect the lung from further ventilator-induced injury (see section on management).

Hemodynamic Profile

Pulmonary Artery and Wedge Pressure. Pulmonary artery systolic and diastolic pressures are elevated. In the absence of left ventricular dysfunction, the PWP is normal to low. The very wide PAd-PWP gradient correlates with the tremendously increased pulmonary vascular resistance. An example of hemodynamic measurements in stage 4 is right atrial pressure (CVP), 10 mm Hg; pulmonary artery systolic pressure, 60 mm Hg; pulmonary artery diastolic pressure, 30 mm Hg; PWP, 5 mm Hg; and PAd-PWP gradient, 25 mm Hg (normal, 1 to 4 mm Hg). As stated earlier, a markedly increased pulmonary vascular resistance reflected in a proportionately increased PAd-PWP gradient indicates a poor prognosis.

Cardiac Output. If the hyperdynamic circulation is maintained, cardiac output is greater than normal. However, if mean pulmonary artery pressures exceed 35 to 45 mm Hg, cardiac output usually falls because of right ventricular failure (acute cor pulmonale).

Laboratory and Other Diagnostic Tests

Chest Radiograph. Within 5 to 7 days, apparent improvement may occur in the x-ray picture. The opaque, whiteout appearance becomes less homogeneous, and the lung fields appear blacker. This may be related to a decrease in the amount of alveolar edema. Although the chest film may "look better," the patient shows no signs of clinical improvement. Hypoxemia is still severe and refractory to oxygen therapy because a thick hyaline membrane is present on the alveolar walls. It is common at this stage for bacterial pneumonia to become radiographically evident in the form of localized infiltrates.

Arterial Blood Gases. Because of massive ventilation/perfusion mismatching, diffusion block, and intrapulmonary shunting, the P_{O_2} progressively decreases with very poor response to higher levels of F_{IO_2}. At this stage, the shunt fraction may be greater than 40% and the Pa_{O_2} may be as low as 40 mm Hg while the patient is receiving 100% oxygen. Vascular microthrombosis increases the alveolar dead space volume (dead space/tidal volume ratios may exceed 0.60) and leads to a progressive rise in P_{CO_2}.

Mixed Venous Oxygen Saturation. The Sv_{O_2} may be decreased if the patient is hypoxemic but may be deceptively high due to the deficit in cellular oxygen uptake and utilization. Pulmonary function studies become increasing abnormal with progression of the disease and reflect the pathphysiologic effects. Changes include decreased total lung capacity, decreased static compliance, decreased functional residual capacity, increased dead space, and decreased diffusion capacity.

The aforementioned time-related progression of pathophysiologic and clinical events does not apply in patients with acute aspiration pneumonitis, smoke inhalation, inhalation of irritant gases, air or aminitoic fluid emboli, and near-drowning. In these cases, catastrophic injury is primarily responsible for lung injury and the clinical and pathophysiologic changes typically occur immediately after or within hours after the event rather than unfolding over a period of days. However, deterioration may progress over time.

Treatment

Despite the tremendous amount of research into the prevention and reversal of SIRS and ARDS, there is currently no generally agreed-on therapy that prevents the development or progression of lung injury or promotes lung healing once injury is established. Given this dismal fact, it is not surprising that the mortality rate remains high. Current management is directed toward removal or control of the inciting event and maintenance of patient support in the hope that the process will spontaneously resolve and the lung will heal and recover normal function.

Management Guidelines

Removal of the Primary Problem. This measure is essential to halting the disease process, as well as reversing the capillary leak and pulmonary fibrosis. All of the following therapies only "buy time" for the body to spontaneously heal; by themselves, these therapies do not cure. Also, the importance of immediate correction of any associated abnormalities and prevention of complications, such as gastric aspiration, periods of hypotension, sepsis, or pneumonia, cannot be overstated because they are additional insults that propagate or worsen the systemic inflammatory response.

Correction of Hypoxemia. This entails the administration of supplemental oxygen. However, pulmonary oxygen toxicity is predicted when an FiO_2 greater than 0.50 to 0.60 mm Hg is administered for an extended period. Ironically, the clinical, histologic, pathophysiologic, and laboratory picture of pulmonary oxygen toxicity is identical to that of ARDS. The length of time that it takes for toxicity to occur is variable and cannot be predicted individually. Depending on the dose of oxygen (FiO_2) and individual susceptibility, this may be clinically significant within a few days. Therefore the lowest FiO_2 that provides an acceptable PaO_2 should be used; an FiO_2 less than 0.5 is preferred. Patients with a high cardiac output and normal hemoglobin usually tolerate lower PaO_2 (approximately 60 mm Hg) fairly well because oxygen transport is only minimally reduced. Patients with perfusion failure or severe anemia tolerate lower than normal PaO_2 values (90 to 100 mm Hg) poorly because of the decreased oxygen transport reserve. Lower levels of FiO_2 may be achieved with applied PEEP.

Mechanical Ventilatory Assistance with Positive End-Expiratory Pressure. Conventional mechanical ventilation with PEEP has been the cornerstone of ventilatory management since the early 1970s. PEEP, compared with ventilatory support using atmospheric end-expiratory pressure, prevents small airway and alveolar collapse and recruits previously collapsed alveoli (see Figure 18-20). These effects maintain or increase the surface area of the lung available for the diffusion of gases and may reduce

compliance. There are, however, several physiologic and monitoring drawbacks to the use of PEEP:

1. *At levels higher than 10 to 15 cm H_2O, PEEP frequently makes determination of accurate pulmonary artery and wedge pressures difficult* (see Chapter 10, section on ventilatory effects on pulmonary artery pressure measurements).
2. *PEEP has the potential to depress cardiac output via several mechanisms:*
   a. Decreasing venous return to the heart by compression of the compliant venae cavae.
   b. Producing a tamponade effect on both ventricles that may interfere with ventricular filling.
   c. Compressing the pulmonary capillaries by PEEP-distended alveoli. Because pulmonary capillary compression may impair right ventricular emptying, high levels of PEEP also have the potential to decrease blood flow to the left heart. Also, at levels of PEEP greater than 15 cm H_2O, equalization of right and left ventricular filling pressures (as measured clinically by right atrial pressure and PWP) may occur. The increase in right ventricular diastolic pressure that results shifts the intraventricular septum toward the left ventricle and reduces its internal dimensions and volume capacity. The change in left ventricular shape and size compromises systolic and diastolic function, and for any given left ventricular end-diastolic filling volume, the left ventricular end-diastolic pressure (PWP) becomes disproportionately high relative to ventricular filling volume.

The aforementioned hemodynamic effects are partially offset by the fact that the stiff lungs of patients with ARDS tend to prevent transmission of high alveolar and airway pressure to the cardiovascular structures. This problem minimizes the pressure effects on hemodynamic measurements and minimizes the depressant effects on cardiac output. It is impossible to generalize to all patients or to accurately predict the magnitude of the effects of PEEP on hemodynamic measurements and cardiac output. The degree of lung stiffness is highly variable from patient to patient, is variable within the same patient during the course of the illness, and is variable regionally within the same lung.

However, the very mechanical ventilator device that is intended for patient support may paradoxically induce further injury. This process has been termed *ventilator-induced lung injury.* There are several mechanisms of injury. *Barotrauma and volutrauma* (pneumothorax, pneumomediastinum, pneumopericardium, air cysts, emphysema, systemic air embolism) are thought to be due to high levels of PEEP and high peak inspiratory pressures or increased lung volume. *Biotrauma* refers to enchanced inflammation caused by airway opening and closing, as well as mechanical ventilator–induced increases in lung cytokine release. The precise mechanism of each cause of lung injury continues to be debated.

Overall, the goals in ventilatory management of ARDS patients are to use the lowest level of PEEP that provides a maximal increase in PaO_2 with a minimal decrease in cardiac output and that maintains sufficient tidal volume and improves lung compliance; decrease mean airway pressure; maintain an inspiratory plateau pressure of 30 cm H_2O to limit barotrauma; and maintain FiO_2 as low as possible.

Several lung-protective approaches have been proposed for the ventilatory management of ARDS patients.[16-19] For example, a large multicenter trial, sponsored by the National Heart, Lung and Blood Institute of the National Institutes of Health in the United States, was designed to study the difference between ventilating ARDS patients with a tidal volume of 6 ml/kg versus the conventional 12 ml/kg and not exceeding an inspiratory plateau of 30 as a means of protecting the lungs from hyperinflation (volutrauma, barotrauma) injury. The resulting hypercapnea was permitted with efforts to maintain the pH above 7.25. The relative reduction in mortality rate in the low-tidal-volume group was 22%, there was no difference in the indicence of baratruma between the two groups, and organ failures were reduced in the low-tidal-volume group. See reference 20 for elaboration of this relatively complex technique.

Provision of Good Tracheobronchial Hygiene. This involves effective suctioning of the intubated patient as needed or frequently encouraging effective coughing and deep breathing in spontaneously breathing patients.

Frequent Change of the Patient's Position. Repositioning patients every hour can significantly reduce the tendency toward pooling of secretions, hypostatic pneumonia, and atelectasis. Position changes also alter the ventilation/perfusion patterns within the lungs. Evaluation of the "best" position for any patient at any point is determined by evaluating the effects of body position on oxygen saturations as monitored by pulse oximetry or mixed venous oxygen saturations with an oximetric pulmonary artery catheter. The "best" position should not be maintained for prolonged periods. Proper and frequent positioning are commonly given low priority in providing patient care because monitoring lines, intravenous tubing, and indwelling catheters and tubes make repositioning difficult. Meticulous attention to this aspect of patient care can have a significant, favorable impact on patient survival.

Reduction of Pulmonary Capillary Hydrostatic Pressure (as Estimated by Pulmonary Artery Wedge Pressure). In ARDS, the pulmonary capillary hydrostatic pressure is the primary force that determines fluid movement out of the pulmonary capillaries into the interstitial and alveolar spaces. Small increases in PWP, even within the normal range, may produce rapid progression in lung edema because of the increased porosity of the capillary membrane. The clinical corollary is that keeping the PWP low should minimize the transudation of water from the vascular to the tissue space. However, if PWP is too low, cardiac output and oxygen delivery may be sacrificed and the cycle—hypoperfusion leading to organ dysfunction leading to organ failure—is accelerated. The optimal level of PWP in the management of ARDS has not yet been established. Attempts are usually made to keep PWP in the low range of normal. Gradual dehydration (versus forced diuresis, which may result in hypovolemia and hypotension) and careful patient monitoring are recommended (see Figure 18-23).

Maintenance of Adequate Cardiac Output. Because efforts are made to keep the PWP in the low-normal range in ARDS, an inotropic agent such as dopamine may be required to increase or maintain an adequate cardiac output.

Keeping the Patient's Oxygen Demands as Low as Possible. Factors that increase systemic oxygen demand, such as fever, pain, restlessness, shivering, and anxiety, should be aggressively treated.

Experimental Therapies. None of the following strategies has been proven generally effective, and all have drawbacks. All are still considered experimental; some are not generally available or recommended for clinical use.

1. *Inhaled pulmonary vasodilators.* Nitric oxide and prostacyclin, in small inhaled doses, result in selective pulmonary vasodilation that reduces pulmonary hypertension. They also have antiinflammatory properties. Ventilation/perfusion mismatching is decreased by inducing local vasodilation of well-ventilated alveoli, thereby "stealing" blood away from nonventilated alveoli. However, no clinical trails have been able to demonstrate improved patient survival.

2. *Prone mechanical ventilation.* Delivering mechanical ventilation to patients maintained in the prone position for extended periods of time (up to 8 hours) has been shown to significantly improve PaO_2 in ARDS patients. This therapeutic approach is based on the fact that computed tomography has shown that the nondependent areas of lung adjacent to the anterior chest wall

are less atelectatic and consolidated when patients are maintained in the supine position. By turning the patient to the prone position, gravitational factors redistribute lung blood flow to these better-ventilated areas of lung, thereby improving the matching of ventilated to perfused alveoli. Because, with the passage of time, atelectasis and consolidation will develop in the new dependent areas of lung, the patient must periodically be turned back to the supine position. Major disadvantages of this technique are that it is highly labor intensive; it is extremely difficult to maintain vascular lines, tubes, and catheters; and pressure areas may develop on the patientís shoulders and pelvis.

3. *High-frequency ventilation.* Small tidal volumes (2 to 3 ml/kg) delivered at high rates (60 to 120 breaths per minute) are thought to limit barotraumas. No controlled studies have confirmed this hypothesis.

4. *Extracorporeal membrane oxygenation.* Systemic venous blood is directed from the lungs to a membrane oxygenator and is then returned to the systemic circulation. Thus the lungs are allowed to rest and recover. This therapy is complex and labor intensive and is available in only a few highly specialized centers. Anticoagulation is required; consequently substantial bleeding may occur.

5. *Inhaled surfactant.* Patients with ARDS have been shown to have dysfunctional pulmonary surfactant that may contribute to the pathogenesis of ARDS. Exogenous pulmonary surfactant prevents atelectasis, facilitates clearance of mucus, scavenges oxygen radicals, and suppresses inflammation. However, no study has shown improvement in mortality rate in adults.

6. *Liquid ventilation.* The lungs are filled with perfluorocarbon, which is a dense, colorless liquid capable of gas transport, and mechanical ventilation proceeds with the perfluorocarbon in place. Benefits include improved oxygenation, decreased barotraumas, clearance of debris, and reduction of inflammation. The effects on survival are unknown; large, controlled trials in ARDS patients are in progress.

7. *Antiinflammatory therapies.* Uncontrolled inflammation plays an important role in the pathogenesis of ARDS. It is hypothesized that agents that suppress inflammation could favorably affect patientoutcome. Corticosteroids, prostaglandin E_1, inhibitors of arachidonic acid metabolism such as ketoconazole, and ibuprofen have been investigated for this purpose. None has demonstrated improved survival to date.

TABLE 18-5

General Anticipated Direction of Change in Hemodynamic Parameters in Patients with Common Acute Pulmonary Disorders

Disorder	Arterial Pressure	Pulse Pressure	Systemic Vascular Resistance	Pulmonary Vascular Resistance	Central Venous Pressure	Pulmonary Artery (PA) Pressure	PA Wedge Pressure	Cardiac Output	Svo$_2$
Chronic obstructive pulmonary disease (COPD)	~	~	~ ↓	↑	~ ↑	↑	~	~	↓
Massive pulmonary embolism	~ ↓	~ ↓	~ ↑	↑	↑	↑	~ ↓	~ ↓	↓
High-pressure (cardiogenic) pulmonary edema	↑ or ↓	~ ↓	↑	↑	~ ↑	↑	↑	↓	↓
Adult respiratory distress Syndrome (ARDS)									
Stage 1—injury				Specific to type of injury					
Stage 2—latent period	~	~	~	~ ↑	~	~ ↑	~	~	~ ↓
Stage 3—respiratory failure	~	~	~ ↓	↑	~	↑	~	~	↓
Stage 4—severe respiratory distress (preterminal)	~	~	~ ↓	↑	~ ↑	↑	~	~ ↓	↓

Key: ↑, increase; ↓, decrease; ~, no change.

Note: The magnitude of direction of change can be modified by coexisting factors or complications (hypovolemia, fluid overload, severity of the primary problem, adequacy of compensatory mechanisms).

SUMMARY

Caring for critically ill or injured patients with isolated or complicated pulmonary disease challenges the intellectual and emotional resources of clinicians. Awareness of each patient's risk factors for pulmonary complications; meticulous physical, hemodynamic, and laboratory assessment; early identification of the pulmonary problem; aggressive and effective therapeutic interventions; and recognition of the patient as a highly physically, emotionally, and spiritually vulnerable human being are essential to a favorable outcome. Table 18-5 illustrates the anticipated direction of change in the hemodynamic measurements of those pulmonary diseases described in this chapter.

REFERENCES

1. Dalen JE, Alper JS: Natural history of pulmonary embolism, *Prog Cardiovasc Dis* 17:259, 1975.
2. Virchow RLK: *Gessammelte zur Wissenschaftlichen,* vol 4, *Thrombose und Emboli,* Berlin, 1862, G. Hamm-Grotesche Buchhandlung.
3. Value of the ventilation/perfusion scan in acute pulmonary embolism: results from the Prospective Investigation of Pulmonary Embolism Diagnosis (PIOPED), *JAMA* 263:2753, 1990.
4. Krivec B, Voga G, Zuran I, et al: Diagnosis and treatment of shock due to massive pulmonary embolism: approach with transesophageal echocardiography and intrapulmonary thrombolysis, *Chest* 112:1310, 1997.
5. McIntyre KM, Sasahara AA: Determinants of cardiovascular responses to pulmonary embolism. In Moser KM, Stein M, editors: *Pulmonary thromboembolism,* Chicago, 1973, Year Book.
6. Anderson FA et al: Physician practices in the prevention of venous thromboembolism, *Ann Intern Med* 115:591, 1991.
7. Gladwin MT, Pierson DJ: Mechanical ventilation of the patient with severe chronic obstructive pulmonary disease, *Intensive Care Med* 24:898, 1998.
8. Hess D, Medoff BD: Mechanical ventilation of the patient with chronic obstructive pulmonary disease, *Respir Clin North Am* 4:439, 1998.
9. Kerley P: In Shanks SC, Kerly P, editors: *A textbook of x-ray diagnosis,* vol 2, ed 3, Philadelphia, 1962, W.B. Saunders.
10. Guyton AC, Lindsey AW: Effect of elevated left atrial pressure and decreased plasma protein concentration on the development of pulmonary edema, *Circ Res* 7:649, 1959.
11. Bernard GR, Brigham KL, Artigas A: The American-European Consensus Conference on ARDS: definitions, mechanisms, relevant outcomes, and clinical trial coordination, *Am J Respir Crit Care Med* 149:818, 1994.
12. Pepe PE, Potkin RT, Reus DH: Clinical predictors of the adult respiratory distress syndrome, *Am J Surg* 144:124, 1982.
13. Villar J, Slutsky AS: The incidence of the adult respiratory distress syndrome, *Am Rev Respir Dis* 140:814, 1989.
14. Ferring M, Vincent JL: Is outcome for ARDS related to the severity of respiratory failure? *Eur Respir J* 10:1297, 1997.
15. Knaus WA, Sun X, Hakim RB, et al: Evaluation of the definitions for adult respiratory distress syndrome, *Am J Respir Crit Care Med* 150:311, 1994.
16. Marini JJ: Ventilation of the acute respiratory distress syndrome: looking for Mr. Goodmode, *Anesthesiology* 80:972, 1994.
17. Marini JJ: Tidal volume, PEEP and barotraumas: an open and shut case, *Chest* 109:302, 1996.
18. Bigatello LM: The acute respiratory distress syndrome (ARDS): mechanical ventilation. In *Critical care handbook of the Massachusetts General Hospital,* ed 3, Philadelphia, 2000, Lippincott Williams & Wilkins.
19. Steward TE, Meade MO, Cook DJ, et al: Evaluation of a ventilation strategy to prevent barotraumas in patients at high risk for acute respiratory distress syndrome, *N Engl J Med* 338:355, 1998.
20. The Acute Respiratory Distress Syndrome Network: Ventilation with lower tidal volumes as compared with traditional tidal volumes for acute lung injury and the acute respiratory distress syndrome, *N Engl J Med* 342:1301, 2000.

SUGGESTED READINGS
General

Banner MJ, Jaeger MJ, Kirby RR: Components of the work of breathing and implications for monitoring ventilator-dependent patients, *Crit Care Med* 22:515, 1994.

D'Alonzo GE, Lodato RF, Fuentes F: Diagnostic approaches in pulmonary hypertension, *J Crit Illness* p 17, August 1987.

Finkbeiner WE: General features of respiratory pathology. In Murray JF, Nadel JA, editors: *Textbook of respiratory medicine,* ed 3, Philadelphia, 2000, W.B. Saunders.

Hurford WE, Zapol WM: The right ventricle and critical illness: a review of anatomy, physiology, and clinical evaluation of its function, *Intensive Care Med* 14:448, 1988.

Janicki JS, Scroff SG, Weber KT: Ventricular interdependence. In Scharf SM, Cassidy SS, editors: *Heart-lung interactions in health and disease,* vol 42, New York, 1989, Marcel Dekker.

Koleff MH: Hemodynamic measurements during a tension pneumothorax, *Crit Care Med* 22:896, 1994.

Murray JF: General principles and diagnostic approach. In Murray JF, Nadel JA, editors: *Textbook of respiratory medicine,* ed 3, Philadelphia, 2000, W.B. Saunders.

Paraport E: Cor pulmonale. In Murray JF, Nadel JA, editors: *Textbook of respiratory medicine,* ed 3, Philadelphia, 2000, W.B. Saunders.

Shepherd KE, Hurford WE: Preoperative evaluation of the patient with pulmonary disese. In Sweitzer BJ, editor: *Preoperative evaluation and management,* Philadelphia, 2000, Lippincott Williams & Wilkins.

A special thank you to R. Phillip Dellinger, MD, FCCP, Professor of Medicine at Rush University and Director of Medical Intensive Care at Rush Presbyterian—St. Luke's Medical Center, Chicago, Illinois, for his review of and suggestions for this chapter.

Ten Eyck LG: The work of breathing in normal and diseased individuals, *Arkos* March 1989.

West JB: *Pulmonary pathophysiology: the essential,* ed 5, Baltimore, 1998, Williams & Wilkins.

Wiedemann HP, Matthay RA: The management of acute and chronic cor pulmonale. In Scharf SM, Cassidy SS, editors: *Heart-lung interactions in health and disease,* vol 42, New York, 1989, Marcel Dekker.

Pulmonary Embolism

Anand SS, Wells PS, Hunt D, et al: Does this patient have deep venous thrombosis? *JAMA* 279:1094, 1998.

Becker DM, Philbrick JR, Walker FB: Axillary and subclavian venous thrombosis, *Arch Intern Med* 151(10):1934, 1991.

Blaisdell FW: Thromboembolic problems. In American College of Surgeons: *Care of the surgical patient,* New York, 1993, Scientific American Medicine.

Carlson JL et al: The clinical course of pulmonary embolism, *N Engl J Med* 326:1240, 1992.

Elliott CG: Pulmonary physiology during pulmonary embolism, *Chest* 101(4 suppl):163S, 1992.

Hirsh J: Antithrombotic therapy in deep vein thrombosis and pulmonary embolism, *Am Heart J* p 123, April 1992.

Hufnagel CA: Deep venous thrombosis: an overview, *Angiology* 41(5):337, 1990.

Hyers TM: Venous thromboembolism, *Am J Respir Crit Care Med* 159:1, 1999.

Jeffery PC, Nicolaides AN: Graduated compression stockings in the prevention of postoperative deep vein thrombosis, *Br J Surg* 77:38, 1990.

Juni JE, Alavi A: Lung scanning in the diagnosis of pulmonary embolism: the emperor redressed, *Semin Nucl Med* 21(4):281, 1991.

Kearon C, Ginsberg JS, Hirsh J: Noninvasive diagnosis of deep venous thrombosis, *Ann Intern Med* 128:663, 1998.

Keith SL et al: Do graduated compression stockings and pneumatic boots have an additive effect on the peak velocity of venous blood flow? *Arch Surg* 127:727, 1992.

Kelley MA: Pulmonary embolism in the critically ill patient. In Carlson RW, Geheb MA, editors: *Principles and practice of medical intensive care,* Philadelphia, 1992, W.B. Saunders.

Marini JJ, Wheeler AP: Venous thrombosis and pulmonary embolism. In *Critical care medicine—the essentials,* Baltimore, 1989, Williams & Wilkins.

Monreal M et al: Upper-extremity deep venous thrombosis and pulmonary embolism. A prospective study, *Chest* 99:280, 1991.

Palevsky HI: The problems of the clinical and laboratory diagnosis of pulmonary embolism, *Semin Nucl Med* 21:276, 1991.

Palevsky HI, Alvai A: A noninvasive strategy for the management of patients suspected of pulmonary embolism, *Semin Nucl Med* 21(4):325, 1991.

Rogers LQ, Lutcher CL: Streptokinase therapy for deep venous thrombosis: a comprehensive review of the English literature, *Am J Med* p 88, April 1990.

Sherman S: Pulmonary embolism update. Lessons for the '90's, *Postgrad Med* 89:195, 1991.

Silver D: An overview of venous thromboembolism prophylaxis, *Am J Surg* p 161, April 1991.

Stein PD, Saltzman HA: Clinical characteristics of patients with acute pulmonary embolism, *Am J Cardiol* 68:1723, 1991.

Tobin MJ: Venous thromboembolic disease. In *Essentials of critical care medicine,* New York, 1989, Churchill Livingstone.

Wilson RF: Pulmonary emboli. In *Critical care manual,* ed 2, Philadelphia, 1992, FA Davis.

Chronic Obstructive Pulmonary Disease

Cicale MJ, Block AJ: Acute respiratory failure in chronic obstructive pulmonary disease. In Civetta JM, Taylor RW, Dirby RR, editors: *Critical care,* ed 2, Philadelphia, 1992, JB Lippincott.

Curtis JR, Hudson LD: Acute respiratory failure in chronic obstructive pulmonary disease. In Carlson RW, Geheb MA, editors: *Principles and practice of medical intensive care,* Philadelphia, 1993, W.B. Saunders.

Demling RH, Goodwin CW: Pulmonary dysfunction. In American College of Surgeons: *Care of the surgical patient,* vol 1, *Critical care,* New York, 1993, Scientific American Medicine.

Fink JB, Tobin MJ, Dhand R: Bronchodilator therapy in mechanically ventilated patients, *Respir Care* 44:53, 1999.

Irwin RS: Chronic obstructive pulmonary disease. In Rippe JM et al, editors: *Intensive care medicine,* ed 2, Boston, 1991, Little, Brown.

Koleff MH: Hemodynamic measurements during a tension pneumothorax, *Crit Care Med* 22:896, 1994.

Lesser BA et al: The diagnosis of acute pulmonary embolism in patients with chronic obstructive pulmonary disease, *Chest* 102:17, 1992.

Piquette CA, Rennard SI, Snider GL: Chronic bronchitis and emphysema. In Murray JF, Nadel JA, editors: *Textbook of respiratory medicine,* ed 3, Philadelphia, 2000, W.B. Saunders.

Rotman HH: Acute exacerbation in chronic obstructive pulmonary disease. In Dantzker DR, editor: *Cardiopulmonary critical care,* ed 2, Philadelphia, 1991, W.B. Saunders.

Sethi S: Infectious exacerbations of chronic bronchitis. Diagnosis and management, *J Antimicrob Chemother* 43(suppl A):97, 1999.

Wilson RF: Chronic respiratory failure. In *Critical care manual,* ed 2, Philadelphia, 1992, FA Davis.

Pulmonary Edema

Allison RC: Initial treatment of pulmonary edema: a physiological approach, *Am J Med Sci* 302:385, 1991.

American Thoracic Society: Round table conference. Acute lung injury, *Am J Respir Crit Care Med* 158:675, 1998.

Anderson BO, Harken AH: Multiple organ failure: inflammatory priming and activation sequences promote autologous tissue injury, *J Trauma* 30(12 suppl):S44, 1990.

Artigas A et al: The American-European Consensus Conference on ARDS. Part 2, *Am J Respir Crit Care Med* 157:1332, 1998.

Bernard GR et al: The American-European Consensus Conference on ARDS. Definitions, mechanisms, relevant outcomes and clinical trial coordination, *Am J Respir Crit Care Med* 149:818, 1994.

Bersten AD et al: Treatment of severe cardiogenic pulmonary edema with continuous positive airway pressure delivered by face mask, *N Engl J Med* 325:1825, 1991.

Blake GJ: Furosemide for pulmonary edema, *Nursing* 20:108, 1990.

Cope DK et al: Pulmonary capillary pressure: a review, *Crit Care Med* 20:1043, 1992.

Cunningham AJ: Acute respiratory distress syndrome—two decades later, *Yale J Biol Med* 64:387, 1991.

Dellinger RP, Simmerman JL, Taylor RW, et al: Effects of inhaled nitric oxide in patients with acute respiratory distress syndrome: results of a randomized phase II trial, *Crit Care Med* 26:15, 1998.

Donnelly TJ, Meade P, Jagels M, et al: Cytokine, complement, and endotoxin profiles associated with the development of the adult respiratory distress syndrome after severe injury, *Crit Care Med* 22:768, 1994.

Dreyfuss D, Saumon G: Overexpansion pulmonary edema, *J Appl Physiol* 71:777, 1991.

Dreyfuss D, Saumon G: Ventilator-induced lung injury, *Am J Respir Crit Care Med* 157:294, 1998.

Ferring M, Vincent JL: Is outcome from ARDS related to the severity of respiratory failure? *Eur Respir J* 10:1297, 1977.

Fishman AP, Renkin EM: *Pulmonary edema,* Bethesda, MD, 1979, American Physiological Society.

Hall JB. Respiratory system mechanics in adult respiratory distress syndrome, *Am J Respir Crit Care Med* 158:1, 1998.

Hall JB, Schmidt GA, Wood MD: Acute hypoxemic respiratory failure. In Murray JF, Nadel JA, editors: *Textbook of respiratory medicine,* ed 3, Philadelphia, 2000, W.B. Saunders.

Humphrey H et al: Improved survival in ARDS associated with a reduction in pulmonary capillary wedge pressure, *Chest* 97:1176, 1990.

Roberts SL: High-permeability pulmonary edema: nursing assessment, diagnosis, and interventions, *Heart Lung* 19:287, 1990.

Ronco JJ, Belzberg A, Phang PT, et al: No difference in hemodynamics, ventricular function, and oxygen delivery in septic and nonseptic patients with the adult respiratory distress syndrome, *Crit Care Med* 22:777, 1994.

Schuller D et al: Fluid balance during pulmonary edema. Is fluid gain a marker or a cause of poor outcome? *Chest* 100:1068, 1991.

Starling EH: On the absorption of fluids from the connective tissue space, *J Physiol* 18:312, 1986.

Staub NC: Pulmonary edema, *Physiol Rev* 54:678, 1974.

Suchyta MR et al: The adult respiratory distress syndrome. A report of survival and modifying factors, *Chest* 101:1074, 1992.

Velazauez M, Schuster DP: Perfusion alters alveolar flooding; vasoconstriction vs vascular decompression, *J Appl Physiol* 70:600, 1991.

Villar J, Slutsky AS: The incidence of the adult respiratory distress syndrome, *Am Rev Respir Dis* 140:814, 1989.

Weil MH et al: Relationship between colloid osmotic pressure and pulmonary artery wedge pressure in patients with acute cardiorespiratory failure, *Am J Med* 64:643, 1978.

White BS, Roberts SL: Pulmonary alveolar edema: preventing complications, *Dimens Crit Care Nurs* 11:90, 1992.

Wickerts CJ, Berg B, Blomqvist H: Influence of positive end-expiratory pressure on extravascular lung water during the formation of experimental hydrostatic pulmonary oedema, *Acta Anaesthesiol Scand* 36:309, 1992.

Wilson RF: Acute respiratory failure. In *Critical care manual,* ed 2, Philadelphia, 1992, FA Davis.

19

MARY FRAN HAZINSKI

Pediatric Evaluation and Monitoring Considerations

The principles of hemodynamic monitoring in children are identical to those in adults. However, equipment and technique must be modified because children differ from adults in size, in organ system development and function, and in metabolic rate and oxygen consumption. The equipment used to monitor pediatric patients must have rapid response times and must be accurate in the detection of the relatively rapid heart rates, as well as in the measurement of the relatively low arterial pressures. Evaluation of hemodynamic measurements requires familiarity with pediatric norms and the ability of clinicians to interpret data in view of disease or injury.[1]

This chapter first discusses the hemodynamic characteristics of the pediatric circulation throughout the perinatal period and during childhood. Clinically relevant differences between children and adults, as well as assessment of hemodynamic competency in pediatric patients and important features of congenital heart disease, are then presented. The remainder of the chapter focuses on specific monitoring techniques with caveats and considerations specific to pediatric patients.

CARDIOPULMONARY PHYSIOLOGY AND MATURATION IN CARDIOVASCULAR FUNCTION

Perinatal Circulatory Changes

The first weeks after birth are a time of circulatory transition. The circulation must be converted from a system oxygenated by the placenta to a system oxygenated by the lungs; this requires both structural and physiologic adaptation. The fetal circulation has relatively inefficient separation of well-oxygenated and poorly oxygenated blood. Immediately after birth, the circulation must convert to a system with complete separation of systemic venous and pulmonary venous blood.

Fetal Circulation

The fetal circulation is designed to divert well-oxygenated blood from the placenta to the fetal brain and away from the lungs and to return fetal blood to the placenta. Following birth, the circulation must adapt to divert systemic venous blood to the lungs and deliver pulmonary venous (oxygenated) blood to the neonate's body.

The fetal arterial oxygen tension (PaO_2) is approximately 22 to 29 mm Hg, and hemoglobin saturation is approximately 60% to 79%.[2] Although the fetus is hypoxemic, tissue oxygen delivery is adequate because cardiac output (per kilogram body weight) is approximately 200 to 300 ml/kg/min. This blood flow rate is much higher than that of older children or adults and, as a result, maintains adequate oxygen delivery despite the hypoxemia.[2-4] In addition, hemoglobin is relatively well saturated at a PaO_2 of 22 to 29 mm Hg because "fetal" hemoglobin contains less 2,3-diphosphoglycerate (2,3-DPG) than "adult" hemoglobin. Decreased 2,3-DPG, in turn, shifts the fetal oxyhemoglobin dissociation curve to the *left* of the normal adult oxyhemoglobin dissociation curve. At any PaO_2, the fetal hemoglobin is more saturated with oxygen than adult hemoglobin. As a consequence, the fetal arterial oxygen content is higher than that of adults at the same hemoglobin saturation.[2,4]

During fetal life, pulmonary vascular resistance is high, because the lungs are fluid filled. The absence of oxygen in the alveoli results in constriction of the small pulmonary arteries. In contrast, fetal systemic vascular resistance is low because some descending aortic blood flow enters the placenta, which is a low-resistance circulatory pathway.

Normal fetal anatomic shunts include the ductus arteriosus, foramen ovale, and ductus venosus. These shunts facilitate diversion of blood from the fetal placenta through the ductus venosus and the foramen ovale to the left heart and ascending aorta and ultimately to the fetal brain. The ductus arterious diverts blood away from the pulmonary artery (away from the nonfunctional lungs) into the descending aorta. Much of the descending aortic blood flow ultimately returns to the placenta (Figure 19-1).[2,5]

Perinatal Circulatory Conversion

At birth, newborns change from oxygenation of the blood by the placenta to oxygenation of the blood by the lungs. The lungs are more efficient oxygenators of blood than the placenta; therefore the arterial oxygen tension rises immediately. The fluid present in alveoli is reabsorbed into the pulmonary capillaries and is also removed by the pulmonary lymphatics.[5] Replacement of alveolar fluid by air eliminates alveolar hypoxia, which, in turn, results in pulmonary vasodilation and a fall in pulmonary

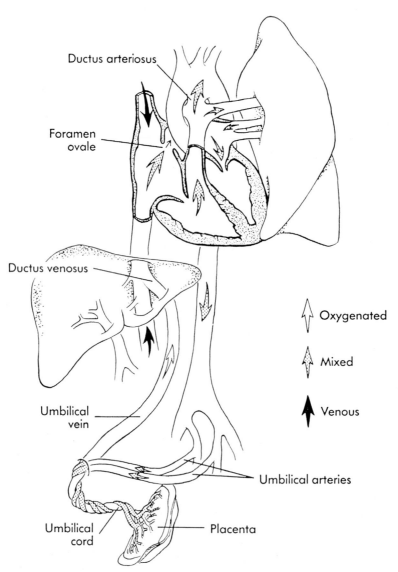

FIGURE 19-1 Fetal circulation. (Reproduced with permission from Hazinski MF: Cardiovascular disorders. In Hazinski MF, editor: *Nursing care of the critically ill child,* ed 2, St Louis, 1992, Mosby.)

vascular resistance.[2,5] These pulmonary vascular changes occur several days after birth.[2,4,5]

The fetal anatomic shunts normally begin to close immediately after birth and are closed within a few days. Closure of the ductus arteriosus is stimulated by a rise in arterial and perivascular oxygen tension following onset of alveolar ventilation. However, ductal closure may be delayed in premature infants, who lack constrictive muscle in the ductus. Ductal closure also may be delayed in neonates with lung disease or in infants living at high altitudes.[2,5]

The fall in pulmonary vascular resistance associated with the onset of alveolar ventilation results in an immediate fall in right ventricular and right atrial pressures. Removal of the low-resistance placenta produces a simultaneous, sudden elevation in systemic vascular resistance, and thus left ventricular and left atrial pressures begin to rise. Once left atrial pressure exceeds right atrial pressure, the foramen ovale closes functionally. Anatomic closure (final sealing of the foramen ovale) occurs during the next several months, although the foramen ovale remains probe patent throughout life in a small number of people. Although this characteristic normally has no circulatory consequences, it may enable passage of a catheter from the right atrium into the left atrium.

Perinatal Pulmonary Vascular Changes

As mentioned, on intake of the first breath, alveolar oxygenation results in pulmonary vasodilation. Consequently, pulmonary vascular resistance begins to fall immediately after birth in infants born at sea level. If the ductus closes normally in these patients, pulmonary artery pressure falls approximately 80% immediately after birth, and mean pulmonary artery pressure falls to approximately one half of mean systemic arterial pressure within 24 hours of birth.[2,5,6] Within the first weeks of life, pulmonary vascular resistance drops to adult levels (Table 19-1), and right ventricular and right atrial pressures likewise fall. In infants born at higher altitudes, the fall in pulmonary vascular resistance and right ventricular changes may be delayed for several weeks.

The pulmonary arteries of neonates are reactive and may intensely constrict in response to alveolar hypoxia, acidosis, alveolar distention, or hypothermia.[2,7] Pulmonary arterial constriction, in turn, results in an increase in pulmonary vascular resistance and pulmonary artery systolic and diastolic pressures. Consequently, these conditions should be avoided because they exacerbate the hemodynamic abnormalities present in patients with preexisting pulmonary hypertension and may cause pulmonary hypertension in patients with previously normal pulmonary artery pressures.

TABLE 19-1
Calculation of Pulmonary Vascular Resistance

Calculations

$$PVR \text{ (Wood units)} = \frac{\text{Mean PA pressure} - \text{Mean LA pressure (mm Hg)}}{\text{Cardiac output (L/min)}}$$

$$PVR \text{ (index units)} = \frac{\text{Mean PA pressure} - \text{Mean LA pressure (mm Hg)}}{\text{Cardiac index (L/min/m}^2 \text{ BSA)}}$$

$$PVR \text{ (dynes-sec-cm)} = \frac{\text{Mean PA pressure} - \text{Mean LA pressure (mm Hg)}}{\text{Cardiac output (L/min)}} \times 80$$

Note: To obtain PVR index in dynes-sec-cm^{-5} multiply substitute cardiac index for cardiac output in denominator.

Normal Values in Infants and Children

Age	PVR (Wood Units)	PVR (Index Units)	PVR (dynes-sec-cm^{-5})
Young infant	25 – 40	7 – 10	2000 – 3200 (indexed: 560 – 800 dynes-sec-cm^{-5}/m^2)
Child	0.5 – 4	1 – 3	40 – 320 (indexed: 80 – 240 dynes-sec-cm^{-5}/m^2)

Potential Causes of Elevated PVR

- Alveolar hypoxia and pulmonary artery constriction: consider all potential causes of alveolar hypoxia, including hypoventilation, endotracheal tube obstruction, and pneumothorax
- Increased blood flow (cardiac output) in the face of unchanged vascular tone
- Obstruction to flow: pulmonary venous obstruction, mitral valve stenosis, or severe left ventricular failure

Adapted from Hazinski MF: *Manual of pediatric critical care,* St Louis, 1999, Mosby.

LA, left atrial; *PA,* pulmonary artery; *PVR,* pulmonary vascular resistance.

TABLE 19-2

Potential Factors Affecting Pulmonary Vascular Resistance

Factor	Potential Constrictors	Potential Dilators
Alveolar oxygenation	Alveolar hypoxia	Alveolar oxygenation
	Reduce Fio_2	Increase Fio_2
Serum pH	Acidosis	Alkalosis
Ventilation	Hypoventilation	Mild hyperventilation
	Alveolar hyperinflation	
Body temperature	Hypothermia	—
Stimulation	Pain, stimulation	Sedation, analgesia
Pharmacologic therapy		Inhaled nitric oxide

Data from Hazinski MF, Barkin RM: Shock. In Barkin RM, editor: *Pediatric emergency medicine: concepts and clinical practice,* ed 2, St Louis, 1997, Mosby.

Factors causing pulmonary vasoconstriction include: alveolar hypoxia, acidosis, hypothermia, hyperinflation, and stimulation.[7] These factors should be avoided or promptly treated in the infant or child with pulmonary hypertension or congenital heart disease with inadequate pulmonary blood flow.

Pulmonary arterial dilation may be facilitated through (1) therapeutic measures that maintain effective alveolar oxygenation, (2) induced alkalosis (usually accomplished through mild hyperventilation or hyperventilation in combination with administration of buffering agents), and (3) avoidance of hypothermia and alveolar distention (Table 19-2).[7-12] Inhaled nitric oxide also promotes pulmonary vasodilation.[10,13,14]

When pulmonary blood flow is excessive (e.g., neonates with single ventricle or single ventricle physiology), pulmonary blood flow can be limited by eliminating factors that cause pulmonary vasodilation and promoting factors that cause vasoconstriction.[8-12,14] Alveolar oxygenation can be reduced by administering room air (eliminating supplemental oxygen). Inspired oxygen can be further reduced by "bleeding in" carbon dioxide or nitrogen into the inspired air circuit to reduce the inspired Fio_2 to less than 0.21.[14]

Perinatal Systemic Vascular Changes

When the placenta is separated from the circulation, systemic vascular resistance (SVR) begins to rise.[2,5,15] SVR continues to rise during childhood and adolescence (Table 19-3). As SVR increases, left ventricular and atrial pressures increase, and left ventricular myocyte growth exceeds that of the right ventricle.[2,16] Within the first year of life, left ventricular muscle thickness exceeds right ventricular muscle thickness. Overall, pediatric intracardiac pressures and oxygen saturations are equivalent to those

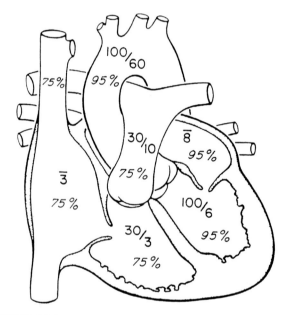

FIGURE 19-2 Normal pressures and saturations in the pediatric heart. (Reproduced with permission from Watson SP, Watson DC Jr: Anatomy, physiology, and hemodynamics of congenital heart disease. In Ream AK, Fogdall RP, editors: *Acute cardiovascular management: anesthesia and intensive care,* Philadelphia, 1982, JB Lippincott.)

of adults by the time the child enters elementary school, unless the child has congenital heart disease or pulmonary hypertension (Figure 19-2).[16]

Perinatal Oxygen Consumption and Cardiac Output

The oxygen consumption of neonates is approximately double the oxygen consumption (per kilogram body weight) of a 2-month-old infant. Because oxygen consumption is

TABLE 19-3
Calculation of Systemic Vascular Resistance

Calculations

$$\text{SVR (Wood units)} = \frac{\text{Mean arterial pressure } - \text{ Mean RA pressure (mm Hg)}}{\text{Cardiac output}}$$

$$\text{SVR (index units)} = \frac{\text{Mean arterial pressure } - \text{ Mean RA pressure (mm Hg)}}{\text{Cardiac index}}$$

$$\text{SVR (dynes-sec-cm}^{-5}) = \frac{\text{Mean arterial pressure } - \text{ Mean RA pressure (mm Hg)}}{\text{Cardiac output}} \times 80$$

Note: To determine SVR index in dynes-sec-cm^{-5} substitute cardiac index for cardiac output in the denominator of this equation.

Normal Values for Infants and Children

Age	SVR (Wood Units)	SVR (Index Units)	SVR (dynes-sec-cm^{-5})
Infant	35–50	10–15	2800–4000 (indexed: 800–1200 dynes-sec-cm^{-5}/m^2)
Toddler	25–35	20	2000–2800 (indexed: 1600 dynes-sec-cm^{-5}/m^2)
Child	15–25	15–30	1200–2000 (indexed: 1200–2400 dynes-sec-cm^{-5}/m^2)

Note: The numerical value of indexed measurements decreases with age because body surface area is very low in infants and gradually increases with growth.

Factors Causing Changes in SVR
Increased
- Compensatory vasoconstriction associated with low cardiac output
- Administration of vasoconstrictive agents
- Adrenergic stimulation

Decreased
- Sepsis, the systemic inflammatory response syndrome
- Anaphylaxis
- Administration of vasodilatory agents
- Sympathetic nervous system blockade (spinal anesthesia, barbiturate overdose); damage to or transection of the spinal cord

Adapted from Hazinski MF: *Manual of pediatric critical care,* St Louis, 1999, Mosby.

RA, right atrial; *SVR,* systemic vascular resistance.

---

near the maximal level at this age, neonates have minimal oxygen reserve. Consequently, factors that further increase oxygen demand or reduce cardiac output or arterial oxygen content (factors in oxygen delivery) are likely to result in a compromise in tissue oxygenation. Pain, infection, and increased work of breathing *must* be promptly treated in all patients, but particularly in neonates, because they all increase oxygen demand and may lead to tissue hypoxia.[1]

Cold stress also increases oxygen demand, because shivering does not occur in the first months of life. Instead, an energy-requiring process termed *nonshivering thermogenesis* is stimulated.[17] Maintenance of a neutral thermal environment through use of overbed warmers or incubators minimizes oxygen demand by preventing nonshivering thermogenesis in neonates and very young infants.

Fetal cardiac output is approximately 200 to 300 ml/kg/min; cardiac output increases substantially immediately after birth and is as high as 300 to 400 ml/kg/min.[2-5] This cardiac output is the equivalent of a 21 to 28 L/min cardiac output in a 70 kg adult. This high postnatal cardiac output parallels the tremendous increase in oxygen consumption during the first weeks of life.[1,2,5,18] Cardiac output is determined by the interplay of heart rate and stroke volume.

Heart Rate

Table 19-4 lists normal heart rate relative to patient age. *During childhood, cardiac output is extremely dependent on the child's heart rate.* Any decrease in heart rate often produces an equivalent decrease in the child's cardiac output.[1,3,18] During the neonatal period, the resting heart rate is near maximal levels at this age. *Increases* in the heart rate above a rate of 160 to 180 beats per minute may not cause significant increases in cardiac output.[1,3,18] In fact, an extremely rapid heart rate in any child (exceeding 180

TABLE 19-4

Normal Awake and Sleeping Heart Rates in Children

Age	Awake Heart Rate (per min)*	Sleeping Heart Rate (per min)*
Neonate	100–180	80–160
Infant (6 months)	100–160	75–160
Toddler	80–110	60–90
Preschooler	70–110	60–90
School-age	65–110	60–90
Adolescent	60–90	50–90

Reproduced with permission from Hazinski MF: Children are different. In Hazinski MF, editor: *Nursing care of the critically ill child,* ed 2, St Louis, 1992, Mosby. All rights reserved. And from Gillette PC et al: Dysrhythmias. In Adams FH, Emmanouilides GC, editors: *Moss' heart disease in infants, children, adolescents,* ed 4, Baltimore, 1989, Williams & Wilkins.

*Always consider patient's normal range and clinical condition. Heart rate will normally increase with critical illness, fever, or pain.

to 200 beats per minute) is undesirable, because ventricular filling and myocardial perfusion time are shortened. Decreased ventricular filling and myocardial perfusion, in turn, may produce a *fall* in cardiac output.[1,18,19]

Stroke Volume

The stroke volume in pediatric patients is very small, and relatively small changes in stroke volume can have a significant impact on cardiac output. Stroke volume, in turn, is influenced by ventricular preload, contractility, and afterload. (See Chapters 10 and 20 for a discussion of the clinical application of these principles, as well as special considerations that are related to patients with heart disease.)

Preload

The term *preload* refers to the presystolic stretch of ventricular muscle fibers as influenced by ventricular end-diastolic volume (also termed *filling volume*). Ventricular end-diastolic volume, in turn, is determined by venous return and circulating blood volume. As ventricular filling volume increases, stroke volume increases; as filling volume decreases, stroke volume decreases.

The Frank-Starling law of the heart describes the curvilinear relationship between the ventricular end-diastolic myocardial fiber length and the stroke volume (Figure 19-3). To a point, an increase in the ventricular end-diastolic myocardial fiber *length* (as a result of an increase in end-diastolic volume) produces an increase in stroke volume and cardiac output. Measurement of ventricular myocardial fiber length is not feasible in the clinical setting, and measure-

ment of ventricular end-diastolic volume is limited in its clinical application. However, when heart function is normal, there is good correlation between ventricular end-diastolic volume and pressure. Therefore ventricular end-diastolic pressure is evaluated and is manipulated through fluid administration to optimize cardiac output.

Ventricular end-diastolic pressure can be measured directly or indirectly. Direct measurement involves placement of a catheter in the right or left ventricle, such as occurs in the cardiac catheterization laboratory. Indirect measurement is performed at the bedside and entails evaluation of right atrial or central venous pressure (right ventricular preload) and left atrial or pulmonary artery wedge pressure (left ventricular preload).

Bedside Measurement of Right Ventricular Preload. Right atrial pressure, which may be measured from the proximal port of a pulmonary artery catheter, is equal to right ventricular end-diastolic pressure (RVEDP) in the absence of tricuspid valve disease. The central venous pressure (CVP), measured via a catheter placed in the superior vena cava, may also be employed to estimate right atrial pressure (and RVEDP), provided there is no obstruction to central venous return, such as that associated with superior vena caval syndrome, tension pneumothorax, or mechanical ventilation using high mean airway pressures. To minimize the effects of positive pressure ventilation on measured right atrial or central venous pressure during mechanical ventilation, the right atrial or CVP pressure measurements should be obtained during end-expiration.

Bedside Measurement of Left Ventricular Preload. Left atrial pressure is equal to the left ventricular end-diastolic pressure (LVEDP) in the absence of mitral valve disease. The pulmonary artery wedge pressure (PWP) approximates the left atrial pressure and, in turn, the LVEDP if there is an unobstructed column or channel of blood from the wedged catheter tip in the pulmonary artery to the left ventricle. Several factors, such as obstruction to blood flow within the cardiopulmonary circulation (e.g., by mechanical ventilatory assistance using high airway pressures or mitral valve defects) and poor dynamic response characteristics of the monitoring system, may cause the measured PWP to correlate poorly with either left atrial or left ventricular filling pressure. These factors must be considered when evaluating hemodynamic measurements (see Chapters 6 and 10).

Use of Central Venous Pressure to Evaluate Left Ventricular Filling

The central venous pressure will reflect right ventricular filling pressure (as a guide to fluid therapy) in the

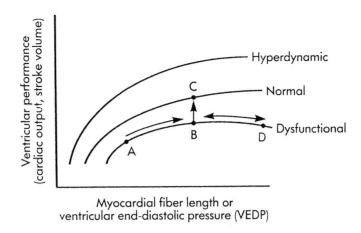

FIGURE 19-3 Frank-Starling curve. In the laboratory description of the Frank-Starling Law (using *isolated normal myocardial fibers*), an increase in the end-diastolic myocardial fiber length increased the tension generated by the myocardial fiber. In the clinical setting, measurement of end-diastolic fiber length is impossible. Therefore the *ventricular end-diastolic pressure* (VEDP), which is a reasonably close correlate in normal hearts, is increased to produce improvement in stroke volume or cardiac output. To a point, an increase in VEDP will produce an improvement in cardiac output *(A → B)*; this increase in VEDP is accomplished through judicious titration of intravenous fluid. The clinician must also recognize that a family of myocardial function curves exists; the patient's myocardial function may be characterized as normal, dysfunctional, or hyperdynamic. If the myocardium is dysfunctional, it generally requires a higher VEDP than the normal myocardium to maximize cardiac output. In addition, excessive volume administration can produce a decrease in cardiac output and myocardial performance if the ventricle is dysfunctional *(B → D)*. In this case, administration of a diuretic or vasodilator may improve cardiac output *(D → B)*. Correction of acid-base imbalances, reduction in afterload, or administration of inotropic medications may improve myocardial function so that cardiac output increases without need for further increase in VEDP *(B → C)*. If the patient's myocardial function is hyperdynamic, cardiac output will be high even at relatively low VEDP. (Reproduced with permission from Hazinski MF: Cardiovascular disorders. In Hazinski MF, editor: *Nursing care of the critically ill child,* ed 2, St Louis, 1992, Mosby. All rights reserved.)

absence of tricuspid stenosis. If right and left ventricular functions and pulmonary and systemic vascular resistances are normal, right and left ventricular end-diastolic pressures may correlate, so the right ventricular end-diastolic pressure (central venous pressure) may approximate the left ventricular end-diastolic pressure. However, *this correlation becomes invalid and unpredictable in patients with cardiopulmonary disease.* For example, a child with severe pulmonary hypertension and right ventricular failure may have a high right ventricular end-diastolic pressure and CVP measurement, while simultaneously the measured PWP may be normal or low, because left ventricular function is normal.

The CVP or right atrial pressure therefore cannot be reliably used to estimate left ventricular end-diastolic pressure in patients with known or suspected cardiopulmonary disease. In such patients, insertion of a pulmonary artery catheter should be considered when accurate evaluation of LVEDP becomes diagnostically or therapeutically necessary.

Effects of Cardiac Dysfunction and Altered Ventricular Compliance on the Starling Curve

Volume administration and augmentation of preload improve stroke volume. Normally, relatively small increases in ventricular end-diastolic filling produce marked increases in stroke volume (the steep, ascending portion of the Starling curve). However, patients with ventricular dysfunction have a blunted stroke volume response to volume loading. In addition, the relationship of ventricular filling volume and ventricular filling pressure to changes in stroke volume are not consistent *between* patients and are not the same over time in the *same* patient, because these relationships are affected by ventricular compliance. The term *ventricular compliance* refers to the distensibility of the ventricle. *Ventricular compliance* is defined as the change in ventricular filling *pressure* that occurs in response to a change in ventricular filling *volume*.[20] For example, if a patient's ventricle is extremely compliant (distensible), a large increase in ventricular end-diastolic volume will be tolerated before end-diastolic pressure increases. In such a patient, a fluid challenge produces minimal changes in measured ventricular filling pressure, although stroke volume may increase significantly. Vasodilator agents tend to increase ventricular compliance, which, in turn, results in a relatively low filling pressure despite a relatively high ventricular filling volume and improvement in stroke volume.

In comparison, if a child has a noncompliant "stiff" ventricle (such as a hypertrophic ventricle), even small increases in ventricular end-diastolic volume (such as those produced by volume administration or heart failure) may produce significant increases in ventricular end-diastolic pressure. High filling pressure, in turn, may be associated with complications such as pulmonary edema and elevated systemic venous pressures (right ventricle) and dependent edema. In such a patient, the increase in stroke volume produced by the increase in ventricular end-diastolic volume may be minimal.

The myocardium of neonates is less compliant than the myocardium of older children and adults, and ventricular end-diastolic pressure is higher in neonates, even at rest. In addition, ventricular end-diastolic pressure may rise more sharply in neonates during volume administration.[16] Myocardial dysfunction and disease may be associated with a further reduction in ventricular compliance. These differences do not mean that neonates are incapable of increasing stroke volume in response to volume administration. Because the compliance of the neonatal ventricle is low, higher ventricular filling pressure may be required to maximize stroke volume and cardiac output in neonates than the filling pressure required to maximize stroke volume and cardiac output the normal pediatric or adult patient.[21] (Box 20-1, Chapter 20, lists causes of increased and decreased ventricular compliance.) It is commonly accepted that a hypertrophic or failing ventricle requires a higher "filling pressure" than the normal ventricle to maximize stroke volume. However, the data supporting this concept in the treatment of adult or pediatric shock are limited.[22-24] A single study of hypovolemic and septic *adult* patients documented significant improvement in stroke volume and cardiac output when left ventricular filling pressure was increased (using volume challenges) from less than 5 to 8 mm Hg to 10 to 12 mm Hg. Little improvement was reported, however, when the LVEDP was increased beyond 12 mm Hg.[23]

Because children with sepsis may demonstrate extensive third-space fluid shifts and evaporative losses caused by fever, they frequently require aggressive volume resuscitation to maintain optimal levels of preload and cardiac output. As much as 60 ml/kg of fluids may be required during the first hour of therapy for children with sepsis.[25] In these patients, the development of pulmonary edema should be anticipated and preparations made to support ventilation. *Do not withhold fluid administration from a patient with septic shock* because pulmonary edema develops—patients with septic shock require volume administration to support cardiac output.

Regardless of patient age, titration of fluid administration to optimize stroke volume and cardiac output must always be individualized, and clinical and hemodynamic responses to therapy must be evaluated frequently. Fluid administration is appropriate if it produces clinical or physiologic improvement. Fluid administration that is not needed and is not associated with clinical improvement may be inappropriate and may predispose the patient to complications such as pulmonary edema.

Construction of Ventricular Function Curves

To determine the optimal ventricular filling pressure of either ventricle for any patient, serial preload measurements can be charted against calculated cardiac output, stroke volume, or stroke work index to construct myocardial function curves for each patient (see Chapter 10, section on construction of ventricular function curves). This enables evaluation of responses to therapy. Optimal ventricular filling pressures may change from hour to hour or day to day if the patient's ventricular compliance and function change.

Contractility

Contractility refers to the efficiency of myocardial fiber shortening regardless of preload and afterload. Although the myocardium of neonates contains less contractile elements and higher water content than does the myocardium of adults,[16] the contractility of the infant myocardium compares favorably with that of adults. In fact, infants have a *higher* ejection fraction than adults.[26] Ventricular contractility may be *depressed* by infection, hypoxia, electrolyte or acid-base imbalance, drug toxicity, or congenital heart disease. Contractility may be *improved* by correction of these factors or administration of inotropic agents.

Although construction of ventricular function curves from hemodynamic measurements provides one means of evaluating contractility, the most reliable method of evaluating ventricular contractility at the bedside is through echocardiographic evaluation of the left ventricular shortening fraction (LVSF) using the following formula:[27]

$$LVSF = \frac{LV \text{ end-diastolic dimension } - \text{ LV end-systolic dimension}}{LV \text{ end-systolic dimension}} \times 100$$

The normal shortening fraction in children is approximately 28% to 44%, and a reduction in shortening fraction indicates decreased ventricular contractility.[27]

Afterload

The term *afterload* refers to the impedance to ventricular ejection or the sum of all forces opposing ventricular emptying. In other words, afterload is equivalent to the sum of all stresses placed on the ventricle (the ventricular wall) during systole.[1,16,20,28]

Afterload is determined primarily by the impedance to ejection determined by pulmonary artery and aortic diastolic pressures, as well as pulmonary and systemic vascular resistance. Because pulmonary and systemic vascular resistance cannot be measured directly, they must be calculated using the inflow minus outflow pressure of each circulation divided by the calculated cardiac output (see Tables 19-1 and 19-3). The calculated measurements should be regarded as merely estimates rather than precise indices of vascular resistance.

Because afterload is equivalent to *ventricular wall stress*,[1,16,20,28] it is also affected by the diameter of the ventricular cavity, the thickness of the ventricular wall, the ventricular intracavity pressure at end-diastole, and any outflow obstruction such as aortic stenosis.

Maturational Changes in Stroke Volume

Initial studies of isolated and nonhuman myocardium suggested that infants cannot increase stroke volume in response to volume administration.[16] However, more recent studies have demonstrated that the neonate's stroke volume *can* increase in response to fluid (volume) administration, provided that ventricular function is good and ventricular afterload is appropriate.[29] If a severe or acute increase in afterload develops, however, stroke volume and cardiac output decrease, particularly in a patient with underlying ventricular dysfunction.

CLINICALLY RELEVANT DIFFERENCES BETWEEN CHILDREN AND ADULTS

There are differences between cardiovascular function in children and adults. These differences affect interpretation of hemodynamic data, as well as management of invasive hemodynamic monitoring devices.

Circulatory Differences

Heart Rate

The resting heart rates of infants and children are greater than those of adults (see Table 19-4). Heart rate is an important measurement in unstable pediatric patients,

and bradycardia is a significant, ominous premonitory finding. Whereas ectopic or reentrant ventricular tachyarrhythmias are common terminal cardiac rhythms in adults, bradycardia is the most common terminal cardiac rhythm in children. Bradycardia typically indicates patient deterioration due to severe hypoxia or cardiorespiratory failure.[1,18,30-34] Persistent or profound bradycardia also may *precipitate* cardiovascular collapse, because a child's stroke volume does not usually increase commensurately with significant decreases in heart rate.[3,15] Sinus tachycardia in infants and children is often a nonspecific sign of distress and may have a variety of causes, such as fever, pain, or cardiorespiratory compromise.

Another significant arrhythmia observed in children is *supraventricular tachycardia*.[1,18] Clinically significant *ventricular* arrhythmias are unusual in children without structural heart disease, electrolyte imbalance, or myocarditis, and they are extremely rare in neonates.[1,18,32-34] Ventricular arrhythmias do, however, occur in children with complex congenital heart disease. In fact, ventricular tachycardia and fibrillation may occur as terminal rhythms in this group of patients.[35] Malignant ventricular arrhythmias also develop in asphyxiated patients, including submersion victims or patients with myocarditis.

A child's heart rate should always be evaluated in light of the clinical condition and sleep-awake state (see Table 19-4). *Normal vital signs are not always appropriate vital signs in critically ill children*.[1,19] A heart rate greater than that anticipated for the child's age *should* be present if the child has cardiorespiratory distress, and the presence of a "normal" heart rate in such a child is inappropriate. As mentioned, the presence of bradycardia in a critically ill child is usually an ominous sign and often indicates that cardiorespiratory arrest is imminent.[1,19]

Cardiac Output, Oxygen Delivery, and Consumption—Pediatric Differences

The cardiac output of children is higher per kilogram of body weight than that of adults, and cardiac index (3.0 to 4.5 $L/min/m^2$ body surface area) typically is slightly higher than that of an adult.[15] The high cardiac output yields a higher oxygen delivery in children than in adults, even when normalized to body surface area.[4,19] Children require a higher cardiac output and oxygen delivery because the metabolic rate and oxygen demands of children are higher than those of adults. Because pediatric oxygen delivery is at near-maximal levels (and oxygen demand is high), infants and children have little oxygen reserve; therefore any compromise in oxygen delivery or increase in oxygen demand may result in tissue hypoxia.

The absolute cardiac output of children, however, is smaller than that of adults. Small changes in calculated cardiac output may therefore be clinically significant. In addition, because heart rate is rapid and stroke volume is small, relatively small decreases in heart rate or stroke volume may be associated with significant decreases in cardiac output.

Circulating Blood Volume

The circulating blood volume of infants and children is higher per kilogram of body weight than that of adults, and total body water is a greater percent of body weight.[4,15] The absolute circulating blood volume of children, however, is smaller than the circulating blood volume of adults, and thus even a small quantity of blood lost or drawn for laboratory analysis may be clinically significant.[19] Total blood volume should be estimated at approximately 80 ml/kg for infants and 75 ml/kg for children.[19] In addition, the quantity of all blood lost or drawn for laboratory analysis should be totaled and calculated as a percent of that volume so that the significance of blood loss can be determined specific to the child's age and size.

Fluid Requirements

Because metabolic rate is more rapid and the surface area-to-volume ratio of children is greater than that in adults,[19] the insensible, evaporative, and metabolic fluid requirements of pediatric patients are higher *per kilogram body of weight.* However, the absolute fluid requirements are small compared with those of adults because the weight of children is less than that of adults. For this reason, the rate of intravenous fluid administration must be strictly controlled in children to avoid inadvertent fluid overload. Fluids used to flush monitoring lines also must be carefully measured and regulated. Typically, the total volume of fluid used to flush monitoring lines should be minimized so that therapeutic nutritional and electrolyte requirements can be met without risk of fluid overload.

Monitoring Differences

Vascular Catheterization

Small catheters must be used to establish vascular access and invasive monitoring in very young patients. These small catheters may be difficult to insert and may easily become obstructed by clots or small kinks. Therefore, whenever catheters are inserted, they must be firmly taped and scrupulously maintained.

Correlation of Physical Assessment Findings and Hemodynamic Measurements

Clinical and hemodynamic signs of deterioration in children may be subtle, and *shock may be present long before the blood pressure falls.*[1,18,19,36] Initially, pediatric patients in shock may simply demonstrate a change in responsiveness, mottled color, and nonspecific signs of distress, including tachycardia and tachypnea.[1,19] However, once the blood pressure does fall, decompensated shock is present and cardiopulmonary arrest is usually imminent.[18,19,33]

The clinical examination of pediatric patients is always more important than any single hemodynamic measurement.[37] Hemodynamic measurements will be useful in the evaluation of patient *trends* over time and in responses to therapy. It is therefore imperative that all measurements be obtained using *exactly the same technique by every member of the health care team.* Consistency ensures that errors are eliminated or standardized so that trends can be evaluated.[37]

Psychosocial Differences

Children are often unable to comprehend the reason for the institution of invasive monitoring and may be unable to cooperate with the maintenance or insertion of noninvasive or invasive devices. As a result, nurses must be prepared to remain at the bedside to support the child and to maintain the catheter position and protect the integrity of equipment. Catheters can be quickly dislodged when the patient moves, and tubing connections may come apart unless the catheters and supporting tubing are taped securely. All connections should be secured using Luer-Lok connections and should be visible on top of bedclothes so that loose connections are prevented or quickly detected.

Psychologic preparation for catheter insertion or monitoring must be accomplished at a level appropriate to the child's degree of distress and his or her cognitive and psychosocial level of development. Teaching, preparation, and support also must be provided for the family, who, in turn, will provide valuable emotional comfort for the patient. Although the parents may be asked to comfort the child during a procedure, family members should not be asked to restrain their child or otherwise assist with a painful procedure.

CLINICAL ASSESSMENT OF HEMODYNAMIC COMPETENCY IN PEDIATRIC PATIENTS

Evaluation of the effectiveness of systemic perfusion is essential, particularly in critically ill or injured pediatric patients. Evaluation of the child's general appearance and assessment of intravascular volume and systemic perfusion are presented here.

General Appearance

Infants and children generally "look good" if the color of the mucous membranes and nailbeds is pink and the

TABLE 19-5
Assessment of the Child: "Looks Good" Versus "Looks Bad"

Responsiveness	"Looks Good"	"Looks Bad"
Color	Pink mucous membranes Color consistent over trunk, extremities	Pallor Mottled color
Skin perfusion	Warm Brisk capillary refill	Cold (peripheral to proximal cooling) Sluggish capillary refill
Activity	Age appropriate (may be frightened, unhappy, unwilling to be separated from parents) Will engage in play	Fretful, then lethargic Will not play
Responsiveness	Age appropriate	Irritable (early), then lethargic; decreased response to painful stimulus is worrisome
Infant feeding	Eats well Demonstrates strong suck	Weak suck Tires during feeding May develop respiratory distress during feedings

From Hazinski MF: Postoperative care of the critically ill child, *Crit Care Nurs Clin North Am* 2:599, 1990.

color of the trunk and extremities is consistent and if the child is appropriately responsive to the environment (Table 19-5).[38,39] Hypoxemia and poor perfusion often produce a mottled appearance to the skin long before cyanosis is observed. Peripheral cyanosis (diffuse bluish discoloration while the conjunctiva and mucous membranes under the tongue remain pink) or pallor may indicate circulatory failure; the patient's skin may also be cool or cold. Central cyanosis (the diffuse bluish discoloration that is observed in the lips and under the tongue and in the conjunctiva) is observed in children with unrepaired cyanotic congenital heart disease or in those with profound hypoxemia due to pulmonary disease. The patient's skin is usually warm.[38]

The child's level of responsiveness reflects the effectiveness of cerebral oxygenation and perfusion. A healthy, stable child will respond in an age-appropriate way to parents and to clinicians during therapeutic interventions. For example, young infants should be oriented to faces and brightly colored objects and should readily make eye contact with parents. Older infants should protest vigorously when the parents depart or when a stranger approaches. Toddlers should be reluctant to lie down and should vigorously resist handling by strangers. Preschool children should be curious about hospital equipment and procedures but apprehensive about painful procedures. School-age children and adolescents typically can discuss specific signs and symptoms and locate pain and should be expected to be self-conscious during examinations. Each child should be approached in a manner appropriate to that child's level of

psychosocial development and stress, and the privacy and sensitivity of each child must be respected.[1,19]

The effects of hypoxemia or inadequate systemic perfusion (such as decompensated shock) on the central nervous system may cause the child to become irritable or lethargic. The child's level of consciousness must always be evaluated in light of age, psychosocial maturity, and clinical condition. *If a previously alert child does not respond to a painful stimulus, severe cardiorespiratory or neurologic deterioration should be suspected.* The patient should be immediately and thoroughly evaluated and appropriate therapy instituted.[1,19,38]

Clinical Assessment of Intravascular Volume

As in adults, the intravascular volume of pediatric patients must be adequate relative to the size of the vascular space. Intravascular volume is certainly diminished in patients with sudden, massive hemorrhage, but patients receiving systemic vasodilator therapy may be relatively hypovolemic, although blood volume and total body water are normal. Classic signs of inadequate intravascular volume relative to the vascular space include tachycardia, low central venous pressure, and inadequate systemic perfusion. The heart size is often small on chest radiograph. The patients are oliguric. The urine specific gravity is typically high and urine sodium low.

Evidence of *dehydration* (due to protracted vomiting, diarrhea, excessive sweating not accompanied by fluid replacement) also may be associated with inadequate intravascular volume. Signs of dehydration include a sunken fontanelle in infants less than 16 to 18 months of age, poor skin turgor (skin remains "tented" after it is pinched into a fold), and dry mucous membranes. Salivary bubbles, which are normally present under the tongue, are not observed, and tearing may not be present when the infant cries. These signs of dehydration will usually *not* be present or be observed in patients with acute blood loss or vasodilator reactions.

Intravascular volume may be inadequate despite the presence of systemic or pulmonary edema. Edema despite hypovolemia or normovolemia is caused by increased capillary permeability or low serum protein concentrations rather than by increased systemic and pulmonary venous pressures. Such edema classically occurs in patients with sepsis and the systemic inflammatory response syndrome (SIRS). Both are characterized by a generalized systemic and pulmonary capillary leak.

If the child is in heart failure, intravascular volume may still be inadequate, normal, or high. It is difficult to determine the need for volume resuscitation in these patients or in any patients with significant differences between right and left ventricular filling pressures due to failure of one ventricle. In these patients, it may be necessary to maintain the end-diastolic pressure of the diseased ventricle at a level somewhat higher than normal to optimize cardiac output.

Assessment of Systemic Perfusion

Cardiovascular deterioration may result from intrinsic cardiovascular disease (usually congenital defects or myocarditis) or from extracardiac causes, such as hypovolemia or sepsis. Risk factors for circulatory failure should be identified, and high-risk patients should be frequently and carefully assessed. Routine assessment of systemic perfusion should be performed on a regular basis throughout any patient's hospitalization.

Noninvasive or invasive hemodynamic monitoring devices are used to obtain measurements or calculations that indicate or confirm *trends* in circulatory function. However, hemodynamic measurements always must be evaluated in conjunction with serial physical assessment findings. *Heart rate, blood pressure, and calculated cardiac output should also be evaluated in terms of the effectiveness of systemic perfusion and oxygen delivery.*[24] It is less important to know if the cardiac output is "normal" or "high" or "low" than if it is *adequate* or *inadequate* to maintain effective systemic perfusion for each patient.[28]

Clinical evaluation of systemic perfusion requires assessment of the child's general appearance and level of responsiveness, as well as evaluation of organ function. Evaluation of organ function is presented followed by

clinical descriptions of pediatric patients with systemic hypoperfusion due to heart failure or shock syndromes.

Evaluation of Organ Function as an Index of Systemic Perfusion

When cardiac output is inadequate, blood flow is often diverted from nonessential organ systems (such as the skin, kidney, and gut) to the heart and brain. This redistribution of blood flow is typically observed with hypovolemic and cardiogenic shock. The severity of organ dysfunction generally reflects the severity of perfusion failure in the organ systems.

Skin. Skin color, capillary refill, temperature, and strength of peripheral pulses can provide information about the adequacy of systemic perfusion.

Capillary refill time should be virtually instantaneous in healthy patients in a warm environment.[1] Perfusion failure usually results in prolonged capillary refill time (longer than 3 to 4 seconds). However, an infant or a child in a cold environment can have a prolonged capillary refill time and peripheral cyanosis even if circulatory function is normal.[1,18,39,40] Shock associated with redistribution of blood flow from the skin will produce cooling of the skin of the extremities in a peripheral-to-proximal direction. The fingers and toes will be cool; if shock progresses, the hands and feet and then lower arms and legs will be cool to the touch. As cardiac output falls, the distal pulses may become difficult to palpate, although central pulses generally will be maintained until circulatory collapse (decompensated shock) develops.[1,18]

Skin blood flow may not consistently correlate with effectiveness of systemic perfusion or cardiac output. For example, patients with heart failure and hypovolemic and cardiogenic shock characteristically demonstrate signs of decreased blood flow to the skin and other nonvital tissue. In contrast, patients with septic, neurogenic, and anaphylactic shock may have warm skin, brisk capillary refill, and bounding pulses despite inadequate blood flow to major organ systems because of a "maldistribution" of cardiac output.[41,42]

Kidneys. Inadequate cardiac output results in a reduction in renal perfusion, glomerular filtration rate, and urine output. When hydration and fluid intake and cardiac output are adequate, normal urine output averages 2 ml/kg/hr in the infant, 1 ml/kg/hr in the child, and 0.5 ml/kg/hr in the adolescent. A urine volume of less than 0.5 to 1.0 ml/kg/hr despite normovolemia and adequate fluid intake in a child with normal renal function may indicate renal hypoperfusion.[1,18,19]

Gut. Poor systemic perfusion results in impaired gastrointestinal perfusion and, as a result, gastrointestinal dysfunction. Decreased gastrointestinal motility, malabsorption of foodstuffs, or paralytic ileus may be observed. Feeding intolerance may be noted in infants; an increase in gastric residuals may be noted in patients receiving gastric tube feedings. Hepatic ischemia may be indicated by a rise in liver enzymes and may occasionally be associated with mild jaundice.

Metabolism. Significant systemic hypoperfusion results in anaerobic metabolism and generation of lactic acid. Uncompensated metabolic acidosis will produce a fall in the arterial pH and a significant base deficit (below -2). The serum lactate level (normally approximately 1 to 2 mmol/L) will rise in the presence of shock. The serum lactate level also rises, and metabolic acidosis develops in patients with seizures and hypermetabolic conditions, such as malignant hyperthermia. However, the rise is *transient* and the serum pH should rapidly return to normal when the underlying condition has been corrected. By comparison, the elevation in serum lactate level and metabolic acidosis is more severe and persistent in cases of shock that are refractory to therapy.[43]

Central Nervous System. When systemic perfusion is significantly compromised, neurologic deterioration is apparent. An infant or a child initially becomes irritable or fretful. An infant usually fails to make eye contact, and a young child may cry or whimper. On further deterioration, lethargy and decreased responsiveness become apparent. When systemic perfusion is severely compromised, the patient responds only to painful stimuli and ultimately may fail to respond to any stimuli. The development of coma in a shock patient is an absolute medical emergency. Aggressive corrective therapy is required.

Assessment of Pediatric Patients at Risk for Shock

In children of all ages, shock may be present despite the presence of a "normal" blood pressure. *Hypotension is a late sign of shock that reflects cardiovascular collapse and indicates that cardiorespiratory arrest may be imminent.* The presence of a "normal" blood pressure therefore does not rule out the presence of shock. If there is probable cause for shock; if other signs of major organ dysfunction are present (e.g., if the level of consciousness deteriorates, if the skin is pale and cool, if the urine output is reduced); or if lactic acidosis is evident on blood gas analysis, the patient should be considered to be in shock.[24]

Compensated (Early) Shock

Compensated shock is present when signs of inadequate organ perfusion, organ dysfunction, and lactic acidosis are present despite normotension. The patient should be tachycardic, but urine output may be low. Therefore children with risk factors for shock, such as severe dehydration, trauma, ventricular dysfunction, or overwhelming sepsis, should be vigilantly assessed and monitored for the subtle signs of shock (e.g., cool hands and feet, skin color changes, mental changes, and possible decreased urine flow rates).

Decompensated (Late) Shock

Decompensated shock occurs when hypotension develops in a child with signs of inadequate systemic perfusion, organ dysfunction, and lactic acidosis. The fall in blood pressure indicates that compensatory mechanisms such as vasoconstriction and redistribution of blood flow have been exhausted and all major organ systems are significantly underperfused. Rapid and perhaps irreversible organ failure follows.

The clinical and hemodynamic manifestations of shock patients may differ considerably depending on whether the cause of shock is characterized by high cardiac output and low SVR or low cardiac output and high SVR.

Clinical Signs of Shock Associated with Low Cardiac Output and High Systemic Vascular Resistance

Signs of *hypovolemic* or *cardiogenic shock* in children are similar to those in adults and include irritability or lethargy, tachycardia, tachypnea, cool skin with prolonged capillary refill despite a warm environment, diminished intensity of peripheral pulses or absent peripheral pulses, oliguria, and lactic acidosis. The development of bradycardia or hypotension indicates the presence of cardiovascular collapse.[1,18,19,24,36]

Clinical Signs of Shock Associated with Normal or High Cardiac Output and Low Systemic Vascular Resistance

Sepsis, spinal cord injury or transection, and anaphylaxis may result in the development of shock characterized by massive vasodilator reaction, maldistribution of blood flow, and normal or even increased cardiac output. See Chapter 16 for descriptions of the pathophysiology, hemodynamics, and clinical presentation of these shock syndromes, which are similar for pediatric and adult patients. Because sepsis, SIRS, and septic shock so commonly complicate the course of critically ill and injured patients, these are briefly described here. See Chapter 17 for an expanded description of SIRS.

Sepsis and SIRS are characterized by "hyperdynamic" cardiovascular function.[39,41,42] The child is tachycardic with high cardiac output, low SVR, and possible increased cutaneous blood flow. The skin is often warm with brisk capillary refill and may have a plethoric appearance. Peripheral pulses are usually bounding. Septic patients require a cardiac output that is higher than normal, because the blood flow is maldistributed through the inappropriately dilated systemic circulation.

Flow in excess of need is present in some tissues, whereas other tissues have flow less than that needed and may be ischemic. Thus laboratory studies may demonstrate lactic acidosis despite a normal or high cardiac output. In fact, the cardiac output may double "normal" values but may still be *inadequate* to maintain perfusion and oxygen delivery to some organ systems, such as the gut.

Septic shock is present when a child with sepsis develops signs of organ dysfunction. These include lactic acidosis, acute alteration in mental status, oliguria, and possibly hypotension. Septic shock is also present despite a "normal" blood pressure if aggressive volume infusion and vasopressors are required to maintain the blood pressure.[41,42] Approximately 90% of adults and children with septic shock have higher than "normal" cardiac output, even when hypotension and lactic acidosis are present. However, late in the septic course, cardiac output may fall to normal or subnormal levels in a small number of patients (10%), thus giving rise to a "hypodynamic" circulation.

Assessment of Pediatric Patients at Risk for Congestive Heart Failure

A reduction in stroke volume is the fundamental defect in heart failure not due to bradyarrhythmias or arteriovenous malformations. The decrease in stroke volume is typically compensated by the increase in heart rate, constriction of the blood vessels that perfuse nonvital organs (which redistributes the available cardiac output to the heart and brain), and retention of salt and water by the kidneys to augment venous return and preload. Generally, pediatric patients with congestive heart failure develop some degree of biventricular failure with evidence of elevated systemic or pulmonary venous pressures. Consistent signs of heart failure include the signs of adrenergic stimulation (Box 19-1).

Signs of adrenergic stimulation include tachycardia, peripheral vasoconstriction (with redistribution of blood flow), decreased urine output, and diaphoresis. The diaphoresis is most easily observed on the head of the infant and is usually worse during feeding or sleep.

Children with congestive heart failure (CHF) and a high central venous pressure frequently have hepatomegaly and periorbital edema. However, ascites is rarely observed in children unless the central venous pressure is extremely high or the serum albumin concentration is extremely low. Jugular venous distention is virtually impossible to appreciate in infants, because their necks are usually very short and fat. As a result, jugular venous distention cannot be effectively evaluated in infants and young children with CHF.[28]

High pulmonary venous pressure measured as PWP exceeding 20 to 25 mm Hg results in pulmonary edema and, as a consequence, tachypnea and increased work of breathing. Crackles and wheezes (formerly called rales or rhonchi), which signify pulmonary edema, are often *not* appreciated in pediatric patients, because lung edema fluid is cleared rapidly by the lymphatics when children become tachypneic. More important, children in pulmonary edema tend to breathe shallowly, and thus adventitial sounds may not be audible.

If pulmonary edema develops when a child is receiving mechanical ventilatory support, the increased work of breathing that typically develops cannot be readily assessed, particularly if the child is being maintained on controlled ventilation. Calculated lung compliance, however, decreases. If a volume-cycled ventilator (MA-1, Bear 2) is used, the decrease in lung compliance will be apparent when the peak inspiratory pressure increases despite a constant tidal volume. If a pressure-cycled ventilator (Bennett PR2) is used, the pressure limit will be reached at a smaller tidal volume and an inadequate alveolar ventilation may result. The audible alarm indicating inadequate inspiratory flow may be activated.

Pulmonary edema increases the fraction of intrapulmonary shunt. The increase in the number of perfused but nonaerated alveoli, in turn, results in hypoxemia unless

---

BOX 19-1

Signs of Congestive Heart Failure in the Infant or Child

Signs of adrenergic stimulation
  Tachycardia
  Tachypnea
  Peripheral vasoconstriction
  Oliguria (urine output less than 1 to 2 ml/kg/hr despite adequate intake)
  Diaphoresis
Signs of systemic venous congestion
  Hepatomegaly
  Periorbital edema
  Ascites (rare)
Signs of pulmonary venous congestion
  Tachypnea
  Increased work of breathing (retractions, nasal flaring)
  Possible crackles (may be impossible to hear)

the inspired oxygen concentration is increased and positive end-expiratory pressure (PEEP) is applied.[28]

CONGENITAL HEART DISEASE

Congenital heart disease is a common cause for prolonged hospitalization of neonates and for their later readmission. Here, an overview of the major forms of congenital heart disease is followed by a discussion of pulmonary hypertension, which may or may not coexist with congenital deformation of the heart.

Intracardiac Pressures and Saturations in Patients with Congenital Heart Disease

In normal patients, systemic blood and pulmonary venous blood are completely separated in the heart. Systemic arterial oxygen saturation is 97% to 100%, whereas systemic venous oxygen saturation is approximately 60% to 80%.

Congenital heart disease may be characterized by intracardiac shunting of blood, which results in abnormalities in the oxygen saturation of the blood in the right or left heart chambers, as well as in flow abnormalities within the pulmonary circulation. For example, right heart oxygen saturation levels are elevated in patients with left-to-right intracardiac shunts, such as an atrial or a ventricular septal defect or an anomalous pulmonary venous return, and pulmonary blood flow is increased. In comparison, left heart and systemic arterial oxygen saturations are decreased in patients with right-to-left intracardiac shunts, such as uncorrected tetralogy of Fallot or tricuspid atresia, and pulmonary blood flow may be decreased.

Children with uncorrected cyanotic heart disease (right-to-left shunts) have a risk of spontaneous cerebral thromboembolic event (stroke) because systemic venous blood is allowed to bypass filtration through the pulmonary circulation and flow directly into the systemic arterial and cerebral circulation. *In patients with uncorrected cyanotic congenital heart disease, absolutely no air can be allowed to enter any intravenous line because the air may produce a cerebral air embolus (stroke).*[1,19,24]

The most common congenital heart defects and associated hemodynamic alterations are listed in Table 19-6. Refer to more comprehensive sources for further information.[28]

Text continued on 492

TABLE 19-6
Common Congenital Heart Defects

Six common congenital heart defects are described. The first three—atrial septal defect, ventricular septal defect, and patent ductus arteriosus—are characterized by left-to-right intracardiac shunts. The fourth, tetralogy of Fallot, is a defect characterized by a valvular or subvalvular lesion and right-to-left intracardiac shunt. The fifth, transposition of the great arteries, is characterized by malposition of the great arteries, and the sixth, coarctation of the aorta, is characterized by malformation of the aorta.

Defect: Atrial Septal Defect

	Description and Abnormalities in Blood Flow and Pressure	Abnormalities in Circulatory Oxygen Saturations	Postoperative Hemodynamics
	There is an abnormal opening in the atrial septum through which blood flows from the left atrium to the right. Increased right atrial flow, in turn, results in an increase in blood flow into the right ventricle, pulmonary artery, and increased return to the left atrium. Despite the increased blood flow, pulmonary arterial and right ventricular systolic pressures are normal or only	The left-to-right atrial shunt produces an increase in right heart and pulmonary arterial oxygen saturations.	Normal intracardiac pressures and saturations should be present unless the patient develops secondary pulmonary vascular changes or heart failure. The right ventricle is usually very compliant, and volume administration usually produces minimal change in right heart pressures (right atrial pressure, CVP).

Continued

TABLE 19-6
Common Congenital Heart Defects—cont'd

Defect: Atrial Septal Defect—cont'd

	Description and Abnormalities in Blood Flow and Pressure	Abnormalities in Circulatory Oxygen Saturations	Postoperative Hemodynamics
	slightly elevated unless pulmonary hypertension develops. Systemic blood flow is normal. The defect is generally well tolerated until adult years when secondary pulmonary vascular changes, pulmonary hypertension, and heart failure may develop. However, during childhood the patient may be easily fatigued and somewhat underdeveloped.		

Defect: Ventricular Septal Defect

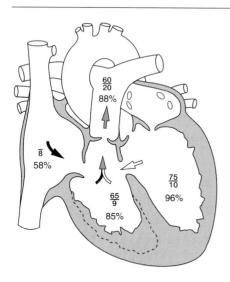

	Description and Abnormalities in Blood Flow and Pressure	Abnormalities in Circulatory Oxygen Saturations	Postoperative Hemodynamics
	A defect in the ventricular septum allows a left-to-right shunt. This, in turn, results in increased flow to the pulmonary circulation and left heart. If the defect is large, there is virtual equalization of ventricular pressures. As a result, the systolic pressures of both ventricles, the aorta, and pulmonary artery are virtually the same. The volume of blood returning to the left atrium is increased. Congestive heart failure results in increased RA/RVEDP and LA/LVEDP. Secondary pulmonary vascular changes are likely to develop over time. Right ventricular	The left-to-right ventricular shunt produces an increase in the oxygen saturations in the right ventricle and pulmonary artery.	The hemodynamic profile may be normal postoperatively. Patients with secondary pulmonary vascular changes may have persistent pulmonary hypertension. If a surgical repair was accomplished through a right ventriculotomy incision, some degree of RV failure should be expected in the immediate postoperative period.

TABLE 19-6
Common Congenital Heart Defects—cont'd

Defect: Ventricular Septal Defect—cont'd

	Description and Abnormalities in Blood Flow and Pressure	Abnormalities in Circulatory Oxygen Saturations	Postoperative Hemodynamics
	failure may eventually develop. If the defect is large (unrestrictive), the amount of blood going into the pulmonary or systemic circulation is determined by the resistance present in each circulation. For example, systemic vasoconstriction or aortic stenosis increases resistance to flow into the systemic circulation and increases the volume of left-to-right shunt. Systemic vasodilation decreases resistance to systemic flow and decreases the volume of left-to-right shunt.		

Defect: Patent Ductus Arteriosus

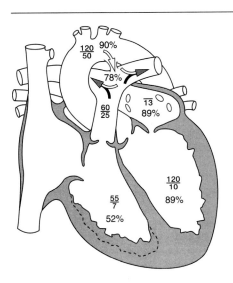

Persistence of this fetal vascular structure allows shunting of oxygenated blood from the aorta directly into the pulmonary artery via the patent ductus. The aortic-to-pulmonary arterial shunt increases the volume of blood flow to the lungs and left heart relative to the size of the patent ductus arteriosus. In patients with a large patent ductus, the aorta and pulmonary artery are essentially the same size, and pulmonary artery systolic pressure is nearly equal to	The aortic-to-pulmonary arterial shunt increases the oxygen saturation within the pulmonary artery. Right ventricular and pulmonary artery pressures increase if the shunt is large and pulmonary hypertension develops.	Most patients have a normal postoperative hemodynamic profile. However, secondary pulmonary vascular changes and pulmonary hypertension may persist postoperatively.

Continued

TABLE 19-6
Common Congenital Heart Defects—cont'd

Defect: Patent Ductus Arteriosus—cont'd

	Description and Abnormalities in Blood Flow and Pressure	Abnormalities in Circulatory Oxygen Saturations	Postoperative Hemodynamics
	aortic systolic pressure. Over time, the pulmonary vasculature responds to the excessive blood flow, with hypertrophic and fibrotic changes. Pulmonary hypertension and pulmonary vascular congestion (due to left ventricular failure caused by flow overload) ensue. The right ventricle eventually becomes overburdened by the pulmonary hypertension and fails. In summary, the child with uncorrected patent ductus arteriosus may eventually develop right ventricular failure because of impedance to ejection and left ventricular failure because of flow overload.		

Defect: Tetralogy of Fallot

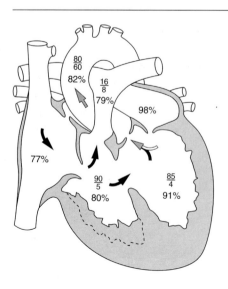

Tetralogy of Fallot is characterized by four intracardiac anomalies: 1. A large ventricular septal defect. 2. Obstruction to right ventricular outflow at the pulmonic valve (pulmonic stenosis) and subvalvular area (termed the infundibulum). 3. A rightwardly deviated aorta. The aorta overrides the ventricular septal defect, which is	The degree of arterial desaturation is related directly to the severity of the right-to-left shunt as influenced by pulmonic outflow tract obstruction. Right ventricular and pulmonary arterial saturations are normal because blood flows from right to left across the septal defect.	If correction of the defect is complete, oxygen saturations and flow patterns within the heart and great vessels will be normal. However, if a right ventriculotomy was required for the correction, some right ventricular failure should be anticipated, as evidenced by increased CVP or right atrial pressures. The right ventricle will also

TABLE 19-6
Common Congenital Heart Defects—cont'd

Defect: Tetralogy of Fallot—cont'd

	Description and Abnormalities in Blood Flow and Pressure	Abnormalities in Circulatory Oxygen Saturations	Postoperative Hemodynamics
	located high in the septum. 4. Right ventricular hypertrophy. The abnormally increased muscularization of the right ventricle is caused by the abnormally high impedance to right ventricular ejection (equal to that of the left ventricle). The primary factor that determines how well patients tolerate this defect is the resistance to right ventricular outflow. If the pulmonic or subpulmonic stenosis is severe, the resistance to right ventricular outflow is high. Deoxygenated right ventricular blood will preferentially shunt into the aorta, and pulmonary blood flow decreases. Because a large volume of desaturated blood enters the aorta, affected children are very cyanotic. Much of pulmonary blood flow may be by way of collateral vessels. On the other hand, if the stenosis to right ventricular outflow is mild, the amount of blood entering the pulmonary artery may be nearly normal, and arterial oxygen		be noncompliant postoperatively. If a large patch is placed over the right ventricular outflow tract and pulmonic valve area, some pulmonic regurgitation and right ventricular failure should be expected postoperatively.

Continued

TABLE 19-6

Common Congenital Heart Defects—cont'd

Defect: Tetrology of Fallot—cont'd

	Description and Abnormalities in Blood Flow and Pressure	Abnormalities in Circulatory Oxygen Saturations	Postoperative Hemodynamics
	saturation may be nearly normal (pink tetralogy of Fallot). Right ventricular outflow obstruction may also be very dynamic. Therefore, some patients may become "blue" only with exertion or hypovolemia.		

Defect: D-Transposition of the Great Arteries

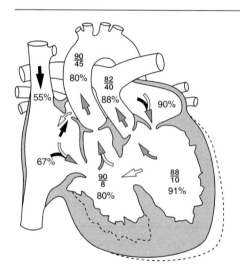

This is a common cyanotic defect that presents in newborns and small infants. The great arteries arise from the incorrect ventricle; the aorta arises from the right ventricles and the pulmonary artery arises from the left ventricle. As a result of the D-transposition, aortic and systemic arterial oxygen saturations are extremely low, whereas richly oxygenated blood continues to recirculate through the left ventricle, the pulmonary artery, and the lungs. The newborn must therefore have a defect between the two circulations, such as an atrial septal defect, a ventricular septal defect, or a patent ductus

As mentioned, a defect that allows mixing of blood between the two circulations must be present for patient survival. Without associated defects, all systemic venous blood would enter the right heart and flow into the aorta; therefore aortic and systemic Pao_2 and oxygen saturations would become intolerably low. At the same time, all pulmonary venous drainage would enter the left heart and then reenter the lungs via the pulmonary artery; pulmonary arterial blood would therefore be maximally saturated.

In patients with D-transposition of the great arteries, the hemodynamics and oxygen saturations depend on the combination of

The individual child's hemodynamics are determined by the type of surgical correction performed. If a complete correction is performed, the child's oxygen saturations should be normalized. If a corrective procedure that redirects blood within the atria (such as the Mustard or Senning operation) is performed, pulmonary and systemic blood oxygenation is normalized but the circulation is still abnormal. For this procedure, the blood flow is diverted within the atria so that pulmonary venous blood is directed toward the right ventricle (which remains the systemic ventricle), and systemic venous blood is directed toward the left ventricle, which continues to serve the pulmonary circulation.

TABLE 19-6
Common Congenital Heart Defects—cont'd

Defect: D-Transposition of the Great Arteries—cont'd

	Description and Abnormalities in Blood Flow and Pressure	Abnormalities in Circulatory Oxygen Saturations	Postoperative Hemodynamics
	arteriosus, to allow arterialized blood to enter the systemic circulation. Otherwise, the newborn will die because of progressive hypoxemia. The right ventricle is the systemic ventricle and its systolic pressure will be equal to the patient's systolic blood pressure. The left ventricular systolic pressure will be equal to pulmonary artery systolic pressure.	defects present, as well as the volume of blood flow through the defects. These factors determine the amount of mixing between the pulmonary and systemic circulations and consequently the degree of arterial desaturation and pulmonary saturation.	As a result, should the child develop ventricular dysfunction, right ventricular failure produces systemic hypoperfusion and pulmonary edema, whereas left ventricular failure results in dilated systemic veins and generalized, dependent edema. If the more common *intraarterial* correction is performed, the great vessels are moved to join their appropriate ventricles. Blood flow pathways are then normalized.

Defect: Coarctation of the Aorta *(Arrow)*

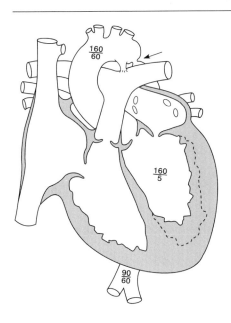

Coarctation of the aorta is a narrowing of the aorta (usually in the vicinity of the ductus arteriosus) that may be mild but is usually severe. The distal aorta usually receives most of its flow by way of collateral vessels, which are typically abundant in older children with uncorrected coarctation. Abnormalities of the aortic valve are present in approximately 80% of cases.
Left ventricular systolic pressure increases to maintain flow through

If the coarctation is present *proximal* to the ductus arteriosus and the ductus remains patent, the descending aorta may be perfused with systemic venous blood from the right ventricle through a patent ductus. In affected patients, right ventricular systolic and diastolic pressures will be elevated and low oxygen saturations will be present in systemic arteries branching from the descending aorta.
If the coarctation is *distal* to the ductus arteriosus, oxygen

Theoretically, postoperative hemodynamics should should be normal, but hypertension may persist into the postoperative period. Occasionally, in small infants, the left subclavian artery is used to reconstruct the resected aortic segment. In these patients, no pulses will be palpable in the left brachial or radial artery postoperatively. The infant's left arm cannot be used for blood pressure monitoring and blood sampling.

Continued

TABLE 19-6
Common Congenital Heart Defects—cont'd

Defect: Coarctation of the Aorta *(Arrow)*—cont'd

	Description and Abnormalities in Blood Flow and Pressure	Abnormalities in Circulatory Oxygen Saturations	Postoperative Hemodynamics
	the partially obstructed aorta. This results in an increase in left ventricular and systemic arterial systolic pressure proximal to the coarctation. (Systolic, as well as diastolic, hypertension is noted in blood pressures obtained from one or both upper extremities.) Distal to the coarctation, the blood pressure is lower than pressure in the upper extremities. The principal intracardiac defect is compensatory left ventricular hypertrophy.	saturations are unaffected by the coarctation.	

Figures redrawn from Watson SP, Watson DC Jr: Anatomy, physiology, and hemodynamics of congenital heart disease. In Ream AK, Fogdall RP, editors: *Acute cardiovascular management and intensive care,* Philadelphia, 1982, JB Lippincott.

CVP, central venous pressure; *LA/LVEDP,* left atrial/left ventricular end-diastolic pressure; *RA/RVEDP,* right atrial/right ventricular end-diastolic pressure; *RV,* right ventricular.

Pulmonary Hypertension

Many forms of congenital heart disease are associated with chronic or episodic hypoxemia, abnormal pulmonary blood flow, or polycythemia. Affected children are vulnerable to the development of pulmonary hypertension. In addition, pulmonary hypertension also may manifest as a primary disease. Significant pulmonary hypertension may result in *cor pulmonale,* right heart failure caused by the increase in pulmonary vascular resistance (see Chapter 18).

Definition

Pulmonary hypertension is defined as a pulmonary artery systolic pressure greater than 25 mm Hg, a diastolic pressure greater than 18 mm Hg, or a mean pulmonary artery pressure greater than 13 mm Hg in infants beyond 1 month of age or children living at sea level. Pulmonary artery hypertension also may be defined by a pulmonary vascular resistance exceeding 10 Wood units or 4 index units in children with normal pulmonary blood flow (see Table 19-1).[44,45]

Causes

There are four major causes of acute and chronic pulmonary hypertension in infants and children: hypoxic vasoconstriction, hypertrophic and fibrotic changes in the pulmonary vascular bed, reduction in the cross-sectional area of the pulmonary vascular bed, and hyperviscosity syndromes.[44-46] Each of these causes is reviewed briefly.

Hypoxic Pulmonary Vasoconstriction. Pulmonary arteries reflexly constrict in response to alveolar hypoxia and may acutely produce pulmonary hypertension or may augment chronic pulmonary hypertension. The chronic type may be the result of chronic lung disease such as bronchopulmonary dysplasia, particularly if adequate supplemental oxygen is not provided. Acutely, low alveolar oxygen tension (alveolar hypoxia) may be produced during suctioning. Alveolar hypoxia may also be the result of hypoventilation caused by diffuse airway disease, depression of the respiratory control centers of the brain, or inadequate ventilatory support (low tidal volume or respiratory rate). Pulmonary arterial constriction also may be induced in lung areas where alveoli are not aerated, such as areas of atelectasis or pneumonia. Respiratory acidosis commonly coexists with and intensifies hypoxic pulmonary vasoconstriction.

Hypertrophic and Fibrotic Changes in the Pulmonary Vascular Bed. This chronic condition is typically the result of congenital heart disease that causes increased pulmonary blood flow. The abnormally increased pulmonary blood flow and pressure, in turn, result in secondary changes in the structure and distribution of the pulmonary vessels.[44]

Not all children with congenital heart disease associated with increased pulmonary blood flow develop pulmonary vascular changes. The rate of development and severity of pulmonary vascular disease cannot always be predicted by the nature and severity of the flow defect. Generally, however, the severity of the pulmonary vascular changes and the pulmonary hypertension is affected by the volume and pressure of increased pulmonary blood flow. Increased pulmonary blood flow that occurs under *high pressure* (such as that caused by a large ventricular septal defect or truncus arteriosus) usually results in structural pulmonary vascular changes within a few months or years. In comparison, increased pulmonary blood flow under *low pressure* (such as that caused by an atrial septal defect) may not result in structural pulmonary vessel changes and pulmonary hypertension for decades. In some patients, pulmonary vascular disease and pulmonary hypertension never develop.

Obstruction to pulmonary venous return also can produce pulmonary vascular disease. This form of pulmonary hypertension typically occurs in an infant with total anomalous pulmonary venous return below the diaphragm. These infants usually develop signs of congestive heart failure and pulmonary edema in the first weeks of life. Hypoxemia for any reason may also obstruct pulmonary venous return by causing pulmonary venoconstriction. Mitral stenosis and hypoplastic left heart syndrome also result in pulmonary venous obstruction.

Patients with cyanotic congenital heart defects associated with decreased pulmonary blood flow may eventually develop secondary pulmonary vascular changes and pulmonary hypertension. One contributing factor is polycythemia, which results in increased blood viscosity and hypercoagulability. Pulmonary hypertension in these patients is thought to be the result of development of pulmonary vascular thromboemboli that obstruct and narrow the pulmonary vascular lumina.[44]

Children with cyanotic congenital heart disease may also have increased pulmonary blood flow (e.g., the child with truncus arteriosus and no pulmonary stenosis). These children may have pulmonary vascular changes caused by both the polycythemia and the increased volume and pressure of pulmonary blood flow.

Reduction in the Cross-Sectional Area of the Pulmonary Vascular Bed. A diminished pulmonary vascular capacity is associated with diaphragm hernia, premature muscularization of the pulmonary vascular bed (so-called persistent pulmonary hypertension of the newborn or persistent fetal circulation), or pulmonary hypoplasia associated with oligohydramnios.[47] Acute reduction in the cross-sectional area of the pulmonary vascular bed and acute pulmonary hypertension also develop in patients with massive pulmonary embolism or massive atelectasis, such as that which occurs in patients with right mainstem bronchus intubation and collapse of the left lung. When normal cardiac output flows through a vascular bed that is small, pulmonary hypertension will be present.

Hyperviscosity of the Blood. Hyperviscosity also may produce pulmonary hypertension. In general, this condition is observed within hours after birth in neonates with a hematocrit value exceeding 55% to 60%.[47]

Therapy

The therapy for pulmonary hypertension is determined by the cause. For example, anatomic lesions that produce abnormalities in pulmonary blood flow or obstruction to pulmonary venous return must be surgically corrected (if possible) or surgically palliated. Until surgical correction or palliation is accomplished, all efforts must be made to prevent or minimize factors known to produce pulmonary vasoconstriction. These factors may exacerbate the underlying pulmonary hypertension, regardless of cause. For example, alveolar hypoxia, acidosis, alveolar distention, hypothermia, and painful stimuli must be avoided.

In unstable patients with severe pulmonary hypertension, controlled mechanical ventilation enables support of oxygenation, as well as maintenance of an alkalotic pH (7.5). In the past, extreme hyperventilation was used to create an alkalotic pH. Currently, significant hypocarbia is avoided because it reduces cerebral blood flow. If hyperventilation is used, only mild hyperventilation is created ($Paco_2$ 32 to 34 mm Hg). An alkalotic pH also may be maintained through administration of small doses of sodium bicarbonate,[7] although the buffering action of the bicarbonate will generate carbon dioxide. This effect, in turn, necessitates an increase in minute ventilation. Inhaled nitric oxide promotes pulmonary vasodilation and may be used as a temporizing measure in patients with severe pulmonary hypertension that is poorly responsive to other measures.[13,14,48-51]

Airway suctioning must be performed carefully and skillfully to prevent alveolar hypoxia. In general, two clinicians are required to suction an unstable infant or child. The first clinician provides supplemental oxygenation before and immediately after each suction attempt and monitors the patient's color, heart rate, and oxygen saturation during the suction attempt. The second clinician suctions quickly but gently. If the child's color, heart rate, or oxygen saturation levels deteriorate during the suctioning effort, it should be discontinued and the child should be ventilated with 100% oxygen until stable.

FLUID-FILLED MONITORING SYSTEMS
Challenges Specific to Pediatric Monitoring

The principles of hemodynamic monitoring using fluid-filled systems are identical for patients of all ages (see Chapter 6). The equipment required is virtually identical to that used for adults, including catheter, noncompliant tubing, pressure transducer, flush system with flow-limiting valve, amplifier, and display monitor. For pressure measurements to be accurate, there must be an unobstructed fluid column between the catheter tip and the transducer, so that the dynamic cardiovascular pressure exerted on the fluid column will be reliably transmitted to the transducer. *The pressure transducer must be zeroed, leveled, and calibrated.* These steps ensure that it will convert a mechanical signal of known quantity to an electrical signal of appropriate waveform magnitude and accurate digital display. The related principles are briefly discussed later in this chapter and are discussed at greater length in Chapter 6.

Although the principles of hemodynamic monitoring are identical in adult and pediatric care, the application of these monitoring principles differs. Some clinically significant considerations are specific to pediatric patients. These are summarized in the following sections.

Reduced Margin of Safety for Unintentional Blood Loss through Leaks in Monitoring Lines

The *circulating blood volume* of a young child is extremely small, averaging 80 ml/kg in infants and 75 ml/kg in children. A small volume of blood loss therefore can constitute a significant hemorrhage for infants and children. For example, a 35 ml blood loss represents 0.6% of the circulating blood volume of an adult and 2% of the blood volume of a 25 kg child, whereas this same volume produces a 12% hemorrhage in a 4 kg infant.

It is unrealistic to expect an alert child to hold a catheterized extremity immobile. The catheter and all connections must be tightly secured so they will not become dislodged or separated. Luer-Lok connections should be used throughout the system. All stopcocks and connections also must be visible on top of bedclothes so that a loose connection is detected before significant blood loss occurs.

Potential Significance of Small Changes in Vital Signs

A child's *heart rate* is normally more rapid than an adult's, and the *arterial pressure* is normally lower than adult arterial pressure. Small quantitative changes in these parameters can indicate clinically significant changes in a child's condition. Therefore the monitoring systems in pediatric patients must be capable of recognizing rapid heart rates and must accurately reflect low arterial pressures. Monitor alarms must be adjustable so that they may be set to sound or signal small quantitative changes in heart rate or arterial pressure.

The high- and low-pressure alarms must be individually set to provide audible and visual signals when the blood pressure changes by 15% or more. *The low-pressure alarm must never be permanently disabled,* because the patient can experience significant hemorrhage within a few minutes if the tubing in the system separates. When blood sampling is performed or when the tubing is changed, the alarms should be *temporarily* disabled so that they will automatically reactivate within 60 to 90 seconds. *The clinician should not leave the bedside of the patient with invasive monitoring equipment in place unless all appropriate alarms are activated.*

Difficulty in Inserting and Maintaining Catheters

The *arteries* and *veins* of infants and children are small and may be extremely difficult to cannulate. Once the small catheter is inserted, it must be carefully maintained and stabilized. The small catheters used in pediatric patients can readily kink, become obstructed by particulate matter, or clot.

Greater Risk of Unintentional Fluid Overload

The *flush system* for continuous irrigation of the monitoring catheter should include a volume-controlled infusion pump. All fluids used to flush monitoring lines must be measured and added to the child's total fluid intake. In general, it is unwise to have a pressure bag joined directly to the monitoring tubing for automatic continuous irrigation of the pediatric catheter. Such a system is not recommended. It will be impossible to determine the precise volume infused during continuous flush and irrigation with this system. Instead, the catheter is continuously irrigated, using a volume-controlled infusion pump.

Additional irrigation is necessary following blood sampling and when the pressure signal becomes damped. Such irrigation should be performed manually, employing a syringe, so that a known quantity of fluid is provided *gently*. Forceful irrigation of an arterial line is not recommended for two reasons: (1) it may result in trauma to the small catheterized vessel, and (2) forceful irrigation of an arterial line can result in retrograde infusion of air, clots, or cellular debris into the aorta and cerebral circulation. Retrograde flow of irrigant fluid to the arch of the aorta has been documented in neonates following forceful irrigation of radial or umbilical artery catheters.[52]

Blood Sampling

Blood sampling should be performed in a manner that minimizes blood loss and avoids the need for irrigation with a large volume of fluid following the sampling. Such a technique is presented later.[37] All blood lost or drawn for laboratory analysis should be recorded on the infant's flow sheet, and blood replacement should be considered if this blood loss approximates 7% to 10% of the circulating blood volume over a short period of time.

Universal precautions must be observed, and thus gloves must be worn during any sampling procedures. Needleless syringes or syringes and stopcocks are typically used to eliminate the risk of needle injuries.

Probably the most popular method of blood sampling in critical care units involves syringe aspiration of 1 to 3 ml of irrigant and blood from a stopcock or sampling port closest to the patient and the catheter. This amount of blood acts as a "discard" sample. The syringe containing this "discard sample" is capped and set aside while the actual blood sample is drawn. The aspirated fluid-blood "discard" solution in the original syringe is commonly reinfused after the sample is obtained. However, this practice is undesirable for two reasons:

1. *Potential for systemic emboli.* Tiny clots may form in the fluid-blood solution, and infusion of these clots into an arterial line may embolize in an antegrade direction into the extremity, as well as retrograde toward the arch of the aorta. When neonatal radial arteries were flushed with bubbled saline, retrograde flow of the irrigant into the carotid artery was documented.[52] In patients in whom it is deemed necessary to reinfuse the originally aspirated fluid-blood mixture, reinfusion via a central or peripheral vein is probably preferable to reinfusion into the artery.

2. *Potential for fluid overload.* Reinfusion of the aspirated fluid-blood mixture results in net fluid administration because the mixture must be followed by additional irrigant to flush the line. For these two reasons, a two-stopcock system (or two-sampling-port system) may be preferable for blood sampling.

Two-Stopcock (or Two-Sampling-Port) System. A two-stopcock system may be assembled from supplies available in unit stock. In addition, several two-stopcock (or two-sampling-port) units are commercially available. The two-sampling-port units use needleless syringes and eliminate potential contact with patient blood (Figure 19-4). These systems contain a proximal stopcock or sampling port and distal stopcock or sampling port. The *distal* stopcock or port is positioned near the transducer, farther from the patient. The syringe in the distal stopcock or port is used to aspirate fluid from the tubing and replace irrigant fluid into the tubing. A syringe (termed the *irrigant syringe*) filled with exactly 2 ml of irrigant fluid is placed in the distal stopcock or in the sampling port.[37]

Some commercially available systems use a small segment of noncompliant microbore tubing between the distal stopcock or port and the irrigant syringe. The addition of this tubing effectively increases the volume of the discard that is aspirated before the patient blood sample is taken.

The *proximal* stopcock or port is located nearer the skin entrance site of the catheter and is used for obtaining the blood sample. Typically, a 6-inch segment of tubing is placed between the catheter and this first stopcock. The rationale for this additional length of tubing is that the

PROCEDURAL REVIEW

The procedure for obtaining blood using the two-stopcock or two-sampling-port method is as follows:[37]

1. Turn the distal stopcock "off" to the transducer and "open" between the irrigant syringe and the patient. (Reset monitor alarms as needed; it is preferable to inactivate the alarm temporarily so that the alarm automatically reactivates within approximately 30 to 90 seconds.) If a sampling port is used, insert a needleless syringe containing exactly 2 ml of irrigant fluid into the distal sampling port. Ensure that exactly 2 ml of irrigant fluid is present in the irrigant syringe joined to the distal stopcock.

2. Aspirate blood from the patient with the irrigant syringe until blood is observed *within the tubing* between the proximal and distal stopcocks, but *has not reached* the distal stopcock or sampling port. It is extremely important to avoid contamination of the distal stopcock and sampling port and the irrigant syringe with blood because such contamination will necessitate irrigation following sampling. If a commercially made sampling system is employed, blood will be aspirated to but not beyond a black line or indicator. Note the final volume of fluid in the irrigant syringe (slightly more than 3 ml). The volume of blood in the tubing between the proximal stopcock or port and the distal stopcock or port (or aspiration black line) will serve as the "discard" blood sample, although it is never removed from this system.

3. Turn the distal stopcock "off" to the patient if a stopcock system is used.

4. Place a 1 ml syringe on the sampling port of the proximal stopcock, and turn this stopcock "off" to the transducer and "open" to the patient. If a 3 or 6 ml syringe is already joined to the proximal stopcock, that syringe may be used. If a sampling port is used, insert a needleless syringe into the proximal sampling port.

5. Withdraw approximately 0.1 to 0.3 ml of blood. If you are using a stopcock, turn the stopcock midway between two positions (so that it is "off" to all positions). This 0.1 to 0.3 ml of blood will be discarded because it contains irrigant fluid from the hub of the sampling port. This discarded amount should be added to the total of blood lost during this sampling.

6. Replace the 1 ml syringe with the actual sampling syringe. If you are using a stopcock system, turn the proximal stopcock "open" between the sampling syringe and the patient, and gently aspirate the necessary sample. When sampling is complete, turn the stopcock "off" to the sampling port and "open" to the transducer. If you are using a sampling port, withdraw the syringe from the sampling port.

7. If you are using a distal stopcock, turn the distal stopcock "off" to the transducer and "open" to the irrigant syringe. With the original irrigant syringe in the distal stopcock or sampling port, gently irrigate the tubing (the flush should move toward the patient), using fluid in the irrigant syringe, until exactly 2 ml of irrigant fluid remains in the irrigant syringe. This irrigation has simply returned the blood from the tubing to the patient and replaced the irrigant fluid into the tubing so that no net fluid administration has occurred. The tubing should be clear of blood at this point.

8. Place a 3 ml syringe on the *proximal* stopcock. Turn the *proximal* stopcock "off" to the patient and "open" to the sampling port, and use the 2 ml in the distal irrigant syringe to irrigate blood from the sampling port into the 3 ml syringe. If a sampling port is used, place a syringe in the proximal sampling port and crimp or obstruct the tubing between this port and the patient, and irrigate from the distal syringe into this proximal syringe. Discard the 3 ml syringe.

9. Turn the sampling stopcock "off" to the sampling port and "open" to the transducer, and turn the distal stopcock "off" to the irrigant syringe and "open" to the transducer. Replace the irrigant syringe with another syringe containing exactly 2 ml of irrigant fluid.

10. Place protective covers or syringes on all stopcock ports. Verify that a clear waveform tracing is observed on the monitor and that all alarms are reset and all tubing connections are tight.

weight of the stopcock is less likely to create tension or torsion on the in situ catheter.

MONITORING SYSTEM SETUP TO ENSURE ACCURATE DISPLAY OF HEMODYNAMIC MEASUREMENTS

Because pediatric patients have a smaller absolute stroke volume and cardiac output and a lower blood pressure, *small quantitative changes in hemodynamic variables can be qualitatively very significant.*[1,28] Consequently, meticulous attention to monitoring system setup is required to ensure fidelity of displayed measurements. Hemodynamic measurements must also be obtained and calculations performed in *exactly* the same way by all caregivers so that small errors are eliminated or standardized. (See Chapter 6 for a more detailed discussion of the following principles.)

First, the pressure transducer stopcock (or zero reference point on a water manometer) must be leveled to the patient's midchest. This step eliminates the effects of hydrostatic pressure on the transducer diaphragm or water manometer.

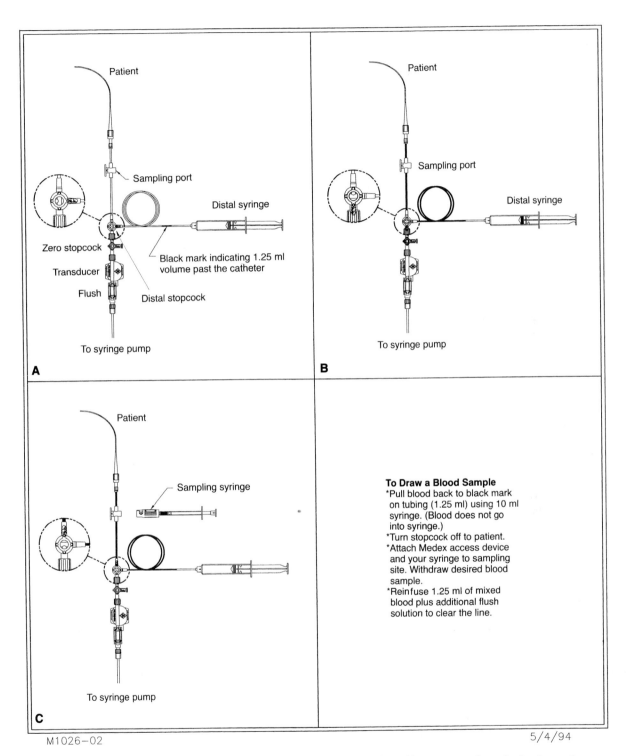

To Draw a Blood Sample
*Pull blood back to black mark on tubing (1.25 ml) using 10 ml syringe. (Blood does not go into syringe.)
*Turn stopcock off to patient.
*Attach Medex access device and your syringe to sampling site. Withdraw desired blood sample.
*Reinfuse 1.25 ml of mixed blood plus additional flush solution to clear the line.

M1026–02   5/4/94

FIGURE 19-4 Blood drawing using commercial pediatric sampling kit with two stopcocks and microbore tubing. **A,** System in "resting" position. **B,** To begin sampling, turn stopcock "off" to transducer and "open" between distal syringe and patient. Begin with 2 ml in distal syringe. Aspirate until patient blood moves into tubing to (but not beyond) black mark. **C,** Turn distal stopcock "off" to patient. Join sampling syringe to proximal (sampling) stopcock. Turn distal stopcock "off" to distal syringe and tubing. Draw sample from sampling port. Then reinfuse blood from tubing to patient and irrigant fluid from microbore tubing into main tubing. If 2 ml remains in the distal syringe, the patient has not received any net fluid administration. (Courtesy of Medex, Inc.)

Second, the pressure transducer must be given a zero reference point to establish a standard for all measured pressures. This procedure eliminates the effects of atmospheric pressure on hemodynamic pressure measurements. When the pressure transducer is zeroed and leveled to midchest, it must remain at the same relationship to midchest throughout monitoring. If the patient's torso is raised or lowered in relationship to the transducer, the transducer must be releveled and rezeroed to reestablish hydrostatic pressure neutrality within the monitoring system.

Third, a calibration check should be performed on the pressure transducer. This is particularly important for reusable transducers because, over time, they may lose pressure sensitivity and accuracy. Testing by activating the "calibration" option on the bedside monitor does not ensure transducer accuracy; rather, an accurate calibration check requires provision of a known mechanical signal to the transducer itself. The mechanical signal may be applied with a mercury or water manometer. The amplifier and the digital and waveform displays also must be included in the test to ensure display of an appropriate signal size or number.

Disposable transducers manufactured today are much more accurate than in the past. For this reason, it is not necessary to mechanically calibrate every transducer before use. If a transducer is significantly "out of calibration," this fact should be detected by the bedside monitor and an error signal should occur. In addition, it may be impossible to "zero" the transducer. However, the clinician should know how to mechanically calibrate a transducer so if there is any question of transducer function or calibration it will be possible to verify the calibration even when the transducer is joined to a patient monitoring system.

Calibration Techniques

Water Manometer Calibration Check

An inexpensive and often preferable alternative to mercury manometer transducer calibration is *water manometer* transducer calibration. The monitoring system is assembled and flushed in a standard fashion, with the addition of a 24-inch piece of noncompliant tubing attached to the transducer stopcock. This additional tubing is flushed with the same solution used to flush the rest of the monitoring system. The distal end of the tubing is then capped. The printer also may be activated during this method of calibration to check the calibration accuracy of the printer.[37]

The transducer is first leveled at the patient's midchest and opened to air. It is then zeroed in the standard fashion (typically a "zero" button must be activated on the bedside

monitor). The 24-inch piece of tubing is then joined to the transducer at the stopcock. The "zeroing" port of the transducer stopcock may be used. This tubing is filled with irrigant fluid. The distal end of the 24-inch tubing is then uncapped and the stopcock is turned "open" between the transducer and tubing. When the open distal end of the tubing is held at the level of the zero reference point, the monitor should display a pressure of 0. The open distal end is then elevated *exactly* 27.2 cm above the zero reference point. This creates a column of water 27.2 cm high, which will exert a pressure of 27.2 cm H_2O on the transducer. By conversion, 27.2 cm H_2O pressure is equal to 20 mm Hg pressure (1.36 cm H_2O pressure = 1 mm Hg pressure). The digital display, waveform, and printout should display a pressure of 20 mm Hg during this maneuver if the transducer, display, and printer are all accurately calibrated (Figure 19-5).

Use of a Commercial Calibrator

Transducer calibration also can be accomplished using an automatic calibrator; several such calibrators are commercially available. Such a calibrator generates a mechanical pressure of specified quantity that can be applied to the transducer. The equipment may be costly, and it may be impossible to check the accuracy of the calibrator, which may become distorted over time.

Ensuring Consistency of Monitoring Technique

As noted earlier, it is imperative that each clinician obtain hemodynamic measurements in exactly the same way so that the measurements can be standardized and used to evaluate *trends* in the patient's condition. The relationship between the transducer and the patient's cardiovascular zero reference point (midchest) must remain constant once the transducer is zeroed (Figure 19-6). Because a child rarely fills the entire bed, the transducer can be placed on the mattress, beside the patient's chest, so that the relationship between the transducer and the patient's midchest can be verified instantly. It is helpful to tape the transducer-stopcock system to a folded disposable diaper or small linen roll to lift the transducer off the mattress to the height of the patient's midchest.

Alternatively, the transducer can be mounted on a transducer pole, and a stopcock for zeroing can be taped to the child's midchest. This stopcock serves as the zero reference point when it is opened to air (see Chapter 6, Figure 6-8, *B*, for a vertical plane stopcock on an adult). The advantage of this arrangement is that the "zeroing" point in the monitoring system will always be at the patient's midchest because it is taped there. The disadvantage of

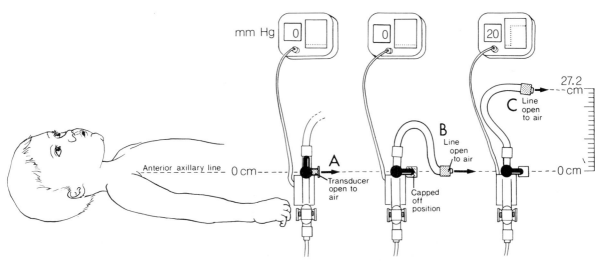

FIGURE 19-5 Mechanical calibration of transducer using a fluid-filled tube. Transducer calibration using 27.2 cm H_2O pressure. One method of calibrating a transducer uses a column of water 27.2 cm high to create a 20 mm Hg signal. The first step to calibration is zeroing of the transducer to air **(A).** The "zeroing" port of the stopcock is then capped, and a 24-inch section of noncompliant tubing is flushed and joined to the transducer at the stopcock. The stopcock is turned "off" to the zeroing port and "open" between the tubing and the transducer. The distal end of this tubing is open to air and is held at the level of the zero reference point **(B);** a zero pressure reading should be displayed on the monitor. The distal (open) end of the tubing is then held 27.2 cm above the zero reference point **(C),** and a 20 mm Hg pressure should be noted by the monitor (1.36 cm H_2O pressure $=$ 1 mm Hg pressure, so 27.2 cm H_2O $=$ 20 mm Hg). (Reproduced with permission from Webster H: Bioinstrumentation: principles and techniques. In Hazinski MF, editor: *Nursing care of the critically ill child,* ed 2, St Louis, 1992, Mosby. All rights reserved.)

this technique is that the relationship between the zero reference point and the transducer changes whenever the transducer-patient relationship changes, such as when raising or lowering the bed. If the transducer-patient relationship changes, the transducer must be rezeroed.

Regardless of which technique is chosen, the transducer and monitoring system should be zeroed on a regular basis (e.g., every 4 or 8 hours) or whenever there is a significant change in hemodynamic measurements without apparent cause.

APPLICATION OF HEMODYNAMIC MONITORING SYSTEMS IN ASSESSMENT OF PEDIATRIC PATIENTS

The principles, techniques, and pitfalls of various hemodynamic monitoring technologies are identical for pediatric and adult patients. A brief discussion of each of these technologies, along with considerations specific to pediatric patients, is presented in the remainder of this chapter. Refer to the chapter specific for the monitoring technique for more comprehensive discussion of each monitoring technique.

NONINVASIVE AND INVASIVE TECHNIQUES OF BLOOD PRESSURE MEASUREMENT

See also Chapter 7. Considerations specific to pediatric patients are presented in this section.

Arterial Pressure Monitoring

Arterial pressure monitoring is a routine part of vital sign evaluation for hospitalized patients. The frequency and the type of monitoring are determined by the patient's underlying condition. When the patient's condition is stable, noninvasive monitoring enables acceptably reliable evaluation of arterial pressure. However, *the accuracy of noninvasive measurements becomes unreliable in hemodynamically unstable patients.* Therefore invasive monitoring should be established in patients at risk of hemodynamic deterioration or in patients actually in an unstable condition, or in patients who require frequent blood sampling.

Evaluation of Pediatric "Norms" Relative to Patient Age

Normal systolic and diastolic blood pressures in children are provided in Table 19-7.[19,53] There are two methods of evaluating pediatric blood pressure in context with

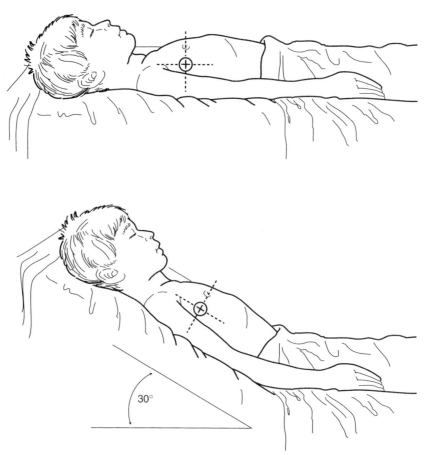

FIGURE 19-6 Placement of transducer at zero reference point (with the patient recumbent and semiupright). (Redrawn with permission from Hazinski MF: *Nursing care of the critically ill child,* ed 2, St Louis, 1992, Mosby.)

the established normal values for a given age—the 50th percentile systolic blood pressure and the 5th percentile systolic blood pressure. Both systolic pressure measurements can be estimated using formulas.

The 50th Percentile Systolic Blood Pressure. This is the median systolic blood pressure for children of a specific age. This means that half of the normal children of that age can be expected to have a systolic blood pressure higher than the number estimated, and half of the normal children of that age can be expected to have a systolic blood pressure lower than the number estimated. An estimate of the median systolic blood pressure for any child from 1 to 10 years of age can be calculated by adding 90 mm Hg to twice the child's age in years. For example, for a 5-year-old child, the 50th percentile systolic blood pressure is estimated as 90 mm Hg + (2 × 5), or 90 mm Hg + 10, or 100 mm Hg.

The 5th Percentile Systolic Blood Pressure. The estimated value of the 5th percentile systolic blood pressure is used as an index of hypotension.[1,18,19] Only 5% of normal children of that age would be expected to have a systolic blood pressure lower than the number estimated. In other words, 95% of normal children of that age will have a systolic blood pressure higher than the estimated value. For children 1 to 10 years of age, the 5th percentile systolic blood pressure is estimated by adding 70 mm Hg plus twice the child's age in years. For example, for a 7-year-old child, the 5th percentile blood pressure is estimated as 70 mm Hg + (2 × 7), or 70 mm Hg + 14, or 84 mm Hg. Because only 5% of normal 7-year-olds are expected to have a systolic blood pressure lower than 84 mm Hg, clinicians should consider this pressure indicative of hypotension and promptly assess an ill or injured patient physically for other indications of systemic hypoperfusion.

TABLE 19-7
Normal Blood Pressures in Children

Age	Systolic Pressure (mm Hg)	Diastolic Pressure (mm Hg)
Birth (12 hr, <1000 g)	39-59	16-36
Birth (12 hours, 3 kg weight)	50-70	25-45
Neonate (96 hr)	60-90	20-60
Infant (6 mo)	87-105	53-66
Toddler (2 yr)	95-105	53-66
School age (7 yr)	97-112	57-71
Adolescent (15 yr)	112-128	66-80

Reproduced with permission from Hazinski MF: Children are different. In Hazinski MF, editor: *Nursing care of the critically ill child,* ed 2, St Louis, 1992, Mosby.

Blood pressure ranges taken from the following sources: *Neonate*—Versmold H et al: Aortic blood pressure during the first 12 hours of life in infants with birth weight 610–4220 gms, *Pediatrics* 67:107, 1981. 10th–90th percentile ranges used. *Others*—Horan MJ, chairman, Task Force on Blood Pressure Control in Children, National Heart, Lung and Blood Institute: Report of the second task force on blood pressure in children—1987, *Pediatrics* 79:1, 1987. 50th–90th percentile ranges indicated.

Noninvasive Monitoring of Arterial Blood Pressure

Noninvasive Pressure Measurements

Measurement of the arterial blood pressure may be accomplished with a cuff and sphygmomanometer. The cuff employed for pressure measurement must be of the appropriate width and length. The width of the cuff should cover three fourths of the length of the child's upper arm (i.e., the segment from the shoulder to the elbow).[53] The bladder of the cuff should encircle the arm completely, with or without overlap. Standard sizes for blood pressure cuffs for children of all ages have been established by the National Heart, Lung, and Blood Institute's Task Force for Blood Pressure Control in Children (Table 19-8).[53]

Several factors may reduce the accuracy of arterial pressure measurement by cuff. For example, if the cuff is too large, a falsely low blood pressure measurement will be obtained. If the cuff is too small, a falsely high arterial pressure measurement will result. If the child is hypotensive, it is likely that a measurement obtained with a cuff and a mercury manometer will *underestimate* the systolic and diastolic blood pressure, even if the cuff is sized appropriately.[53] Overall, noninvasive methods of blood pressure measurement provide convenient, risk-free methods to monitor the blood pressure in stable, *normotensive* neonates and children. However, when patients are

TABLE 19-8
Commonly Available Blood Pressure Cuff Sizes

Cuff Name*	Bladder Width (cm)	Bladder Length (cm)
Newborn	2.5-4.0	5.0-9.0
Infant	4.0-6.0	11.5-18.0
Child	7.5-9.0	17.0-19.0
Adult	11.5-13.0	22.0-26.0
Large arm	14.0-15.0	30.5-33.0
Thigh	18.0-19.0	36.0-38.0

Reproduced from Task Force on Blood Pressure Control in Children, National Heart, Lung and Blood Institute: Report of the second task force on blood pressure control in children—1987, *Pediatrics* 79:3, 1987. Reproduced by permission of *Pediatrics.*

*Cuff name does not guarantee that the cuff will be appropriate size for a child within that age range.

hemodynamically unstable, the noninvasive methods may be inaccurate, and intraarterial pressure monitoring should be strongly considered. Regardless of the technique for blood pressure measurements, the accuracy of the measurements and all sources of error must be considered when evaluating data.

Oscillometric blood pressure monitoring devices were validated using normotensive children.[54,55] These devices may yield inaccurate blood pressure readings when they are used in hypotensive or hypertensive children.[56-58] If the child is unstable or hypotensive or hypertensive, intraarterial blood pressure monitoring remains the "gold standard" for evaluation and continuous monitoring.

Intraarterial (Direct) Pressure Monitoring

Intraarterial pressure monitoring enables continuous display of the child's arterial pressure and provides arterial access for blood sampling. This form of monitoring should be used when the child's blood pressure is unstable, vasoactive drugs are being administered, or continuous and accurate determinations of blood pressure are required (e.g., treatment of increased intracranial pressure and intracranial pressure monitoring). Insertion of an intraarterial catheter should also be considered if the patient requires frequent blood sampling or evaluation of arterial blood gases, particularly if pulse oximetry and end-tidal carbon dioxide (PETCO$_2$) monitoring cannot be employed or if noninvasive blood gas measurements or calculations display measurements thought to be questionable or unreliable. For example, PETCO$_2$ monitoring can be unreliable in infants or children during spontaneous breathing.[28]

Overall, intraarterial blood pressure measurement enables the most accurate determination of the arterial pressure, provided the transducer is appropriately zeroed, leveled, and calibrated and the fluid-filled monitoring system is intact and in direct contact with the arterial stream.

Sites for Arterial Catheter Insertion in Pediatric Patients

The site most frequently chosen for pediatric intraarterial pressure monitoring is the radial artery, although the femoral, dorsalis pedis, brachial, and posterior tibial arteries are also commonly chosen. Femoral artery cannulation is often reserved for emergencies, because this site is difficult to immobilize, and there is a high risk of contamination with urine and feces in incontinent patients. Temporal artery cannulation is no longer recommended because of the risk for significant complications, such as cerebral thromboembolic events.[59]

Potential complications of arterial catheterization at any site include local or systemic infection, embolization of air or particulate matter, and arterial occlusion and thrombosis with associated tissue necrosis.[18] If these complications develop in a neonate, limb growth may be affected.[60-68]

Central Venous and Right Atrial Pressure Monitoring

Pediatric central venous access provides a reliable intravascular site for the rapid infusion of intravenous fluid, administration of hypertonic or irritant fluids (e.g., parenteral nutrition, concentrated electrolyte solutions, and medications), or CVP monitoring. In the absence of vena caval obstruction, CVP is equal to right atrial pressure. These pressures also correlate with right ventricular end-diastolic pressure in patients without tricuspid valve disease (see Chapter 9).

Sites for Venous Access in Pediatric Patients

The site chosen for central venous access is determined by operator preference and experience, as well as the age and clinical condition of the child. Umbilical venous catheterization is possible only during the first weeks of life. The umbilical vein may be readily catheterized during the first days of life, but access in a neonate after this period may require cutdown of the umbilical stump.

The most popular sites for central venous catheterization in infants and children include the femoral vein, the subclavian vein, and the internal jugular vein.[18] Each of these sites has distinct advantages and disadvantages.

The *femoral vein* is located well away from the chest, and thus it may be the best central vein to catheterize during resuscitation of patients with trauma to the head, neck, or chest. Catheterization of this site is associated with a relatively low rate of complications; however, the urine and feces may easily contaminate the femoral site if the infant or child is incontinent.[69] In addition, the presence of the femoral catheter in the relatively small veins of infants and small children also may compromise venous return. Venous stasis, in turn, predisposes the patient to edema of the leg and to deep vein thrombus formation.

The *subclavian vein* is a popular site for central venous access. The left subclavian vein also is frequently employed for the insertion of a pulmonary artery catheter. The skin entrance site may be covered with a bio-occlusive dressing and can be visualized during routine care.[70] The subclavian catheter can be secured easily, and movement restriction may not be necessary. This site is unlikely to be contaminated unless the patient has wounds or burns of the chest or neck. Subclavian vein catheterization should be attempted *only* by operators experienced in the technique, however, because it is associated with a high risk for pneumothorax or hemothorax.

Catheterization of the *internal jugular vein* should be attempted only by operators skilled in the technique, because the potential for complications in unskilled hands is unacceptably high. The incidence of inadvertent puncture of the right carotid artery is approximately 8%, even in skilled hands.[71] If bleeding develops during or after venous catheterization (as a result of vascular laceration or through-and-through puncture), hemorrhage may be very difficult to control. If the internal jugular vein will be used, the right internal jugular vein is selected more than the left because it is a direct pathway to the superior vena cava and avoids the thoracic duct. Pneumothorax is less likely because the apex of the right lung is lower than the apex of the left lung.[18] The internal jugular catheter is more difficult to secure than the subclavian or femoral venous catheter, and flow through the catheter can be altered by a change in the patient's head position.

The *external jugular vein* is a popular site for central venous cannulation in children.[18] This vein is superficial and visible through the skin and can be entered rapidly. However, catheters inserted at this site may be inadvertently advanced upward and toward the head rather than downward and toward the heart because of the anatomic relationship of the external jugular vein relative to the subclavian vein and internal jugular vein.

CVP catheters may be inserted percutaneously, via cutdown, or catheters may be placed transthoracically at the time of cardiovascular surgery. Any transthoracic catheter should be labeled at the exit site from the chest, and the distance from the exit site to the first connection should be measured so that catheter migration will be more easily detected.

Causes of Alterations in Central Venous Pressure Measurements

The normal CVP in an infant is 0 to 4 mm Hg and in a child is 2 to 6 mm Hg, with a mean CVP of 3 mm Hg.[6] Hemorrhage, dehydration, or extravascular fluid shifts all can cause a *fall* in the CVP. In addition, vasodilation, such as that associated with sepsis or rewarming after hypothermic cardiovascular surgery, produces a relative hypovolemia and a fall in the CVP.

Elevations in the CVP occur in pediatric patients with right ventricular failure, hypervolemia, extreme tachycardia (because true diastolic pressures are not observed when the heart rate is extremely rapid), tricuspid stenosis or insufficiency, or positive pressure ventilation (particularly with PEEP). An increase in the CVP or right atrial pressure should be anticipated following surgical correction of congenital heart disease when the corrective procedure includes a right ventriculotomy incision or when it results in a significant increase in right ventricular afterload, such as that from insertion of a pulmonary artery conduit in a child with pulmonic stenosis or insufficiency.

Pulmonary Artery Pressure Monitoring

Indications for pediatric pulmonary artery catheterization are identical to those for adults and include the following:[72]

- Need to assess patient responses to therapeutic interventions, including titration of PEEP
- Shock unresponsive to volume resuscitation
- Titration of therapy for pulmonary hypertension in children with congenital or acquired heart disease
- Need to determine fluid and vasoactive drug therapy requirements in patients with severe, multiple trauma; severe burn injury; sepsis; or multiple organ failure
- Perioperative monitoring of patients with major surgical procedures
- Clinical research studies

Pulmonary artery catheterization is contraindicated whenever the potential risks outweigh the possible benefits. Such risks include severe arrhythmias, large intracardiac shunts, and coagulopathies (see Chapter 10).

Preferred Sites and Technique of Pulmonary Artery Catheter Insertion in Pediatric Patients

The vessels for insertion of a pulmonary artery catheter in children are the left subclavian vein, the right internal jugular vein, and the right femoral vein. The left subclavian vein is preferred over the right subclavian vein because approach from the left side appears to facilitate curvature and passage of the catheter through the right ventricle and pulmonary artery. The right subclavian vein may be used as an alternative site if the left subclavian vein is not suitable for cannulation (e.g., as the result of areas of burn or traumatic injury).

Transthoracic placement of a pulmonary artery catheter may be accomplished during cardiovascular surgery. A 4-French pulmonary artery catheter may be brought through the chest wall and placed directly into the pulmonary artery.[73] The catheter is sutured into place at the skin. The 4-French transthoracic pulmonary artery catheter does not contain a balloon tip and may contain a thermistor that enables calculation of cardiac output.

The most popular pulmonary artery catheter sizes available commercially for pediatric patients are 5-, 5.5-, and 7-French pulmonary artery catheters; 7- and 7.5-French catheters are used for older children and adolescents. Each of these catheters is available with four ports (right atrial port, pulmonary artery port, pulmonary artery balloon inflation port, and thermistor) to enable calculation of thermodilution cardiac output.

The 5- and 5.5-French catheters are usually inserted in children who weigh less than 15 to 18 kg, whereas the 7-French catheter is generally used in children weighing more than 18 to 20 kg. The 5- and 5.5-French catheters are considerably more difficult to insert, advance, use, and maintain than the larger-diameter catheters. A small catheter does not float easily into the pulmonary artery, and the tiny lumina contained within the catheter can readily become occluded by cellular debris. In addition, injection of the thermal indicator into the injection port of the 5- or 5.5-French catheter can be difficult because the right atrial lumen is very narrow and provides a great deal of resistance to fluid flow during injection.

As in adult patients, the pulmonary artery catheter is inserted through an introducer. A 6-French introducer is used for the 5- and 5.5-French catheters, and an 8.5-French introducer is used for the 7- and 7.5-French catheters.

If possible, infusion of medications through the pulmonary artery port should be avoided for two reasons: (1) crystallization of drugs (particularly antibiotics) may contribute to lumen occlusion, and (2) a concentrated drug effect in a portion of the pulmonary circulation may produce tissue injury. Occasionally, vasodilators may be preferentially infused into the pulmonary artery lumen to provide direct effects on the pulmonary vascular bed. The pulmonary artery port should not be used for bolus fluid administration because rapid flow rates may injure the relatively small, thin-walled vessels.

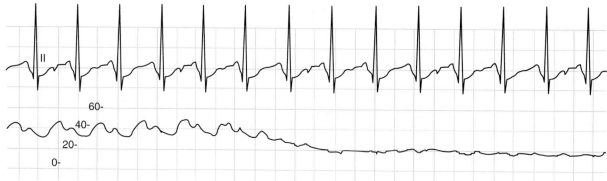

FIGURE 19-7 Relationship between pulmonary artery end-diastolic pressure and pulmonary wedge pressure (PWP). As the balloon is inflated and the tracing converts from a pulmonary artery to a PWP tracing, the difference between the pulmonary artery end-diastolic pressure of 26 to 30 mm Hg and the PWP of 18 mm Hg is apparent. This discrepancy is observed when pulmonary vascular resistance is elevated. This adolescent's pulmonary vascular resistance was slightly elevated at 332 dynes-sec-cm^{-5}/m^2 (normal pulmonary vascular resistance for a child is 80 to 240 dynes-sec-cm^{-5}/m^2, and normal pulmonary vascular resistance for an adult is 45 to 225 dynes-sec-cm^{-5}/m^2).

The techniques for catheter flotation, maintenance, and evaluation of obtained measurements are identical to those for adults (Figure 19-7). Many patient-related and technical factors may result in displayed pressure measurements that bear no relationship to the patient's true hemodynamic status. Correct in situ catheter tip placement is one factor that can be documented by postinsertion anteroposterior and lateral chest radiographs. Unless proper placement is confirmed, the validity of pulmonary artery pressure measurements is in question (Figure 19-8).

Chapter 10 includes a detailed discussion of the many other variables that may affect accuracy of obtained measurements. Meticulous attention to monitoring system setup and maintenance and consideration of these factors are of critical importance so that diagnosis and therapy are based on physiologic fact rather than patient- or instrumentation-related artifacts.

Since 1996, reports of complications related to pulmonary artery catheterization in adults have raised concerns about the usefulness and complications of this form of hemodynamic monitoring.[74-76] In addition, several studies have documented that health care providers often lack information needed to appropriately interpret the measurements and calculations derived from the use of the pulmonary artery catheter or to troubleshoot the device itself.[77,78] Pulmonary artery catheters are still used relatively infrequently in children, making it difficult for pediatric nurses to maintain expertise in their use. In addition, there is a paucity of data regarding complications associated with their use.[72] For these reasons, nurses involved in the care of children with pulmonary artery catheters should develop educational materials, setup policies (with step-by-step instructions and

illustrations), and team teaching to ensure consistency in the use and maintenance of these catheters.[1]

Reported Complications of Pulmonary Artery Catheterization in Children

Complications associated with pulmonary artery catheterization in infants and children include those of insertion and those related to the catheter itself. Those complications associated with insertion are related to the insertion site and the experience of the technician and include bleeding, pneumothorax (for subclavian approach), and infection. Most complications related to the use of the catheter itself in children are similar to those reported in the adult population. However, the risk of *thrombosis* and *infection* appear to be higher in children than in adults. These risks are interrelated, because there is a link between the development of thrombosis and the development of later infection.[72]

The greater risk of thrombosis appears to be explained by the small vessel size of the infant and child and the large ratio of catheter to vessel size. Heparin-bonded catheters used for femoral venous catheterization appear to be associated with fewer thrombotic complications and lower rates of infection, despite the fact that the heparin coating lasts less than 24 hours.[72,79] Replication of this study using a heparin-bonded pulmonary artery catheter has not been reported. Infection has been reported in approximately 8% to 10% of pediatric uses, with a frequency of 1.4 septic episodes per 100 catheter days. Most infections have been reported in infants and most with catheters in situ more than 1 week after placement.[69,72,80] Additional complications include supraventricular and

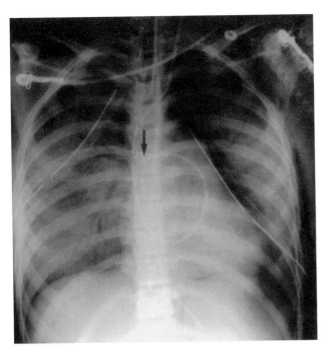

FIGURE 19-8 Radiographic evaluation of pulmonary artery catheter tip location by anteroposterior portable film. The catheter tip is in good position in a main pulmonary artery (although the vertical relationship to the heart cannot be determined on the anteroposterior film). A good zone III pulmonary artery wedge pressure tracing was obtained.

ventricular arrhythmias, with one reported formation of a knot. Catheter lumen occlusion and balloon rupture have also been reported.[69,72,80] Although the frequency of pulmonary artery rupture was described as "extremely rare" in a review article, the article cited *no* reports of this complication in infants and children.[72]

Thermodilution Cardiac Output Measurements

Serial cardiac output determinations using the thermodilution technique are useful in the evaluation and management of critically ill and injured pediatric patients. Thermodilution pulmonary artery catheters are commercially available in sizes 5, 5.5, 7.0, and 7.5 French. A 4-French catheter with a thermistor is occasionally used in cardiac catheterization laboratories and cardiovascular surgical suites,[71] but is not often used in clinical situations. The 4-French catheter does not contain a balloon, and thus PWP measurements are not possible.

Occasionally, a small pulmonary artery thermistor is placed through the chest wall and into the pulmonary artery at the time of cardiovascular surgery.[73] The thermistor is used to calculate a thermodilution cardiac output following

injection of an iced fluid through a right atrial line. The injectate volumes for these thermodilution cardiac output measurements vary slightly from those of the standard thermodilution catheters; therefore the clinician must follow the manufacturer's recommendations for injectate volumes specific to this catheter.

The principle underlying thermodilution pediatric cardiac output calculation is identical to that of adults. The patient's core temperature is first evaluated by the cardiac output computer. A known quantity of cold fluid (5% dextrose in water or normal saline) is then injected into the right atrial port within 4 seconds. The cold injectate thoroughly mixes within the right ventricle and flows into the pulmonary artery, where a temperature change will be detected by the thermistor bead located near the tip of the catheter positioned in a main pulmonary artery branch. A microprocessor in the cardiac output computer or bedside monitor module registers the magnitude and duration of the temperature change over time and calculates a time-temperature curve. The area under the curve is inversely related to the flow rate in the pulmonary artery, which normally correlates with left ventricular output and systemic blood flow (Figure 19-9).

For example, *if the patient's cardiac output is high,* the cold injectate will appear almost immediately in the pulmonary artery. The rapid flow of blood from the right atrium to the pulmonary artery will then wash out the cold injectate quickly and restore the baseline temperature of pulmonary arterial blood rapidly. Consequently, *the slope of the curve will be steep, the temperature change in the pulmonary artery will be brief, and the area under the cardiac output curve will be small.*

If, conversely, the patient's *cardiac output is low,* the appearance of the cold injectate in the pulmonary artery will be delayed, and the temperature change in the pulmonary artery will be large and will be prolonged. Consequently, the slope of the curve will be slurred, and the area under the cardiac output curve will be large (see Chapter 11, Figure 11-4).

Considerations for Accurate Cardiac Output Calculations

Clinicians must remember that the cardiac output calculation obtained via the thermodilution technique is based on many variables, but it is a *calculation* rather than a true *measurement of blood flow* over 1 minute. Poor technique, as well as numerous uncontrollable factors, may result in displayed calculations that do not reflect the child's true cardiac output. Therefore it is essential that correct technique be used to perform the calculation so that trends in the calculated cardiac output reflect real trends in the patient's condition. For example, a conversion factor must

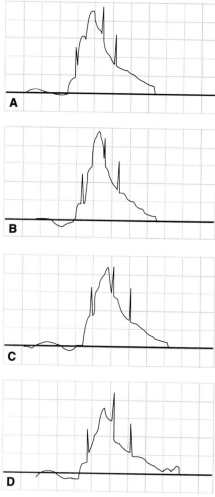

FIGURE 19-9 Cardiac output injection curves. Four cardiac output injection curves are depicted here. Each is performed by the same clinician within minutes of the other to determine cardiac output in an adolescent with sepsis. Calculation is based on 5 ml iced injectate. The adolescent's body surface area (BSA) is 1.71 m^2. **A,** The first injection resulted in a calculated cardiac output of 7.9 L/min and a calculated cardiac index of 4.62 L/min/m^2 BSA. This calculation was discarded because it is the first injection; loss of thermal indicator in the catheter ("priming" the catheter with cold injectate) results in a falsely high cardiac output calculation. **B,** The second injection resulted in a calculated cardiac output of 7.4 L/min and a calculated cardiac index of 4.33 L/min/m^2 BSA. **C,** The third injection resulted in a calculated cardiac output of 7.0 L/min and a calculated cardiac index of 4.09 L/min/m^2 BSA. This injection is extremely close in appearance to the previous two injections; the magnitude of the temperature change (height of the curve) is similar in all three curves, and the duration of the temperature change (length of the curve) is similar. The cardiac outputs and indexes calculated by injections 2 and 3 differ by only 6%, and thus these two injections were averaged to provide a calculated cardiac output of 7.2 L/min and a calculated cardiac index of 4.2 L/min/m^2 BSA. **D,** The fourth curve differs markedly in appearance from the previous curves for several reasons. The injection volume used for this curve was only 4.9 ml, so that the magnitude of the temperature change is smaller (the curve is not as high), and a falsely high cardiac output calculation results (7.9 L/min). In addition, the injection technique is inconsistent with that of the previous injections. The injection was slow, prolonging the duration of the temperature change (lengthening the curve). This injection was not used for cardiac output calculations.

be programmed into the computer or bedside monitor module based on the size of the catheter (5.0, 5.5, or 7.0 French), as well as the volume and temperature of the injectate solution. Changes in the volume or temperature of injectate solution mandate that the conversion factors or injectate description be appropriately changed. If an incorrect calibration constant, catheter size, or injectate volume is programmed into a bedside computer, the resulting cardiac output calculation will be inaccurate.

Factors That Affect the Strength of the Thermal Signal and Accuracy of Cardiac Output Calculations

Thermodilution cardiac output calculation is determined from the magnitude of the temperature change in the pulmonary artery over time. As a result, the injectate volume, injectate temperature, and cardiac output all profoundly influence the accuracy of the calculation.

Three factors *reduce* the magnitude of the thermal signal—room temperature injectate, small injectate volume, and low cardiac output. (Note that "low cardiac output" does not mean low for age, but low in absolute volume.) A reduced thermal signal means that the microprocessor must magnify the signal and thus may compromise the accuracy and reproducibility of the calculation. Poor injection technique (erratic, slow) also has a greater effect on the calculated cardiac output when the signal is magnified by the microprocessor over 4 seconds.

Although 10 ml *room temperature* injections can produce adequate correlation with 10 ml iced injections in *adult* patients with normal or high cardiac output, the accuracy and reproducibility of obtained measurements is still highest with iced injection.[1,81, 82] Ten-milliliter room temperature injections can be used for *adult* and *adolescent* patients because administration of this volume usually does not risk fluid overload. However, the use of 10 ml room temperature injectates is not recommended for thermodilution cardiac output calculations in children for several reasons. First, large-volume (10 ml) injectates should *not* be given to infants and small children because they will contribute to fluid overload if frequent serial cardiac output calculations are performed throughout the day. Second, the small (3 to 5 ml) injections recommended for small pediatric patients result in a lower thermal signal than larger injections. When the signal must be magnified, any error in technique is also magnified. Third, the absolute cardiac output of a small child is small, and low cardiac output may be overestimated by the computer when small injectate volumes are used.

To optimize the thermal signal created during cardiac output injections and to maximize accuracy and reproducibility of thermodilution cardiac output calculations in infants and small children, *all leading manufacturers of thermodilution cardiac output catheters recommend the use of iced injectate for 3 ml injections and strongly suggest iced injectate for 5 ml injections.* Iced injections produce a stronger thermal signal (greater difference between the child's body temperature and the injectate temperature), which yields more accurate and reproducible results when the injection volume is small and cardiac output is relatively small or actually low.[1,82] Of course, all fluids injected for the calculations should be added to the patient's total fluid intake.

When possible, the cold solution should be injected at end-expiration to standardize technique and minimize the effects of slight changes in pulmonary arterial blood temperature relative to the respiratory cycle (pulmonary artery temperature drops slightly during inspiration). The printer should record the thermal injections with a paper speed of 5 mm per second. At this speed, each dark vertical line indicates 1 second of time. Analysis of the cardiac output curve helps identify faulty injection technique, as well as other factors that may cause inaccurate calculations (see Figure 19-9; see also Chapter 11, Figure 11-7). Because the cardiac output of infants and small children is very small, it is extremely important to detect even small variations in injection technique, and thus analysis of the injection recordings is extremely important.

In general, a minimum of three injections is required for each cardiac output calculation. The cardiac output calculated from the first injection is usually higher than that obtained from subsequent injections because a portion of the first injectate merely displaces the fluid contained within the lumen of the catheter, so that volume does not enter the right atrium. This reduces the effective volume of cold thermal indicator actually entering the right atrium; a false-high cardiac output calculation usually results. In some units, the catheter is flushed with iced injectate once just before the cardiac output calculation. Usually, however, the results of the first injection are ignored if they vary by more than 10% from the results of subsequent injections, and a fourth injection is occasionally necessary. Either process may be used, provided the technique is consistent from clinician to clinician. The results of at least two injections that do not vary by more than 10% are averaged for final cardiac output and cardiac index calculation.

Cardiac index (cardiac output divided by the body surface area in square meters) is generally used (instead of cardiac output) to evaluate pediatric patient hemodynamics because normal cardiac index is the same for all pediatric patients beyond the first weeks of life. A "normal" pediatric cardiac index is approximately 3.0 to 4.5 L/min/m^2 body surface area (BSA). A low pediatric cardiac index is considered to be less than 2.0 to 2.5 L/min/m^2 BSA. Some patients may *require* a cardiac output or a cardiac index that is higher than normal. In these patients (those with sepsis or severe traumatic or burn injury), consideration of the underlying problem, as well as clinical evaluation of systemic perfusion and hemodynamic trends, should be taken into account when making diagnostic or therapeutic judgments. *The appropriate cardiac output or cardiac index for any patient is that which is required to maintain effective tissue perfusion and organ function.*

Factors That Result in Changes in Cardiac Output Calculations

The patient's cardiac output calculations may change in response to changes in the patient's metabolic oxygen requirements, as well as deterioration or improvement in cardiovascular or respiratory function. These changes are a hemodynamic reality and generally correlate with the underlying condition and what the child "looks like." Many technical factors may result in changes in the calculated cardiac output that bear no relationship to the patient's condition (i.e., inaccurate calculations).

The most common causes of inaccurate cardiac output calculations include an inaccurate calibration constant or inaccurate programming of the bedside monitor module. Programming of the bedside monitor or calibration constant must be accurate for the catheter size, injectate volume, and injectate temperature. Error may also be introduced during injection if an incorrect injectate volume is used (e.g., lost through a loose connection), if the operator uses room temperature injectate (e.g., drawn from the portion of the coil that is between the cooler and the patient) when the computer is programmed for iced injectate, or if the operator uses poor injection technique.

Causes of Inaccurate Low Cardiac Output Calculations. In general, any factor that artificially *increases* the magnitude of the temperature change in the pulmonary artery will result in a falsely low cardiac output calculation. If the computer or bedside monitor is programmed for room temperature injectate and iced injectate is used (e.g., for the adolescent patient with 10 ml injectates), the resulting cardiac output calculation will be falsely low. If the calibration constant or bedside module is programmed for a 7-French catheter and a 5.0- or 5.5-French catheter is used, a falsely low cardiac output calculation will result.

When an inappropriately large injectate volume is used, the temperature change in the pulmonary artery will be increased, and a falsely low cardiac output calculation will result. For example, if a 5 ml injection is provided when the computer or bedside monitor is calibrated for a 3 ml injection, the resulting cardiac output calculation will be inappropriately low.

Causes of Falsely High Cardiac Output Calculations. Falsely high cardiac output calculations also may result from inappropriate setting of the calibration constant or inaccurate setting of the bedside monitor module, faulty injection volume or temperature, and faulty injection technique. In general, any factor that artificially *decreases* the magnitude of the temperature change in the pulmonary artery will result in a falsely high cardiac output calculation.

If the calibration constant is set for iced injectate and room temperature injectate is used (remember that room temperature injectate should not be used in small children but may be used in adolescents), a falsely high cardiac output calculation will result. Falsely high cardiac output calculations also result, for example, if the calibration constant or bedside monitor module is programmed for a 5-French catheter and a 7-French catheter is used.

Inadequate injectate volume results in a decrease in the magnitude of the pulmonary artery temperature change and will produce a falsely high cardiac output calculation. Loss of injectate volume may occur through an error in injection, a loose connection, or an increased tubing dead space between the injectate syringe and the right atrial port.

If the injectate is warmed in the syringe or tubing before injection, a falsely high cardiac output calculation results. The injectate syringe should be insulated, and the fingers of the hand should not surround the syringe during preparation for injection. There should be no delay between determination of appropriate injectate temperature and actual injections.

If the iced fluid is injected too slowly into the right atrial port, the magnitude of the temperature change in the pulmonary artery may be reduced. Faulty injection technique will be detected through examination of the printout of the thermodilution curve (see Figure 19-9).

Continuous Monitoring of Mixed Venous Oxygen Saturation

Mixed venous oxygen saturation (Svo$_2$) can be monitored continuously via a fiberoptic pulmonary artery catheter. Continuous monitoring of mixed venous oxygen saturation is now possible in pediatric patients, because fiberoptic catheters are now commercially available in 5.5-French size.

The principles of Svo$_2$ monitoring are virtually identical for pediatric and adult patients (see Chapter 12); that is, a light-transmitting optic device located in the tip of the fiberoptic catheter emits light of varying narrow wavebands into the blood within the pulmonary artery. Oxygenated hemoglobin reflects red light well, whereas desaturated hemoglobin does not. Reflected light is then captured by the receiving optic device and is used to determine the percent of hemoglobin that is oxygenated (oxyhemoglobin).[83,84] This process is termed *reflective spectrophotometry* and correlates well with determination of the percent of mixed venous oxyhemoglobin by blood gas analysis. However, this technique is susceptible to more artifact and error than pulse oximetry, which measures light *absorption* across a tissue bed (see Pulse Oximetry, later in this chapter).

Catheter Insertion and Calibration Technique

The pulmonary artery catheter with Svo_2 fiberoptics is inserted in a manner identical to that required for pulmonary artery catheterization. However, before insertion, the Svo_2 processor and monitor must be turned on (with adequate warm-up time allowed), and the optical module must be joined to the connector plug and the processor.

In Vitro Calibration. Fiberoptic catheters must be calibrated *before* insertion into the patient (in vitro calibration). To calibrate the catheter, the optical module is connected to the computer, and the computer is turned on. The catheter is packaged so that the distal end of the catheter can be joined to the optical module without removing the catheter from the sterile tray. The computer multifunction buttons are employed to select in vitro calibration.

If *two* wavelengths of light are used by the monitor, different calibration curves are required for different hematocrit values. Therefore, during any calibration of the monitor, the patient's hemoglobin and hematocrit values must be entered into the computer. *If incorrect hemoglobin and hematocrit values have been entered or the patient's hemoglobin and hematocrit values change after calibration, the Svo_2 calculation will be inaccurate.*

If *three* wavelengths of light are used by the monitor, the third wavelength automatically recalibrates the optical modules with changes in the patient's hemoglobin and hematocrit values.

In Vivo Calibration. At regular intervals, an in vivo calibration of the Svo_2 monitor is required. Most manufacturers suggest that such calibration be done only every 24 to 48 hours; however, unit policy may require more frequent calibration checks. To perform the in vivo calibration, the Svo_2 computer must be switched to the in vivo calibration function, and a blood sample is *slowly and gently* drawn from the pulmonary artery. The pulmonary artery catheter lumen should be irrigated gently after the blood sample is drawn. The blood sample is then sent for laboratory measurement of Svo_2 by co-oximetry. When the results are available, the monitored Svo_2 and the pulmonary artery blood sample Svo_2 are compared.

Use and Maintenance of the Svo₂ Monitor

When the pulmonary artery catheter is placed, Svo_2 calculations are immediately visible on the Svo_2 processor screen. Light intensity also should be indicated. Once the catheter is in place, the processor should be programmed for baseline light intensity, and alarm limits should be set for 10% above and below the patient's baseline Svo_2.

The Svo_2 should be recorded hourly and with any changes in the child's condition. Continuous hard copy of Svo_2 calculations should be recorded. Significant clinical events, such as airway suctioning or episodes of hypotension or pneumothorax, should be indicated on the hard copy with a label indicating the unusual event. Significant or sustained changes in the Svo_2 should be investigated immediately and, if possible, appropriately treated.

During continuous Svo_2 monitoring, the light signal strength must be closely monitored. If the signal strength is weak, the catheter tip may be covered with clot or the fiberoptic catheter may be malfunctioning. If the signal strength is too strong, the catheter may be positioned against a vessel wall, which results in falsely high Svo_2 calculations.

Interpretation of Changes in the Svo₂

The Svo_2 is normally 60% to 80%, but it should never be evaluated as an isolated physiologic variable. It is affected by uncompensated changes in systemic oxygen delivery (Do_2) or oxygen consumption (Vo_2). *Systemic oxygen delivery* indexed to body surface area (Do_2I) averages 550 to 750 ml/min/m² in children[37] and is determined by hemoglobin concentration and its oxygen saturation and by cardiac index. *Oxygen consumption* indexed to body surface area (Vo_2I) averages 120 to 270 ml/min/m² in children[37] and can be raised by factors that increase oxygen demand. Oxygen consumption by tissues is normally one fourth of oxygen delivery in adults (i.e., the oxygen extraction ratio is approximately 25%). Oxygen consumption, however, constitutes a higher percent of oxygen delivery in infants and children. As a result, pediatric patients have smaller oxygen reserves than do adults. In children, any factor that decreases oxygen delivery or increases oxygen consumption may rapidly produce generalized tissue hypoxia.

Decrease in Oxygen Delivery. Oxygen delivery may decrease as the result of anemia, hypoxemia, or decrease in cardiac output. If the hemoglobin or oxygen saturation level falls, the effect on oxygen delivery and Svo_2 will depend on the cardiac output response. If cardiac output increases commensurately, oxygen delivery and Svo_2 do not change. If, however, either hemoglobin concentration or oxygen saturation falls without a commensurate increase in cardiac output, oxygen delivery falls, as does the Svo_2. If the cardiac output decreases, oxygen delivery decreases and the Svo_2 likewise decreases.[1]

Increase in Oxygen Demand. Examples of conditions causing systemic increase in oxygen demand include fever, pain, shivering, and cold stress in neonates. Anesthesia may *reduce* oxygen demand.[81,85] The Svo_2 decreases if systemic oxygen demand increases without a commensurate rise in oxygen delivery.

Sepsis may affect the Svo_2 in several ways. Although sepsis may increase tissue oxygen requirements, it also may decrease the ability of cells to take up and use oxygen. Although sepsis is associated with high cardiac output and oxygen delivery, maldistribution of blood flow results in hypoperfusion of some tissue beds and excessive blood flow to others. The Svo_2 is typically high and the oxygen extraction ratio is typically low. If treatment of the septic patient is successful, the distribution of blood flow becomes more appropriate and cellular oxygen metabolism normalizes. The Svo_2 then decreases as the oxygen extraction ratio increases to normal levels.

Response to Decrease in Svo_2. If the Svo_2 decreases acutely, the clinician should immediately explore and identify the causes and institute appropriate therapy. A sudden fall in hemoglobin is unlikely because even massive hemorrhage does not produce an acute (within minutes) drop in the hemoglobin level. Acute decreases in Svo_2 may be produced by hypoventilation (inadequate tidal volume or respiratory rate), airway obstruction, endotracheal tube displacement or kinking, massive simple pneumothorax or tension pneumothorax, or unintentional disconnection from the oxygen supply. Endotracheal suctioning may be associated with a decrease in oxygen delivery and Svo_2 An acute fall in cardiac output (caused by bradyarrhythmias or tachyarrhythmias or ventricular dysfunction) also may cause a sudden decrease in Svo_2. In addition, factors that suddenly increase oxygen demand (fever, shivering, increased work of breathing, fear, infection, pain, cold stress in neonates) may result in an acute fall in the Svo_2 (Box 19-2).

BOX 19-2
Causes of Acute Changes in the Mixed Venous Oxygen Saturation (Svo_2)

Decreases in Svo_2
Decreased Arterial Oxygen Content
Anemia (decreased hemoglobin/hematocrit)
Hypoxemia
Hypoventilation
Airway obstruction
Pulmonary edema
Atelectasis
Pneumothorax
Endotracheal tube displacement

Decreased Cardiac Output
Bradycardia
Tachyarrhythmias
Decreased stroke volume
Relative hypovolemia
Cardiac dysfunction
Increased afterload

Increased Oxygen Demand
Fever
Shivering
Pain
Anxiety
Increased work of breathing
Cold stress (in neonates and young infants)

Increases in Svo_2
Increased Arterial Oxygen Content
Transfusion
Improved arterial oxygen saturation (e.g., with PEEP or mechanical ventilation)

Increased Cardiac Output
Increased heart rate
Correction of arrhythmia
Increased stroke volume
Volume therapy
Inotropic support
Vasodilator therapy

Decreased Oxygen Demand
Treatment of fever
Elimination of pain or increase in comfort
Sedation
Support of ventilation
Anesthesia
Provision of neutral thermal environment

Falsely high Sv_{O_2} measurements may be obtained if the catheter is lodged against a vessel wall or if a clot forms around the tip of the thermistor. Falsely low Sv_{O_2} values may be recorded if the fiberoptic catheter is damaged or if a kink or clot forms in the catheter.

Pulse Oximetry

Indications

Pulse oximetry is a noninvasive technique that enables continuous monitoring of arterial oxyhemoglobin saturation. It should be used for any patient at risk for the development of hypoxemia. Pulse oximetry evaluates arterial *oxygenation,* but it does *not* evaluate *ventilation* (carbon dioxide elimination). Furthermore, hypoxemia may be only a late sign of deterioration in some children with respiratory failure, particularly when blood gas concentrations have been maintained at normal levels by compensatory tachypnea (e.g., in status asthmaticus).

Function

The pulse oximeter has two diodes that emit a red and an infrared light. These diodes are located in a probe that can be placed on the finger, toe, or earlobe. The light-emitting diodes are typically placed directly *across* a pulsatile tissue bed from the photodetectors, also located within the probe. The photodetectors capture the red and infrared light after they have traversed the pulsatile tissue bed. Oxygenated hemoglobin absorbs very little red light but large amounts of infrared light. Conversely, deoxygenated hemoglobin absorbs a large amount of red but very little infrared light. A microprocessor determines the relative absorption of red and infrared light and then calculates the relative amount (percent) of oxygenated versus deoxygenated hemoglobin present in the pulsatile tissue bed. Pulse oximeters also indicate the pulse rate, and alarms may be set to signal low or high heart rate.

Use and Maintenance of the Pulse Oximeter

The pulse oximeter requires no calibration and little maintenance. However, care must be taken to use the oximeter processor and probe as specified by the manufacturer. Probes should be used *only* with the oximeter processor from the *same* manufacturer. Use of probes from one manufacturer with oximeter processors from another manufacturer can result in equipment malfunction or excessive probe light intensity and patient burns.[86] Before the probe is placed, it should be inspected for signs of casing fracture; breaks in the casing also can produce burns of the skin under the probe.[86]

The pulse oximetry probe must be carefully placed so that the light-emitting diodes are directly across a pulsatile tissue bed from the photodetectors. A strong pulsatile signal must be present for accurate determination of hemoglobin saturation. Because methemoglobin and carboxyhemoglobin do not influence red or infrared light absorption, *most pulse oximeters do not accurately reflect total hemoglobin saturation in patients with methemoglobinemia or carbon monoxide poisoning.* For example, a child with carbon monoxide poisoning may have 20% carboxyhemoglobin, but the pulse oximeter may indicate a saturation of 97%. The pulse oximeter cannot distinguish normal from abnormal hemoglobins. The pulse oximeter indicates only the percentage of normal hemoglobin that is saturated with oxygen. Children with either methemoglobinemia or carbon monoxide poisoning require *laboratory measurement* of hemoglobin saturation using a co-oximeter to determine hemoglobin saturation.

Occasionally, intense ambient lighting can produce artifact during pulse oximetry. In this case, loose wrapping of the extremity in gauze may sufficiently eliminate the effects of the ambient light.

Movement artifact can interfere with accurate pulse oximetry monitoring. The more distal the placement of the probe, the more susceptible it will be to movement artifact. When the probe is placed on a fingertip or toe, slight movement may interfere with pulse oximetry. Movement of the probe to the edge of the hand or foot may reduce this artifact.

The commercially available pulse oximeters vary widely in their response times to the development of hypoxemia.[87,88] A delay may occur between the onset of hypoxemia in the patient and a decrease in displayed hemoglobin saturation by the pulse oximeter. Therefore the hemoglobin saturation determined by pulse oximetry should always be evaluated in light of the patient's clinical condition. If the patient's clinical condition deteriorates, hypoxemia may be present even if it is not yet reflected by the pulse oximeter. Whenever pulse oximetry estimations are in question, evaluation of arterial oxygenation through arterial blood gas analysis may be necessary.

CONCLUSIONS

The principles of hemodynamic monitoring in children are virtually the same as those in adults. However, pediatric patients have more rapid heart rates and lower arterial blood pressures and absolute lower cardiac outputs than do adults. It is important to detect small changes in the cardiovascular function of these small patients. Because trending of hemodynamic data is more important than any single measurement, it is essential that each member of the health care team perform the measurements in exactly the same way so that errors can be standardized or eliminated.

REFERENCES

1. Hazinski MF, editor: *Manual of pediatric critical care,* St Louis, 1999, Mosby.
2. Heymann MA: Fetal and neonatal circulation. In Adams FH, Emmanouilides GC, Riemenschneider TA, editors: *Moss' heart disease in infants, children, and adolescents,* ed 4, Baltimore, 1989, Williams & Wilkins.
3. Rudolph AM, Heymann MA: Cardiac output in the fetal lamb: the effects of spontaneous and induced changes of heart rate on right and left ventricular output, *Am J Obstet Gynecol* 124:183, 1976.
4. Lister G et al: Oxygen delivery in lambs; cardiovascular and hematologic development, *Am J Physiol* 237:H668, 1979.
5. Teitel DF: Circulatory adjustments to postnatal life, *Semin Perinatol* 12:96, 1988.
6. Rudolph AM: Cardiac catheterization and angiocardiography. In Rudolph AM, editor: *Congenital diseases of the heart,* Chicago, 1974, Year Book.
7. Schrieber MD, Heymann MA, Soifer SJ: Increased arterial pH, not decreased $Paco_2$ attenuates hypoxia-induced pulmonary vasoconstriction in newborn lambs, *Pediatr Res* 20:113, 1986.
8. Barnea O, Austin EH, Richman B, et al: Balancing the circulation: theoretic optimization of pulmonary/systemic flow ratio in hypoplastic left heart syndrome, *J Am Coll Cardiol* 24:1376, 1994.
9. Chang AC et al: Pulmonary vascular resistance in infants after cardiac surgery: role of carbon dioxide and hydrogen ion, *Crit Care Med* 23:568, 1995.
10. Reddy VM et al: fetal model of single ventricle physiology; hemodynamic effects of oxygen, nitric oxide, carbon dioxide and hypoxia in the early postnatal period, *J Thorac Cardiovasc Surg* 112:437, 1996.
11. Riordan CH et al: Effects of oxygen, positive end-expiratory pressure, and carbon dioxide on oxygen delivery in an animal model of the univentricular heart, *J Thorac Cardiovasc Surg* 112:644, 1996.
12. Riordan CJ et al: Monitoring systemic venous oxygen saturations in the hypoplastic left heart syndrome, *Ann Thorac Surg* 63(3):835, 1997.
13. Kinsella JP et al: Selective and sustained pulmonary vasodilation with inhalational nitric oxide therapy in a child with idiopathic pulmonary hypertension, *J Pediatr* 122:803, 1993.
14. Shine N et al: Hypoxic gas therapy using nitrogen in the preoperative management of neonates with hypoplastic left heart syndrome, *Pediatr Crit Care Med* 1:38, 2000.
15. Rudolph AM: *Congenital diseases of the heart,* Chicago, 1974, Year Book.
16. Riemenschneider TA, Brenner RA, Mason DT: Maturational changes in myocardial contractile state of newborn lambs, *Pediatr Res* 15:349, 1981.
17. Aherne W, Hull D: Brown adipose tissue and heat production in the newborn infant, *J Pathol Bacteriol* 91:223, 1966.

18. Chameides L, Hazinski MF, Nadkarni V, editors: *Textbook of pediatric advanced life support,* ed 2, Dallas, 1997, American Heart Association.
19. Hazinski MF: Children are different. In Hazinski MF, editor: *Nursing care of the critically ill child,* ed 2, St Louis, 1992, Mosby.
20. Perloff WH: Physiology of the heart and circulation. In Swedlow DB, Raphaely RC, editors: *Cardiovascular problems in pediatric critical care,* vol 10, *Clinics in critical care medicine,* New York, 1986, Churchill Livingstone.
21. Fanaroff AA, Martin RJ: *Neonatal-perinatal medicine,* ed 6, St Louis, 1997, Mosby.
22. Rackow EC et al: Fluid resuscitation in circulatory shock: a comparison of the cardiorespiratory effects of albumin, hetastarch, and saline solutions in patients with hypovolemic and septic shock, *Crit Care Med* 11:839, 1983.
23. Packman MI, Rackow EC: Optimum left heart filling pressure during fluid resuscitation of patients with hypovolemic and septic shock, *Crit Care Med* 11:156, 1983.
24. Hazinski MF, Barkin RM: Shock. In Barkin RM, editor-in-chief: *Pediatric emergency medicine: concepts and clinical practice,* St Louis, 1992, Mosby.
25. Carcillo JA, Davis AL, Zaritsky A: Role of early fluid resuscitation in pediatric septic shock, *JAMA* 266:1242, 1991.
26. Graham TP et al: Right ventricular volume determinations in children: normal values and observations with volume or pressure overload, *Circulation* 47:144, 1973.
27. Meyer RA: Echocardiography. In Adams FH, Emmanouilides GC, Riemenschneider TA, editors: *Moss' heart disease in infants, children, and adolescents,* ed 4, Baltimore, 1989, Williams & Wilkins.
28. Hazinski MF: Cardiovascular disorders. In Hazinski MF, editor: *Nursing care of the critically ill child,* ed 2, St Louis, 1992, Mosby.
29. Clyman RI et al: How a patent ductus arteriosus affects the premature lamb's ability to handle additional volume loads, *Pediatr Res* 22:531, 1987.
30. Eisenberg M, Bergner L, Halstrom A: Epidemiology of cardiac arrest and resuscitation in children, *Ann Emerg Med* 12:672, 1983.
31. Walsh CK, Krongard E: Terminal cardiac electrical activity in pediatric patients, *Am J Cardiol* 51:557, 1983.
32. Coffing CR, Quan L, Graves JR, et al: Etiologies and outcomes of the pulseless, nonbreathing pediatric patient presenting with ventricular fibrillation, *Ann Emerg Med* 21:1046, 1992 (abstract).
33. Hazinski MF et al: Outcome of cardiovascular collapse in pediatric blunt trauma, *Ann Emerg Med* 23:1229, 1994.
34. Chandra NC, Krischer JP: The demographics of cardiac arrest support "phone fast" for children, *Circulation* 88(suppl):I-193, 1994 (abstract).
35. Gillis J, Dickson D, Rieder M, et al: Results of inpatient pediatric resuscitation, *Crit Care Med* 14:469, 1986.
36. Perkin RM, Levin DL: Shock in the pediatric patient. I, *J Pediatr* 101:163, 1982.

37. Hazinski MF: Hemodynamic monitoring of children. In Daily EK, Schroeder J, editors: *Techniques in bedside hemodynamic monitoring,* ed 5, St Louis, 1994, Mosby.

38. Hazinski MF: Nursing care of the critically ill child: the 7-point check, *Pediatr Nurs* 11:453, 1985.

39. Hazinski MF: Shock in the pediatric patient, *Crit Care Nurs Clin North Am* 2:309, 1990.

40. Gorlick MH, Shaw KN, Maker EM: Effect of ambient temperature on capillary refill in healthy children, *Pediatrics* 92:699, 1993.

41. ACCP/SCCM Consensus Conference Committee, American College of Chest Physicians/Society of Critical Care Medicine Consensus Conference: Definitions for sepsis and organ failure and guidelines for the use of innovative therapies in sepsis, *Crit Care Med* 20:864, 1992.

42. Hazinski MF, Iberti TJ, MacIntyre NR, et al: Epidemiology, pathophysiology, and clinical presentation of gram-negative sepsis, *Am J Crit Care* 2:224, 1993.

43. Weil MH, Michaels S, Rackow EC: Comparison of blood lactate concentrations in central venous, pulmonary artery and arterial blood, *Crit Care Med* 15:489, 1987.

44. Rabinovitch M, Reid LM: Quantitative structural analysis of the pulmonary vascular bed in congenital heart defects. In Engle MA, editor: *Pediatric cardiovascular disease,* vol 11, *Cardiovascular clinics,* Philadelphia, 1981, FA Davis.

45. Hoffman JIE, Heymann MA: The normal pulmonary circulation. In Scarpelli EM, editor: *Pulmonary physiology of the fetus, newborn, and child,* Philadelphia, 1989, Lea & Febiger.

46. West JB, Dollery CT, Naimark A: Distribution of blood flow in isolated lung: relation to vascular and alveolar pressures, *J Appl Physiol* 19:713, 1964.

47. Philips JB, editor: Symposium on neonatal pulmonary hypertension, *Clin Perinatol* 11:1, 1984.

48. Dellinger RP et al: Effects of inhaled nitric oxide in patients with acute respiratory distress syndrome: results of a randomized phase II trial, *Crit Care Med* 26:15, 1996.

49. Demirakca SM et al: Inhaled nitric oxide in neonatal and pediatric acute respiratory distress syndrome: dose response, prolonged inhalation and weaning, *Crit Care Med* 24:1913, 1996.

50. Hoffman GM et al: Inhaled nitric oxide reduces the utilization of extracorporeal membrane oxygenation in persistent pulmonary hypertension of the newborn, *Crit Care Med* 15:352, 1997.

51. Mc Hugh J, Cheek DJ: Nitric oxide and regulation of vascular tone: pharmacologic and physiological considerations, *Am J Crit Care* 7:131, 1998.

52. Butt WW et al: Complications resulting from use of arterial catheters: retrograde flow and rapid elevation in blood pressure, *Pediatrics* 76:250, 1985.

53. Task Force on Blood Pressure Control in Children: Report of the second task force on blood pressure in children, *Pediatrics* 79:1, 1987.

54. Carroll GC: Blood pressure monitoring, *Crit Care Clin* 4:411, 1988.

55. Park MK, Manard SM: Accuracy of blood pressure measurement by the Dinamap monitor in infants and children, *Pediatrics* 79:907, 1987.

56. Wareham JA et al: Prediction of arterial blood pressure in the premature neonate using the oscillometric method, *Am J Dis Child* 141:1108, 1987.

57. Diprose GK et al: Dinamap fails to detect hypotension in very low birthweight infants, *Arch Dis Child* 61:771, 1986.

58. Hazinski MF et al: Noninvasive blood pressure measurements overestimate arterial blood pressure in hypotensive adolescent. Unpublished manuscript, Vanderbilt University Children's Hospital, 1994.

59. Bull MJ, Schreiner RL, Garg BP, et al: Neurologic complications following temporal artery catheterization, *J Pediatr* 96:1071, 1980.

60. Guy RL et al: Limb shortening secondary to complications of vascular cannulae in the neonatal period, *Skeletal Radiol* 19:423, 1990.

61. Sellden H et al: Radial arterial catheters in children and neonates: a prospective study, *Crit Care Med* 15:1106, 1987.

62. Miyasaka K, Edmonds JF, Conn AW: Complications of radial artery lines in the paediatric patient, *Can Anaesth Soc J* 23:9, 1976.

63. Hack WW et al: Incidence and duration of total occlusion of the radial artery in newborn infants after catheter removal, *Eur J Pediatr* 149:275, 1990.

64. Butt WW et al: Effect of heparin concentration and infusion rate on the patency of arterial catheters, *Crit Care Med* 15:230, 1987.

65. Mozersky DJ, Buckley CJ, Hagood CO Jr, et al: Ultrasound evaluation of the palmar circulation: a useful adjunct to radial artery cannulation, *Am J Surg* 126:810, 1973.

66. Allen EV: Thromboangiitis obliterans: methods of diagnosis of chronic occlusive arterial lesions distal to the wrist with illustrative cases, *Am J Med Sci* 178:237, 1929.

67. Morray JP, Brandford HG, Barnes LF, et al: Doppler-assisted radial artery cannulation in infants and children, *Anesth Analg* 63:346, 1984.

68. Kamienski RW, Barnes RW: Critique of the Allen test for continuity of the palmar arch assessed by Doppler ultrasound, *Surg Gynecol Obstet* 142:861, 1976.

69. Damen J, Van Der Twell I: Positive tip cultures and related risk factors associated with intravascular catheterization in pediatric cardiac patients, *Crit Care Med* 16:221, 1988.

70. Byington K: Guidelines for central venous catheter maintenance [Appendix]. In Hazinski MF, editor: *Nursing care of the critically ill child,* ed 2, St Louis, 1992, Mosby.

71. Nicolson SC et al: Comparison of internal and external jugular cannulation of the central circulation in the pediatric patient, *Crit Care Med* 13:747, 1985.

72. Thompson AE: Pulmonary artery catheterization in children, *New Horiz* 5:244, 1997.

73. Introna RP et al: Percutaneous pulmonary artery catheterization in pediatric cardiovascular anesthesia: insertion techniques and use, *Anesth Analg* 70:562, 1990.

74. Connors AF Jr, Speroff T, Dawson NV, et al: The effectiveness of right heart catheterization in the initial care of critically ill patients, *JAMA* 276:889, 1996.

75. Pulmonary Artery Catheter Consensus Conference Participants: Pulmonary artery catheter consensus conference: consensus statement, *Crit Care Med* 25:910, 1997.

76. Bernard GR et al: Pulmonary artery catheterization and clinical outcomes: National Heart, Lung and Blood Institute and Food and Drug Administration Workshop Report, *JAMA* 283:2568, 2000.

77. Iberti TJ, Daily EK, Leibowitz AB, and others: Assessment of critical care nurses' knowledge of the pulmonary artery catheter, *Crit Care Med* 22:1674, 1994.

78. Gnaegi A, Feihl F, Perret C: Intensive care physicians' insufficient knowledge of right-heart catheterization at the bedside, *Crit Care Med* 25:213, 1997.

79. Krafte-Jacobs B, Sivit CJ, Mejia R, and others: Catheter-related thrombosis in critically ill children: comparison of catheters with and without heparin bonding, *J Pediatr* 126:50, 1995.

80. Damen J, Wever JEAT: The use of balloon-tipped pulmonary artery catheters in children undergoing cardiac surgery, *Intensive Care Med* 13:266, 1987.

81. Kadota L: Theory and application of the thermodilution cardiac output measurement: a review, *Heart Lung* 14:605, 1985.

82. Renner LE, Morton MJ, Sakuma GY: Indicator amount, temperature, and intrinsic cardiac output affect thermodilution cardiac output accuracy and reproducibility, *Crit Care Med* 21:586, 1993.

83. White KM et al: The physiologic basis for continuous mixed venous oxygen saturation monitoring, *Heart Lung* 19:548, 1990.

84. Nelson LD: Continuous monitoring of O_2 saturation, *Chest* 96:956, 1989.

85. Fahey JT, Lister G: Oxygen transport in low cardiac output states, *J Crit Care* 2:288, 1987.

86. Sobel DB: Burning of a neonate due to a pulse oximeter: arterial saturation monitoring, *Pediatrics* 89:154, 1992.

87. Severinghaus JW, Naifeh KH: Accuracy of response of six pulse oximeters to profound hypoxia, *Anesthesiology* 67:551, 1987.

88. Verhoeff F, Sykes MK: Delayed detection of hypoxic events by pulse oximeters: computer simulations, *Anesthesia* 45:103, 1990.

20

ROBERT J. HENNING and GLORIA OBLOUK DAROVIC

Specific Monitoring Considerations for Patients with Cardiac Disease

Cardiovascular disease is the leading cause of death in the industrialized world. Despite major advances in diagnostic and therapeutic methods, approximately 900,000 people die annually from cardiovascular disease in the United States. People with chronic disorders of the heart and blood vessels commonly have major disabilities and impaired lifestyles. The physical, emotional, and financial toll that acute and chronic cardiovascular disease extracts from society is of enormous proportion.

Normal cardiac function is dependent on adequate oxygen supply/demand balance, preload, afterload, contractile state of the myocardium, and heart rate. Acute or chronic heart disease changes the response of the heart to these factors because disease alters the type and magnitude of cardioadaptive responses. This chapter discusses the clinical and monitoring implications of altered cardioadaptive responses that occur in patients with heart disease or failure.

Ischemic heart disease, valvular heart disease, and cardiomyopathy are presented in the next three chapters. In general, the clinical picture of patients with heart disease is dependent on the amount of cardiac reserve. In patients with little or no cardiac reserve, minor cardiac or other organ system problems can be associated with significant circulatory compromise. Consideration of this fact and of the altered dynamics of cardiac function is of paramount importance in the evaluation and management of patients with cardiovascular disease.

FACTORS AFFECTING CARDIAC FUNCTION AND STROKE VOLUME

The factors that may profoundly affect heart function, particularly in patients with cardiovascular disease, include the myocardial oxygen supply and demand balance; preload; afterload; contractile state of the myocardium; coordinated pattern of ventricular contraction (muscular synchrony); and heart rate. These factors are discussed next.

Myocardial Oxygen Supply and Demand

Myocardial oxygen supply must equal or exceed demand to maintain myocardial contractile force and normal ventricular function. In other words, normal myocardial contractility is directly dependent on adequate oxygen availability. Oxygen deprivation to a portion of the myocardium decreases contractility. Depending on the severity of oxygen deprivation, the involved myocardium may become weakly contractile (hypokinetic); may become noncontractile (akinetic); or may move in a direction opposite the surrounding, normally contracting, myocardium (dyskinetic). The metabolic changes in myocardial cells that produce these functional abnormalities occur within 30 to 60 seconds of the reduction in oxygenated blood supply. The wall motion abnormalities may be localized to a specific area or may involve the entire ventricle. Localized or generalized coronary hypoperfusion or severely decreased arterial oxygen content

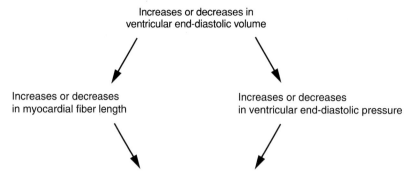

FIGURE 20-1 Schematic representation of the relationship between ventricular end-diastolic volume, myocardial fiber length, end-diastolic pressure, and stroke volume assuming normal ventricular compliance.

therefore causes the heart to become a less efficient pump and may cause electrical instability.

Many patients with cardiovascular disease due to cardiomyopathy and valvular, hypertensive, and coronary artery disease have some degree of cardiac dysfunction but may not have functional disability. However, patients with compensated cardiovascular disease can deteriorate into acute, and often life-threatening, heart failure because of focal or global myocardial hypoxia if their cardiovascular system is stressed by (1) increased oxygen demands due to tachyarrhythmias, hypertension, exercise, trauma, anemia, sepsis, or pregnancy or (2) decreased oxygen supply due to a significant drop in blood pressure or a coronary artery lesion that obstructs blood flow. Most therapeutic interventions for patients with cardiovascular disease, such as vasodilating and inotropic drugs, supplemental oxygen administration, and intraaortic balloon pumping, are directed toward bringing cardiac oxygen supply and demand into a more favorable balance.

Preload

Preload refers to the amount of stretch on myocardial muscle fibers at end-diastole, which is determined by the amount of ventricular end-diastolic (also termed *filling*) volume. According to Starling's law of the heart, increased myofibrillar stretch, within physiologic limits, causes a more forceful contraction and therefore a greater stroke volume. In other words, *the larger the ventricular filling volume (cardiac input), the greater the stroke volume (cardiac output); the smaller the ventricular filling volume, the smaller the cardiac output.*

Myocardial fiber length is impossible to measure at the bedside. In the normal heart, however, ventricular muscle fiber length is proportional to the end-diastolic volume, which correlates well with the hemodynamically monitored end-diastolic pressure in normal individuals (Figure 20-1).

Ventricular filling pressures are estimated at the bedside by monitoring pulmonary artery wedge pressure (PWP) for the left ventricle and right atrium or central venous pressure (CVP) for the right ventricle. The preload relationship between left ventricular diastolic volume (as inferred by PWP) and stroke volume is graphically illustrated in the ventricular function curve (Figure 20-2, A).

As shown in Figure 20-2, in the normal left ventricle (over a left ventricular end-diastolic pressure range of 4 to 12 mm Hg), relatively large increases in stroke volume and cardiac output occur with small increases in ventricular filling pressure. Maximal preload-dependent ventricular performance is attained in normal individuals when an end-diastolic blood volume is associated with a PWP of approximately 8 to 10 mm Hg. Beyond this preload level, ventricular performance in the healthy heart no longer increases but rather plateaus. The preload characteristics in the diseased heart differ from those in the normal heart. Understanding these differences is essential to good patient management, particularly in the intensive care unit. These differences include the following.

Decreased Preload Reserve

The normal heart has a large preload reserve to meet the demands of life's activities that vary from rest to strenuous exercise and can also tolerate hypovolemia relatively well. Patients with severe heart failure have very little cardiac reserve. Large *increases in preload* produce only small increases in stroke volume. The ventricular function curve in such a patient is significantly depressed and can be flattened (Figure 20-2, *B*). In fact, severely failing, dilated hearts may have no preload reserve because their muscle fibers at rest are chronically maximally stretched

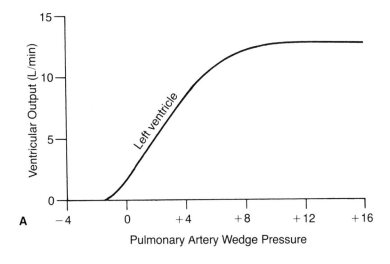

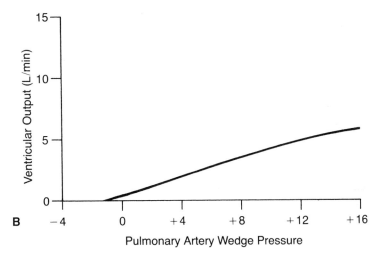

FIGURE 20-2 A, Peak left ventricular performance is attained with a level of preload, as measured by pulmonary artery wedge pressure (PWP), of 8 to 10mm Hg in a patient with known coronary artery disease, no myocardial ischemia, and baseline normal ventricular function. A PWP of 4 mm Hg still produces a cardiac output that is acceptable under a varied range of activities. **B,** In the same patient during an acute ischemic attack, the sudden onset of left ventricular dysfunction and decreased compliance acutely alters the ventricular function curve so that a PWP of 16 mm Hg is required to optimize left ventricular performance. Note that even at this level of preload, maximal cardiac output is far less than that under normal circumstances and may be inadequate for many activities.

to their peak performance. If the venous return and ventricular filling are increased, such hearts are unable to respond with greater force of contraction. In affected patients, any stress may precipitate sudden onset or worsening of heart failure.

On the other hand, *decreases in preload* may also have disastrous cardiovascular consequences in patients with a diseased ventricle. For example, a diseased left ventricle typically requires a greater than normal ventricular filling volume to maintain stroke volume. In patients with severe heart failure, stroke volume may be subnormal despite a PWP greater than 20 mm Hg. In such patients, even small reductions in preload due to diuresis, vasodilator drugs, hemorrhage, or third-space fluid shifts may be associated with significant reductions in stroke volume and consequent systemic hypotension.

Effects of Preload on Ventricular Transmural Perfusion Pressure

Perfusion of ventricular muscle is directly dependent on the difference (gradient) between systemic arterial diastolic pressure and ventricular end-diastolic pressure.

Large increases in PWP, such as those in left ventricular failure, or decreases in blood pressure will therefore reduce the perfusion pressure across the ventricular wall and compromise myocardial blood flow (Figure 20-3).

Systemic hypotension is particularly dangerous to patients with severe coronary artery disease because coronary flow reserve is compromised or may be absent.

Hemodynamic Effects of Changes in Ventricular Compliance

Acute or chronic changes in ventricular compliance (wall stiffness, distensibility) alter the ventricular filling volume/pressure relationship (Box 20-1). These changes have important hemodynamic and monitoring implications.

In patients with decreased compliance (increased wall stiffness) due to myocardial ischemia or fibrosis, small increases in venous return and ventricular filling may produce disproportionately large increases in ventricular end-diastolic pressure. In this instance, the stiff cardiac ventricle cannot yield to accommodate an increase in blood volume.

If venous return and ventricular filling volume remain constant, a sudden decrease in ventricular compliance due to acute myocardial ischemia is associated with an acute increase in end-diastolic pressure. Therefore an acute increase in PWP, in the absence of a fluid challenge or the administration of vasopressor drugs, is an early indication of left ventricular ischemia and often occurs before

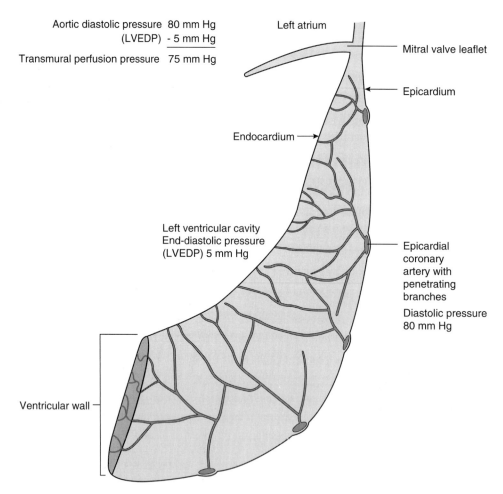

Aortic diastolic pressure 80 mm Hg
(LVEDP) - 5 mm Hg
_____
Transmural perfusion pressure 75 mm Hg

Left atrium

Mitral valve leaflet

Epicardium

Endocardium

Left ventricular cavity
End-diastolic pressure
(LVEDP) 5 mm Hg

Epicardial coronary artery with penetrating branches

Diastolic pressure 80 mm Hg

Ventricular wall

FIGURE 20-3 The transmyocardial pressure gradient. This schematic illustrates that the volume of left ventricular myocardial blood flow is dependent on the transmyocardial pressure gradient—that is, the difference between the arterial diastolic pressure and the left ventricular end-diastolic pressure (PWP). A decrease in arterial diastolic pressure or an increase in left ventricular end-diastolic pressure may reduce myocardial perfusion by narrowing the pressure gradient.

electrocardiographic ST segment changes or patient complaints of chest pain (Figure 20-4).

In general, patients with noncompliant ventricles may have a normal ventricular end-diastolic volume, but the measured end-diastolic pressure (PWP and CVP for the left and right ventricles, respectively) is disproportionately and deceptively high. The stiff muscle fibers, however, are highly dependent on ventricular filling volume to produce adequate myofibrillar stretch at end-diastole. Consequently, a noncompliant heart is very sensitive to decreases in venous return, and mild hypovolemia may produce significant decreases in stroke volume. In contrast, patients with nonischemic dilated cardiomyopathy may have *decreased* wall stiffness, and a larger than normal end-diastolic volume may be associated with a disproportionately low end-diastolic pressure.

Increases in Preload Increase Myocardial Oxygen Requirements

As the radius of the ventricle increases, more systolic tension must be developed by each muscle fiber to produce and maintain a given peak systolic pressure according to the law of LaPlace. Because myocardial oxygen requirements rise in proportion to systolic wall tension, ventricular dilation directly increases myocardial oxygen consumption.

Cardiomegaly is the hallmark of systolic heart failure. As the ventricle dilates and fails, stroke volume decreases, while end-systolic and diastolic volumes, cardiac chamber dimensions, systolic and diastolic wall tension, and myocardial oxygen requirements increase. The greater the increase in tension that the failing, dilated ventricle must

---

BOX 20-1
Factors That Alter Ventricular Compliance

Decreased Compliance

Ventricular hypertrophy
Myocardial fibrosis
Infiltrative disease
Pericardial tamponade
Pericardial constrictive disease
Disease or dilation of the contralateral ventricle
Advanced age
Hypoxia
Ventricular ischemia
Acidosis

Increased Compliance

Ventricular dilation
Any drug that significantly decreases ventricular diastolic pressure ultimately alters ventricular compliance (e.g., nitroglycerin, calcium antagonists)

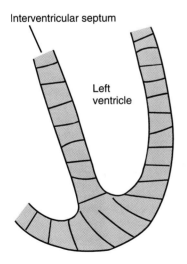
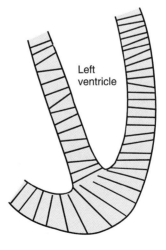

A Normal compliance
End-diastolic volume 120 ml
End-diastolic pressure 8 mm Hg

B Reduced compliance
End-diastolic volume 120 ml
End-diastolic pressure 18 mm Hg

FIGURE 20-4 Effect of decreased compliance on left ventricular end-diastolic pressure as measured by PWP. **A,** A normal left ventricular end-diastolic volume of approximately 120 ml is associated with an end-diastolic pressure of 8 mm Hg. **B,** With the advent of an ischemic-induced reduction in ventricular compliance (illustrated by decreased cavity size and denser myocardial fibers), an identical end-diastolic volume may be associated with an end-diastolic pressure of 18 mm Hg.

BOX 20-2
Effect of Preload on Ventricular Function and Myocardial Oxygen Requirements

Increased Preload
Increased stroke volume
Increased ventricular work
Increased myocardial oxygen requirements

Decreased Preload
Decreased stroke volume
Decreased ventricular work
Decreased myocardial oxygen requirements

BOX 20-3
Effect of Afterload on Ventricular Function and Myocardial Oxygen Requirements

Increased Afterload
Increased ventricular work
Increased myocardial oxygen requirements
Decreased stroke volume

Decreased Afterload
Decreased ventricular work
Decreased myocardial oxygen requirements
Increased stroke volume

---

develop during systole, the greater the decrease in the rate of ventricular muscle fiber shortening and the velocity of ejection. This further limits the failing ventricle's ability to eject blood.

In summary, ventricular dilation due to heart failure may significantly increase myocardial work and oxygen consumption and further reduce stroke volume (Box 20-2).

The important clinical point of the preceding discussion is that the filling *volume* of the ventricle, not the filling *pressure,* affects muscle fiber length and the quantity of blood the ventricle ejects. As a result of changes in ventricular compliance or contractility imposed by cardiac disease, each patient has an optimal point on the ventricular function curve. It is at this point that stroke volume is maximized at a particular end-diastolic pressure. This particular "number," which is appropriate for the patient's condition, may not be within the standard normal range, which is 4 to 12 mm Hg for the left ventricle and 0 to 8 mm Hg for the right ventricle. In other words, *the standard hemodynamic measurements (which are derived from healthy humans) may not be optimal or even marginally acceptable measurements for critically ill or injured patients.* In addition, an optimal or acceptable "number" may suddenly change in the same patient—in response to acute pathophysiologic alterations in the myocardium or because of therapeutic correction of these alterations (see Figure 20-2).

The effect of preload on stroke volume is therefore an important consideration in managing acutely ill patients, particularly those with cardiovascular disease. By serially assessing preload and its relationship to stroke volume and constructing a pressure/volume Starling curve, a patient's optimal level of stroke volume and cardiac output can be determined. In patients who are

volume overloaded, preload reduction with diuretics or vasodilator drugs, with resultant decrease in ventricular radius, may be associated with a decrease in myocardial oxygen requirements.

Afterload

Afterload is the sum of all the forces against which the myocardial fibers must shorten during systole. These loads include the aortic diastolic pressure, systemic vascular resistance, intraventricular pressure, and mass and viscosity of blood in the aorta and great arteries. For the left ventricle, outflow resistance is imposed primarily by aortic diastolic pressure and systemic vascular resistance. The corresponding factors for the right ventricle are pulmonary artery diastolic pressure and pulmonary vascular resistance. If the impedance to ventricular ejection is increased, ejection velocity and stroke volume can fall while ventricular work and oxygen consumption proportionately rise. Conversely, if impedance to ejection is reduced, ejection velocity and stroke volume increase and heart work and oxygen consumption decrease (Box 20-3).

Diseased ventricles are exquisitely sensitive to abrupt changes in afterload; the greater the baseline ventricular dysfunction, the more sensitive the ventricle is to sudden changes in afterload. Applied clinically, vasopressors used to treat hypotension may increase blood pressure by increasing systemic vascular resistance. However, because of the increased afterload, heart work and myocardial oxygen consumption rise while stroke volume and systemic blood flow may actually fall.

Conversely, arterial vasodilators help "open the door" to ventricular ejection by decreasing aortic impedance and systemic vascular resistance. Stroke volume and systemic blood flow may increase while heart work and myocardial oxygen consumption fall. By the careful administration of vasodilator drugs, right and left ventricular performance may be optimized through evaluation and manipulation of pulmonary artery and aortic diastolic pressures, as well as pulmonary and systemic vascular resistance.

Contractile (Inotropic) State of the Myocardium

Stroke volume, heart work, and myocardial oxygen consumption increase or decrease with proportionate increases or decreases in the force and velocity of myocardial contraction. Inotropy is affected by the presence and severity of disease, drugs, and autonomic nervous system effects.

Ischemic heart disease, cardiomyopathy, and negative inotropic agents, such as beta blockers in large doses, reduce contractility. In this instance, myocardial oxygen consumption and stroke volume decrease and the Starling function curve can be shifted downward and to the right.

Negative inotropic agents are frequently used to reduce myocardial oxygen demands and the frequency and severity of anginal attacks. The price paid for the reduction in oxygen demand, however, may be a reduction in cardiac output. Therefore patients treated with negative inotropic agents must be carefully monitored to ensure that the reduction in cardiac output does not exceed the reductions in myocardial oxygen consumption and myocardial ischemia.

Stimulation of the sympathetic nervous system or administration of potent positive inotropic agents increases the force and velocity of myocardial contraction and stroke volume. As a consequence, the Starling function curve is shifted upward and to the left. In patients with occlusive coronary artery disease, the concomitant increase in myocardial work and oxygen consumption may precipitate an acute ischemic episode and may require discontinuation of the positive inotropic drug. An increase in myocardial contractility also may predispose the patient with a hypertrophic heart to ischemia because the blood supply may be inadequate for the augmented oxygen requirements of the increased muscle mass.

Pattern of Ventricular Contraction

The normal left ventricular contractile pattern is a globally inward movement. This is termed *normal muscular synergy.* Uncoordinated ventricular contraction, termed *dyssynergy,* may seriously impair pump function and cardiac output and may waste contractile energy. Causes of uncoordinated ventricular contraction include (1) regional ventricular wall motion abnormalities due to ischemic disease, aneurysm, or trauma; (2) abnormal sequence of ventricular depolarization due to ventricular ectopic beats or abnormalities in electrical

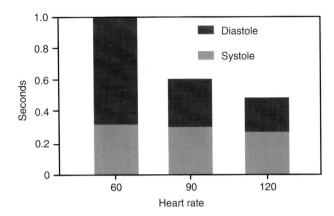

FIGURE 20-5 Changing systolic/diastolic time ratio with increases in heart rate. Note that as heart rate increases, diastole becomes progressively shortened and systole occupies more of the cardiac cycle.

conduction secondary to bundle branch blocks; and (3) marked ventricular fibrosis and dilation.

Heart Rate

Healthy hearts tolerate wide ranges of heart rate without hemodynamic compromise. In patients with severe acute or chronic heart disease, abrupt or sustained changes in heart rate may result in severe hemodynamic compromise.

For example, if the patient's ability to increase stroke volume is limited by myocardial fibrosis or heart failure, *bradycardia* may be associated with severe reductions in cardiac output. Circulatory failure may also occur if venous return is reduced because of hypovolemia or administration of venodilator agents and the patient cannot appropriately increase the heart rate (sinus node ischemia, beta-adrenergic receptor blockade, heart block).

Tachyarrhythmias are particularly threatening to patients with cardiac disease. As the heart rate increases, ventricular diastolic filling, cardiac output, and coronary blood flow are reduced (Figure 20-5). With arrhythmias associated with loss of the atrial contribution to ventricular filling, an additional 10% to 30% decrease in ventricular filling occurs.

Increases in heart rate also cause proportionate increases in myocardial oxygen demand. In people with a normal coronary circulation, the coronary arteries easily dilate to allow increased blood flow proportionate to the metabolic needs of a heart stressed by exercise, fever, seizure activity, or shivering. However, a severely diseased coronary circulation cannot dilate to accommodate increased flow demands. Acute myocardial ischemia may result. Overall, the rapidly beating diseased heart requires more oxygen but paradoxically may be getting less. Therefore, *tachyarrhythmias tend to ravage the ischemia-prone myocardium.*

In summary, changes in ventricular preload, afterload, contractile force, muscular synergy, and heart rate may produce significant hemodynamic deterioration or acute imbalances in myocardial oxygen supply and demand in patients with acute or chronic heart disease. Susceptible patients are thus predisposed to increased myocardial ischemia. In the clinical setting, myocardial ischemia may be the result of hypovolemia, loss of the atrial contribution to ventricular filling with resultant decrease in cardiac output (atrial fibrillation, ventricular demand pacing, ventricular ectopy), systemic or pulmonary hypertension, or emotional or physiologic stress. Only by treating the inciting event and instituting therapy to optimize ventricular performance can improved cardiac performance and tissue perfusion be achieved.

HEART FAILURE

Congestive heart failure is a major health problem worldwide. Approximately 400,000 new cases are diagnosed annually in the United States.[1] The 5-year mortality rate is 62% for women and 75% for men.[2] Most current medical and surgical therapies are only palliative.

Heart failure is a pathophysiologic condition in which the heart is unable to maintain an output of blood sufficient to meet the metabolic needs of the body. Any form of cardiovascular disease may be complicated by heart failure.

In some patients, the heart may be normal but the output of the heart may be inadequate if the metabolic needs of the body are abnormally high (malignant hyperthermia, thyroid storm). In these patients, the primary abnormality is metabolic.

Whether heart failure is due to primary disturbances in myocardial contractility, an excessive workload placed on the ventricle, or both, an extremely complex interplay of structural adaptive (ventricular hypertrophy, dilation, and remodeling), neurohumoral, and subcellular (molecular) adjustments ensue. Specific changes occur in the neurohumoral system, sympathetic nervous system, renin-angiotensin-aldosterone system, and vasopressin system activation. It is well beyond the scope of this chapter and purpose of this text to discuss these complex mechanisms. See references 3 through 6 for a more detailed description of these pathophysiologic adaptations.

Initially, these adaptive changes may maintain a compensated cardiovascular status. However, over time, if the underlying problem is not corrected, progressive deterioration in heart function occurs (Figure 20-6).

Although both ventricles share the interventricular septum, one ventricle typically fails before the other. The terms *left heart failure* and *right heart failure* are used to designate

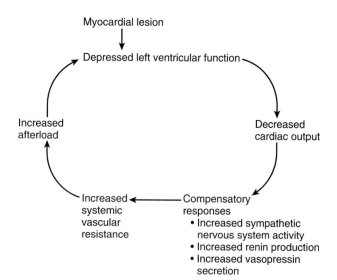

FIGURE 20-6 Self-perpetuating cycle of cardiac damage and heart failure.

the side of the heart that is primarily diseased or that produces the predominance of physical signs and symptoms.

Left Heart Failure

Heart failure most commonly begins with disease of the left ventricle due to damage or stress. This is because ischemic or valvular disease most frequently affects the left ventricle. Also, hypertension, which is epidemic in industrialized society, adversely affects the left ventricle.

Causes

Conditions that damage or distort the ventricular musculature, such as ischemic disease and cardiomyopathy, result in primary contractile failure. Left ventricular failure also may result from conditions that stress the normal left ventricle beyond its physiologic pumping capacity. Stress-induced failure may occur secondary to arterial pressure overload (severe systemic hypertension, aortic stenosis) or diastolic blood volume overload (severe aortic regurgitation).

Hemodynamic Effects and Clinical Presentation

The terms *systolic dysfunction* and *diastolic dysfunction* describe the dynamics of heart failure specific to the patient's condition and are used most commonly with reference to the left ventricle. One third of all patients with "heart failure" have primary diastolic dysfunction. However, left ventricular systolic and diastolic dysfunction more commonly occur together. See Box 20-4 for compar-

---

BOX 20-4

Causes, Hemodynamic Effects, and Signs and Symptoms of Systolic and Diastolic Dysfunction

Systolic Dysfunction

Common in Patients With
- Ischemic heart disease
- Dilated cardiomyopathy
- Myocardial contusion
- Severe aortic stenosis
- Chronic, severe aortic regurgitation
- Severe mitral regurgitation

Physical Characteristics
- Dilated, enlarged ventricle
- Large end-diastolic volume

Hemodynamic Characteristics
- Decreased ejection fraction
- Typically a decreased stroke volume
- Typically an increased ventricular end-diastolic pressure
- Possible vascular congestion proximal to failing ventricle
- Increased systemic vascular resistance

Signs and Symptoms
- Hypoperfusion of the circulation distal to the failing ventricle (forward components of failure)
- S_3 audible over the apex

Diastolic Dysfunction

Common in Patients With
- Ischemic heart disease
- Ventricular hypertrophy
- Cardiac tamponade
- Constrictive pericarditis
- Advanced age
- Advanced aortic stenosis (secondary to ventricular hypertrophy)

Physical Characteristics
- Thickened (hypertrophic) or stiff ventricular walls
- May have a normal ventricular end-diastolic volume

Hemodynamic Characteristics
- Impaired ventricular filling (noncompliant ventricle resists filling)
- Increased ventricular end-diastolic pressure
- Vascular congestion proximal to failing ventricle

Signs and Symptoms
- Volume/pressure overload of the cardiovascular structures proximal to the failing ventricle (congestive failure)
- S_4 audible

---

ison of the causes, hemodynamic effects, and signs and symptoms of systolic and diastolic dysfunction.

Systolic heart dysfunction is characterized primarily by failure of forward blood flow (decreasing stroke volume) and inadequate systemic perfusion. However, systolic failure also may also be associated with pulmonary vascular congestion and edema.

Diastolic heart dysfunction is characterized by a significant decrease in myocardial compliance and a "stiff" ventricle that resists filling. This commonly occurs in patients with myocardial ischemia or severe ventricular hypertrophy. Impaired left ventricular filling results in blood volume/pressure overload in the lungs. The clinical and hemodynamic abnormalities of left heart failure are further described as follows and are illustrated in Figure 20-7.

The signs and symptoms of *left ventricular systolic dysfunction* can be related to specific organ systems. Subnormal perfusion to the gastrointestinal tract is manifest clinically and pathologically as anorexia, nausea and indigestion, and poor absorption of nutrients; in the kidneys

as salt and water retention; in the skin as pallor and cool extremities; and in skeletal muscle as weakness, fatigue, and exercise intolerance. In response to a decrease in cardiac output, the systemic arterioles constrict. Compensatory systemic vasoconstriction helps maintain mean aortic pressure and cerebral and coronary blood flow; however, perfusion to less vital organs is diminished. In a patient with severe left ventricular systolic failure, systemic blood flow may be so severely impaired that the patient develops cardiogenic shock.

The signs and symptoms of *left ventricular diastolic dysfunction* are related to the passive accumulation of blood in the pulmonary circulation due to impaired ventricular filling. This results in increased pulmonary capillary hydrostatic pressures (which correlate with PWP) greater than 18 to 20 mm Hg. The elevated pulmonary intravascular pressures result in extravasion of fluid into the lungs. Pulmonary edema is clinically manifested as tachypnea, dyspnea, cough, hypoxia, and auscultatory crackles and wheezes.

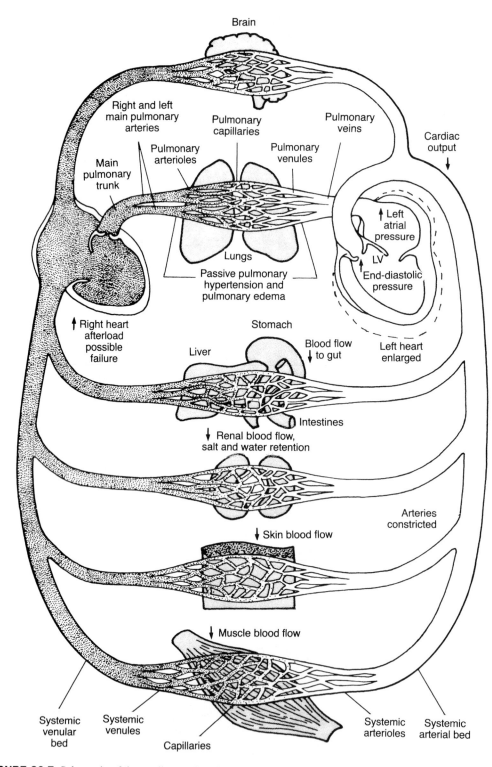

FIGURE 20-7 Schematic of the cardiovascular circuit in left heart failure. Cardiac output is decreased, resulting in decreased systemic perfusion. Pulmonary vascular congestion and hypertension can result from the decrease in forward blood flow.

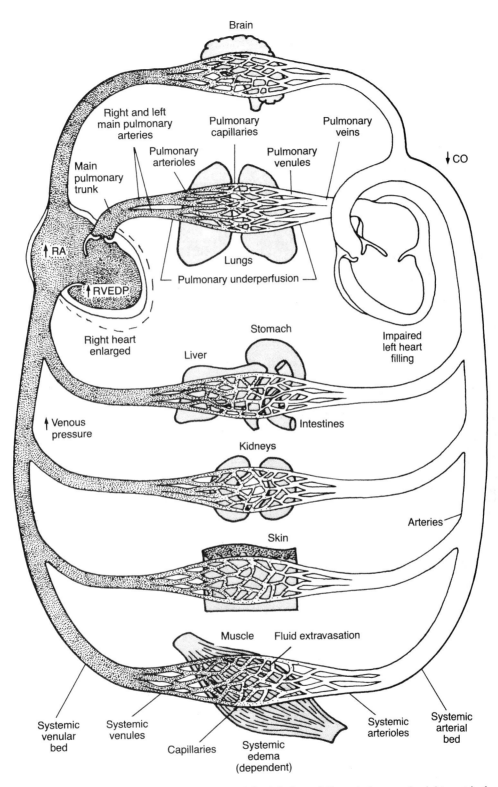

FIGURE 20-8 Schematic of the cardiovascular circuit in right heart failure. A decrease in right ventricular output results in venous congestion and hypertension, causing edema, which is most evident in the lower extremities. A corresponding decrease in pulmonary blood flow, left heart filling, and cardiac output may also occur.

Higher right ventricular systolic pressures are required to propel blood through the volume-loaded, high-pressure pulmonary circuit. When right ventricular afterload exceeds the physiologic reserve of the right ventricle, the right ventricle fails. The signs and symptoms of pulmonary edema may then *decrease* because the volume of blood entering the pulmonary circuit decreases. As a consequence, the pulmonary circulation is partially unloaded and fluid extravasation into the lungs diminishes.

Right Heart Failure

Right ventricular failure may occur because of increased pulmonary artery pressures secondary to left heart failure or primary disease of the lung such as massive pulmonary embolism, idiopathic pulmonary hypertension, or pulmonary hypertension due to chronic obstructive lung disease. In these diseases, pulmonary hypertension increases the systolic work of the right ventricle, which fails when stressed beyond its physiologic capacity. Right heart failure also may result from damage to the right ventricular myocardium because of ischemia, cardiomyopathy, or right ventricular contusion. In general, left heart failure is the most common cause of right heart failure. The hemodynamic and clinical abnormalities are illustrated in Figure 20-8.

The signs and symptoms of right heart failure are due to systemic venous congestion and elevated venous pressures as blood passively accumulates in the structures in back of the failing right ventricle. The internal jugular veins become visibly distended. The liver becomes engorged with blood, enlarged, tender, and variably compromised. Manual compression of the liver often results in distention of the internal jugular veins (the hepatojugular reflux). Extravasation of fluid from engorged venules and capillaries results in abdominal ascites and pitting, dependent edema. Decreased pulmonary perfusion results in decreased left ventricular filling and reductions in cardiac output.

Ventricular Interdependence

The right and left ventricles are part of a continuous, closed circulation. Consequently, in the absence of abnormal congenital shunts in the heart, the right or left ventricle cannot pump more or less blood than the other ventricle for any significant time. The right and left ventricles share a common pliable septum. Right ventricular failure can cause deviation of the interventricular septum into the left ventricle, and this deviation can significantly affect left ventricular dynamics. Because of the ventricular and anatomic interdependence, pure failure of one side of the heart will ultimately produce hemodynamic and anatomic abnormalities in the contralateral ventricle. This will result in biventricular failure.

CONCLUSION

A major concern underlying any cardiac disturbance or disease is that it will produce heart failure. Mild cardiac disease (valvular disease, a small myocardial infarction) not associated with heart failure is generally well tolerated, and the patient typically leads a normal lifestyle. The development of heart failure is typically associated with progressive disability, discomfort due to symptoms such as dyspnea, and shortened life expectancy. In fact, the development of heart failure in patients with severe aortic stenosis is a grave prognostic sign. Corrective measures for the underlying disease (e.g., valve surgery, myocardial revascularization) offer the greatest hope for the patient's survival. When correction is not possible, measures to preserve myocardial function, as well as early detection and treatment of heart failure, are essential to preserving the quality and quantity of the patient's life. Hemodynamic profiles of patients in right and left heart failure are described and illustrated in the sections relating to specific types of heart disease.

REFERENCES

1. Gillum RF: Epidemiology of heart failure in the United States, *Am Heart J* 126:1042, 1993.
2. Ho KKL, Anderson KM, Kannel WB, et al: Survival after the onset of congestive heart failure in Framingham Heart Study subjects, *Circulation* 88:107, 1993.
3. Antman EM, Braunwald E: Acute myocardial infarction. In *Heart disease: a textbook of cardiovascular medicine,* ed 6, Philadelphia, 2001, W.B. Saunders.
4. Cohn JN: Pathophysiology and clinical recognition of heart failure. In Willerson JT, Cohn JN, editors: *Cardiovascular medicine,* ed 2, New York, 2000, Churchill Livingstone.
5. Solomon SD, Pfeffer MA: The decreasing incidence of left ventricular remodeling following myocardial infarction, *Basic Res Cardiol* 92:61, 1997.
6. St John SM et al: Cardiovascular death and left ventricular remodeling two years after myocardial infarction: baseline predictors and impact of long-term use of captopril: information from the Survival And Ventricular Enlargement (SAVE) trial, *Circulation* 96:3294, 1997.

SUGGESTED READINGS

Alexander RW, Schlant RC, Fuster V: *Hurst's the heart,* ed 9, New York, 1998, McGraw-Hill.

Berne RM, Levy MN: *Cardiovascular physiology,* ed 7, St Louis, 1997, Mosby.

Braunwald E: *Heart disease,* ed 6, Philadelphia, 2001, W.B. Saunders.

Henning RJ, Grenvik A: *Critical care cardiology,* New York, 1989, Churchill Livingstone.

Pepine CJ, Hill JA, Lambert CR: *Diagnostic and therapeutic cardiac catheterization,* Baltimore, 1998, Williams & Wilkins.

21

ROBERT J.HENNING and GLORIA OBLOUK DAROVIC

Ischemic Heart Disease

Ischemic heart disease is characterized by changes in cardiac muscle that occur when coronary arterial oxygen supply significantly decreases below myocardial oxygen demand. Ischemic heart disease has a wide pathophysiologic and clinical spectrum. In some patients, the initial presentation may be primary ventricular fibrillation and sudden cardiac death. Acute myocardial infarction may be the first indication of ischemic heart disease in other patients. Still other patients develop angina pectoris, which warns them of the presence of significant obstructive coronary artery disease. Other groups of patients are relatively asymptomatic during their lives and are found incidentally at autopsy to have severe coronary artery disease while the cause of death is due to cancer, major infection, or trauma. This latter group may have experienced "silent ischemia" or "anginal equivalents" during their lives.

EPIDEMIOLOGY AND CAUSES

Ischemic heart disease resulting from coronary thrombosis and atherosclerosis is the most common cause of death in the industrialized world. Of the approximately 12 million people affected with the disease in the United States, approximately 500,000 die annually.[1] Coronary artery disease most often becomes clinically significant during middle age, with men being more vulnerable than premenopausal women. Following menopause, however, the incidence is nearly equal in both sexes. The major risk factors for ischemic heart disease include hypertension, diabetes mellitus, cigarette smoking, hyperlipidemia with increased concentrations of low-density lipoproteins and

triglycerides, and psychologic stress. Obesity and sedentary lifestyle have also been implicated.

Box 21-1 presents a summary of the causes of myocardial ischemia. Myocardial ischemic events most commonly result from atherosclerotic and thrombotic obstructive coronary artery disease, but ischemia also may be the result of coronary artery vasoconstriction due to spontaneous or drug-induced (cocaine, ergotamine) spasm. Myocardial ischemia also may occur due to severe hypoxemia due to pulmonary disease. Alternatively, ischemia may develop if a patient becomes hypotensive as a result of major blood loss, sepsis, or obstruction to blood flow due to massive pulmonary embolism, cardiac tamponade, or aortic dissection.

PATHOPHYSIOLOGY

Myocardial oxygen demands vary considerably depending on the person's emotions and activity. Figure 21-1 shows the myocardial oxygen supply/demand balance. The actual requirements of the myocardial cells for oxygen depend on the force of contractility, ventricular filling volume (preload), heart rate, and pressure work imposed on the heart (afterload). All are affected by physiologic and psychologic stress. Because the myocardium at rest normally extracts 70% to 80% of the oxygen from the coronary arterial blood, increased myocardial oxygen requirements *must* be met by appropriately increased coronary blood flow mediated by coronary vasodilation (Table 21-1).

Generally, coronary blood flow during *rest* does not decrease until coronary intraluminal diameter is decreased to 80% of normal. When the narrowing of the coronary

527

BOX 21-1
Causes of Myocardial Ischemia

Major Causes of Myocardial Ischemia
Atheromatous Plaque
May be smooth or rough, eccentric or concentric, variable in length, single or in series.

Incidence: Most frequent cause of decreased coronary blood flow and myocardial ischemia.

Consequence: Thrombus formation with atherosclerotic plaque rupture is a frequent cause of acute, persistant myocardial ischemia and also myocardial infarction. Atheromatous plaque, when narrowing the coronary intraluminal diameter by 50%, limits blood flow only to subendocardium, particularly during stress. When a platelet thrombus forms as a result of a coronary atherosclerotic plaque rupture or fissure and occludes the vessel, transmural ischemia and possibly myocardial infarction result.

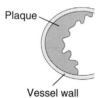

Plaque

Vessel wall

Coronary Vasoconstriction or Spasm
Typically occurs at or near an atheromatous plaque but may occur in a normal coronary artery segment.

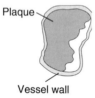

Plaque

Vessel wall

Incidence: Frequently coexists with fixed stenotic lesions resulting in the mixed contribution of fixed and dynamic

coronary artery obstruction. This results in ischemic events occurring variably at rest or with exercise.

Consequences: Spasm may cause transient transmural ischemia or myocardial infarction. Platelet thrombi may form from stasis of blood in the involved vessel segment.

Less Common Causes of Myocardial Ischemia
Coronary Emboli
Emboli may be the result of pieces of left ventricular thrombi, clots from prosthetic mitral or aortic valves, valvular vegetations, or fragments of calcium from a calcified aortic valve. Microemboli may result in minor ischemic damage to the myocardium, whereas large emboli may occlude coronary ostia and result in transmural infarction or sudden death.

Severe Hypotension
It is estimated that when the mean arterial pressure falls below 45 to 55 mm Hg in people with a normal coronary circulation, coronary autoregulation is lost and blood flow becomes pressure dependent. People with fixed stenotic lesions may require higher mean arterial pressures to maintain coronary blood flow. Consequently, mean arterial pressures should be maintained above 70 mm Hg or at even higher levels in persons with known coronary artery disease.

Aortic Valvular Stenosis
Hypertrophic Cardiomyopathy
Inflammatory Disease of the Coronary Arteries
Congenital Anomalies of the Coronary Circulation
Extremely Rapid Heart Rates
Extreme tachyarrhythmias significantly compromise coronary artery diastolic flow. This condition may be seen in patients with major systemic infections, severe blood loss, or cocaine abuse.

---

intraluminal diameter exceeds 50%, coronary blood flow is not able to meet the myocardial oxygen demands of strenuous physical activity or strong emotion and the patient may experience chest pain (classic angina). With progression of the coronary obstructive disease, critical reductions in blood flow to the myocardium eventually occur with minimal exertion and then, perhaps, even at rest. Acute thrombus formation on atherosclerotic plaque also may critically reduce myocardial blood flow and produce acute myocardial ischemia.

Patients with minimally obstructive coronary disease who also develop coronary vasospasm may exhibit angina that varies in severity and with circumstances. This symptomatic variability is due to differing contributions of fixed and dynamic coronary artery obstruction (mixed angina). Even in the absence of atherosclerotic plaque, coronary artery spasm may result in transient myocardial ischemia. In this instance, the anginal attacks typically occur at rest and in the early morning hours (Prinzmetal's or variant angina). In some patients, transient coronary vasoconstriction or

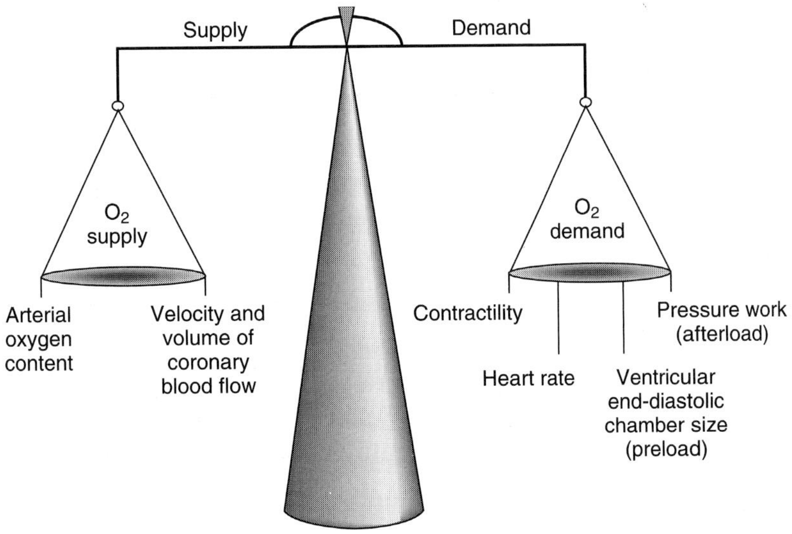

FIGURE 21-1 Myocardial oxygen supply/demand balance. Patients may develop myocardial ischemia if (1) myocardial oxygen supply falls short of normal demand or (2) myocardial oxygen demand exceeds upper limits of supply.

TABLE 21-1
Myocardial Oxygen Requirements and Coronary Blood Flow at Rest and Exercise

	Left Ventricle Oxygen Requirements (ml/min/100 g myocardium)	Coronary Blood Flow (ml/min/100 g myocardium)
Rest	8–10	80
Exercise	40	300

From Melvin Marcus M: *The coronary circulation in health and disease,* New York, 1983, McGraw-Hill.

spasm may acutely result in a critical reduction in the artery's intraluminal diameter and may cause acute myocardial ischemia.

When oxygen supply falls short of demand, compensatory mechanisms attempt to maintain the function and viability of the myocardium. These mechanisms include the following:

1. *Dilation of the coronary arterioles distal to the obstructive lesion caused by autoregulation.* Vasodilation decreases resistance to blood flow. However, autoregulatory changes may not be beneficial during an acute ischemic attack if the vasculature of the ischemic myocardium is chronically maximally dilated.

2. *The development of a coronary collateral circulation within the portion of the ventricle vulnerable to*

ischemia. This mechanism may increase regional blood flow but is a slowly developing adaptation to chronic coronary artery obstruction and myocardial ischemia. Furthermore, the development and extent of collateral circulation is unpredictable and varies among individuals.

3. *Anaerobic metabolism of the involved ischemic tissue.* Anaerobic metabolism is energy inefficient and ineffective in maintaining tissue viability. In fact, anaerobic metabolism can sustain the myocardium for only a few minutes before profound metabolic changes and severe functional deficits occur. These changes include increased myocardial cell membrane permeability, cellular edema, decreased cellular function, lactic acid production, and decreased contractility of the involved area of myocardium.

Hemodynamic Effects of Myocardial Ischemia

Systolic and diastolic abnormalities causing varying degrees of hemodynamic change may develop in patients with myocardial ischemia (Table 21-2).

Systolic Abnormalities

The force of myocardial contraction is directly dependent on oxygen availability. Generally, a global or local reduction in coronary flow results in a similar percentage deficit in myocardial contractility, which occurs almost immediately. Ischemia-induced contractile abnormalities are thought to result from an impairment in the mitochondrial

TABLE 21-2

Guidelines to Anticipated Hemodynamic Changes in Two Types of Ischemic Heart Disease

Disorder	Arterial Pressure	Pulse Pressure	Systemic Vascular Resistance	Pulmonary Vascular Resistance	Central Venous Pressure	Pulmonary Artery Pressure	Pulmonary Wedge Pressure	Cardiac Output	Svo$_2$
Angina pectoris	↓ ~ ↑	~ ↓	↑	~	~	~ ↑	~ ↑	~ ↓	~ ↓
Acute myocardial infarction (AMI)	↓ ~ ↑	~ ↓	↑ ↓	~ ↑	↓ ~ ↑	↓ ~ ↑	↓ ~ ↑	~ ↓	~ ↓

KEY: ↑ = increase; ~ = no change; ↓ = decrease.

NOTE: The magnitude or direction of change in hemodynamic measurements can be modified by coexisting factors or complications (hypovolemia, fluid overload) or the adequacy of compensatory mechanisms.

generation of high-energy compounds (adenosine triphosphate) and an accumulation of cellular hydrogen ions that then interfere with the interaction of calcium ions with the myocardial contractile proteins—actin and myosin.

With an approximately 20% reduction in coronary blood flow, the involved area of myocardium continues to contract, but with slightly less force (termed *hypokinesis*). With approximately 50% reduction in coronary blood flow, the force of contraction becomes markedly weaker, and the myocardium begins to produce lactic acid. With an approximately 80% to 90% reduction in coronary blood flow, the myocardium ceases to contract (termed *akinesis*); and with a 95% reduction in regional blood flow, the ischemic nonfunctional ventricular muscle segment may paradoxically bulge outward in systole (termed *dyskinesis*). The paradoxic ventricular wall motion may profoundly impair ventricular emptying and is wasteful of contractile energy (Figure 21-2). Although these events develop with ischemia of any cause, persistent wall motion abnormalities usually indicate varying degrees of infarction.

If the ischemic damage is localized, the remaining adequately perfused myocardium may contract normally or with increased force (termed *hyperkinesis*), thereby maintaining a normal ejection fraction. Clinical evidence of heart failure occurs when the ischemic wall motion abnormalities are so severe or include such a large area that the uninvolved myocardium cannot maintain acceptable pump function. Table 21-3 lists clinical and hemodynamic manifestations of left ventricular muscle loss.

The metabolic changes in myocardial cells that produce these functional abnormalities occur within 30 to 60 seconds of the reduction in oxygenated blood flow.

Following brief ischemia, myocardial dysfunction may persist for hours to days depending on the severity and the

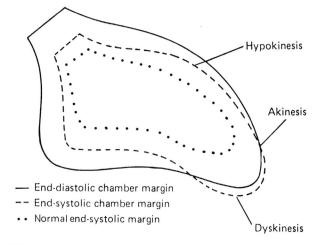

- — End-diastolic chamber margin
- -- End-systolic chamber margin
- •• Normal end-systolic margin

FIGURE 21-2 A left ventricular wall motion study from a patient who experienced a large anterior-lateral wall myocardial infarction. In the right anterior oblique view of the left ventricle, the apex moves paradoxically during systole (dyskinetic) while the anterior wall systolic motion is reduced (hypokinetic) or absent (akinetic).

duration of the ischemic attack, a condition termed *myocardial stunning*. Return to normal function is gradual. If, however, ischemia is chronic, myocardial function may remain chronically depressed, a condition termed *myocardial hibernation*. In this situation, the myocardium may return to normal function if the coronary blood flow is reestablished by surgical revascularization or angioplasty.

Diastolic Abnormalities

Diastolic abnormalities often occur before any changes in systolic function. Ischemic myocardial fibers become poorly compliant and resist filling. When more than 15% of

TABLE 21-3

Clinical and Hemodynamic Manifestations of Left Ventricular Muscle Loss

Left Ventricular Muscle Loss	Clinical or Hemodynamic Manifestation
Greater than 8%	Decreased compliance
Greater than 10%	Decreased ejection fraction
Greater than 15%	Increased ventricular end-diastolic pressure
Greater than 20%	Increased ventricular end-diastolic volume (systolic failure)
Greater than 25%	Clinical evidence of heart failure
Greater than 40%	Cardiogenic shock or death

From Henning RJ, Ake G: *Critical care cardiology,* New York, 1989, Churchill Livingstone.

the left ventricular mass is ischemic, the end-diastolic volume/pressure relationship also becomes distorted. The left ventricular end-diastolic pressures (pulmonary artery wedge pressure [PWP]) increases while the ventricular end-diastolic filling volume remains unchanged. Many patients with acute myocardial ischemia or infarction, particularly acute anterior wall infarction, require left ventricular end-diastolic pressures in the range of 15 to 18 mm Hg (normal is 4 to 12 mm Hg) to maintain normal stroke volume.

If the acutely ischemic myocardium is reperfused within 20 to 60 minutes, the function of the myocardium gradually returns to normal, and the PWP returns to baseline values. In this instance, permanent damage to the myocardial cells may not occur.

In summary, myocardial ischemia may result in contractile dysfunction and incomplete ventricular emptying (systolic dysfunction). Ischemia also impairs ventricular filling because the stiffer left ventricular chamber cannot accommodate the diastolic inflow (diastolic dysfunction). The combination of systolic and diastolic abnormalities, if severe, may lead to systemic perfusion failure and pulmonary edema (congestive heart failure).

Autonomic Nervous System Responses to Acute Myocardial Ischemia

Sympathetic Hyperactivity

Increased sympathetic nervous system discharge occurs more commonly in patients with anterior wall ischemia than in patients with inferior wall ischemia. However, increased sympathetic nerve discharge may also occur in patients with inferior wall ischemia. During an episode of acute myocardial ischemia, the primary compensatory mechanism, which

attempts to maintain cardiac output and mean systemic arterial pressure within a normal range, is the release of epinephrine from the adrenal glands, as well as the release of norepinephrine from the sympathetic nerves. The release of these cardiac excitatory hormones increases the force and velocity of myocardial contraction and the rate of ventricular relaxation. Both actions increase the efficiency of the heart. However, if myocardial oxygen supply is significantly limited, myocardial work cannot increase because oxygen consumption cannot increase in proportion to the work demand.

Norepinephrine and epinephrine maintain or increase the mean arterial pressure by causing arteriolar constriction, but these catecholamines also increase left ventricular afterload and oxygen requirements. As a consequence, the severity and size of the ischemic injury may increase. Increased concentrations of circulating catecholamines also predispose the patient to ectopic cardiac arrhythmias. Indeed, many patients with acute myocardial ischemia die from ventricular fibrillation without having suffered any permanent damage to the ventricular muscle.

Parasympathetic Hyperactivity

Some patients with acute inferior wall ischemia or infarction develop increased parasympathetic activity. This is clinically manifest as sinus bradycardia and, on occasion, as an inappropriate decrease in systemic vascular resistance. These changes may be associated with significant systemic hypotension.

ANGINA PECTORIS

Angina pectoris is pain or discomfort that results from transient myocardial ischemia. Angina pectoris may be either stable or unstable.

Stable angina pectoris is usually caused by significant increases in myocardial oxygen requirements, which are usually the result of physical stress or strong emotional stimuli. Patients typically have greater than 60% to 70% intraluminal coronary artery obstruction. Stable angina pectoris is relieved within 10 to 20 minutes by rest or administration of sublingual nitroglycerin (or both). Many patients with chronic, stable angina lead relatively normal lives for years and either eventually develop an acute coronary syndrome or die of an unrelated illness or injury.

Angina is considered *unstable* if the pattern of pain or discomfort progressively increases in frequency, severity, intensity, or ease of provocation. Unstable angina is also termed *crescendo angina* or *preinfarction angina* and may occur during minimal exertion or rest. It is not relieved promptly by rest or administration of sublingual nitroglycerin. Unstable angina is the result of transient coronary artery occlusion mediated by platelet aggregation that occurs secondary to atherosclerotic plaque rupture or fissure. *Patients with unstable angina should be hospitalized and assessed for the appropriateness of reperfusion therapies.* Unstable angina is an important component of *acute coronary syndromes* (unstable angina, non–Q wave infarction, Q wave infarction).

In a *non–Q wave infarction,* necrosis involves the subendocardium, the intramural myocardium, or both. The myocardium immediately adjacent to the epicardium is spared ischemic death. Q waves are not likely to evolve on the electrocardiogram (ECG).

The necrotic damage of a *Q wave infarction* usually extends through the full thickness of the ventricular wall and is evidenced by the development of Q waves on the ECG in contiguous leads. Overall, the term *acute coronary syndrome* emphasizes the fact that patients can progress quickly from unstable angina to myocardial infarction. *The importance of immediate patient evaluation and institution of reperfusion therapies (thrombolytic agents, angioplasty, stent placement, coronary revascularization surgery), when indicated, cannot be overstated.*

For patients with acute myocardial infarction, the greater the amount of time that lapses from the onset of chest pain to initiation of reperfusion therapies, the greater the loss of viable, functional ventricular mass. The loss of a critical mass of functional ventricular muscle, in turn, translates into increased morbidity, decreased short- and long-term survival, and a decrease in the quality of life in long-term survivors (see Table 21-3).

Consequently, if a patient comes to the emergency department with a complaint of chest pain and a history suggestive of unstable angina or an acute myocardial infarction, physical assessment, laboratory studies (including ECG) with immediate interpretation, and risk factor evaluation must be performed within 10 minutes of arrival (door-to-data interval). Within the following 10 minutes, a treatment decision must be made (data-to-decision interval). The ultimate goal in patients who are within 6 to 12 hours of the onset of symptoms of acute infarction is initiation of fibrinolytic therapy within 30 minutes of arrival or, for patients in whom coronary balloon angioplasty is the selected therapy, the door-to-balloon time is within 90 minutes of hospital admission.

Clinical Presentation

The intensity of anginal discomfort or pain is variable and may range from a vague substernal sensation to intolerable pain. The character of the discomfort may be described as a heaviness, pressure, choking, burning, or a tight sensation

in the retrosternal region. The discomfort also may radiate to or be limited to the left shoulder, arm, wrist, or elbow; the throat, jaw, or teeth; or the back or abdomen. Patients usually remain immobile because activity increases the discomfort; however, some patients merely slow their activity to obtain relief. A minority of patients become restless.

Some patients with angina pectoris may *not* complain of discomfort but may have substantial ST-T wave changes on their ECGs. As many as 80% of the ST-T wave changes that occur on a 24-hour electrocardiographic record may not be associated with symptoms. This process is termed *silent myocardial ischemia.*

Mentation

There is usually no change in mentation in patients with stable angina. Patients with unstable angina may complain of dizziness, light-headedness, or weakness and may appear anxious.

Cutaneous Manifestations

Skin color is usually normal, and the skin is usually warm and dry. With unstable angina the skin may be pale, cool, diaphoretic, or even cyanotic if cardiac output is significantly reduced.

Heart Rate and Character of Pulse

The heart rate is usually increased above the patient's baseline value and may be weak if the stroke volume is significantly decreased. Bradycardia may occur in patients with angina due to severe right coronary or left main coronary artery obstruction. The pulse also may be irregular because of frequent atrial or ventricular ectopic beats.

Heart Sounds

When the patient's left ventricle is stiff or failing, there may be an audible and a palpable S_4 due to decreased ventricular compliance during atrial contraction and an S_3 sound due to ventricular failure. In patients with transient papillary muscle ischemia, there also may be a transient systolic mitral regurgitant murmur.

Palpation of the Precordium

Third and fourth heart sounds may be palpable at the apical area. This feature helps distinguish these sounds from the S_3 sounds heard in young patients and the S_4 sounds sometimes heard in athletes with ventricular hypertrophy. In healthy individuals, these sounds are not associated with abnormal precordial movements.

There may be a palpable abnormality in left ventricular wall motion. This abnormality may be perceived by the examiner as a distinct double impulse, separated by a few centimeters, which is caused by the apex beat and a dyskinetic portion of the ventricular wall.

Neck Veins

The jugular veins are typically not distended.

Respiratory Rate and Character of Breathing

Pain and anxiety are both potent stimuli to breathing and thus, during the painful ischemic attack, the patient's respiratory rate may be greater than the baseline value. The depth of ventilatory movements may be normal or splinted because patients with angina often limit movement.

Lung Sounds

In patients with short episodes of stable angina pectoris, the lungs are usually clear to auscultation. In contrast, patients with prolonged episodes of unstable angina may have diffuse crackles present in the dependent areas of the lungs. The association of pulmonary edema with unstable angina is often indicative of severe multivessel coronary artery disease.

Acid-Base Values

Acid-base values are usually maintained within the normal range unless persistent perfusion failure produces metabolic acidosis (lactic acidosis) or pulmonary edema produces respiratory alkalosis and hypoxemia. In this setting, patients may ultimately develop a combined metabolic acidosis with a respiratory alkalosis.

Hemodynamic Profile

Invasive hemodynamic monitoring is usually not required in patients with unstable angina pectoris. If, however, anginal pain is not promptly relieved by medical therapy, or if the hemodynamic condition deteriorates, invasive hemodynamic monitoring may be helpful in titrating medical therapy.

Arterial Pressure

This measurement may decrease and the pulse pressure may narrow if there is a significant reduction in stroke volume. This finding is particularly likely to occur in a patient with unstable angina (Figure 21-3). Often, however, the arterial pressure is normal or elevated because of systemic arteriolar constriction due to sympathetic nervous system stimulation.

Systemic Vascular Resistance

Vascular resistance is often increased, reflecting generalized vasoconstriction due to increased circulating norepinephrine and epinephrine.

Pulmonary Vascular Resistance

There is typically no change in pulmonary vascular resistance.

Central Venous Pressure or Right Atrial Pressure

This measurement is usually in the normal range of 0 to 8 mm Hg. In patients with right coronary artery disease, the central venous pressure may become elevated during prolonged periods of unstable angina because of decreased right ventricular compliance or contractile failure.

Pulmonary Artery and Wedge Pressures

In patients with unstable angina, the pulmonary artery systolic and diastolic pressures increase in tandem with elevations in the PWP. The PWP is increased above the patient's baseline normal value because of the acutely noncompliant or hypocontractile left ventricle (Figure 21-4).

Pulmonary Artery Wedge Pressure Waveform

Because atrial contraction significantly contributes to the end-diastolic filling of a stiff or failing ventricle, the atrial *a* wave (end-diastolic wave) may be of increased amplitude. The mean PWP, which is the average of both *a* and *v* waves, may be significantly lower than left ventricular end-diastolic pressure. When possible, measurements should be taken from the crest of the *a* wave, which approximates the left ventricular end-diastolic pressure.

Although relatively uncommon, a prominent *v* wave may appear if acute mitral regurgitation develops. The magnitude of the *a* and *v* waves is significantly increased in these patients if the atrium is normal in size and noncompliant (Figure 21-5). Conversely, if the left atrium is markedly enlarged and compliant, due to preexisting chronic mitral valve regurgitation, the *a* and *v* waves may not be pronounced on the PWP tracing.

Cardiac Output

Cardiac output may be decreased if significant wall motion abnormalities are present and involve a large area. Cardiac output, however, may be maintained in the low-normal range by compensatory tachycardia mediated by increased circulating catecholamines.

Mixed Venous Oxygen Saturation

In patients with stable angina pectoris, the mixed venous oxygen saturation is normally greater than 70%. If systemic tissue perfusion decreases as a result of

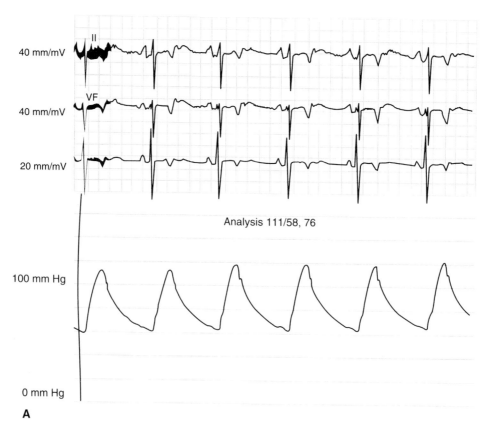

40 mm/mV — II

40 mm/mV — VF

20 mm/mV

Analysis 111/58, 76

100 mm Hg

0 mm Hg

A

FIGURE 21-3 Electrocardiographic and arterial blood pressure changes before *(panel A)* and during *(panel B)* acute myocardial ischemia. Marked ST segment elevation is present in leads II and aVF, in panel B, and is associated with a reduction in both the peak systemic arterial pressure and the pulse pressure. Electrocardiographic and arterial pressure changes often precede the patient's subjective complaints of pain or discomfort.

severe left ventricular dysfunction, as may occur in patients with unstable angina, mixed venous oxygen saturation values decrease relative to the degree of circulatory failure.

Laboratory Examination and Diagnostic Testing

Electrocardiogram

A 12-lead ECG must be obtained and interpreted within 10 minutes of arrival at the hospital. With acute myocardial ischemia, the ECG may reveal either ST segment depression that occurs in approximately 30% of patients (suggestive of unstable angina) or elevation (suggestive of myocardial infarction). The T waves may be peaked or inverted (Figures 21-6 and 21-7).

With relief of ischemia, the ST-T wave changes return to the previous morphology. Ventricular ectopic beats may accompany acute ischemic episodes. *The resting ECG may be normal in approximately one half of patients with myocardial ischemia.* Consequently, a normal ECG does not rule out acute coronary syndrome. Figure 21-8 shows a summary of physical, hemodynamic, and ECG changes associated with myocardial ischemia.

Echocardiogram

Transient hypokinesis, akinesis, or occasionally dyskinetic wall motion abnormalities may be observed in the area of ischemia during echocardiographic examination. Occasionally patients have normal systolic function and ejection fractions but abnormal diastolic function with impairment of ventricular filling detectable on echo-Doppler examination. These patients may have a poorly compliant ventricle because of intermittent myocardial ischemia or a

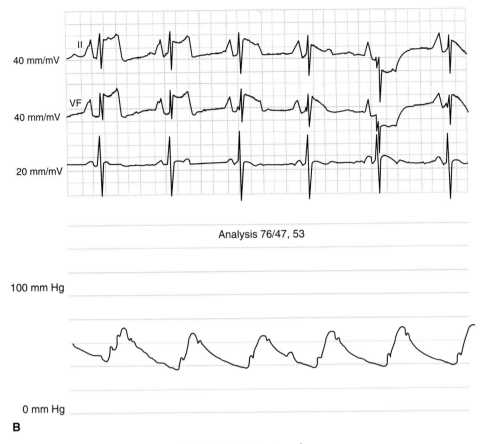

FIGURE 21-3 *Continued*

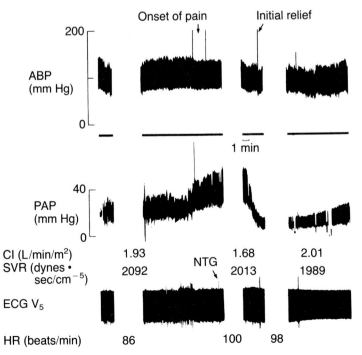

FIGURE 21-4 Simultaneous systemic and pulmonary arterial pressure tracings obtained during an acute ischemic episode from a patient with unstable angina. The level of arterial systolic and diastolic pressures remained unremarkable throughout the ischemic episode. The first evidence of a change from normal was the abrupt increase in pulmonary artery diastolic pressure (a close correlate to left ventricular end-diastolic pressure) from approximately 15 mm Hg to greater than 25 mm Hg. In patients without pulmonary disease, hypoxemia, or acidemia, this pressure increase relates to sudden-onset decreased ventricular compliance or heart failure or both. The increase in pressure was then followed by the patient's complaint of chest pain; the pain was a relatively late symptom of the ischemic attack. Because of nitroglycerin-induced venodilation and decreased venous return to the heart *(arrow),* ventricular end-diastolic pressure, pulmonary artery pressure (PAP), heart size, and myocardial oxygen consumption were reduced, and the patient experienced relief from pain. (Courtesy of HJC Swan, MD, Cedars-Sinai Medical Center, Los Angeles.)

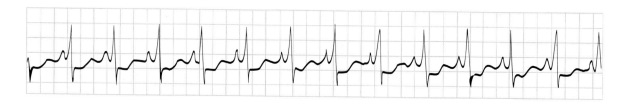

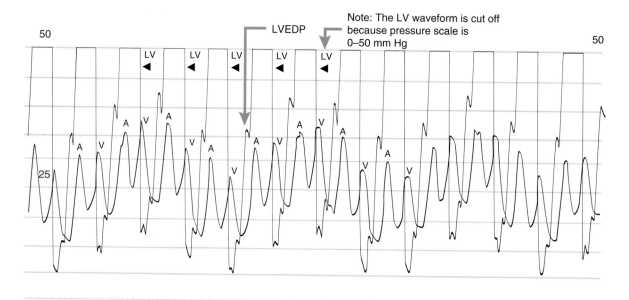

FIGURE 21-5 Left ventricular pressure and pulmonary artery wedge pressure tracing correlated with an ECG rhythm strip in a patient with an acute anterior wall myocardial infarction. The scale is 0 to 50 mm Hg. The left ventricular end-diastolic pressure is increased because of decreased left ventricular compliance. Part of the left ventricular pressure tracing *(arrows)* is cut off. Prominent *a* and *v* waves are present in the pulmonary artery wedge pressure tracing. The increased-amplitude *a* wave is the result of impaired end-diastolic filling because of decreased ventricular compliance, and the increased-amplitude *v* wave is the result of mitral regurgitant flow because of ischemic papillary muscle dysfunction. Note that the PWP *a* wave approximates but does not exactly equal the left ventricular end-diastolic pressure.

chronically stiff (hypertrophied or fibrotic) ventricle. Chronic abnormal left ventricular diastolic performance may lead to a substantial, chronic elevation in the end-diastolic pressure, which predisposes the patient to pulmonary edema.

Thallium Scan

Radionuclide thallium is preferentially taken up by the perfused, normally functioning myocardial cells. When the heart is scanned after the intravenous injection of thallium, areas of myocardial ischemia, termed *cold spots,* appear as an absence of thallium uptake. These cold spots may not be visualized on subsequent repeat imaging if, following the acute ischemic attack, reperfusion of the myocardium occurs.

Cardiac Biochemical Markers

See the section on acute myocardial infarction, laboratory examination and other diagnostic tests. In patients being treated at the emergency department with a history and symptoms suggestive of an acute coronary syndrome, these laboratory markers may be helpful in ruling out acute myocardial infarction.

Cardiac Catheterization

Coronary angiography is the only definitive means of localizing the site and extent of coronary artery obstructions. Coronary angiography also may distinguish a fixed obstructive lesion from coronary artery spasm. *Cardiac catheterization and coronary angiography are indicated in patients with unstable angina or in*

Nomenclature for Determination
of ST-Segment Abnormalities

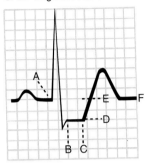

A = PQ junction
B = J point
C = 80 msec from J point
D–E = 2 mm ST-segment
 depression
F = Isoelectric line

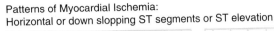
Patterns of Myocardial Ischemia:
Horizontal or down slopping ST segments or ST elevation

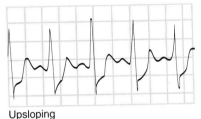

Horizontal

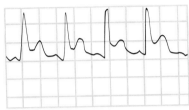

Downsloping

Upsloping

Elevation

FIGURE 21-6 Electrocardiographic ST segment abnormalities commonly seen with acute myocardial ischemia. Myocardial ischemia is definitely present if there is 1 mm or more horizontal or downsloping depression of the ST segment when measured at 80 ms from the J point or 1.5 mm or more upsloping ST segment depression. ST segment elevation equal to or greater than 1 mm at 80 ms from the J point suggests that the ischemia is the result of high-grade coronary artery disease or coronary artery spasm. (From *Quick reference guides to cardiovascular medicine,* 1986, Physicians World Communications Group.)

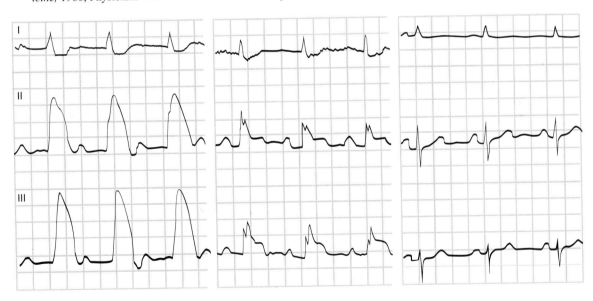

A. Onset of pain   B. Pain subsiding   C. After the attack

FIGURE 21-7 Marked electrocardiographic ST segment elevation in a patient with coronary artery spasm. As the pain resolves, the ECG returns to a normal pattern.

patients with angina that occurs with minimal exertion or with low-level exercise that does not respond to medical therapy. When indicated and possible, definitive therapies (angioplasty, stent placement) may then be undertaken.

Differential Diagnosis of Acute Coronary Syndromes

Conditions in which the clinical presentation may be identical to that of acute coronary syndromes include dissecting aortic aneurysm; pulmonary embolism; acute

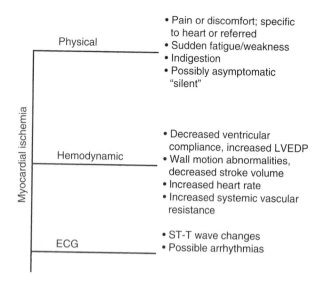

FIGURE 21-8 Correlation of physical, hemodynamic, and ECG changes with myocardial ischemic attack.

pericarditis, costochondritis; gastroesophageal reflux disease; spontaneous pneumothorax; acute cholecyctitis; and panic attack.

Treatment

The goal in managing patients with angina pectoris is to optimize the myocardial oxygen supply/demand balance and prevent myocardial infarction. In patients with *stable angina pectoris,* treatment consists of the administration of aspirin, nitroglycerin, and beta-adrenergic receptor blocking agents or calcium-channel antagonists. The medications should be titrated on a regular basis to control the patient's symptoms.

Patients with unstable angina must be aggressively treated in the hospital while on bed rest with continuous ECG monitoring and frequent assessment of vital signs. Immediate (within less than 10 minutes) general measures for patients admitted to the hospital with chest pain suggestive of myocardial ischemia include oxygen therapy, aspirin in a dose of 160 to 325 mg, nitroglycerin (sublingually or spray), and intravenous morphine if the pain is not relieved with nitroglycerin. In addition, patients with unstable angina or non–Q wave myocardial infarction are candidates for glycoprotein IIb-IIIa platelet receptor antagonists. These patients are also given intravenous heparin, nitroglycerin, and beta-adrenergic blocking agents following the 12-lead ECG if there are changes suggestive of ischemia, injury, or infarction.

The patient is given no food by mouth until the condition is stabilized because emergent cardiac catheterization or revascularization surgery may be indicated if medical therapy does not relieve the pain or if the patient's condition deteriorates.

Oxygen Therapy

Supplemental oxygen is advocated to maximize oxygen delivery and thereby increase the oxygen supply to the myocardium.

Medications

Nitroglycerin is one of the mainstays of therapy for acute myocardial ischemia. The primary mode of action is dilation of the systemic veins, which promotes venous pooling. This produces an immediate reduction in ventricular volume and therefore ventricular radius. By the law of LaPlace, myocardial oxygen consumption decreases (see Figure 21-4).

Nitroglycerin also produces some coronary and systemic arterial dilation because it contributes to nitric oxide formation, which causes vasodilation. The vasodilator properties of nitroglycerin may relieve myocardial ischemia and thereby improve regional, as well as global, ventricular function. The reduction in systemic and pulmonary vascular resistance reduces afterload for both ventricles. Nitroglycerin may be given sublingually, orally, topically, or intravenously. Intravenous nitroglycerin is most useful for the treatment of patients with unstable angina. It may be safely given to patients who are normovolemic and closely monitored. Continuous intravenous dosing allows moment-to-moment drug titration to optimize ischemic pain relief while assessing the drug's hemodynamic effect. Therapy is directed at relief of myocardial ischemia without decreasing the preload-dependent cardiac output of the ischemic heart.

In general, low concentrations of intravenous nitroglycerin may be administered to patients with systolic arterial pressures greater than 100 mm Hg without the necessity for invasive monitoring of systemic or pulmonary arterial pressures. However, blood pressure should be determined at frequent intervals manually or automatically with external blood pressure devices. Patients with arterial pressures less than 100 mm Hg, and especially patients with arterial hypotension (a systolic pressure less than 90 mm Hg in a previously normotensive person or a systolic pressure that has decreased more than 40 mm Hg in a previously hypertensive person), often require invasive arterial pressure monitoring during intravenous nitroglycerin administration. In patients with hypotension, cardiac output and pulmonary artery and wedge pressures should be monitored. A reduction in pulmonary artery pressures may be noted with nitroglycerin administration because nitroglycerin causes dilation of the systemic veins and the pulmonary arterioles.

Opiate Analgesia. Morphine sulfate is indicated for treatment of continuing chest pain despite nitrate administration. By depressing the central and sympathetic nervous systems, morphine sulfate induces mild arteriolar dilation and venodilation; therefore this drug reduces both afterload and preload. Opiate analgesics also decrease circulating catecholamines and therefore the tendency for arrhythmias. Although bradycardia, hypotension, respiratory depression, and nausea may result from morphine sulfate, these untoward effects can be minimized by cautious "mini-dosing" and avoiding jostling the patient during routine care and transport. Morphine is administered intravenously in 2 to 5 mg increments every 5 to 30 minutes based on the patient's clinical and hemodynamic response.

The importance of relieving ischemic myocardial pain cannot be overemphasized. Failure to do so results in the further release of endogenous catecholamines, which then increases myocardial work and oxygen consumption. Catecholamines also predispose patients to ventricular and atrial arrhythmias. Because continuing chest pain indicates *ongoing ischemia,* definitive anti-ischemic therapy should be immediately undertaken. *If the ischemic pain is not relieved by aspirin, heparin, nitroglycerin, beta-adrenergic blocking agents, or calcium-channel blocking agents, patients should receive glycoprotein IIb-IIIa platelet receptor antagonists or undergo emergency coronary angiography.* Angiographic evaluation of the coronary arteries permits the determination of the appropriate definitive approach for reperfusion of the persistently ischemic myocardium, such as angioplasty and placement of intracoronary stents, which are placed in greater than 70% of patients who undergo angioplasty, or coronary bypass surgery.

Beta-Adrenergic Receptor Antagonists (Beta-Blockers). This group of drugs lowers myocardial oxygen requirements by decreasing arterial pressure, heart rate, and myocardial contractility by preventing norepinephrine and epinephrine from combining with and stimulating the beta-adrenergic receptors. Beta-blockers have the additional benefits of decreasing platelet adhesiveness, and therefore thrombus formation, and decreasing the incidence of primary ventricular fibrillation. In general, beta-blockers may be administered if there are no contraindications such as left ventricular failure, reactive airway disease (chronic obstructive pulmonary disease or asthma), or second- or third-degree atrioventricular block. Because stroke volume may decrease due to the negative inotropic effects of these drugs, patients should be closely observed for signs and symptoms of heart failure such as orthopnea, tachypnea, tachycardia, S_3 gallop rhythms, positive hepatojugular reflux, and radiographic evidence of pulmonary congestion or edema.

Patients who continue to experience angina at rest, those who do not tolerate beta-blockade therapy, or those who experience primary diastolic ventricular dysfunction should receive calcium channel blocking agents.

Calcium Channel Blocking Agents. These agents increase myocardial oxygen supply by dilating coronary arteries. They are most helpful in patients with coronary artery spasm. These drugs may also decrease myocardial oxygen consumption by reducing contractility and systemic vascular resistance. Short-acting calcium channel blocking agents, such as nifedipine, should be avoided because they may cause significant swings in systemic blood pressure. Second-generation calcium channel blocking agents, such as felodipine or amlodipine, should be used if this class of drugs is prescribed.

Anticoagulation. Systemic heparinization is indicated in the treatment of patients with unstable angina pectoris to inhibit propagation of the coronary artery thrombus and prevent formation of deep venous or ventricular wall thrombi. In some medical centers, unfractionated heparin has been replaced by fractionated (low-molecular-weight) heparin, which does not require repeated measurements of the partial thromboplastin time and rarely causes heparin-induced thrombocytopenia. Aspirin in doses of 325 mg is also given daily.

Gylcoprotein IIb-IIIa Platelet Receptors Antagonists. Patients with unstable angina are candidates for glycoprotein IIb-IIIa platelet receptor antagonists. These drugs inhibit the binding of fibrinogen or von Willebrand factor to activated platelets, thereby preventing intracoronary platelet aggregation and clot propagation. A platelet receptor antagonist is administered intravenously for approximately 48 hours. Because these drugs inhibit platelet aggregation and they are also given with intravenous heparin, *patients are at increased risk for bleeding.* Contraindications to the administration of a glycoprotein platelet receptor inhibitor include significant hypertension (blood pressure 180/110 or greater), anemia (hemoglobin less than 10 g), thrombocytopenia (platelet count less than 130,000), active bleeding, surgery within the past 30 days, or stroke within the past 30 days. If the patient is persistently symptomatic, cardiac catheterization and coronary angiography is performed and the patient is evaluated for angioplasty and stent placement, or possibly coronary bypass surgery.

Treatment of Arrhythmias. Rhythm diagnosis of hemodynamically stable (no signs of cerebral or systemic hypoperfusion) wide QRS tachyarrhythmias (aberrantly conducted supraventricular tachycardia [SVT] versus ventricular tachycardia [VT]) enables selection of appropriate antiarrhythmic drugs or other specific therapies, such as vagal maneuvers for SVT. Intravenous diltiazem or amiodarone can be used in patients with SVT. Amiodarone is recommended in patients with supraventricular tachyarrythmias and ejection fractions less than 40%.

However, hemodynamically unstable tachyarrhythmias with heart rates greater than 150 beats per minute must be immediately treated with direct current cardioversion. For heart rates less than 150 beats per minute, intravenous amiodarone or procainamide may be used in patients with ejection fractions greater than 40% and no clinical evidence of heart failure. Only amiodarone is recommended for patients with poor ventricular function. Although lidocaine still appears in the advanced cardiac life support algorithm for monomorphic or polymorphic stable VT, amiodarone is currently the first-line drug of choice.[2]

Stool Softeners. Stool softeners are prescribed because straining at stool (Valsalva maneuver) may cause bradycardia and hypotension in patients with acute ischemic heart disease. Stable patients are commonly permitted to use the bedside commode because it is more comfortable and less stressful than the bedpan.

ACUTE MYOCARDIAL INFARCTION
Pathophysiology

Acute myocardial infarction (AMI) is myocardial necrosis that results from prolonged ischemia. The lay expression is "heart attack." If acute, severe ischemia persists for more than approximately 1 hour, myocardial cells begin to die within the blighted ischemic zone, and the infarct formation begins. After 4 to 6 hours, there is usually massive cellular necrosis with swelling and functional impairment of the ischemic myocardium surrounding the infarcted area. The rate of progression and the extent of necrotic damage are related to the degree of coronary artery occlusion, the size of the involved vascular bed, the presence or absence of collateral circulation, and the balance between myocardial oxygen demand and supply. For example, if the patient is stressed by persistent hypertension, tachycardia, or continued pain, myocardial oxygen demand significantly exceeds the fixed, reduced oxygen supply, and infarct formation occurs more rapidly and extensively.

The ischemic process begins and is most severe in the inner one third of the myocardium (subendocardium). There are several reasons:

1. Systolic myocardial tension and oxygen demands are greatest in this area.

2. Diastolic coronary blood flow is limited within the subendocardium because intramyocardial pressure (determined, in part, by ventricular end-diastolic pressure) is greatest in this area.

3. Systolic compression of the penetrating coronary artery branches is most severe in the subendocardium and normally allows no systolic blood flow.

In other words, even under normal conditions the subendocardium consumes the most oxygen but receives the least coronary arterial flow.

A myocardial infarction may be limited to the subendocardium, or a wavefront of cell death may move outward progressively to include the epicardial layer of the myocardium, ultimately producing a transmural myocardial infarction.

Transitional Zones of Ischemic Myocardial Damage and Dysfunction

In a fully developed acute transmural myocardial infarction, three zones of functional and electrophysiologic abnormalities are determined by the regional severity of myocardial oxygen deprivation. These zones are not sharply defined anatomic or functional areas.

1. *The area of necrosis.* The central area of *necrosis* receives little or no blood supply and is unable to sustain life. This area is noncontractile, devoid of viable nerve fibers (and therefore does not contribute to perception of pain), and is electrically inert. The necrotic area (myocardial infarction) is depicted by a deep, wide Q wave in ECG leads oriented to this area in 80% of patients on the standard surface ECG.

2. *The area of injury.* This area is immediately adjacent to the necrotic area and undergoes severe metabolic derangements. These include increases in cell membrane permeability, influx of sodium and water, and efflux of potassium and hydrogen ions. The resulting cellular edema contributes to decreased ventricular compliance, as well as decreased or absent wall motion. The electrophysiologic instability of this tissue predisposes the patient to reentrant arrhythmias. ECG leads oriented to the injured region record ST segment elevation.

3. *The area of ischemia.* The oxygen-deprived area surrounding the area of injury undergoes less severe metabolic alterations, is electrically unstable, and can be hypokinetic. ECG leads oriented to the area of ischemia often show symmetric T wave inversion. Figure 21-9 illustrates the total constellation of typical ECG changes in a myocardial infarction as demonstrated in electrocardiographic leads oriented to the infarcted area.

Nerve fibers generally remain intact in the areas of injury and ischemia and are responsible for the patient's

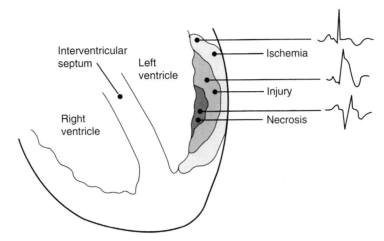

FIGURE 21-9 Electrocardiographic evidence of acute non–Q wave myocardial infarction correlated with schematic illustration of transitional zones of ischemic damage. The Q wave reflects the area of necrosis, the ST segment elevation reflects the area of injury, and the T wave inversion reflects the most peripheral area of ischemia.

complaint of chest pain or discomfort. The presence of persistent ischemic pain indicates that viable areas of ischemic and injured myocardium are in jeopardy of necrosis.

Variables Affecting Patient Presentation

The hemodynamic status and clinical status of the patient are related to the size of the infarcted and ischemic myocardium, the functional status of the noninvolved myocardium and the heart valves, and the severity of coronary artery disease. A cumulative loss of more than 40% of the left ventricular muscle mass usually results in cardiogenic shock. In patients with previous myocardial infarction or cardiac dysfunction, a relatively small infarct superimposed on a previously compromised heart may precipitate a hemodynamic disaster.

Patients with AMI are categorized as either uncomplicated or complicated. Within these general categories, patients may seek treatment either early (within minutes or up to 12 hours of the onset of symptoms) or late (after 12 hours of the onset of symptoms), at which time salvage of jeopardized myocardium may not be possible. Public education directed toward recognition of the signs and symptoms of a "heart attack" leading to *early* admission to the hospital (less than 4 hours from onset of symptoms) is critical to preserving myocardial viability and saving lives.

Patients with *complicated* AMI have (1) persistent or recurrent chest pain poorly responsive to medical therapy; (2) low cardiac output and pulmonary edema; (3) recurrent or persistent bradyarrhythmias or tach-yarrhythmias or ventricular ectopy; and (4) cardiogenic shock that may be the result of extensive myocardial infarction, papillary muscle dysfunction or rupture, right ventricular infarction, or interventricular septal or left ventricular free wall rupture.

Clinical Presentation

Patients who are treated within 12 hours of the onset of symptoms often complain of chest pain or discomfort. However, some patients with persistent pain for more than 12 hours may have "stuttering infarction" and should be considered for thrombolytic therapy, coronary angioplasty, or surgical revascularization.

The character of AMI pain is similar to that of angina. However, the pain is usually more severe and prolonged until it resolves because of either myocardial cell death, restoration of adequate oxygenated blood flow to the ischemic area, a reduction in myocardial oxygen demand (such as preload reduction), or opiate analgesia. The pain may be associated with diaphoresis, shortness of breath, gastrointestinal upset, or generalized weakness and fatigue. However, 15% to 30% of patients with acute myocardial infarction experience no pain. In these patients, myocardial infarction may not be detected immediately or may be associated only with syncope, gastrointestinal upset, arrhythmias, extreme weakness or fatigue, or sudden-onset pulmonary edema. These patients often have a history of diabetes mellitus.

Patients who are treated more than 12 hours after the onset of symptoms may be free of pain and may have experienced a complete myocardial infarction.

Clinical Features

Mentation

Most commonly, mentation is normal. Patients may become extremely anxious during periods of acute pain. A decrease in the cardiac output may result in light-headedness, anxiety, restlessness, or depressed mentation.

Cutaneous Manifestations

Some patients maintain a normal complexion even during an acute attack. Severe pain or perfusion failure may be associated with pale, cold, and diaphoretic skin.

Heart Rate and Character of Pulse

Sinus tachycardia may be produced by anxiety, fever, circulating catecholamines, or low cardiac output due to hypovolemia or heart failure. Sinus bradycardia may be present in (1) patients with obstruction of the right coronary artery in which the blood supply to the sinoatrial node is compromised, or (2) patients with obstruction of the left main coronary artery that results in left ventricular distention and activation of ventricular stretch receptors and reflex parasympathetic stimulation. Right or left coronary artery obstruction may be associated with ectopic arrhythmias or conduction disturbances. With significant decreases in stroke volume, the peripheral arterial pulses are of low volume.

Heart Sounds

The first heart sound may be diminished due to a decrease in left ventricular contractile force. An atrial gallop sound, or S_4, is frequently audible. If systolic failure is present with elevation of the left ventricular end-diastolic pressure (PWP) to 20 mm Hg or greater, a ventricular gallop sound, or S_3, is frequently audible. A systolic mitral regurgitant murmur may result from ischemic dysfunction of a left ventricular papillary muscle or from ischemic dysfunction of the myocardium that anchors the papillary muscles.

Palpation of the Precordium

Rarely is the apical impulse completely normal in patients with acute ischemic heart disease. Both an atrial gallop (S_4) and a ventricular gallop (S_3) may be palpable at the apex, particularly if the patient is examined while on the left side. The examiner also may perceive paradoxic ventricular wall motion (dyskinesis) as an extra impulse at a site a few centimeters away from the apex beat.

Left ventricular dilation tends to displace the apex beat downward and to the left toward the axilla. This may take days to occur following the advent of heart failure because the normally stiff pericardium tends to resist the acute dilation of the heart. A decrease in the force and an increase in the duration (because of prolonged left ventricular ejection time) of the apex beat are also characteristic of left ventricular failure due to ischemic disease.

Neck Veins

The superficial, easily visible external jugular veins are collapsed in patients with hypovolemia who are examined while in the supine position. Conversely, in patients with severe biventricular failure or right ventricular failure who are examined while in the 30- to 40-degree semirecumbent position, the internal jugular veins are visibly distended to a level relative to the elevation in systemic venous pressure (see Chapter 5).

Respiratory Rate

Hyperventilation commonly accompanies pain. Otherwise, the rate and character of breathing are normal in the absence of pulmonary edema. In patients with severe pulmonary edema as a result of left ventricular failure, deep, rapid respirations or episodes of Cheyne-Stokes respirations can occur.

Lung Sounds

If severe left ventricular failure produces acute pulmonary edema, expiratory wheezing termed *cardiac asthma* occurs as a result of bronchial narrowing due to peribronchial fluid accumulation. When alveoli begin to flood with fluid, inspiratory crackles that sound like Velcro opening are heard at the gravity-dependent areas of lung. With progression of alveolar and airway flooding, coarse crackles are heard over at least half of the dependent lung fields.

Urine Output

The urine volume is usually well maintained unless the patient is in significant heart failure or cardiogenic shock. Diuretic therapy invalidates urine flow rates as an indicator of renal and systemic perfusion.

Acid-Base Values

A mild-to-moderate respiratory alkalosis may occur due to hyperventilation associated with anxiety, pain, or acute pulmonary edema. Metabolic acidosis results from lactic acid production due to severe hypoxemia and low cardiac output causing significant tissue hypoperfusion.

Hemodynamic Profile

Invasive hemodynamic monitoring is indicated in less than 20% of patients with AMI because most patients are hemodynamically stable or have only mild-to-moderate left ventricular failure. When differentiation of moderate and severe heart failure is difficult based on clinical assessment alone, or when the patient is in severe heart failure or cardiogenic shock, invasive hemodynamic monitoring is indicated. Other considerations for invasive monitoring in AMI are listed in Box 21-2.

Arterial Pressure

In patients with uncomplicated acute myocardial infarction, the arterial pressure is often within the normal range. If, however, the blood catecholamine concentrations are increased as a result of an acute stress response

---

BOX 21-2

Considerations for Invasive Hemodynamic Monitoring in Acute Myocardial Infarction

Persistent chest pain
Persistent tachycardia
Hypertension
Hypotension
Significant left ventricular failure
Suspicion of significant right ventricular infarction
Use of vasoactive or inotropic agents for the management of any of the above
Development of a new systolic murmur

From Grauer K, Cavallara D: *ACLS certification preparation and a comprehensive review,* ed 3, St Louis, 1993, Mosby.

and sympathoadrenal discharge, the patient may be hypertensive. Conversely, if ventricular function and cardiac output are severely depressed, the patient may experience a significant decrease in blood pressure and become hypotensive. Between 10% and 20% of patients with acute myocardial infarction and hypotension are hypovolemic secondary to nausea and vomiting, diaphoresis, hyperventilation, or excessive diuresis. In these patients, careful physical assessment and hemodynamic monitoring indicate that the narrowed pulse pressure and hypotension are the result of volume depletion.

Arterial Waveform

If left ventricular ejection velocity and stroke volume decrease, the rate of the rise of the upstroke of the arterial waveform is slowed and the pulse pressure is narrowed. These give a "damped" appearance to the waveform. Pulsus alternans, with alternate weak and strong beats, indicates severe left ventricular dysfunction and heart failure (Figure 21-10).

Systemic Vascular Resistance

Systemic vascular resistance is commonly elevated due to norepinephrine- and epinephrine-induced systemic vasoconstriction. A small percentage of patients with hypotension or cardiogenic shock exhibit an inappropriate vascular response and decreased systemic vascular resistance. Such inappropriate vasodilation predicts a poor patient outcome.

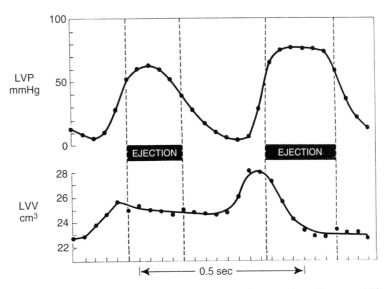

FIGURE 21-10 Alternating weak and strong left ventricular systoles, or pulsus alternans. Although a left ventricular pressure wave is recorded during the weak beat, very little blood volume is actually ejected from the left ventricle. *LVP,* left ventricular pressure; *LVV,* left ventricular volume.

Pulmonary Vascular Resistance

This calculated measurement is usually normal unless hypoxemia, pulmonary edema, or pulmonary embolism complicate the patient's clinical picture. In these circumstances, pulmonary vascular resistance is increased.

Central Venous Pressure and Right Atrial Pressure

Volume depletion, such as may occur with excessive furosemide diuresis, decreases this measurement. In contrast, right ventricular failure or infarction, which often is the result of occlusion of the right coronary artery, increases this measurement. Therefore these pressures may equal or exceed the left ventricular end-diastolic (PWP) pressure (Figure 21-11).

Pulmonary Artery Pressures

These measurements are increased commensurate with elevations in pulmonary artery wedge pressure in patients with pulmonary edema, hypoxemia, or acidemia. The elevations in pulmonary vascular resistance are associated with greater elevations in the pulmonary artery systolic and diastolic pressures relative to PWP. This results in a widening of the pulmonary artery diastolic to wedge pressure gradient.

Pulmonary Artery Wedge Pressure

This measurement may be in the normal range of 4 to 12 mm Hg in patients who maintain relatively normal left ventricular function. Patients with hypovolemia may have significant reductions in the PWP. Clinicians must remain mindful, however, that "numbers" are relative to the patient's ventricular compliance. In patients with decreased ventricular compliance, a "normal" wedge pressure of 8 mm Hg may be associated with a suboptimal ventricular filling volume. A normal wedge pressure associated with a low cardiac index suggests a need for volume loading.

The PWP is elevated in proportion to the degree of left ventricular dysfunction in patients with a significant reduction in left ventricular compliance or left ventricular failure. In general, *patients with an elevated PWP have more severe coronary artery disease and wall motion abnormalities than patients with normal PWP measurements.*

Cardiac Output

Output is maintained within normal limits in patients with uncomplicated myocardial infarction but is decreased when ventricular dysfunction or other abnormalities (papillary muscle ischemia, papillary muscle or

interventricular septal rupture) complicate the myocardial infarction.

Mixed Venous Oxygen Saturation

Compensation for hypoperfusion consists of increased tissue oxygen extraction; therefore mixed venous oxygen saturation is decreased. As a result, a decreased mixed venous oxygen saturation (SvO_2) in a patient with AMI indicates significantly decreased tissue perfusion. A severe decrease in mixed venous oxygen saturation associated with a significant increase in PWP and a decrease in cardiac output has two important implications: (1) the patient has severe cardiac dysfunction, and (2) oxygen transport is severely compromised, which will further jeopardize myocardial function and systemic tissue oxygenation. Both implications suggest a poor patient outcome.

Several studies have demonstrated that, after careful physical examination of critically ill patients, experienced clinicians correctly predicted PWP, cardiac output, and other hemodynamic parameters less than 50% of the time.[3-5] Following pulmonary artery catheterization, the therapeutic plan was changed in almost 50% of cases. Echocardiography and invasive hemodynamic monitoring have significantly improved the evaluation of patients and have allowed the development of prognostic indices, as well as the design of specific therapeutic interventions relative to each hemodynamic subset (Table 21-4). As a consequence, the mortality and morbidity rates of critically ill patients with ischemic heart disease have declined.

Laboratory Examination and Other Diagnostic Tests

The diagnosis of AMI should be based on a combination of the patient's history and clinical presentation, ECG, and laboratory results.

The white blood cell count and erythrocyte sedimentation rate are elevated in patients with AMI by the second day. The degree of elevation roughly correlates with the extent of myocardial damage and inflammation. The hematocrit value often rises slightly because of hemoconcentration. The blood glucose level is initially elevated as part of the general sympathoadrenal (stress) response.

Although the ECG provides confirmation of the presence of AMI, special caveats related to the initial diagnosis of patients with an acute ischemic event include the following: (1) the initial ECG may be completely normal (see later), and (2) the signs and symptoms of AMI may be atypical or absent. The patient may appear remarkably well although a potentially lethal process is evolving in the patient's heart.

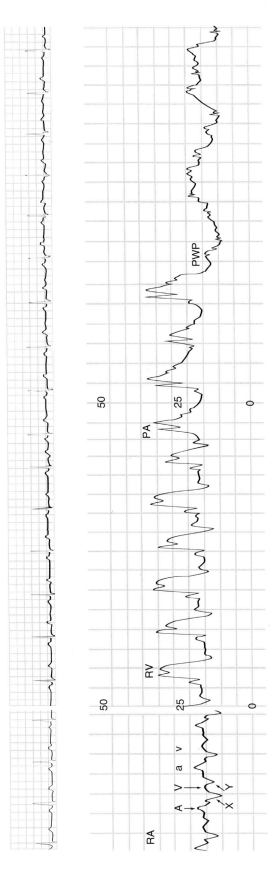

FIGURE 21-11 Right atrial, right ventricular, pulmonary artery, and pulmonary artery wedge pressure tracings from a patient with left ventricular inferior-posterior wall and right ventricular infarctions. The right heart pressures are increased, and there is a prominent a wave from increased force of right atrial contraction. The right ventricle is dilated but "constrained" by the pericardium. Consequently, there is equalization of right heart diastolic pressures. Pericardial fluid with tamponade is excluded because of the prominent Y descent. The Y descent is due to tricuspid valve opening and rapid inflow of blood into the ventricle. In cardiac tamponade, the Y descent is significantly reduced or absent. The positive, normal v wave is produced by right atrial filling. Constrictive pericarditis is unlikely because of the slow heart rate of 54 beats per minute.

545

TABLE 21-4

Therapeutic Intervention in Acute Myocardial Infarction

Hemodynamic Subset	PWP (mm Hg)	Cardiac Index	Intervention
Normal	≤12	2.7–3.5	Aspirin, heparin, nitrates, beta blockade; thrombolytic therapy or angioplasty if within 6-12 hours of symptoms and onset of Q wave infarction; IIB-IIIA platelet receptor antagonists are given to patients with non–Q wave or ST segment depression infarction
Hyperdynamic state	≤12	≥3.0	Beta-adrenergic receptor blockade, then normal subset protocol
Hypoperfusion due to hypovolemia	≤7	≥2.7	Fluid challenge, then normal subset protocol
Left ventricular failure			
Moderate	18–22	≤2.5	Intravenous furosemide + nitroglycerin
Severe	≥23	≤2.0	Intravenous furosemide + nitroglycerin + dobutamine
Cardiogenic shock	>18–25	≤1.8	Intravenous nitroglycerin, dopamine, furosemide, circulatory assistance, angioplasty, or surgical revascularization

PWP, pulmonary artery wedge pressure.

Electrocardiogram

Figures 21-12 and 21-13 show classic evolutionary changes in the standard 12-lead ECG.

Although the ECG is important in the diagnosis of AMI, pitfalls must be emphasized:

1. Significant myocardial injury and necrosis may be associated with only slight ST segment changes or T wave inversion.
2. T wave abnormalities may be delayed for more than a week after the infarction.
3. ST and T wave changes may be caused by pericarditis, medications, electrolyte imbalance, anxiety, and hyperventilation.

The resting ECG may initially be normal in one half of patients with myocardial ischemia. On the other hand, isolated J-point elevation may be present as a normal variant in young, healthy adults.

Cardiac Biochemical Markers

The diagnosis of AMI should be confirmed by an increase in the plasma concentration of troponin T or I and the myocardial band (MB) fraction of the creatine kinase (CK). However, troponin is a more sensitive and specific indicator of myocardial damage than CK-MB. For example, troponin levels may be elevated in patients with unstable angina, although CK-MB levels are normal. Elevations in troponin I have also been shown to predict increased risk of death in patients with non–Q wave AMI or unstable angina.[6] However, *troponin levels may be normal in patients within the first 6 hours of onset of the acute event.* The plasma concentrations of troponin

T or I and CK-MB elevate within 12 to 24 hours in more than 90% of patients with AMI. These are the best tests to diagnosis AMI 12 to 24 hours after the onset of symptoms (Table 21-5). In patients treated within 6 hours of the onset of symptoms, the laboratory diagnosis of AMI is best made by measurements of CK-MB subforms (MB2/MB1 ratio) or by measurements of plasma myoglobin. Although myoglobin rises early in AMI and is highly sensitive, it is not specific (false-positive values may occur in patients with renal disease or skeletal muscle disease or injury).

The plasma concentration of troponin and CK-MB should be determined on admission and at least every 8 hours for 24 hours. An increase in the plasma concentration of troponin or CK-MB more than 3 standard deviations (99th percentile) from the normal value or an increase in CK-MB by more than 50% over a 4-hour period is indicative of myocardial infarction. The plasma concentration of troponin I remains elevated for 5 to 14 days.

Chest Radiograph

In the absence of heart failure, the lung fields are normal. As the left ventricle fails and dilates, signs of pulmonary congestion and interstitial edema (perihilar haze, pulmonary vascular redistribution with prominence of the upper lobe pulmonary veins, and Kerley B lines) appear on the chest radiograph. Cardiac enlargement and signs of pulmonary congestion may be present even when other clinical signs and symptoms of heart failure are absent.

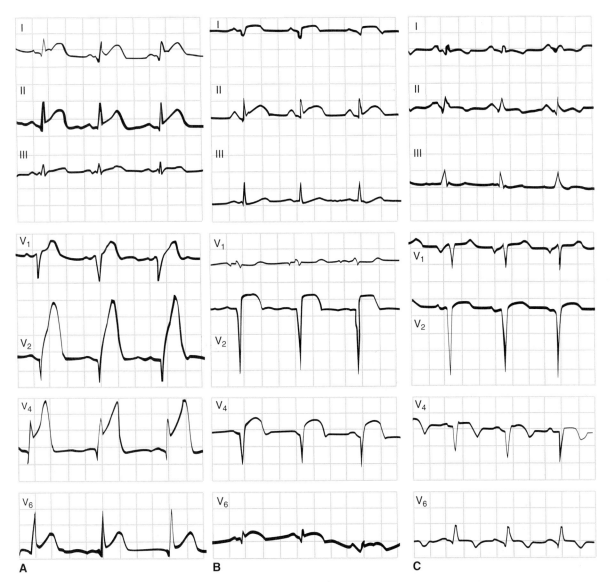

FIGURE 21-12 Acute anterior-lateral wall myocardial infarction. Note the deep, wide Q wave and ST-T wave changes in the leads oriented to the anterior-lateral walls, predominantly V₁ through V₆. **A,** One hour after AMI. **B,** Twenty-four hours after AMI. **C,** Ten days after AMI. (Courtesy of Dr. Erik Sandoe and Dr. Bjarne Sigurd: *Arrhythmias,* 1984, Fachmed AG Verlag fur Fachmedien.)

Regions of lungs that are airless due to exudate (pneumonia), fluid (pulmonary edema), or collapse (atelectasis) appear white on the chest radiograph. Consequently, diffuse, fluffy-appearing "whiteouts" become evident on the chest radiograph. Pulmonary edema "opacities" are often more extensive at the hilar regions with sparing of the peripheral lung fields (butterfly-wing distribution) (see Chapter 18, Figure 18-19). There may be a time lag, however, between the appearance of an elevated pulmonary artery wedge pressure and the radiographic evidence of acute pulmonary edema. Similarly, after normalization of the PWP, 12 to 24 hours may be required for the radiographic evidence of pulmonary edema to subside.

Echocardiogram-Doppler Examination

Hypokinesia or akinesia of the involved ischemic myocardium and the resultant reduction of the ejection fraction are frequently evident on the echocardiogram. Wall motion abnormalities detected by echocardiography, in fact, often precede electrocardiographic changes of AMI. Occasionally, paradoxic systolic expansion (dyskinesis) of severely ischemic or necrotic myocardium is visualized. Expansion of a myocardial infarct may be demonstrated on serial echocardiograms by progressive regional hypokinesis or akinesis, transmural diastolic thinning of the ventricular wall, and ventricular dilation. In addition, left ventricular mural thrombi are frequently visualized in patients with large anterior wall infarctions. The echo-Doppler examina-

tion is also useful for diagnosing the mechanical complications of AMI (see later in this chapter).

Radionuclide Studies

Technetium scans are useful in confirming the diagnosis of AMI, especially in patients with left bundle branch block on the electrocardiogram or in patients in whom the history, electrocardiographic changes, and plasma markers are unavailable or unreliable. The radionuclide technetium

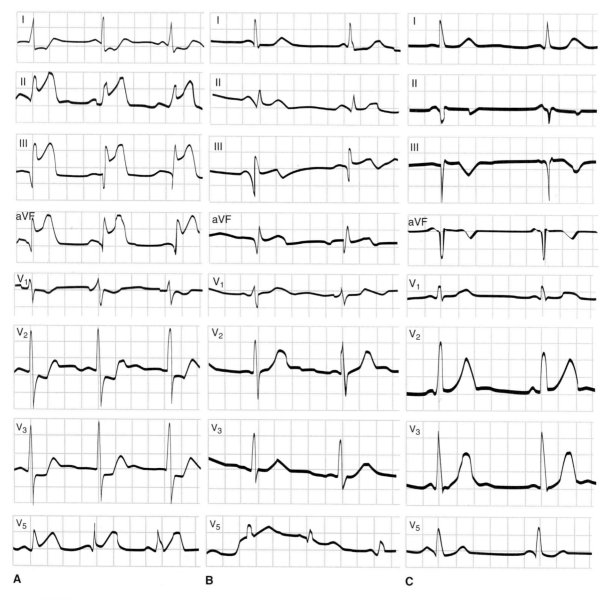

A   **B**   **C**

FIGURE 21-13 Acute inferior-posterior wall myocardial infarction. Note the classic ischemia/injury/necrosis–induced ECG changes in the leads oriented to the inferior left ventricular wall—leads II, III, and aVF. **A,** One hour after AMI. **B,** Twenty-four hours after AMI. **C,** Ten days after AMI. (Courtesy of Dr. Erik Sandoe and Dr. Bjarne Sigurd. *Arrhythmias,* 1984, Fachmed AG Verlag fur Fachmedien.)

pyrophosphate is taken up by calcium in the acutely damaged cells and results in a "hot spot" when the myocardium is scanned with a scintillation camera. The scan becomes positive within 12 to 36 hours after AMI and remains positive for approximately 6 to 10 days. Radionuclide ventriculograms, when gated (timed) to the electrocardiogram, make possible the noninvasive assessment of right and left ventricular ejection fractions, as well as the evaluation of right and left ventricular wall motion. Serial thallium scans may be useful in demonstrating changes in myocardial perfusion abnormalities in patients who are successfully revascularized with either angioplasty or thrombolytic therapy.

Cardiac Catheterization

Visualization of the coronary arteries helps guide therapy by localizing the site and extent of the coronary lesions in patients with persistent chest pain who are not promptly responsive to medical therapy, who have ST elevation or a new bundle branch block, or who have complicated AMI. When personnel and proper catheterization facilities are available, percutaneous transluminal coronary angioplasty (PTCA) and stenting opens the obstructive coronary lesion, improves the ventricular function, and salvages viable myocardium. Ischemia-induced anatomic defects, such as papillary muscle rupture or ventricular septal defect, as well as the need for emergency revascularization surgery, can also be more carefully defined.

Treatment

The goals of therapy for AMI patients are to limit infarct size by increasing myocardial oxygen supply and decreasing myocardial oxygen demand (Figure 21-14), promoting electrical stability, ensuring patient comfort, and preventing or managing complications. Routine treatment measures are similar to those used for management of patients with unstable angina pectoris. Other treatment decisions relate to the amount of time that has passed from the onset of chest pain to admission to hospital, as well as the patient's clinical and hemodynamic picture.

In patients with uncomplicated AMI admitted more than 12 to 24 hours after the onset of symptoms, fundamental treatment measures include bed rest, supplemental oxygen therapy, and aspirin and heparin to prevent reinfarction and left ventricular and deep venous thrombus formation. Beta-adrenergic blockade therapy and nitroglycerin are begun in patients without contraindications to this therapy on admission to the critical care unit. Other therapies that may be selected based on the patient's risk profile, clinical picture, and laboratory results include ventricular unloading agents, inotropic agents, angiotensin-converting enzyme inhibitors, control of arrhythmias, opiate analgesia, lipid-lowering agents, and glycoprotein IIb-IIIa platelet antagonists.

TABLE 21-5
Cardiac Biochemical Markers of Acute Myocardial Infarction

Myoglobin	CK-MB	CK-MB Subforms	cTnT	cTnI
First detectable	1-2 hr	2-4 hr	2-6 hr	2-6 hr
>85% sensitivity	6-10 hr	6 hr	10-12 hr	10-12 hr
Peak	4-8 hr	6-12 hr	10-24 hr	10-24 hr
Duration (days)	0.5-1.0	0.5-1.0	5-14	5-14

Adapted in part from Adams J, Abendschein D, Jaffe A: Biochemical markers of myocardial injury, *Circulation* 88:750, 1993; Zimmerman J, Fromm R, Meyer D, et al: Diagnostic marker cooperative study for diagnosis of myocardial infarction, *Circulation* 99:1671, 1999.
cTnT, cardiac troponin T; *cTnI,* cardiac troponin I.

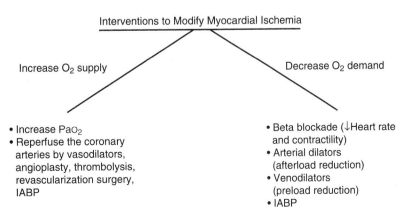

FIGURE 21-14 Therapeutic interventions to prevent or modify myocardial ischemia. *IABP,* Intraaortic balloon counterpulsation.

Antiarrhythmic Therapy

Cardiac arrhythmias are common and may be controlled by the correction of electrolyte imbalances, provision of adequate systemic and myocardial oxygenation, reduction of sympathetic nervous stimulation, and diminution of myocardial oxygen demands. Although it was routinely used for the prophylaxis of ventricular arrhythmias from the 1960s through the 1990s, lidocaine (Xylocaine) is currently not recommended for prophylaxis of ventricular arrhythymias in the setting of AMI.[7] Lidocaine suppresses ventricular arrhythmias due to myocardial ischemia once they occur but is second in choice to amiodarone or procainamide. Antiarrhythmic agents, electrical countershock, or cardiac pacing is required when systemic organ perfusion and function are significantly compromised by cardiac arrhythmias.

Beta Blockade. Patients with excessive sympathetic nervous system stimulation are tachycardic, hypertensive, and more vulnerable to primary ventricular fibrillation. An early intravenous administration of a beta-blocking agent, such as metoprolol (Lopressor), is given in increments of 1 to 5 mg intravenously; the dose is repeated until a total 15 mg loading dose is delivered or bradycardia occurs. During the intravenous administration of metoprolol, the patient's blood pressure, heart rate, and ECG should be carefully monitored. In patients who tolerate the full intravenous dose, an oral dose of 50 mg is started 15 minutes after the last injection and is administered every 12 hours for 48 hours. Thereafter, patients should receive a maintenance dose of 50 to 100 mg twice daily. Beta-blockade therapy should not be used in patients with heart rates less than 60 beats per minute, second- or third-degree heart block, hypotension (less than 100 mm Hg systolic pressure) or shock, heart failure, or severe pulmonary or peripheral vascular disease.

Atropine Sulfate for Parasympathetic Nervous System Hyperactivity. Patients with inferior wall infarction may have significant bradycardia. Atropine counteracts vagal activity and may be useful in treating patients who are hypotensive or those who have significant ventricular ectopy or chest pain as a consequence of the inappropriately slow heart rate. The drug should be given cautiously, in 0.5 mg increments repeated every 5 minutes, until the patient's clinical response improves or a maximum total dose of 0.04 mg/kg (approximately 2 mg) is given.

Angiotensin-Converting Enzyme Inhibition. Patients with AMI and left ventricular dysfunction, especially patients with hypertension and congestive heart failure, should be treated within the first 24 hours with angiotensin-converting enzyme (ACE) inhibition therapy (captopril, lisinopril, fosinopril, ramipril, or benazepril) to reduce left ventricular dysfunction and congestive heart failure and limit or prevent left ventricular remodeling. The efficacy of this class of drugs is greatest in patients with prior myocardial infarction, anterior wall myocardial infarction, congestive heart failure, or tachycardia. An ACE inhibitor should not be given if the patient has hypotension (systolic blood pressure less than 100 mm Hg), bilateral renal artery stenosis, renal failure, or a history of angioedema with previous ACE treatment.

Pharmacologic Manipulation of Preload, Afterload, and Contractility

In patients with complicated AMI, pharmacologic manipulation of preload, afterload, and contractility is required, and medications are selected and titrated according to the patient's hemodynamic profile and clinical response. However, these drugs are typically a means of patient support and not a therapeutic end-point. Mechanical and surgical interventions, such as intraaortic balloon counterpulsation and coronary angioplasty, emergency aortocoronary bypass surgery, or corrective surgery for mechanical complications of AMI, are often required to optimize cardiac function and prevent further complications. In complicated cases, the safe and efficacious use of preload- and afterload-reducing agents, inotropic agents, and mechanical interventions requires pulmonary and systemic arterial pressure monitoring, as well as the measurement of cardiac output. The practitioner must remember that the "best hemodynamic numbers" vary from patient to patient. Therapy is directed at determining and maintaining hemodynamic measurements that optimize cardiac output and tissue perfusion and prevent pulmonary edema, while reducing heart work and oxygen consumption. PWP measurements and cardiac output studies also provide data for plotting ventricular function curves (see Chapter 10) by which pharmacologic therapy can be evaluated and optimized.

Preload Reduction. Acute left heart failure signifies that more than 25% of the left ventricular myocardium is dysfunctional. The presence of heart failure implies a poor prognosis. However, preload reduction may relieve symptoms of pulmonary congestion (Figure 21-15, point A to point B, furosemide).

By diminishing the volume of blood returning to the ischemic ventricle, chamber size and oxygen requirements are decreased and transmural perfusion pressure (mean arterial pressure minus left ventricular end-diastolic pressure—see Chapter 20, Figure 20-3) is increased. If the PWP is greater than 20 mm Hg, preload reduction is of additional benefit in treating acute pulmonary edema. Two

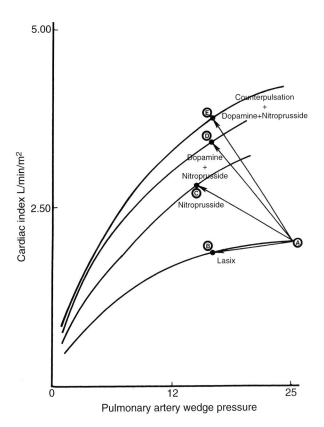

FIGURE 21-15 The relationship between the cardiac index and the pulmonary artery wedge pressure in a patient with an acute myocardial infarction and pulmonary edema. *Point A* illustrates the patient's initial hemodynamic status. The administration of a diuretic (preload reduction) decreased the PWP and relieved the pulmonary vascular congestion but did not improve the cardiac index. In terms of cardiac function, the patient's condition remained at the same peak level on the Starling curve and moved from *point A* to *point B*. Intravenous nitroprusside reduced the impedance to left ventricular ejection (reduced left ventricular afterload), improved cardiac index, and decreased PWP by causing venodilation (preload reduction). The overall effect is a shift to *point C* on an improved Starling curve.

The addition of intravenous dopamine increased cardiac index by improving myocardial contractility, but the inotrope also slightly raised the PWP via the drug's venoconstrictor effect. Consequently, a shift to *point D* occurred.

Finally, the addition of intraaortic balloon counterpulsation to the patient's therapy improved myocardial contractility and cardiac index by increasing coronary perfusion pressure and decreasing afterload. As a consequence, balloon counterpulsation resulted in a shift to *point E* on an optimal Starling curve.

commonly administered preload-reducing agents are furosemide (Lasix) and nitroglycerin.

Furosemide (Lasix). The initial effect of furosemide on preload reduction is venodilation. This effect is achieved within the first 5 minutes of administration; furosemide results in the pooling of significant amounts of blood in the systemic veins. Thereafter the drug's diuretic effect facilitates the excretion of sodium and water by the kidney.

Nitroglycerin. This drug, typically titrated by continuous intravenous drip, is given to reduce myocardial oxygen requirements by reducing ventricular end-diastolic volume and myocardial wall tension. Nitroglycerin should be titrated to maximally decrease ischemic pain without compromising stroke volume. Preload reduction with nitroglycerin is achieved by dilating and pooling blood in the systemic venous bed.

Morphine Sulfate. Although nitroglycerin relieves myocardial ischemic pain, supplementation with morphine sulfate given intravenously, *cautiously titrated to effect,* is commonly necessary (see also section on opiate analgesia for unstable angina). Adverse effects include hypotension, particularly in hypovolemic patients (treated with the supine position or fluid administration); vagally mediated bradycardia (treated with atropine); and respiratory depression (treated with naloxone or mechanical ventilatory support).

Afterload Reduction. In patients with significant vasoconstriction, arteriolar dilating agents such as nitroprusside (Nipride) or nitroglycerin, when given in larger doses, decrease the impedance to left ventricular ejection and therefore increase the stroke volume and tissue perfusion (see Figure 21-15, point A to point C). The ventricular function curve is shifted upward and to the left, indicating a more efficient pump. Because myocardial work is reduced, oxygen requirements also are reduced. Because an ischemic, failing ventricle is extremely sensitive to changes in afterload, a reduction in significantly elevated systemic vascular resistance can increase cardiac output by as much as 25%.

Afterload reduction also is beneficial in patients with acute mitral regurgitation or acute ventricular septal rupture that may complicate AMI. In these patients, a reduction in the systemic vascular resistance facilitates forward systemic blood flow and decreases regurgitant volume (acute mitral regurgitation) or left-to-right interventricular shunt (acute septal rupture). These conditions may also require the intraaortic balloon pump (IABP), which mechanically reduces afterload, facilitates systemic tissue perfusion, and increases coronary perfusion.

Nitroprusside also causes venodilation and therefore is a preload-reducing agent. Consequently, the clinician should expect the pulmonary artery pressure, the PWP, and the signs and symptoms of pulmonary edema to decrease with the use of this drug.

Inotropic Agents. Patients with low cardiac output and hypotension require drugs that improve contractility and systemic blood flow (see Figure 21-15, point A to point D). These pharmacologic agents include dopamine (Intropin) and dobutamine (Dobutrex) (see Chapter 14 for specific properties of each agent). Milrinone is an inotropic drug of third choice. Generally, dopamine and dobutamine should be titrated to doses less than 10 µg/kg/min for optimal therapeutic effect. When used in concentrations greater than 10 µg/kg/min, dopamine and dobutamine may significantly increase myocardial oxygen demands because of elevations in heart rate. Dopamine at higher dose levels (approximately greater than 20 µg/kg/min) also increases systemic and pulmonary vascular resistance. These effects may actually extend the infarction.

Combination therapy, which is the concomitant use of a vasodilating agent and an inotropic agent (see Figure 21-15, point A to point E), optimizes stroke volume while limiting heart work and oxygen requirements. This type of "mixed" pharmacologic therapy requires careful titration of both drugs and continuous bedside physical assessment and hemodynamic monitoring. The IABP (see Chapter 15) further assists ventricular emptying by increasing coronary and systemic blood flow.

Glycoprotein IIb-IIIa Platelet Receptor Inhibitors. Patients with acute chest pain without ST segment eleva-

tion but abnormal biochemical markers, who have high-risk features (prior AMI, widespread ECG changes, impaired left ventricular function, or recurrent ischemia), should be evaluated for glycoprotein IIb-IIIa receptor inhibitor therapy. Patients with contraindications due to risk of bleeding (see glycoprotein IIb-IIIa section, treatment of angina pectoris) are excluded from consideration for this treatment.

Intraaortic Balloon Pump

If ventricular unloading and inotropic therapy do not promptly stabilize the condition of patients with complicated AMI, IABP counterpulsation should be instituted when available. Balloon inflation during diastole augments aortic diastolic pressure, thereby augmenting coronary perfusion pressure and coronary blood flow. Deflation of the balloon during systole decreases ventricular afterload, which facilitates ventricular ejection and systemic tissue perfusion (Figure 21-16).

The IABP may improve cardiac function by as much as 25%. Balloon counterpulsation is useful also in stabilizing the patient's condition before and during cardiac catheterization, before and during induction of anesthesia, and during and following required surgical interventions (coronary revascularization, repair of ruptured

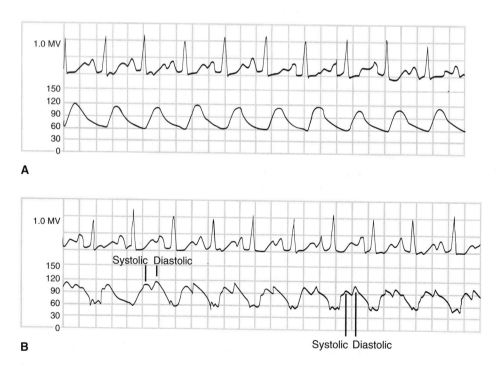

FIGURE 21-16 Simultaneous electrocardiographic and arterial blood pressure recordings before *(panel A)* and during *(panel B)* intraaortic balloon counterpulsation. The peak diastolic (coronary perfusion) pressure is increased and the peak systolic pressure is decreased during counterpulsation. Overall, myocardial oxygen supply is augmented whereas myocardial oxygen demand is reduced.

ventricular septum or papillary muscle) (see Chapters 15 and 16).

Patients who are within 6 to 12 hours of the onset of symptoms, have ST segment elevation or a new bundle branch block, or have intermittent symptoms for less than 24 hours are candidates for reperfusion therapies. These include fibrinolytic therapy and mechanical restoration of the patency of the diseased artery or arteries with primary angioplasty (PTCA) and stenting or surgical myocardial revascularization.

Fibrinolytic Therapy

Thrombolysis produces the greatest benefit when given within 6 hours of the onset of symptoms, although the patient may still benefit if the drug is given within 12 hours. *The time goal for the administration of thrombolytic therapy is less than 30 minutes after the patient enters the hospital (door-to-needle time).* Contraindica-

tions include a history of poorly controlled severe hypertension, cerebrovascular pathology, major surgery or trauma within the preceding 2 months, aortic dissection, active peptic ulcer disease, and predisposition to bleeding (Box 21-3). In patients who have contraindications to thrombolytic therapy and in centers where physician preference is to use angioplasty as a first-line measure, thrombolysis may be deferred. Angioplasty should be reserved for centers with skilled, high-volume (more than 75 cases per year), invasive cardiologists who are practicing at a high-volume center (200 to 300 cases per year). If the patient is admitted to an institution where these angiographic requirements are not met, the patient should be transferred to such an institution, preferably one with the capacity to do emergency surgical revascularization if necessary.

Thromboytic therapy is in a continued state of evolution. For any patient with AMI who is a potential candidate for

---

BOX 21-3
Thrombolytic Therapy for Patients with Acute Myocardial Infarction

Patient Eligibility

1. Symptoms compatible with acute myocardial infarction of less than 12 hours and in some instances 12 to 24 hours in duration if chest pain and electrocardiographic ST segment elevations are persistent
2. ST elevation equal to or greater than 1 mm in two or more contiguous electrocardiographic leads that is not relieved by nitroglycerin or new-onset left bundle branch block
3. Patient able to give informed consent

Exclusions

1. Active internal bleeding or history of recent gastrointestinal bleeding, active peptic ulcer disease, or ulcerative colitis
2. Severe liver disease, renal failure, or a bleeding diathesis
3. Recent stroke (within 1 year), head trauma, or known intracranial neoplasm, aneurysm, or arteriovenous malformation
4. Surgery, invasive procedure, or trauma within past 2 months
5. Aortic dissection
6. Acute pericarditis
7. Prolonged or traumatic cardiopulmonary resuscitation
8. Pregnancy
9. Unstable angina with ST segment depression or non−Q wave myocardial infarction

Relative Exclusions

1. Age greater than 75 years
2. Uncontrolled hypertension (greater than 180/110 mm Hg)
3. Diabetic proliferative retinopathy
4. History of cerebrovascular accident
5. Previous allergy to or prior treatment with thrombolytic agent (streptokinase, reptilase, or anistreplase); does not apply to recombinant tissue−type plasminogen activator (rt-PA)
6. High likelihood of left heart thrombus
7. Bacterial endocarditis
8. Vascular puncture in a noncompressible site
9. Current use of anticoagulants in therapeutic doses (international normalized ratio [INR] 2 to 3)

Baseline Studies

1. Complete blood count, prothrombin time, INR, partial thromboplastin time, fibrinogen, and complete metabolic panel
2. MB creatine kinase cardiac biochemical marker at baseline, then every 12 hours for 24 hours, then every day for 2 days; troponin I or T drawn on admission and at 6- to 8-hour intervals to a total of three specimens
3. Electrocardiogram at baseline, immediately after thrombolytic therapy, 4 hours after thrombolytic therapy, then every day; ECGs also taken whenever clinically indicated
4. Blood specimen to blood bank for blood typing

thrombolytic therapy, cardiology consultation should be *immediately* obtained regarding the indications, contraindications, choice of a specific thrombolytic drug, and dosage. Choices include the following:

- Alteplase (Activase), recombinant tissue–type plasminogen activator (rt-PA)
- Tenecteplase (TNKase)
- Anistreplase (Eminase), anisolated plasminogen streptokinase activator complex
- Reteplase, recombinant (Retavase)
- Streptokinase (Streptase)

Cardiac Catheterization, Percutaneous Transluminal Coronary Angioplasty, Placement of Stents, and Revascularization Surgery

The patient may be taken directly to the cardiac catheterization laboratory for mechanical restoration of coronary patency if there are contraindications to thrombolytic therapy or if it is the philosophy of the cardiology department to bypass thrombolytics and take the patient directly to the cardiac catheterization laboratory for evaluation of the coronary circulation and mechanical revascularization. Drug therapies are only *palliative* procedures that "buy time" when coronary blood supply is limited. The coronary arterial obstruction must be relieved. Cardiac catheterization is therefore indicated in patients with complicated AMI who do not respond promptly to medical therapy or in those who are dependent on the IABP. In the catheterization laboratory, high-grade coronary vascular obstructions may be delineated and dilated with balloon angioplasty, or the decision may be made to surgically revascularize the patient's coronary arteries. Mechanical defects such as papillary muscle rupture or ventricular septal rupture can be readily identified and treated surgically.

Combination Reperfusion Therapies

Combination reperfusion therapies are also currently being investigated. These include coadministration of a glycoprotein IIb-IIIa receptor inhibitor and a fibrinolytic agent, fibrinolysis and PTCA, and glycoprotein IIb-IIIa receptor inhibition with PTCA with or without stenting.

Mechanical Complications of Acute Myocardial Infarction

Complications that decrease the integrity of the cardiac musculature or architecture of the cardiac structures may occur at any time in the periinfarction period. Mechanical complications occur most frequently in the initial 7 to 10 days after the AMI. Complications may range from those that produce transient or minor hemodynamic dysfunction to those that may prove fatal if not promptly diagnosed and treated. Potentially fatal mechanical complications

include papillary muscle dysfunction or rupture, acute ventricular septal defect, cardiac rupture, and massive right ventricular infarction.

Postmyocardial infarction pericarditis is discussed in Chapter 23.

Papillary Muscle Dysfunction or Rupture

Normal papillary muscle function is essential to proper closure of the mitral valve leaflets. Ischemic dysfunction or rupture of a papillary muscle results in failure of normal mitral valve closure, thereby permitting systolic regurgitant flow from the left ventricle to left atrium (see Chapter 22, section on acute mitral regurgitation).

The posterior papillary muscle is more commonly affected because its only blood supply is from the posterior descending branch of the right or left coronary artery. The anterior papillary muscle normally has a dual blood supply from tributaries of the diagonal branch of the left anterior descending coronary artery and the marginal branch of circumflex artery.

Ischemic papillary muscle dysfunction, or dysfunction of the myocardium that anchors the papillary muscle, may be transient and may be present only during acute episodes of angina pectoris. Depending on the severity of the papillary muscle ischemia and resultant dysfunction, symptoms may be mild or profound. If the ischemia is intermittent, the patient may have periods of hemodynamic stability punctuated by episodes of acute-onset hemodynamic deterioration with an accompanying sudden-onset systolic mitral regurgitant murmur and "flash pulmonary edema."

Complete rupture of a left ventricular papillary muscle causes a flail mitral valve leaflet and produces overwhelming regurgitation of blood into the left atrium with sudden elevation of left atrial and pulmonary vascular pressures and profoundly decreases cardiac outflow into the systemic circulation. Complete papillary muscle rupture is characterized clinically by low cardiac output and acute pulmonary edema, which are most often associated with sudden death.

Complete or partial rupture of a papillary muscle should be suspected when shock, acute pulmonary edema, apical palpable thrill, and high-pitched pansystolic murmur develop in a patient with a recent myocardial infarction.

A large regurgitant mitral orifice and a poorly contractile left ventricle may make the murmur inaudible and may prevent auscultatory detection. Emergency echo-Doppler examination or cardiac catheterization is often necessary to diagnose this potentially lethal complication. If the patient has a pulmonary artery catheter in place, the detection of large *v* waves in the PWP tracing may be the first indication of mitral regurgitation. The amplitude of the left atrial *v* wave may reach levels of 50 to 70 mm Hg (Figure 21-17).

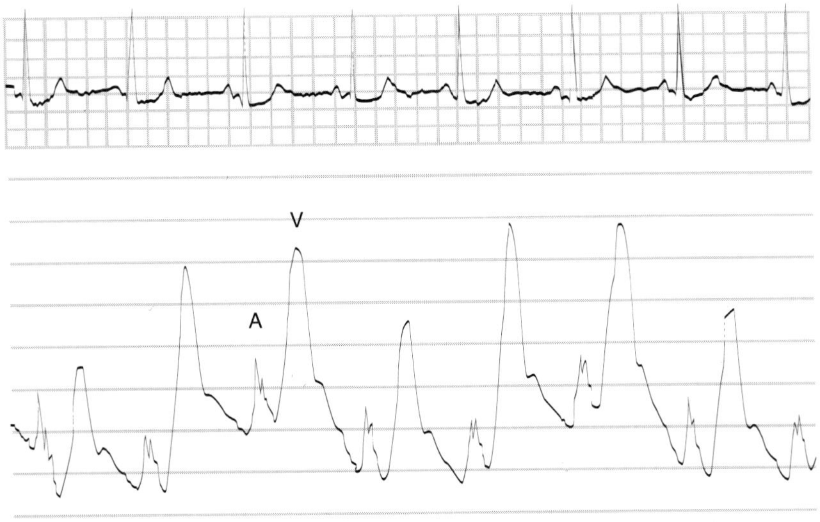

FIGURE 21-17 Large regurgitant v waves on the PWP tracing in a patient with papillary muscle dysfunction and acute mitral regurgitation. Left atrial and pulmonary artery pressures are elevated because of the large regurgitant v wave. The v waves visually reflect the systolic backflow from the left ventricle through the left atrium and into the pulmonary veins.

Complete papillary muscle rupture is an *absolute emergency for surgical repair of the papillary muscle or replacement of the mitral valve;* otherwise, rapid clinical deterioration and death occur. Rapid diagnosis is essential and lifesaving, if followed by supportive medical management as the patient is being prepared for emergency valve repair or replacement.

For the patient with severe ischemic papillary muscle dysfunction, medical management is used for initial support. However, definitive therapy consists of coronary angioplasty or coronary revascularization to improve the blood supply to the involved papillary muscle and relieve the dysfunction.

Preoperative medical management for papillary muscle rupture or supportive therapy for papillary dysfunction is directed at reducing or eliminating the regurgitant stream and increasing systemic perfusion with vasodilator drugs such as nitroglycerin or nitroprusside. Reduction in systemic resistance to left ventricular outflow (afterload) decreases the mitral regurgitant volume and enhances systemic perfusion. Reduction in left ventricular end-diastolic volume (preload) results in an improvement in the alignment of papillary muscles. Therefore reduction in preload may decrease the size of the regurgitant mitral valve orifice and consequently reduce the regurgitant volume into the left atrium due to an ischemic papillary muscle. Inotropic support with dobutamine can be given to further improve left ventricular performance without increasing systemic vascular resistance.

Reduction of systemic vascular resistance is critical to the management of papillary muscle dysfunction or rupture. Afterload reduction facilitates ejection of blood into the aorta, thereby decreasing the volume of regurgitant flow into the left atrium. Conversely, vasopressor agents such as norepinephrine (Levophed) and phenylephrine (Neo-Synephrine) increase aortic outflow resistance and therefore increase regurgitant flow from the left ventricle into the left atrium.

If the patient has significant hypotension (mean arterial pressure less than 70 mm Hg, which contraindicates the use of vasodilating agents), the IABP provides hemodynamic support in conjunction with pharmacologic therapy. The IABP mechanically reduces left ventricular outflow resistance while augmenting aortic diastolic and coronary perfusion pressure.

Acute Ventricular Septal Defect

Rupture of the intraventricular septum is a potentially lethal event that complicates the hospital course of 1% to 3% of patients with anterior or inferior wall AMI. Patients experiencing their first infarction, in whom collateral blood flow to the septum is limited, are particularly vulnerable. The majority of septal ruptures occur within the first week, and 20% of all ruptures occur as early as the first 24 hours after the onset of symptoms of myocardial infarction. Sixty percent of septal ruptures develop with infarction of the anterior ventricular wall, and 40% occur with infarction of the posterior or inferior ventricular wall.

Septal rupture with anterior infarction is usually apical in location. Inferior infarction may be associated with a perforation of the basal portion of the septum and a worse prognosis.

During systole, left ventricular blood that is 97% to 99% saturated with oxygen is shunted through the ventricular septal defect (VSD) into the right ventricle (Figure 21-18). There, the oxygenated blood mixes with venous deoxygenated blood. The pure venous blood is variably saturated (75% or lower) relative to the degree of circulatory failure. However, the volume-overloaded right ventricle then ejects a supernormal volume of blood with an increased oxygen saturation into the pulmonary circulation. Flow overload of the pulmonary circulation and left heart eventually causes acute pulmonary edema. At the same time, systemic perfusion decreases because the left ventricular output into the aorta is decreased and eventually leads to shock. The volume of the shunted blood and therefore the severity of the hemodynamic abnormality depend on the size of the septal defect and the systolic pressure difference between the two ventricles. Another factor that influences patient outcome is the

functional state of the right heart. This determines the right ventricle's capacity to meet the abnormal, acute systolic volume challenge.

Hemodynamic deterioration is sudden in onset and often relentless as the shunted blood continues to erode the walls of the defect and progressively enlarge the size of the septal defect. The arterial pressure and pulse pressure progressively fall relative to the decrease in volume ejected into the aorta. Right ventricular and pulmonary artery pressures rise in proportion to the size of the defect and the blood flow through the defect. The PWP also is elevated because of the abnormally high blood flow through the pulmonary vasculature, which empties into the left atrium. When pulmonary blood flow increases, the PWP *v* wave may increase in amplitude, in the absence of mitral regurgitation, because of the additional amount of blood entering the normally small, relatively noncompliant left atrium during left ventricular systole.

The presence of a pansystolic decrescendo murmur accompanied by a palpable thrill, in a patient with low cardiac output that progresses to acute pulmonary edema and cardiogenic shock, is a typical finding due to an acute VSD. Early recognition of this consellation of symptoms followed by immediate diagnostic studies and aggressive treatment may be lifesaving. The murmur is characteristically loudest at the lower left and right sternal borders; however, the murmur may be loudest at the left ventricular apex. Overall, the clinical picture may be indistinguishable from that of patients with acute, severe mitral regurgitation.

The pulmonary artery catheter is a useful diagnostic tool in differentiating acute VSD from acute mitral regurgitation because these conditions commonly are difficult to distinguish by physical assessment. Patients with acute VSD may have an oxygen saturation "step-up" in excess of 10% when sequential blood samples are obtained from the right atrium, the right ventricle, and the pulmonary artery. Table 21-6 gives an example of oxygen saturations from blood drawn from the right atrium, right ventricle, and pulmonary artery during flotation of a pulmonary artery catheter in a patient with a large VSD.

Echo-Doppler examination is the most helpful noninvasive tool in distinguishing mitral regurgitant flow from the left-to-right ventricular shunt of acute VSD.

When pulmonary blood flow is more than two times systemic blood flow, as assessed by echo-Doppler cardiac study or cardiac catheterization, circulatory assistance and emergency surgery are necessary. Emergency temporizing medical therapy is directed toward reducing the impedance to left ventricular outflow. This reduces the shunt volume and increases the systemic blood flow. If available, IABP counterpulsation should be instituted

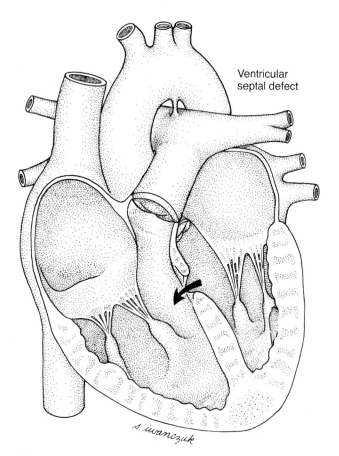

FIGURE 21-18 Flow abnormality in ventricular septal defect.

immediately. Nitroprusside also may improve hemodynamics by (1) lowering systemic vascular resistance and improving left ventricular outflow, thus decreasing the severity of the shunt; and (2) decreasing pulmonary vascular congestion by promoting venous pooling. Another temporizing emergency maneuver consists of inflation of the pulmonary artery catheter balloon to 1.5 to 2.0 ml immediately above the pulmonic valve and maintaining the balloon in that position. This increases the resistance to blood flow through the pulmonary artery and temporarily decreases the severity of the left-to-right shunt. The desired catheter tip location is best determined by chest radiograph examination.

Cardiac Rupture

Rupture of the left ventricular free wall occurs in 1% to 3% of patients with acute transmural infarctions and accounts for 10% to 15% of all deaths following AMI. The lethal event typically occurs within the first 3 to 6 days after an acute infarction. This is the time period when the necrotic tissue is the most friable, but rupture may occur later. The rupture typically develops at the peripheral border of a large transmural infarcton that involves more than 20% of the anterior wall. AMI patients at greatest risk include the elderly; females; those with sustained hypertension; and those with recurrent, severe chest pain.

The rate of progression and the severity of symptoms are determined by the rate and volume of blood flow through the ventricular tear into the pericardial sac. A rapid progression to death due to tamponade is common with acute, severe rupture. However, a slow leak may occur and may be associated with hematoma formation and subsequent pericardial adhesions.

TABLE 21-6

Right Heart Oxygen Saturations in a Patient with Acute Ventricular Septal Defect

Sample Site		Saturation (%)
Systemic arterial		97
Right atrium		40
Right ventricle		87
Proximal pulmonary artery		88
Pulmonary artery pressure	50/30 mm Hg	
Left-to-right shunt calculation	4.5:1	

The very low right atrial oxygen saturation (normal 70%-75%) indicates the very low systemic tissue perfusion in this patient with a very large ventricular septal defect. Blood flow through the pulmonary artery exceeded systemic blood flow by 4.5-fold.

The hemodynamic profile and clinical presentation are identical to those of a patient with an acute cardiac tamponade. The time course and clinical presentation of the tamponade may be condensed into a few minutes or may be prolonged with a slower leak. The patient becomes hypotensive and experiences elevated venous pressures, distended neck veins, dyspnea, distant heart sounds, equalization of right and left heart pressures during diastole (diastolic plateau), and pulsus paradoxus (see also Chapter 23, section on cardiac tamponade). The sudden onset of sinus bradycardia followed by a junctional or idioventricular rhythm and decreased-amplitude QRS complexes may precede electromechanical dissociation and death. Emergency surgical repair can be lifesaving in patients with a small ventricular tear and slow leak.

Right Ventricular Infarction

The right coronary artery supplies blood to both the inferior wall of the left ventricle and the right ventricular wall. Consequently, total occlusion of the proximal right coronary artery produces right ventricular infarction in many patients. Right ventricular infarction may occur in 19% to 43% of all patients with acute inferoposterior wall myocardial infarction. The area of damage is generally the posterior right ventricular wall, but in a small number of patients the damage also involves the anterolateral right ventricular wall. There is almost always damage to the inferior wall of the left ventricle as well.

The damaged right ventricle may be unable to generate sufficient contractile power to eject enough blood to adequately fill the left ventricle. As a result, left ventricular stroke volume and systemic blood pressure fall.

The normally rigid parietal pericardium limits outward expansion of the acutely dilated, infarcted right ventricle. The enlarged right ventricle then encroaches on the limited pericardial space and increases intrapericardial pressure. Consequently, the patient's hemodynamic profile may be similar to that of patients with constrictive pericardial disease, which is characterized by equalization of diastolic pressures of the right and left ventricles (see Chapter 23). Other hemodynamic findings include decreased right ventricular systolic and pulse pressures. In the right ventricular pressure waveform, the right ventricular diastolic descent is well preserved but there is an early diastolic plateau (Figure 21-19).

With large right ventricular infarctions, the diastolic pressures in the right and left ventricles may rapidly equalize. In patients with smaller right ventricular infarctions, the right atrial and right ventricular end-diastolic pressures may *gradually* increase to levels that are equal

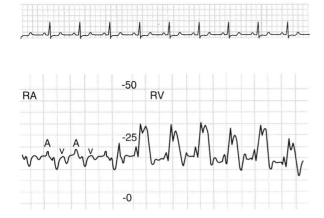

FIGURE 21-19 Square root sign in a patient with inferior-posterior wall and right ventricular myocardial infarction. The right ventricular diastolic pressure rises rapidly and reaches a plateau (the "square root configuration") before atrial contraction because of the restriction of right ventricular filling by the pericardium

to or occasionally greater than the left ventricular end-diastolic pressure. The left ventricular end-diastolic pressure may be low, normal, or elevated depending on the functional state of the left ventricle and the adequacy of left ventricular filling. If right heart pressures become greater than those of the left heart, the intraventricular septum may shift into the left ventricular cavity, thereby altering left ventricular geometry and reducing the internal diameter of the left ventricle. As a result, for any given left ventricular end-diastolic volume, the end-diastolic pressure (PWP) is disproportionately and deceptively high.

The clinical spectrum of right ventricular infarction ranges from less than 10 mm Hg reduction in systemic arterial pressure in patients with minimal right ventricular contractile failure to significant hypotension in patients with severe right ventricular dysfunction. In these latter patients, marked systemic *venous* hypertension, venous distention, and right ventricular third and fourth heart sounds are present. In many cases, the lungs are clear to auscultation; in fact, the pulmonary circulation is subnormally perfused. In patients with inferior wall infarction, a Kussmaul sign (a fall greater than 10 mm Hg in systemic arterial pressure during patient inspiration) is highly predictive of right ventricular infarction. The standard 12-lead ECG indicates damage to the inferior wall of the left ventricle. More specific information about the right ventricle can be obtained from the right precordial ECG leads such as V_4R (whose lead position is identical to that of V_4 but is recorded on the right chest), as well as V_5R or V_6R. An ST segment elevation of 1 mm or more in the right precordial leads is a highly sensitive and

specific sign for the diagnosis of acute right ventricular infarction.

Two-dimensional echocardiography is helpful in distinguishing right ventricular infarction from pericardial tamponade. On the two-dimensional echocardiogram, right ventricular dilation and abnormal wall motion, as well as depression of the right ventricular ejection fraction, are frequently observed.

Treatment is directed toward increasing left heart filling so that cardiac output and arterial pressure are restored to levels that sustain systemic perfusion. Intravascular volume is expanded until the cardiac output and arterial pressure normalize or fail to increase further with intravenous fluid infusion. Inotropic drugs such as dobutamine or dopamine may be required when hypoperfusion persists after adequate fluid has been given. Temporary transvenous pacing is important in patients with bradycardia or atrioventricular block. Patients who require pacing should have atrioventricular sequential pacing to maintain the atrial contribution (atrial kick) to cardiac output. In fact, arteriovenous sequential pacing may increase cardiac output by 10% to 30%.

REFERENCES

1. American Heart Association: *Cardiovascular diseases,* accessed October 2001. Available at www.americanheart.org/statistics/03cardio.html.
2. A guide to the international ACLS algorithms, *Circulation* 102(8, suppl): 2000.
3. Connors AF, McCaffree DR, Gray BA: Evaluation of right heart catheterization in the critically ill patient without acute myocardial infarction, *Am J Cardiol* 39:137, 1983.
4. Eisenburg PR, Jaffe AS, Schuster DP: Clinical evaluation compared to pulmonary artery catheterization in the hemodynamic management of critically ill patients, *Crit Care Med* 12:549, 1984.
5. Forrester JS, Diamond G, McHugh TJ, et al: Filling pressures in the right and left sides of the heart in acute myocardial infarction, *N Engl J Med* 285:190, 1971.
6. Antman E, Tanasijevic M, Thompson B, et al: Cardiac-specific troponin I levels to predict the risk of mortality in patients with acute coronary syndromes, *N Engl J Med* 335:1342, 1996.
7. Advanced cardiovascular life support. Section 1. Introduction to ACLS 2000: overview of recommended changes in ACLS, *Circulation* 102(8, suppl): I1, 2000.

SUGGESTED READINGS
General

Braunwald E: *Heart disease,* ed 6, Philadelphia, 2001, W.B. Saunders.
Henning RJ, Grenvik A: *Critical care cardiology,* New York, 1989, Churchill Livingstone.

Hurst's the heart, ed 9, New York, 1998, McGraw-Hill.

Willerson JT, Cohn JN: Coronary artery disease. In Willerson JT, Cohn JN, editors: *Cardiovascular medicine,* ed 2, Churchill Livingstone, 2000, New York.

Ischemic Heart Disease

Adams J, Abendschein D, Jaffe A: Biochemical markers of myocardial injury: is MB creatine kinase the choice for the 1990s? *Circulation* 88:760, 1993.

Anderson HN, Willerson JT: Thrombolysis in acute myocardial infarction, *N Engl J Med* 329:703, 1993.

Antman EM et al: Cardiac-specific troponin levels to predict the risk of mortality in patients with acute coronary syndromes, *N Engl J Med* 335:1342, 1996.

Bolooki H: *Clinical application of the intra-aortic balloon pump,* Mount Kisco, 1984, Futura.

Califf RM et al: One year results from the global utilization of streptokinase and TPA for occluded coronary arteries (GUSTO-1) trial, *Circulation* 94:1233, 1996.

DeWood MA, Stifter WF, Simpson CS, et al: Coronary arteriographic findings soon after non−Q wave myocardial infarction, *N Engl J Med* 315:417, 1986.

First International Study of Infarct Survival Collaborative Group: Randomized trial of intravenous atenolol among 16027 cases of suspected acute myocardial infarction: ISIS-1, *Lancet* 2:57, 1986.

Forrester JS, Diamond G, Chatterjee K: Medical therapy of acute myocardial infarction by application of hemodynamic subsets, *N Engl J Med* 295:1356, 1976.

Forrester JS, Diamond GA, Swan HJC: Correlation classification of clinical and hemodynamic function after acute myocardial infarction, *Am J Cardiol* 39:137, 1977.

Fuster V, Badimon L, Cohen M, et al: Insights into the pathogenesis of acute ischemic syndromes, *Circulation* 77:1213, 1988.

Goldberg RJ, Gore JM, Alpert JS, et al: Cardiogenic shock after acute myocardial infarction, *N Engl J Med* 325:1118, 1991.

International Consensus on Science−American Heart Association in collaboration with the International Liaison Committee on Resuscitation (ILCOR): Acute coronary syndromes (acute myocardial infarction), *Circulation* 102(8 suppl): I172, 2000.

ISIS-2 (Second International Study of Infarct Survival) Collaborative Group: Randomized trial of intravenous streptokinase, oral aspirin, both, or neither among 17187 cases of suspected acute myocardial infarction, *J Am Coll Cardiol* 12:3A, 1988.

ISIS-3 Collaborative Group: A randomized comparison of streptokinase vs tissue plasminogen activator vs anistreplase and of aspirin plus heparin vs aspirin alone among 41,299 cases of suspected acute myocardial infarction, *Lancet* 339:753, 1992.

ISIS-4: A randomized factorial trial assessing early oral captopril, oral mononitrate, and intravenous magneiusm sulphate

in 58050 patients with suspected acute myocardial infarction, *Lancet* 345:669, 1995.

Kinch JW, Ryan TJ: Right ventricular infarction, *N Engl J Med* 330:1211, 1994.

Lee L et al: Multicenter registry of angioplasty therapy of cardiogenic shock: initial and long-term survival, *J Am Coll Cardiol* 17:599, 1991.

Lilavie CJ, Gersh PJ: Mechanical and electrical complication of acute myocardial infarction, *Mayo Clin Proc* 65:709, 1990.

Maseri A et al: Coronary vasospasm as a possible cause of myocardial infarction, *N Engl J Med* 299:1271, 1978.

Moore CA, Nygaard TW, Kaiser DL, et al: Post infarction ventricular septal rupture: the importance of location of infarction and right ventricular function in determining survival, *Circulation* 74:45, 1986.

Nishimura RA: Acute myocardial infarction: the role of echocardiography. In Fuster V, Ross R, Topol EJ, editors: *Atherosclerosis and coronary artery disease,* Philadelphia, 1996, Lippincott-Raven.

Nishimura RA, Schaff HV, Shub C, et al: Papillary muscle rupture complicating acute myocardial infarction, *Am J Cardiol* 57:373, 1983.

Normand SL et al: Using admission characteristics to predict short-term mortality from myocardial infarction in elderly patients: results from the Cooperative Cardiovascular Project, *JAMA* 275:1322, 1996.

Parker AB, Waller BF, Gering LE: Usefulness of the 12-lead electrocardiogram in detection of myocardial infarction: electrocardiographic-anatomic correlations, *Clin Cardiol* 19:55, 1996.

Pfeffer MA et al: Effect of captopril on mortality and morbidity in patients with left ventricular dysfunction after myocardial infarction. Results of the survival and ventricular enlargement trial, *N Engl J Med* 327:669, 1992.

Rackley CE, Satler LF, Pearle DL, et al: Use of hemodynamic measurements for management of acute myocardial infarction. In Rackley CE, editor: *Advances in critical care cardiology,* Philadelphia, 1986, FA Davis.

Roberts R: Inotropic therapy for cardiac failure associated with acute myocardial infarction, *Chest* 93:22S, 1988.

Rodgers WJ et al: Comparison of primary angioplasty versus thrombolytic therapy for acute myocardial infarction, *Am J Cardiol* 74:111, 1994.

Schreiber TL, Miller DH, Zola B: Management of myocardial infarction shock: current status, *Am Heart J* 117:435, 1989.

Stone GW et al: Clinical and angiographic follow-up after primary stenting in acute myocardial infarction: the Primary Angioplasty in Myocardial Infarction (PAMI) trial, *Circulation* 99:1548, 1999.

Zimmerman J et al: Diagnostic marker cooperative study for the diagnosis of myocardial infarction, *Circulation* 99:1671, 1999.

22

GREGORY L. FREEMAN, LLOYD W. KLEIN, and GLORIA OBLOUK DAROVIC

Valvular Heart Disease

Under normal conditions, the four cardiac valves maintain unimpaired, unidirectional flow of blood from the atria to the ventricles and from the ventricles to the pulmonary and systemic circulations. Valvular heart disease results when structural changes or functional abnormalities of one or more heart valves lead to disturbances of cardiac performance. The two ways in which a valve can malfunction are (1) failure to open sufficiently, thereby impairing forward blood flow (stenosis); and (2) failure to close completely, thereby permitting flow in the wrong direction (regurgitation).

Because the manner in which the pathologic process that deforms the valve structure is patient variable, the valvular lesion may be pure (stenosis or regurgitation) or mixed (variable degrees of stenosis and regurgitation). Furthermore, the underlying disease, such as rheumatic fever or endocarditis, may damage more than one heart valve. Patients with mixed or multiple valve involvement typically have complex clinical and hemodynamic abnormalities that challenge both assessment and management strategies.

In this chapter, the hemodynamic and clinical effects, laboratory findings, and therapies of pure and mixed lesions of the aortic and mitral valves are discussed. Tricuspid regurgitation is also discussed, both as a primary lesion and as a secondary consequence of right ventricular failure.

AORTIC STENOSIS

The aortic valve is a thin, pliable semilunar structure that flattens against the aortic wall during ventricular ejection. The normal valve provides no resistance to left ventricular outflow. *Aortic stenosis* is a valvular disorder characterized by progressive narrowing of the valve orifice and obstruction to left ventricular outflow, adaptive left ventricular hypertrophy, and left atrial dilation. Although initially well tolerated because of the power of the hypertrophic left ventricle, significant stenosis is hemodynamically characterized by a marked difference between left ventricular and aortic systolic pressure, an elevated left ventricular end-diastolic pressure, and a decreased stroke volume (Figure 22-1).

Clinical features of severe stenosis include signs and symptoms of perfusion failure, predisposition to pulmonary edema, and potential for myocardial ischemia even in the absence of coronary artery disease. Although obstruction to left ventricular ejection can occur at valvular, subvalvular, or supravalvular locations, this discussion focuses on valvular aortic stenosis, which is the most common type in adults.

Causes

In adult patients, valvular aortic stenosis has three primary causes: congenital, rheumatic, and degenerative.

Congenital Aortic Stenosis

The initial anatomic defect is due to abnormal valvular development, which usually results in the presence of two unequally sized cusps (bicuspid aortic valve). Typically, the patient remains asymptomatic during childhood and early adulthood, although a systolic murmur can be detected. Symptoms usually develop between 40 and 60 years of age as the abnormal valve cusps thicken and

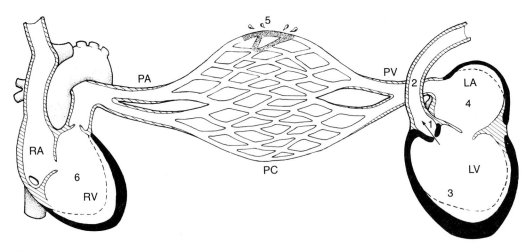

FIGURE 22-1 Schematic of the chambers of the left heart and pulmonary circulation drawn end to end for conceptual purposes. Note the alteration in architecture of the atrium and ventricle in decompensated aortic stenosis *(solid lines)* compared with that of the normal heart *(broken lines)*. *1,* Left ventricular outflow obstruction. *2,* Reduction in stroke volume. *3,* Hypertrophic and dilated left ventricle. *4,* Dilated left atrium, atrial contribution to ventricular filling of critical importance. *5,* Potential for pulmonary edema. *6,* Possible right heart failure (unusual).

perhaps become calcific. No other associated congenital heart defects are usually present. However, bicuspid aortic valves are present in 80% of patients with coarctation of the aorta, and bicuspid aortic valves also are frequently associated with patent ductus arteriosus. Rarely, a unicuspid valve is present, which produces severe aortic stenosis in infants and children.

Degenerative Aortic Stenosis

This lesion occurs in patients 65 years of age or older because of cusp fibrosis and calcium deposition in the sinuses of Valsalva. These changes develop secondary to the ordinary mechanical stress on the valve (normal closing pressure of 80 mm Hg is 10 times greater than that of the pulmonic valve). In degenerative aortic stenosis, the commissures of the valve cusps are not fused; however, cusp fibrosis impairs the mobility of the cusps, and valve calcification creates a stone-hard, fixed obstruction. Degenerative aortic stenosis is more common in females. The process may result in hemodynamically insignificant "aortic sclerosis" or may eventually progress to a point at which significant left ventricular outflow obstruction and pressure overload impair circulatory function.

Rheumatic Aortic Stenosis

Rheumatic involvement of the aortic valve results in progressive cusp fibrosis, fusion of one or more of the aortic commissures, and possibly valve calcification. The rigid valve structures are frequently both stenotic and regurgitant. A history of rheumatic fever is present in 30%

to 50% of patients with rheumatic aortic valve disease; the other patients presumably have suffered a subclinical streptococcal infection. Isolated rheumatic aortic valve disease almost never occurs; some involvement of the mitral valve is typically present.

Less common causes of aortic stenosis include hyperlipidemia, infective endocarditis, metabolic abnormalities, and systemic lupus erythematosus (SLE).

Hemodynamic Effects

Three factors determine the hemodynamic significance of aortic stenosis: (1) the severity of valvular obstruction to left ventricular outflow, (2) the adequacy of compensatory left ventricular hypertrophy that enables adequate chamber emptying, and (3) the preservation of the atrial contribution to ventricular filling.

With progressive reduction in the aortic valve orifice size, a constellation of pathophysiologic and hemodynamic abnormalities develops that may jeopardize ventricular performance and threaten myocardial ischemia even if the coronary arteries are normal.

Systolic Abnormalities

The initial and primary hemodynamic abnormality of aortic stenosis occurs during systole when blood is ejected through the narrowed aortic valve orifice. Obstruction to left ventricular outflow demands the generation of a higher left ventricular systolic pressure to maintain adequate stroke volume and systemic arterial pressure. A pressure difference develops between the left ventricular

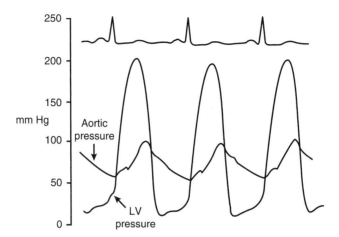

FIGURE 22-2 Simultaneous measurement of left ventricular and aortic pressures in a patient with critical aortic stenosis. Note the wide transaortic pressure gradient: left ventricular systolic pressure is 200 mm Hg, aortic systolic pressure is 100 mm Hg. Observe the slurred upstroke of the aortic pressure curve, narrow pulse pressure, and poorly defined dicrotic notch. These features give a damped appearance to the arterial waveform.

and aortic systolic pressure, which is termed the aortic valve gradient. The aortic valve gradient is a classic hemodynamic feature of aortic stenosis (Figure 22-2).

With a critical reduction of the size of the valve orifice, left ventricular systolic pressure may reach levels as high as 300 mm Hg, whereas the aortic systolic pressure may be lower than 100 mm Hg (greater than 200 mm Hg gradient). The left ventricular pressure overload also results in proportionate increases in myocardial oxygen demand.

If, for any reason, significant depression in contractility develops, the resultant drop in stroke volume is associated with compensatory systemic vasoconstriction, which maintains mean arterial pressure. The hemodynamic and physiologic disadvantage is that increased systemic vascular resistance further increases left ventricular pressure work and oxygen consumption. This finding may worsen the ventricular failure, decrease stroke volume, and increase the likelihood of myocardial ischemia.

Adaptive Ventricular Hypertrophy and Diastolic Dysfunction

The reduction in valve orifice size worsens over a prolonged period. As an adaptation to the increased systolic pressure requirements and cardiac work, the left ventricle progressively hypertrophies. This type of hypertrophy is termed *concentric hypertrophy,* which is structurally characterized by an increase in ventricular wall thickness and mass with no increase in left ventricular chamber diameter.

This hypertropy has important effects on diastolic performance of the heart. The passive distensibility of the left

ventricle varies with the volume of blood in the chamber. The lower curve shows the passive length-tension relation of a normal heart: less tension is required to distend the fully relaxed (passive) ventricle to larger volumes. Near the left-hand side of the curve, substantial filling can take place with a relatively small increase in pressure. In this range the ventricle is compliant (the flat slope of the tangent line segment reflects compliance at that length). Once the chamber is filled further than this, even a small increase in length requires a significant increase in tension (illustrated by the steeper slope of the tangent line segment). After concentric hypertrophy has occurred, filling the heart to any given volume requires higher distending pressure. At any given volume, the stiffness of the heart is less, illustrated by the steeper slope of the tangent line in the upper curve.

The adaptive increase in left ventricular muscle mass has several significant drawbacks, however. The stiff, hypertrophied left ventricle resists diastolic filling and is associated with a disproportionately high end-diastolic pressure for any given end-diastolic volume. Maintenance of atrial contraction is crucial to adequately fill the nondistensible ventricle and may contribute as much as 40% to diastolic filling and stroke volume (normal 10% to 30%) (Figure 22-3). Because end-diastolic pressures are out of proportion to filling volume, the importance of the atrial contribution to filling is further increased.

Mild-to-moderate aortic stenosis may be well tolerated, and the patient may remain asymptomatic for decades owing to the ability of the hypertrophied ventricle to maintain a normal ejection fraction and cardiac output.

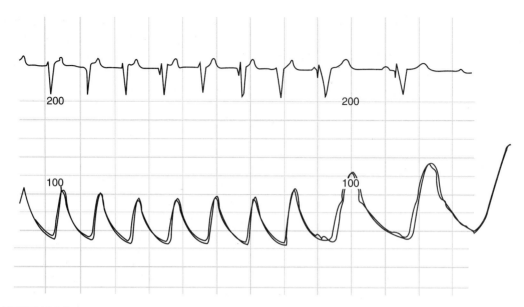

FIGURE 22-3 Hemodynamic significance of atrioventricular synchrony in a patient with critical aortic stenosis. Note that the paced beats are associated with an arterial systolic pressure of less than 100 mm Hg. With restoration of sinus rhythm (beats now preceded by atrial contraction) the systolic pressure immediately rises to approximately 130 mm Hg. (Courtesy of Dr. David J. Hale, Foster G. McGaw Medical Center of Loyola University, Maywood, Illinois.)

Secondary Left Atrial Enlargement

The increased left atrial systolic pressure (measured as the crest of the *a* wave in the pulmonary artery wedge pressure [PWP] waveform) produces progressive left atrial enlargement, although *mean* left atrial pressure is not high enough to produce pulmonary edema. When left ventricular function deteriorates because of either ischemia or decompensation of the hypertrophied myocardium, ventricular end-diastolic pressure may then increase sufficiently to raise the mean left atrial pressure to levels greater than 18 mm Hg. The patient is thus prone to pulmonary edema because the left ventricle is noncompliant.

Effects on Myocardial Oxygen Supply and Demand

The thickened left ventricular muscle mass, elevated systolic pressure work, and prolonged ejection time increase myocardial oxygen demand. At the same time, excessive intramyocardial systolic and diastolic wall tension may reduce myocardial blood flow by compression of the elongated, thin, penetrating coronary artery branches and coronary microcirculation. As a consequence of the increased oxygen demands and decreased oxygen supply, the patient's myocardium, particularly the subendocardium, is susceptible to ischemia. Even in the absence of coronary artery disease, anginal pain, myocardial in-

farction, and sudden cardiac death may occur. This is a particularly severe problem in patients with obstructive coronary lesions. In these patients, acute myocardial infarction or sudden death may be the first sign of aortic stenosis.

Important Implications in Caring for Patients with Aortic Stenosis

The heart of the patient with critical aortic stenosis (calculated valve area of less than 0.7 cm^2) requires a fine balance of preload and afterload to maintain cardiac output while simultaneously preventing pulmonary edema. Myocardial oxygen supply and demand are likewise in a particularly precarious balance. Several factors may produce sudden hemodynamic deterioration or myocardial ischemia in patients with severe aortic stenosis.

Alterations in Preload

Because the hypertrophic ventricle is highly preload dependent for adequate myofibrillar stretch, critical reductions in the ventricular filling volume and, consequently stroke volume may result from relatively small amounts of blood loss, excessive diuresis, third-space fluid shifts, dehydration, venodilator agents, and protracted vomiting or diarrhea. Measured filling pressure (PWP) is disproportionately elevated, however, and may be in the clinically established "normal" range despite hypovolemia.

Because atrial contraction contributes significantly to left ventricular filling, loss of the "atrial kick" (atrial fibrillation, atrioventricular dissociation, or ventricular pacing) also may produce a critical reduction in left ventricular end-diastolic volume with resultant circulatory collapse (see Figure 22-3).

Alternatively, the stiff, hypertrophied left ventricle of patients with aortic stenosis is highly sensitive to volume loading. A relatively small intravenous fluid challenge may cause the left ventricular end-diastolic pressure to rise sharply to levels that predispose the patient to pulmonary edema.

Alterations in Afterload

Systemic hypotension decreases coronary perfusion pressure, but because the stenotic valve lesion is fixed in size, the ventricular systolic pressure and oxygen demand remain elevated. A severe myocardial ischemic attack may result secondary to the sudden decrease in oxygen supply relative to the consistently high oxygen demand. As a clinical counterpoint, systemic hypertension further increases heart work and myocardial oxygen demand without producing proportionate elevations in coronary blood flow. Severe ischemic attacks and sudden heart failure commonly result.

Cardiac Arrhythmias

Tachyarrhythmias reduce coronary perfusion and ventricular filling time, while myocardial oxygen consumption rises in proportion to increases in heart rate. Therefore reductions in stroke volume and the ischemic risk rise in proportion to increases in heart rate. *Atrial fibrillation* and *ventricular tachycardia* are especially threatening arrhythmias because loss of the atrial contribution to ventricular filling in conjunction with the rapid ventricular rates may lead to precipitous hypotension and pulmonary edema.

In summary, patients with severe aortic stenosis are "hemodynamically and clinically brittle." Relatively small alterations in preload, afterload, heart rate, or heart rhythm may produce pulmonary edema, hypotension, or myocardial ischemic attacks.

Clinical Presentation

Most patients with mild-to-moderate aortic stenosis are asymptomatic and develop symptoms only when valve obstruction becomes severe. Clinical deterioration typically occurs when the aortic valve area is reduced to less than 0.7 cm². (Normal valve orifice size is 1.6 to 2.5 cm².) Patients then develop the following symptoms:

1. *Syncope and light-headedness* due to decreased cerebral perfusion when cardiac output cannot increase commensurate with stress or postural change. This finding may occur with or immediately following physical exertion or when the patient suddenly assumes an upright position (orthostatic syncope).
2. *Angina pectoris* is related to the excessive oxygen needs of the myocardium that coexists with reduced myocardial oxygen supply.
3. *Dyspnea and fatigue* are related to pulmonary edema and systemic underperfusion. Fatigue, dyspnea, or exercise intolerance may develop gradually in some patients, whereas in other patients symptoms develop suddenly. In fact, significant hemodynamic deterioration may occur over a period of only a few weeks.

The development of syncope, angina, or heart failure as a result of aortic stenosis is a sign that the patient's prognosis is poor. An approximately 50% mortality rate occurs within 2 years for patients having congestive heart failure, within 3 years for patients having syncope, and within 5 years for patients having angina. In some patients, the outlook is even more dismal, and sudden death may occur within days to weeks from the onset of symptoms; in others, sudden death is the first sign of aortic stenosis. Definitive treatment by surgical valve replacement should be strongly considered as soon as symptoms appear.

Clinical Features

Mentation. The level of mentation is normal except for possible episodes of fainting, light-headedness, or "fading out" spells. These symptoms relate to transient cerebral underperfusion in patients with critical aortic stenosis.

Cutaneous Manifestation. With critical disease the skin is pale and the patient's hands and feet may be cool.

Heart Rate and Rhythm. The heart rate is normal in compensated patients and increases as cardiac output falls. Irregularities in the pulse may occur owing to transient arrhythmias, some of which predispose the individual to sudden cardiac death. In fact, some syncopal episodes are thought to be the result of transient ventricular fibrillation. Sudden cardiac death occurs in 15% to 20% of patients with severe aortic stenosis.

Character of Pulse. The arterial pulse rises slowly and peaks late. This is termed *pulsus parvus et tardus*. *Pulsus alternans* (i.e., the force of contraction of the alternate beats varies) is a common finding in patients with left ventricular failure.

Heart Sounds. The first heart sound is normal or soft. Paradoxic splitting of the second heart sound may occur as a result of prolonged left ventricular systole and delayed aortic valve closure. The aortic component of the S_2 sound is soft. Atrial (S_4) and ventricular (S_3) gallops are commonly heard in patients with advanced disease. The murmur of aortic stenosis is systolic, harsh, with a crescendo-decrescendo (diamond-shaped) configuration. The murmur is accentuated in the beat following an extrasystole (post-extrasystolic potentiation). As the outflow obstruction worsens, the peak of the murmur shifts toward late systole; therefore a "late peaking" murmur correlates with severe aortic stenosis. The murmur is loudest at the aortic area and is well transmitted to the neck, upper back, and apex, where it may have a musical quality. The following factors may make auscultatory diagnosis difficult. The murmur may be faint or inaudible in barrel-chested, obese, or muscular people, particularly when the left ventricle fails. With the advent of heart failure, the murmur, which results from forceful ejection of blood from the left ventricle across the obstructing valve, becomes softer.

Palpation of the Precordium. The apical pulse is in the normal position if the left ventricle is not dilated, but the pulse may be sustained in duration. As the ventricle dilates in response to failure, the apical impulse becomes laterally and inferiorly displaced. A systolic thrill may be palpated over the aortic area and carotid arteries. A precordial *a* wave (the atrial thrust) may be both visible and palpable and corresponds to the fourth heart sound.

Neck Veins. An increased internal jugular *a* wave is often observed secondary to the reduction in right ventricular compliance due to the hypertrophied septum.

Respiratory Rate and Character of Breathing. Respiratory effects typically are unremarkable unless the patient has pulmonary edema.

Breath Sounds. Breath sounds are typically normal. An episode of acute pulmonary edema is an ominous sign and is associated with rapid clinical deterioration. However, other signs and symptoms of left ventricular failure typically develop well before pulmonary edema becomes a problem.

Acid-Base Values. These measurements are normal unless pulmonary edema or systemic perfusion failure develops.

Hemodynamic Profile

Hemodynamic measurements are usually in the normal range until compensatory mechanisms are no longer adequate to maintain left ventricular function and circulatory status. Decompensation typically occurs in patients with critical aortic stenosis.

Arterial Pressure

The arterial pressure may be maintained at a normal level until significant left ventricular outflow obstruction occurs. The systolic pressure is then decreased while the diastolic pressure remains within the normal range. The narrowed pulse pressure correlates with the decreased stroke volume. The arterial pressure waveform shows a sloped upstroke and delayed rate of rise, termed *pulsus parvus et tardus,* which is Latin for a small and late pulse. Because systole is prolonged, closure of the aortic valve is delayed and the dicrotic notch may be observed farther down on the descending limb of the arterial pressure waveform. Owing to abnormal valve movement at closure, the dicrotic notch also may be poorly defined. Overall, the waveform of aortic stenosis appears damped (Figure 22-4).

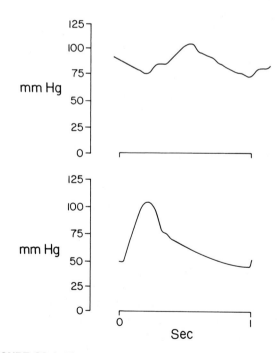

FIGURE 22-4 The *upper panel* is the aortic pressure wave of a patient with severe aortic stenosis; the *lower panel* is the aortic pressure wave in a patient with a normal valve. Note the reduced amplitude and late peaking of the aortic wave in the *upper panel,* a pattern termed *pulsus parvus et tardus.*

Cuff Technique. An auscultatory gap between systolic and diastolic pressure may be present. Therefore the systolic pressure must be estimated by palpation while inflating the cuff, or the cuff should be inflated until the pressure gauge registers a value well above the anticipated systolic pressure (see Chapter 7). Left ventricular systolic pressure is significantly higher than systemic arterial systolic pressure, but this pressure difference can be determined only on left heart catheterization.

Systemic Vascular Resistance

This calculated value is usually within the normal range until late in the disease when cardiac output falls. Any factor (compensatory vasoconstriction, vasopressor therapy, chilling, anxiety) that increases systemic vascular resistance increases the hemodynamic burden on the constantly systolic pressure-overloaded left ventricle.

Pulmonary Vascular Resistance

This calculated value is usually normal or slightly decreased. During episodes of acute pulmonary edema, values increase in response to the perivascular edema and the hypoxemic pulmonary vasoconstrictor stimulus.

Central Venous Pressure or Right Atrial Pressure

These values are usually normal. Right ventricular failure may develop late in the course of aortic stenosis (if at all), and it is an *ominous* prognostic sign. The right atrial *a* wave may be prominent because of a reduction in right ventricular compliance that results from hypertrophy of the intraventricular septum, which is shared by both ventricles.

Pulmonary Artery Pressure

Pulmonary artery systolic and diastolic pressures remain normal until late in the disease when critical aortic stenosis and left ventricular failure cause these measurements to rise in tandem with elevated mean left atrial pressures (passive pulmonary hypertension).

Pulmonary Artery Wedge Pressure

This measurement may be normal or slightly elevated in patients with mild-to-moderate disease. With the development of left ventricular failure, the mean PWP rises to levels that may produce pulmonary edema.

Cardiac Output

The cardiac output is normal at rest in most patients with aortic stenosis, but in patients with moderate-to-severe stenosis, cardiac output may fail to increase appropriately with emotional or physical stress (exercise, shivering, fever, sepsis) or postural changes. Resting cardiac output and ejection fraction are usually subnormal in patients with critical aortic stenosis.

Mixed Venous Oxygen Saturation

With the advent of systemic underperfusion or pulmonary edema, this measurement falls.

Laboratory and Other Diagnostic Studies

Electrocardiograph

A pattern of left ventricular hypertrophy and strain gradually evolves (Figure 22-5).

Conduction defects may be present, including left anterior hemiblock or left bundle branch block. These may arise from calcific invasion of conduction tissue in patients with calcific aortic stenosis. Complete heart block is rare. P wave abnormalities signify left atrial enlargement. *Atrial fibrillation is a late, poorly tolerated, and ominous sign in patients with aortic stenosis because it may lead to cardiovascular collapse.* Ventricular ectopy also may be noted.

Chest Radiograph

The chest film may be normal in the early stages of aortic stenosis. Cardiomegaly as a result of left ventricular dilation and left atrial enlargement is a common finding in patients with critical aortic stenosis. There is often calcium in the area of the aortic valve (best seen on the lateral chest X-ray), as well as prominence of the ascending aorta in patients with advanced disease. Radiographic evidence of pulmonary vascular congestion occurs in concert with development of heart failure.

Echocardiogram

This diagnostic procedure is useful in delineating valve mobility and structure and assessing left ventricular function. Left ventricular hypertrophy and chamber size also can be quantified echocardiographically. Doppler echocardiography provides helpful information on the velocity of blood flow through the narrowed orifice, allowing accurate assessment of the pressure gradient and valve area.

Cardiac Catheterization

The systolic pressure gradient between left ventricle and aorta, left ventricular end-diastolic pressure, and cross-sectional area of the valve can be determined. This procedure also is used to assess the coronary arteries and left ventricular function.

Valve Area Calculation. The normal cardiac valves allow free flow of blood even at high cardiac outputs. As the valve opening narrows, the valve orifice offers progressively increasing resistance to flow, resulting in a pressure difference (gradient) across the valve. For any narrowed orifice size, the pressure gradient increases as cardiac output increases. Dr. Richard Gorlin[1] developed a means of calculating the cross-sectional area of stenotic valves, taking into account the relationship of cardiac output and the pressure gradient for use in the catheterization laboratory.

There are major limitations to the Gorlin formula, and these must be kept in mind when interpreting or acquiring hemodynamic data. These include transducer calibration, cardiac output measurement method, operator technique (see Chapter 6), and factors discussed in the following paragraphs.

Measured cardiac output represents only forward flow; therefore, if the patient has a coexisting regurgitant lesion, the calculation assessment may yield a deceptively small valve area. In patients with low cardiac output, the inherent errors in measuring both valve gradient and flow are high and the calculated valve area may be inaccurate. In addition, in patients with low cardiac output, a sclerotic valve may fail to open fully, which may result in a smaller effective valve area at that point. This may mislead clinicians to believe that the degree of aortic stenosis is worse than it actually is.

Nevertheless, advocates of both noninvasive and invasive tests continue to use the valve area as the standard method to assess the severity of a stenotic lesion. For example, with a normal cardiac output, an actual aortic

valve area of less than 0.7 cm^2 is usually associated with a mean systolic aortic gradient of 50 mm Hg. At this level of disease, valve replacement is indicated.

Treatment

Aortic stenosis with minimal obstruction requires no specific therapy. Prophylactic antibiotic coverage is recommended before all dental and most instrumentation or surgical procedures (not cardiac catheterization, not cardiac surgery) to protect against bacterial endocarditis.

Medical therapy usually is not justified in the asymptomatic patient. Once symptoms appear, the clinical course rapidly deteriorates and patient mortality rates are high. Many clinicians advocate surgery for patients who demonstrate aortic gradients greater than 50 mm Hg, even in the absence of symptoms, because of the increased susceptibility to sudden death and the likelihood that some patients will develop symptoms within a short period. Two surgical options are available.

Aortic Commissurotomy

This procedure may be somewhat effective in relieving the left ventricular outflow obstruction in younger patients who do not have calcific disease. Attempts have been made to perform commissurotomy by means of balloon valvuloplasty. The long-term results of this approach have been uniformly disappointing, however, and it is doubtful that it will achieve general acceptance. Aortic valvuloplasty may have a place in management of the rare

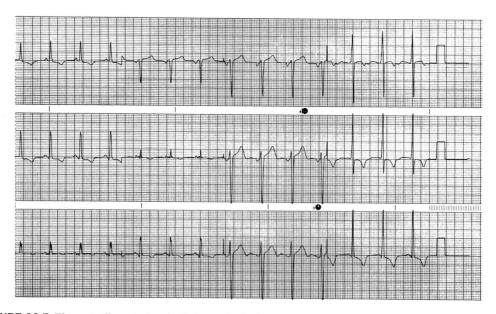

FIGURE 22-5 Electrocardiogram showing left ventricular hypertrophy with strain in a patient with critical aortic stenosis. Note the increased QRS voltage in the precordial leads (V1 through V6).

elderly patient who has acute hemodynamic compromise. In such a patient, this procedure may offer temporary hemodynamic stabilization as a bridge to ultimate aortic valve replacement.

Aortic Valve Replacement

All patients with severe aortic stenosis should receive corrective valvular surgery regardless of left ventricular function because removal of the impedance to aortic outflow is the sole remedy for elevated left ventricular wall stress and systemic underperfusion, when present. Operative mortality rate in elective surgery for patients with no other cardiac illness and a nondilated left ventricle is approximately 3% to 5%; the risk increases with age and worsening hemodynamic status.

The overall response to valve replacement is excellent. If left ventricular performance is depressed before surgery, an improvement in function can be anticipated after surgery because the obstruction to ejection is removed. The hypertrophy also regresses over the course of the following few months or years.

In cases with concomitant, severe, or symptomatic coronary artery disease, bypass surgery should be performed for both perioperative and long-term benefit. However, combined valve and bypass surgery increases the cardiopulmonary bypass and aortic cross-clamp time, which tends to increase perioperative morbidity and mortality rates.

All patients with metallic prosthetic valves require long-term anticoagulation. In patients with absolute contraindications to anticoagulation, a heterograft (bioprosthetic) valve may be considered. Unfortunately, within 7 to 10 years these valves degenerate and calcify, leading to recurrence of aortic valve disease. Thromboemboli also may occur in the absence of anticoagulation with bioprosthetic valves, and thus an antiplatelet regimen should be instituted for these patients.

AORTIC REGURGITATION (INSUFFICIENCY)

The aortic valve cusps normally close in diastole to provide a fluid-tight seal that prevents backflow of blood from the aorta into the left ventricle.

Aortic regurgitation is a valvular disorder in which incompetence of the aortic valve results in a reflux of blood from the aorta to the left ventricle during diastole. In contrast to causes of aortic stenosis, there are many possible causes of aortic regurgitation. The onset may be acute or chronic, and the clinical signs and hemodynamic profile may vary enormously among patients depending on the cause and severity of regurgitant flow. Patients with chronic disease typically have an adaptively dilated, hypertrophied left ventricle and a "hyperdynamic" circulation (Figure 22-6). In comparison, patients with an acute regurgitant lesion are usually in profound circulatory failure and pulmonary edema.

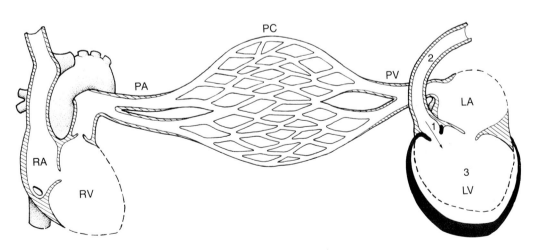

FIGURE 22-6 Schematic illustrating the flow abnormality and left heart changes that accompany chronic, decompensated aortic regurgitation. The *arrow* indicates the abnormal direction of blood flow across the aortic valve. Note the physical adaptive changes in the left ventricle *(solid lines)* as compared with shape and size of a normal left ventricle *(broken lines)*. *1,* Diastolic regurgitant flow through aortic valve. *2,* Stroke volume increases until late in the disease, when stroke volume and systemic blood flow decrease. *3,* Volume-overloaded, hypertrophic, and dilated left ventricle.

Causes

The many causes of aortic regurgitation can be subclassified as being the result of primary valve deformity or disruption or the result of dilation of the aortic root, which prevents complete valve closure. The valvular etiologies include rheumatic fever; infectious endocarditis; collagen vascular diseases, such as ankylosing spondylitis, SLE, and Reiter's disease; valve damage consequent to blunt trauma (particularly steering-wheel injury); and congenital bicuspid valves. Aortic root etiologies include hypertension; cystic medial necrosis of the aorta, which is common in patients with Marfan syndrome; acute aortic dissection; and sinus of Valsalva aneurysms.

Some of these conditions create acute, severe aortic regurgitation; others are associated with a slowly developing regurgitant lesion. The underlying cause and the rapidity of onset of the defect are crucial in determining the patient's prognosis, hemodynamic tolerance, and severity of signs and symptoms.

Hemodynamic Effects

The flow abnormality in aortic regurgitation occurs in diastole when the aortic valve fails to close completely. Because diastolic pressure in the aorta is normally 70 to 80 mm Hg and the diastolic pressure in the left ventricle is normally 4 to 12 mm Hg, a substantial pressure gradient exists between the two chambers. Any opening within the aortic valve therefore allows a "regurgitant jet" of blood into the left ventricle that results in an increase in left ventricular end-diastolic volume and subsequent increase in stroke volume. During systole, the left ventricle empties into a poorly filled thoracic aorta, which facilitates the rapid ejection of a large volume of blood. However, in the following diastole, part of the blood leaks back into the left ventricle.

The hemodynamic effects of *compensated* and *decompensated* chronic aortic regurgitation and *acute aortic regurgitation* are presented. Among these extremes are many possible clinical and hemodynamic gradations that are related to the size of the regurgitant orifice, the pressure difference between the aorta and left ventricle in diastole, the duration of diastole, the preexisting state of the left ventricle, the presence or absence of coexisting disease, and the time period over which the defect developed (Table 22-1).

Chronic Aortic Regurgitation, Compensated

When aortic regurgitation develops over a prolonged period, progressive valve dysfunction or progressive dilation of the aortic root is associated with gradual increases in the regurgitant leak. To maintain a normal circulatory status, the left ventricle must eject the usual stroke volume plus the regurgitant volume delivered from the aorta. Of crucial importance to maintaining acceptable pump function is the time period over which the left ventricle is able to adapt to the diastolic volume overload.

To protect the heart and pulmonary circulation from increases in left ventricular end-diastolic pressure despite the supernormal end-diastolic volume, the left ventricle adaptively enlarges and increases chamber diameter. To increase the power of the left ventricle and maintain normal ventricular wall stress, the myocytes hypertrophy to allow a proportionate increase in wall thickness. These adaptive changes enable greater total left ventricular output (stroke volume can be two times greater than normal) with no significant change in ventricular end-diastolic pressure or wall stress. Systemic vascular resistance also decreases and helps maintain forward blood flow by reducing left ventricular afterload. Over time, the hearts of

---

TABLE 22-1

Hemodynamic Profile in Chronic Compensated, Decompensated, and Acute Aortic Regurgitation

Hemodynamic Parameter	Chronic Compensated Aortic Regurgitation	Chronic Decompensated Aortic Regurgitation	Acute Aortic Regurgitation
Right atrial pressure	~	↑	~ ↑
Systemic vascular resistance	~ ↓	~ ↑	↑
Pulmonary vascular resistance	~	~ ↑	↑
Pulmonary artery pressure	~	↑	↑
Pulmonary artery wedge pressure	~ or ↑	↑	↑
Cardiac output	↑ or ~	~ ↓	↓
Ejection fraction	↑, ~, or ↓	↓	~ ↓
Mixed venous oxygen saturation	~ or ↑	~ ↓	↓

KEY: ↑ Increased; ↓ decreased; ~ no change.

patients with chronic aortic regurgitation adaptively become the largest in cardiac pathology. Such massively enlarged hearts are referred to as *cor bovinum,* or cow heart.

The large stroke volume entering the aorta produces a high systolic pressure (sometimes in excess of 200 mm Hg), and the decreased systemic vascular resistance and diastolic regurgitation produce a low aortic diastolic pressure (approaching left ventricular end-diastolic pressure) (Figure 22-7). These features are characteristic of a *hyperdynamic circulation,* which is also clinically distinguished by bounding pulses; warm, moist skin; visible arterial pulsations; flushed complexion; and reddish mucous membranes.

Chronic Aortic Regurgitation, Decompensated

With progression of the valve defect and volume of regurgitant flow, the limits of compensation are eventually exceeded. When chamber distention exceeds proportional increases in wall thickness, pathologic dilation occurs. Ultimately, contractile depression ensues and signs of congestive heart failure develop. Patients with aortic regurgitation are particularly vulnerable to myocardial ischemia because aortic diastolic pressure, the primary determinant of coronary perfusion pressure and blood flow, is reduced while myocardial oxygen requirements simultaneously rise.

As left ventricular function deteriorates, forward stroke volume decreases and left ventricular end-systolic and end-diastolic blood volumes increase. With severe disease, the regurgitant volume is often 40% to 60% of the stroke volume; this results in severe left ventricular

diastolic volume overload. The left ventricular myocardium also becomes less distensible. As a result, the left ventricular end-diastolic pressure increases. The pressure increases may be transmitted to the left atrium and pulmonary circulation. This, in turn, predisposes patients to pulmonary edema and right ventricular failure. More often, however, the regurgitant flow causes premature mitral valve closure, which prevents end-diastolic pressure equilibration across the mitral valve. This has the beneficial effect of maintaining left atrial pressure below that of the elevated left ventricular end-diastolic pressure; therefore the effects of high pressure on the pulmonary circulation are minimized. The level of pressure protection is not uniform, however, and some patients with severe disease may have considerable elevation of the left atrial (PWP), pulmonary arterial, right ventricular, and right atrial pressures. Other patients maintain mildly elevated left atrial and pulmonary vascular pressures.

Systemic vascular resistance increases as a reflex response to the decreasing forward stroke volume. Vasoconstriction increases impedance to left ventricular ejection; stroke volume falls farther, and the regurgitant volume increases. Thus a self-perpetuating cycle of circulatory failure and worsening regurgitant flow is set in motion.

In summary, the once relatively efficient hyperdynamic circulation of patients with mild-to-moderate aortic regurgitation gradually deteriorates into a circulation characterized by congestive heart failure. A hemodynamic hallmark of severe decompensated aortic regurgitation is that the aortic and left ventricular diastolic pressures nearly equalize in late diastole (Figure 22-8).

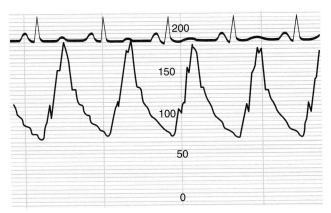

FIGURE 22-7 Arterial pressure waveform from a patient with compensated aortic regurgitation. Note the increased amplitude of the waveform (wide pulse pressure). In a bisferious pulse, shown here, the two systolic peaks may be equal or one or the other may be larger. The initial upstroke relates to the early pressure wave from forceful ventricular ejection, and the second peak relates to reflections propagated back from the vasodilated arterial circulation.

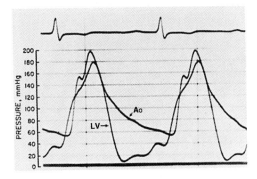

FIGURE 22-8 Superimposed left ventricular and aortic pressure tracings in a patient with severe aortic regurgitation due to rheumatic heart disease. Note the near equilibration of left ventricular and aortic pressures occurring in late diastole. This is termed *diastasis.* (From Grossman W, Baim DS: *Cardiac catheterization, angiography and intervention,* ed 4, Philadelphia, 1991, Lea & Febiger.)

Acute Aortic Regurgitation

A patient with infective endocarditis, aortic dissection, and traumatic disruption of the valve structure incurs an abrupt hemodynamic burden. A substantial regurgitant volume load is suddenly imposed on a left ventricle unable to dilate and hypertrophy acutely to accommodate the regurgitant flow and hemodynamic demands. The patient usually has intense vasoconstriction to distribute the diminished cardiac output to organs necessary for immediate survival. However, the increase in left ventricular afterload usually worsens the regurgitant flow and systemic perfusion failure.

Patients with acute, severe aortic regurgitation develop sudden-onset circulatory failure that can quickly progress to shock and death. Pulmonary edema usually is not present because premature mitral valve closure protects the pulmonary circulation from the volume- and pressure-overloaded left ventricle. Recognition of acute aortic regurgitation is of critical importance because emergency valve replacement is required to save the patient's life.

Clinical Presentation

In the early phases of chronic aortic regurgitation, the patient is asymptomatic, and the physical examination findings are unremarkable except for a characteristic blowing decrescendo diastolic murmur. Symptoms indicative of deterioration (dyspnea on exertion, arrhythmias, paroxysmal nocturnal dyspnea, and angina) develop over a period of several years, by which time significant ventricular dysfunction has occurred. Patients also may complain of nocturnal and rest angina. Syncope and sudden death occasionally occur but are less common than with aortic stenosis.

Mentation

Mentation is normal, except in patients with severe acute aortic regurgitation, who are usually in shock.

Cutaneous Manifestations

In mild-to-moderate aortic regurgitation, the skin is typically flushed and moist; ruddy mucous membranes and flushed palms (palmar erythema) also are characteristic of the hyperdynamic circulation. In severe decompensated or acute disease, the patient's complexion may be pale and the hands and feet cool.

Heart Rate and Character of Pulse

With chronic, compensated disease, the pulses reflect the rapid ejection of an increased volume of blood from the left ventricle. Patients may be aware of their heartbeat, especially when recumbent. They also may complain of a pulsatile sensation in their heads. On palpation, the peripheral pulses are bounding and of a water hammer-like quality, which is characterized by a quick upstroke followed by a rapid collapse (Corrigan's pulse). Careful palpation of the peripheral pulse and inspection of the arterial waveform (see Figure 22-7) shows two distinctly palpable pulsations in systole, termed *bisferiens* (from the Latin, *twice beating*). The supraclavicular and carotid areas, as well as the suprasternal notch, also may show active pulsations and, on palpation, may have a thumping quality. The pulse pressure is wide, and Korotkoff sounds may be audible to zero, although true intraarterial pressure rarely falls below 30 mm Hg. Loud pistol shot-like systolic sounds may be heard over medium-sized arteries (Traube's sign). Duroziez's sign, a biphasic femoral artery bruit, is often heard. As the left ventricle fails, the pulse pressure progressively narrows, and the force of the pulses weakens.

In patients with acute aortic regurgitation, the findings are those of cardiogenic shock, tachycardia with weakened pulses, and intense systemic vasoconstriction.

Heart Sounds

Classically, the high-pitched early diastolic, decrescendo murmur of aortic regurgitation is loudest along the left sternal border in patients with valvular deformity or disruption and loudest along the right sternal border in patients with aortic dilation. The duration of the diastolic murmur correlates with chronicity and severity, except with acute, severe regurgitation, when the murmur may be short, soft, or even inaudible. Correlation of the severity of aortic regurgitation by the loudness of the murmur is notoriously inaccurate because as blood flow rates decrease, the level of turbulence producing the murmur and the audibility of the murmur diminish. A systolic ejection murmur may be the result of coexisting aortic stenosis or turbulence from the rapid ejection of the increased stroke volume. An S_3 gallop indicates ventricular failure. The Austin-Flint murmur, which is a mid- to late-diastolic murmur, is easily confused with diastolic rumble of mitral stenosis and may be present. This murmur is the result of a severe regurgitant jet that restricts opening of the anterior mitral leaflet and that may cause a fluttering of the mitral valve leaflets. This phenomenon may be observed on cardiac ultrasound.

Palpation of the Precordium

In general, regurgitant valve lesions lead to an active precordium. The position and character of the apex beat are important in assessing aortic regurgitation. With significant aortic regurgitation the impulse becomes forceful, lifting, and sustained; it is displaced downward and to the left. With acute aortic regurgitation, the apex beat is in the normal position or moderately displaced and is not forceful.

Neck Veins

Jugular venous distention may be observed if the patient is in right ventricular failure.

Respiratory Rate and Character of Breathing

The breathing pattern and rate are normal unless pulmonary edema is present. Tachypnea and dyspnea therefore are suggestive of a failing circulation. Auscultatory findings are unremarkable unless pulmonary edema is present.

Acid-Base Values

In decompensated states, patients are hypoxemic and may have a mild respiratory alkalosis secondary to hyperventilation as a result of pulmonary vascular congestion or edema. Severe perfusion failure and anaerobic metabolism are associated with metabolic acidosis.

Hemodynamic Profile

Significant variations exist between the hemodynamic profile seen in patients with chronic compensated, decompensated, and acute aortic regurgitation. These differences are illustrated in Table 22-1.

Laboratory and Other Diagnostic Studies

Electrocardiograph

The electrocardiograph (ECG) may be normal in mild aortic regurgitation, but left ventricular hypertrophy with strain is common in patients with significant disease. P wave abnormalities related to left atrial enlargement may be noted. Atrial fibrillation is rare if there is no associated mitral valve disease.

Chest Radiograph

Cardiac size is related to the duration and severity of the regurgitant flow and left ventricular function. In acute aortic regurgitation, there is little, if any, cardiac enlargement, and radiologic evidence of pulmonary edema may be present. In chronic regurgitation, the enlarging heart assumes an ovoid, oblong shape. Patients with severe disease commonly have a cardiothoracic ratio greater than 60%. Signs of pulmonary venous congestion and edema may be present in patients with left ventricular failure (Figure 22-9). Dilation of the ascending aorta and aortic valve ring are diagnostic in patients with aortic dissection, Marfan syndrome, cystic medial necrosis, or syphilitic aortitis.

Echocardiogram

This test may be useful in determining the etiology of the regurgitant flow. For example, vegetations are evidence of infective endocarditis, whereas disruption of the

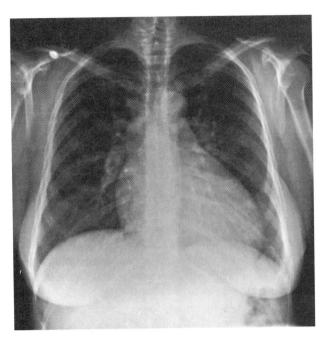

FIGURE 22-9 Chest radiograph of a patient with chronic aortic regurgitation. Note the enlarged cardiac silhouette, the appearance of the apex drooping below the level of the diaphragm (indicative of left ventricular enlargement), and increased pulmonary vascular markings.

valve cusps may be seen in aortic dissection or blunt anterior chest trauma. The regurgitant fraction can be approximated by echocardiogram, and Doppler studies allow an excellent estimate of severity based on how far back into the left ventricle (toward the apex) the regurgitant jet reaches. Increased left ventricular volume and chamber size are common echocardiographic findings.

Cardiac Catheterization

Aortography is the standard to assess severity as based on the degree of contrast reflux into the left ventricle following injection in the aorta. An assessment of ventricular function also is crucial in determining the prognosis and the urgency of surgical intervention. In the absence of left ventricular dysfunction, the ejection fraction should be greater than 70% because the higher preload (end-diastolic volume) increases contractility and stroke volume, as defined by Starling's law. When the ejection fraction diminishes to the 50% to 70% range, early ventricular dysfunction will probably reverse with valve replacement. However, some degree of dysfunction is irreversible in patients with ejection fractions less than 50%, and the risk of operative mortality is also increased.

Treatment

Treatment is related to symptoms and to the severity of aortic regurgitation. Asymptomatic patients with mild-to-moderate aortic regurgitation may lead an entirely normal life but should avoid strenuous isometric exercise or competitive sports. Antibiotic prophylaxis is necessary for dental procedures and for many surgical and instrumentation procedures.

The mildly symptomatic patient with chronic aortic regurgitation should be instructed to avoid exercise or exhausting activity. Digitalis and diuretics are used to treat symptoms of heart failure. By reducing left ventricular afterload, arterial vasodilators increase the volume of blood flowing into the systemic circulation and decrease the volume of regurgitant flow.

It remains controversial as to when, or if, asymptomatic patients should have valve replacement. A fall in ejection fraction with exercise, a left ventricular systolic dimension greater than 55 mm on echocardiography, cardiomegaly noted on chest radiograph, and a diminished exercise capacity have been variably advocated indications by investigators. As mentioned earlier, long-term outcome and risk of operative mortality worsen proportionately as the ejection fraction diminishes because this implies myocardial damage. An ejection fraction of less than 20% implies a severely, irreversibly damaged myocardium. In these patients, nonsurgical therapy should be strongly considered because left ventricular function occasionally worsens with valve replacement. Because it is possible that the left ventricular ejection fraction could diminish up to 5% following valve replacement, surgery in such patients may worsen outcome by exchanging chronic aortic regurgitation for a more severely compromised ventricle. In either case, progressive impairment of cardiac function can be expected, and sudden death is not rare in patients with severe disease.

Patients with acute, severe aortic regurgitation are supported clinically with inotropic agents, diuretics, and vasodilator agents while diagnostic tests and preparations for emergency aortic valve replacement are underway. Intraaortic balloon pumping, for perioperative stabilization, is contraindicated because it increases the volume of regurgitant flow.

MITRAL STENOSIS

The mitral valve apparatus consists of two pliable valve leaflets and a network of chordal attachments to papillary muscles. The valve leaflets open widely during diastole and allow unrestricted blood flow from the left atrium into the left ventricle.

Mitral stenosis is a chronic, progressive valvular disorder in which impairment of valve function and narrowing of the valve orifice restricts the free flow of blood from the left atrium to the left ventricle. As a consequence, the left atrium becomes enlarged and the left ventricle may be smaller in size with reduced wall thickness. Hemodynamic features include a progressive rise in left atrial pressure, a progressive reduction in left ventricular filling and stroke volume, and an end-diastolic pressure gradient across the mitral valve. Clinical features include chronic fatigue, decreasing exercise tolerance, and dyspnea with progressively less provocation.

Causes

The only common cause of mitral stenosis is *rheumatic fever.* Progressive endocardial inflammatory changes eventually cause scarring and fusion of the chordae tendineae, fibrotic thickening and rigidity of the leaflets, and adhesions between the two valve leaflets. Calcium, which also may be deposited on the valve leaflets, further impairs valve movement and narrows the valve opening. Altogether, these physical changes result in progressive obstruction to blood flow across the mitral valve. Because valve scarring and deformity occur slowly, functional impairment sufficient to produce symptoms typically does not develop for many years after the episode of rheumatic fever.

Uncommon causes of mitral stenosis include congenital abnormalities (seen occasionally in infants and children); carcinoid; and calcium accumulation in the mitral valve annulus (ring) associated with diabetes, hyperparathyroidism, or advanced age.

Hemodynamic Effects

The main factors that determine the patient's hemodynamic and clinical status are (1) the severity of valvular obstruction, (2) the heart rate and rhythm, and (3) the severity of secondary pulmonary arteriolar change that increases pulmonary vascular resistance.

Valvular Obstruction

Blood ordinarily flows freely across the mitral valve through a central principal orifice and several secondary orifices that lie between the chordae (Figure 22-10, *A*). Rheumatic inflammation of the endocardium and subsequent fibrotic and calcific changes obliterate the secondary orifices and reduce the size of the principal orifice. As the valve opening becomes narrowed, obstruction to blood flow results in a persistent progressive rise in left atrial pressure, a reduction in left ventricular filling, and consequently a diastolic pressure gradient between the left atrium and ventricle. The elevated left atrial pressure is transmitted to the pulmonary circulation, and it predisposes patients to episodes of acute

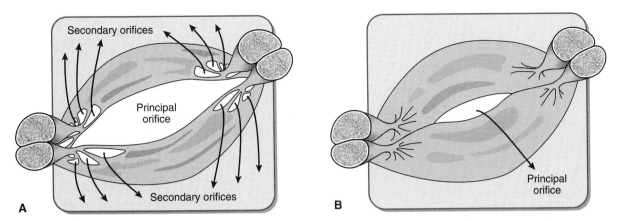

FIGURE 22-10 Schematic drawing of the normal mitral valve as viewed from below. **A,** Transmitral blood flow may occur through the principal orifice (between the anterior and posterior valve leaflets) or may flow through the secondary orifices (the spaces between the chordae tendineae). **B,** Schematic drawing of a rheumatic, stenotic mitral valve viewed from below. The primary orifice is reduced to a slitlike opening, due to commissural fusion, and the secondary orifices are obliterated due to chordal fusion. (Adapted from Sonnabeau RV, Stevenson JE, Edwards JE: Obliteration of the principal orifice of the stenotic mitral valve: a rare form of restenosis, *J Thorac Cardiovasc Surg* 49:265, 1965.)

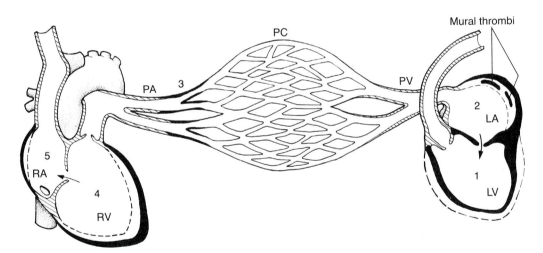

FIGURE 22-11 Schematic illustrating the central circulatory changes that accompany severe mitral stenosis. The *small arrow* indicates the subnormal blood flow across the narrowed valve orifice. *Dashed lines* indicate normal cardiac structures; *solid lines,* structural cardiac changes. Note the structural changes in the left atrium and ventricle as a consequence of the progressive flow obstruction across the valve. *1,* Decreased left ventricular filling; decreased, fixed cardiac output. *2,* Elevated left atrial pressure and pulmonary vascular pressures (passive pulmonary hypertension). Left atrial enlargement and atrial fibrillation are common, as are mural thrombi. *3,* Possible pulmonary arteriolar hypertrophy and hyperplasia (second stenosis) associated with a widened PAd-PWP gradient (active pulmonary hypertension). *4,* Right ventricular hypertrophy; possible dilation and failure leading to tricuspid regurgitation. *5,* Possible right atrial enlargement.

pulmonary edema. Pulmonary hypertension, in turn, increases resistance to right ventricular ejection and may eventually result in right ventricular failure. Figure 22-11 illustrates the anatomic and hemodynamic changes characteristic of mitral stenosis (Figure 22-12).

A reduction in the mitral orifice size from the normal 4 to 6 cm^2 to less than 1.0 cm^2, termed *critical mitral stenosis,* requires a left atrial pressure of approximately 35 mm Hg to maintain acceptable ventricular filling and resting cardiac output. With progressive valve

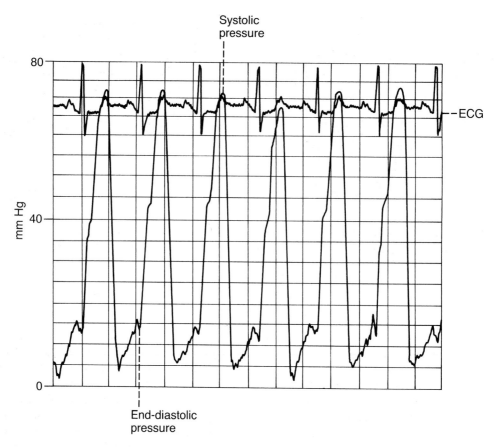

FIGURE 22-12 In the presence of pulmonary hypertension from any cause, an abnormally high afterload is imposed on the right ventricle. With gradually increasing pulmonary artery pressures, the right ventricle hypertrophies and is able to meet the abnormally high pressure demand but may eventually fail. In this tracing, right ventricular systolic pressure approaches 75 mm Hg. Right ventricular end-diastolic pressure is approximately 15 mm Hg; this abnormally high filling pressure indicates right ventricular failure.

narrowing, cardiac output becomes inadequate even at rest.

The chronically elevated left atrial pressure results in left atrial enlargement, whereas the left ventricular musculature may become somewhat atrophic as a result of the reduction in diastolic filling and therefore contractile work.

Rate of Blood Flow across the Mitral Valve

The left atrial pressure, and therefore the pressure gradient across the mitral valve, is highly dependent on the moment-by-moment rate of blood flow between the left heart chambers. If venous return increases because of exercise or postural changes, blood flow through the central circulation likewise increases. However, the stenotic valve cannot accommodate the greater blood flow. Consequently, left atrial pressures may acutely rise to physiolog-ically intolerable levels, predisposing the patient to acute pulmonary edema (Figure 22-13).

Heart Rate and Rhythm

Heart rate and rhythm also are crucial determinants of valve gradient and hemodynamic stability. Tachycardia increases the rate of blood flow entering the left atrium, but because the stenotic mitral valve restricts ventricular inflow, left atrial pressure increases. In addition, the time for ventricular filling is shortened proportionate to increases in heart rate; therefore preload and stroke volume cannot rise appropriately to body need.

Another important consideration influencing transmitral blood flow is the atrial contribution to ventricular filling. In early to mid diastole, flow is passive but substantial flow occurs. Normally, as left atrial and

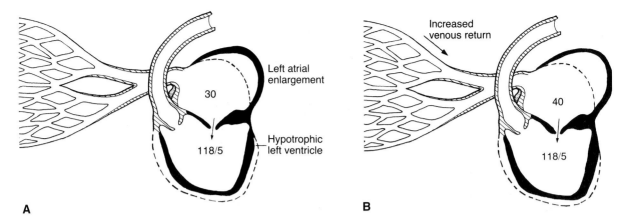

FIGURE 22-13 Mitral stenosis. Schematic of the left heart and pulmonary veins with the patient under resting conditions **(A)** and on increasing venous return (physical or emotional stress or recumbency) **(B).** Note that the left atrial pressure and mitral valve gradient increase by 10 mm Hg, which will likely be associated with shortness of breath due to the acute onset of pulmonary edema.

ventricular pressures equalize at the end of diastole, no further flow occurs unless atrial contraction actively pushes blood through the valve opening. In patients with severe mitral stenosis, ventricular filling is especially dependent on atrial contraction to force additional blood past the narrowed valve. Therefore the development of a tachyarrhythmia (particularly with atrioventricular asynchrony) is usually associated with hemodynamic deterioration. Atrial fibrillation, with its associated rapid ventricular rate, variably shortened ventricular filling period, and loss of atrial contraction, can precipitate the patient's first symptoms of mitral stenosis or a worsening of preexisting symptoms. Atrial fibrillation is particularly threatening to patients with preexisting left ventricular dysfunction. Ventricular tachycardia also may have disastrous hemodynamic consequences for patients with critical mitral stenosis.

Left Atrial Enlargement and Pulmonary Vascular Changes

Progressive increases in left atrial pressure are associated with simultaneous increases in pulmonary vascular pressures, termed *passive pulmonary hypertension.* The patient thus is predisposed to pulmonary edema. However, compensatory changes develop to protect patients from pulmonary edema; the changes are distinctive anatomic characteristics of mitral stenosis.

Left Atrial Enlargement. To accommodate increasing left atrial blood volume without increasing left atrial pressure, the left atrium enlarges. This protects the pul-

monary circulation from abnormally high pressure. With progressive dilation, however, the distorted atrial musculature becomes prone to frequent premature atrial contractions; then to transient supraventricular tachyarrhythmias; and, finally, to permanent atrial fibrillation, which may compromise the patient's hemodynamic status.

Stasis of blood in the dilated, fibrillating atrial chambers favors formation of blood clots that cling to the atrial walls (mural thrombi). These clots may detach or fragment, predisposing the patient to pulmonary or systemic emboli. Ultimately, the limit of left atrial distensibility is exceeded and left atrial and pulmonary vascular pressures rise.

Pulmonary Vascular Changes. As pulmonary vascular pressures rise, changes occur within the lungs that elevate the threshold level necessary to produce pulmonary edema. These occur variably among individuals and include several components:
1. The development of supernormal pulmonary lymph flow, which enables the removal of excess fluid that sequesters into the lung
2. Diminished permeability of the alveolar capillary membrane, which reduces the rate of fluid movement into the lung
3. Hypertrophy and hyperplasia of the pulmonary arterioles, which become capable of intense constriction
Pulmonary capillary hydrostatic pressure (the prime determinant of fluid movement into the lung) is influenced by pulmonary venous or left atrial pressure, as well as the amount of blood flowing into the pulmonary capillary

bed. Pulmonary arteriolar constriction reduces the amount of blood flowing into the pulmonary capillary bed and therefore may lower the hydrostatic pressures distal to the pulmonary arterioles. This compensatory mechanism helps protect against pulmonary edema.

Pulmonary arteriolar constriction and hyperplasia, however, increase resistance to blood flow between the larger pulmonary arteries and the pulmonary capillaries and cause greater elevations in pulmonary artery pressures. This is termed *precapillary pulmonary hypertension* or *active pulmonary hypertension*. It is reflected on pulmonary artery pressure measurements as a widening of the pulmonary artery diastolic to pulmonary artery wedge pressure (PAd-PWP) gradient. Precapillary pulmonary hypertension results in an even greater pressure load on the right ventricle, which adaptively hypertrophies and often ultimately fails (Figure 22-14).

The pulmonary arteriolar constriction and hyperplastic narrowing are sometimes referred to as the "second stenosis" in patients with mitral stenosis. Once developed, the pulmonary vascular changes may not reverse completely or even substantially with medical or surgical therapy. Indeed, when pulmonary arterial pressures attain systemic levels, the condition is considered inoperable because

experience has shown that these patients cannot be weaned from inotropic or ventilator support postoperatively. Preexisting right ventricular dysfunction made worse by the trauma and stress of surgery may make weaning from cardiopulmonary bypass impossible. This "second stenosis" as a result of pulmonary arteriolar constriction generally occurs after critical narrowing of the valve area; however, in any patient, there is no clear relationship between the transmitral pressure gradient and the severity of pulmonary vascular change. Therefore each patient responds individually, giving rise to great variability in clinical presentations.

Clinical Presentation

Symptoms do not usually appear until the mitral valve orifice is reduced to 1.0 cm^2 or less. Symptoms, which are usually related to exertion, can develop so gradually that the patient may automatically modify activity and may not be aware of progressive disability. Anything that increases venous return or heart rate may precipitate symptoms; examples are pregnancy, atrial fibrillation, respiratory infection, shivering, exercise, emotional stress, or assuming a supine position. The principal symptoms of mitral stenosis and their causes are shown in Table 22-2.

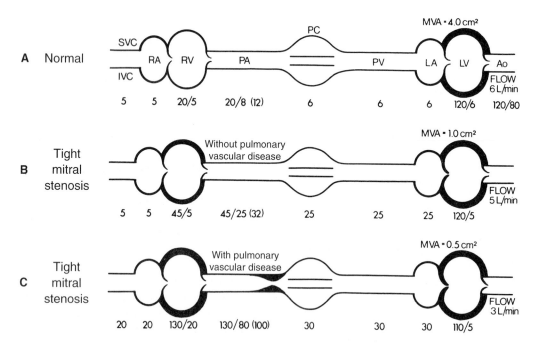

FIGURE 22-14 The structures of the central circulation drawn end to end. **A,** The circulation of a person with a normal heart and hemodynamics. **B,** Tight mitral stenosis with no pulmonary vascular change. **C,** Tight mitral stenosis with secondary pulmonary vascular change resulting in a "second stenosis" at the pulmonary arteriolar level. (From Grossman W, Baim DS: *Cardiac catheterization, angiography and intervention,* ed 4, Philadelphia, 1991, Lea & Febiger.)

Mentation

Mentation is usually normal unless embolization from a left atrial thrombus has resulted in cerebral infarction.

Cutaneous Manifestations

A pinkish-purple discoloration of the cheeks is common in patients with severe disease, the so-called mitral facies. Generally, the complexion is pale, the skin is warm, and peripheral cyanosis may be present on exertion. Generalized, pitting edema indicates right ventricular failure.

Heart Rate and Character of Pulse

Heart rate is normal or slightly tachycardic unless the patient is in uncontrolled atrial fibrillation (ventricular rate greater than 100 beats per minute). In more advanced disease, the pulse is small and, in the presence of atrial fibrillation, totally irregular and variable in volume. A pulse deficit is typical of atrial fibrillation (the apical pulse is greater than the simultaneously counted radial pulse) because some cardiac contractions do not generate a noticeable peripheral pulse.

Heart Sounds

The typical auscultatory findings occur in the following sequence with progression of the valvular deformity.

TABLE 22-2

Major Symptoms of Mitral Stenosis and Their Causes

Symptom	Cause
Dyspnea	Pulmonary venous hypertension
Fatigue	Low cardiac output
Paroxysmal nocturnal dyspnea; orthopnea; night cough	Redistribution of fluid from the lower extremities and trunk to the lungs with recumbency
Hemoptysis	Palmonary venous hypertension causing rupture of some vessels
Palpitations	Atrial fibrillation with a rapid ventricular response
Hoarseness	Enlargement of the left atrium and compression of the laryngeal nerve
Hepatic congestion, ascites dependent edema, and jugular venous distention	Right ventricular failure
Chest pain	Right ventricular hypertension, concomitant coronary artery disease, or coronary embolization
Cerebral findings (stroke or seizures)	Systemic embolization of mural thrombus from the left atrium

---

The initial finding is that the first heart sound (S_1) is accentuated because the thickened, less mobile mitral valve leaflets remain maximally open at the onset of systole. The valve leaflets must then swing through a wide arc to close and consequently produce a louder closing (S_1) sound. The second heart sound (S_2) is normal unless pulmonary hypertension is present. If pulmonary artery pressures are elevated, the P_2 is loud and may be closely split. As right ventricular failure occurs and ejection time is prolonged, P_2 may be delayed, resulting in a widely split second heart sound.

Following the second heart sound there is a characteristic opening snap, which is attributed to the abrupt cessation of the outward movement of the rigid mitral valve leaflets early in diastole. The opening snap is high-pitched and is best heard at the apex with the diaphragm of the stethoscope.

As the valve opening becomes narrowed, a diastolic rumble may be audible. It is a low-pitched murmur best heard with the bell of the stethoscope held over the apical impulse and with the patient in the left lateral position. The murmur is produced by turbulence when the jet of blood, flowing through the narrowed valve, impinges on the endocardium at the apex of the left ventricle. The loudness of the murmur does not accurately correlate with the severity of the stenosis because decreased flow across the narrowed orifice, as a result of low cardiac output, decreases turbulence and audibility of the murmur. A long diastolic rumble indicates that the gradient between the left atrium and ventricle is maintained throughout diastole. If the rumble becomes shortened, it suggests that left ventricular end-diastolic pressure is increasing because of either fluid overload or heart failure from coexisting disease of the left ventricle or aortic valve.

Palpation of the Precordium

The precordium is generally quiet. The impulse of the suboptimally filled, somewhat atrophic left ventricle is of short duration and lightly tapping. A left parasternal lift may be present and is indicative of right ventricular pressure overload due to pulmonary hypertension.

Neck Veins

The jugular veins become distended when right ventricular function deteriorates. A visible internal jugular *a* wave also may be visible.

Respiratory Rate and Character of Breathing

The resting respiratory rate is slightly increased (22 to 24 breaths per minute) in patients with chronic interstitial pulmonary edema, but rest dyspnea is not present.

Increasing tachypnea and dyspnea develop with the onset of acute severe pulmonary edema. Patients with severe mitral stenosis usually sleep in a chair or on several pillows because the supine position increases venous return and precipitates acute pulmonary edema. Orthopnea, paroxysmal nocturnal dyspnea, or dyspnea precipitated by physical or emotional stress may be the first symptom noted by the patient.

Breath Sounds

The breath sounds are normal. With the onset of acute pulmonary edema and alveolar flooding, crackles and wheezes are audible.

Acid-Base Values

These values are normal unless acute pulmonary edema or a marked reduction in cardiac output is present.

Hemodynamic Profile

The hemodynamic features of mitral stenosis at any level of severity and any point in time are acutely determined by venous return and by heart rate and rhythm.

Arterial Pressure

The blood pressure remains normal unless left ventricular output falls significantly. This may occur during uncontrolled atrial fibrillation or ventricular tachycardia. Alternatively, this finding is noted in patients with complicating heart disease such as acute myocardial infarction.

Systemic Vascular Resistance

As stroke volume decreases, systemic vascular resistance reflexively increases.

Pulmonary Vascular Resistance

This value may be normal in patients with few or no pulmonary arteriolar changes. Patients with severe pulmonary arteriolar constriction or sclerosis may have values as high as 2000 dynes/sec/cm^{-5}.

Central Venous Pressure or Right Atrial Pressure

These measurements may be normal in the early stages of the disease but increase when prolonged, severe pulmonary hypertension results in right ventricular failure. In patients with sinus rhythm, the right atrial waveform shows a prominent *a* wave that graphically reflects greater resistance to end-diastolic filling of the hypertrophied or failing right ventricle. In atrial fibrillation there is only one crest, the *v* or *c-v* wave.

Pulmonary Artery Pressure

This measurement is normal in patients with mild mitral stenosis. In patients with moderate-to-severe disease, pulmonary artery systolic and diastolic pressures are raised in proportion to the elevations in left atrial pressure (passive pulmonary hypertension). If patients have severe pulmonary vascular changes, pulmonary artery systolic and diastolic pressures may exceed systemic arterial pressure. In these patients, there is a proportionate increase in the PAd-PWP gradient (active pulmonary hypertension).

Pulmonary Artery Wedge Pressure

This measurement is classically elevated. The measured value correlates with left atrial pressure but is greater than left ventricular end-diastolic pressure (as measured in the cardiac catheterization laboratory). The transmitral valve gradient is the hemodynamic hallmark of mitral stenosis (Figure 22-15).

Cardiac Output

In patients with severe disease, stroke volume and cardiac output are fixed and low.

Laboratory and Other Diagnostic Studies

Electrocardiograph

The ECG may be normal in the early stages of the disease. Left atrial enlargement is usually manifest by P wave abnormalities (P mitrale). If the mean pulmonary artery pressure is greater than 35 mm Hg, signs of right ventricular hypertrophy, such as right axis deviation, also are common. Atrial fibrillation with coarse fibrillation waves is commonly observed in patients with mitral stenosis severe enough to warrant hospitalization.

Chest Radiograph

The appearance of the chest film is related to the severity of anatomic distortion of the heart, as well as the degree of pulmonary hypertension. In patients with mild mitral stenosis, the chest film is usually normal. In more severe cases, there may be increased prominence of the pulmonary arteries (secondary to pulmonary hypertension) and visibility of the upper lobe vasculature, which is related to distribution of blood flow toward the apices of the lungs. The enlarged left atrium may extend farther from the right heart border than does the right atrium; this gives the right atrial shadow the appearance of a "double density." Left atrial enlargement also causes an elevation of the left mainstem bronchus (Figure 22-16).

Radiographic signs of interstitial pulmonary edema may be present in patients with critical mitral stenosis.

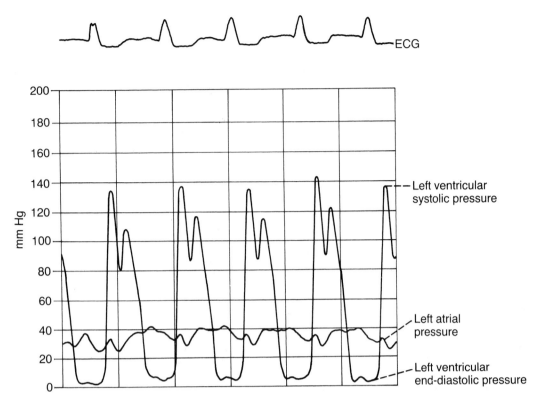

FIGURE 22-15 A left atrial and left ventricular end-diastolic pressure gradient of approximately 30 mm Hg determined from simultaneously obtained tracings obtained in a cardiac catheterization laboratory from a 56-year-old woman with mitral stenosis. The patient is in atrial fibrillation.

Kerley B lines and increased prominence of the horizontal fissure are the radiographic hallmarks of interstitial pulmonary edema. In severe disease, subclinical pulmonary edema is typically the patient's resting, steady state.

Echocardiogram

Motion of the mitral valve leaflets is diminished, and calcium deposits may be visualized. The left atrium is enlarged, and left atrial thrombi may be noted. Doppler studies estimate the velocity of blood flow across the narrowed orifice and allow evaluation of lesion severity. Echocardiography is also useful in evaluating patients' response to medical therapy.

Radionuclide Studies

These techniques are used with the patient at rest or during exercise to determine left ventricular end-diastolic volume, left ventricular ejection fraction, and cardiac output. These studies may also be chosen to follow the patient's response to medical therapy.

Cardiac Catheterization

This diagnostic technique measures the gradient across the valve and other central circulatory pressures, calculates valve orifice size, assesses ventricular function and cardiac output, and detects concomitant valvular or coronary artery disease (see also the section on valve area calculation).

Treatment

Asymptomatic patients with only auscultatory or laboratory signs of mild mitral stenosis require no treatment except for endocarditis prophylaxis. However, some patients who claim to be asymptomatic may be severely limiting their activities with major lifestyle changes and therefore may claim no symptoms despite severe disease.

Medical Treatment

Endocarditis Prophylaxis. Antibiotic therapy is indicated in any patient with anatomic distortion of an endocardial structure who requires a surgical procedure, dental manipulation, or instrumentation that may produce bacteremia. Rheumatic fever prophylaxis, with long-term

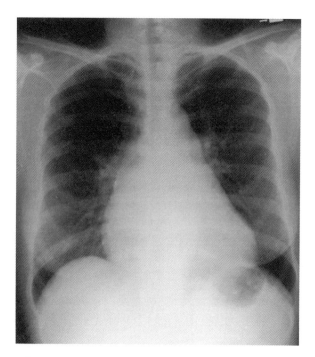

FIGURE 22-16 Chest radiograph of a patient with mitral stenosis. Note the elevation of the left mainstem bronchus (due to the enlarged left atrium), the straightening of the left heart border by the enlarging left atrium, and the double density noted along the right heart border (enlarged left atrium).

administration of either penicillin or sulfadiazine, is suggested in all patients younger than 35 years of age.

With progression of disease and appearance of symptoms, the following therapeutic interventions are added.

Digitalis. Once atrial fibrillation has developed, cardiac glycosides are given to maintain the ventricular response below 100 beats per minute. Some patients depend on a sinus mechanism to maintain hemodynamic stability. In such people, cardioversion may restore sinus rhythm if the left atrium is not too dilated and distorted. Beta blockers are useful for patients in normal sinus rhythm to prevent the adverse consequences of tachycardia. Beta blockade also is useful in managing the course of postoperative patients whose ventricular response to atrial fibrillation cannot be adequately controlled with digitalis because of high levels of adrenergic activity.

Systemic Anticoagulation. In patients with rheumatic mitral valve disease, regardless of cardiac rhythm, long-term anticoagulation with warfarin sodium (Coumadin) is indicated to diminish the high likelihood of stroke and systemic emboli.

Diuretics and Salt Restriction. Because most symptoms are related to the congestive components of left- and right-sided failure, diuretics and salt restriction may reduce plasma volume and therefore pulmonary and systemic venous pressures.

Patient Instruction. Strenuous activity or any factors that induce tachycardia or increased venous return should be avoided.

Surgical Therapy

Surgery should be considered when the patient becomes symptomatic despite optimal medical therapy. This usually correlates with a valve area less than 1.0 cm^2 and a PWP of approximately 30 to 35 mm Hg. When exertional dyspnea affects lifestyle, the patient has experienced episodes of pulmonary edema, or right heart failure develops, valve replacement is indicated.

Mitral Commissurotomy. For this procedure, either the surgeon's finger or a knife is used to create a larger opening at the mitral valve commissure (site of junction between the valve cusps). This is the procedure of choice for patients with pure mitral stenosis and relatively pliable, noncalcific valves with no mitral regurgitation. This procedure is only palliative, and patients usually require reoperation at 5 to 20 years.

This procedure is used less frequently since the advent of balloon valvuloplasty.

Mitral Valvuloplasty. The results of this procedure are more gratifying than those of balloon valvuloplasty of the aortic valve. There are reasonable short- and long-term results reported when valvuloplasty is performed by experienced operators at some medical centers. The procedure requires a physician experienced in transseptal catheterization. Suboptimal results are predictable if the left atrium is very dilated, the valve is calcified, the subvalvular apparatus is thickened, mitral regurgitation is present, or left ventricular function is abnormal (Figure 22-17).

Mitral Valve Replacement. For this procedure, the diseased valve is resected and the prosthetic valve is inserted in its place. This is the procedure of choice in patients with combined mitral regurgitation and stenosis and for patients with extensive valvular calcification. Long-term anticoagulation is required. The prosthetic valve may become defective because of ordinary "wear and tear" and may require replacement within 7 to 12 years.

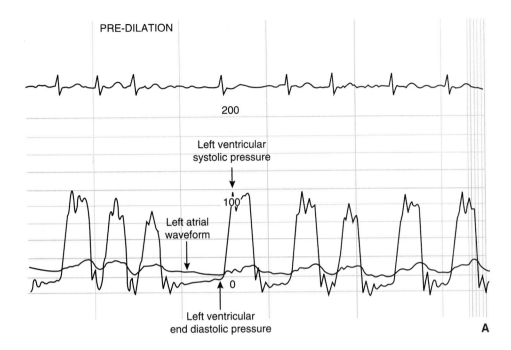

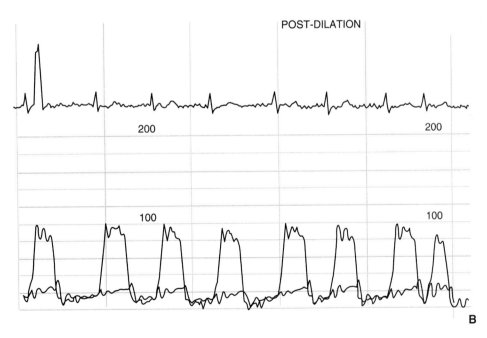

FIGURE 22-17 A, Simultaneously obtained left ventricular and left atrial pressure in an 18-year-old woman with mitral stenosis. At the time of cardiac catheterization, she is near term in pregnancy and very symptomatic. The patient is in atrial fibrillation; the pressure gradient across the mitral valve is 22 mm Hg. The physiologic stress imposed by impending labor and delivery pose a grave threat to this already symptomatic patient. **B,** Immediately following balloon valvuloplasty. There is essentially no gradient across the mitral valve. The woman went on to be safely delivered of a healthy infant. (Courtesy of Dr. David J. Hale, Foster G. McGaw Medical Center of Loyola University, Maywood, Illinois.)

MITRAL REGURGITATION (INSUFFICIENCY)

The mitral valve leaflets approximate and close at the onset of systole as left ventricular contraction causes ventricular cavity pressures to exceed those of the left atrium. The papillary-chordal apparatus applies traction on the valve leaflets to maintain the closed position and size of the valve while the ventricular chamber becomes smaller during ejection.

Mitral regurgitation is either an acute or a chronic valve lesion that occurs when inadequate closure or incompetence of the mitral valve results in the entry of a "regurgitant jet" into the left atrium and pulmonary circulation during ventricular systole. Patients with chronic, progressive disease usually have an enlarged, hypertrophic left ventricle and an enlarged left atrium (Figure 22-18).

Hemodynamic hallmarks of severe mitral regurgitation include increased left atrial and pulmonary vascular pressures and decreased systemic blood flow. The signs and symptoms of severe mitral regurgitation are the result of pulmonary congestion and edema and systemic perfusion failure.

Causes

Competence of the mitral valve apparatus depends on normal anatomy of the valve leaflets, integrity and proper length of the chordae tendineae, integrity and contractile dynamics of the papillary muscles, normal function of the myocardium adjacent to the papillary muscles, and proportionate size of the left ventricle to the mitral valve annulus (ring). Abnormalities in any of these factors may prevent the two valve leaflets from making complete contact in systole, with consequent regurgitant flow into the left atrial chamber and pulmonary circulation. There are numerous causes of mitral regurgitation.

Mitral Valve Prolapse

Prolapse of the mitral valve leaflets into the left atrium during ventricular systole may be the result of a floppy structure of the valve leaflets and chordae secondary to myxomatous degeneration of the valve tissue; an excessive length of the chordae tendineae; or an enlarged valve annulus. Mitral valve prolapse is the most common cause of mild mitral regurgitation in adults, particularly young women. The reasons for this gender/age distribution are not known.

Rheumatic Heart Disease

In patients who develop mitral regurgitation, rheumatic valvulitis leads to progressive fibrotic shortening of the mitral valve leaflets and chordal structures. Valvulitis may also lead to calcification of the valve commissure in a fixed, open position. Further distortion of the valve orifice geometry may result from progressive left atrial

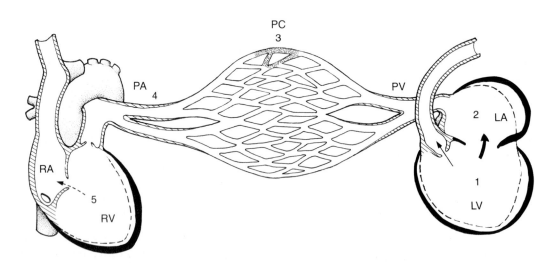

FIGURE 22-18 Schematic of the central circulation with chronic mitral regurgitation; the *arrow* indicates the direction of abnormal blood flow. Note the characteristic enlargement of the left atrium and ventricle *(heavy, black lines)*. *1,* Dilated left ventricle, subnormal forward stroke volume *(thin arrow)* and larger regurgitant volume *(thick arrow)*. *2,* Elevated left atrial and pulmonary venous pressures. *3,* Predisposition to pulmonary edema. *4,* Pulmonary hypertension. *5,* Dilated, failing right ventricle with possible tricuspid regurgitation (late stages). *Broken lines* represent normal heart contour. *Solid lines* represent adaptive structural change.

enlargement that displaces the posterior leaflet over the base of the left ventricular wall. Because secondary left atrial enlargement may accentuate the incompetence of the valve, mitral regurgitation eventually leads to worsening of valve function and greater regurgitant volume.

Bacterial Endocarditis

In patients with sepsis, blood-borne bacteria may become implanted on the valve, leading to destruction of the leaflets or chordae. Bacterial infection of a valve is more likely to occur in an abnormal valve, but it also may occur in the absence of anatomic abnormalities.

Ischemic Heart Disease

Ischemic dysfunction or rupture of the papillary muscle may cause transient or permanent, mild or severe mitral regurgitation.

Left Ventricular Dilation or Dilation of the Mitral Valve Annulus

Dilation of a failing left ventricle, from any cause, may distort the alignment of the chordae and papillary muscles and may increase the size of the valve annulus. The valve leaflets are thus prevented from closing completely in systole. This usually occurs when the ventricle is significantly dilated. Thus heart failure begets more heart failure. Dilation of the mitral valve annulus out of proportion to the left ventricle may also occur in patients with Marfan syndrome or mitral valve prolapse.

Trauma

Cardiac injury secondary to thoracic trauma on rare occasions may result in traumatic rupture of the papillary muscle or chordae.

Hypertrophic Cardiomyopathy

Mitral regurgitant flow is caused by the systolic anterior motion of the anterior valve leaflet and is a characteristic unique to this condition.

Hemodynamic Effects

The primary systolic and secondary diastolic flow abnormalities are discussed separately. Chronic compensatory systolic and diastolic changes, as well as the effects of acute mitral regurgitation, are presented.

Systolic Abnormalities

The primary abnormality of mitral regurgitation is best described if the left ventricle is understood as a pump with a double outlet; blood may exit through either the aortic or the mitral valves. In patients with mitral regurgitation,

throughout left ventricular systole, the total left ventricular output is divided between the systemic stroke volume and the regurgitant volume into the relaxed left atrium. Blood preferentially flows into the area of least resistance; consequently, in patients with severe mitral regurgitation, greater than 50% of left ventricular stroke volume may be ejected into the low-resistance left atrium rather than the high-resistance systemic circulation. The regurgitant left atrial volume and pressure also are reflected back to the pulmonary veins, capillaries, and arteries. These elevated pressures predispose patients to acute pulmonary edema and right ventricular failure. In chronic disease, however, marked left atrial dilation damps the pressure effects so that significant regurgitation may be present for years with relatively normal left atrial and pulmonary venous pressures.

To maintain adequate systemic blood flow, the total blood volume pumped by the left ventricle must increase. With chronic disease, the left ventricle hypertrophies and enlarges in a globular manner, and total output significantly rises. In acute disease, the normal left ventricle cannot adjust to the sudden hemodynamic burden, and profound systemic perfusion failure typically occurs.

Diastolic Abnormalities

During ventricular diastole, the blood that refluxes into the left atrium and pulmonary circulation during the previous systole returns to the left ventricle in addition to the normal pulmonary venous flow. This results in left ventricular diastolic volume overload and, in acute disease, sudden elevations in left ventricular end-diastolic pressure. When the valve defect develops slowly, compensatory left ventricular enlargement and increased distensibility maintain a normal or minimally elevated left ventricular end-diastolic pressure.

Factors That Affect the Regurgitant Volume and the Magnitude of Hemodynamic Consequences

Several factors are interrelated, and they determine the severity of mitral regurgitation. The first two may be therapeutically manipulated for patient stabilization; the last is unalterable.

Size of the Regurgitant Orifice. The most important factor is the size of the mitral regurgitant orifice; the larger the orifice, the greater the volume of regurgitant flow. The mitral valve orifice may increase in size with progression of the primary valve disease, such as rheumatic fever. Left ventricular dilation, which increases with the development of heart failure, also enlarges the mitral orifice and may acutely produce or increase mitral regurgitant flow. Conversely, preload reduction may diminish the size or may entirely eliminate the regurgitant orifice and regurgitant flow.

Left Ventricular Systolic Pressure. The systolic pressure difference between the left atrium and left ventricle also determines the volume of regurgitant flow; the higher the ventricular systolic pressure relative to left atrial pressure, the greater the volume of regurgitant flow. Left ventricular systolic pressure (afterload) is a clinically important and a therapeutically alterable factor in modifying mitral regurgitation. Ventricular systolic pressure and the regurgitant volume proportionately rise or fall in response to increases or decreases in systemic vascular resistance. For example, by raising blood pressure, vasopressor therapy aggravates mitral regurgitation, whereas vasodilator therapy lessens mitral regurgitation by lowering blood pressure (Figure 22-19).

Left Atrial Compliance. In patients with acute mitral regurgitation, the normally small, nondistensible left atrium is unable to damp the pressure effects of the "regurgitant jet." Left atrial (PWP) waveform morphology is characterized by giant regurgitant *v* waves (see section on pulmonary artery waveform analysis). The giant *v* waves contribute to elevating mean left atrial and pulmonary artery pressures, which, in turn, leads to acute pulmonary edema.

If the mitral regurgitant lesion is chronic, the left atrium progressively enlarges and becomes more distensible so that the systolic regurgitant jet can be accommodated with a minimal pressure elevation. The left atrial *v* waves may not thereby be significantly enlarged, although a significant volume of regurgitant flow exists. When the extent of left atrial dilation is maximized and the regurgitant volume continues to increase, left atrial and

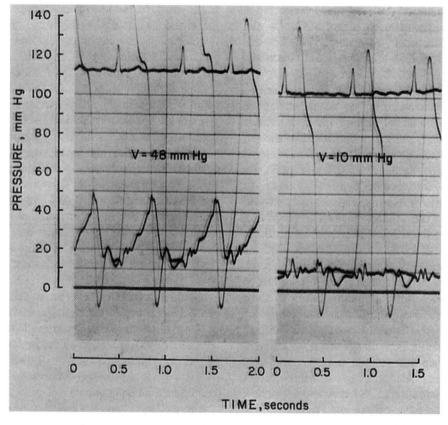

FIGURE 22-19 Left ventricular and pulmonary artery wedge pressure (PWP) tracing before **(A)** and during **(B)** administration of sodium nitroprusside in a patient with severe mitral regurgitation. Note the marked reduction in *v* wave amplitude with afterload reduction. These tracings clearly illustrate the extremely sensitive relationship of afterload to the volume of regurgitant flow. (From Harshaw CW et al: Reduced systemic vascular resistance as therapy for severe mitral regurgitation of valvular origin, *Ann Intern Med* 83:312, 1975.)

pulmonary vascular pressures rise, predisposing patients to pulmonary congestion and edema. In patients with severe disease, the enlarged left atrium also becomes vulnerable to atrial flutter and fibrillation, which may significantly worsen hemodynamics.

Hemodynamic Effects of Chronic versus Acute Mitral Regurgitation

Slowly progressive mitral regurgitation is well tolerated because cardiovascular compensation can maintain forward stroke volume and near-normal left atrial pressure. Conversely, the hemodynamic consequences of acute mitral regurgitation are poorly tolerated and clinically dramatic. The time-related onset of disease is crucial to patient tolerance, and these two very different syndromes are discussed separately.

Chronic Mitral Regurgitation

The condition of patients with mild-to-moderate mitral regurgitation is usually highly stable and relatively symptom free for decades or life. Progressive left atrial enlargement develops to damp the pressure effects of the regurgitant flow. In response to chronic diastolic volume overload, the left ventricle dilates and becomes more compliant. Overall, left ventricular systolic function is enhanced and the effects of rapid, supernormal diastolic filling are minimized so that significant regurgitation may be present with only mild elevations in mean left atrial and pulmonary vascular pressures.

When the volume of regurgitant flow increases beyond a tolerable level with progression of the valve lesion, or another cardiac disorder such as acute myocardial infarction complicates the patient's clinical course, left ventricular function quickly deteriorates and left ventricular end-diastolic volume and pressure progressively rise. With increased ventricular dilation, the mitral regurgitant orifice may enlarge and allow increased regurgitant flow into the left atrium. The rising left atrial and pulmonary vascular pressures predispose the patient to pulmonary edema, and the resulting increase in right ventricular afterload predisposes to right ventricular failure. Decreases in aortic blood flow cause systemic perfusion failure. These interrelating adverse hemodynamic changes cause the patient's condition to spiral downward.

Hemodynamic Profile

Arterial Pressure. The arterial pressure is usually maintained within the normal range.

Systemic Vascular Resistance. This calculated value is usually normal. Any increase in systemic vascular resistance mediated by stress, heart failure, or cold increases

the left ventricular outflow resistance and thereby worsens the regurgitant flow.

Pulmonary Vascular Resistance. This value may be normal or slightly decreased if the patient has a large, compliant left atrium and relatively mild left atrial pressure elevations. Pulmonary vascular resistance may be slightly decreased because mild elevations in left atrial pressure result in the opening of pulmonary vessels at the uppermost portions of the lung (West zones I and II). This increases the functional cross-sectional area of the pulmonary circulation. When the left atrial pressure exceeds 18 to 20 mm Hg, however, pulmonary edema and associated hypoxemia result. Perivascular cuffs of edema fluid narrow the vessels, and hypoxemic vasoconstriction jointly increases pulmonary vascular resistance.

Central Venous Pressure or Right Atrial Pressure. These measurements may be normal if the right ventricle maintains normal function.

Pulmonary Artery and Pulmonary Artery Wedge Pressures. The pulmonary artery systolic and diastolic pressures increase in proportion to the elevation in mean left atrial pressure (PWP). The severity of PWP elevation is related to the volume of regurgitant flow, the compliance and size of the left atrium, and the functional state of the left ventricle. For example, the amplitude of the PWP regurgitant v waves (see section on waveform morphology) may be deceptively low relative to a large regurgitant volume if an enlarged, compliant left atrium absorbs and accommodates the large regurgitant stream (chronic disease). Alternatively, higher-amplitude v waves may be present for a similar volume of regurgitant flow if the patient has a normal, relatively noncompliant left atrium (acute disease). Increases or decreases in left ventricular end-diastolic pressure also directly affect left atrial pressure.

Mitral regurgitation is the only clinical situation in which the mean left atrial pressure (PWP) is actually greater than the pulmonary artery diastolic pressure. The reversal of the normal hemodynamic relationship is due to the regurgitant jet. Blood is literally flowing backward during systole from the left ventricle through the left atrium and pulmonary circulation. The driving (higher) pressure is therefore on the left side of the heart.

The normally close relationship between left atrial pressure (PWP) and left ventricular end-diastolic pressure no longer exists because of the presence of giant v waves. Measured PWP overestimates the left ventricular end-diastolic pressure. Left ventricular end-diastolic pressure is best estimated by measuring the crest of the a wave if the patient is in sinus rhythm, or measuring the pre−v wave area (which correlates with end-diastole) if the patient is in atrial fibrillation (see Chapter 10, section on potential problems and pitfalls in obtaining accurate pressure measurements).

The hemodynamic hallmark of severe, decompensated, or acute mitral regurgitation is an increased-amplitude *v* wave on the left atrial and PWP waveform. Although neither its presence nor its absence can be considered absolutely diagnostic, its importance in the diagnosis and assessment of therapy warrants discussion of the following considerations.

Evolution and Timing of the Normal v Wave

The upstroke of the *v* wave occurs in synchrony with late ventricular systole when the maximal volume of pulmonary venous blood flows into the left atrium. The resulting increase in left atrial blood volume is observed as the upstroke, to the crest, of the *v* wave. The crest of the left atrial *v* wave, which heralds the onset of diastole, is normally approximately 5 to 15 mm Hg in amplitude. At that point, left atrial pressure exceeds left ventricular pressure, and the mitral valve passively opens to allow ventricular filling. As a result, left atrial pressure falls. This correlates with the descending portion of the *v* wave (the *y* descent). On a strip-chart recording with the left atrial (PWP) waveform simultaneously recorded with an ECG rhythm strip, the *v* wave roughly corresponds with the terminal portion of the T wave. *The exact relationship of the* v *wave to the ECG varies among patients because the time required for the pressure wave to reach the sensing transducer depends on the length of the connecting tubing used on a given patient.* Increased length of tubing is associated with a *v* wave recorded farther from the T wave (on the isoelectric line or on the P wave of the succeeding heartbeat).

Timing of the v Wave in Mitral Regurgitation

In patients with acute or chronic mitral regurgitation, the ascending portion of the *v* wave begins with the onset of ventricular systole and becomes superimposed on the *c* wave and therefore obliterates the *x* descent. The *v* wave is also abnormally large and dominates the mean PWP pressure tracing. The initial portion of the *v* wave will appear earlier in the cardiac cycle on a simultaneously recorded ECG than would a normal *v* wave. The peak of the *v* wave usually appears following the T wave because of the prolonged upstroke of the giant *v* wave (Figure 22-20).

This difference in *v* wave position relative to the ECG can be determined only if the patient is having acute periods of mitral regurgitation during which the changing position of the regurgitant *v* wave may be noted relative to that of the normal *v* waves.

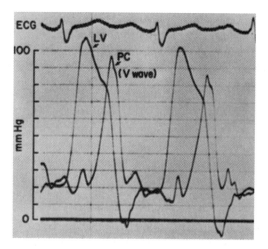

FIGURE 22-20 Left ventricular *(LV)* and pulmonary artery wedge *(PC)* pressure tracing taken from a patient with acute mitral regurgitation due to ruptured chordae tendineae. The giant *v* waves result from regurgitation of blood into a relatively small and noncompliant left atrium. (From Grossman W, Baim DS: Profiles in valvular heart disease. In *Cardiac catheterization, angiography and intervention,* ed 4, Philadelphia, 1991, Lea & Febiger.)

Clinical Relevance

The sudden appearance of large *v* waves suggests acute mitral regurgitation. These large *v* waves may even cause the PWP tracing to take on the appearance of a pulmonary artery waveform, possibly leading the clinician to assume that the balloon will not wedge. One risk is that repeated back-to-back inflations of a distally placed catheter may rupture the involved pulmonary artery branch. Moreover, failure to recognize this sign, usually present in highly unstable patients, may lead to delay in proper treatment.

A large *v* wave may diminish several days after the onset of acute mitral regurgitation as the left atrium compensates for the sudden volume and pressure overload by dilation. Arterial vasodilator therapy may be guided by monitoring the size of the *v* wave. Diminution in amplitude indicates adequate afterload reduction and normalization of intracardiac blood flow, whereas increased-amplitude *v* waves indicate an increase in regurgitant flow (see Figure 22-19).

Interpretation of v Waves in Pulmonary Artery Wedge Pressure Tracings

Two criteria for clinically significant large *v* waves diagnostic of severe mitral regurgitant flow are as follows:

1. *A v wave peak 10 mm Hg above the mean PWP.* This criterion is not always specific for mitral regurgitation. Other conditions in which a large *v* wave may be observed, although rarely, include aortic stenosis or insufficiency, cardiomyopathy, and hypertensive heart disease. Patients with these conditions all have a stiff, noncompliant left atrium, which may not be able to accommodate normal pulmonary venous inflow. Thus a large *v* wave is inscribed with normal left atrial filling during ventricular systole. Increased-amplitude *v* waves also may be observed in patients with acute ventricular septal defect because the systolic left-to-right intracardiac shunt increases pulmonary venous flow and left atrial systolic filling.
2. *A v wave peaks at least twice the value of the mean PWP.* This criterion is more specific for mitral regurgitation and should yield few false-positive results.

Cardiac Output. Systemic blood flow remains normal if the left ventricle remains compensated and the volume of the regurgitant flow is not large. However, systemic blood flow is less than total left ventricular output; therefore these become two different and distinct hemodynamic measurements. Furthermore, all invasive measurements of cardiac output, which measure pulmonary blood flow, may be inaccurate because of the contamination of pulmonary arterial blood by the regurgitant jet. As a consequence, accurate analysis of arteriovenous oxygen content difference (Fick's formula), dye concentration (dye dilution), or blood temperature changes (thermodilution) is impossible. Results of all of the cardiac output measurement techniques are invalid. In most cardiac catheterization laboratories, the oxygen content difference between the vena cava and aorta is used to estimate forward cardiac output. Total cardiac output (forward and regurgitant) is determined from the left ventricular angiogram. These data can then be used to estimate a regurgitant fraction (i.e., what percent of ejection is moving backward).

Mixed Venous Oxygen Saturation. In compensated patients, this value (Svo_2) is normal.

Acute Mitral Regurgitation

Acute mitral regurgitation is a potentially lethal condition characterized by sudden-onset pulmonary edema and severe perfusion failure. It often results from acute bacterial endocarditis, transient ischemic dysfunction of a papillary muscle, rupture of the head of a papillary muscle, or rupture of chordae tendineae.

Hemodynamic disturbances are profound because the regurgitant flow is suddenly imposed on a normal left atrium and supernormal flow demands are levied on a normal left ventricle. The left ventricular musculature cannot accommodate the excessive systolic blood flow demands, and systemic perfusion may be low enough to produce shock. The inability of the left atrium and ventricle to acutely dilate and increase compliance results in marked increases in left ventricular end-diastolic pressure and left atrial pressure. The amplitude of the left atrial *v* wave may reach levels of 50 to 70 mm Hg, although mean left atrial pressure is considerably less. The pulmonary artery systolic and diastolic pressures abruptly rise and cause acute pulmonary edema. As a consequence, right ventricular pressure overload may result in acute right ventricular failure.

Hemodynamic Profile

Arterial Pressure. The blood pressure initially may be normal, but, with progressive hemodynamic deterioration, the patient becomes hypotensive. The pulse pressure is likely to be narrowed.

Systemic Vascular Resistance. This calculated value increases relative to the degree of perfusion failure. The compensatory rise in systemic vascular resistance worsens the regurgitant leak by increasing the impedance to aortic outflow.

Pulmonary Vascular Resistance. This calculated value increases when the patient develops pulmonary edema.

Central Venous Pressure or Right Atrial Pressure. These measurements increase with the onset of right ventricular failure, as may the amplitude of the right atrial *a* wave.

Pulmonary Artery Pressure. Pulmonary artery systolic and diastolic pressures increase in proportion to increases in left atrial pressure. If the regurgitation is severe, the regurgitant waves may be transmitted back to the pulmonary artery and may distort the pulmonary artery waveform (see Chapter 10, Figure 10-16).

Pulmonary Artery Wedge Pressure. This measurement is elevated, and prominent *v* waves are noted. Patients with acute mitral regurgitation usually have sinus tachycardia. The *a* waves may also be of increased amplitude because of increased resistance to the end-diastolic filling of the acutely volume overloaded failing left ventricle (Figure 22-21).

Cardiac Output. Systemic blood flow can be expected to fall relative to the regurgitant fraction (measured in a cardiac catheterization laboratory). A regurgitant

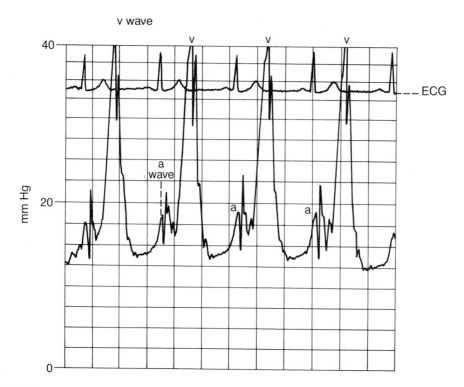

FIGURE 22-21 Pulmonary artery wedge tracing from a patient with acute mitral regurgitation. Note the increased amplitude *a* waves suggestive of impaired ventricular end-diastolic filling, as well as the characteristic giant *v* waves that result from the regurgitation stream into a normally small, nondistensible left atrium.

fraction less than 20% is mild and usually is associated with no symptoms; a fraction of 20% to 40% is moderate, 40% to 60% is moderately severe, and greater than 60% is very severe and usually associated with significant signs of perfusion failure and pulmonary edema. Underlying myocardial disease, such as acute myocardial infarction, may further compromise cardiac function and systemic blood flow. All invasive measurements of cardiac output may be inaccurate (usually underestimating true pulmonary arterial blood flow) because of the regurgitant stream. The greater the volume of regurgitant flow, the greater the likelihood for inaccuracy of obtained values (see section on cardiac output measurements in regurgitant valvular lesions, p. 597).

Mixed Venous Oxygen Saturation. This value decreases relative to the perfusion status and coexisting hypoxemia.

Clinical Presentation

People with a minimal to mild degree of chronic mitral regurgitation appear healthy and lead normal lives with no restrictions on activities. On physical examination, the only abnormality noted may be a systolic murmur at the apex that may radiate to the axilla. This is sometimes accompanied by a third heart sound that is related to rapid diastolic filling of the ventricle and does not necessarily indicate failure. Because of the low pressure against which the left ventricle ejects into the left atrium, the valve defect is well tolerated and the asymptomatic clinical course may extend over many decades or even a lifetime.

Symptoms are a function of the severity of the regurgitation, the rate of progression, the level of pulmonary artery pressure, and the presence of associated valvular or coronary artery disease. The clinical features of moderate to severe mitral regurgitation and acute mitral regurgitation are discussed in the following sections.

Mentation

Patients with *chronic disease* complain of weakness and fatigue, but mentation is normal. In *acute, severe mitral regurgitation*, patients may have signs of cerebral underperfusion such as obtundation, confusion, or irritability.

Cutaneous Manifestations

Patients with *chronic, decompensated disease* appear pale, but the skin is likely to be warm except for the hands and feet, which may be cool. In *acute, severe mitral regurgitation,* patients are typically ashen with peripheral cyanosis, and the skin also is cool and clammy.

Heart Rate and Character of Pulse

Early in the course of the disease when mild atrial dilation is present, the patient has occasional premature atrial contractions. With progression of the valve defect and degree of atrial dilation, atrial ectopy becomes more complex, such as bouts of atrial tachycardia. Atrial fibrillation is common in patients with *severe, chronic* disease. With severe left ventricular dysfunction, pulsus alternans also may be detected. In *acute, severe mitral regurgitation,* the amplitude of the pulse is reduced and the heart rate is rapid. Possible rhythm disturbances include sinus arrhythmia, premature ventricular beats, and possibly atrial fibrillation.

Heart Sounds

The classic auscultatory finding is a pansystolic, blowing, high-pitched murmur, which is best heard at the apex and may radiate to the left axilla and left back. In patients with *acute, severe mitral regurgitation,* the murmur may last only through the first half of systole or may be decrescendo, diminishing before the S_2 sound. This auscultatory characteristic of acute, severe mitral regurgitation is due to the fact that the regurgitant jet cannot be accommodated throughout systole by a normal-sized, relatively nondistensible left atrium. An atrial gallop and a ventricular gallop are commonly present, but usually only a summation gallop is heard because the patient is tachycardic.

Palpation of the Precordium

In *acute, severe mitral regurgitation,* the apex beat is in the normal position and is usually hyperactive. A systolic thrill may be felt over the apex. With *chronic, severe regurgitation,* the apex beat is active, laterally displaced, and sustained, and it covers a large area.

Neck Veins

The jugular venous distention is clinically suggestive of right ventricular failure in patients with both acute and chronic disease.

Respiratory Rate and Character of Breathing

Patients with pulmonary edema are tachypneic and prefer to sit upright. Breathing is labored relative to the severity of the pulmonary edema.

Acid-Base Values

Respiratory alkalosis is the result of acute pulmonary edema. With severe perfusion failure, the accumulation of lactic acid produces metabolic acidosis. Both problems commonly coexist in patients with *acute mitral regurgitation;* consequently, these patients have blood gas analysis findings of combined respiratory alkalosis and metabolic acidosis.

Laboratory and Other Diagnostic Studies

Electrocardiograph

In *acute mitral regurgitation,* the ECG is usually normal, unless the lesion is caused by myocardial ischemia or infarction. There also may be frequent ectopy. In *chronic mitral regurgitation,* the ECG shows evidence of left atrial enlargement with P wave abnormalities. The incidence of left ventricular hypertrophy is 50%, right ventricular hypertrophy is 15%, and atrial fibrillation is 75%. Coarse fibrillatory waves are common.

Chest Radiograph

In patients with *acute mitral regurgitation,* the heart size is normal, with only mild left atrial enlargement; however, typically there is evidence of pulmonary edema with alveolar flooding. Patients with severe *chronic mitral regurgitation* may have massive dilation of all four cardiac chambers. The first chamber to enlarge is the left atrium; this is followed by left ventricular enlargement. Right heart and pulmonary artery enlargement are seen in patients with pulmonary hypertension. The lung fields are clear if pulmonary vascular pressures are not sufficiently high to produce clinically overt pulmonary edema. Kerley B lines, most commonly noted at the right lung base, and increased prominence of the horizontal fissure are present in patients with interstitial (subclinical) pulmonary edema. Interstitial edema may be the steady state of patients with severe, decompensated disease.

Echocardiogram

This laboratory test reveals left atrial and ventricular enlargement and hyperdynamic wall motion. The cause of the valve dysfunction may be diagnosed by visualization of ruptured chordae tendineae, mitral valve prolapse, flail leaflets, or a rheumatic mitral valve. Doppler studies allow an estimate of how far back in the left atrium the regurgitant jet reaches. This finding is an index of lesion severity. Reverse flow in the pulmonary veins during systole is another sign of severity.

Cardiac Catheterization

This procedure is performed to confirm the diagnosis and to assess the ventricular function. The regurgitant fraction and the ejection fraction are measured, as are pressures in the various heart chambers. Coexisting coronary artery or other valvular abnormalities also can be assessed.

Treatment

Medical Therapy

Medical therapy for asymptomatic patients with mild-to-moderate mitral regurgitation and good ventricular function has not proved beneficial in delaying the onset of ventricular dysfunction, but regular follow-up is mandatory so that early signs of decompensation can be identified and appropriately managed. Prophylactic antibiotics are required before dental manipulations or invasive medical or surgical procedures. No restriction of activity is necessary.

With the development of symptoms, the patient should be instructed to avoid strenuous physical exercise. The following therapeutic interventions help relieve symptoms and maintain hemodynamic stability.

Vasodilators. Arterial and venous dilators reduce the end-systolic and diastolic volumes of the left ventricle and reduce systemic vascular resistance. Both interventions help decrease the size of the regurgitant opening, which, in turn, decreases the volume of regurgitant flow. Afterload reduction improves systemic blood flow and decreases regurgitant flow by reducing systemic vascular resistance. Vasodilators are the therapeutic mainstay for patients with symptomatic mitral regurgitation. In fact, afterload reduction with angiotensin-converting enzyme inhibitors is recommended for patients with minimal symptoms (American Heart Association, class I disease), along with 6-month to yearly follow-up with noninvasive tests as a guide to the need for surgical intervention (before left ventricular dilation becomes marked). With acute disease, sodium nitroprusside (Nipride) is titrated to give maximal hemodynamic benefit (see Figure 22-19).

Digitalis and Anticoagulants. If atrial fibrillation develops, these pharmacologic agents can help control the ventricular rate and decrease the embolic complications, respectively.

Salt Restriction and Diuretics. These measures help relieve the congestive symptoms of heart failure.

Surgical Replacement of the Mitral Valve

Because the patient's clinical course rapidly deteriorates when left ventricular dysfunction develops, and because ventricular dysfunction can be reversible if the cardiac lesion is treated early on, it is recommended that patients undergo operation when they become sympto-

matic with heavy exercise or when there is laboratory documentation of increased left ventricular dilation or left ventricular dysfunction. Following valve replacement, patients should be carefully observed for the development of left ventricular failure. If the left ventricle was compromised before surgery, valve replacement can result in worsening failure because the left ventricle is suddenly required to eject its entire contents into the high-resistance systemic circulation. The abrupt change in afterload can produce transient deterioration in left ventricular function, and ejection fraction usually falls 5% to 10%. When the ejection fraction is less than 20%, conservative therapy is usually recommended because further postoperative systolic dysfunction may not be compatible with life.

Mitral Valve Repair

In selected cases, when redundant tissue is easily resected, scar easily removed, or orifice dilation corrected with placement of a ring, repair may be undertaken with an excellent outcome.

TRICUSPID REGURGITATION (INSUFFICIENCY)

At the onset of systole, the tricuspid valve leaflets float to a closed position as right ventricular contraction causes intraventricular pressure to exceed right atrial pressure. Throughout ventricular systole, the papillary chordal structures apply traction to the valve leaflets to maintain valve alignment and complete closure.

Tricuspid regurgitation occurs when any portion of the tricuspid valve apparatus becomes incompetent. Incomplete valve closure then allows retrograde flow of blood from the right ventricle to the right atrium and central veins during systole (Figure 22-22).

Hemodynamic features of pure tricuspid regurgitation include a large systolic *(v)* wave in central venous pressure or right atrial pressure tracings, elevated right atrial and central venous pressures, and normal or decreased pulmonary artery wedge pressures and cardiac output. Clinical hallmarks include systemic venous distention and large systolic pulsations of the jugular veins, clear lungs, systemic edema, and signs and symptoms of systemic underperfusion.

Causes and Pathophysiology

Tricuspid regurgitation may result from primary disease or disruption of the tricuspid apparatus because of rheumatic heart disease, severe blunt thoracic trauma, metastatic carcinoid tumor, infectious endocarditis, or right ventricular infarction. The most common cause of tricuspid

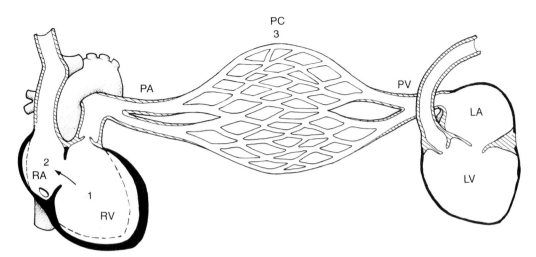

FIGURE 22-22 Schematic drawing of the central circulation with primary tricuspid regurgitation; *arrow* indicates direction of abnormal systolic flow. *1,* Right ventricle dilated due to diastolic volume overload. *2,* Right atrium enlarged. *3,* Subnormal pulmonary blood flow and left heart filling. *Broken lines* represent normal right heart contour.

regurgitation is right ventricular dilation and failure, termed *functional tricuspid regurgitation.* Dilation of the right ventricle distorts the ventricular-valve spatial relationship, and this results in "functional" incompetence of the valve. Right ventricular failure is most commonly the result of increased afterload due to left ventricular failure or mitral stenosis. Other relatively common causes include pulmonary hypertension because of massive pulmonary embolism or chronic lung disease. Right ventricular failure also may be the result of primary right ventricular disease such as infarction or myopathy. Functional tricuspid regurgitation may diminish or even disappear with successful treatment of heart failure.

Hemodynamic Effects

The situation parallels that of mitral regurgitation; the total right ventricular stroke volume is divided between the pulmonary circulation (forward stroke volume) and the right atrium (regurgitant flow). Therefore the right ventricle must perform increased work to maintain forward blood flow. When adequate forward flow is not maintained, left ventricular filling is reduced and, consequently, cardiac output decreases.

The increase in right atrial pressure, induced by the systolic regurgitant flow, is transmitted throughout the venous system and is graphically illustrated on right atrial pressure or central venous pressure tracings as a prominent *v* wave. Systemic venous hypertension and congestion, as well as dependent tissue edema, result.

Clinical Presentation

Signs and symptoms of systemic venous hypertension are present in all patients with moderate-to-severe tricuspid regurgitation. Because tricuspid regurgitation is most often the result of left ventricular failure or mitral stenosis, dyspnea, orthopnea, weakness, and chronic fatigue are common. By delivering less blood into the pulmonary circulation, the development of right heart failure may modify the pulmonary congestive symptoms of left heart failure. If tricuspid regurgitation is the result of infective endocarditis, fever usually accompanies fatigue and systemic edema.

Mentation

The level of consciousness and cognition is typically normal.

Cutaneous Manifestations

In patients with functional tricuspid regurgitation, skin color and temperature relate to the underlying disease. The level of systemic edema is related to the acuity of the process, the severity of right ventricular failure, and the size of the regurgitant volume.

Heart Rate and Character of Pulse

Atrial fibrillation is common because of right atrial distention or coexisting mitral stenosis. The pulses therefore are of variable volume and are irregularly irregular.

Heart Sounds

A pansystolic murmur at the left sternal border that increases with inspiration is a characteristic auscultatory finding of tricuspid regurgitation. The inspiratory effect distinguishes the murmur from that of mitral regurgitation, which is not affected by inspiration.

Neck Veins

Signs of peripheral venous congestion are common, with substantial jugular venous distention being typical. Evaluation of the jugular venous pulse shows a prominent *v* wave produced by the systolic regurgitant flow into the right atrium and venous system.

Breath Sounds

In patients with pure tricuspid regurgitation, the chest is clear. In patients with left ventricular failure, bilateral rales and wheezes are typically present.

Hemodynamic Profile
Arterial Pressure

Because tricuspid regurgitation most commonly occurs as a secondary phenomenon to other cardiopulmonary disease (mitral stenosis, left ventricular failure, massive pulmonary embolism), the blood pressure is related to the interplay of the primary problem and the severity of the regurgitant flow.

Systemic Vascular Resistance

This calculated value usually is proportionately elevated if cardiac output is decreased.

Pulmonary Vascular Resistance

This value is normal in patients with primary tricuspid regurgitation and is increased in patients with functional tricuspid regurgitation as a result of mitral stenosis or pulmonary disease.

Central Venous Pressure or Right Atrial Pressure

Mean measurements are classically elevated because of the increased-amplitude regurgitant *(v)* wave. Measurements chronically exceeding 10 mm Hg usually lead to the development of systemic edema. The height of the central venous or right atrial regurgitant *v* wave usually correlates with the magnitude of the regurgitant volume (Figure 22-23).

Right Ventricular Systolic Pressure

If a patient with severe tricuspid regurgitation has a right ventricular systolic pressure less than 40 mm Hg, the tricuspid regurgitation is usually the result of primary disease of the valve apparatus. Conversely, if the right ventricular systolic pressure is greater than 60 mm Hg, the tricuspid regurgitation is usually "functional." This distinction is of practical therapeutic importance because the former is usually treated with tricuspid valve replacement or annuloplasty. In the latter case, therapy is directed toward the primary problem, such as mitral stenosis, left heart failure, or massive pulmonary embolism.

Pulmonary Artery and Pulmonary Artery Wedge Pressures

These measurements may be normal or decreased in patients with primary tricuspid regurgitation. In patients with mitral stenosis or left ventricular failure, these values are elevated. If tricuspid regurgitation is due to pulmonary hypertensive disease such as chronic obstructive pulmonary disease, massive pulmonary embolism, primary pulmonary hypertension, or mitral stenosis with secondary pulmonary vascular changes, the PAd-PWP gradient is increased proportionate to the severity of pulmonary disease.

Cardiac Output

This measurement is affected by the severity of coexisting problems and by the volume of tricuspid regurgitant flow. Invasive measurements of cardiac output may be invalid because of the recirculation of blood in the right heart chambers (see section on complex valvular heart disease, p. 597).

Mixed Venous Oxygen Saturation

Coexisting primary disease and regurgitant flow volume determine the adequacy of the circulation and mixed venous oxygen saturation.

Laboratory and Other Diagnostic Studies
Electrocardiograph

Acute tricuspid regurgitation may be associated with atrial ectopy or the sudden onset of atrial tachyarrhythmias because of acute right atrial distention. If the patient is in sinus rhythm, a characteristic finding of tricuspid regurgitation is a large P wave (due to right atrial enlargement) in the absence of right ventricular hypertrophy. Atrial fibrillation is common in patients with chronic disease.

Chest Radiograph

Right atrial enlargement is the rule, and right ventricular enlargement is common. Ventricular enlargement is best seen as a loss of the anterior clear space on the lateral view.

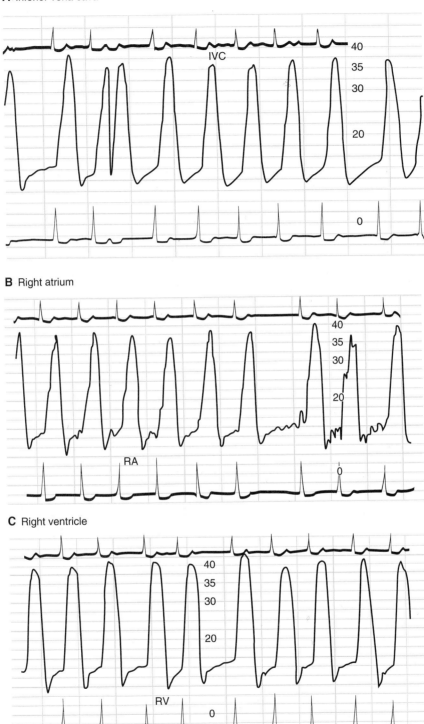

A Inferior vena cava

B Right atrium

C Right ventricle

FIGURE 22-23 Severe tricuspid regurgitation secondary to pulmonary hypertension in a patient with severe mitral stenosis. This 68-year-old man is inoperable because severe right heart dysfunction may render the patient nonweanable from cardiopulmonary bypass or postoperative ventilatory support. Note that the inferior vena caval **(A)**, right atrial **(B)**, and right ventricular **(C)** waveform morphology are nearly identical. (Courtesy of Cheryl Finkl, RN, Medical Center Hospital, Largo, Florida.)

Echocardiogram

Right atrial enlargement is the rule, whereas right ventricular enlargement indicates dilation and the likelihood of secondary "functional" tricuspid regurgitation. Doppler studies show regurgitant flow across the tricuspid valve. The depth in the right atrium at which this flow can be seen reflects the magnitude of the regurgitant flow.

Cardiac Catheterization

This invasive procedure provides quantitative evaluation of the right and left heart pressures. It may be difficult to assess the degree of tricuspid regurgitation on right ventricular angiography because of the tendency for significant ectopy to develop during injection of contrast media. Another difficulty is that a right ventricular catheter positioned across the tricuspid valve *causes* tricuspid regurgitation. However, catheterization also provides evaluation of the structural abnormalities and functional capacity of the left ventricle, which is often causally linked to the tricuspid regurgitation, as well as the degree of concomitant coronary artery disease.

Treatment

Medical Therapy

Medical therapy depends on the cause of the lesion; if tricuspid regurgitation is the result of left heart failure, standard treatment regimens, including diuretics, inotropic drugs, and vasodilators, are valuable. If right heart failure is the result of exacerbation of chronic lung disease or acute lung disease, management is directed at primary support of the pulmonary system. In patients with isolated tricuspid regurgitation, the mainstay of treatment is diuresis. Some benefit may be gained from venodilating agents, but afterload reducers are usually poorly tolerated in patients with right-sided heart disease. Hypotension is likely to occur when the arterial circulation dilates in patients with an underfilled left ventricle.

Surgical Replacement of the Tricuspid Valve

This is not a commonly undertaken surgical procedure. It may be useful, however, in patients with severe, primary tricuspid regurgitation, particularly in cases due to trauma or infectious endocarditis. Valve annuloplasty is indicated in patients with severe functional tricuspid regurgitation. This is a surgical procedure in which the valve annulus is therapeutically narrowed and involves a supporting ring sewn into the tricuspid annulus, a purse-string suture, or plication of the posterior valve leaflet. When the tricuspid regurgitation is the result of mitral stenosis, some surgeons advocate performing tricuspid annuloplasty at the time of mitral valve repair or replacement.

Table 22-3 summarizes the anticipated hemodynamic findings in patients with several types of valvular heart disease.

TABLE 22-3

Guidelines to Anticipated Hemodynamic Changes in Several Types of Valvular Heart Disease

Disorder	Arterial Pressure	Pulse Pressure	Systemic Vascular Resistance	Pulmonary Vascular Resistance	Central Venous Pressure	Pulmonary Artery Pressure	Pulmonary Wedge Pressure	Cardiac Output	Svo$_2$
Aortic stenosis	~	↓	~ ↑	~	~	~ ↑	~ ↑	~ ↓	~ ↓
Aortic regurgitation									
Chronic compensated	↑	↑	~ ↓	~	~	~	~ ↑	↑ or ~	~ or ↑
Chronic decompensated	↑	↓ or ↑	~ ↑	~ or ↑	↑	↑	↑	~ ↓	~ ↓
Acute	~ ↑	↓ or ↑	↑	↑	~ ↑	↑	↑	↓	↓
Mitral stenosis	~	↓	~ ↑	~ ↑	~ ↑	↑	↑	↓	↓
Mitral regurgitation									
Chronic	~	~	~	~	~	↑	↑	~	~
Acute	~ ↓	↓	↑	↑	~ ↑	↑	↑	↓	↓
Tricuspid regurgitation	~ ↓	~ ↓	~	↑ or ↓	↑	↑ or ↓	↑ or ↓	↓	↓

KEY: ↑ increase, ↓ decrease, ~ normal or no change.

Note: The magnitude of the direction of change is affected by the severity of the valve defect, as well as by coexisting factors or complications such as hypovolemia or fluid overload.

COMPLEX VALVULAR HEART DISEASE

It is not uncommon to find patients with multiple valvular lesions because the majority of pathologic processes may affect mitral, aortic, and, rarely, right heart valves. A combination of stenosis and regurgitation usually accompanies rheumatic and degenerative valvular processes, typically with one lesion predominating in the deformed valve. Overall, the left heart valves are more commonly affected; primary right heart lesions are relatively uncommon. Depending on the defects, multivalvular disease of the mitral and aortic valves may be associated with left ventricular pressure overload, volume overload, or combinations of the two.

Tricuspid regurgitation, because of right ventricular dilation and failure, may complicate any disease (cardiac or noncardiac) that is associated with elevated pulmonary artery pressures, but it almost invariably is associated with serious disease of the mitral valve.

Different combinations of valvular abnormalities are associated with a variety of physical assessment and hemodynamic syndromes. As a general rule, when the valve deformities are of nearly equal severity, the hemodynamic and clinical manifestations of the more proximally located diseased valve, such as the mitral valve in patients with combined mitral and aortic valvular disease, dominate the hemodynamic and clinical picture. When the aortic valve pathology is dominant, however, the hemodynamic and clinical consequences of the mitral valve process are usually mild.

Clinical Presentation

In all patients with multivalvular aortic and mitral valve lesions, significantly decreased left ventricular contractile force (systolic dysfunction) is associated with diastolic dysfunction, as well as with elevated pulmonary vascular pressures and predisposition to pulmonary edema. Therefore dyspnea is the most common complaint of people with mitral and aortic valve lesions. The enlarged left atrium of severe mitral valve disease is vulnerable also to atrial fibrillation, and thus palpitations are a common symptom. Fluid retention, chronic fatigue, and exercise intolerance accompany heart failure as a result of any combination of valve defects. Syncope may be associated with regurgitation of both mitral and aortic valves or mitral regurgitation when it is accompanied by aortic stenosis.

Unreliability of Invasive Cardiac Output Measurements in Patients with Regurgitant Lesions

Normally, in health, right ventricular output, pulmonary blood flow, left ventricular output, and systemic blood flow are equal. Therefore cardiac output measurements obtained by any invasive method (Fick's formula, dye dilution, thermodilution) are representative of forward blood flow at all points in the circulation. Even though all methods measure only pulmonary blood flow, the assumption can be made that left ventricular output and systemic blood flow are correlated.

This correlation becomes invalid in patients with regurgitant valve lesions, because the regurgitant (backward) flow goes unmeasured. This complicates hemodynamic assessment of valvular heart disease. The greater the volume of regurgitant flow, the greater the total stroke volume (ventricular output) that goes unmeasured and the less the blood flow that goes into the receiving circulation. For example, in mitral regurgitation, the total left ventricular output as assessed in the cardiac catheterization laboratory may be 10 L/min. Pulmonary blood flow, however, as measured by thermodilution, may be 4.5 L/min. The clinically immeasurable regurgitant volume is 5.5 L/min.

To complicate matters further, a severe mitral regurgitant jet, which may have beat-by-beat volume variability in acute disease, contaminates the blood at the pulmonary artery sampling site. This renders accuracy of any single reading by thermodilution cardiac output completely unreliable and evaluation of trends over time equally unreliable.

Tricuspid regurgitation is associated with such significant recirculation of blood in the right heart chambers that accurate cardiac output measurements are essentially impossible. Overall, regurgitant lesions of the right heart and severe regurgitant lesions of the mitral valve impose serious and unpredictable limitations to the accuracy of cardiac output measurements so that even trend-based evaluation may be misleading.

Basic Principles Applicable to Patients with Both Aortic and Mitral Valve Lesions

- Because a proximal valve lesion may overshadow an equally severe distal lesion, significant aortic regurgitation may be overlooked in patients with severe mitral stenosis. Mitral stenosis reduces the left ventricular volume overload and therefore minimizes the widened pulse pressure characteristic of aortic regurgitation.
- Mitral stenosis masks many of the manifestations of coexisting aortic stenosis. The atrial contribution to ventricular filling, which is so important to maximize left ventricular preload in patients with aortic stenosis, has minimal impact and even may be absent in patients with severe mitral stenosis with atrial fibrillation. In such patients, the stroke volume (and cardiac output) is lower than that for any given level of pure aortic stenosis. Thus affected patients have a lower left ventricular systolic pressure and narrower transaortic pressure gradient.

- Preoperative recognition of significant aortic regurgitation or stenosis is of paramount importance for patients with mitral stenosis. Surgical restoration of normal flow across the mitral orifice may impose a sudden, intolerable volume load on the left ventricle and precipitate acute pulmonary edema.

- Mitral regurgitation tends to dilate and eventually damage the left ventricular musculature. Aortic stenosis is associated with extraordinary left ventricular work and oxygen demands. Because of the secondary cardiomyopathy that weakens the left ventricle, and because of the left ventricular outflow obstruction that increases the volume of mitral regurgitant flow, *mitral regurgitation that coexists with aortic stenosis is the worst possible scenario of coexisting valve defects.* Hemodynamic and clinical toleration of this combination of valve defects is very poor. Patients have severely reduced systemic blood flow and marked elevations in left atrial and pulmonary vascular pressures. Clinically, it may be difficult to differentiate and recognize the two distinct systolic murmurs.

- Mild mitral regurgitation that coexists with mild aortic regurgitation is usually well tolerated for a time, but once left ventricular failure occurs, the downhill course is rapid. If both valvular leaks are severe, this combination of defects is very poorly tolerated. In pure aortic regurgitation, the normal mitral valve usually protects the left atrium and the pulmonary circulation from overload by premature closure. With combined aortic and mitral regurgitant lesions, blood may reflux from the aorta through both left heart chambers to the pulmonary circulation in diastole. Affected patients are thus disposed to acute pulmonary edema.

In analyzing echocardiographic, angiographic, and hemodynamic data, these principles should be remembered for the accurate assessment of valve dysfunction in each patient with complex valve disease.

REFERENCES

1. Gorlin R, Gorlin G: Hydraulic formula for calculation of area of stenotic mitral valve, other cardiac valves and central circulatory shunts, *Am Heart J* 41:1, 1951.

SUGGESTED READINGS
General

Braunwald E: Valvular heart disease. In Braunwald E, editor: *Textbook of cardiovascular disease,* ed 6, Philadelphia, 2001, W.B. Saunders.

Grossman W: Profiles in valvular heart disease. In Grossman W, Baim DS, editors: *Cardiac catheterization, angioplasty and intervention,* ed 4, Philadelphia, 1991, Lea & Febiger.

Henning RJ, Grenvik A: Valvular heart disease. In Henning RJ, Grenvik A, editors: *Critical care cardiology,* New York, 1989, Churchill Livingstone.

Hirshfeld JW: Valve function: stenosis and regurgitation. In Pepine CJ, editor: *Diagnostic and therapeutic cardiac catheterization,* Baltimore, 1989, Williams & Wilkins.

Rackley C et al: Valvular heart disease. In Fuster V, editor: *The heart,* ed 10, New York, 2001, McGraw-Hill.

Mitral Regurgitation

Baxley WA et al: Hemodynamics in ruptured chordae tendineae and chronic rheumatic mitral regurgitation, *Circulation* 48:1288, 1973.

Braunwald E: Mitral regurgitation. Physiologic, clinical and surgical considerations, *N Engl J Med* 281:425, 1969.

Braunwald E, Awe WC: The syndrome of severe mitral regurgitation with normal left atrial pressure, *Circulation* 27:29, 1963.

Brody W, Criley JM: Intermittent severe mitral regurgitation. Hemodynamic studies in a patient with recurrent acute left-sided heart failure, *N Engl J Med* 1983:673, 1970.

Burch GE, DePasquale NP, Phillips JH: The syndrome of papillary muscle dysfunction, *Am Heart J* 75:399, 1968.

Chatterjee K, Parmley WW, Swan HJC, et al: Beneficial effects of vasodilator agents in severe mitral regurgitation due to dysfunction of subvalvular apparatus, *Circulation* 48:684, 1973.

DeBusk RF, Harrison DC: The clinical spectrum of papillary-muscle disease, *N Engl J Med* 281:1458, 1969.

Fuchs RM et al: Limitations of pulmonary wedge v waves in diagnosing mitral regurgitation, *Am J Cardiol* 49:840, 1982.

Grose R, Strain J, Cohen MV: Pulmonary arterial v waves in mitral regurgitation: clinical and experimental observations, *Circulation* 69:214, 1984.

Grossman W et al: Lowered aortic impedance as therapy for severe mitral regurgitation, *JAMA* 230:1011, 1974.

Harshaw CW et al: Reduced systemic vascular resistance as therapy for severe mitral regurgitation of valvular origin, *Ann Intern Med* 83:312, 1975.

Korn D, Sell S, DeSanctis RW: Massive calcification of mitral annulus, *N Engl J Med* 267:900, 1962.

Lewis BM et al: Clinical and physiological correlations in patients with mitral stenosis, *Am Heart J* 43:2, 1952.

Libanoff AJ, Rodbard S: Evaluation of the severity of stenosis and regurgitation, *Circulation* 33:281, 1966.

Pichard AD, Kay R, Smith H, et al: Large v waves in the pulmonary wedge pressure tracing in the absence of mitral regurgitation, *Am J Cardiol* 50:1044, 1982.

Pocock WA, Barlow JB: Etiology and electrocardiographic features of the billowing posterior mitral leaflet syndrome, *Am J Med* 51:731, 1971.

Samet P, Litwak RW, Bernstein WH, et al: Clinical and physiological relationships in mitral valve disease, *Circulation* 19:517, 1959.

Selzer A, Kohn KE: Natural history of mitral stenosis: a review, *Circulation* 45:878, 1972.

Wood P: An appreciation of mitral stenosis. I. Clinical features. II. Investigations and results, *BMJ* 1:1051, 1113, 1954.

Tricuspid Regurgitation

Lingamneni R et al: Tricuspid regurgitation: clinical and angiographic assessment, *Cathet Cardiovasc Diagn* 5:7, 1979.

Mitral Stenosis

Fredman CS et al: Comparison of hemodynamic pressure half-time method and Gorlin formula with Doppler and echocardiographic determinations of mitral valve area in patients with combined mitral stenosis and regurgitation, *Am Heart J* 119:121, 1990.

Gorlin R, Gorlin G: Hydraulic formula for calculation of the area of the stenotic mitral valve, other cardiac valves, and central circulatory shunts, *Am Heart J* 41:1, 1951.

Heller SJ, Carleton RA: Abnormal left ventricular contraction in patients with mitral stenoses, *Circulation* 42:1099, 1970.

McKay CR, Kawanishi DT, Kotlewski A, et al: Improvement in exercise capacity and exercise hemodynamics 3 months after double-balloon catheter balloon valvuloplasty treatment of patients with symptomatic mitral stenosis, *Circulation* 77:1013, 1988.

Thomas JD, Wilkins GT, Choong CYP, et al: Inaccuracy of mitral valvotomy: dependence on transmitral gradient and left atrial and ventricular compliance, *Circulation* 78:980, 1988.

Aortic Stenosis

Finegan RE, Gianelly RE, Harrison DC: Aortic stenosis in the elderly, *N Engl J Med* 281:1261, 1969.

Frank S, Johnson A, Ross J Jr: Natural history of aortic valvular stenosis, *Br Heart J* 35:41, 1973.

Frank S, Ross J Jr: The natural history of severe acquired valvular aortic stenosis, *Am J Cardiol* 19:128, 1967.

Gorlin WB, Gorlin R: A generalized formulation of the Gorlin formula for calculating the area of the stenotic mitral valve and other stenotic cardiac valves, *J Am Coll Cardiol* 15:246, 1990.

Oh JK, Taliercio CP, Holmes DR Jr, et al: Prediction of the severity of aortic stenosis by Doppler aortic valve area determination: prospective Doppler-catheterization correlation in 100 patients, *J Am Coll Cardiol* 11:1227, 1988.

Roberts WC: The structure of the aortic valve in clinically isolated aortic stenosis, *Circulation* 42:91, 1970.

Aortic Regurgitation

Bolger AF, Eigler NL, Maurer G: Quantifying valvular regurgitation: limitations and inherent assumptions of Doppler techniques, *Circulation* 78:1316, 1988.

Croft CH et al: Limitations of qualitative angiographic grading in aortic or mitral regurgitation, *Am J Cardiol* 53:1593, 1984.

Gaasch WH, Andrias CW, Levine HJ: Chronic aortic regurgitation: the effect of aortic valve replacement on left ventricular volume, mass and function, *Circulation* 58:825, 1978.

Goldschlager N, Pfeifer J, Cohn K, et al: The natural history of aortic regurgitation: a clinical and hemodynamic study, *Am J Med* 54:577, 1973.

Labovitz AJ, Ferrara RP, Kern MJ, et al: Quantitative evaluation of aortic insufficiency by continuous wave Doppler echocardiography, *J Am Coll Cardiol* 8:1341, 1986.

Mann T et al: Assessing the hemodynamic severity of acute aortic regurgitation due to infective endocarditis, *N Engl J Med* 293:108, 1975.

Morganroth J et al: Acute severe aortic regurgitation: pathophysiology, clinical recognition, and management, *Ann Intern Med* 87:223, 1977.

Segal J, Harvey WP, Hufnagel C: A clinical study of one hundred cases of severe aortic insufficiency, *Am J Med* 21:200, 1956.

23

SHAUL ATAR, GLORIA OBLOUK DAROVIC, and ROBERT J. SIEGEL

Cardiomyopathies and Pericardial Disease

Several circulatory disorders are discussed in this chapter. Among the cardiomyopathies, the circulatory disturbances are related primarily to intrinsic disease of the heart muscle. In constrictive pericarditis and tamponade, the heart is typically normal, but external cardiac restriction to normal heart action produces circulatory compromise.

CARDIOMYOPATHIES

The term *cardiomyopathy* refers to disease of the heart muscle that occurs in the absence of congenital, ischemic, valvular, hypertensive, or pericardial disease. The cause frequently is not known. The word "cardiomyopathy" is sometimes loosely applied to end-stage myocardial dysfunction due to hypertensive, ischemic, or valvular heart disease, although these do not represent intrinsic diseases of the heart muscle. The true cardiomyopathies are classified into three types based on their structural and pathophysiologic features: dilated, hypertrophic, and restrictive cardiomyopathy (Figure 23-1).

Dilated cardiomyopathy is characterized by bilateral atrial and ventricular dilation and diffuse contractile failure (systolic dysfunction). *Hypertrophic cardiomyopathy* is associated with an inappropriate increase in ventricular mass, restricted and impaired ventricular filling, and normal or increased contractile function. *Restrictive cardiomyopathy* is characterized by restricted biventricular filling as a result of endocardial or myocardial fibrosis or infiltration. The incidence of cardiomyopathies is 0.7 to 7.5 cases per 100,000 people per year in the United States.

As with all forms of heart disease, the cardiomyopathies may be present and progressing but the patient may be asymptomatic for years. The person so afflicted, but undiagnosed, may enter the hospital for elective surgery, trauma, or unrelated illness. Because of the stress of the primary disease or injury, the patient may then exhibit signs and symptoms of cardiac disease, such as heart failure or arrhythmias, despite the absence of an immediately apparent organic cause. The disease also may be discovered when abnormalities are detected on a routine chest radiograph or electrocardiogram (ECG). However, the diagnosis usually is made when patients seek medical consultation when progression of the disease finally produces symptoms and disability.

Invasive hemodynamic monitoring is indicated in patients with cardiomyopathies in the following circumstances:
1. Coexisting disease or injury is associated with hemodynamic instability.
2. Therapy for coexisting disease is in conflict with the management of the specific cardiomyopathy, and the patient therefore requires close hemodynamic observation for guidance of drug therapy (e.g., patients with status asthmaticus with hypertrophic cardiomyopathy).
3. Patients with severe disease in whom parenteral drug therapy is indicated (e.g., patients with dilated cardiomyopathy receiving potent vasodilator or inotropic therapy).

Dilated Cardiomyopathy

Dilated cardiomyopathy (DCM), formerly termed *congestive cardiomyopathy,* is defined as a primary myocardial disease physically characterized by dilated ventricular chambers, secondary biatrial dilation, and diffuse systolic dysfunction. Dilated cardiomyopathy clinically manifests with signs and symptoms of low cardiac output, systemic and pulmonary venous congestion, and possibly embolic episodes. This disease accounts for approximately 80% of all primary myocardial diseases.

Causes

The etiology of dilated cardiomyopathy is often unknown. It is likely that this disease represents a final pathophysiologic expression of progressive myocardial injury that results from a variety of toxic, metabolic, or infectious agents. However, familial transmission is reported in approximately 10% of cases. The following conditions or factors are related to or identified with dilated cardiomyopathy.

Drugs, Toxins, and Deficiencies

Alcoholic Cardiomyopathy. Consumption of excessive quantities of alcoholic beverages over a long period of time (more than 8 oz/day for longer than 6 months) is a major cause of dilated cardiomyopathy. Individual susceptibility is variable. Those more vulnerable to alcohol-induced myocardial damage may have associated myocardial damaging factors such as nutritional deficiencies or hypertension. Abstinence may be associated with resolution in the early stages, but the disease recurs if drinking is resumed. Persistent myocardial dysfunction and deterioration occur with continued alcohol abuse. Approximately 50% of patients have resolution of cardiac dysfunction with abstinence from alcohol.

Drug-Induced Cardiomyopathy. Consumption of cocaine, lithium salts, doxorubicin (Adriamycin), and interferon has been suggested as a cause of DCM. This type of cardiomyopathy is usually reversible after discontinuance of the drug.

Pregnancy and the Puerperium. Symptoms of heart failure, chest pain, palpitations, or systemic and pulmonary embolism may occur any time during the last 3 months of pregnancy or the first 6 months postpartum. The precise mechanism that induces disease is unknown, but DCM occurs most commonly in women over 30 years of age, in multiparous women, in those with twin pregnancies, in those with a history of toxemia, in those of African descent, and among poorly nourished mothers. Approximately 50% of women recover; the rest experience continuous deterioration, with high morbidity and

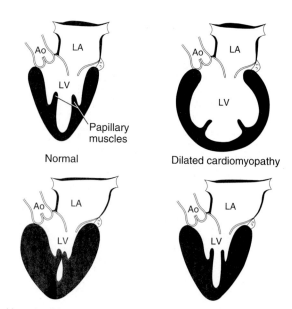

FIGURE 23-1 Diagram comparing three morphologic types of cardiomyopathies. *Ao,* aorta; *LA,* left atrium; *LV,* left ventricle. In the normal heart, the left intraventricular chamber is cone shaped, tapering at the apex. In dilated (congestive) cardiomyopathy, the left ventricular chamber becomes dilated and nearly spherical in diastole; the atria also are dilated. In hypertrophic cardiomyopathy, the left ventricular cavity is small in diastole and becomes slit shaped and partly obliterated in systole. In restrictive cardiomyopathy, the intraventricular cavities are smaller than normal in size, and the atria are dilated. (From Waller BF: Pathology of the cardiomyopathies, *J Am Echocardiol* 1:4, 1988.)

mortality rates. There is a tendency for symptoms to recur with subsequent pregnancies.

Viral Infections. In some cases, signs of cardiovascular deterioration surface in the weeks following a viral illness such as influenza. It is postulated that dilated cardiomyopathy occurs as a consequence of viral-mediated immunologic myocardial damage.

Idiopathic. Dilated cardiomyopathy, in which no cause or risk factor can be identified, occurs in people of all ages and races but is more common in persons of African descent and men. The course is characterized by progressive deterioration leading to death after an average of approximately 5 years of illness.

Other varied causes of DCM include endocrine disease, such as pheochromocytoma and hypothyroidism or hyperthyroidism; metabolic disorders, such as uremia; infectious diseases, such as toxoplasmosis and mycoplasma; hypersensitivity reactions; and collagen-vascular disease.

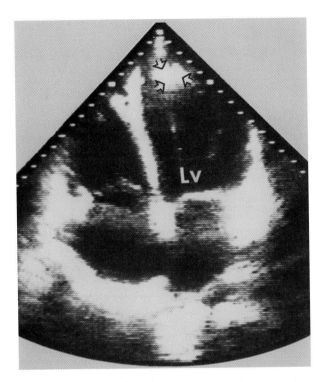

FIGURE 23-2 A two-dimensional echocardiogram demonstrates a bright echo dense mass, a thrombus *(arrows)*, in the left ventricular *(Lv)* apex of a patient with idiopathic dilated cardiomyopathy.

Cigarette smoking, independent of the risk of ischemic heart disease, also has been implicated with DCM.

Pathophysiology

There are several pathophysiologic features of DCM; however, the primary pathologic features are dilation of both ventricles and contractile failure. It is generally presumed that diffuse systolic dysfunction is primary, and as a result of the reduced ejection fraction there is a consequent increase in the end-systolic and diastolic blood volumes of both ventricles. The abnormally large ventricular diastolic volumes (associated with increased ventricular end-diastolic pressures), in turn, limit atrial emptying. This results in a passive diastolic increase in atrial pressures and subsequent atrial dilation.

Overall, DCM is associated with a globally enlarged, sphere-shaped heart. Stasis of blood in the enlarged, poorly contractile ventricles and dilated atria also predisposes patients to intracavitary thrombi, particularly in the left ventricular apex (Figure 23-2). Systemic emboli that dislodge from the left heart, as well as pulmonary emboli that originate in the right heart or deep veins of the legs, are complications of DCM.

The thickness of the ventricular musculature also may increase as a compensatory mechanism to maintain cardiac function, although the degree of hypertrophy usually does not parallel the degree of dilation. If such an increase in left ventricular wall thickness does occur in patients with DCM, it has been shown to be a good prognostic sign, perhaps because the increase in wall thickness helps reduce hemodynamic left ventricular wall stress. In such patients, diastolic relaxation may be slow and incomplete, and ventricular compliance may be decreased, causing *diastolic dysfunction.*

Structurally, the leaflets of all four cardiac valves are usually normal. "Functional" mitral and tricuspid regurgitation often occur because of dilation of the valve annulus that supports the valve leaflets or because ventricular dilation may result in papillary muscle dysfunction. The coronary arteries are usually normal in younger patients, and, in older patients, the degree of ventricular dysfunction is disproportionate to existing coronary artery disease. The chest pain some patients experience in the absence of coronary artery disease may be the result of myocardial ischemia. This is caused by underperfusion due to the relative increase in ventricular muscle mass compared with the size of the coronary vascular bed. The chest pain also may be caused by a reduced perfusion pressure across the ventricular wall due to the elevated ventricular end-diastolic pressures. Ventricular dilation also is accompanied by greater wall tension and pressure work, which increase myocardial oxygen demand.

Activation of the neurohormonal system in patients with myocardial failure has been of major interest in the last decade. The renin-angiotensin-aldosterone system is activated as a result of the low cardiac output, leading to a detrimental increase in afterload through systemic arterial vasoconstriction, as well as an increase in water and salt retention. Increased levels of angiotensin II are being studied as a risk factor for the development of atherosclerosis. Angiotensin II was found to have a detrimental effect on endothelial function and to increase low-density lipoprotein oxidation, inflammation, and coagulation, thus leading to increased risk of myocardial infarction. Moreover, primarily elevated levels of angiotensin II increase systemic blood pressure, leading to the development of hypertensive cardiomyopathy. Thus activation of the renin-angiotensin-aldosterone system may be a cause, and not only the result, of heart failure. Elevated levels of endothelins, the most potent vasoconstrictors known, are produced by cardiac myocytes and endothelial cells in patients with cardiac failure and are currently being explored as a potential therapeutic target.

Hemodynamic Effects

In the earlier stages of the disease, resting cardiac output may be maintained near normal despite progressive systolic dysfunction and decreasing ejection fraction by two compensatory mechanisms:

1. *An increase in end-diastolic muscle fiber length.* With mild disease, increased myofibrillar stretch increases the force of myocardial contraction, and an adequate stroke volume may be ejected. However, because of the intrinsic systolic (contractile) dysfunction, the heart cannot appropriately increase stroke volume during stress, such as exercise (Table 23-1). With progressive dilation, however, the disadvantages of increased end-diastolic fiber length ultimately outweigh the advantages. Ventricular dilation is associated with a decreased rate of muscle fiber shortening and decreased velocity of ejection. This effect eventually further compromises cardiac function.

   Because cardiac output does not increase normally in any stage of the disease, if the patient is stressed (strenuous activity, shivering, sepsis, respiratory failure), ventricular end-diastolic pressures suddenly increase and, when reflected back to the pulmonary and systemic veins, result in systemic venous hypertension.

2. *An increase in heart rate.* In the early stages of DCM, an increase in resting heart rate may compensate for a reduced stroke volume. With advanced disease, tachycardia can no longer compensate for the contractile defect, and the patient develops symptoms of perfusion failure.

Clinical Presentation

The clinical manifestations of DCM are related to the degree of cardiac dysfunction. Unrecognized, mild myocardial disease may exist for years and produce no noticeable symptoms. Sudden-onset cardiac arrhythmias (atrial fibrillation is common) may be the first indication of the disease. However, the most common symptom is exertional dyspnea, which occurs in more than 75% of patients. As left ventricular function deteriorates and left ventricular end-diastolic pressure rises, dyspnea occurs at progressively lower levels of exertion. Chest pain is noted in one quarter to one half of patients because of concomitant ischemic heart disease. With progression of DCM and cardiac dysfunction, orthopnea, paroxysmal nocturnal dyspnea, chronic fatigue, and weakness become common complaints, although left ventricular function and symptoms are not always well correlated. Indications of right ventricular failure, such as peripheral edema; an enlarged,

TABLE 23-1

Rest and Exercise Hemodynamics in Idiopathic Dilated Cardiomyopathy

	Rest	Exercise
Heart rate	Normal or increased	Subnormal increase
LV end-diastolic pressure	Increased	Further increase
LV end-systolic volume	Increased	Further increase
LV end-diastolic pressure	Increased	Further increase
LV ejection fraction	Low	No significant change
Stroke volume	Low or normal	Subnormal increase

LV, Left ventricle.

pulsatile liver (a reflection of severe tricuspid regurgitation); and ascites are late and ominous symptoms of severe disease. In end-stage cardiac failure, patients may be severely debilitated and bedridden.

Mentation. The patient is typically alert and mentally sound. However, cerebral embolization may produce varying degrees of neurologic impairment. In advanced disease, prolonged reduction in cerebral perfusion may lead to lethargy, decreased ability to concentrate, and irritability. Stress or posturally induced periods of cerebral underperfusion may produce light-headedness, altered mentation, or syncope.

Cutaneous Manifestations. In patients with cardiac decompensation and overt heart failure, the skin is pale, cool at the extremities, and slightly cyanotic.

Heart Rate and Character of Pulse. With severe DCM, compensatory tachycardia may elevate resting heart rates to levels as great as 140 beats per minute. The pulse is of small volume, and pulsus alternans is sometimes present and reflects severe left ventricular dysfunction (Figure 23-3). There may be irregularities in the pulse because of atrial arrhythmias such as atrial fibrillation. Ventricular arrhythmias may further reduce cardiac output and predispose the patient to syncopal attacks or sudden death.

Palpation of the Precordium. Because cardiac enlargement is the primary characteristic of the disease, the

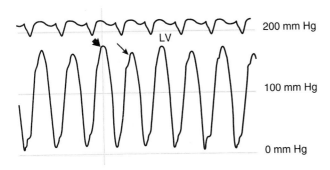

200 mm Hg

100 mm Hg

0 mm Hg

FIGURE 23-3 Pulsus alternans. Left ventricular pressure tracing from a patient with idiopathic dilated cardiomyopathy. Note the left ventricular systolic pressure alternating from 160 mm Hg *(thin arrow)* to 175 mm Hg *(thick arrow)*. Pulsus alternans reflects severe left ventricular dysfunction. On left ventricular catheterization, this patient's left ventricular end-diastolic pressure was 24 to 28 mm Hg, and, on angiogram, the patient has a left ventricular ejection fraction of 15% to 20%. The coronary arteries were normal.

apex beat is displaced inferolaterally and is diminished in force. A nonsustained right ventricular impulse may be palpated along the left lower sternal border.

Heart Sounds. The first heart sound is normal or soft in intensity, the latter of which reflects impaired contractility and reduced rate of ventricular systolic pressure rise. Systolic murmurs secondary to mitral and tricuspid regurgitation are often present (see portion of Figure 23-4 indicating heart sounds). The volume of regurgitant flow progressively diminishes during systole as the ventricular cavity and valve annulus become smaller, which then allows complete valve closure. Therefore the mitral and tricuspid murmurs are usually decrescendo and usually end before S_2 (Figure 23-4). A third and fourth heart sound are frequently present.

Gallop sounds and regurgitant murmurs often can be brought out or enhanced by isometric hand grips (squeezing the examiner's hand). This assessment maneuver increases afterload, which in turn increases regurgitant flow and murmur audibility.

Neck Veins. Jugular venous distention with prominent *a* and *v* waves is usually present in patients with right ventricular dysfunction.

Respiratory Rate and Character of Breathing. Respiratory difficulty usually occurs only with exertion in patients with mild to moderate disease. Tachypnea and dyspnea at rest are usually present in the patient with end-stage DCM.

Lung Sounds. The lungs are clear to auscultation in the early stages of DCM. Wheezes and crackles indicate the presence of pulmonary edema. Pulmonary edema may be expected to occur when left ventricular end-diastolic pressure exceeds 20 to 25 mm Hg.

Acid-Base Values. Acid-base values are normal in patients with mild disease. Severe disease is usually associated with hypoxemia and hypocapnea (secondary to hyperventilation).

Hemodynamic Profile

The hemodynamic findings are a reflection of diffuse systolic dysfunction and heart failure. The changes described are related to patients with moderate to severe DCM.

Arterial Pressure. The systolic values are usually in the normal to low range, and the pulse pressure, which is narrowed, reflects the decreased stroke volume.

Systemic Vascular Resistance. In severe disease, this value is usually elevated beyond 1500 dynes/sec/cm^{-5}. This is because of compensatory stimulation of the renin-angiotensin-aldosterone system and enhanced sympathetic nervous system activity. Unfortunately, the compensatory vasoconstriction increases left ventricular afterload, which in turn increases mitral regurgitant flow and further decreases stroke volume. It is speculated that the sympathetic nervous system stimulation and increased circulating catecholamine levels also may potentiate myocardial damage.

Pulmonary Vascular Resistance. With advanced disease, measurements may increase to greater than 150 dynes/sec/cm^{-5}.

Pulmonary Artery Pressures. Pulmonary artery pressures may be elevated as a result of left ventricular failure. Increases in mean pulmonary artery pressure, which commonly reach values of 30 mm Hg, worsen right ventricular function.

Pulmonary Artery Wedge Pressure. This measurement is usually elevated and reflects the higher left ventricular end-diastolic pressure (Figure 23-5). With symptomatic disease, mean values greater than 20 mm Hg are common. The *a* wave may be of increased amplitude, and a large *v* wave often indicates mitral regurgitation but also may indicate reduced left atrial compliance.

Cardiac Output and Ejection Fraction. The resting cardiac output measurement may be normal or reduced

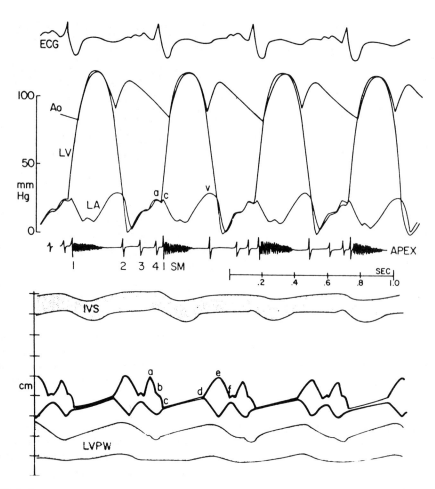

FIGURE 23-4 Schematic showing the electrocardiographic, hemodynamic, auscultatory, and M-mode echocardiographic findings from a patient with dilated cardiomyopathy (DCM). The top panel is the electrocardiogram *(EKG),* below which are the aortic *(Ao),* left ventricular *(LV),* and left atrial *(LA)* pressure tracings. Note the elevated left ventricular and left atrial diastolic pressures, as well as the increased-amplitude *a* and *v* waves in the left atrial pressure tracing. Beneath the pressure tracings are the typical auscultatory findings in DCM, namely a third and fourth heart sound and a decrescendo systolic murmur of mitral regurgitation. The M-mode echocardiogram reveals a dilated and hypocontractile left ventricular interventricular septum *(IVS)* and posterior wall *(LVPW).* The distance between the mitral valve after the onset of diastole *e* point and the IVS also reflects the poorly contractile state of the left ventricle. (From Criley JM: Valvular heart disease. In Ross G et al, editors: *Pathophysiology of the heart,* New York, 1982, Masson.)

relative to the severity of the disease and effectiveness of the compensatory mechanisms. Resting cardiac output may be maintained at or near normal despite a low ejection fraction because of ventricular dilation and a compensatory increase in heart rate. With advanced disease, the ejection fraction may be as low as 10% to 15% and the patient is typically symptomatic, even at rest.

Mixed Venous Oxygen Saturation. In symptomatic patients, the severity of the reduction in oxygen saturation of mixed venous blood correlates with the severity of heart failure.

Laboratory and Other Diagnostic Studies
Electrocardiograph. Sinus tachycardia is common, and the entire range of atrial or ventricular arrhythmias, as well as conduction disturbances, may be noted. Atrial fibrillation occurs in approximately 20% to 25% of patients and is an ominous complication because the loss of the atrial contribution to ventricular filling usually leads to a further decrease in cardiac output. The QRS complex is

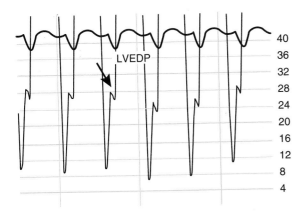

FIGURE 23-5 Left ventricular *(LV)* tracing, with an arrow showing the end-diastolic pressure *(EDP),* which is markedly elevated to levels of 24 to 28 mm Hg in this patient with DCM, who also had pulsus alternans as shown in Figure 23-3. Pressure scale 4 mm Hg per line. The top of the LV wave form is cut off in this illustration.

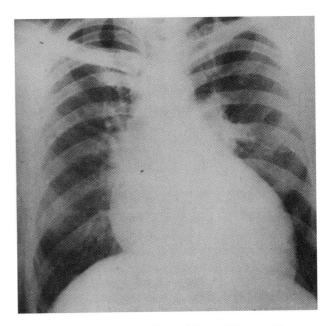

FIGURE 23-6 This chest radiograph from a 75-year-old woman with idiopathic dilated cardiomyopathy demonstrates an enlarged cardiac silhouette with a slight increase in blood flow to the upper lobes, suggesting mild pulmonary congestion.

often prolonged to greater than 0.10 seconds. Left ventricular hypertrophy is present in nearly 50% of cases, and a left bundle branch block pattern occurs in approximately 20% to 30% of patients. When there is extensive myocardial fibrosis, a pseudoinfarct pattern consisting of Q waves in the inferior and anterolateral leads commonly is seen in patients without past myocardial infarction.

Chest Radiograph. Multichamber enlargement and an overall enlarged cardiac silhouette are common (Figure 23-6).

The pulmonary vasculature is often congested with blood and is prominent. Distribution of blood flow to the upper lobe vessels occurs because of the elevated pulmonary venous volume and pressures. Interstitial and alveolar edema are late manifestations, or they may occur acutely with episodes of stress.

M-Mode and Two-Dimensional Echocardiogram with Doppler. These studies are useful in assessing the degree of left ventricular dysfunction and in detecting possible coexisting valvular or pericardial disease. Four-chamber enlargement is the classic finding; the left ventricle is often the most dilated and sometimes is the only chamber enlarged. Diffuse hypokinesis of the left ventricle is the most common finding, but occasionally patients have segmental wall motion abnormalities. The latter are associated with a better patient prognosis. Left ventricular mass is invariably increased, even though wall thickness may be normal. Compensatory hypertrophy and wall thickening are generally not seen because the primary

abnormality is a volume, *not* pressure, overload of the left ventricle. As stated earlier, however, increases in left ventricular wall thickness have been associated with an improved prognosis (see Figure 23-4).

Radionuclide Angiographic Techniques. Biventricular dilation with a global decrease in contractility is typical. However, the left ventricle contractility is usually more depressed than the right.

Endomyocardial Biopsy. In patients with new-onset (less than 6 months) cardiomyopathy, endomyocardial biopsy is recommended by some practitioners to exclude myocarditis and infiltrative disorders (Figures 23-7 and 23-8). However, the yield of a positive biopsy sample is generally present in less than 10% of patients with DCM, and the appropriate, effective treatment of myocarditis is still uncertain.

This procedure may be performed in the procedure room of the coronary care unit or cardiac catheterization laboratory using fluoroscopy or two-dimensional echo guidance (or both). Experienced operators have complication rates that are similar to those of routine cardiac catheterization. However, cardiac perforation with tamponade is a potential hazard that limits use of this procedure to hospitals where experienced teams are available.

Two-dimensional echo guidance may reduce this risk by ensuring that the myocardial biopsy samples are taken from the right ventricular septum rather than the right ventricular free wall, which, due to its relative thinness, is more subject to perforation.

Cardiac Catheterization. Left ventriculography demonstrates left ventricular enlargement and diffuse reduction in wall motion. Although segmental wall motion abnormalities may occur in patients with DCM, localized wall motion abnormalities are more characteristic of ischemic heart disease, whereas diffuse contractile dysfunction is more typical of DCM. Coronary angiography is important in patients with segmental wall motion abnormalities for the purpose of excluding underlying coronary atherosclerosis or anomalous coronary artery. In patients with a diseased or anomalous coronary circulation, correction of the coronary arterial defects may be curative.

Management

The goals of therapy are to preserve the myocardium, reduce the elevated ventricular end-diastolic pressures, maximize the stroke volume and cardiac output, and eliminate the underlying cause, if it is known.

Medical Therapies. Physical, dietary, and pharmacologic therapies are palliative.

Oxygen Therapy. Oxygen therapy is always warranted in severe cases and usually in mild cases to improve tissue oxygenation and relieve dyspnea.

Prolonged Bed Rest or Reduction in Activity. Marked reductions in activity have been advocated to delay the onset of heart failure or relapse into heart failure. With recuperation, patients may be enrolled in outpatient cardiac rehabilitation programs for a graded exercise plan or home exercise program. This frequently results in an improved exercise tolerance.

Dietary Modifications. Salt restriction may help relieve the congestive symptoms of heart failure. Vitamin and coenzyme Q10 supplementation and a nutritious diet may improve general health and help the patient feel better but have no effect on the outcome of the disease. It is imperative that alcohol intake be abandoned completely.

Diuretics. Diuretics are a mainstay of therapy to reduce the symptoms of pulmonary and systemic venous congestion. Optimal diuresis and consequent preload reduction also may decrease the size of the ventricles and may thereby (1) decrease the magnitude of mitral or tricuspid regurgitation and (2) decrease the ventricular wall tension and, consequently, myocardial oxygen demand. It is important to maintain normal serum magnesium and potassium levels for

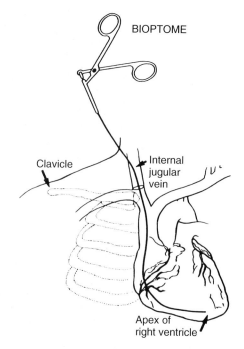

FIGURE 23-7 Schematic of a bioptome entering the right internal jugular vein and apex of the right ventricle to obtain an endomyocardial biopsy. (From O'Connell JB et al: Dilated cardiomyopathy: emerging role of endomyocardial biopsy, *Curr Probl Cardiol* 7:459, 1986.)

patients with DCM. Serum potassium levels greater than 4.0 mEq/L and serum magnesium levels greater than 2.0 mEq/L may reduce the incidence of ventricular ectopy, whereas low levels may potentiate arrhythmias. In the RALES (Randomized Aldactone Evaluation Study)[1] trial, it has been demonstrated that the administration of spironolactone, an aldosterone antagonist, to patients with severe heart failure significantly reduces mortality rate and improves symptoms without additional side effects.

Vasodilator Agents. Reduction in the impedance of left ventricular ejection (afterload) is pivotal to vasodilator therapy and may provide dramatic hemodynamic and clinical benefits. Hydralazine's (Apresoline) pure arterial dilator effects decrease systemic and pulmonary vascular resistance, increase stroke volume, and decrease myocardial oxygen consumption, all of which result in an overall improvement in circulatory function. Balanced arterial and venodilator agents such as nitroprusside (Nipride) and captopril (Capoten) also lower systemic and pulmonary venous pressures and biventricular preload. Pure preload-reducing agents, such as nitroglycerin (Tridil) or isosorbide dinitrite (Isordil), used in conjunction with other vasodilators, such as captopril, appear synergistic and

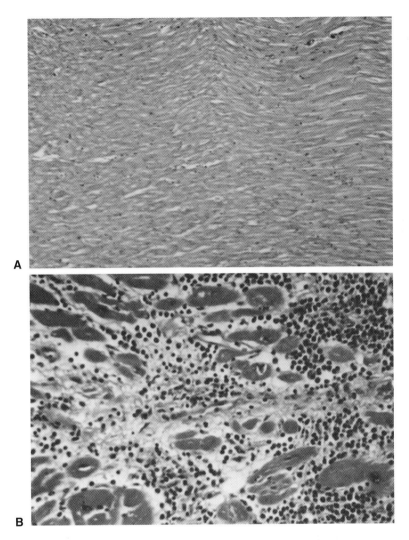

FIGURE 23-8 Photomicrograph of **(A)** normal myocardial tissue and **(B)** active myocarditis with extensive mononuclear cell infiltrate. Muscle damage may eventually occur as the result of myocardial inflammation.

have been associated with improved short-term survival. Nitroprusside and intravenous nitroglycerin can be given only in the acute care setting.

Titration of parenteral vasodilator therapy is guided by careful assessment of the patient's hemodynamic measurements. Once therapeutic end-points are optimized for the individual patient, oral vasodilators are begun and the patient is gradually weaned from parenteral medications. The angiotensin-converting enzyme (ACE) inhibitors are considered the oral vasodilators of choice because of their proven reduction in mortality rate, improvement in symptoms, and reduction in rehospitalization frequency for congestive heart failure. Alternatively, the angiotensin receptor blockers (valsartan, losartan) may be used in patients intolerant to ACE inhibitors. These agents have been

proven (ELITE II study)[2] to have similar efficacy to ACE inhibitors in patients with DCM. A newer agent currently being studied in multicenter trials with a potential of being effective in these patients is omapatrilat, which combines vasopeptidase inhibition with ACE inhibition. Endothelin-1 antagonists (e.g., tezosentan) have been shown to relieve symptoms, improve hemodynamics, and reduce mortality rates in various subsets of patients with heart failure (RITZ II study).[3]

Selective Beta-Adrenergic Blockade. Although seemingly paradoxic, beta-adrenergic blockade with agents such as metoprolol (Lopressor) has been administered to treat DCM. Beginning with low doses and increasing cautiously according to patient response, beta-adrenergic blocking agents are generally well tolerated and have been shown in some series to improve both myocardial function and survival.[4-8] The combined beta- and alpha-adrenergic blocking agent carvedilol (Coreg) has been found to be superior to metoprolol in patients with severe heart failure regardless of the etiology of DCM (the CAPRICORN[9] and COPERNICUS[10] trials). The mechanism of improvement is thought to be due to several factors, including upregulation of beta receptors, which are depressed and decreased in density in a chronically failing heart, and reduction in catecholamine-induced myocardial damage. The drug-induced reduction in heart work and oxygen consumption can be likened to "pharmacologic bed rest."

Antiarrhythmic Agents. Although there is no evidence that antiarrhythmic agents improve survival or prevent sudden death in patients with DCM, most clinicians treat symptomatically disabling or life-threatening arrhythmias. However, because of the potential adverse effects of these drugs, such as myocardial depression, treatment must be individualized while vigilantly weighing efficacy against deleterious effects, such as worsening of heart failure. Agents such as mexiletine and quinidine seem to have the least negative inotropic effects, but patients must be watched carefully for prolongation of the Q-T interval because it may predispose them to ventricular tachyarrhythmias. An automatic implantable cardiac defibrillator should be given to patients with life-threatening ventricular arrhythmias or nonsustained ventricular tachycardia (VT) and an inducible VT in electrophysiologic study. These devices have been proven to improve survival in patients with DCM.

Biventricular pacing, performed by placing an electrode in the right ventricular apex and a second electrode in the coronary sinus or great cardiac vein (for left ventricular pacing), has been proven to improve symptoms and quality of life in patients with DCM and complete left bundle branch block or intraventricular conduction delay (Multisite Stimulation in Cardiomyopathies [MUSTIC][11] and Multicenter InSync Randomized Clinical Evaluation [MIRACLE][12] studies).

Anticoagulation. There is a significant increase in the frequency of systemic and pulmonary emboli in patients with DCM, even in those without echocardiographic or clinical evidence of thrombus formation. The thrombotic and embolic risk is increased in patients with atrial fibrillation and those on bed rest. The incidence of embolic events in non-anticoagulated patients is from 10% to 20% over a variable follow-up period. The autopsy finding of pulmonary or systemic emboli is from 25% to 40%. Patients should therefore be given anticoagulation therapy as long as there are no contraindications. A less than standard dose may be required because of the decreased hepatic clearance of the drugs as a result of heart failure.

Inotropic Therapy. Digitalis may be used in the long term, especially in patients with atrial fibrillation, to control the heart rate and improve exercise tolerance. The more potent parenteral inotropic agents may be given during hospitalization. However, patients with severe heart failure hospitalized specifically for parenteral therapy with agents such as dobutamine, amrinone, dopamine, or epinephrine were found to have an increased mortality rate despite temporary improvement in symptoms.

Surgical Therapy. Cardiac transplantation should be considered in patients with end-stage heart failure. Cardiac transplantation usually has a 1-year survival rate in excess of 80%, and 3- to 5-year survival rates are now in the range of 70% to 80%. Improved cardiac transplantation survival rates reflect better methods of organ procurement, improved regimens of immunosuppression, and greater clinical expertise. A new surgical form of therapy, cardiac myoplasty, is being performed on an experimental basis in some centers in the United States and Europe. This procedure entails wrapping the heart in the latissimus dorsi muscle and pacing this muscle along with the heart as a sort of "booster pump." The future role of this form of therapy is currently uncertain. Left ventricular reduction surgery (partial left ventriculectomy, the Batista procedure) has recently gained interest for treatment of end-stage DCM. Although immediate and short-term results seemed promising, the long-term effects still have been disappointing. Left ventricular assist devices (LVADs) have been studied in the last decade and are currently approved by the Food and Drug Administration and in use as a bridge to cardiac transplantation. LVADs are also used as a final optional treatment of end-stage heart failure. At the time of this publication, mechanical hearts are being implanted with good short-term success.

Hypertrophic Cardiomyopathy

Hypertrophic cardiomyopathy (HCM) is a primary myocardial disease physically characterized by generalized hypertrophy and a hypercontractile left ventricle. Hypertrophic cardiomyopathy is clinically expressed as signs and symptoms of pulmonary venous congestion (dyspnea), myocardial ischemic chest pain, syncope, and sometimes sudden death. The primary hemodynamic feature is related to impairment of left ventricular filling (diastolic dysfunction). Since its original description in the 1950s, HCM has been known by numerous other descriptive names (Box 23-1).

Causes

In most patients, causes are usually familial with autosomal dominant inheritance. A series of gene loci has now

---

BOX 23-1
Eponyms for Hypertrophic Cardiomyopathy

Eponym	Year
Functional obstruction of the left ventricle	1957
Asymmetric hypertrophy of the heart	1958
Idiopathic hypertrophic subaortic stenosis	1960
Idiopathic myocardial hypertrophy	1963
Hypertrophic obstructive cardiomyopathy	1964
Hypertrophic hyperkinetic cardiomyopathy	1965
Stenosing hypertrophy of the left ventricle	1966
Obstructive myocardiopathy	1968
Hypertrophic cardiomyopathy	1970
Dynamic hypertrophic subaortic stenosis	1971
Asymmetric hypertrophic cardiomyopathy	1972
Idiopathic hypertrophic cardiomyopathy	1972
Diffuse muscular subaortic stenosis	1973

BOX 23-2
Pathologic Anatomy of Hypertrophic Cardiomyopathy; Morphologic Criteria for Diagnosis

1. Idiopathic primary ventricular hypertrophy
   A. Usually asymmetric
      1. LV > RV
      2. Septum > free wall
      3. Regional variants (including apical)
   B. Nondilated ventricular cavities
   C. "Crowded" and traumatized mitral valve
      1. Disproportionate elongation of leaflets
      2. Thickened leaflets
      3. Impact endocardial lesions (plaques)
         a. Septal (opposite anterior leaflet)
         b. Mural (beneath posterior leaflet)
      4. Calcified annulus
2. Atrial dilatation (LA > RA)
3. Microscopic features
   A. Focal myofiber disarray
   B. Myocyte hypertrophy
   C. Interstitial fibrosis
   D. Thickened intramural coronary arteries

From Siegel RJ et al: Echo-Doppler in hypertrophic cardiomyopathy. In Schapira JN, Harold JG, editors: *Two-dimensional echocardiography and cardiac Doppler,* Baltimore, 1990, Williams & Wilkins.

been identified on chromosomal mapping leading to abnormal hypertrophy of cardiac muscle. Abnormalities in the β-myosin heavy chain account for 35% of cases, myosin-binding protein C for 15%, troponin T for 15%, α-tropomyosin for 5%, and myosin light chain for 1% of cases. Other suggested causes include (1) abnormalities in sympathetic nervous system responsiveness of the heart, (2) abnormalities in catecholamine levels or metabolism, and (3) systemic hypertension. Hypertrophic cardiomyopathy also may occur after a variable period following surgical treatment of valvular aortic stenosis.

Morphologic Characteristics

Because of generalized myocardial hypertrophy and stiffness, the intraventricular cavities are small and resist filling. The left ventricle is typically more involved in the hypertrophic process than the right. The hypertrophic changes may symmetrically involve all areas of the left ventricle (see Figure 23-1). However, in most patients, there is more extensive involvement of the intraventricular septum, which is approximately twice normal thickness. In some patients, the muscular hypertrophy may be highly inconsistent, and adjoining myocardial regions vary greatly in thickness.

The atria are often dilated because of impaired ventricular diastolic relaxation and filling and the associated increase in left ventricular end-diastolic pressure. The mitral valve apparatus tends to be crowded with disproportionate elongation and thickening of the leaflets. The mitral valve annulus also may be calcified. Fibrous plaque is generally present on the endocardial surface of the left ventricular outflow tract (Box 23-2).

Pathophysiology and Hemodynamic Effects

The structural changes produce systolic and diastolic abnormalities in cardiac function, as well as imbalances in myocardial oxygen supply and demand, which predispose patients to myocardial ischemia. However, the predominant hemodynamic problems of HCM are related to the impairment to left ventricular filling (diastolic dysfunction). Box 23-3 outlines the pathologic abnormalities of HCM.

Systolic Abnormalities. The smaller left ventricular cavity is banana shaped rather than the normal cone shape (broader at the mitral area and tapering at the apex). Because of hypercontractility of the left ventricle, the abnormally shaped intraventricular cavity becomes narrowed to a slit in systole. This effect, in turn, results in narrowing of the left ventricular outflow tract (see Figure 23-1). When the hyperdynamic ventricle contracts, high-velocity blood flow through the narrowed ventricular outflow channel produces flow currents that draw both mitral valve leaflets toward the intraventricular septum. Shifting of the mitral leaflets may not allow complete valve closure, which results in mid- to late-systolic regurgitant blood

From Siegel RJ et al: Echo-Doppler in hypertrophic cardiomyopathy. In Schapira JN, Harold JG, editors: *Two-dimensional echocardiography and cardiac Doppler,* Baltimore, 1990, Williams & Wilkins.

BOX 23-3
Pathologic Anatomy of Hypertrophic Cardiomyopathy

1. Systolic features
   A. "Hyperdynamic" ventricular contractions
      1. Increased ejection fraction (degree of emptying)
      2. Increased rate of ventricular emptying
         a. Ventricle "empty" by mid systole
         b. Aortic valve "preclosure"
      3. Sustained contraction (after emptying)
      4. Intracavitary pressure gradients
      5. Brisk aortic upstroke (increased dP/dT)
   B. Mitral valve dysfunction
      1. Mitral regurgitation
         a. Holosystolic
         b. Late systolic augmentation
      2. Systolic anterior motion
2. Diastolic features
   A. Delayed rate of isovolumic relaxation
   B. Decreased diastolic compliance
   C. Increased atrial transport function (increased "atrial kick")

---

flow. The mitral regurgitant flow is usually mild, but in some people it may become hemodynamically significant.

In normal persons, there is no difference in ventricular intracavitary pressure during systole. However, in approximately 25% of patients with HCM, a left ventricular intracavitary systolic pressure gradient can be documented in the cardiac catheterization laboratory. The pressure gradient, which typically occurs across the left ventricular outflow tract just below the aortic valve, is a hemodynamic characteristic unique to HCM. Two mechanisms have been proposed for this intracavitary gradient: (1) midsystolic intracavitary *obstruction* by the flow-shifted mitral valve leaflets and hypertrophied septum; and (2) excessive and rapid early systolic emptying of the small left ventricular cavity, which results in complete cavity *obliteration* (closure).

Hemodynamic and Clinical Distinctions between Patients with HCM versus Obstructive Pressure Gradients such as Aortic Stenosis

Differences in Aortic Waveform Morphology. In patients with aortic stenosis, there is a decreased slope and delayed rate of rise of the pressure waveform distal to the obstruction. Conversely, in patients with an obliterative gradient such as HCM, the aortic pressure waveform is characterized by a brisk, rapid upstroke (Figure 23-9).

Differences in Ejection Fractions and Rates of Ventricular Emptying. Patients with HCM with outflow tract gradients tend to have ejection fractions that are higher than those without gradients. The rate of ventricular emptying and the completeness of emptying are enhanced when an outflow gradient is induced or increased. This finding is the opposite of that which occurs with outflow obstruction (aortic stenosis), in which there is an impaired rate of ventricular ejection and degree of emptying (Figure 23-10). The nonobstructed concept is further supported by the following clinical observations.

Correlation with Development of Ventricular Hypertrophy. The presence of left ventricular outflow gradients in HCM is not related to the progression of left ventricular hypertrophy, whereas outflow gradients due to obstruction always are. In patients with HCM, development of left ventricular hypertrophy is independent of a left ventricular outflow gradient.

Correlation with Clinical Presentation. Outflow tract gradients with HCM do not correlate with cardiac symptoms, survival, or incidence of sudden death, whereas obstructive gradients, such as those in aortic stenosis, typically do.

The presence of an intracavitary systolic gradient is time variable, and a patient may have no outflow gradient at one time and a large one at another time. Three mechanisms provoke or increase the outflow gradient by reducing intraventricular blood volume at end-diastole: (1) inotropic stimulation of the ventricle, (2) reduction in preload, and (3) reduction in afterload.

Diastolic Abnormalities. Increased stiffness of the hypertrophic left ventricle results in diminished ventricular relaxation and distensibility. These result in impaired filling, which in turn reduces or limits stroke volume. The massive, nondistensible ventricle also is associated with elevated left ventricular end-diastolic pressures and correlated increases in left atrial and pulmonary venous pressures. Pulmonary venous hypertension predisposes the patient to pulmonary vascular congestion and episodes of acute pulmonary edema. The stiff, hypertrophic myocardium also is highly dependent on the atrial contribution to ventricular filling to maximize end-diastolic volume, myofibrillar stretch, and stroke volume. Therefore any arrhythmia associated with a loss of the "atrial kick" may precipitate hemodynamic deterioration. There also is an impairment to peak diastolic filling associated with exercise. This may seriously limit the ambulatory outpatient's exercise capacity or may worsen a patient's hemodynamic status if suddenly stressed by seizure activity, shivering, sepsis, or chemical withdrawal such as from alcohol.

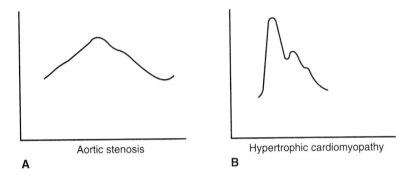

FIGURE 23-9 Comparison of the arterial waveform of a patient with aortic stenosis (obstructive pressure gradient) versus that of a patient with hypertrophic cardiomyopathy (obliterative pressure gradient). In aortic stenosis the upstroke of the pulse wave is slow and late peaking, whereas in hypertrophic cardiomyopathy the upstroke is rapid rising and nearly vertical.

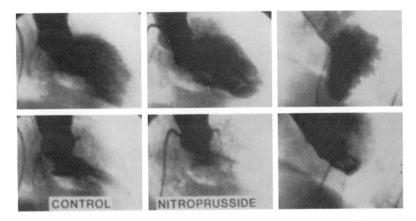

FIGURE 23-10 Angiograms, *left panel* without a left ventricular outflow tract pressure gradient, *far right panels* after an 87 mm Hg left ventricular outflow tract gradient induced by decreasing systemic vascular resistance with the administration of nitroprusside (Nipride). *Top panels* are end-diastole; *bottom panels* are end-systole. The left ventricle emptied more rapidly and more completely with the induction of the dynamic pressure gradient. The left ventricular ejection fraction rose from 89% to 94%. (Adapted from Siegel RJ, Criley JM: Left ventricular emptying in hypertrophic cardiomyopathy, *Br Heart J* 53:283, 1985.)

Effect of Hypertrophic Cardiomyopathy on Myocardial Oxygen Supply and Demand. As with all hypertrophic or hyperdynamic hearts, the balance of myocardial oxygen supply and demand is threatened because (1) the hypercontractile heart has a supernormal oxygen demand, and (2) the elevated left ventricular end-diastolic pressure reduces the perfusion pressure gradient and blood flow rates across the ventricular wall. Thus the patient with HCM is vulnerable to diffuse myocardial ischemia and fibrosis. In unusual cases (less than 15%), the previously *hyper*contractile left ventricle can become *hypo*contractile. Systolic dysfunction may then complicate the hemodynamic and clinical picture.

In summary, the hemodynamic and pathophysiologic abnormalities observed in patients with the overmuscled, stiff, hypercontractile ventricle of HCM are reduced intraventricular diastolic volume capacity that limits or decreases stroke volume; elevated ventricular end-diastolic pressures and pulmonary venous hypertension; rapid, vigorous systolic emptying; mitral regurgitation; and potential imbalances in myocardial oxygen supply and demand even without coronary artery disease.

Clinical Presentation

The spectrum of symptoms varies so that some patients may be asymptomatic whereas other patients may be disabled by HCM. The clinical presentation generally is related to the extent of hypertrophy. However, this relationship is not always consistent. In other words, some patients have severe symptoms with relatively mild hypertrophy, whereas patients with severe hypertrophy may be relatively symptom free. The patient's age, rate of progression of disease, course typical of affected family members in inherited disease, and daily activity level also may affect frequency and severity of symptoms. Other factors that may contribute to symptoms are (1) magnitude of mitral regurgitant flow, (2) autonomic dysfunction, (3) frequency of supraventricular and ventricular arrhythmias, and (4) disease-related medial hypertrophy of the coronary arteries with abnormalities, such as narrowing of the septal perforating coronary branches of the left anterior descending coronary artery.

The most common symptoms of dyspnea, chest pain, and syncope can be explained on the basis of excessive ventricular muscle mass. Namely, inordinate myocardial hypertrophy has the potential to produce an imbalance in myocardial oxygen supply and demand, which then predisposes the patient to myocardial ischemia. This results in further reductions in ventricular distensibility and consequent further reductions in end-diastolic volume and stroke volume, as well as arrhythmias. Physical or emotional stress may exacerbate this process and may cause further clinical deterioration.

Dyspnea is a clinical signal of acute pulmonary edema. Patients with HCM are predisposed to stress-induced pulmonary edema due to the elevated left ventricular end-diastolic pressure, which reflects back to the pulmonary circulation. *Chest pain* because of myocardial ischemia may be present in both children and adults. *Syncope* is often exertionally related and may result from ischemia-induced supraventricular or ventricular arrhythmias; syncope also may result from the inability of the heart to increase cardiac output in proportion to the level demanded by physical activity.

The most serious and sometimes the first indication of HCM is *sudden death.* Death-producing arrhythmias occur at a rate of 4% to 5% annually and tend to occur in patients less than 40 years of age. This fatal event can occur when affected people engage in strenuous physical activity. In fact, HCM is one of the most common causes of sudden death in young athletes. The magnitude of left ventricular hypertrophy highly correlates with the risk of sudden death. Patients with wall thickness greater than 30 mm have an 18 per 1000 person-years risk of sudden death, whereas those with wall thickness less than 15 mm have almost no risk.

Mentation. Near-syncopal or syncopal episodes may occur when the patient is upright or exercising, and they are relieved when the patient lies down. Otherwise, mentation is normal.

Heart Rate and Character of the Pulse. The heart rate is usually normal. The peripheral arterial pulse is of normal volume, and the initial ejection phase is perceived by the examiner's fingers as an abrupt upstroke, which is jerky in quality, followed by collapse. The carotid upstroke is likewise brisk and then declines in midsystole. The internal jugular venous pulse may demonstrate a prominent *a* wave. This reflects diminished right ventricular compliance due to the massively hypertrophied intraventricular septum.

Palpation of the Precordium. The precordium is usually active, with a palpable atrial gallop and a sustained ventricular impulse. A systolic thrill, most frequently palpable at the apex or the left lower sternal border, may be present in patients with mitral regurgitation.

Heart Sounds. There is a normal S_1 that often is preceded by a fourth heart sound. A harsh, mid- to late-peaking systolic murmur is typically present and is the result of mitral regurgitation or left ventricular outflow tract turbulence. The murmur is best heard between the apex and the left sternal border and often radiates to the lower sternum and axilla. The audibility of the murmur varies inversely with the size of the left ventricular cavity. In other words, as the left ventricular cavity gets smaller, the murmur gets louder and vice versa. For example, factors that decrease the left ventricular cavity size by preload reduction, such as standing, Valsalva maneuver during strain, tachycardia, venodilating drugs such as nitroglycerin, or hypovolemia, intensify the murmur. Isoproterenol (Isuprel), digitalis, and exercise, which increase contractility, result in a smaller end-systolic volume and intensify the murmur. Alternatively, squatting, leg elevation, isometric hand grip, phenylephrine (Neo-Synephrine), and beta blockade all decrease the intensity of the murmur by enhancing ventricular filling and increasing left ventricular cavity size.

Respiratory Rate and Character of Breathing. As stated previously, dyspnea is a common complaint and occurs in up to 90% of symptomatic patients. Tachypnea typically coexists with dyspnea.

Hemodynamic Profile

The hemodynamic measurements reflect the aforementioned abnormalities in systolic and diastolic ventricular function.

Arterial Pressure. The blood pressure is usually normal. A minority of patients (approximately 25%) have moderate systemic hypertension.

Arterial Waveform. In patients with HCM, 90% of stroke volume is ejected during the first half of systole and only 10% during the second half of systole (in normal persons, 50% to 55% of stroke volume is ejected during the first half of systole). The initial high-volume, high-velocity outflow produces a steep, rapid upstroke of the arterial waveform. This prominent early "percussion" wave may produce an exaggerated reflected wave that results in a double arterial systolic peak termed *pulsus bisferiens.*

Systemic Vascular Resistance. This calculated measurement is usually normal but may increase late in the disease if heart failure develops as a result of myocardial ischemia and fibrosis.

Pulmonary Vascular Resistance. This value increases secondary to hypoxemia and perivascular swelling if the patient develops pulmonary edema.

Pulmonary Artery Pressure. Pulmonary artery systolic and diastolic pressures are elevated in approximately 25% of patients.

Pulmonary Artery Wedge Pressure. This measurement is usually elevated and reflects the reduced left ventricular distensibility that accompanies ventricular wall thickening, as well as the decreased rate and extent of ventricular relaxation. The *a* wave in the pulmonary artery wedge pressure (PWP) tracing is exaggerated. After opening of the atrioventricular valves, the *y* descent,

which correlates with the rate of decline in the left atrial pressure, may be diminished.

Cardiac Output and Ejection Fraction. The resting cardiac output is usually normal until late in the disease course when contractile failure may occur. Ventricular systolic emptying is rapid and nearly complete; therefore the ejection fraction is greater than normal—in the range of 75% to 90%.

Laboratory and Other Diagnostic Studies

Electrocardiograph. This test may be normal in a minority of patients. ST segment and T wave (repolarization) abnormalities and increased QRS voltage, greatest in the mid-precordial leads, are electrocardiographic evidence of left ventricular hypertrophy (Figure 23-11).

Prominent abnormal Q waves involving the inferior or lateral leads, reflective of septal hypertrophy, are seen in up to 25% of cases. In patients with predominantly apical hypertrophy (an HCM variant) giant inverted precordial T waves are commonly present. Premature ventricular contractions are detected in approximately 75% of patients who have continuous ambulatory monitoring. Ventricular tachycardia is noted in as many as 25% of patients studied and is associated with an eightfold increase in the risk of sudden cardiac death over those patients without ventricular tachycardia. Supraventricular tachycardia occurs in 25% to 50% of patients; atrial fibrillation occurs in 5% to 10% of patients.[13]

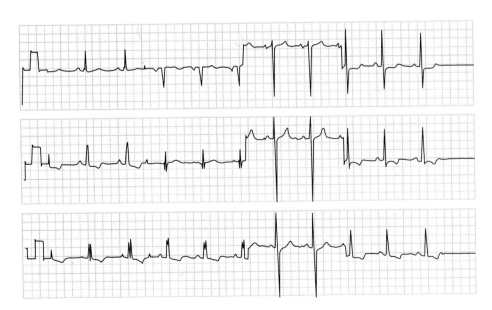

FIGURE 23-11 Twelve-lead ECG from a patient with hypertrophic cardiomyopathy. Note the increased QRS voltage over the precordial leads that reflects the left ventricular hypertrophy.

Chest Radiograph. Heart size may be normal or markedly enlarged. In patients with severe diastolic dysfunction or severe mitral regurgitation, left atrial enlargement and evidence of pulmonary venous congestion may be present.

Cardiac Catheterization. Left ventriculography demonstrates a hyperdynamic left ventricle with rapid emptying and increased ejection fraction. Mid- to late-systolic mitral regurgitation, due to abnormal movement of the mitral leaflets, also may be apparent. Coronary artery disease may be present in older patients or those with a high risk profile for coronary artery disease.

Echocardiogram-Doppler Studies. These studies are extremely useful in diagnosing HCM and are based on documenting left ventricular hypertrophy in the absence of identifiable factors such as aortic stenosis and systemic hypertension. Echocardiography demonstrates asymmetric septal hypertrophy in two thirds to three fourths of patients. In one half or more of the patients, there is systolic motion of the mitral apparatus toward the ventricular septum. Left atrial enlargement is common, and a hypercontractile left ventricle is demonstrated in more than 90% of cases. Doppler studies are useful to identify mitral regurgitation, assess the magnitude of left ventricular outflow tract gradients, and evaluate the degree of diastolic dysfunction.

Treatment

It is important to focus therapy on the central role of diastolic dysfunction in the pathophysiologic dynamics of HCM. In the hypercontractile left ventricle with a high ejection fraction characteristic of patients with HCM, "what gets into the ventricle gets out." Stroke volume is limited only by abnormal diastolic filling, *not* reduced or impaired left ventricular ejection. Consequently, the therapeutic maintenance of adequate diastolic filling is important in patients with HCM. Hypovolemia due to excessive diuresis, fluid shifts, and blood loss may be hemodynamically disastrous to critically ill or injured patients with coexistent HCM. The patient with HCM also requires a controlled heart rate less than 120 beats per minute and preferably less than 70 beats per minute to allow time for adequate ventricular filling. Maintenance of sinus rhythm is important because atrial contraction may account for 30% to 35% of left ventricular filling.

Because of the massive and hypercontractile left ventricular musculature characteristic of HCM, it is extremely important to maintain an adequate coronary perfusion pressure to supply the supernormal oxygen needs of the thick, hypercontractile myocardium. The mean arterial pressure should be maintained in the normal range, with diastolic pressures greater than 60 mm Hg (preferably 70 to 90 mm Hg), with alpha-adrenergic agents such as ephedrine or methoxamine (Vasoxyl). However, the specific vasopressor used is not as important as is the goal of maintaining mean normal arterial pressure, normal systemic vascular resistance, and adequate aortic diastolic (coronary perfusion) pressure while also carefully controlling heart rate.

Unlike patients with cardiac disease characterized by systolic dysfunction, a reduction in left ventricular afterload may worsen hemodynamics in patients with HCM by exacerbating mitral regurgitation. This is in direct opposition to the effects of afterload reduction in patients with mitral regurgitation of other causes (dilated cardiomyopathy, rheumatic valve disease, papillary muscle dysfunction or rupture) in which afterload reduction decreases the regurgitant volume. In all patients with mitral regurgitation, increases in the mitral regurgitant volume worsen circulatory failure and promote myocardial ischemia by decreasing forward stroke volume.

Beta-Adrenergic Blockade. Beta-adrenergic blockers are the mainstay of medical therapy. The mechanisms of their beneficial therapeutic effects appear to be mediated by a reduction in heart rate that prolongs and improves diastolic filling, reduction in contractility, inhibition of sympathetic stimulation of the heart during physical or emotional stress, and overall reduction in myocardial oxygen demand. Beta blockade also may exert antiarrhythmic benefits. Ventricular relaxation also is enhanced with propranolol (Inderal) at doses greater than 300 mg per day. Symptoms are satisfactorily improved in approximately 50% of patients after initiating standard doses of beta-adrenergic blockers (equivalent to 160 to 320 mg of propranolol per day).

Many patients develop recurring symptoms during long-term therapy. In these patients, or in those who do not initially respond, higher doses (up to 1 g per day of propranolol) may be required.

Calcium Channel Blocking Agents. These pharmacologic agents are therapeutic options in symptomatic patients. Verapamil (Calan, Isoptin) reduces symptoms and increases exercise tolerance in the majority of patients during short-term therapy. Sustained clinical improvement has been reported during long-term therapy in over 50% of patients.

Possible therapeutic drug actions in patients with HCM include negative chronotropic and inotropic effects and enhancement of left ventricular filling by reducing the asynchronous regional ventricular relaxation that is one of the features of the disease. Verapamil should be started at a low dose and increased, as needed, progressively over days or weeks, according to patient tolerance. Verapamil should be given with caution to patients who have conduction defects (due to the potential for bradycardia, atrioventricular block), or to patients who are also on beta-adrenergic blockers. Because of the drug's vasodilator and negative inotropic effects, it should not be given or given only with extreme caution in patients with PWP greater than 20 mm Hg. In these patients, the drug effects predispose them to pulmonary edema, systemic hypotension, and death.

In some patients, nifidipine (Procardia) may be better tolerated than verapamil. By improving left ventricular relaxation and filling, the drug improves diastolic function without depressing systolic function. It is, however, a more potent vasodilator than verapamil, and this effect may predispose the patient to a drop in blood pressure and associated reflex tachycardia. To prevent the reflex tachycardia, which has undesirable hemodynamic effects, nifedipine should be administered in conjunction with a beta-adrenergic blocker. Diltiazem (Cardizem) also can be an effective and a well-tolerated drug in older patients, who often have significant adverse effects from the other two calcium channel blocking agents. Disopyramide (Norpace) may be a helpful adjunct in patients to reduce excessive left ventricular contractility and the severity of mitral regurgitation.

Endocarditis Prophylaxis. Because of the presence of mitral regurgitation, patients with HCM should receive appropriate prophylaxis for bacterial endocarditis as recommended by the American Heart Association guidelines before undergoing operative, endoscopic, or dental procedures.

Antiarrhythmic Therapy. Disopyramide (Norpace) produces symptomatic improvement in a number of patients with HCM with atrial or ventricular arrhythmias. Its negative inotropic effects have been associated with a reduction in the outflow gradient and in some cases with a decrease in mitral regurgitation (see previous discussion). Arrhythmias associated with the loss of atrial contraction (atrial fibrillation, ventricular tachycardia) should be electrically or pharmacologically cardioverted. Loss of the atrial contribution to ventricular filling and rapid ventricular rates are often associated with acute hemodynamic deterioration.

For slowing of the ventricular rate, beta-adrenergic blockers or calcium channel blockers with atrioventricular nodal blocking effects are preferred. Amiodarone may be chosen for the management of both ventricular and atrial tachyarrhythmias. Because ventricular tachycardia or

fibrillation appears to be the principal mechanism of sudden death in patients with HCM, recently there has been an increasing use of implantable automatic defibrillators in high-risk patients. Recent studies demonstrate that for patients with severe left ventricular hypertrophy (wall thickness greater than 30 mm), the use of prophylactic defibrillators appears to reduce the incidence of sudden death.

Exercise and Stress Limitation. Patients must clearly understand that strenuous exercise and competitive sports are absolutely prohibited because of the risk of sudden death. Likewise, in hospitalized patients with co-existing illness or injury, measures should be aggressively taken to reduce the physical stress imposed by factors such as seizure activity, shivering, chemical withdrawal, and sepsis.

Dual-Chamber Pacing. Dual-chamber pacing, using a short programmed atrioventricular delay to ensure constant activation of the right ventricle from its apex, reduces intraventricular gradient and improves symptoms in patients with obstructive hypertrophic cardiomyopathy. However, there is often a mismatch between reduction in gradient and subjective improvement.

Nonsurgical Septal Reduction. Transcoronary injection of ethanol into the first septal perforator of the left anterior descending coronary artery induces a controlled infarction of the basal anterior septum. The new septal motion abnormality immediately reduces left ventricular outflow gradient in 85% to 90% of patients. Symptomatic improvement has been noted in many of the patients on follow-up of 1 year.

Surgical Therapy. Surgical enlargement of the left ventricular outflow tract was commonly performed in the past for severely symptomatic patients. Today, a preference for the surgical approach to therapy remains variable by institution; however, we do not recommend this form of therapy. Surgical intervention is usually in the form of transaortic septal myotomy and myectomy. This procedure often relieves the outflow tract pressure gradient and may reduce the degree of mitral regurgitation. The ejection fraction routinely falls postoperatively and reflects a surgically induced reduction in left ventricular contractility. The operative mortality rate ranges from 5% to 10%, although in experienced centers it is now probably as low as 1% to 2%. Long-term postoperative follow-up studies reported that approximately 70% of patients had substantial symptomatic improvement during a follow-up period of 5 years; however, most of these patients remained on medication.[14] There has never been a controlled study documenting the efficacy of pure surgical therapy. Consequently, postoperative survival rate has not been shown to be higher than that of medically treated patients. However, in patients with severe mitral regurgitation or infective endocarditis, mitral valve replacement may be warranted.

Restrictive Cardiomyopathy

Restrictive cardiomyopathy (RCM) is a primary myocardial disease physically characterized by poorly compliant (stiff) ventricular walls that impair diastolic filling. Systolic function is usually normal early in the course of the disease. Restrictive cardiomyopathy is clinically manifest by signs and symptoms of systemic and pulmonary venous congestion, such as generalized edema and a predisposition to pulmonary edema. Hemodynamically, the disease is characterized by elevated and nearly equal left and right ventricular filling pressures. This form of heart disease often mimics and may be clinically indistinguishable from constrictive pericardial disease.

Incidence and Causes

Of the three categories of cardiomyopathies, the restrictive type is the least common. Causes are diverse. For example, one form is the result of iron overload and deposition of the element in body tissue (hemochromatosis), whereas in some cases the cause cannot be determined (idiopathic RCM). However, in North America, 90% of cases occur as the result of systemic amyloidosis. Amyloidosis is an infiltrative disease of various causes characterized by the deposition of insoluble, twisted protein fibrils (amyloid) in various tissues of the body. Vital organ function, such as heart function, may ultimately become impaired (Box 23-4).

Morphologic Characteristics and Hemodynamic Effects

At autopsy, the heart generally has biatrial dilation with normal or small ventricular cavities (see Figure 23-1). When the condition is long-standing, the ventricles may be dilated secondary to systolic failure. The ventricular walls may be normal or mildly to markedly increased in thickness and are firm and rubbery.

The fundamental hemodynamic abnormality is impaired diastolic filling due to the stiff nature of the ventricular musculature. As a consequence of subnormal ventricular filling, stroke volume is reduced and fixed, although contractile function is usually normal. However, if RCM is due to amyloidosis, systolic dysfunction may develop as the infiltrative process progresses. Elevated right- and left-sided ventricular filling pressures, clinically measured as right atrial or central venous pressure and PWP, respectively, are

---

BOX 23-4
Causes of Restrictive Cardiomyopathy

1. Infiltrative disorders
   A. Amyloidosis
   B. Hemochromatosis
   C. Neoplastic infiltration
   D. Glycogen storage disease
   E. Mucopolysaccharidosis
   F. Sarcoidosis
2. Collagen-vascular diseases
3. Endocardial diseases
   A. Endomyocardial fibrosis
      1. With eosinophilia
      2. Without eosinophilia
   B. Endocardial fibroelastosis
4. Idiopathic

From Criley JM, Siegel RJ: The patient with known or suspect cardiomyopathy. In Pepine C, editor: *Diagnostic and therapeutic cardiac catheterization,* Baltimore, 1989, Williams & Wilkins.

---

the result of the stiff, nondistensible ventricular walls. Bilateral atrial dilation develops over time because of the restriction to ventricular end-diastolic filling.

Clinical Presentation

Symptoms of right-sided systemic venous congestion predominate over those of left-sided pulmonary venous congestion. The elevated systemic venous pressures result in generalized, dependent edema; an enlarged, tender liver; ascites; and distention of the visible veins. Prominent x and y descents are noted in the jugular venous pulsations. However, dyspnea is also a common complaint and is related to pulmonary venous hypertension and consequent predisposition to pulmonary edema.

Other clinical findings are related to the low, fixed cardiac output. Chronic fatigue and dyspnea are the most common complaints. Intolerance to exercise or physical stress (shivering, severe injury, fever) is common because of the restricted heart's inability to increase cardiac output by tachycardia without further diminishing ventricular filling. In the setting of amyloidosis, systemic hypotension, as well as syncope, may be present because of neural involvement. Orthostatic hypotension occurs in approximately 10% of patients with amyloidosis.

On physical examination, the apex beat is usually palpable, in contrast to *constrictive pericarditis* wherein it is nonpalpable. The apical impulse may be shifted inferiorily and laterally because of moderate cardiomegaly. A third (S_3) and fourth (S_4) heart sound may be present on auscultation, and the sounds are representative of reduced ventricular

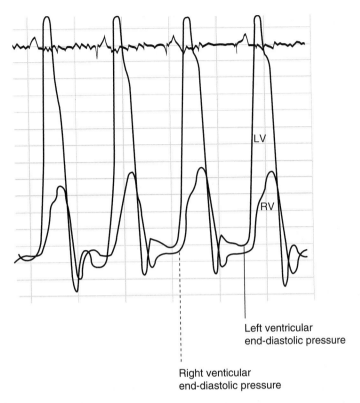

LV

RV

Left ventricular
end-diastolic pressure

Right venticular
end-diastolic pressure

FIGURE 23-12 Elevated and nearly equal right ventricular *(RV)* and left ventricular *(LV)* diastolic pressures from a patient with idiopathic restrictive cardiomyopathy. Also note the "dip and plateau" diastolic waveform that is present in both the right and left ventricular pressure tracings; 4 mm Hg scale.

compliance, not necessarily contractile failure. Tricuspid and mitral regurgitation are relatively common because of atrial dilation and amyloid involvement of the papillary muscles.

Hemodynamic Profile

The obtained values and waveform morphology reflect the abnormal dynamics of ventricular filling. Points of hemodynamic differentiation between restrictive and constrictive cardiomyopathy are included in this discussion because of the clinical similarity between the two diseases.

Arterial Pressure. The blood pressure is reduced below the patient's previous values; systolic arterial pressures of 80 to 100 mm Hg are not unusual. The pulse pressure is narrow. Prior hypertension is often reversed in patients with RCM that results from amyloidosis. As stated, orthostatic hypotension occurs in approximately 10% of patients with amyloid disease.

Systemic Vascular Resistance. This value is increased because of compensatory vasoconstriction secondary to reduced stroke volume.

Pulmonary Vascular Resistance. This value is elevated in patients with RCM as a result of pulmonary venous hypertension or, less commonly, amyloid lung infiltration. In *constrictive pericardial disease* this calculated value is usually normal.

Pulmonary Artery Pressure. Measurements are elevated in tandem with increases in left atrial and pulmonary venous pressures. If pulmonary vascular resistance is elevated because of amyloid lung infiltration, widening of the pulmonary artery diastolic to wedge pressure gradient occurs proportionate to the degree of pulmonary involvement and vascular resistance. With *constrictive pericardial disease,* the pulmonary artery systolic pressure is rarely elevated.

Right Atrial and Pulmonary Artery Wedge Pressures. These values are elevated and correlate with the elevated and nearly equal right and left ventricular end-diastolic pressures. Right atrial or central venous pressure measurements are in the approximate range of 12 to 22 mm Hg, and the PWP is usually slightly higher (Figure 23-12). If the patient is stressed (exercise, shivering, etc.), or if the patient receives a fluid volume load, the left ventricular end-diastolic pressure often rises to a greater extent than that in the right ventricle. This finding also helps differentiate RCM from *pericardial constriction,* in which ventricular end-diastolic pressures rise equally because both ventricles are equally constrained by the rigid pericardium that limits left ventricular and right ventricular diastolic expansion.

Atrial and Ventricular Waveform Morphology. The dynamics of resistive ventricular filling produce characteristic changes in both atrial and ventricular waveform morphology.

Atrial Waveform. The right and left atrial waveforms are characterized by prominent *a* waves that reflect the increased atrial force required to fill the noncompliant ventricles at end-diastole. As the atria relax at the onset of ventricular systole, atrial pressures drop abruptly and produce an exaggerated *x* descent. As the atria fill during systole, intraatrial pressures rise, inscribing the ascending limb of the *v* wave. Then, as the mitral and tricuspid valves open at the onset of diastole (crest of the *v* wave), blood flows rapidly into the ventricle. The graphically correlated *y* descent is even more pronounced than the exaggerated *x* descent and is followed by the upstroke of the *a* wave of the next beat (Figure 23-13).

An inspiratory increase in right atrial pressure, termed *Kussmaul sign,* is often present in RCM. The right atrial pressure rises on inspiration because the noncompliant right ventricle is unable to accept the normal inspiratory-induced increase in venous return without a significant increase in end-diastolic pressure. Kussmaul sign is present in other cardiac diseases such as constrictive pericarditis and right ventricular infarction (Figure 23-14).

Ventricular Waveform. In the ventricular pressure tracings, a deep and rapid decline in pressure occurs at the onset of diastole followed by a rapid rise to a mid- to end-diastolic plateau. This imparts a square root–like shape to the diastolic portion of the waveform, termed the *square root* sign (Figure 23-15).

Cardiac Output and Ejection Fraction. Resting cardiac output tends to be below normal because of the limitation to ventricular filling. There is a serious limitation to the blood flow increases demanded by stress or exercise. The ejection fraction is usually normal.

Mixed Venous Oxygen Saturation. This measurement (SvO_2) falls in proportion to the level of perfusion failure.

Laboratory and Other Diagnostic Studies
Electrocardiograph. Electrocardiographic findings may reflect the underlying cause of RCM. In idiopathic RCM, atrial arrhythmias are common. In patients with RCM due to amyloidosis, the ECG abnormalities include generalized low voltage of the QRS complex, as well as myocardial infarction patterns, bundle branch blocks, and axis deviations (Figure 23-16). Sinus bradycardia may be present because of amyloid infiltration of the sinus node. Complex ventricular arrhythmias may be present in patients with amyloidosis and are a poor prognostic sign.

Chest Radiograph. Cardiomegaly, when present, is in large part the result of the biatrial dilation. Pleural effusions are common, whereas pulmonary vascular congestion is uncommon in compensated patients.

Echocardiography. The echocardiogram assesses ventricular contractility, which is typically normal in patients with RCM. The test also is useful for exclusion of pericardial effusions as a possible cause of restricted ventricular filling. With amyloidosis, an increase in the left ventricular wall thickness is noted (Figure 23-17). The increase in ventricular muscle mass associated with amyloid disease is characterized by an abnormal voltage/mass relationship. Reduced QRS voltage is noted on ECG recordings, although there is an increased ventricular mass

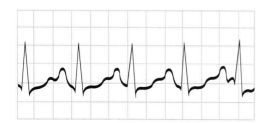

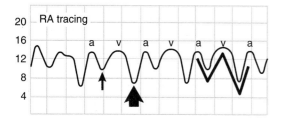

FIGURE 23-13 Right atrial pressure tracing in a patient with restrictive cardiomyopathy. The top panel is the ECG tracing. The bottom panel is the right atrial *(RA)* pressure tracing (4 mm Hg scale). Note the prominent *x (small arrow)* and *y (large arrow)* descents in this patient. Note also the W appearance to the waveform inscribed during one cardiac cycle *(solid line).*

defined by echo examination. Normally, ventricular hypertrophy is associated with increased QRS voltage, which correlates with increased muscle mass noted on echocardiography. When RCM is the result of amyloid disease, a "scintillating" (bright and speckled) myocardium is sometimes detected by two-dimensional echocardiography.

Radionuclide Angiographic Techniques. In the early stages of RCM, results of these studies are generally normal, but ultimately systolic dysfunction ensues if amyloid infiltrates cause the disease. Technetium pyrophosphate scans (also called *hot spot scans*), which are typically used for the diagnosis of acute myocardial infarction, often reveal diffusely positive findings in the setting of cardiac amyloidosis.

Myocardial Biopsy. See Figure 23-7. Tissue sampling is extremely helpful for identifying causes of RCM. The biopsy sample is generally diagnostic for amyloidosis and hemochromatosis, as well as other infiltrative disorders and endocardial diseases. In fact, one of the authors (RJS) believes that endomyocardial biopsy has its greatest use in RCM with the exception of use for patients after cardiac transplantation.

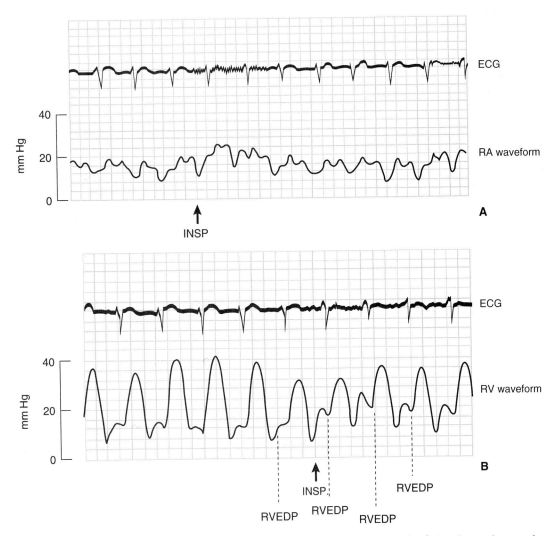

FIGURE 23-14 Kussmaul sign in a patient with idiopathic restrictive cardiomyopathy. **A,** Inspiratory increase in right atrial pressure at *arrow.* **B,** Inspiratory increase in right ventricular diastolic pressure (4 mm Hg scale). (Courtesy of Prediman K. Shah, MD, Cedars-Sinai Medical Center, Los Angeles, California.)

Cardiac Catheterization. Coronary angiography and cardiac catheterization usually are not indicated in this condition. However, invasively obtained hemodynamic measurements assist in the diagnosis.

Magnetic Resonance Imaging. Magnetic resonance imaging (MRI) is particularly useful in differentiating restrictive cardiomyopathy from constrictive pericarditis, as well as defining abnormal diastolic flow patterns. More recently, MRI was found to have a potential role in the noninvasive diagnosis of cardiac amyloidosis identifying typical morphologic markers and suggesting the presence of infiltrative disease using tissue characterization.

Treatment

Patient outcome is directly related to the underlying cause of RCM and the potential for cure. Iron overload is a potentially reversible condition with desferoxamine chelation therapy or phlebotomy, depending on the cause of the iron overload. Treatment of amyloidosis is

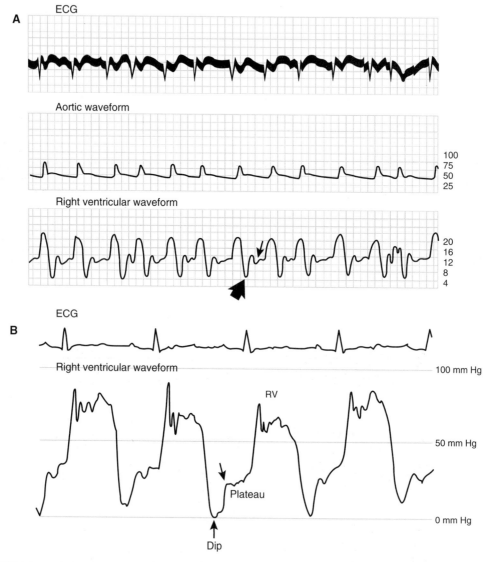

FIGURE 23-15 A, Electrocardiogram *(ECG; top),* aortic pressure *(middle,* 25 mm Hg scale), and right ventricular pressure *(bottom,* 4 mm Hg scale). Note the hypotensive values of the arterial pressure and the narrow pulse pressure from this patient with restrictive cardiomyopathy. Note also the prominent dip *(thick arrow)* and plateau *(thin arrow)* in the right ventricular pressure tracing. **B,** Right ventricular pressure tracing showing the classic dip and plateau or "square root" pattern from another patient with hemodynamic findings suggestive of restrictive cardiomyopathy.

usually not effective because the cause cannot be eliminated and progression of the disease cannot be halted. From the onset of congestive symptoms, the 2-year mortality rate is greater than 80%. Idiopathic RCM, although debilitating, is not as rapidly progressive as amyloid cardiomyopathy.

Treatment of RCM is primarily directed at providing symptomatic relief by reducing systemic or pulmonary vascular congestion. This is best accomplished with low-dose diuretics with or without vasodilators. However, there is a risk of hypotension with these agents, because excessive volume depletion or vasodilator-induced preload reduction may result in hemodynamically significant reduction in stroke volume and hypotension. Therefore institution of these drug therapies should be in the low-dose range and increased according to tolerance while the patient is being vigilantly assessed.

When patients on these medications go home, they must understand that the drugs should not be taken without the physician's knowledge and sanction when dehydration (due to gastroenteritis, excessive sweating) or hypovolemia (hemorrhagic blood loss) are present. *In patients with amyloidosis, both digitalis and calcium channel blocking agents are contraindicated.* Digitalis should not be used or should be used only with extreme caution because patients with amyloid RCM are particularly prone to digitalis-induced arrhythmias and heart block. Likewise, calcium channel blocking agents may predispose to refractory hypotension in patients with amyloid infiltration.

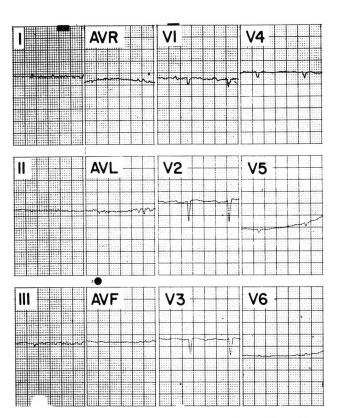

FIGURE 23-16 This 12-lead ECG from a patient with cardiac amyloidosis demonstrates marked, diffuse low voltage and inferior and anterior myocardial infarction patterns (Q waves), as well as first-degree atrioventricular block (PR interval, 0.22 second).

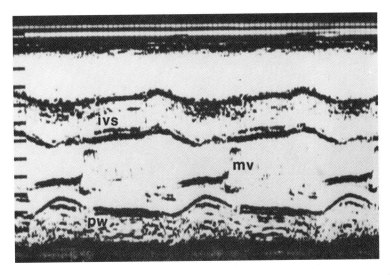

FIGURE 23-17 M-mode echocardiogram from a patient with amyloid disease demonstrates a thickened interventricular septum *(ivs)* and posterior wall *(pw)* with preserved left ventricular contractility. Measured lines to left represent 1 cm marks. *mv,* Mitral valve.

CONSTRICTIVE PERICARDIAL DISEASE (CONSTRICTIVE PERICARDITIS)

Constrictive pericardial disease is characterized by a thick, rigid, scarred pericardium that restricts filling of all four chambers of the heart. The clinical features include signs and symptoms of circulatory failure and systemic and pulmonary venous congestion. The hemodynamic hallmarks are subnormal ventricular filling volume, consequent reduction in stroke volume, and elevation and equalization of ventricular end-diastolic pressures.

Causes

Constrictive pericardial disease is thought to begin with an episode of acute pericarditis. This has a variety of causes (Box 23-5). However, in many patients, no precipitating factor can be identified. These "idiopathic" cases have been theorized to be the result of antecedent subclinical viral infections involving the pericardium. In underdeveloped countries, tuberculosis accounts for a large number of cases. With the proliferation of cardiac surgery in the past few decades in the United States, there has been an increase in postcardiac surgery pericarditis and constrictive pericardial disease. No specific agent or aspect of surgical trauma has been identified as the inciting factor. These cases may or may not be typical of the postcardiotomy syndrome. Recently, cases have been identified following placement of automatic implantable cardiac defibrillator patches.[15]

Pathophysiology

Initially, pericardial inflammation is associated with progressive fibrin deposition and fluid accumulation in the pericardial space that may be clinically undetectable. Over time, however, the fluid is reabsorbed as progressive pericardial scarring and thickening render the pericardial sac stiff and unyielding. The visceral and parietal pericardium eventually become completely fused, and calcium deposition contributes to making the normally protective, supportive pericardial sac an adherent, oppressive, hard shell that encases a healthy heart.

Hemodynamic Effects

As previously stated, the normal heart is constrained by the rigid pericardium. As a result, all four cardiac chambers are forced within a circumscribed space in diastole. The uniform, symmetrically constricting effect produces a mid- to late-diastolic filling restriction of all four cardiac chambers, an elevation and equilibration of diastolic pressures, and an impediment to systemic and pulmonary venous return. In fact, all of ventricular filling occurs *only* in early diastole. Because of the abruptly limited ventricular

---

BOX 23-5
Causes of Constrictive Pericardial Disease
Infectious—tuberculous, bacterial, viral
Traumatic
Postcardiotomy
Postirradiation
Collagen-vascular disease—rheumatoid arthritis, systemic lupus erythematosus
Neoplastic
Idiopathic*

*Most common in the United States.

---

filling time, ventricular end-diastolic volume and stroke volume are decreased as systemic and pulmonary venous pressures become elevated. Compensatory tachycardia initially maintains cardiac output, but with progressive pericardial restriction, cardiac output and, eventually, blood pressure gradually fall.

In patients with constrictive pericarditis, the dynamics of ventricular filling are as follows. At the onset of diastole, intraventricular blood volume and pressures are at their lowest level and right atrial and central venous pressures, as well as left atrial and pulmonary venous pressures, are abnormally elevated. As a result of the large atrial-to-ventricular pressure gradient, when the atrioventricular valves open, initial diastolic filling is very rapid. On the ventricular waveform, this is noted as the lowest recorded pressure, which then abruptly rises. When the ventricular walls attain the maximal distention allowed by the restraining pericardium, the abnormally rapid early ventricular filling is suddenly halted. At this time, ventricular pressures rise steeply to a plateau that is maintained to end-diastole.

The graphically recorded ventricular filling pressure pattern produces a waveform in both ventricles with a characteristic early dip followed by a plateau, termed the *square root sign* (Figure 23-18). This ventricular waveform morphology is similar to that noted in restrictive cardiomyopathy because in both diseases there is abrupt limitation to ventricular filling. In RCM, however, the diastolic filling limitation is imposed by scarred, stiff ventricular walls, whereas in constrictive pericardial disease the normal heart is constrained by the fibrotic, scarred, or calcific pericardium (Figure 23-19).

Clinical Presentation

The most common initial symptom of acute or subacute pericarditis is sharp, knifelike chest pain that is usually

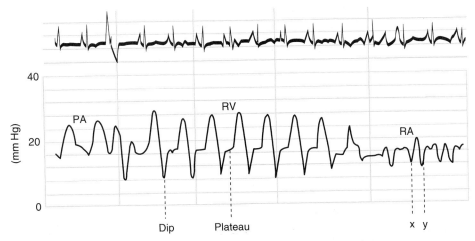

FIGURE 23-18 Equalization of the pulmonary artery *(PA)* diastolic pressure, right ventricular *(RV)* end-diastolic pressure, and right atrial *(RA)* pressure in a patient with pericardial constriction. A dip and plateau "square root" is present in the RV pressure tracing, and prominent *x* and *y* descents are noted in the atrial pressure tracing. This tracing was obtained as the pulmonary artery catheter was "pulled back" through the right heart from the pulmonary artery position.

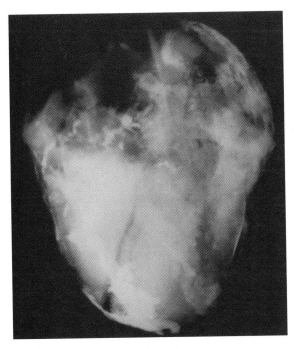

FIGURE 23-19 Postmortem radiograph of the heart from a patient with constrictive pericardial disease. Note the extensive radiographic calcification of the pericardium *(white)*.

substernal and is made worse by deep breathing, coughing, or motion. In patients with chronic disease, pain is uncommon. Overall, the typical signs and symptoms of constrictive pericardial disease are those of perfusion failure and systemic and pulmonary venous congestion. Chronic fatigue and exercise intolerance are common complaints. When the biventricular end-diastolic pressures become elevated to 10 to 15 mm Hg, symptoms are related primarily to systemic venous hypertension. These include distention of the jugular veins; dependent edema; ascites; enlarged liver; and gastrointestinal upsets, such as anorexia and indigestion. When ventricular end-diastolic pressures exceed 18 mm Hg, signs and symptoms of pulmonary congestion such as dyspnea on exertion, tachypnea, orthopnea, and cough develop. These occur if patients attempt to exercise, have an increased circulatory fluid load, or suffer progression of the disease. Disabling weakness and fatigue, weight loss, and muscle wasting (termed *cardiac cachexia*) are noted in patients with advanced disease and are related to the chronically subnormal delivery of oxygen and nutrients to body tissue.

The apex beat is usually not palpable, but systolic retraction of the chest wall may be observed. A pericardial friction rub, which occurs with acute pericarditis, is not expected with chronic pericardial constriction. Rather, a pericardial knock, which occurs in approximately 30% of patients, is diagnostic. The knock occurs early in diastole and is usually heard best along the left sternal border with the diaphragm of the stethoscope. The knock, which has a higher frequency sound than a gallop, corresponds to the sudden, early diastolic cessation to ventricular filling.

The external jugular veins are distended to a level relative to increases in venous pressure, and rapidly collapsing *x* and *y* waves may be observed in the internal jugular venous pulsations. The Kussmaul sign, which is an inspiratory rise in venous pressure, may be observed at the bedside as inspiratory distention or lack of an inspiratory drop in the height of the jugular venous pulsations.

Hemodynamic Profile

Ordinarily, the combination of a low stroke volume and increased ventricular end-diastolic pressure indicates heart failure because of intrinsic cardiac dysfunction. However, in constrictive pericardial disease, the heart is usually normal, and circulatory failure is the result of pericardial restriction to normal ventricular filling.

Arterial Pressure

The arterial pressure may be normal or lower than the patient's previous normal level. The level of the drop is relative to the severity of the disease. The narrowed pulse pressure reflects the decreased stroke volume. Unlike pericardial tamponade, constrictive pericardial disease is rarely associated with a paradoxic arterial systolic pressure (pulsus paradoxus).

Right and Left Arterial Pressures

The key to the hemodynamic diagnosis of constrictive pericardial disease is elevated and equal right- and left-sided intracardiac end-diastolic pressures. With moderate disease, right atrial pressure and PWP are between 10 and 15 mm Hg. With severe disease, measurements may be as high as 25 mm Hg. For clinical purposes, *equal* is defined as mean pressures within 4 to 5 mm Hg from one cardiac chamber to the other because fluid-filled monitoring systems may not faithfully document the true chamber-to-chamber equilibration.

Atrial Waveform

The most highly characteristic features of the atrial waveforms are the prominent *x* and *y* descents. As the atria relax at the onset of ventricular systole, atrial pressures drop sharply and produce an exaggerated *x* descent. The upstroke and amplitude of the *v* wave are normal. When the mitral and tricuspid valves open at the onset of diastole (the crest of the *v* wave), atrial pressures again drop precipitously, graphically indicating that atrial emptying is very rapid. On the atrial waveform this feature is noted as an exaggerated *y* descent (see Figure 23-18, right atrial waveform). Overall, the steep *x* and *y* descents impart an M or W pattern to the atrial waveform morphology

similar to that observed with restrictive cardiomyopathy (see Figure 23-13).

Ventricular Waveform. On flotation of a pulmonary artery catheter, the right ventricular pressure tracing reveals the classic *dip and plateau* or *square root sign* described earlier. The left ventricular waveform (obtained in the cardiac catheterization laboratory) is similar in shape to, although greater in amplitude than, that in the right ventricle.

Pulmonary Artery Pressures. These measurements are increased in tandem with elevations in left atrial pressure (PWP). Pulmonary artery and right ventricular systolic pressures are usually between 25 and 40 mm Hg. Increases in pulmonary vascular resistance are not expected in pure constrictive pericarditis. Although mild increases in pulmonary artery pressures may be noted, pulmonary hypertension is uncommon, which serves as a point of distinction from restrictive cardiomyopathy.

Cardiac Output

Constrictive pericardial disease is associated with a fixed stroke volume because ventricular filling volume is absolutely limited by the nonyielding pericardium. Under no circumstances (exercise, stress) can the heart exceed the fixed stroke volume. In the early stages of constrictive pericarditis, compensatory tachycardia may maintain a normal resting cardiac output, but appropriate increases in cardiac output during exercise are impossible. Eventually tachycardia can no longer compensate for the progressively constrained heart, and the fixed cardiac output decreases.

Laboratory and Other Diagnostic Studies

Electrocardiograph

Electrocardiographic findings include nonspecific ST-T wave changes and low QRS voltage. Atrial fibrillation may be present and may be related to the progressive, long-standing elevations in atrial pressure or inflammatory changes in the atrial wall or conduction system.

Chest Radiograph

Pericardial calcification increases in frequency with the duration of the disease and is best seen on an overpenetrated lateral or oblique chest radiograph (see Figure 23-19).

Echocardiography

This laboratory test is generally nondiagnostic in pericardial constrictive disease and is typically not useful in assessing pericardial thickness.

Computed Tomography Scanning and Magnetic Resonance Imaging

With the advent of cardiac computed tomography scanning and MRI, it became feasible to accurately detect pericardial thickening. Both of these methods are highly sensitive and specific for assessing pericardial thickness. Detection of pericardial thickening in the setting of suggestive hemodynamic measurements is indicative of constrictive pericarditis.

Cardiac Catheterization and Coronary Angiography

Cardiac catheterization is useful in documenting the four-chamber diastolic pressure elevation and equalization, determining stroke volume, assessing systolic function, and evaluating the coronary circulation for intrinsic disease. Coronary angiography may demonstrate that the coronary arteries are "veiled." Rather than appearing to be on the epicardial surface they appear to be beneath tissue, which is the thickened pericardium. Systolic ventricular function is generally well preserved.

Treatment

Constrictive pericarditis is a progressive disease without remission or reversal of pericardial constriction and hemodynamic compromise. In a small group of patients, survival is 20 years or more with medical management, such as careful use of diuretics, limitation of activity, and sodium-restricted diet. However, the majority of patients become slowly disabled from the chronically low and progressively decreasing cardiac output.

Complete surgical resection of the pericardium is the treatment of choice and is curative. Because of the relative rarity of this condition, optimal surgical results are best obtained at medical centers that are experienced in performing pericardiectomy. Some patients show significant hemodynamic and symptomatic improvement in the immediate postoperative period, whereas in others there may be a lag time of weeks to months before cardiac function returns to normal.

PERICARDIAL TAMPONADE (CARDIAC TAMPONADE)

Pericardial tamponade is a condition in which an abnormal accumulation of fluid within the pericardial space compresses the heart and impairs diastolic filling and cardiac function. Signs and symptoms of perfusion failure, jugular venous distention, and a "quiet heart" are classic clinical features. The hemodynamic characteristics include hypotension, elevated systemic venous pressure, and

equalization of central circulatory diastolic pressure. The magnitude of hemodynamic dysfunction and severity of the clinical presentation depend on the rate and volume of fluid accumulation.

Causes

The accumulation of fluid within the pericardium, termed *pericardial effusion*, may result from several sources:

1. *Iatrogenic.* Postpericardiotomy, after percutaneous transluminal coronary angioplasty, pacemaker implantation, or electrophysiologic testing, was recently found to be a common cause of pericardial tamponade in the Western world.
2. *Infectious processes.* Viral, bacterial, or fungal pericarditis may lead to effusion and tamponade.
3. *Neoplastic disease.* Metastatic carcinoma of the breast or lung is a common cause of effusion and possible tamponade.
4. *Trauma.* Gunshot wounds, stab wounds, perforation of a cardiac chamber by a vascular catheter, surgery, or blunt chest trauma may result in intrapericardial bleeding. Penetrating injury in the precordial area may result in cardiac laceration and tamponade; however, patients with penetrating injury *anywhere* in the thorax or epigastrium should be assessed for possible tamponade.
5. *Nontraumatic hemorrhage.* Leaking aneurysms, dissection of the ascending aorta, or anticoagulant therapy may result in pericardial effusion and tamponade.
6. *Rupture of the left ventricular free wall complicating myocardial infarction.* This lethal event is due to sudden, massive accumulation of blood in the pericardial sac, which produces a rapid tamponade death (Figure 23-20) (see Chapter 21, section on mechanical complications of acute myocardial infarction).
7. *Other causes.* Radiation pericarditis, connective tissue disease (rheumatic arthritis, systemic lupus erythematosus), or uremic pericarditis may result in progressive effusion and, eventually, tamponade.

Morphology and Hemodynamic Effects

The fibrous pericardium is a double-walled sac that completely encases the heart and attaches at its junctions to the great arteries and veins. The pericardial space normally contains approximately 20 to 50 ml of fluid that provides a friction-free surface for the beating heart.

Pericardial pressure is less than atmospheric pressure and is also 3 to 5 mm Hg less than pressure in the central veins and right atrium. This relatively low intrapericardial pressure maintains slight distention of the right atrium and central veins. Central venous pressure is approximately 3

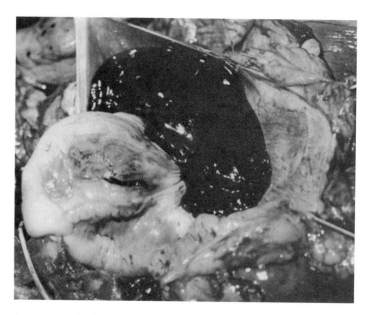

FIGURE 23-20 A large hemorrhagic pericardial effusion was present in this patient, who died of pericardial tamponade secondary to myocardial rupture. In addition, a large intrapericardial hematoma *(black)* was present on the surface of the heart at the time of autopsy.

to 5 mm Hg less than the pressure in the peripheral systemic veins. This pressure gradient maintains continuous blood flow from the systemic veins to the right atrium. As fluid begins to accumulate in the pericardial space, pericardial pressure rises until it equilibrates with central venous and right atrial pressures. Further accumulation of pericardial fluid then causes both pressures to rise together to the level of the left atrial and left ventricular end-diastolic pressures. As the pericardial effusion increases in volume, all pressures continue to rise together. Thus, in tamponade, pulmonary artery wedge pressure (a correlate of left ventricular end-diastolic pressure), pulmonary artery diastolic pressure, and central venous pressure (a correlate of right ventricular end-diastolic pressure) eventually equilibrate. The elevation and equilibration in central circulatory diastolic pressures is the result of the uniform compression of the heart by the fluid-filled pericardium.

The physical effects of cardiac tamponade produce two unfavorable hemodynamic consequences:

1. *First, both ventricles cannot distend and fill normally in diastole.* However, the thin-walled right ventricle is more vulnerable to filling impairment due to external compression and may even collapse in diastole. Less blood is then delivered to the left ventricle. With severe tamponade, ventricular end-diastolic volume may fall to as little as 25 to 30 ml, which is significantly less than normal end-diastolic volume (100 to 180 ml) or normal stroke volume (60 to 120 ml). As a result of severely impaired ventricular end-diastolic filling, stroke volume and cardiac output eventually fall to levels that may be incompatible with life. The end-diastolic volume/pressure relationship of both ventricles is completely distorted; as filling pressures rise, filling volumes fall. Normally, ventricular filling volumes and pressures rise and fall nearly proportionately.

2. *Second, venous return is reduced.* Elevated pericardial pressures impede venous return. In severe tamponade, there may be no diastolic venous return because pericardial pressures are at their highest level in diastole. Because the heart can pump out only that which it receives, stroke volume progressively falls and eventually the systemic blood pressure also falls. Impaired venous return also results in systemic venous congestion and hypertension.

Systemic *arterial hypotension* with concomitantly developing systemic *venous hypertension* causes critical reductions in the pressure gradient (mean arterial pressure minus central venous pressure) across the systemic circulation. As a result, systemic blood flow may ultimately fall to levels inadequate to sustain life.

Three sympathetic nervous system–mediated mechanisms are quickly activated to compensate for these defects:

1. *The ejection fraction, which is normally 55% to 70%, increases to 70% to 80%.* The heart then empties more

completely with each beat, stroke volume increases, and intraventricular diastolic suction may draw blood from the systemic and pulmonary veins to facilitate ventricular filling.

2. *The heart rate increases.* Hence, cardiac output initially may be maintained despite the decreasing stroke volume.

3. *Systemic vascular resistance increases in nonvital tissue such as skeletal muscle.* Vasoconstriction helps maintain mean arterial pressure and shunts the available cardiac output to the vital heart and brain.

As the tamponade worsens, however, compensatory mechanisms are no longer able to maintain blood pressure, and hypoperfusion of all organ systems ensues. *Cardiac tamponade is a medical emergency because effective cardiac function and circulation of blood may ultimately cease. Early clinical recognition of this life-threatening condition is of paramount importance because it is readily treatable.*

Factors That Affect Individual Patient Responses

Individual hemodynamic responses may be modified by several factors.

Hypovolemia. The anticipated rise in intracardiac and central venous pressures and venous distention may be blunted in hypovolemic patients. For example, patients with severe trauma with significant blood loss may have significant signs of tamponade unmasked only after restoration of intravascular volume.

Rapidity of Fluid Accumulation. If fluid accumulation occurs over weeks or months (slow tamponade), 1 to 2 L of pericardial fluid may be present without significant increases in central circulatory pressures and without hemodynamic compromise. This is possible because the pericardium is able to gradually stretch. As a result, pericardial pressure remains low, cardiac compression does not occur, and venous return remains normal. The pericardium cannot distend acutely. Therefore, if accumulation of fluid is rapid (acute tamponade), cardiac compression may occur with as little as 100 ml of fluid.

Magnitude of Sympathetic Nervous System Response. Disease or drug-related (beta blockade, vasodilators, opiates) alterations in autonomic nervous system activity may profoundly affect the patient's hemodynamic response. Hypotension may develop precipitously in patients with blunt or depressed sympathetic nervous system responses with relatively lesser degrees of pericardial effusion and tamponade.

Clinical Presentation

The symptoms of cardiac tamponade are related to the rate and volume of fluid accumulation. The classic clinical findings, termed *Beck's triad,* are (1) hypotension; (2) elevated venous pressures with jugular venous distention; and (3) a small, quiet heart with cardiac activity being nonpalpable. In sudden, massive tamponade, which occurs with cardiac rupture, patients having rapid deterioration may not be able to complain of symptoms, and precipitous hypotension may quickly usher in death. In "slow tamponade," which occurs in neoplastic disease, viral pericarditis, uremia, or radiation injury, the patient may not appear acutely ill. Typically, the major complaint is dyspnea. Other symptoms of temponade include dizziness, a feeling of fullness in the head, a retrosternal pain, or an oppressive feeling in the chest. Dysphagia, cough, or hiccoughs, as well as other symptoms related to the cause of the tamponade (pericarditis, trauma, aortic dissection), also may be present.

Mentation

The patient may be lucid but anxious in mild tamponade. With progressive fluid accumulation and hemodynamic deterioration, patients are likely to become restless and may display altered behaviors such as confusion or combativeness, and their level of consciousness then may deteriorate to stupor or coma.

Cutaneous Manifestations

Initially, the skin may be slightly pale and warm and only the hands and feet may be cool. With the development of severe circulatory failure, the skin is generally cool, moist, and ashen with peripheral cyanosis.

Heart Rate and Character of Pulse

Tachycardia is an important compensatory mechanism to maintain cardiac output. In severe tamponade, bradycardia heralds electrical-mechanical dissociation and death. Pulsus paradoxus is a classic finding in tamponade (see the section on arterial pressure, hemodynamic profile). On palpation of an artery, a cyclic variation in amplitude of the peripheral pulses (diminishes on inspiration and strengthens on expiration) is noted. If, however, the patient is hypotensive, the changing volume of the pulse may not be appreciated. In some patients, the weakened pulse may disappear completely during inspiration. This is termed *total paradox* and is commonly associated with combined cardiac tamponade and hypovolemia. Blood pressure measurement with a sphygmomanometer may be useful for numeric confirmation of the paradoxic pulse (see Chapter 5). However, a palpable paradoxus is a clinically significant paradoxus. In a rapidly deteriorating, hemodynamically unstable patient, the time wasted attempting to confirm a numeric paradoxus by cuff technique may assume life-or-death significance. In this situation, immediate, definitive therapy is indicated. Diagnosis is based on patient history, presence of Beck's triad, and other indicative hemodynamic and clinical findings.

Heart Sounds and Palpation of the Precordium

Heart sounds are muffled or totally inaudible because of the damping effect of the pericardial fluid on the transmission of heart sounds. The apex beat is usually weak or even may be imperceptible.

Neck Veins

With severe tamponade, the external jugular veins may be distended up to the level of the jaw, even with the patient sitting upright. If tamponade is accompanied by hypovolemia, jugular venous distention may be noted only after intravascular volume is restored to normal.

Respiratory Rate and Character of Breathing

The patient is typically tachypneic and dyspneic. If not hypotensive, the patient typically prefers to sit upright, leaning slightly forward.

Lung Sounds

The lungs are usually clear to auscultation. The complaint of dyspnea expressed by many patients may be the result of interstitial pulmonary edema due to elevations in left atrial and pulmonary venous pressures. Although interstitial pulmonary edema results in stiff lungs that increase the work of breathing, there are no auscultatory findings.

Acid-Base Values

Respiratory alkalosis because of tachypnea is typically present until severe perfusion failure produces lactic acidosis. At this time, a combined respiratory alkalosis and metabolic acidosis are noted on blood gas analysis.

Hemodynamic Profile

Arterial Pressure

Initially, sympathetic nervous system stimulation may elevate the systolic pressure to levels as high as 150 mm Hg. More commonly, however, the systolic pressure is in the range of 90 to 100 mm Hg. A normal to slightly elevated diastolic pressure is typical and is maintained at this level by compensatory systemic vasoconstriction. The pulse pressure may be narrowed to 10 to 20 mm Hg because of the greatly reduced stroke volume. The arterial waveform reveals a narrowed pulse pressure.

Pulsus paradoxus, defined as a drop in systolic pressure greater than 10 mm Hg in inspiration, gives a roller-coaster appearance to the systolic peaks in a continuous arterial tracing (Figure 23-21). Pulsus paradoxus is an exaggeration of the normal phasic changes in right and left heart filling because of respiratory-related changes in intrathoracic pressure. Normally, with inspiration, there is an increase in systemic venous return and right heart filling while simultaneously the volume of blood returning to the left heart is reduced because of lung inflation.

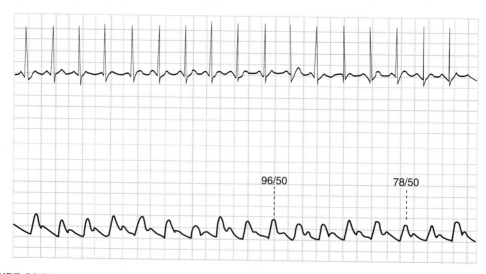

FIGURE 23-21 Pulsus paradoxus. Note the cyclic variation in systolic pressure. An increased systolic pressure is associated with expiration, and a decreased systolic pressure is associated with inspiration. (In gratitude to and in memory of the late Barbara J. Agnew, RN.)

Therefore the inspiratory left ventricular stroke volume falls slightly, and the inspiratory systolic pressure falls less than 10 mm Hg. During expiration, the opposite occurs. In patients with tamponade, the already compromised left heart filling and stroke volume are further reduced by inhaling. This results in an inspiratory systolic pressure fall greater than 15 mm Hg (see Chapter 5, section on pulsus paradoxus).

Systemic Vascular Resistance

This calculated measurement usually increases proportionate to progressive reductions in stroke volume.

Pulmonary Vascular Resistance

This parameter increases if hypoxemia or acidemia complicates the patient's condition.

Pulmonary Artery Pressure

The pulmonary artery systolic pressure is usually normal, and the pulmonary artery diastolic pressure is equal (within 4 to 5 mm Hg) to right atrial pressure. Fluid-filled monitoring systems may not precisely document the true intracardiac pressure equilibration.

Right Atrial and Pulmonary Artery Wedge Pressures

These measurements are elevated and closely approximate the aforementioned pulmonary artery diastolic pressure. The atrial pressures are usually in excess of 15 mm Hg in patients with acute tamponade. If tamponade occurs as a result of trauma and the patient is hypovolemic, the venous pressures may be in the normal to low range and the neck veins may not be distended. Once intravascular volume is restored with fluid therapy, venous pressures rise to greater than normal and the patient displays neck vein distention.

Arterial Waveform Morphology and Hemodynamic Differentiation of Cardiac Tamponade and Constrictive Pericarditis

Both cardiac tamponade and constrictive pericardial disease (see preceding section) are associated with equilibration of central circulatory diastolic pressures, systemic venous hypertension, and systemic venous distention, as well as a reduction in cardiac output. Knowledge of the various cardiac dynamics is essential to understanding the differences in atrial and ventricular waveform morphology. Knowledge of cardiac dynamics is also necessary for distinguishing the patient with subacute tamponade from the patient with constrictive pericardial disease.

The mechanism of diastolic restriction to cardiac filling in tamponade is very different from that of pericardial

constriction. In *pericardial constrictive disease,* there is no limitation to early ventricular filling, but, rather, there is mid- to late-diastolic constraint of the ventricle by the scarred, rigid pericardium. The atrial waveform is characterized by exaggerated *x* and *y* descents, which produces an M or W pattern to the atrial waveform. The ventricular waveform is distinguished by a dip and plateau or square root morphology, which reflects the rapid initial ventricular filling followed by an abrupt mid- to late-diastolic cessation of filling (see Figure 23-18).

In *cardiac tamponade,* the fluid is mobile within the pericardial space and is displaced by changes in intracardiac blood volume relative to the phases of the cardiac cycle. At the onset of systole, ventricular contraction is associated with a diminution in cardiac size. This results in a decrease in the pericardial pressure and therefore decreases compression of the atria. This event, in turn, is associated with the drop in right and left atrial pressures and corresponds with a marked *x* descent on the atrial pressure waveform. This fall in atrial pressure then permits a surge of venous return and enhanced atrial filling. However, atrial filling during the remainder of ventricular systole (coincident with the upstroke of the *v* wave) displaces pericardial fluid and increases pericardial pressure.

On opening of the tricuspid and mitral valves at the onset of ventricular diastole (the crest of the *v* wave), the elevated intrapericardial pressure compresses both atria and ventricles. As a result, the normal *y* descent is markedly blunt or lost on the atrial pressure tracings.

In summary, unlike constrictive pericarditis wherein ventricular filling is rapid in early diastole and is halted in mid to late diastole, in cardiac tamponade ventricular filling is slow throughout diastole. As a consequence, in the ventricular waveforms of patients with tamponade, the early diastolic dip, which reflects rapid early filling, is absent.

Cardiac Output

Initially, compensatory mechanisms may maintain cardiac output within a normal range. However, with continued increases in pericardial volume and pressure, these mechanisms are overwhelmed and cardiac output falls.

Mixed Venous Oxygen Saturation

This value falls relative to the severity of perfusion failure or hypoxemia.

Laboratory and Other Diagnostic Studies

Electrocardiograph

The ECG often shows reduced QRS amplitude in the limb leads because the excess pericardial fluid tends to lower the recorded QRS voltage. With very large volumes of pericardial fluid, which are often due to metastatic cancer, alternating amplitude of the QRS complexes (electrical alternans) or alternating amplitude of the entire PQRST sequence (total alternans) is an indicator of cardiac tamponade. This ECG phenomenon represents the swinging movement of the heart within the effusion and results in beat-to-beat changes in the electrical axis. Typically, patients are in sinus tachycardia. As mentioned earlier, bradyarrhythmias are an ominous and frequently preterminal sign. Arrest of the circulation is usually noted as pulseless electrical activity that deteriorates to asystole.

Chest Radiograph

Patients in acute tamponade may not show an enlarged cardiac silhouette, and serial chest films may be helpful in detecting progressive enlargement of the cardiac silhouette. In patients with chronic pericardial effusions with or without tamponade, the cardiac silhouette is large with a "water bottle" contour. Patients with effusion and tamponade have clear lung fields, which is helpful in distinguishing tamponade from heart failure. Fluoroscopy reveals absence or near absence of cardiac motion due to fluid surrounding the heart.

Echocardiography

This is the major clinical tool to assess patients in impending tamponade, as well as to exclude it. This noninvasive test is easily performed, even on an emergency basis, anywhere in the hospital. The echocardiogram can document the presence and magnitude of pericardial fluid and can rapidly differentiate between pericardial tamponade and other causes of systemic venous hypertension and arterial hypotension, such as right ventricular infarction and biventricular failure. Echocardiography may also be performed during pericardiocentesis to monitor the procedure and may help guard against inadvertent needle puncture of a cardiac chamber.

In tamponade, fluid almost always surrounds the entire heart so that there is both an anterior and a posterior effusion (Figure 23-22). Exceptions are localized effusions that selectively compress one heart chamber. Localized effusions may be seen in patients following cardiac surgery or in trauma patients whose cardiac injury is localized. Other echocardiographic signs suggestive of tamponade include inspiratory increases in right ventricular filling with decreases in left heart filling, diastolic collapse of the right atrium or ventricle, and swinging of the heart within the fluid-filled pericardial sac.

In some instances, a trauma patient with tamponade may enter the emergency department moribund, or the rapidly deteriorating hemodynamic status of the patient

may obviate laboratory tests. The diagnosis is then based solely on the patient's history and physical findings, and definitive therapy is immediately instituted.

Treatment

Medical Therapy

Medical therapy, which is directed at patient support and maximizing cardiac function, is only a temporizing measure. The only definitive therapy for cardiac tamponade is to remove the pericardial fluid, thereby normalizing pericardial pressure and cardiac function.

1. *Intravascular volume expanders.* The most important aspect of medical therapy is to expand the intravascular volume to maximize venous return, left ventricular filling, and stroke volume. Volume expansion may be accomplished with colloids, normal saline, or Ringer's lactate.

2. *Isoproterenol (Isuprel).* The use of this drug is controversial, but its use has been prompted by some because it increases myocardial contractility and decreases systemic vascular resistance. Isoproterenol, however, is known to produce a marked increase in myocardial oxygen requirements, and it predisposes patients to arrhythmias. Therefore continuous monitoring of the hemodynamic measurements, ECG, and clinical status during drug titration is essential.

It should be stressed, however, that volume expansion and isoproterenol are inadequate therapy for tamponade

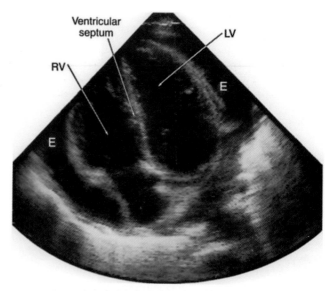

FIGURE   23-22 Two-dimensional echocardiogram, four-chamber view, demonstrating a large pericardial effusion *(E)* surrounding the heart in a patient with pericardial tamponade.

and are, at best, useful only for "buying time" pending definitive therapy.

Surgical Therapy

The only effective treatment of cardiac tamponade is to drain the pericardial fluid. Surgical approaches include the following.

Pericardiocentesis. Needle aspiration of the pericardial fluid is used to relieve cardiac compression. Pericardiocentesis is usually reserved for those patients with life-threatening symptoms or effusions with evidence of hemodynamic compromise. The procedure carries the risk of ventricular puncture, ventricular arrhythmias, trauma to the myocardium, and coronary artery laceration or pleural tear. Constant monitoring of hemodynamic measurements may be obtained during pericardiocentesis in a patient in whom a pulmonary artery catheter has been previously placed. It is recommended that pericardiocentesis be guided by electrocardiographic, fluoroscopic, or echocardiographic monitoring. It is our preference to use electrocardiographic and echocardiographic monitoring simultaneously. Echocardiographic monitoring allows on-line assessment of the size of the effusion during the procedure. The ECG is continuously monitored by attaching the pericardiocentesis needle to an ECG electrode with an alligator clip. The ECG demonstrates an injury pattern (ST segment elevation) if the needle contacts the ventricular epicardium. We also assess intrapericardial

pressure serially by attaching a pressure manometer to the pericardiocentesis needle with a three-way stopcock. This step permits documentation that intrapericardial pressure corresponds with intracardiac diastolic pressure, which further confirms the presence of pericardial tamponade.

Surgical Evacuation of the Pericardial Fluid and Repair of the Traumatic Defect. This may be accomplished either by extensive pericardiectomy or by limited pericardiectomy. Total pericardiectomy is indicated when extensive exploration is required.

Alternatively, a surgical pericardial "window," made through a 3 to 4 cm subxiphoid incision, may be performed using general or local anesthesia for drainage of the pericardial space.

Recurrent, chronic effusions may be treated by repeat pericardiocentesis, surgical window, sclerosis therapy, or (more recently) a balloon catheter that makes a hole in the pericardial space large enough for drainage into the adjoining pleural space or abdominal cavity. Although the patient with drainage into the pleural space may develop pleural effusions, the pleural effusions are not life threatening and may be more easily tapped (as required) than pericardial effusions.

Table 23-2 provides a summary of the anticipated direction of change in hemodynamic measurements in patients with severe cardiomyopathy or pericardial disease.

TABLE 23-2
Guidelines to Anticipated Hemodynamic Changes in Patients with Severe Cardiomyopathy and Pericardial Disease

Disorder	Arterial Pressure	Pulse Pressure	Systemic Vascular Resistance	Pulmonary Vascular Resistance	Central Venous Pressure	Pulmonary Artery Pressure	Pulmonary Wedge Pressure	Cardiac Output	Svo$_2$
Dilated cardiomyopathy	~	↓	↑	↑	↑	↑	↑	↓	↓
Hypertrophic cardiomyopathy	~	~	~	~	~	~	↑	~↓	~
Restrictive cardiomyopathy	↓	↓	↑	↑	↑	↑	↑	↓	↓
Constrictive pericarditis	~↓	↓	↑	~	↑	↑	↑	↓	↓
Pericardiac tamponade	~↓	↓	↑	~	↑	↑	↑	↓	↓

KEY: ↑ increase, ↓ decrease, ~ normal or no change.

Note: The magnitude of the direction of change is affected by the severity of the defect, as well as by coexisting factors or complications, such as hypovolemia.

REFERENCES

1. Effectiveness of spironolactone added to an angiotensin-converting enzyme inhibitor and a loop diuretic for severe chronic congestive heart failure (the Randomized Aldactone Evaluation Study [RALES], *Am J Cardiol* 78(8):902, 1996.

2. Pitt B, Poole-Wilson PA, Segal R, et al: Randomized trial of losartan versus captopril on mortality in patients with symptomatic heart failure, *Lancet* 355:1582, 2000.

3. Louis A, Cleland JG, Crabbe S, et al: Clinical trials update: CAPRICORN, COPERNICUS, MIRACLE, STAF, RITZ-2, RECOVER, and RENAISSANCE and cachexia and cholesterol in heart failure: highlights of the Scientific Sessions of the American College of Cardiology, 2001, *Lancet* 357:1385, 2001.

4. Eichhorn EJ et al: Effect of beta-adrenergic blockade on myocardial function and energetics in congestive heart failure, *Circulation* 82:473, 1990.

5. Engelmeier RS et al: Improvements in symptoms and exercise tolerance by metoprolol in patients with dilated cardiomyopathy: a double-blind, randomized, placebo-controlled trial, *Circulation* 3:536, 1985.

6. Gilbert EM et al: Long term beta-blocker vasodilator therapy improves cardiac function in idiopathic dilated cardiomyopathy: a double blind, randomized study of bucindolol versus placebo, *Am J Med* 88:223, 1990.

7. Waagstein F et al: Beta-blockers in cardiomyopathies: they work, *Eur Heart J* 4:173, 1983.

8. Woodley SL et al: Beta-blockade with bucindolol in heart failure caused by ischemic versus idiopathic dilated cardiomyopathy, *Circulation* 84:2426, 1991.

9. Dargie HJ: Effect of carvedilol on outcome after myocardial infarction in patients with left ventricular dysfunction: the CAPRICORN randomised trial, *Lancet* 357:1385, 2001.

10. Packer M, Coats AJ, Fowler MB, et al: Effect of carvedilol on survival in severe chronic heart failure, *N Engl J Med* 344:1651, 2001.

11. Cazeau S, Leclercq C, Lavergne T, et al: Effects of multisite biventricular pacing in patients with heart failure and intraventricular conduction delay, *N Engl J Med* 344:873, 2001.

12. *Multicenter InSync Randomized Clinical Evaluation*, unpublished results presented at European Society of Cardiology meeting in Stockholm, September 2001.

13. Maron BJ, Bonow RO, Cannon RO III, et al: Hypertrophic cardiomyopathy: interrelations of clinical manifestations, pathophysiology, and therapy—part II, *N Engl J Med* 316:844, 1987.

14. Maron BJ, Epstein SE, Morrow AG: Symptomatic status and prognosis of patients after operation for hypertrophic obstructive cardiomyopathy: efficacy of ventricular septal myotomy and myectomy, *Eur Heart J* 4(suppl F):175, 1983.

15. Chevalier P, Moncada E, Canu G, et al: Symptomatic pericardial disease associated with patch electrodes of the automatic implantable cardioverter defibrillator: an underestimated complication? *Pacing Clin Electrophysiol* 19:2150, 1996.

SUGGESTED READINGS
General

Felker MG, Hu W, Hare JM, et al: The spectrum of dilated cardiomyopathy. the Johns Hopkins experience with 1,278 patients, *Medicine* 78:270, 1999.

Goodwin JF: The frontiers of cardiomyopathy, *Br Heart J* 48:1, 1982.

Goodwin JF: Cardiomyopathies and specific heart muscle diseases. Definitions, terminology, classifications and new and old approaches, *Postgrad Med J* 618(suppl):S3, 1992.

MacLellan WR. Advances in molecular mechanisms of heart failure, *Curr Opin Cardiol* 15:128, 2000.

Mohr R, Schaff H, Danielson GK: The outcome of surgical treatment for hypertrophic obstructive cardiomyopathy: experience over 15 years, *J Thorac Cardiovasc Surg* 97:666, 1998.

Roberts WC, Ferrans VJ: Morphologic observations in the cardiomyopathies. In Fowler NO, editor: *Myocardial diseases,* New York, 1973, Grune & Stratton.

Shabetai R: Cardiomyopathy: how far have we come in 25 years, how far yet to go? *J Am Coll Cardiol* 1:252, 1983.

Dilated Cardiomyopathy

American college of cardiology consensus conference report: Mechanical cardiac support 2000: current applications and future trial design, *J Am Coll Cardiol* 37:340, 2001.

Batista RJV, Verde J, Nery P, et al: Partial left ventriculectomy to treat end-stage heart failure, *Ann Thorac Surg* 64:634, 1997.

Blanc P, Girard C, Vedrinne C, et al: Latissimus dorsi cardiomyoplasty. Perioperative management and postoperative evolution, *Chest* 103:214, 1993.

Captopril Digoxin Multicenter Research Group: Comparative effects of therapy with captopril and digoxin in patients with mild to moderate heart failure, *JAMA* 259:539, 1988.

Constanzo MR, Augostine S, Bourge R, et al: Selection and treatment of candidates for heart transplantation. A statement for health professionals from the Committee on Heart Failure and Cardiac Transplantation of the Council on Clinical Cardiology, American Heart Association, *Circulation* 92:3593, 1995.

Diaz RA, Obasohan A, Oakley CM: Prediction of outcome in dilated cardiomyopathy, *Br Heart J* 58:393, 1987.

Duchman SM, Thohan V, Kalra D, et al: Endothelin-1: a new target of therapeutic intervention for treatment of heart failure, *Curr Opin Cardiol* 15:136, 2000.

Farmer JA. Renin angiotensin system and ASCVD, *Curr Opin Cardiol* 15:141, 2000.

Figulla HR, Kellerman AB, Stille-Siegener M, et al: Significance of coronary angiography, left heart catheterization, and endomyocardial biopsy for the diagnosis of idiopathic dilated cardiomyopathy, *Am Heart J* 124:1251, 1992.

Fowler MB: Controlled trials with beta blockers in heart failure: metoprolol as the prototype, *Am J Cardiol* 71:45C, 1993.

Fuster V, Gersh BJ, Guiliani ER, et al: The natural history of idiopathic dilated cardiomyopathy, *Am J Cardiol* 47:525, 1981.

Gaudio C, Tanzilli G, Mazzarotto P, et al: Comparison of left ventricular ejection fraction by magnetic resonance imaging and radionuclide ventriculography in idiopathic dilated cardiomyopathy, *Am J Cardiol* 67:411, 1991.

Gilbert EM et al: Beta-adrenergic receptor regulation and left ventricular function in idiopathic dilated cardiomyopathy, *Am J Cardiol* 71:23C, 1993.

Guyatt GH, Sullivan MJJ, Fallen EL, et al: A controlled trial of digoxin in congestive heart failure, *Am J Cardiol* 61:371, 1988.

Hardy CJ et al: Altered myocardial high-energy phosphate metabolites in patients with dilated cardiomyopathy, *Am Heart J* 122:795, 1991.

Johnson RA, Palacios I: Dilated cardiomyopathy of the adult, *N Engl J Med* 307:1051, 1982.

Kelly TL et al: Prediction of outcome in late-stage cardiomyopathy, *Am Heart J* 119:1111, 1990.

Keogh AM et al: Timing of cardiac transplantation in idiopathic dilated cardiomyopathy, *Am J Cardiol* 61:418, 1988.

Magovern JA, Furnary AP, Christlieb IY, et al: Right latissimus dorsi cardiomyoplasty for left ventricular failure, *Ann Thorac Surg* 53:1120, 1992.

Manolio TA, Baughman KL, Rodeheffer R, et al: Prevalence and etiology of idiopathic dilated cardiomyopathy (summary of a National Heart, Lung, and Blood Institute workshop), *Am J Cardiol* 69:1458, 1992.

Olshausen KV, Stienen U, Math D, et al: Long-term prognostic significance of ventricular arrhythmias in idiopathic dilated cardiomyopathy, *Am J Cardiol* 61:146, 1988.

Packer M: Vasodilator and inotropic drugs for the treatment of chronic heart failure: distinguishing hype from hope, *J Am Coll Cardiol* 12:1299, 1988.

Packer M, Bristow MR, Cohn JN, et al: The effect of carvedilol on morbidity and mortality in patients with chronic heart failure, *N Engl J Med* 334:1349, 1996.

Pitt B, Zannad F, Remme WJ, et al: The effect of spironolactone on morbidity and mortality in patients with severe heart failure, *N Engl J Med* 341:709, 1999.

Poll DS, Marchlinski FE, Buxton AE, et al: Sustained ventricular tachycardia in patients with idiopathic dilated cardiomyopathy: electrophysiologic testing and lack of response to antiarrhythmic drug therapy, *Circulation* 70:451, 1984.

Richardson PJ, Why HJ, Archard LC: Virus infection and dilated cardiomyopathy, *Postgrad Med J* 68(suppl 1):17, 1992.

Roberts WC, Siegel RJ, McManus BM: Idiopathic dilated cardiomyopathy: analysis of 152 necropsy patients, *Am J Cardiol* 60:1340, 1987.

Sugrue DD, Rodeheffer RJ, Codd MB, et al: The clinical course of idiopathic dilated cardiomyopathy. A population-based study, *Ann Intern Med* 117:117, 1992.

Swedberg K: Initial experience with beta blockers in dilated cardiomyopathy, *Am J Cardiol* 71:30C, 1993.

Swedberg K et al: Beneficial effects of long-term beta-blockade in congestive cardiomyopathy, *Br Heart J* 44:117, 1980.

Tavel ME: Problem of management of obstructive cardiomyopathy, *Chest* 101:558, 1992.

Unverferth DV, Magorien RD, Moeschberg ML, et al: Factors influencing the one-year mortality of dilated cardiomyopathy, *Am J Cardiol* 54:147, 1984.

Volpe M, Tritto C, DeLuca N, et al: Angiotensin converting enzyme inhibition restores cardiac and hormonal responses to volume overload in patients with dilated cardiomyopathy, *Circulation* 86:1800, 1992.

Wang RY et al: Alcohol abuse in patients with dilated cardiomyopathy. Laboratory vs clinical detection, *Arch Intern Med* 150:1079, 1990.

Hypertrophic Cardiomyopathy

Aron LA, Hertzeanu HL, Fisman EZ, et al: Prognosis of nonobstructive hypertrophic cardiomyopathy, *Am J Cardiol* 67:215, 1991.

Bonow RO, Dilsizian V, Rosing DR, et al: Verapamil-induced improvement in left ventricular diastolic filling and increased exercise tolerance in patients with hypertrophic cardiomyopathy: short and long-term effects, *Circulation* 72:853, 1985.

Braunwald E, Lambrew CT, Morrow AG, et al: Idiopathic hypertrophic subaortic stenosis, *Circulation* 30:1, 1964.

Chan WL et al: Effect of preload change on resting and exercise cardiac performance in hypertrophic cardiomyopathy, *Am J Cardiol* 66:746, 1990.

Cohn LH, Trehan H, Collins JJ Jr: Long-term follow-up of patients undergoing myotomy/myectomy for obstructive hypertrophic cardiomyopathy, *Am J Cardiol* 70:657, 1992.

Criley JM, Siegel RJ: Has "obstruction" hindered our understanding of hypertrophic cardiomyopathy? *Circulation* 72:1148, 1985.

Epstein SE, Rosing DR: Verapamil: its potential for causing serious complications in patients with hypertrophic cardiomyopathy, *Circulation* 64:437, 1981.

Grose R et al: Production of left ventricular cavitary obliteration in normal man, *Circulation* 64:448, 1981.

Koga Y, Kihara K, Yamaguchi R, et al: Therapeutic effect of oral dipyridamole on myocardial perfusion and cardiac performance in patients with hypertrophic cardiomyopathy, *Am Heart J* 123:433, 1992.

Lakkis NM, Nagueh SF, Kleiman SF, et al: Echocardiography-guided ethanol septal reduction for hypertrophic obstructive cardiomyopathy, *Circulation* 98:1750, 1998.

Lorell BH, Paulus WJ, Grossman W, et al: Modification of abnormal left ventricular diastolic properties by nifedipine in patients with hypertrophic cardiomyopathy, *Circulation* 65:499, 1982.

Maron BJ, Bonow RO, Cannon RO III, et al: Hypertrophic cardiomyopathy: interrelations of clinical manifestations, pathophysiology and therapy, *N Engl J Med* 316:780, 1987.

Maron BJ, Olivotto I, Spirito P, et al: Epidemiology of hypertrophic cardiomyopathy-related death: revision of large non-referral-based population, *Circulation* 102:858, 2000.

Maron BJ, Shen WK, Link MS, et al: Efficacy of implantable cardioverter-defibrillator for the prevention of sudden death in patients with hypertrophic cardiomyopathy, *N Engl J Med* 342:365, 2000.

Messerli FH: Left ventricular hypertrophy: impact of calcium channel blocker therapy, *Am J Med* 90:27S, 1991.

Murgo JP, Alter BR, Dorethy JF, et al: Dynamics of left ventricular ejection in obstructive and nonobstructive hypertrophic cardiomyopathy, *J Clin Invest* 66:1369, 1980.

Roberts CS, Gertz SD, Klues HG, et al: Appearance of or persistence of severe mitral regurgitation without left ventricular outflow obstruction after partial ventricular septal myotomy-myectomy in hypertrophic cardiomyopathy, *Am J Cardiol* 68:1726, 1991.

Sanderson JE et al: Left ventricular filling in hypertrophic cardiomyopathy: an angiographic study, *Br Heart J* 39:661, 1977.

Siegel RJ, Criley JM: Comparison of ventricular emptying with and without a pressure gradient in patients with hypertrophic cardiomyopathy, *Br Heart J* 53:283, 1985.

Spirito P, Bellone P, Harris KM, et al: Magnitude of left ventricular hypertrophy and risk of sudden death in hypertrophic cardiomyopathy, *N Engl J Med* 342:1778, 2000.

Restrictive Cardiomyopathy

Appleton CP, Hatle LK, Popp RL: Demonstration of restrictive ventricular physiology by Doppler echocardiography, *J Am Coll Cardiol* 11:757, 1988.

Benotti JR, Grossman W, Cohn PF: Clinical profile of restrictive cardiomyopathy, *Circulation* 61:6, 1980.

Cutler DJ, Isner JM, Bracey AW, et al: Hemochromatosis heart disease: an unemphasized cause of potentially reversible restrictive cardiomyopathy, *Am J Med* 69:923, 1980.

Fattori R, Rocchi G, Celleti F, et al: Contribution of magnetic resonance imaging in the differential diagnosis of cardiac amyloidosis and symmetric hypertrophic cardiomyopathy, *Am Heart J* 136:824, 1998.

Meaney E, Shabetai R, Bhargana V, et al: Cardiac amyloidosis, constrictive pericarditis and restrictive cardiomyopathy, *Am J Cardiol* 38:547, 1976.

Pellikka PA, Holmes DR Jr, Edwards WD, et al: Endomyocardial biopsy in 30 patients with primary amyloidosis and suspected cardiac involvement, *Arch Intern Med* 148:662, 1988.

Plehn JF, Friedman BJ: Diastolic dysfunction in amyloid heart disease: restrictive cardiomyopathy or not? *J Am Coll Cardiol* 13:54, 1989.

Shebetai R: Controversial issues in restrictive cardiomyopathy, *Postgrad Med J* 68(suppl):S47, 1992.

Siegel RJ, Shah PK, Fishbein MC: Idiopathic restrictive cardiomyopathy, *Circulation* 70:165, 1984.

Pericardial Disease

Atar S, Chiu J, Forrester JS, et al: Bloody pericardial effusion in patients with cardiac tamponade: is the cause cancerous, tuberculous, or iatrogenic in the 1990s? *Chest* 116:1564, 1999.

Bush CA et al: Occult constrictive pericardial disease: diagnosis by rapid volume expansion and correction by pericardiectomy, *Circulation* 56:924, 1977.

Guberman B, Fowler NO, Engel PJ, et al: Cardiac tamponade in medical patients, *Circulation* 664:633, 1981.

Hirschmann JV: Pericardial constriction, *Am Heart J* 96:110, 1978.

Nishimura RA et al: Constrictive pericarditis: assessment of current diagnostic procedures, *Mayo Clin Proc* 60:397, 1985.

Pandian NG, Brockway B, Simonetti J, et al: Pericardiocentesis under two-dimensional echocardiographic guidance in loculated pericardial effusion, *Ann Thorac Surg* 45:99, 1988.

Sagrista-Sauleda J, Permanyer-Miralda G, Soler-Soler J: Tuberculous pericarditis: ten year experience with a prospective protocol for diagnosis and treatment, *J Am Coll Cardiol* 11:724, 1988.

Shabetai R, Fowler NO, Guntheroth WG: The hemodynamics of cardiac tamponade and constrictive pericarditis, *Am J Cardiol* 26:479, 1970.

Spodick DH: The normal and diseased pericardium: current concepts of pericardial physiology, diagnosis and treatment, *J Am Coll Cardiol* 1:240, 1983.

Vaitkus PT, Kussmaul WG: Constrictive pericarditis versus restrictive cardiomyopathy: a reappraisal and update of diagnostic criteria, *Am Heart J* 122:1431, 1991.

Additional Reading of General Interest

Criley JM, Siegel RJ: The patient with known or suspected cardiomyopathy. In Pepine CJ, editor: *Diagnostic and therapeutic cardiac catheterization,* Baltimore, 1989, Williams & Wilkins.

Grossman W: Profiles in dilated (congestive) and hypertrophic cardiomyopathies. In Grossman W, Baim DS, editors: *Cardiac catheterization, angiography, and intervention,* Philadelphia, 1991, Lea & Febiger.

Lorell BH, Grossman W: Profiles in constrictive pericarditis, restrictive cardiomyopathy and cardiac tamponade. In Grossman W, Baim DS, editors: *Cardiac catheterization, angiography, and intervention,* Philadelphia, 1991, Lea & Febiger.

Wenger NK, Abelmann WH, Roberts WC: Cardiomyopathy and specific heart muscle disease. In Hurst JW, editor: *The heart,* ed 7, New York, 1990, McGraw-Hill.

Wynne J, Braunwald E: The cardiomyopathies and myocarditis: toxic, chemical and physical damage to the heart. In Braunwald E, editor: *Heart disease: textbook of cardiovascular medicine,* Philadelphia, 1992, W.B. Saunders.

24

ROBERT J. MARCH, DONNA STEL, and GLORIA OBLOUK DAROVIC

Monitoring the Patient Following Open Heart Surgery

HISTORICAL PERSPECTIVE

Ancient physicians believed the living heart to be sacred and untouchable. They also observed that wounds of the heart were nearly always fatal. Consequently, throughout history, it was believed to be ill advised, if not impossible, to surgically repair a beating heart. Christian Albert Billroth, the great surgical innovator of the late nineteenth century, warned, "a surgeon who tries to suture a heart wound deserves to lose the esteem of his colleagues."[1] Despite Billroth's admonition, the first case of successful suture repair of a cardiac wound was reported at the turn of the twentieth century. Thus the era of cardiac surgery began and brought the hope for a longer and improved life to countless people suffering from disease or deformities of the heart and its circulation.

Several landmarks are provided that tell the story of cardiovascular surgery. More could be discussed, but the 14 chosen are those that were so innovative and pivotal that special attention must be given to them. They are listed in approximate chronologic order, although many occurred nearly simultaneously.

- **1896.** Ludwig Rehn performed the first successful surgical repair of torn myocardium and subsequently performed suture repair of 124 cardiac wounds.[2]
- **1920s to 1940s.** "Closed" cardiac valve repair, such as valvulotomy using a valvulotome or commissurotomy, was developed and introduced to palliate stenotic valve defects.
- **1946.** Arthur Vineberg performed the first successful myocardial revascularization procedure. Vineberg im-

planted an internal mammary artery, distally dissected from the chest wall and bleeding from its side branches, into a surgically created myocardial tunnel.[3] This implanted vessel ultimately perfuses ischemia-jeopardized myocardium by developing anastomosis with the coronary circulation.

- **1947.** Zimmerman, Scott, and Becker developed the technique that enabled them to catheterize the left side of the heart.[4] This allows assessment of preoperative left ventricular function, a diagnostically valuable and important predictor of surgical risk and outcome.
- **1951.** Charles Hufnagel placed a ball-valve prosthesis in the descending thoracic aorta.[5] The extracardiac approach for aortic valve replacement was used because, at that time, there was no method available to work within the beating heart.
- **1953.** John Gibbon developed and introduced a pump-oxygenator to divert blood from the heart and was then able to successfully close an atrial septal defect.[6] The landmark introduction of *cardiopulmonary bypass* now allows surgeons to stop the heart safely, thereby allowing the time and a motionless heart for the definitive correction of cardiac or coronary artery lesions.
- **1962.** Bahnson and Hufnagel developed a single-leaflet valve prosthesis, and in 1961 Albert Starr successfully replaced a mitral valve.[7] Total valve replacement makes possible the prolongation of life and improvement in the quality of life for patients with calcific, regurgitant, or complex (regurgitant and stenotic) valve defects.

- **1962.** Mason Sones, at the Cleveland Clinic, developed selective coronary arteriography.[8] Before his contribution, diagnosis of coronary artery disease was based on the presence of chest pain and suspected electrocardiograph (ECG) changes, neither of which is diagnostically reliable or lesion specific. Coronary angiography provides the surgeon with accurate preoperative knowledge of the extent and sites of coronary lesions. Coronary angiography also allows postoperative evaluation of myocardial revascularization procedures.
- **1964.** Michael DeBakey used a saphenous vein to bypass an obstructive coronary arterosclerotic lesion.[9]
- **The late 1960s.** Rene Favaloro and Dudley Johnson refined techniques by utilizing vein conduits to bypass an obstructive lesion from the root of the aorta to a coronary arterial site distal to the plaque (aortocoronary bypass). Newer conduits used today include gastroepiploic arteries, inferior epigastric arteries, cephalic veins, and cadaver veins.[10,11]
- **The 1960s.** Norman Shumway and co-workers at Stanford University did invaluable research in cardiac transplantation. Techniques of myocardial preservation, physiologic response to cardiac denervation, and course and modification of recipient rejection paved the way to the first cardiac transplantation. The introduction in 1970 of cyclosporin A improved long-term survival in heart transplants by dramatically increasing the control of rejection. Cyclosporin A also led to the success of all other tissue transplants.[12]
- **The 1960s.** Mouloupoulos developed the intraaortic balloon pump, and Buckley refined its clinical application in the management of the cardiac surgical patient.[13] The counterpulsation device facilitates weaning from cardiopulmonary bypass and assists surgically stunned and failing hearts in the immediate postoperative period. The intraaortic balloon pump also may be inserted preoperatively to help stabilize the condition of patients during the induction of anesthesia.
- **1967.** Christian Barnard performed the first human heart transplant. This procedure is now established as the treatment of choice for end-stage ischemic and nonischemic cardiomyopathy for patients under age 65.[14]
- **1980s.** Surgical treatment of supraventricular and ventricular arrhythmias was introduced. Direct ablation by surgical incisions or cryoblation of an irritable myocardial focus or foci is one of the newest and fastest growing aspect of cardiac surgery. Implantable cardioverters/defibrillators have been invaluable therapeutic additions to this field.

Over the past 100 years, the art and science of cardiac surgery has expanded exponentially in both the number of cases performed and the complexity and sophistication of the surgical procedures. More than 100 years after the first surgical cardiac repair, there is no acquired cardiac lesion that cannot be surgically corrected or palliated.

This chapter briefly discusses preoperative evaluation, indications, and preparation of the patient who is about to undergo open heart surgery, as well as preparation of the patient's family. The remainder of the chapter focuses on postoperative hemodynamic and clinical assessment, as well as on the management of the major disturbances in organ system function in patients having had major cardiac surgical procedures.

PREOPERATIVE EVALUATION

Assessment of the patient begins with a meticulously obtained history and physical examination. The patient's story details the chronicity or acuteness of the presenting problem and thus determines the need for an immediate or delayed workup.

Routine laboratory tests, electrocardiogram, chest radiographs, exercise stress electrocardiogram, coronary angiography, cardiac catheterization, echocardiogram, and possibly electrophysiology studies help define the patient's hemodynamic and physiologic profile. When this information is gathered, the treatment format and urgency of definitive therapy can be identified.

Indications

The current indications for valvular surgery, myocardial revascularization, cardiac transplantation, and surgical intervention for arrhythmias are outlined.

Valvular Surgery

A discussion of cause, hemodynamic effects, clinical findings, diagnostic evaluation, and management of patients with left heart valve disease and tricuspid regurgitation appears in Chapter 21.

Mitral Stenosis. The normal cross-sectional area of the mitral valve orifice is 4 to 6 cm². Significant hemodynamic changes occur when the valve orifice is reduced to 2.0 to 2.5 cm². When the area drops below 1.5 cm² to 1 cm², the patient becomes symptomatic at rest; 0.5 cm² is the smallest valve area compatible with life.

The clinical indications for valve surgery are episodes of pulmonary edema, pulmonary artery pressures greater than about 40/20 mm Hg, right ventricular failure, secondary tricuspid regurgitation, or systemic embolization. The physiologic measurements corresponding to the clinical indications are a valve area less than 1.5 cm², even if the patient is asymptomatic, and a mean left atrial pressure (pulmonary artery wedge pressure [PWP]) exceeding 30 mm Hg.

Mitral Regurgitation. Patients with chronic, asymptomatic mitral regurgitation should be followed for clinical signs of heart failure such as shortness of breath, weakness, and fatigability. Echocardiography scheduled every 6 months to 1 year, unless a change in symptoms occurs, is helpful in detecting increased diameter of the left ventricle.

When ventricular dysfunction and dilation develop in a patient with chronic mitral regurgitation, the clinical course quickly deteriorates. Because a significant portion of ventricular dysfunction is irreversible, the patient should not be allowed to experience severe heart failure before the valve is replaced. Because surgical treatment has become safer than in the past, it is indicated as soon as the patient becomes symptomatic or the laboratory documentation of ventricular dysfunction and dilation is positive.

Aortic Stenosis. The development of symptoms such as angina, weakness, fatigue, shortness of breath, and light-headedness is an indication for rapidly scheduled elective surgery. Classic teaching states that significant clinical symptoms do not develop until the normal valve area of 3 cm^2 is reduced to 0.5 cm^2, or until a pressure gradient greater than 70 mm Hg exists across the aortic valve. However, a lower pressure gradient may be associated with a significantly reduced valve area if there is a significant decrease in left ventricular ejection fraction.

Determinants of operative risk include overt heart failure. A pulmonary artery systolic pressure exceeding 100 mm Hg has been associated with increased risk of sudden death, and patients with this condition should undergo surgery as soon as possible (within days). If the patient can be fully anticoagulated postoperatively, a prosthetic mechanical valve is used for replacement. Otherwise, a tissue valve is placed, and, after 3 months, anticoagulation with warfarin sodium (Coumadin) can be discontinued. Mechanical aortic valves require lifelong anticoagulation with Coumadin plus low-dose aspirin (81 mg daily).

Aortic Regurgitation. Until recently, surgery was indicated primarily on a clinical basis—increased heart size on echocardiogram or chest radiograph, increased heart failure despite adequate medical therapy, and angina pectoris. Because valve replacement has become such a safe and well-established procedure, we recommend surgery before these signs or symptoms appear to minimize irreversible left ventricular muscle damage and dysfunction.

Coronary Artery Disease

The gold standard for diagnosis of coronary artery disease remains coronary angiography. Indications for coronary angiography include sudden-onset angina, crescendo angina, postinfarction angina, and coexisting development of heart failure. Medical management is the therapy of choice for single-vessel disease. If one or two coronary arteries have 70% or greater blockage, balloon angioplasty or atherectomy is considered. Aortocoronary bypass is reserved for patients with triple-vessel disease (particularly when the ejection fraction is less than 35%), left main or right ostial coronary disease, failed angioplasty, and unstable angina, as well as for those needing concomitant cardiac surgery, such as valve replacement. If, however, the patient has severe two-vessel disease (90% to 100% occlusion) and is symptomatic, surgical revascularization may be undertaken.

Cardiac Transplantation

Cardiac transplantation is indicated for end-stage cardiac disease no longer responsive to medical therapy. The two most common etiologies are ischemic and nonischemic cardiomyopathies.

Long-term survival for orthotopic heart transplant patients has improved steadily. Currently, at Rush–Presbyterian–St. Luke's Medical Center, 1-year patient survival is approximately 90%, and the 5-year survival is approximately 70%.

Arrhythmia Surgery

The *supraventricular arrhythmias* that have been treated surgically include Wolff-Parkinson-White pathways, atrioventricular node reentrant pathways, and primary atrial tachyarrhythmias. Although these arrhythmias have been treated successfully with surgery in more than 95% of cases, the majority of patients are treated without surgery using radiofrequency ablation of the atrioventricular node in the electrophysiology laboratory followed by pacemaker insertion.

Ventricular arrhythmias, however, are increasingly treated by surgical intervention. Drug therapy has a high failure rate. Failure of pharmacologic therapy in this group of patients is typically and unfortunately primarily manifested as sudden death. Three modes of surgical intervention are currently available: surgical ablation, antitachycardia pacing, and automatic implantable cardioverter/defibrillator.

Patients who are considered for *surgical ablation* have a monomorphic tachycardia; an ejection fraction of 30% or more; and, in most cases, a distinct ventricular aneurysm. The procedure currently done in our institution is endocardial resection with cryoblation as directed by intraoperative myocardial mapping. Candidates for *antitachycardia pacing* have monomorphic tachycardia, and they can be reproducibly "paced out" of this rhythm in the electrophysiology laboratory. The most common surgical treatment today is the *implantable cardioverter/defibrillator.* The current criteria for its use include presence of all left ventricular ejection fractions, drug failure, and presence of multiple monomorphic or polymorphic tachycardias causing syncope or cardiac arrest.

The group of patients with ventricular arrhythmias represents a double-edged management sword for medical and nursing personnel. The first edge is that most patients have depressed left ventricular ejection fractions, commonly below 35%. This finding portends hemodynamic compromise in the perioperative period. The second edge is that the ventricular arrhythmias may be very unstable in the perioperative period and may require multiple cardioversions or defibrillations. Inotropic support of the heart; use of the intraaortic balloon pump; and administration of antiarrhythmic medications, such as procainamide (Pronestyl), amiodarone, and lidocaine (Xylocaine), may be required postoperatively.

PREOPERATIVE PREPARATION OF THE PATIENT AND FAMILY

The reality of impending open heart surgery is often perceived as overwhelming to the patient and family because people generally think of the heart as the essence of life, as well as the seat of emotions. Patient and family response to imminent surgery may be fear, anxiety, anger, disbelief, depression, isolation, and, paradoxically, hope and anticipated relief that incapacitating chest pain will be relieved or disability minimized or eliminated.

The intensity of emotional responses may be minimized, although never eliminated, by encouraging the patient and family to talk about their feelings and by patiently and simply (in nontechnical language) answering all questions.

Patient and Family Teaching

Knowledge of what is about to happen helps dispel the insecurity and fear that comes with facing the unknown. Patients are advised about their postoperative circumstances and about how it will feel on awakening in the recovery area. The need for possible continued endotracheal intubation and ventilatory support is discussed. Patients are informed that speech will not be possible until the tube is removed, but they will be able to communicate by writing notes. They can be assured that the tube can be

removed as they awake and become aware of it. Other support and monitoring devices that may be used are discussed. Very simply, their purpose is described. It should be stressed to the patient and family that life is *not* dependent on these devices but that these devices lend support to or monitor the patient only.

If soft wrist restraints are routinely applied at your institution, the rationale for their use and the fact that they will be removed as soon as possible should be discussed. The patient should be made aware of the availability of pain medication and told that analgesics may be given at the patient's request or on the discretion of the staff. When possible, the patient and family are taken to the open heart surgery recovery area to be shown the equipment and introduced to the intensive care team. The preoperative establishment of "personal anchors" with the staff may minimize patient and family anxiety.

The clinician must remember to honor the sanctity and needs of the human being. If denial is manifest by preoccupation with seemingly irrelevant issues or by an apparently distracted appearance during instruction, teaching should not be forced on patients "for their own good." Denial may be the only coping mechanism available to the patient.

POSTOPERATIVE MANAGEMENT

Factors Affecting the Postoperative Course

The patient's physiologic and hemodynamic status following cardiac surgery is related to three major factors:

1. The completeness of repair of the cardiac or coronary defect
2. The intraoperative course as determined by the patient's response to induction of anesthesia, duration and type of anesthesia, duration of aortic cross-clamp "ischemic time," duration of cardiopulmonary bypass "pump time," and any unexpected findings during the course of the procedure
3. The degree of preexisting dysfunction; the urgency of the procedure; the reserve of major organ systems; and the individual patient's constitution, history, sex, and age (Table 24-1)

To effectively manage the course of the postoperative cardiac surgical patient's recovery and to achieve the best possible outcome, knowledge of the presence, severity, and effects of preexisting disease; understanding of the physiologic abnormalities inherent to cardiopulmonary bypass and major surgery; consideration of intraoperative time and course; and knowledge of appropriate supportive and corrective therapies are essential.

TABLE 24-1
Patient Risk Factors for Cardiac Surgery

Overall, patients undergoing cardiac surgery within the last 10 to 15 years tend to be older, with more chronic diseases, and have greater severity of heart failure and coronary artery disease.

Risk	Comment
Left ventricular dysfunction	Variables that reflect left ventricular dysfunction include the following: 1. An ejection fraction less than 50% 2. A left ventricular end-diastolic pressure (PWP) greater than 20 mm Hg 3. A cardiothoracic ratio greater than 0.50
Advanced age	Morbidity and mortality rates increase in patients older than 70 years of age
Female gender	At any age, operative mortality rate is higher in women due to smaller body habitus and target vessel size and later referral for cardiologic testing (possibly due to atypical symptoms)
Extent and severity of coronary artery disease	Particularly patients with left main coronary artery stenosis greater than 70% with a left dominant circulation
Urgency of surgery and preoperative stability	The preoperative presence of pulmonary edema, cardiogenic shock, and unstable preoperative angina pectoris adversely alters postoperative morbidity and mortality rates
Preoperative use of platelet inhibitors or abnormalities in the coagulation or fibrinolytic mechanisms	It is recommended that aspirin be discontinued 10 days before surgery Other antiplatelet agents such as dipyridamole and nonsteroidal antiinflammatory agents should be discontinued 72 hours before surgery There is slightly higher incidence of postoperative bleeding in patients with cyanotic heart disease or right heart failure, presumably due to hepatic congestion resulting in impaired synthesis of clotting factors Congenital clotting deficiencies should be defined and corrected preoperatively by blood component replacement therapy In patients predisposed to postoperative bleeding, the blood bank should be informed several days before the operation so that appropriate blood component therapy (platelets, fresh frozen plasma, cryoprecipitate) can be made available Fibrinolytic deficiencies such as antithrombin (heparin cofactor) deficiency should be identified and treated with replacement (fresh frozen plasma); otherwise, it will be difficult to anticoagulate patients for cardiopulmonary bypass or when anticoagulation is indicated postoperatively (prosthetic valve replacement)

On admission of the patient from the operating room to the recovery area, the nurse assigned to manage the patient's care should obtain a brief but thorough overview of the patient's health and intraoperative history, as well as the desired range of postoperative hemodynamic measurements (Box 24-1).

Overall, patients undergoing cardiac surgery within the last 10 to 15 years tend to be older, with more chronic diseases and greater severity of heart failure and coronary artery disease.

In this section, assessment and management of each organ system is addressed separately. Although a systems analysis approach is used to set guidelines for patient evaluation and management, caregivers must never lose sight of the fact that a sensitive human being having had open heart surgery, rather than a "valve replacement with pulmonary dysfunction" or an "aortocoronary bypass in cardiogenic shock," is in their care. The patient with excessive anxiety and fear may have increased morbidity postoperatively because of the direct effect of psychologic stress on major organ systems.

Assessment and Management of the Cardiovascular System

Pulmonary Artery Catheter versus Left Atrial Line

Before the induction of anesthesia, it is customary in our institutions to insert a pulmonary artery catheter. This facilitates the intraoperative and postoperative measurement of pulmonaary artery pressures, right

---

BOX 24-1
Clinical Assessment in the Immediate Postoperative Period

Level of consciousness, movement of extremities, symmetry of facial movement.

Skin color, temperature, capillary refill.

Dressings—intact, clean, bloody.

Peripheral pulses—strength of radial, posterior tibial, and pedal pulses.

Color, character, and amount of chest tube drainage.

Distribution and character of breath sounds.

Heart sounds—because the pericardium is left open, friction rubs are frequently present. Heart sounds tend to be muffled and difficult to auscultate. It may be possible to hear the S_1 and S_2 sounds, but it is unlikely that an atrial or ventricular gallop, if present, will be audible. The sounds made by an intraaortic balloon pump tend to obscure all other heart sounds.

Precordial movements—note position and character.

Chest wall movement—depth and symmetry.

Presence or absence of abdominal distention and bowel sounds.

Assessment of a 3-inch cardiac rhythm strip on admission, each shift, and as necessary.

Patient's history, presence of chronic lung disease, chronic hypertension, alcoholism, renal disease, etc.

Discussion of expected left ventricular performance with the surgeon and expected and desired pulmonary artery and systemic pressures.

Determination of whether there were technical problems in the operation (e.g., vessels that could not be bypassed; what was the cardiopulmonary bypass "pump" time and aortic cross-clamp "ischemic" time?).

---

atrial pressure, cardiac index, core temperature, continuous mixed venous saturation monitoring, and calculation of pulmonary and systemic vascular resistance. We prefer the pulmonary artery catheter to the left atrial line because it provides more monitoring information and it is available during the induction of anesthesia. Drawbacks to the left atrial line include the following: (1) it can be inserted only after the chest is opened; (2) it provides only limited monitoring information (left atrial pressure); (3) it holds the potential for the accidental entry of air or fibrin into the systemic circulation, which may result in brain and other major organ infarction; (4) and it poses the small risk of bleeding from the left atrial wall after removal of the catheter.

General Considerations Related to Postoperative Cardiac Function

Following open heart surgery, impaired left ventricular performance, as evidenced by a PWP (left atrial and left ventricular end-diastolic pressures) greater than 20 mm Hg and cardiac index less than 2.2 L/min/m², occurs in approximately 10% of patients. Approximately 2% of patients require temporary support with the intraaortic balloon pump. *Diastolic dysfunction,* characterized by ventricular wall stiffness and resistance of filling, is noted in all patients following cardiopulmonary bypass and may result from myocardial ischemia or edema, as well as the presence of toxic oxygen radicals. Transient, variable degrees of *systolic dysfunction* (contractile failure) also occur in all patients for the same reasons (see Chapter 20). Significant postoperative cardiac dysfunction is more likely to be present in patients in whom the preoperative ejection fraction was less than 35%, when intraoperative technical difficulties occurred, and when the aortic cross-clamp or total bypass time was prolonged.

Significant contractile failure is first manifest in the operating room by difficulty to wean the patient from cardiopulmonary bypass. Generally, a few minutes of additional support with cardiopulmonary bypass will allow the heart to recover sufficiently for weaning. When the heart is unable to sustain an adequate mean arterial pressure without the pump, inotropic support is indicated. The drugs administered include dobutamine (Dobutrex), norepinephrine (Levophed), epinephrine (Adrenalin), dopamine (Intropin), amrinone (Inocor), and Neo-Synephrine. If inotropic support fails, intraaortic balloon pumping is instituted. If, after these measures, a patient still cannot be weaned from cardiopulmonary bypass, cardiac assist devices, such as the Biomedicus biopump, are employed.

Additional factors that may precipitate or worsen the patient's low cardiac output at any time in the postoperative period include acid-base disturbances, hypoxemia, electrolyte imbalances, cardiodepressant anesthetic/sedative drugs (such as morphine sulfate or benzodiazepines), endocrine dysfunction, hypovolemia, or cardiac tamponade due to incomplete mediastinal chest tube drainage. Many of these factors are addressed later in the chapter and must be considered and rapidly investigated so that appropriate corrective therapy can be immediately instituted.

Postoperative Assessment

The patient admitted to the recovery area following open heart surgery is to be considered hemodynamically and physiologically unstable until proved otherwise. Continuous bedside vigilance is imperative for at least the initial 24 postoperative hours because life-threatening complications may occur within seconds. We recommend that a 1:1 nurse/patient ratio be maintained for the initial 8 to 12 postoperative hours. If, after that time, the patient has maintained clinical and hemodynamic stability, the nurse may be assigned another stable, nonventilator patient. Unstable patients require one-on-one patient care until they have been stable for at least 12 hours.

Parameters that assess the function of the cardiovascular system in the immediate postoperative period include continuous measurements of intraarterial and pulmonary artery pressures. (Box 24-2 has other serially monitored values.) If a good correlation between the pulmonary artery diastolic and wedge pressures is noted, the pulmonary artery diastolic pressure may be used to continuously track the left heart pressures.

Patients are physically assessed frequently; however, clinical signs of low cardiac output such as restlessness; cool, pale skin; weak peripheral pulses; poor capillary refill; and low urine output are generally difficult to evaluate in the recently admitted open heart patient. Residual anesthesia or morphine analgesia clouds evaluation of restlessness; the recent administration of potent diuretics invalidates urine output as an indicator of systemic perfusion. The vasoconstrictive responses that occur secondary to cardiopulmonary bypass, induced hypothermia, and excessive sympathetic nervous system activity and increased catecholamine levels (part of the stress response) render evaluation of skin temperature, color, and capillary refill difficult. *Any physical changes that imply patient deterioration, however, should be immediately reported and investigated.*

The patient's blood pressure may not be a reliable indicator of cardiac function. If hypotension is present (systolic pressure less than 70 to 80 mm Hg), cardiac function is generally severely impaired. If, however, the blood pressure is normal or greater than normal, cardiac output may be high, normal, or low. A normal or an elevated blood pressure may be the result of intense systemic vasoconstriction mediated by sympathetic nervous system stimulation or hypothermia. *The arterial pressure is not an infallible indicator of cardiac performance. A normal blood pressure implies, but does not guarantee, an acceptable hemodynamic status.* Serial measurements of cardiac index combined with serial measurements of left ventricular end-diastolic pressures (PWP) (construction of ventricular function curves), correlated with the patient's appearance and response to various therapeutic interventions, are more sensitive and reliable means of assessing cardiac function.

Physiologic Variables Affecting Pump Performance

The effects of afterload, preload, contractility, and heart rate and rhythm are presented, with discussion of related postoperative complications and management (see Chapter 10, section on assessment of variables in circulatory function using the pulmonary artery catheter, and Chapter 20.)

Afterload. Because performance of an impaired ventricle is exquisitely afterload dependent, careful management of afterload in the perioperative period is extremely important. *Afterload* is the resistance to right or left ventricular ejection imposed by arterial diastolic pressures and the resistance to blood flow through the two circulatory beds.

Many factors influence afterload in the perioperative period and, through their secondary effect on ventricular function, may severely compromise the patient's circulatory status. For example, circulating catecholamines and sympathetic nervous system stimulation are elevated because of physiologic and psychologic surgical stress, cardiopulmonary bypass, hypoperfusion, withdrawal or administration of beta-adrenergic blocking agents, and hypothermia. These factors predispose patients to generalized vasoconstriction, thereby increasing systemic vascular resistance and possibly blood pressure. Consequently, stroke volume decreases while heart work and myocardial oxygen consumption increase. This may predispose the patient to systemic hypoperfusion and subendocardial ischemia during the perioperative period.

Cardiopulmonary bypass also triggers activation of the kinin and complement systems as well as histamine release, which result in decreased systemic vascular resistance. If significant, generalized vasodilation may be associated with hypotension.

During the initial hours following open heart surgery, the afterload needs may suddenly change. When being

---

BOX 24-2
Serially Monitored Postoperative Values

Core temperature; heart and respiratory rate; pulmonary artery systolic, diastolic, and wedge pressures.

Chest tube drainage, urine output.

Determination every 15 minutes until stable, then every 30 minutes for 2 hours, then every hour for 24 hours. If the patient's condition becomes unstable later in the postoperative course, vital signs are taken every 15 minutes or more often, as necessary.

weaned from cardiopulmonary bypass, vasodilation occurs from the warming process and patients may become hypotensive. To increase systemic vascular resistance and arterial pressure, Neo-Synephrine, norepinephrine (Levophed), or, rarely, vasopressin is generally given. Alternatively, when the patient is cold because of premature weaning, the systemic vascular resistance may be high, and, consequently, the cardiac index is low. In this situation, the patient is rewarmed with hyperthermia blankets, warming lights, or reflective insulated blankets. As the systemic circulation dilates and the impedance to ventricular ejection is relieved, cardiac index and systemic blood flow improve. The expanded size of the systemic circulatory bed, however, may require volume loading to maintain an acceptable cardiac index and mean arterial pressure.

The most critical group needing meticulous afterload management is those patients with ejection fractions of less than 35%. It is not unusual for these patients to have a systemic vascular resistance that is twice normal and a cardiac output one half its potential. Pharmacologic management consists of an afterload-reducing agent such as nitroprusside (Nipride), volume loading to optimize preload for the left ventricle, and an inotrope such as dobutamine (Dobutrex) to enhance contractility. Nitroprusside should be started cautiously, at a few drops per minute (to assess the patient's hemodynamic tolerance and therapeutic response) and then carefully increased as needed. The intraaortic balloon pump also may be used for the afterload reduction and the additional benefits of increasing coronary and systemic blood flow.

Acute Postoperative Hypertension as a Cause of Increased Afterload and Other Complications. This complication usually develops immediately or within the initial 1 to 2 hours after surgery and, on an average, lasts 5 hours. Patients with a preoperative history of hypertension or preoperative propranolol (Inderal) administration seem to be more predisposed to this postoperative complication. Diagnostic criteria include a mean arterial pressure greater than 95 to 105 mm Hg and a systolic pressure greater than 130 to 140 mm Hg. Other hemodynamic measurements disclose a moderate to severe elevation in systemic vascular resistance and a normal or reduced cardiac index. Acute postoperative hypertension is estimated to occur in one third to two thirds of all open heart patients and tends to be more common in patients having had cardiac valve surgery.

Problems imposed by acute hypertension can be immediately life threatening or associated with permanent sequelae. These include increased capillary oozing and increased vascular shear forces, which predispose the patient to vascular or myocardial suture line bleeding or rupture. Blood pressure elevations also may result in a cerebrovascular accident. Furthermore, the inordinate increase in afterload places a proportionately higher metabolic demand on a heart newly recovering from surgical trauma. Perioperative myocardial infarction may result.

Any form of hypertension may be exacerbated by stimulation of the sympathetic nervous system, or a previously normotensive patient may be catapulted into a hypertensive state by any noxious stimulus or stress. Pressor stimuli include hypoxia, endotracheal suctioning, pain, strong emotional stimuli associated with intolerance to endotracheal intubation or mechanical ventilation, or arousal from general anesthesia. The clinician must therefore attempt to minimize or eliminate triggers to the pressor response by taking care to minimize pressor stimuli and by administering sedation and analgesia before the anticipated stimulus, such as suctioning. Intravenous morphine sulfate may be effective in reducing the blood pressure if given at the onset of hypertensive episodes precipitated by pain or arousal from anesthesia. If morphine is not immediately effective, specific antihypertensive agents include the following.

Sodium Nitroprusside (Nipride). This is the most commonly administered drug for acute postoperative hypertension because of its low side effect profile and its rapid onset and rapid cessation of action, which allow minute-by-minute drug titration. Potential weak points for this drug include the following:

1. Increase in intrapulmonary shunting noted clinically as a decrease in PaO_2 and an increase in the calculated shunt fraction. Nitroprusside has potent vasodilator effects on the pulmonary arterioles. Generalized pulmonary vasodilation may result in increased perfusion to poorly ventilated or nonventilated areas of lung.

2. Excessive drop in systemic arterial diastolic pressure and consequent reduction in coronary blood flow.

3. Difficulty in titrating the drug to an acceptable stable arterial pressure range, particularly if the patient has intravascular volume depletion. In patients who are even mildly hypovolemic, wide and potentially dangerous swings in blood pressure may occur with even minimal changes in drug dosing. Such patients should receive volume replacement.

Overall, nitroprusside in the management of postoperative hypertension mandates *vigilant* monitoring of systemic arterial pressure and careful evaluation of blood gas values.

Nitroglycerin. Nitroglycerin is less potent as an antihypertensive agent than nitroprusside, but it does not result in worsening of intrapulmonary shunting and it does have a coronary artery dilator effect. Because of its primary systemic venodilator and preload-reducing effect, patients with elevated ventricular filling pressures do particularly well with this drug. If, however, the patient also is hypovolemic, nitroglycerin administration may be associated with a precipitous drop in blood pressure.

Esmolol (Brevibloc). This beta blocker has a short half-life and may be particularly efficacious in acute hypertension triggered by excessive catecholamines. Esmolol has no effect on arterial oxygenation but decreases cardiac index by a negative inotropic effect and slowing of heart rate. Consequently, esmolol is indicated when elevated systolic pressures, tachycardia, and elevated cardiac output are present. Conversely, it is not suited for hypertensive patients in whom the cardiac index is low.

Preload. Very few cardiac surgical candidates have normal preload measurements (i.e., a right atrial pressure of 0 to 8 mm Hg for the right ventricle and PWP of 8 to 12 mm Hg for the left ventricle). The ventricular myocardium altered by ischemic or valvular disease tends to have abnormal compliance and abnormal inotropic characteristics. The one exception is the ventricle that is reversibly ischemic and noncompliant and that returns to normal function and compliance shortly after revascularization.

Preload characteristics specific to the patient's operable pathology are discussed in the following sections. Directives for specific recommended numeric preload measurements are avoided; each patient presents an individual case, and acute and chronic myocardial compliance changes may alter the ventricular volume/pressure relationship. The best preload values for patients are those that result in optimal stretching of the myofibrils and optimal stroke volume, but do not produce pulmonary edema.

Aortic Stenosis and Regurgitation. Patients with aortic stenosis have a thickened, noncompliant left ventricle, whereas patients with aortic regurgitation have a dilated, fibrosed ventricle. In both of these valve defects, requirements for an elevated end-diastolic volume continue even after surgery to maintain a normal stroke volume. A general rule is that the preload requirements immediately after surgery approximate the preanesthesia levels. For example, if a patient with aortic stenosis had preoperative wedge pressure of 23 mm Hg, the postoperative wedge pressure requirement is probably in the range of 18 to 20 mm Hg.

Mitral Stenosis. One characteristic of this valve defect is that the left ventricle musculature tends to be atrophic and the left ventricular cavity smaller than normal. This structural change is secondary to a chronically subnormal diastolic filling volume and, consequently, subnormal systolic

work. After the stenotic valve is replaced, the ventricular cavity remains small and a suddenly imposed normal filling volume is associated with a disproportionately elevated filling pressure (PWP). Consequently, the measured PWP remains nearly identical to the preoperative values. In fact, this particular group of patients also may require inotropic support for 3 to 7 days until the small, atrophic ventricle starts to enlarge and adapts to a normal filling volume. Generally, patients with mitral stenosis tolerate markedly elevated left atrial pressures without developing acute pulmonary edema because of compensatory pulmonary vascular changes that developed with progression of the valve defect (see Chapter 22, section on mitral stenosis).

If the patient has significant compensatory pulmonary arteriolar hypertrophy and hyperplasia, pulmonary vascular resistance remains elevated postoperatively. This is reflected in elevated pulmonary artery pressures and in increased pulmonary artery diastolic to wedge pressure gradient.

Mitral Regurgitation. The differences in preoperative and postoperative left atrial pressure (PWP) should be pronounced. Because the preoperative mean wedge pressure is elevated by the beat-by-beat regurgitant volume (noted in the wedge waveform as giant *v* waves), it is not unusual for the wedge pressure to drop significantly (e.g., from 25 mm Hg to 15 mm Hg) when the defective mitral valve is replaced. The pulmonary artery pressures may be less affected postoperatively than the wedge pressure. Because the ventricle is adaptively dilated, ventricular compliance continues to be abnormal postoperatively; therefore support with vasopressor drugs may be required. If the valve is repaired (not replaced), a small *v* wave may be present postoperatively. These patients may benefit from agents such as nitroprusside in the immediate postoperative period. Captopril (Capoten) may be given when the patient can take oral medications.

In the clinical context of *acute mitral regurgitation,* the pulmonary artery pressure returns to a normal value postoperatively. If, however, the left ventricle was impaired because of preexisting disease or if a large myocardial infarction is the cause of mitral regurgitation, the pulmonary artery pressures are lower than the preoperative values but remain above "standard" normal values.

Coronary Artery Disease. The optimal level of left ventricular preload is greatly influenced by the level of left ventricular function, which is best gauged by the ejection fraction. Except in patients with preinfarction ischemia and a normal left ventricle, pulmonary artery wedge pressures cannot be expected to return to normal postoperatively. A general rule is that after revascularization, the left ventricular end-diastolic pressure (PWP) is somewhat reduced, but not to the normal range of 4 to 12 mm Hg.

Cardiac Transplantation. Preload requirements are variable and are gauged for the individual patient.

Factors That May Compromise Optimal Preload. Intravascular volume depletion is a frequent cause of impaired cardiac function in the immediate postoperative period. The extent of the circulatory volume deficit depends on the adequacy of volume replacement at the end of operation, the degree of vasoconstriction present, the magnitude of the postoperative forced diuresis, and the volume of blood lost relative to the volume of fluids replaced. The factors that are related to the decreased circulating blood volume, as well as management, are discussed next.

Vascular Tone. Intense vasoconstriction resulting from sympathetic nervous stimulation, vasopressor agents, or hypothermia may mask the presence or true extent of intravascular volume depletion by maintaining arterial pressure and central circulatory pressures within an acceptable range. In other words, the size of the intravascular space may be contracted to a degree nearly proportionate to the blood volume deficit. In adult patients with chronic valvular heart disease, blood volume may be decreased and whole body venous tone may be increased during the initial 24 to 48 hours following operation. Rapid rewarming, seating the patient upright for a chest radiograph, or vasodilator therapy may suddenly unmask the previously occult hypovolemia and may result in a precipitous drop in blood pressure. Generally, a patient whose blood pressure swings widely and is difficult to control on nitroprusside (Nipride) or any vasodilator agent should be strongly considered to be hypovolemic.

Excessive Diuresis. Loop diuretics promote uncontrolled diuresis. Following the administration of loop diuretics such as furosemide (Lasix), fluid losses may greatly exceed the amount intended, predisposing the patients to significant decreases in preload. Consequently, urine flow rates should be carefully monitored within the first few hours following diuretic administration. If brisk diuresis is observed, ventricular filling pressures should be evaluated every 5 to 15 minutes. If a trend toward a significant decrease in right and left atrial pressure occurs, immediate fluid replacement should begin.

Hemorrhage. The potential for bleeding problems exists for every patient undergoing open heart surgery. Hemorrhagic risk is related to the vascular and tissue trauma from the surgical incisions, the coagulation abnormalities that result from cardiopulmonary bypass and preoperative factors (e.g., medications that increase the risk of bleeding), and the patient's baseline coagulation profile.

Patients who have had prior cardiac surgery also have an increased hemorrhagic risk because adhesions that develop between the sternum and heart are well vascularized and tend to bleed excessively when incised.

An initial preoperative evaluation should identify high-risk patients (see Table 24-1), and thus appropriate preoperative measures may be taken to reduce the risk of operative and postoperative "medical bleeding." Following open heart surgery, iatrogenic disturbances in the clotting mechanism may occur for the following reasons.

Cardiopulmonary Bypass Disturbs the Coagulation Mechanism. Bypass results in damage to the labile coagulation proteins and platelets, dilution of the clotting factors by the priming of the pump-oxygenator with nonblood solutions, reduction of the number of circulating platelets due to the adhesion of platelets to the oxygenator and pump tubing, and consumption of the coagulation factors by fibrinolytic system activation. Of these, platelet damage and dysfunction are probably the most significant and common factors predisposing patients to postoperative hemorrhage. Platelet function disturbances are proportional to the duration of the pump run and the depth of the hypothermia.

Cardiopulmonary Bypass Requires High-Dose Systemic Heparinization. This prevents clotting in the extracorporeal cardiopulmonary bypass circuit. Following cardiopulmonary bypass, the heparin effect is reversed by the administration of protamine, which binds and neutralizes heparin. Inadequate heparin neutralization or heparin rebound rarely may predispose the patient to hemorrhage. If excessive blood loss is noted in the immediate postoperative period, additional protamine may be required to return the activated clotting time to control levels.

Evaluation of Extent and Type of Bleeding. When the patient is admitted to the recovery unit, the chest tube drainage is monitored carefully. Indications for surgical reexploration include the following.

Chest tube drainage that exceeds 100 ml/hr for the first 4 to 5 hours or if the chest tube drainage totals 1000 ml. A significant fall in hematocrit (greater than 3%) or hemoglobin (1 g/dl) also may be observed. These bleeding rates exclude dark, pooled blood that may suddenly drain when the patient is positioned upright for a chest radiograph or is turned.

A patient who has chest tube drainage that stops suddenly or has diminished chest tube drainage and then has a sudden decrease in arterial pressure. In this circumstance, the patient may have cardiac tamponade and should immediately have surgical exploration. Drainage of blood may be impaired or obstructed by clotted chest tubes or by adhesions. The delayed surgical tamponade, however, is a far more common occurrence. This manifests 7 to 15 days postoperatively, most commonly in patients receiving heparin or warfarin (Coumadin). The early clinical presentation includes confusion, anxiety or restlessness, abdominal discomfort because of increased pressure in the pericardium, shortness of breath, sudden-onset supraventricular tachyarrhythmias, and general signs of low cardiac output. An emergent echocardiogram aids diagnosis followed by emergent decompression through the lower sternotomy wound.

The appropriate nursing response for a suspected tamponade is to notify the surgeon immediately and provide rapid intravenous fluid infusion to maintain ventricular filling. One critical mistake is to administer sedation for restlessness. This is because sedative agents may produce vasodilation and therefore further reduce any blood pressure the patient may have.

The patient whose chest tube drainage has been minimal to moderate when suddenly bright red blood pours from the tube. Hypertension may result in excessive vascular shear forces and may cause fresh vascular anastomoses to bleed or rupture (see section on acute postoperative hypertension, earlier in this chapter). In this circumstance, vigorous volume repletion and immediate surgical exploration are required because blood loss may be massive and may result in exsanguination within 10 to 15 minutes.

Excessive chest tube drainage and appearance of blood at three unrelated sites, such as on wound dressings and intravenous catheter dressings, indicate a coagulation abnormality (medical bleeding) (Box 24-3). Abnormalities in the prothrombin time (factor VII) and partial prothrombin time (factors VIII, IX, XI, and XII) may be corrected with fresh frozen plasma or cryoprecipitate. A platelet count less than 80,000 mm^3 or an abnormal bleeding time because of antiplatelet drug therapy may require transfusion with platelet concentrates. Low levels of fibrinogen also may require administration of cryoprecipitate.

BOX 24-3
Laboratory Studies Indicating Coagulation Abnormalities (Medical Bleeding)

Platelet count less than 80,000 mm^3
Prothrombin time more than 1.2 seconds prolonged
Partial thromboplastin time more than 1.2 seconds prolonged
Bleeding time more than 10 minutes prolonged if more than 2 hours has elapsed following termination of cardiopulmonary bypass

---

In patients in whom excessive fibrinolysis is present, epsilon aminocaproic acid (Amicar) may be used to control bleeding. By preventing the conversion of plasminogen to plasmin, this drug prevents propagation of the fibrinolytic cascade. During and following administration, patients should be carefully monitored for hyperkalemia, hypotension, central nervous system symptoms that may lead to grand mal seizure, and localized or diffuse thrombosis.

Aprotinin is a serine protease inhibitor used as an antifibrinolytic agent in reoperative cardiac surgery. Administered as an infusion during cardiopulmonary bypass, it is thought to have antifibrinolytic and, in certain doses, anti-inflammatory activity and is thought to preserve platelet function. Desmopressin (DDAVP) is helpful in patients with uremia and abnormal bleeding times.

Blood pressure control (see section on acute postoperative hypertension, earlier in this chapter) is another important aspect of postoperative care in reducing or preventing bleeding. Elevations in arterial pressure enhance capillary oozing, may cause vascular suture line rupture or bleeding, or may disrupt friable portions of the heart. At Rush Presbyterian—St. Luke's Medical Center, patients who have had patches placed for acute septal defect repair or for aortic dissection are often narcotized and paralyzed for 2 to 3 days to avoid activity- or emotion-associated hypertensive swings and related bleeding. This precaution also allows friable portions of the heart to stabilize.

If all nonsurgical factors are corrected and the patient continues to bleed excessively, surgical correction of the bleeding site and evacuation of clots are indicated. Evacuation of clots stops both consumption of clotting factors and accelerated fibrinolytic activity, and therefore it generally stops hemorrhage. Despite medical attempts to decrease bleeding in the postoperative patient, reexploration is necessary in approximately 5% of patients.

Maintaining Patency of Chest Drainage Tubing. The patency of chest drainage tubing is checked every 5 to 15 minutes in the immediate postoperative period. Care must be taken that the patient is not lying on the tubing, that it is not kinked, and that it is positioned so that gravity will direct the flow of blood into the drainage collection chamber. For example, dependent loops of drainage tubing may create back pressure and may impair evacuation of blood. If the patient is not in shock, 30-degree elevation of the head of the bed promotes evacuation and drainage of blood from the thorax.

Early in the postoperative period, it may be necessary to gently "strip" or "milk" the chest drainage tubes to dislodge clots and move them toward the drainage collection chamber (Figure 24-1). Vigorous stripping of the chest tubes is generally avoided unless used as a temporizing measure when the patient is readied for reoperation for bleeding.

Research has demonstrated that excessively high negative pressures (-400 cm H_2O or more) may be transiently generated by chest tube stripping.[15] These pressures may cause the patient pain, may pull and trap lung tissue in the catheter eyelets, or may exacerbate bleeding by dislodging stabilizing clots. Consequently, chest tube milking is preferable to stripping. Stripping should never be done vigorously and is done only when the chest tube has thick, immobilized clots. *Gravity drainage is the preferred method to keep the chest tubes clear of blood.*

Postoperative Fluid Management. The fluids used for volume replacement in the immediate postoperative period are variable among institutions but are generally D_5W or 0.9 normal saline. The use of blood and blood products for volume repletion has come under greater scrutiny because of the potential for transmitting infectious diseases for which there is no known cure, such as hepatitis B; non-A, non-B hepatitis; or the viral-mediated immune deficiency syndromes. Therefore, when patients need rapid fluid loading, synthetic volume expanders such as 6% hetastarch in 0.9% sodium chloride (Hespan) or 5% albumin may be given.

Generally, transfusion of packed red blood cells is indicated when the hematocrit value is less than 30%. Each unit of packed red blood cells should raise the 70 kg adult's hematocrit value by approximately 3% and the hemoglobin by approximately 1 g/dl. If, however, a patient is tolerating a hematocrit of 24% to 30%, has reasonable cardiac reserve, and has received no transfusions, conservative restoration of red blood cell mass and hemoglobin with vitamins and iron supplementation is undertaken.

Contractility. Contractility is related to the capability of the myocardium to increase the rate and force of muscle fiber shortening, regardless of preload and afterload. Postoperatively, contractility may be variably affected depending on the cardiac defects and the patient's physiologic and metabolic state. For example, excessive contractility occurs in patients with preexisting left ventricular hypertrophy secondary to systemic hypertension or aortic stenosis. A hypercontractile, hypertrophic ventricle is particularly vulnerable to ischemic injury following cardiopulmonary bypass. In these patients, inotropic agents may provoke hypercontractility and should be avoided.

As stated previously, myocardial performance following extracorporeal circulation is usually impaired to a certain degree and usually returns to normal within the first 12 to 24 hours. Common factors that may exacerbate contractile failure are metabolic acidosis, arterial hypoxemia, respiratory alkalosis, electrolyte imbalances, perioperative myocardial infarction, and antiarrhythmic medications. These are discussed as follows.

Metabolic Acidosis. Lactic acidosis may be present in the immediate postoperative period, particularly if the bypass time was prolonged. Because of improved pump techniques, however, this is rare.

A "wash-out" metabolic acidosis may occur if rewarming is rapid because accumulated lactic acid trapped in the extremities is mobilized as the peripheral blood ves-

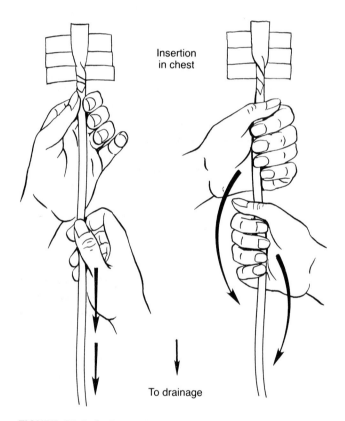

Insertion in chest

To drainage

FIGURE 24-1 **A,** For "stripping," the tube is grasped with one hand just below the connection with the thoracotomy tube. The second hand then compresses the tube and slides over the tubing toward the collection chamber so that the drainage tubing contents are moved along. This process is repeated, using a slide-and-release technique, until the length of the tube is cleared. Care must be taken to stabilize the tubing with the nonstripping hand so that the thoracotomy is not displaced or pulled from the chest. **B,** For "milking," one hand is clasped and squeezed around the tube as close to the chest as possible, and the process is repeated hand-over-hand toward the collection chamber. (From Nursing people experiencing chest surgery. In Luckman J, Sorenson KC, editors: *Medical-surgical nursing,* ed 3, Philadelphia, 1987, W.B. Saunders.)

sels dilate. Mobilized lactate is then circulated throughout the body. More often, metabolic acidosis results from low cardiac output and poor systemic perfusion.

In normal people, a pH of less than 7.25 tends to impair contractility and predisposes patients to arrhythmias. Consequently, low cardiac output predisposes them to anaerobic metabolism and lactic acidosis. The resulting acidosis may then worsen cardiovascular function and perfusion failure. Severe acidosis may also be associated with systemic arterial dilation and venous constriction. Both of these increase capillary stasis and may perpetuate hypoxic acidosis. A surgically stunned, ischemic, or failing heart may be more sensitive to shifts in pH, and correction of moderate to severe acidemia may be associated with a dramatic improvement in cardiac function (Figure 24-2).

Metabolic acidosis is best corrected by maneuvers that increase cardiac output and tissue perfusion. However, infusion of sodium bicarbonate or other buffering agents and ventilator control to create a compensatory respiratory alkalosis may be required in some patients. Vasopressors and inotropic agents may be more effective in the treatment of low cardiac output when acidemia is corrected.

Arterial Hypoxemia. This is rarely encountered postoperatively because of today's effective ventilatory man-

agement. If present, hypoxemia should be immediately corrected to ensure oxygen delivery to the myocardium and other body tissues. Hypoxemia may be associated with contractility failure and predisposition to arrhythmias and conduction defects.

Respiratory Alkalosis. This may be noted initially during the postoperative rewarming process. Respiratory alkalosis is the result of a relative hyperventilation when compared with the low carbon dioxide production common in hypothermia. An arterial PCO_2 less than 30 mm Hg and an arterial pH greater than 7.60 may impair myocardial contractility. Respiratory alkalosis also reduces serum potassium levels.

Electrolyte Imbalances. Electrolyte imbalances may have profound effects on cardiovascular function. The most commonly observed electrolyte imbalances in the immediate postoperative period are hypokalemia and hypomagnesemia; however, imbalances in ionized calcium also may occur and may strongly affect cardiac function. In fact, potassium, calcium, and magnesium deficiencies frequently coexist.

Hypokalemia is defined as a serum potassium concentration of less than 3.5 mEq/L. Several factors may predispose patients to hypokalemia in the early postop-

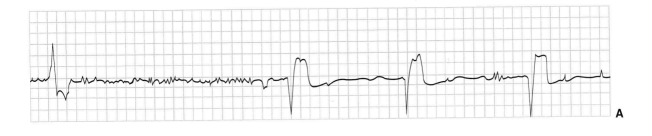

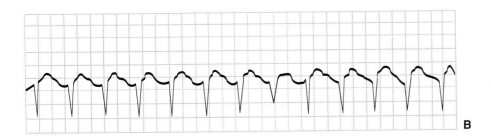

FIGURE 24-2 Tracing *A,* taken at 11:30 AM, is from a 68-year-old man brought into the emergency department by paramedics following resuscitation from ventricular fibrillation complicating acute myocardial infarction. The patient was ashen and minimally responsive to noxious stimuli; peripheral pulses were absent, and blood pressure was unobtainable by cuff technique. Respirations were agonal and arterial blood gas analysis revealed pH of 7.10. Tracing *B,* taken 15 minutes after the administration of sodium bicarbonate with correction of the pH to 7.35 and no other supportive therapy. The arterial pressure was 80/60, the patient became responsive enough to answer questions, and color improved to become pale.

erative period: (1) the infusion of epinephrine, used for inotropic support, may cause the serum potassium level to fall by more than 0.5 mEq/L; (2) a rise in pH of 0.10, because of respiratory alkalosis or administration of alkalizing agents, is associated with a fall in serum potassium of approximately 0.5 mEq/L; and (3) loop diuretics may cause urinary potassium losses to exceed 100 mEq/L (normal 40 to 80 mEq/L). Consequently, a serum potassium level should be obtained 1 hour after diuretic administration.

Low serum potassium levels cause muscle weakness, increase sensitivity of the heart to digitalis toxicity, and predispose patients to major arrhythmias that may significantly impair cardiac function and may increase perioperative mortality rate. The surgically traumatized heart seems to be particularly vulnerable to the effects of hypokalemia. Therefore standing orders for potassium administration are generally directed at maintaining serum potassium levels in the high-normal range. Box 24-4 outlines sample standing orders for electrolyte administration.

BOX 24-4
Electrolyte Therapy in the Postoperative Period

Potassium Therapy*

If the potassium is 3.0 to 3.9 mEq/L, infuse 40 mEq KCl in 250 ml 5% D/W over 1 hour provided there is a normal creatinine and urine output is in a normal range.

If the potassium is 4.0 to 4.5 mEq/L, infuse 20 mEq/L in 100 ml 5% D/W over 1 hour.

If the potassium is greater than 5.0 mEq/L, repeat the serum potassium.

If the repeat potassium is greater than 5.0 mEq/L, remove any added KCl from the intravenous fluids and notify the resident.

Calcium Therapy

Calcium chloride, 1 g, is to be given via slow intravenous push for ionized calcium less than 1.0 mEq/L.

Magnesium Therapy

Magnesium sulfate, 1 g, given via intravenous push for serum magnesium less than 1.5 mEq/L or 2 g in 100 ml 5% D/W over 2 hours.

---

*Central line–administered potassium can be at a concentration of 20 to 40 mEq KCl per 100 ml carrier solution. Peripheral intravenously administered potassium should be diluted to 40 mEq KCl in 500 ml for non-fluid-restricted patients and in 250 ml for fluid-restricted patients. Peripheral administration rate is 10 mEq/hr.

Hypocalcemia is defined as an ionized calcium less than 2.0 mEq/L. The inotropic state of the heart is related to the amount of ionic calcium available for the myocardial contractile system. As ionic calcium rises, myocardial contractility increases. As ionized calcium levels fall, myocardial contractile dynamics decrease. The patient's ionized calcium concentration may be decreased within the initial 24 hours of surgery secondary to hemodilution from electrolyte solutions employed to prime the cardiopulmonary bypass pump. Ionized calcium concentration also may be decreased at any time in the postoperative course because of hypomagnesemia or hypoperfusion or the use of cimetidine (Tagamet).

Hypomagnesemia is defined as a serum magnesium level less than 1.5 mEq/L. Magnesium is essential to the function of enzyme systems that regulate fat, protein, and carbohydrate metabolism. Consequently, hypomagnesemia may be manifested as multisystem dysfunction. Neuromuscular signs include seizures, muscle weakness, obtundation, confusion, or coma. Cardiovascular signs of hypomagnesemia include myocardial contractile failure, hypotension, and arrhythmias. Postoperative factors that may predispose patients to hypomagnesemia include urinary losses from use of loop diuretics and the use of aminoglycosides. Alcohol-addicted patients may develop significant hypomagnesemia early in alcohol withdrawal, which usually coincides with the early postoperative period.

Perioperative Myocardial Infarction. The generally accepted diagnostic definition is the occurrence of a new Q wave in the postoperative electrocardiogram. Enzyme-release myocardial injuries continue to have varied definitions in the literature. The expected incidence of operative myocardial ischemic injury is in the range of 4% to 14%. Multiple studies indicate that the overall incidence of perioperative myocardial infarction is decreasing. Patients at greatest risk include those having unstable angina, those having emergency operation (within 24 hours of catheterization), and those having had previous coronary artery bypass procedures and are currently having "re-do" procedures.

The maintenance of good perioperative coronary blood flow is crucial to optimize heart function and prevent ischemic myocardial injury. Because the perfusion gradient across the penetrating coronary arteries depends on the difference between aortic diastolic pressure and left ventricular end-diastolic pressure (PWP), measures to support an adequate and a stable aortic diastolic pressure while maintaining the lowest level of preload possible to ensure an adequate stroke volume are pivotal in protecting the patient from ischemic ventricular injury or infarction.

The patient having internal mammary artery revascularization needs special mention. The vessels are prone to spasm, particularly in response to hypotension or low-flow states. Therefore a normal blood pressure and cardiac output must be scrupulously maintained during the first 24 hours. Intravenous nitroglycerin as prophylaxis against coronary artery spasm also may be given in the immediate postoperative period.

If the patient develops marked S-T segment elevation and is hemodynamically *unstable,* the surgeon must be notified *immediately* so that the patient may be returned to the operating room for reexploration. The bypass graft may have become kinked or clotted, there may be debris or air obstructing the graft, or the revascularization may have been incomplete.

When the patient has an S-T segment elevation and is hemodynamically *stable,* the alternatives for treatment are best determined by the surgeon who is familiar with the coronary anatomy and problems that may be related to the procedure. The patient may have entered the operation during infarction, and the electrocardiographic changes may simply reflect evolution of the original injury. Alternatively, the vessel in question may have been technically impossible to bypass or vein graft debris may have entered a distal vessel and may have been unretrievable. In these situations, the surgeon may elect to treat the patient as guided by the ECG changes with intravenous nitroglycerin or intraaortic balloon pumping.

Antiarrhythmic Medications. This group of drugs must be used judiciously in the postoperative period because nearly all have direct negative inotropic effects.

Heart Rate and Rhythm. Optimal cardiac output occurs between heart rates of 80 and 110 beats per minute and is dependent on normal contractile sequence and dynamics. Arrhythmias are common following cardiac surgery and may impair cardiac function by producing inappropriate changes in heart rate, altering normal atrioventricular contractile sequence, or distorting ventricular contractile dynamics (muscular asynergy). Significant cardiovascular decompensation is particularly likely during the arrhythmia if the patient had preexisting heart failure.

Risk Factors Predisposing Patients to Arrhythmias. Extracardiac factors that predispose patients to arrhythmias include acid-base disturbances; electrolyte imbalances; hypoxemia; certain drug toxicities, such as to digitalis or quinidine; and sympathetic nervous system stimulation. These abnormalities should be identified and corrected as quickly as possible.

Cardiac factors that predispose individuals to arrhythmias or conduction defects may occur singly or may occur with other arrhythmia risk factors. The presence of several arrhythmia risk factors complicates

arrhythmia management. In patients having had valve surgery, conduction disturbances are common. The proximity of the atrioventricular node to all valve tissue renders it susceptible to trauma and, consequently, to varying degrees of atrioventricular block in the postoperative period. Acute or chronic ischemic myocardial or conduction tissue injury may set the stage for postoperative conduction or rhythm disturbances. Patients with distended cardiac chambers secondary to ischemic disease, cardiomyopathy, or valvular disease frequently have atrial fibrillation and may also have significant ventricular ectopy or conduction disturbances.

Types of Arrhythmias in the Postoperative Period. *Supraventricular arrhythmias* are the most common arrhythmias following cardiac surgery. If the patient's ejection fraction is greater than 40%, atrial fibrillation or flutter seldom is associated with hemodynamic instability, and the patient's condition may be managed pharmacologically. If, however, the ejection fraction is less than 35%, atrial tachyarrhythmias may be associated with perfusion failure. If the patient is becoming hypotensive, it is necessary to cardiovert with synchronized cardioversion starting with 50 to 100 joules. If unsuccessful, this may be repeated in increments of 50 to 100 joules until sinus rhythm is restored.

Ventricular arrhythmias are a complex aspect of cardiac surgical management. As noted earlier in this chapter, many patients currently undergo operations for this problem alone or concomitantly with coronary artery bypass. Although ventricular arrhythmias may be provoked by hypoxemia, acidosis, and electrolyte imbalances, the most common predisposing factor is an unstable metabolite in heart muscle that has been acutely or chronically injured by a myocardial infarction.

Immediate identification and management of ventricular arrhythmias may do much to reduce postoperative morbidity and mortality rates. This occurrence demands a vigilant and rapidly responsive bedside staff. Hemodynamically unstable ventricular tachycardia requires immediate synchronous cardioversion starting with 100 to 200 joules and, if this fails, going immediately to 360 joules. If successful, cardioversion is followed by a lidocaine (Xylocaine) bolus of 1 mg/kg and a drip beginning at 2 mg/min. If the patient continues to repeat the arrhythmia, procainamide, bretylium, and amiodarone are employed. Additional therapy includes patient sedation to reduce circulating catecholamines, which, in turn, tend to increase automaticity. Intraaortic balloon pumping, by its ventricular unloading effects, decreases ventricular distention and, by improving coronary blood flow, increases myocardial oxygenation. Both actions reduce arrhythmogenicity.

Persistent ischemic ECG changes following cardioversion/defibrillation may indicate a problem with a bypass graft, and the patient may have to be returned to the operating room for revascularization.

Conduction Disturbances. Conduction disturbances may occur spontaneously, as a result of the underlying disease, or may be surgically induced. Disturbances are usually transient, although occasionally they may be lasting and require permanent pacing. Because the potential for conduction disturbances exists or because tachyarrhythmia suppression may be necessary for all types of open heart surgery, the surgical placement of ventricular pacing wires is appropriate for all patients. If the patient's left ventricle is strongly dependent on the atrial kick for maximal function, atrial pacing wires also should be placed during operation.

As stated previously, atrioventricular blocks are most common following valvular surgery, particularly aortic valve surgery. Coronary artery disease also may result in ischemic injury of the conduction pathways. For example, right coronary artery disease may affect sinus and atrioventricular nodal function. Likewise, lesions of the left anterior descending coronary artery may be associated with complete heart block or varying types of bundle branch block in the postoperative period. The 10% of patients with a left dominant circulation (the circumflex branch of the left coronary circulation perfuses the atrioventricular node) also may develop atrioventricular block.

Although it is beyond the scope of this text to discuss the varied pharmacologic therapies of cardiac arrhythmias, the important clinical points related to arrhythmia management are these. First, any correctable factor known to produce arrhythmias, such as electrolyte imbalances, should be identified and corrected. Second, the arrhythmic threat to the patient is not necessarily related to the specific arrhythmia but, rather, to how the patient is tolerating it hemodynamically. For example, in some patients a rapid sinus tachycardia may precipitate ischemic myocardial pain and hemodynamic deterioration. In this context, sinus tachycardia is a major arrhythmia and must be aggressively managed. Third, wide QRS tachyarrhythmias *must* be identified as supraventricular with aberrant conduction or ventricular because pharmacologic management of each arrhythmia differs. If, however, the patient's condition is hemodynamically unstable or rapidly deteriorating with the wide QRS tachyarrhythmia, immediate cardioversion is required. It is imperative that the arrhythmia be documented by the bedside staff on rhythm strips, preferably using more than one lead. Precordial leads V_1 and V_6 are most useful in evaluating QRS morphology for distinguishing ventricular ectopic rhythms from aberrantly

conducted supraventricular arrhythmias. See Marriott[16] for techniques in QRS morphology analysis. These measures allow the cardiologist to identify the rhythm and institute appropriate prophylactic drug therapy.

Some patients coming out of surgery may have an implantable defibrillator. The nurse admitting the patient should be informed that the device has been placed and is activated. If the patient develops a rapid ventricular tachycardia or fibrillation, the device will fire within approximately 14 to 18 seconds and the patient will have a generalized muscular contraction. The staff may safely touch the patient because only 2 joules are delivered to the skin. If the device fails to terminate the arrhythmia after four attempts noted by four generalized convulsive movements, the patient should undergo cardioversion/defibrillation in the conventional manner with 360 joules.

Assessment and Management of the Pulmonary System

The operative management of pulmonary function begins with a preoperative assessment and history. Patients who smoke are instructed to stop because even a few days of smoking cessation reduces bronchial secretions. Patients with chronic lung disease should be evaluated preoperatively by a pulmonologist and should have pulmonary function studies performed.

Patients with chronic lung disease generally tolerate cardiac surgery well; however, if pulmonary complications occur, the hospitalization is prolonged and the patient may not survive. This potential must be discussed with the patient and family preoperatively. A question frequently asked by the patient with chronic lung disease is whether surgical correction of the cardiac problem will decrease shortness of breath. The most realistic approach is that the final answer will be given by the patient after recovery from the surgery.

Postoperative Pulmonary Management

Postoperative pulmonary management requires (1) adequate alveolar ventilation; (2) adequate tissue oxygen delivery based on evaluation of the adequacy of blood oxygen content, mixed venous oxygen saturation, and cardiac output; and (3) ongoing evaluation of the patient's overall pulmonary function (pulmonary function tests) and metabolic needs (arterial blood gas).

Assisted (mechanical) ventilation provides the following benefits in the early postoperative period: (1) control of tidal volume and positive end-expiratory pressure to reduce the incidence of atelectasis (a variable degree of atelectasis is present secondary to nonventilation if cardiopulmonary bypass is used during the course of the operation);

(2) control of arterial oxygenation and pH through ventilation ($PaCO_2$); (3) decreased metabolic demands through control of the work of breathing; and (4) clearance of secretions through direct tracheal suctioning via the endotracheal tube. Reoperation for bleeding or tamponade is facilitated if the patient does not require reintubation.

The patient is generally receiving oxygen (FiO_2 of 50% to 100%) on transfer from the operating room. In most institutions, there is a trend toward earlier extubation provided specific parameters are met. Provided the patient is hemodymically stable, normothermic, neurologically intact, and without evidence of mediastinal bleeding, a standard ventilation weaning protocol is initiated. Specific parameters that must be present before weaning include signs of adequate tissue perfusion with minimal inotropic support (normal mentation, warm extremities with good urine output, absence of metabolic acidosis, cardiac index greater than 2.0 $L/min/m^2$); chest tube output less than 100 ml/hr; adequate oxygenation (PaO_2 greater than 80 mm Hg with positive end-expiratory pressure 5 cm or greater); respiratory rate (synchronous intermittent mandatory ventilation [SIMV] and spontaneous) less than 24 breaths per minute; and minimal tracheal secretions. The SIMU rate is decreased at a rate of 2 to 4 breaths per minute every 15 minutes provided the total respiratory rate remains less than 24 breaths per minute and greater than 10 breaths per minute while maintaining a cutaneous oxygen saturation greater than 95%. The patient is closely observed for new agitation, restlessness, diaphoresis, arrhythmias, or significant change in heart rate or blood pressure. Endotracheal suctioning should reveal no excessive airway secretions. At the end of the tolerated wean, the patient is placed on continuous positive airway pressure with +5 cm H_2O. Pressure support is then weaned to 5 cm H_2O. An arterial blood gas is drawn, and if adequate (pH greater than 7.35, PaO_2 greater than mm Hg, $PaCO_2$ 35 to 45 mm Hg), the patient undergoes an assessment of mechanical ventilatory function. Provided the negative inspiratory force is less than −25 cm H_2O, the tidal volume is 5 ml/kg or greater, and the vital capacity is 10 to 15 ml/kg, the patient can be extubated to a 50% O_2 humidified face mask. A postextubation arterial blood gas is obtained. Our institution uses continuous oximetric Swan-Ganz catheters, which allows recognition of a significant change in mixed venous oxygen saturation during the course of the ventilatory weaning process. If the patient had a difficult airway or a fiberoptic intubation was required, an attending anesthesiologist is present for the extubation with prior arrangements made for a flexible bronchoscope at bedside. Following extubation, additional arterial blood gas samples are obtained and the patient is vigilantly assessed for the development of a decrease in cutaneous oxygen saturation of less than 92%, a change in systemic blood pressure of ± 20 mm Hg, arrhythmias or ST segment changes, agitation or disorientation, signs of airway obstruction, or bronchospasm.

Pulmonary Embolism

Patients at particularly high risk of pulmonary embolism are those with a history of thromboembolic disease, prolonged bed rest, heart failure, atrial fibrillation, obesity, advanced age, and hypercoagulable states (see Chapter 18, section on acute respiratory failure). Pulmonary embolism is usually associated with hemodynamic compromise only if greater than 40% to 50% of the cross-sectional area of the pulmonary circulation is obstructed by the clot. Patients with massive pulmonary embolism and hypotension may require percutaneous suction catheter or operative pulmonary embolectomy followed by inferior vena cava filter placement.

Pulmonary Edema

Some patients have pathophysiologic fluid overload before surgery, and all patients take on at least 2 L of fluid from cardiopulmonary bypass. Liberal use of diuretics may be required during the first few postoperative days to prevent severe circulatory overload and pulmonary edema when the fluid is mobilized from body tissue and returns to the vascular space. At our institution, twice-daily diuretics are instituted on postoperative day 2 until the patient returns to his or her preoperative weight.

Fluid management should limit total intravenous fluid intake (maintenance, medication piggybacks, electrolyte boluses) to a maximum of 100 ml/hr.

Nervous System and Psychologic Changes

Neurologic Injury

The most dreaded type of neurologic injury is cerebrovascular accident (CVA). Patients with a history of cerebrovascular disease or peripheral vascular disease tend to have a higher incidence of CVA following open heart surgery. Other, less severe, types of injury also may occur. Abnormalities of intellect may manifest postoperatively as short-term memory disturbances, inability to perform complex mental tasks, poor coordination, and slow reaction time. Fortunately, in most patients, improvement with restoration of faculties occurs in approximately 6 weeks. Damage also may occur to peripheral nerves; nerve damage usually results in transient functional impairment.

Changes in Mood and Thought Process

Depression. Depression is common and typically begins a few days after cardiac surgery. This is not surprising considering the importance attributed to the heart not only physiologically, but also in religion, philosophy, and art. Patients hospitalized for major surgery or illness also find themselves stripped of any sense of autonomy and privacy. Unexpressed or unresolved feelings of anger, fear, or grief may ultimately result in depression. Psychologic depression may manifest as irritability or anger expressed toward hospital staff or family members, refusal to cooperate with treatment, feelings of helplessness or hopelessness, or isolation. Postoperative depression is usually self-limiting and requires only an understanding approach with nontechnical explanations of the purpose of treatments, acceptance of the patient's expressions of frustration or pain, and assurance that the patient will again gain control of his or her life.

Dramatic Changes in Thought and Perception. Dramatic changes in thought and perception, such as disorientation, delirium, or other forms of psychosis, may begin within the first 5 days of surgery. These may begin subtly with an inappropriate remark or may begin with sudden, grossly abnormal behavior.

There are two types of delirium. The first is termed *quiet delirium* in which the patient may be disoriented in some or all spheres, may be unable to recognize family members, or may have inappropriate ideation. Periods of lucidity may alternate with disorientation, which is typically worse at night or in the early-morning hours. This may persist for 3 to 4 days; the medical or psychiatric mechanisms are unknown. *Agitated delirium* is more dramatic and has been referred to as *intensive care unit psychosis*. The patient may be incoherent and shouting, may have paranoid ideation, may have violent outbursts, and may attempt to get out of bed and disconnect or pull out all tubes and catheters. There is the potential for self-harm, as well as harm to others. However, alternatives should be attempted before restraining the patient. These include weaning from the ventilator and discontinuing invasive lines. Give frequent explanation of treatment. Include family support and participation with instruction and education. Try to decrease patient stimulation from the environment (bright lights, noise). When alternatives to modify the patients' behavior fail, apply the least restrictive restraints and closely follow the restraint policy and procedures of your hospital.

The cause of delirium is not known, although sleep deprivation, sensory overload or deprivation, and absence of daytime and nighttime clues have been implicated. Alcohol or recreational drug withdrawal and electrolyte imbalance must also be ruled out because these may produce behavior and neurologic changes and because both are treatable causes of delirium. In patients in whom the cause of delirium cannot be identified, complete resolution usually occurs within 3 to 5 days with no psychologic sequelae.

Renal System

Urine flow rates decrease progressively during induction to anesthesia and thoracotomy as a result of the effects of anesthetic agents on cardiac output and renal vascular resistance. During cardiopulmonary bypass, mean arterial pressure is lowered to 50 to 90 mm Hg, and nonpulsatile blood flow is maintained at 2.2 to 2.4 L/min/m². Levels of circulating vasoconstricting catecholamines and angiotensin II also rise and increase renal vascular resistance. Consequent to the renal vasoconstrictor effect, renal blood flow decreases further. Urine flow rates typically fall to 2 to 3 ml/hr during cardiopulmonary bypass.

During the initial first hours after surgery, urine output is considerably higher than normal. Each patient having cardiopulmonary bypass absorbs several liters of extracellular fluid. The initial diuresis is the result of the osmotic effect of glucose or mannitol used in the perfusate, as well as the loop diuretic often used when the patient is coming off bypass. The remainder of the excess fluid is removed by spontaneous or drug-induced diuresis during the first 1 to 3 days following surgery. Urine output should be maintained at a minimum of 1 ml/kg/hr.

A low urine output should alert the clinician to the possibility of low cardiac output, which should be immediately treated. This consideration is particularly significant in protecting the kidney from postoperative injury because acute renal dysfunction following open heart surgery is almost always the result of renal ischemia. Low postoperative cardiac output is the most common factor. Other risk factors for ischemic renal injury include a bypass time greater than 160 minutes or aortic cross-clamp time greater than 40 minutes.

The incidence of oliguric renal failure after open heart surgery has fallen dramatically over the past 20 years because of improved surgical anesthetic and cardiopulmonary bypass techniques. If, however, the patient develops oliguric renal failure, patient mortality rates rise to 65% to 90%. This finding emphasizes the importance of prevention of renal injury in the operative and postoperative period.

As the age of patients undergoing open heart surgery increases, many more enter operation with slightly decreased renal function. The insult of cardiopulmonary bypass may increase the creatinine and blood urea nitrogen transiently. If severe renal dysfunction develops, renal dialysis becomes necessary if fluid overload or profound acidosis occurs or if hyperkalemia cannot be resolved by medical management. These patients are restricted in fluid intake, and dialysis is performed daily or every other day through a central catheter.

Another group of patients requiring mention are those on long-term renal dialysis. These patients develop significant coronary artery disease owing to chronic renal failure. Generally, these patients undergo dialysis the day before surgery. The postoperative fluid management is guided by the central circulatory pressures, and management in the first 24 hours is usually no different than that for people with normal kidneys. These patients generally have dialysis the day after surgery; however, dialysis may be performed on the day of surgery if fluid overload or altered blood chemistry test results indicate that it is necessary.

A STRING OF CLINICAL PEARLS

Observations of technique and outcome in an extremely busy postoperative open heart care unit over the years have inspired the authors to pass on these hints relating to patient management.

PEARL 1. *Each heart needs 6 to 12 hours to recover from the insult of surgical trauma and cardiopulmonary bypass.* Many staff members make efforts to wean the patient from vasoactive or antiarrhythmic drips shortly after admission to the recovery area. Rather, weaning should begin gradually and with vigilant monitoring after a minimum of 6 hours following discharge from the operating room.

PEARL 2. *Patients admitted to the recovery area should be considered hemodynamically and physiologically unstable until proved otherwise.* In the immediate postoperative period, patients should therefore remain in an uninterrupted supine position until time and serial evaluations determine hemodynamic stability. Soiled linen produces no physiologic derangements; moving unstable patients does. Rolling a patient for bed linen changes may precipitate hypertensive crisis or hypotension in a marginally compensated patient. Likewise, sitting the patient up for an upright chest radiograph in the initial postoperative hours may unmask hypovolemia, and the patient may "crash."

PEARL 3. *Patients having sustained major surgical trauma or illness need rest.* Not every patient needs a bath in the early-morning hours. For that matter, not every patient needs a complete bath every day. The number of baths a patient receives during hospitalization has no beneficial effect on patient outcome. However, sleep deprivation and sensory overload may increase postoperative morbidity rates. When people are exhausted, a bath does not make them feel better; only sleep does. The time spent for the bath might be better spent allowing the patient a period of uninterrupted rest.

PEARL 4. When the patient is admitted to the recovery unit and is placed on the mechanical ventilator, do not assume that the ventilator was hooked up properly. Visually document that the patient's chest moves with each machine ventilation. More important, listen for the presence of bilateral breath sounds and immediately connect the patient to pulse oximetry.

PEARL 5. Double-check that the monitors and monitoring lines function and are connected properly.

PEARL 6. *If unsure about what to do in any circumstance (nurse or physician), ask for consultation or help.* No one was born with an intuitive sense or immediate cognition of how to care for the critically ill. The established experts gained their knowledge through extensive and ongoing study and by asking questions. There is no academic or clinical end-point at which *any* clinician knows everything there is to know about patient care. Any patient may present a challenge to even the most seasoned practitioner; the act of seeking counsel and the help of others acknowledges our human limitations. There is no reward for watching a patient deteriorate by one's self; a collaborative approach to a patient problem may literally make the difference between life and death.

PEARL 7. *Administer morphine analgesia or sedation before performing any potentially noxious stimulus such as suctioning.* This helps modify the pressor response and may prevent an acute hypertensive episode and the associated risks of stroke, increased bleeding, suture line rupture, and myocardial ischemia.

PEARL 8. *The patient should not be left unattended for at least the initial 12 hours.* Life-threatening complications occur within seconds to minutes; the clinician must be at the bedside to identify the potential problems before they become a full-blown crisis. Patients do not suddenly get into trouble; there are usually subtle warning signs that, if treated, avert major complications.

PEARL 9. *There is no monitoring or alarm system that can replace a vigilant caregiver.* Frequently observe, auscultate, and touch the patient. The information gathered from these methods is far more important to an optimal patient outcome than all the technology in the world.

REFERENCES

1. Nisson R: Billroth and cardiac surgery, *Lancet* 2:250, 1963.
2. Rehn L: Uber Penetrierende Herzwunden und Herznaht, *Arch Klin Chir* 55:315, 1897.
3. Vineberg AM: Development of anastomosis between coronary vessels and transplanted internal mammary artery, *Can Med Assoc J* 55:117, 1946.
4. Zimmerman HA, Scott RW, Becker NO: Catheterization of the left side of the heart in man, *Circulation* 1:357, 1950.

5. Hufnagel CA: Aortic plastic valvular prosthesis, *Bull Georgetown Med Ctr* 4:128, 1951.

6. Gibbon JH Jr: Application of a mechanical heart and lung apparatus to cardiac surgery, *Minn Med* 37:171, 1954.

7. Starr A, Edwards ML: Mitral replacement. Clinical experience with a ball-valve prosthesis, *Ann Surg* 154:726, 1961.

8. Sones FM Jr, Shirley EK: Cine coronary arteriography, *Mod Concepts Cardiovasc Dis* 31:735, 1962.

9. Garrett HE, Dennis EW, DeBakey ME: Aortocoronary bypass with saphenous vein graft. Seven year follow up, *JAMA* 223:792, 1973.

10. Favaloro RG: *Surgical treatment of coronary atherosclerosis,* Baltimore, 1970, Williams & Wilkins.

11. Johnson WD, Lepley D Jr: An aggressive surgical approach to coronary disease, *J Thorac Cardiovasc Surg* 59:128, 1970.

12. Borel JF: The history of cyclosporin A and its significance. In White DJG, editor: *Cyclosporin A. Proceedings of an international conference on cyclosporin A,* New York, 1982, Elsevier Biomedical.

13. Moulopoulos SD, Topaz S, Kolff W: Diastolic balloon pumping (with carbon dioxide) in the aorta. Mechanical assistance to the failing circulation, *Am Heart J* 63:669, 1962.

14. Barnard CN: The operation: a human heart transplantation. An interim report of the successful operation performed at Groot Schuur Hospital, Capetown, South Africa, *Afr Med J* 41:1271, 1967.

15. Duncan C, Erickson R: Pressures associated with chest tube stripping, *Heart Lung* 11:166, 1982.

16. Marriott HJL: Aberrant ventricular conduction and the diagnosis of wide-QRS tachycardias. In *Practical electrocardiography,* ed 8, Baltimore, 1988, Williams & Wilkins.

SUGGESTED READINGS

Alcan KE et al: Management of acute cardiac tamponade by subxiphoid pericardiotomy, *JAMA* 247:1143, 1982.

Barden C, Hansen M: Cold versus warm cardioplegia: recognizing hemodynamic variations, *Dimens Crit Care Nurs* 14:114, 1995.

Beggs VL et al: Factors related to hospitalization within thirty days of discharge after coronary artery bypass grafting, *Best Practices and Benchmarking in Healthcare* 1:180, 1996.

Bigger J Jr: Mechanism and diagnosis of arrhythmias. In Braunwald E, editor: *Heart disease,* Philadelphia, 1994, W.B. Saunders.

Blakeman BP, Pifarre R, Sullivan HJ, et al: Cardiac surgery for chronic renal dialysis patients, *Chest* 95:509, 1989.

Blakeman BP et al: Surgical ablation of ventricular tachycardia in the normothermic heart, *J Cardiac Surg* 5:115, 1990.

Blakeman BP, Wilber D, Pifarre R: Median sternotomy for implantable cardioverter/defibrillator, *Arch Surg* 124:1065, 1989.

Braunwald E: Unstable angina, *Circulation* 80:410, 1989.

Brewer DL, Bobbro R, Bartel AG: Myocardial infarction as a complication of coronary bypass surgery, *Circulation* 47:58, 1973.

Chong JL, Pillai R, Fisher A, et al: Cardiac surgery: moving away from intensive care, *Br Heart J* 68:430, 1992.

Christakis CT, Koch JP, Deemer CCP: A randomized study of the systemic effects of warm heart surgery, *Ann Thorac Surg* 54:449, 1992.

Coroso PJ, Hockstein MJ: New techniques in management of the cardiac surgery patient. In Shoemaker WC et al, editors: *Textbook of critical care,* Philadelphia, 2000, W.B. Saunders.

Dam V, Wild MC, Baun MM: Effect of oxygen insufflation during endotracheal suctioning on arterial pressure and oxygenation in coronary artery bypass patients, *Am J Crit Care* 3:191, 1994.

Dipardo JA: *Anesthesia for cardiac surgery,* Stamford, CT, 1998, Appleton & Lange.

Fowler MB, Alderman EL, Oesterly SN, et al: Dobutamine and dopamine after cardiac surgery; greater augmentation of myocardial blood flow with dobutamine, *Circulation* 70(suppl 1):103, 1984.

Hahm MA: Collaborative care: improving patient outcomes in cardiovascular sugery, *Prog Cardiovasc Nurs* 12:15, 1997.

Harder MP, Eijsman L, Roozendaal KJ: Aprotinin reduces intraoperative and postoperative blood loss in membrane oxygenator cardiopulmonary bypass, *Ann Thorac Surg* 51:936, 1991.

Hauser AM et al: Percutaneous intraaortic balloon counterpulsation. Clinical effectiveness and hazards, *Chest* 82:422, 1982.

Hogue CW et al: Risk factors for early or delayed stroke after cardiac surgery, *Circulation* 100:642, 1999.

Imrie MM, Ward M, Hall GM: A comparison of patient rewarming devices after cardiac surgery, *Anaesthesia* 46:44, 1991.

Koller MN, Alfer A, editors: *Cardiac and noncardiac complications of open heart surgery: prevention, diagnosis, and treatment,* Mount Kisco, NY, 1992, Futura.

LoCicero J III et al: Prolonged ventilatory support after open-heart surgery, *Crit Care Med* 20:990, 1992.

Lyn-McHale DJ, Riggs KL, Thurman L: Epicardial pacing after cardiac surgery, *Crit Care Nurse* 11:68, 1991.

Mora CT, editor: *Cardiopulmonary bypass: principles and techniques of extracorporeal circulation,* New York, 1995, Springer.

Mravinac CM: Neurologic dysfunctions following cardiac surgery, *Crit Care Clin North Am* 3(4):691, 1991.

Nikas DJ et al: Use of a national data base to assess perioperative risk, morbidity, mortality, and cost savings in coronary artery bypass grafting, *South Med J* 89:1074, 1996.

O'Connell JB, Wallis D, Johnson SA, et al: Transient branch block following use of hypothermia cardioplegia in coronary artery bypass surgery: high incidence without perioperative myocardial infarction, *Am Heart J* 103:85, 1982.

Pires LA et al: Arrhythmias and conduction disturbances after coronary artery bypass graft surgery: epidemiology, management, and prognosis, *Am Heart J* 129:799, 1995.

Russo AM et al: A typical presentations and echocardiographic findings in patients with cardiac tamponade occurring early and later after cardiac surgery, *Circulation* 104:71, 1993.

Sladen RN: Management of the adult cardiac patient in the intensive care unit. In Ream AK, Fogdall RP, editors: *Acute cardiovascular management,* Philadelphia, 1982, Lippincott.

Smith GH: *Complications of cardiopulmonary surgery,* London, 1984, Bailliere Tindall.

Souza MHL: Weaning from cardiopulmonary bypass: a practical and simplified overview, *Internet Journal of Perfusionists* 1:1, 1997. Available at www.ispub.com.

Steinberg JS et al: New-onset sustained ventricular tachycardia after cardiac surgery, *Circulation* 99:903, 1999.

Tack BB, Gilliss CL: Nurse-monitored cardiac recovery: a description of the first 8 weeks, *Heart Lung* 19:491, 1990.

Tennant DF, Evans MM: Minimizing blood usage after open heart surgery. Nurses play a key role, *Focus Crit Care* 17:308, 1990.

Turner JS et al: Acute physiology and chronic health evaluation (APACHE II) scoring in a cardiothoracic intensive care unit, *Crit Care Med* 19:1266, 1991.

Whitman GR: Hypertension and hypothermia in the acute postoperative period, *Crit Care Clin North Am* 3(4):661, 1991.

Wolman RL et al: Cerebral injury after cardiac surgery: identification of a group at extraordinary risk, *Stroke* 30(3):514, 1999.

Index

Page numbers followed by f indicate figures; t, tables; and b, boxes.